Adult Audiology

Editor

Dafydd Stephens FRCP
Consultant Audiological Physician, Welsh Hearing Institute, University Hospital of Wales, Cardiff

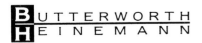
BUTTERWORTH
HEINEMANN

Butterworth-Heinemann
Linacre House, Jordan Hill, Oxford OX2 8DP
A division of Reed Educational and Professional Publishing Ltd

 A member of the Reed Elsevier plc group

OXFORD   BOSTON   JOHANNESBURG
MELBOURNE   NEW DELHI   SINGAPORE

First published 1952
Second edition 1965
Third edition 1971
Fourth edition 1979
Fifth edition 1987
Sixth edition 1997

British Library Cataloguing in Publication Data
A catalogue record for this book is
available from the British Library

Library of Congress Cataloguing in Publication Data
A catalogue record for this book is
available from the Library of Congress

ISBN 0 7506 0595 2 (Volume 1)
     0 7506 0596 0 (Volume 2)
     0 7506 0597 9 (Volume 3)
     0 7506 0598 7 (Volume 4)
     0 7506 0599 5 (Volume 5)
     0 7506 0600 2 (Volume 6)
     0 7506 1935 X (set of six volumes)
     0 7506 2368 3 (Butterworth-Heinemann International Edition, set of six volumes)

Printed and bound in Great Britain by Bath Press, Bath

Contents

Contributors to this volume

Peter W. Alberti PhD, FRCS
Professor of Otolaryngology, Faculty of Medicine, University of Toronto, Canada

Susan Bellman FRCSI
Consultant Audiological Physician, The Hospitals for Sick Children, Great Ormond Street, London

Johanna Beyts BSc
Vestibular Scientist, Royal National Throat, Nose and Ear Hospital, London

Mazal Cohen BA
Lecturer in Audiology, Institute of Laryngology and Otology

R. R. A. Coles FRCP
Emeritus Consultant in Audiological Medicine, MRC Institute of Hearing Research, Nottingham

Rosalyn A. Davies PhD, FRCP
Consultant Physician in Neuro-otology, The National Hospital for Neurology and Neurosurgery, London

Adrian Davis PhD
Medical Research Council Senior Scientist, MRC Institute of Hearing Research, Nottingham

S. Gatehouse PhD
Professor of Audiological Science and Scientist-in-Charge, Scottish Section, MRC Institute of Hearing Research, Royal Infirmary, Glasgow

Ronald Hinchcliffe MD, PhD, FRCP
Emeritus Professor of Audiological Medicine, University of London

Katherine Harrop-Griffiths FRCS
Consultant Audiological Physician, Royal National Throat, Nose and Ear Hospital, London

S. Jakes MPhil
Consultant Clinical Psychologist, Homerton Hospital, London

M. E. Lutman PhD
Professor of Audiology, Institute of Sound and Vibration Research, Southampton University

Linda M. Luxon FRCP
Professor of Audiological Medicine, The Institute of Laryngology and Otology and the National Hospital for Neurology and Neurosurgery, London

Gary J. McKee FRCS
Senior Registrar in Otolaryngology, Royal Victoria Hospital, Belfast

Cliodna F. O Mahoney MRCP
Consultant Audiological Physician, The Hospitals for Sick Children, Great Ormond Street, London

Stuart Rosen PhD
Professor of Speech and Hearing Science, Department of Phonetics and Linguistics, University College, London

Peter A. Savundra MRCP
Senior Registrar in Audiological Medicine, The National Hospital for Neurology and Neurosurgery, London

Dafydd Stephens FRCP
Consultant Audiological Physician, Welsh Hearing Institute, University Hospital of Wales, Cardiff

John C. Stevens DPhil
Consultant Clinical Scientist, Department of Medical
Physics and Clinical Engineering, Royal Hallamshire
Hospital, Sheffield

I. R. C. Swan FRCS
Senior Lecturer in Otolaryngology, University of
Glasgow

A. R. D. Thornton PhD
MRC Institute of Hearing Research, Royal South
Hants Hospital, Southampton

Lam Hoe Yeoh FRCS
Consultant Audiological Physician, St Helier
Hospital, Carshalton, Surrey

Introduction

When I started work on this Sixth Edition I did so in the belief that my experience with the Fifth Edition would make it straightforward. I was wrong. The production of the Fifth Edition was hectic and the available time short. The contributors and volume editors were very productive and in under two and a half years we produced what we, and happily most reviewers, considered to be a worthwhile academic work. On this occasion, with a similar team, we allowed ourselves more time and yet have struggled to produce in four years. One is tempted to blame the health service reforms but that would be unfair. They may have contributed but the problems were certainly much wider than these.

The volume editors, already fully committed clinically, have again been outstanding both in their work and in their understanding of the difficulties we have encountered. Once again there was an excellent social spirit among the editors. They have been very tolerant of the innumerable telephone calls and it has always been a pleasure to work with them. The contributors have also been consistently pleasant to deal with, even those who kept us waiting.

There have been technical problems in the production of this work and I want to pay tribute to the patience of all those who suffered under these, not least the publishing staff at Butterworth-Heinemann. One of the solutions to the problems has been the use of a system of pagination that I consider to be ugly and inefficient for the user and I wish to apologize in advance for this. Unfortunately anything else would have resulted in undue delay in the publication date.

Medicine is a conservative profession and many of us dislike change. Some will feel that we have moved forward in that most Latin plurals have been replaced by English, for example we now have polyps rather than polypi. We have also buried acoustic neuromata, with an appropriate headstone, and now talk about vestibular schwannomas. It has taken about two decades for this to become established in otological circles and may take even longer again, to gain everyday usage in the world of general medicine.

I am pleased with what has been produced. Some chapters have altered very little because there have been few advances in those subjects and we have resisted the temptation of change for change's sake. There have been big strides forward in other areas and these have been reflected in the appropriate chapters.

Despite, and because of, the problems in the production of these volumes, the staff at Butterworth-Heinemann have worked hard and have always been pleasant to deal with. I wish to acknowledge the co-operation from Geoff Smaldon, Deena Burgess, Anne Powell, Mary Seager and Chris Jarvis.

It would be impossible to name all those others who have helped, especially my colleagues in Belfast, but I want to pay tribute to the forbearance of my wife Paddy who graciously accepted the long hours that were needed for this work.

As I stated in my introduction to the Fifth Edition, I was very impressed by the goodwill and generosity of spirit among my Otolaryngological colleagues and am pleased that there has been no evidence of any diminution of this during the nine years between the editions. I remain pleased and proud to be a British Otolaryngologist and to have been entrusted with the production of this latest edition of our standard textbook.

Alan G. Kerr

Preface

Within this volume we endeavour to cover all aspects of audiological medicine relevant to adults with hearing and balance disorders. It links in with Volumes 1, 3 and 6 and there are a number of cross-references in some of the chapters. As such it should be of particular relevance to Audiological Physicians, Otologists and non-medical personnel working within the field.

In this edition, the volume has been restructured as compared with the Fifth Edition of 1987. The main difference has been to split the volume into three sections. The first section deals with general aspects of acoustics, epidemiology, computers, psychology, preventive audiology and medico-legal matters applicable to both hearing and balance disorders. The second section covers different aspects of auditory disorders and the third, balance disorders. We have endeavoured to draw different aspects of the last two sections together by beginning each section with a short overview chapter, linking in as well with the earlier background chapters.

The eight background chapters supplement those from Volume 1 on the anatomy and physiology of hearing and balance and the radiology of the ear. Within this volume we concentrate on aspects more specific to this field, particularly acoustics and the use of computers in audiology. The epidemiological base of hearing disorders is more extensive than in other aspects of the field and that is reflected in the third chapter, which also indicates our dearth of good knowledge with regard to the epidemiology of balance disorders.

The other background chapters on clinical tests, preventive audiology, psychological matters and the use of drugs in this field take us into the more clinical domain, the last of these being a new and important chapter in this volume. Finally, the medico-legal chapter puts the field of audiological legal problems into a broader legal perspective.

The second section on hearing disorders follows broadly the contents of the previous edition. With the integration of test procedures, the evoked response chapter has been amalgamated into the chapter on behavioural and admittance tests. There is a brief new chapter on tactile aids, which have a limited but definite role in the rehabilitation of profoundly deafened individuals. The final chapter in this section is also new, covering aspects of central auditory dysfunction.

The balance section starts again with an overview followed by three chapters along the same lines as in the previous edition. However, as with the other chapters in this book on the same topics as before, all have been completely rewritten and updated, in many cases by different authors, who will inevitably have different approaches.

In certain cases there will be cross-referral to chapters in the previous edition where authors feel that the thrust of recent developments has been in a somewhat different direction but that the background information from the previous edition still has some relevance.

I am grateful to all the contributors for their dedicated efforts and also to Drs Cliodna O Mahoney and Mary Francis who did a final check on the page proofs.

Dafydd Stephens

1

Acoustics

John C. Stevens

This chapter provides an introduction to acoustics. The nature of sound and its physical properties will only be described briefly with more space devoted to the measurement of sound, particularly in relation to the assessment of hearing. In addition, areas of practical importance to professional staff involved in the provision of audiology services will be covered in detail.

The reader is referred to Hall (1993) and Kinsler, et al (1983) for more comprehensive texts on acoustics. In addition, there are many excellent publications from the various professional organizations. *The Journal of the Acoustical Society of America, Acustica* and the *Journal of the Audio Engineering Society* are particularly well respected. Manufacturers of acoustical equipment also produce many good technical publications which can provide an excellent source of practical information. National standards laboratories and national institutes of acoustics and vibration research are also a very good source for up to date information.

Properties of sound

Nature of sound and wave propagation

Sound is used to describe a mechanical disturbance propagated in a solid or fluid elastic medium whether audible or not. Where the sound is of higher frequencies than the audible range it is described as ultrasonic and where it is below the audible range as infrasonic. This chapter will concentrate on the properties and measurement of sound within the audible range. Acoustics is the study of sound and its behaviour in the transmitting medium. The medium is usually treated as being made up of 'particles' which are large compared with the molecular dimensions but small compared to the wavelength of sound.

Idealized examples of sound sources are a point, a line or a plane. In the first of these the sound radiates equally in all directions. In general, sources of sound and the resulting sound fields are complex and not amenable to simple analysis. Readers are referred to standard texts on acoustics for a detailed mathematical treatment, e.g. Kinsler *et al*. (1983).

Some definitions

Sound pressure (P) is the alternating component of the pressure at a point in a sound field.

Particle velocity (u) is the alternating component of the velocity of movement of the medium at a point in a sound field.

Volume velocity (U) is the rate of flow of the alternating component through a specified area.

Intensity (I) of a sound in a specified direction is the average rate of flow of acoustic energy through a unit area normal to the direction specified.

Acoustic impedance

Acoustic impedance is an important parameter in audiology, particularly in relation to the assessment of middle ear function.

The acoustic impedance (Za) is defined as the ratio of the sound pressure (P) to the volume velocity (U) in the transmitting medium. This is analogous to electrical impedance being the ratio of voltage to the current flow through an electrically conductive medium.

$$\text{Thus } Za = P/U$$

In the measurement of acoustic impedance of the middle ear it is normal practice to use the reciprocal of impedance – the admittance (Y).

$$Ya = 1/Za = Ga + iBa$$

where *Ga* is the acoustic conductance and *Ba* is the acoustic susceptance.

In addition, acoustic impedance instruments usually use equivalent volume as the unit of measurement. The equivalent volume of an acoustic impedance *Za* or admittance *Ya* (at a given frequency) is the volume of a hard-walled cavity containing air at standard temperature and pressure which has an impedance whose magnitude is equal to *Za*.

The specific acoustic impedance, also termed characteristic impedance, is the ratio of pressure and the particle velocity.

$$Zs = P/u$$

It is useful in calculations involving transmission of sound from one medium to another. Table 1.1 gives some characteristic impedances. Note the large differences between the two solids, water and air.

Table 1.1 Characteristic acoustic impedances for some common media

Medium	Characteristic impedance (Pa s/m $\times 10^6$)
Steel	47.0
Wood	1.57
Water	1.48
Air	0.000415

Reflection and transmission at a boundary between two media

It can be shown that the relationship between transmitted and reflected waves at a boundary between two acoustic media depends on their characteristic impedances (Z_1, Z_2) thus,

$$\frac{\text{intensity reflected sound}}{\text{intensity incident sound}} = \frac{(Z_2 - Z_1)^2}{(Z_2 + Z_1)^2}$$

$$\frac{\text{intensity transmitted sound}}{\text{intensity incident sound}} = \frac{4Z_2Z_1}{(Z_2 + Z_1)^2}$$

It can be seen from the above equations that maximum transmission occurs when the two impedances are equal and the amount of reflected sound increases as the difference in characteristic impedances increases.

Absorption at a boundary

When a sound wave meets a surface, some of the sound energy may be absorbed. The term *absorption coefficient* is used to describe the ability of the surface to absorb sound having a range from 0 to 1. The value of the coefficient depends on many parameters of the material, e.g. the porosity and density. It is usually frequency-dependent and so it is necessary to make measurements across the full spectrum of sound energy. In the construction of audiometric test rooms and rooms used for fitting hearing aids it is important to design the room to provide an acceptable acoustic environment. The choice of absorptive materials for the floors, walls and ceiling as well as the furniture will determine the amount of sound energy absorbed and in turn the time it takes for sound energy to decay. The term used for the latter is reverberation time. This is discussed further in the last section of this chapter on architectural acoustics.

Diffraction at a boundary

It is important to be aware that sound waves can be diffracted at apertures or edges in a boundary. This is illustrated in Figure 1.1. Acoustic shadows are formed

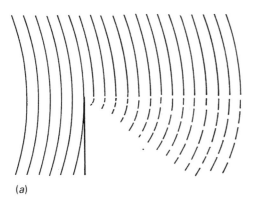
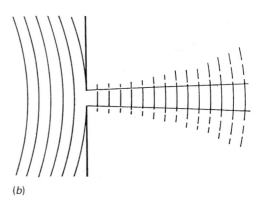

(a)   (b)

Figure 1.1 Effects of diffraction at high frequencies. (*a*) Past an obstacle, forming a shadow; (*b*) through an opening, forming a beam. (Courtesy of Bruel and Kjaer)

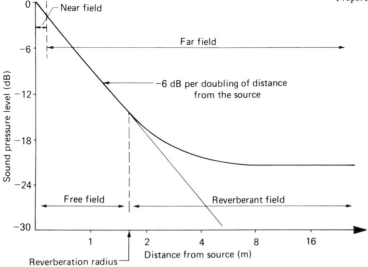

Figure 1.2 Sound field resulting from a combination of direct sound from a spherical source, and reverberant sound, in an enclosure. (Courtesy of Bruel and Kjaer)

by the obstacle but the nature of the shadow depends on the wavelength of the sound in relation to size of the obstacle. In general, the amount of diffraction increases with longer wavelength, so that the obstacle is less able to cut out lower frequency sounds. An example of this, relevant to audiology, is where a sound is presented to one ear, e.g. in behavioural audiometry. The difference in sound level between the test and the non-test ear will be less at low frequencies.

Other factors that affect sound propagation

Other physical factors such as wind, temperature gradients, and humidity can affect the propagation of sound. However, these are not normally of relevance to audiology and the reader is referred to Hassall and Zaveri (1988) for a more detailed description.

Sound levels within a room

The concept of a point source radiating sounds equally in all directions has already been introduced. However, this situation only exists in practice in a room with no reflections – an anechoic chamber. Such rooms are difficult and expensive to construct and would not form an acceptable environment in the audiology clinic. As sound-field testing in audiology uses sound sources that can often be considered as point sources, it is important to be aware of the variation of sound within the typical test room. This is also very important when sound measurements are being made. An illustration of how the sound will vary in a room is given in Figure 1.2. It can be seen that the sound pressure initially obeys an inverse

square law (see next section) as the environment can be considered to be a free field. The rate of drop in sound level with distance then reduces due to the added sound energy from reflections from the walls.

Relationship between intensity and distance from source

In order to develop the equations, the properties of a spherical sound source that radiates equally in all directions (omnidirectional) are used, since this is the simplest possible case. Let us designate the acoustic power radiated by the source as W watts. Assuming that there are no power losses in the air, then all the power radiated must pass through any surface that encloses the source completely. The amount of power flowing through a unit area ($1 m^2$) is designated as the intensity, I. Therefore, intensity is defined in units of watts per square metre (W/m^2). Moving away from the source, the power passing through a unit area decreases.

If a sphere is drawn around the omnidirectional sound source, by definition the intensity at every point on the surface of the sphere is the same. Therefore, if the intensity at the surface of the sphere is known, the source power is:

$$W = I \times 4\pi r^2$$

where r is the radius of the sphere. Rearrangement of this equation gives:

$$I = \frac{W}{4\pi r^2}$$

showing that the intensity is in proportion to the

inverse square of the distance from the omnidirectional source.

Measurement of sound

All the quantities above can be thought of as expressing the amount of sound that is present in various ways. However, in practice the quantities have to be measured. Direct measurement of acoustic power is impractical as it is necessary to measure the sound over a complete closed surface, such as the sphere. Acoustic intensity meters have been constructed, and are being increasingly applied in acoustic diagnosis since they have the virtue that the origin of the sound can be located. However, they are expensive and require some care in use. In general, it is more convenient to measure the sound pressure associated with the acoustic wave since this is easily carried out with a single microphone.

Decibels

The unit bel, and hence the decibel (dB), is named after Sir Alexander Graham Bell, inventor of the telephone, who first derived the concept to facilitate calculations of telegraph performance. The decibel is not an absolute quantity, but the logarithm of the ratio of the measured value to a reference value. It is used in many areas of physics and engineering where a logarithmic scale is more convenient. Sound power ranges from 1 nW (10^{-9}W) in a very soft whisper, to over 1 MW (10^6W) from a large rocket engine. Expressed on a linear scale, this corresponds to 0.000000001 W to 1 000 000 W. It can be seen that due to the large numerical range, calculations could rapidly become difficult.

However, in the decibel scale, the same range corresponds to 30–180 dB sound power level, a much more convenient range of numbers. In this case, the sound power reference level used to make the decibel calculation is 1.0 pW (10^{-12}W). A chart of typical powers together with the sound power levels is given in Figure 1.3. A second reason for using a logarithmic scale is that the ear perceives loudness more closely to a logarithmic change in

Table 1.2 Subjective effect of changes in noise levels

Change in level (dB)	Subjective effect
3	Just perceptible
5	Clearly perceptible
10	Twice as loud

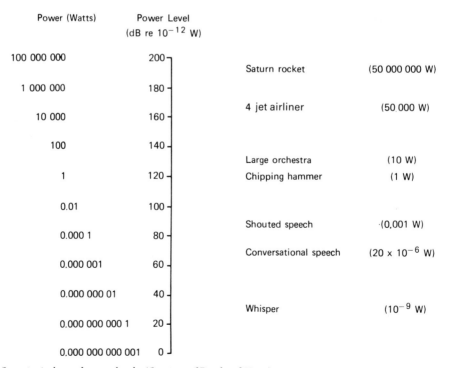

Figure 1.3 Some typical sound power levels. (Courtesy of Bruel and Kjaer)

sound power rather than a linear change. Table 1.2 shows the subjective effect of changes in decibels sound pressure level.

To distinguish between the two ways of expressing the same quantity, the decibel version is always appended by the word 'level'. As an example, therefore, it is usual to see sound power (W), and sound power level (dB) quoted. Often, the reference level is not quoted since it is assumed that an international standard level is used. However, if the wrong reference level is assumed, the result can be markedly different. To eliminate confusion the reference level should be quoted explicity, e.g. 23 dB re. 1 pW.

Decibel formulae

The equation which relates the sound power level (PWL) to the sound power, W, including the reference power, W_0 is defined as:

Sound power level (PWL) = $10\log_{10}(W/W_0)$ dB

Note the multiplying factor of 10, which gives rise to the name decibel. In the same way, the equation for intensity level is defined

Intensity level (IL) = $10\log_{10}(I/I_0)$ dB

As noted above, for practical reasons, the majority of sound measurements are made in terms of pressure. For the equation for sound pressure level (SPL), the convention of defining decibel quantities in terms of the acoustic power is followed. This is done because it is then possible to relate the decibel scales together. For example, if the sound power level of the source increases by 23 dB, then it is not necessary to recalculate the figures to establish that both intensity level and sound pressure level increase by the same number of decibels. Acoustic power in the far field is proportional to the square of the pressure. Therefore, the ratios of the squares of the pressures can normally be used in the calculation of decibel sound pressure level.

Sound pressure level (SPL) = $10\log_{10}(P/P_0)^2$ dB
= $20\log_{10}P/P_0$

where P is the measured pressure and P_0 the reference pressure (see below).

Decibel sound pressure level – summary

For practical reasons, the majority of sound measurements are made by measuring pressure. A logarithmic (decibel) scale is normally used to reduce the range of values needed to describe sound levels. The value in decibels relates the measurement to a reference value and is defined as 20 times the *logarithm of the ratio of the sound pressure measured to the reference pressure*.

Reference levels

An internationally agreed set of reference levels exists for the calculation of decibels of sound. These are:

Scale	Abbreviation	Reference quantity
Power level	PWL	1.0 pW (10^{-12} W)
Intensity level	IL	10^{-12} W/m²
Pressure level	SPL	20 μPa (20×10^{-6} N/m²)

These reference levels have superseded a large number of previous standards and, therefore, when reading older literature it is important to be aware of the particular standard used so that the appropriate corrections can be applied. The standards above apply to sound in air only.

The reference point for sound pressure level was chosen to coincide approximately with the threshold of hearing of normal subjects at 1 kHz.

To gain an appreciation of the scale of sound oscillations, it is interesting to recall that atmospheric pressure is approximately 10^5 Pa. Figure 1.4 gives some examples of sound pressure levels experienced in the environment. Even for a loud sound of 94 dB SPL the oscillation in the air pressure of about 1 pascal is very small compared with the static atmospheric pressure.

Sound pressure (μPa)	Sound pressure level (dB re 2×10^{-5} Pa)	
	140	
100 000 000	130	
		Near to a jet aircraft taking off
	120	
10 000 000	110	
	100	Near a pneumatic drill
1 000 000	90	
		Inside a motor car
	80	
100 000	70	
	60	General office
10 000	50	
	40	Quiet living room
1000	30	
	20	
100		Quiet countryside
	10	
20	0	Threshold of hearing

Figure 1.4 Some typical sound pressure levels. (Courtesy of Bruel and Kjaer)

Relation between units of intensity level and sound pressure level

Some confusion has arisen (particularly in audiology) between intensity level and sound pressure level, where the terms are interchanged freely. As mentioned previously, these quantities are physically quite different and therefore direct interchanging is incorrect. The practice has been caused in part by the standard reference levels that have been defined. In the special case of air acoustics, this has been especially done so that the numbers in the decibel scales for intensity level and pressure level for a given sound are similar. This emphasizes the need in all acoustic measurements to specify carefully the units that are being used.

Hearing level scale

An important modification is made to the decibel scale in the case of audiometry. We have already seen that the sound pressure level scale is defined without reference to frequency, i.e the pressures at for example 20 Hz and 15 kHz required to create a certain sound pressure level are identical. However, it is known that, in the case of the human ear, the threshold of hearing varies with frequency as shown in Figure 1.5. For the purpose of pure tone audiometry a practical scale is required which enables the hearing threshold of an individual to be easily compared with the normal average value. The decibel hearing level scale is therefore used in which the median normal hearing threshold at each frequency is used as the reference level (0 dBHL). Values for the reference level are given in ISO 389 (1991). This is discussed further under audiometric equipment calibration later in this chapter.

Frequency weighting

We have already seen how the threshold of hearing varies with frequency. In the measurement of sound it is useful to measure values which relate to the subjective level perceived by the listener. It is therefore necessary to apply a correction factor which varies with frequency. A further complication is that the correction factor at each frequency varies with sound pressure level as illustrated by the changing shape of the curves in Figure 1.5.

Many such correction curves or weightings have been produced. The principal one in international use is called the 'A' weighting scale (defined in ISO 131) (Figure 1.6). This is because, in the majority of cases, the 'A' weighting correlates measured and perceived noise levels better than other weightings and therefore is a fairly reliable measure of perceived sound. The 'A' weighting curve corresponds approximately to the equal loudness contour passing through 40 dB SPL at 1 kHz (see Figure 1.5). Sound measurement equipment often provides other weightings such as B, C and D. These are shown in Figure 1.6. The B and C weightings relate to equal loudness contours passing through 70 and 100 dB SPL at 1 kHz and were intended for use when sounds with a mean sound pressure level around these values were being recorded. Levels measured using the 'A' weighting should always be suffixed thus: 23 dB(A) SPL to prevent confusion. Similarly any other weighting curve used should be included in the unit description.

Temporal integration

If the duration of a sound is less than about 200 ms, its perceived loudness is less than when the sound is

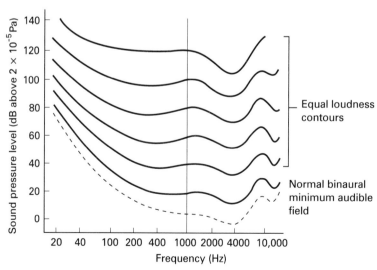

Figure 1.5 Normal equal-loudness contours for pure tones heard binaurally in a free field, from BS 3383. The dashed line shows the minimum audible level

heard continuously. Sound level meters incorporate circuits to simulate this. Figure 1.7 shows the results from different researchers for the subjective perception of short tone impulses and the standardized sound level meter characteristics in the IEC standard 651. L_i-L_D is the sound pressure level difference between the short tone impulses and a continuous tone. In the assessment of hearing it is particularly important to be aware of this as many stimuli used in behavioural testing and electrophysiological testing are of short duration and the use of an appropriate sound level meter is required.

Other scales

Many other scales exist to express measurements of sound. Some are used for objective measurement such as for aircraft noise, while others are intended for subjective applications such as predicting the amount of annoyance caused by a noise source. Therefore, it is important to recognize which scale is being used and the advantages and limitations of each, so that the appropriate one may be used in the correct fashion and circumstances. Some of the more frequently used scales are: sone, phon, noise rating (NR), perceived noise (PNdB), perceived noisiness (Noy), equivalent noise level (Leq). The last of these, with A weighting applied, is frequently used to assess noise over a period of time and in many countries as the unit for assessing the risk of noise-induced hearing loss. It can be considered as the continuous steady noise level which would have the same total A weighted acoustic energy as the actual noise measured over a set period of time. Mathematically:

$$L_{Aeq} = 10\log_{10} \frac{1}{T} \int_0^T \left[\left(\frac{Pa(t)}{Po} \right)^2 \right] dt$$

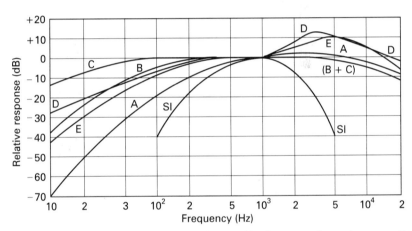

Figure 1.6 The internationally standardized weighting curves for sound level meters and recently suggested E (ear) and SI (speech interference) weighting. (Courtesy of Bruel and Kjaer)

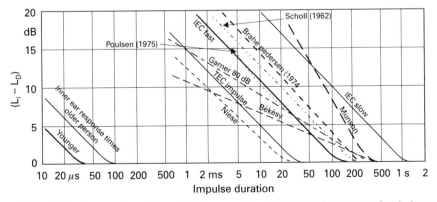

Figure 1.7 Results from different researchers of the subjective perception of short impulses compared with the standardized sound level meter characteristics and inner ear response times. (Courtesy of Bruel and Kjaer)

where $Pa(t)$ is the instantaneous sound pressure level.

For further information, the reader is referred to Burns (1973) and Kinsler *et al.* (1983).

Amplitude measures – average, peak and root mean square

It is possible to measure the amplitude of an arbitrary waveform in a number of ways (each equally valid). For example, we may take the largest amplitude that the waveform attains (the peak value). Alternatively, it may be more useful to ignore the short-term variations and measure the average amplitude instead. The most widely used is the root mean square (RMS) value, which has certain advantages since it is directly related to the energy content of the signal in linear systems. The various measures are shown in Figure 1.8 for a sinusoidal waveform which would be produced by a pure tone. In this case the relationships are well defined as follows:

$$A_{RMS} = \frac{A_{peak}}{\sqrt{2}}$$

$$A_{average} = \frac{2(A_{peak})}{\pi}$$

Many sounds are not pure sinusoids, but contain many frequency components and simple relationships between these descriptive measures do not exist.

Frequency analysis

A very useful method of analysis is to consider that the sound is made up of superimposed sinusoidal waveforms, known as Fourier analysis. The energy at each frequency is plotted against frequency to give a frequency spectrum. Many sound sources are periodic in nature and are particularly suited to this type of analysis. For signals that are not periodic in nature, alternative methods of description are required. Examples of such signals are certain types of background noise, noise from amplifiers and some electrophysiological signals.

The probability density function is one useful measure to describe this type of signal. For a given duration of the signal, the probability that the signal has a particular amplitude is plotted against the range of possible amplitudes. The reader is referred to texts such as Lynn (1989) and Randall (1987) for a more detailed description of these techniques.

Statistical analysis

Many sources of sound, particularly sources of noise in the environment, vary continuously in loudness with time. An instantaneous reading of the sound pressure level does not give an accurate description of the sound. In this case the sound is recorded for a representative period of time and analysed to determine the proportion of time the sound is at each level. An example is shown in Figure 1.9. This method is commonly used in the specification for environmental noise levels. For example, it might be specified that the noise level in a hospital ward should not exceed 40 dB(A)SPL for more than 10% of the time during the working day.

Multiple sources

In practical situations, problems frequently arise involving several sound sources, each of which contributes to the overall sound field. We may wish to know the overall sound pressure level produced by these multiple sources. Since the decibel scale is logarithmic, it is not valid simply to add two levels together. The absolute sound pressures must be calculated by inverting the equation thus:

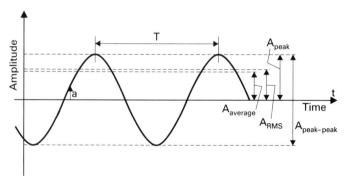

Figure 1.8 Sinusoidal signal showing various measures of signal amplitude

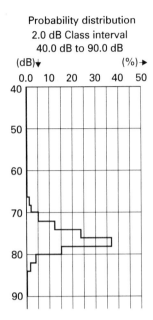

Figure 1.9 Probability distribution plot for motorway noise. (Courtesy of Bruel and Kjaer)

Sound pressure = Antilog$_{10}$ (SPL/20) × reference level

which is:

$$\text{Sound pressure} = 10^{\text{SPL}/20} \times 0.00002 \text{ Pa}$$

(a similar equation with different constants is used for power and intensity). For independent noise sources that are not coherent, and do not therefore produce significant interference of one wave front by another, the contributions can be combined on an energy (or power) basis. The power is proportional to the square of the pressure. Therefore, the squares of the sound pressures are added together:

Total pressure (squared) = $p_1^2 + p_2^2 + \dots$

The square root of this value is then taken, and finally converted back to decibels SPL once more. Where the sound sources produce waves that could interfere destructively or constructively more information is required. It can be seen that addition of sound levels is slightly laborious and often it is possible to simplify the process by charts such as that shown in Figure 1.10. In practice, the addition of contributions from multiple sources is complicated by the environment (e.g. whether reverberant, absorbent) and the type of noise. Therefore, to obtain accurate results it is usually necessary to have knowledge of more than just the levels of the sources.

Background noise can be considered as a second noise source when making sound level measurements. It is important to be aware that an error will be produced by the summation with the measured sound. This becomes significant when the difference in the sound levels is small.

Standards and calibration

The accuracy of a measurement is the 'closeness' of the measured quantity to the true value. The error inherent in a measurement is the difference between the measured and true values. The true value is defined as the measured value obtained with a standard of ultimate accuracy, with zero error. Therefore, in order to make any meaningful measurement, it is necessary to have a reference standard.

The need for universal references has been apparent since the reign of Henry VIII, when he recognized the serious confusion that resulted from the use of many different standards of length. This culminated in the famous royal decree which states that the yard was to be the distance between the King's nose and his fingertips. An immediate problem arose

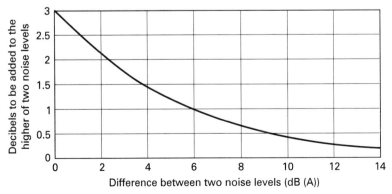

Figure 1.10 Noise level addition chart. (Courtesy of Bruel and Kjaer)

for the innovative monarch, since presumably he did not wish to be consulted every time a merchant wanted to measure cloth. To overcome this limitation, it was necessary to make copies of the standard distance which could be distributed widely for general use.

It was important to ensure these copies (secondary references) were as close to the original prototype (or primary) standard as possible, or the situation would rapidly revert. It was also important that copies were made so that variations in environment did not affect the measurement. This was important in a rapidly growing maritime nation for trade reasons, so for example a yard of material manufactured and measured in Scandinavia was the same as a yard when the same material was exported to hot climates. This was the beginning of the need for international agreement on standards. The same principle is carried on today, with the rapidly growing scientific community being served by secondary standards being distributed and derived from primary standards (see Table 1.3).

Henry VIII's choice of the length of the yard is at first sight a rather arbitrary measure, but in fact was just as arbitrary as any other standard then in use. Even today, international standards are often somewhat nebulous in origin.

The idea of a decimal system of units was conceived by Simon Stevin (1548–1620). Decimal units were also considered in the early days of the French Academy of Sciences founded in 1666, but the adoption of the metric system as a practical measure came later in the general increase in administrative activity in Europe following the French Revolution. The initial basis was the metre (intended to be one ten-millionth of the distance from the North Pole to the Equator through Paris) and the gramme which was the mass of one cubic centimetre of water at 0°C. In 1873 the British Association for the Advancement of Science selected the centimetre and gramme as basic units of length and mass, which together with the later adoption of the second for time, led to the c.g.s. system. About 1900 the metre, kilogramme, second were adopted for practical measures. To link electromagnetic units with these basic mechanical units the ampere was adopted by the International Electrotechnical Commission in 1950. In 1960 the General Conference of Weights and Measures added two further base units, the Kelvin and Candela giving rise to the International System of Units (SI) which has now been almost universally adopted. To supplement the base units, 'derived' units have been generated such as those for force and pressure. A full description can be found in Kaye and Laby (1986).

Coordination of international standards

In order to coordinate the fundamental units of measurement at an international level, it has been necessary to maintain extremely close liaison between the authorities of many countries. The central body for standards is the International Bureau of Weights and Measures (BIPM) in Paris. Every country has its own specialist body whose function is to supervise the definition and distribution of standards. In the UK, this activity is covered by the British Standards Institution (BSI). In Europe, the International Electrotechnical Commission (IEC) produces data, while in the USA, the American Standards Authority (ASA) performs a similar function.

Fundamental and primary standards are usually maintained by the central Government Laboratory and in the case of the UK this is the National Physical Laboratory (NPL). Such laboratories are also responsible for the production of secondary standards, which are then used to manufacture a large number of tertiary (transfer standards) and lower level references for ordinary laboratory use (Bentley, 1988). Great importance is attached to the methods used to compare standards. The central laboratories carry out investigations in this area and many other measurement-related activities.

Calibration and accuracy

In everyday life, we calibrate quantities every time we measure objects, e.g. weighing a parcel. In effect we are comparing a 'known' reference with an 'unknown' and can then state the quantity or magnitude of something with a degree of confidence. In the case of a parcel, the accuracy of measurement required to determine the correct amount of postage is not particularly high and an error of several per cent is probably permissible.

In the laboratory, the degree of accuracy to which comparisons can be made is crucial. For example, if a voltmeter gave wrong readings, the performance of every item of electronic equipment calibrated against it would introduce a systematic error into all measurements subsequently made. The culmination of several such errors could have serious consequences, particularly for example in a medical or nuclear field.

This highlights the importance of ensuring that the measuring instrument is in itself accurate (i.e. it can be stated to be in calibration). The way in which this is done is important. For example, if the reference standard (used to calibrate the measuring instrument) has degraded for some reason, then the overall accuracy is degraded despite the recalibration. Therefore, it is important to ensure that reference standards are as stable as possible with respect to all environmental and usage factors. In addition, it is vitally important to recalibrate measuring instruments regularly, to check for errors caused by ageing, drift, shocks etc.

Traceability

In order to ensure that measurements made with instruments are correct, it is important that each calibration right from the primary standard is as accurate as possible and that the entire chain can be traced back to the primary standard.

As an example, the traceability chain for the mass standard, the kilogram (and the derived standard weight), is shown in simplified form in Table 1.3.

In the UK, in order to maintain traceability to acceptably high standards, with good accessibility to calibrated standards, the National Physical Laboratory (NPL) operates several schemes whereby the capability of calibration laboratories is stringently assessed and, if acceptable, they are granted approval to provide a calibration facility as a service on a commercial basis. This is known as the British Calibration Service (BCS). Other NPL-supervised calibration schemes exist, such as the National Measurement Accreditation Scheme (NAMAS), and similar schemes exist in other countries.

Quoted accuracy and tolerances

Having made the calibration, the immediate question that arises concerns the quality of the result. How accurate is it? In practice, it is not possible to make measurements completely accurately, and it is necessary to allow variations due to the inaccuracies that creep in as a process of errors which accumulate during the calibrations down the traceability chain, and also permit departures from this due to local effects such as variations in temperature and pressure. This range of uncertainty is termed the 'tolerance'. For anyone involved in a calibration service it is essential that the tolerance levels are determined and given with each measurement.

Standards

For any professional involved in acoustic measurements and calibration, it is essential to be familiar with the relevant standards. There are many hundreds of standards relating to acoustics produced by the various organizations, many of which are equivalent. They are being continuously updated and any laboratory should ensure that it is notified of revisions as they appear. A list of those frequently used in

audiology is given in Appendix 1.1. For a more comprehensive list the reader is referred to Chapter 7 of Hassall and Zaveri (1988).

Limitations

Values given in standards refer to measurements made under a highly specified conditions. In audiological practice clinical measurements can be subject to many factors which introduce errors and the professional audiologist should be aware of this. One common problem is the error caused by background noise when measuring the thresholds of hearing particularly in a free-field situation without a noise-excluding headset. Examples of less obvious sources of error are the effect of ear canal size on the sound level presented to the eardrum by earphones and the effect of the coupling force when carrying out bone conduction audiometry.

Equipment for sound level measurement

Sound level meters

The sound level meter is probably the single most important piece of instrumentation available for general acoustical work. A thorough understanding of its construction, principles of use, capabilities and limitations is therefore fundamental to the practising acoustician. Sound level meters are produced in a large variety of types and a detailed reading of the manual is essential to reveal the precise nature of the equipment that is being used. However, all meters have a number of fundamental elements in common, which are covered in this section.

A diagram showing the elements of a typical sound level meter is shown in Figure 1.11. Perhaps the most important element of the sound level meter is the microphone. It is important to have a good knowledge of the characteristics of microphones used for sound level measurement and for this reason they will be covered in detail in the following section.

A microphone is a device which transduces sound energy into electrical energy. There are many different physical principles that have been used in the

Table 1.3 Traceability ladder for the kilogram

Standard	Where held
International prototype kilogram	International Bureau of Weights and Measures
National primary standard	National Physical Laboratory
National secondary standard weight	National Physical Laboratory/British Calibration Service
National transfer standard weight	Portable
Local standard weight	Weights and Measures department
Laboratory standard weight	Calibration laboratory
Weighing instrument	Field

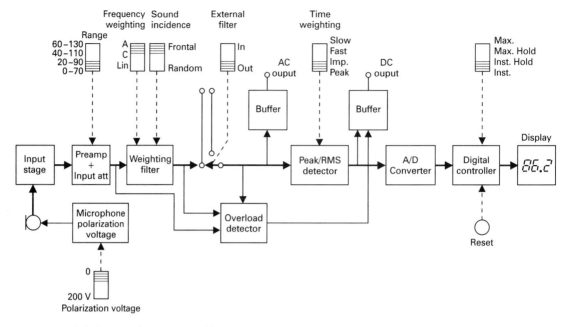

Figure 1.11 Block diagram of a typical sound level meter. (Courtesy of Bruel and Kjaer)

design of microphones, the most common of which are given in Table 1.4. The ideal microphone transduces sound pressure variations into variation in electrical potential without distortion. Table 1.5 lists the main desirable characteristics of a microphone.

The capacitor microphone

In its simplest form, this device consists of a very thin metallic diaphragm stretched across a frame, with a plate parallel to and very close behind it (Figure 1.12). This forms a capacitor, with the air gap acting as an insulating dielectric. The impinging sound waves cause the diaphragm to vibrate. As the membrane moves, the separation between it and the plate

changes microscopically. The capacitance is described by the following simple equation:

$$C = \frac{\varepsilon A}{d}$$

where A is the area of the diaphragm, d is the separation between it and the plate, and ε is the dielectric constant or permittivity (a number, which expresses the quality of the capacitive material in the gap). Therefore, if any of the factors on the right hand side of the equation is changed, the capacitance will change accordingly.

A polarizing voltage (Vp) is applied to the plates forming the capacitor, typically in the region of 200

Table 1.4 Different principles used in design and construction of microphones

Class	Principal cause/effect
Capacitor	Varying capacitor plate separation varies electrical potential on capacitor plates
Electret	Similar to capacitor but with permanent source of electrical potential
Piezoelectric (electrostrictive)	Sound pressure waves stress material and create charge
Electrodynamic	Sound pressure on diaphragm causes movement of coil in magnetic field which generates current

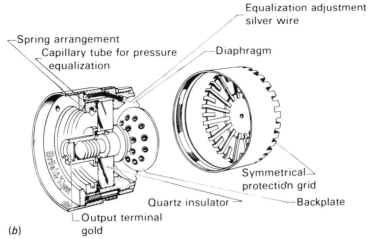

Equalization adjustment
silver wire

Spring arrangement
Capillary tube for pressure
equalization

Diaphragm

Symmetrical
protection grid

Quartz insulator

Backplate

(b)

Output terminal
gold

Figure 1.12 Sectional view of a 1-inch capacitor microphone cartridge. (Courtesy of Bruel and Kjaer)

Table 1.5 Desirable microphone characteristics

Parameter	Characteristic
Frequency response	Wide range, flat response
Sensitivity	High
Stability	Immune to temperature variation, humidity and other environmental factors
Robustness	Withstands shock and variation without damage or change in properties
Dynamic range	Low noise level, with high saturation level
Distortion	Low

V DC. The change in output voltage $V_0(t)$ is proportional to the impinging sound pressure and is given by:

$$V_0(t) = \frac{C(t)}{C_0} \times V_p$$

where $C(t)$ is the change in capacitance with time due to the sound pressure and C_0 is the capacitance of the microphone with no sound present.

Therefore, the higher the polarization voltage, the greater the sensitivity of the microphone. However, it is not practical to make the voltage too high or else it is possible that an arc could be generated between the plates.

For practical design considerations, the size of the microphone is usually increased in order to achieve high sensitivity. However, this conflicts with the requirement for a high frequency response and omni-

directivity. In practice therefore, a range of microphones is used, the selection being dependent on the nature of the sound that is to be measured. Figure 1.13 shows a comparison of frequency response ranges for various Bruel and Kjaer microphones. It is important to note that the output is linear only if the change in capacitance $C(t)$ is small compared with C_0. At very high sound levels this is not the case and distortion will be introduced. Examples are given in Figure 1.14.

In practice it is necessary to remove the polarization voltage (DC component) from the microphone output voltage, leaving the small AC signal. The DC component is isolated by the blocking capacitor, which lets only the AC signal through. The AC signal is then passed to the preamplifier. The fact that the AC signal is small imposes stringent requirements on the regulation of the polarization voltage supply, since if it has hum or noise superimposed upon it, this will appear at the output of the microphone as an AC signal and therefore degrade performance. This can determine the noise level of the device. In addition, there are other factors, such as the diffraction constant, which are much more complex and have a great effect on performance at high frequencies. This factor contributes to the directionality of the microphone, which becomes more pronounced as the frequency increases (Figure 1.15). This is usually described in terms of a polar plot of sensitivity with respect to angle.

Once optimized, the capacitor microphone possesses outstanding performance and is why it is universally used for precision measurements. This type of microphone is nearly always used on precision sound level meters. However, there is a number of disadvantages associated with the capacitor microphone, which limit its field of application. The thin diaphragm is delicate and easily damaged by shock, dirt and probing fingers, which limits its use to fairly benign environments.

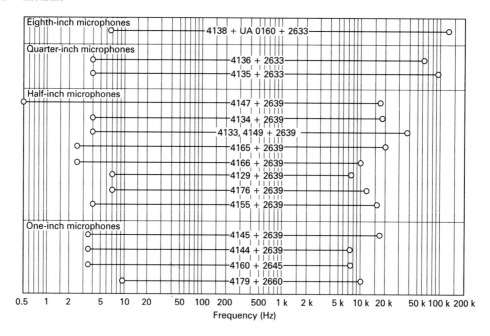

Figure 1.13 Comparison of the frequency response ranges (± 2dB) of recommended microphone and preamplifier combinations. (Courtesy of Bruel and Kjaer)

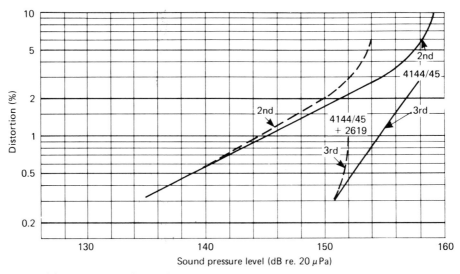

Figure 1.14 Typical distortion curves of one inch microphones at high sound pressure levels. (Courtesy of Bruel and Kjaer)

Standard microphone sizes

The international standards in acoustics are closely related to the 1-inch (25 mm) diameter microphone, since this size has been found to meet most of the basic requirements for acoustical measurements. Three types are in common use, the Bruel and Kjaer 1-inch types 4145 and 4144, and the Western Electric type WE640A.

Free-field and pressure microphones

As noted earlier, when an object, such as a microphone, is placed in a sound field the field is disturbed by a process known as diffraction. Diffraction is caused by the scattering of the incident sound field by the microphone, and is dependent on the microphone size in relation to the wavelength of sound. This is yet another manifestation of the fact that, if

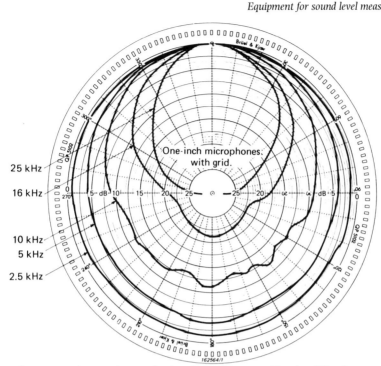

Figure 1.15 Directional properties of a typical one inch microphone. (Courtesy of Bruel and Kjaer)

an object is introduced to measure a physical process, the process is disturbed and therefore the measurement will not be true. In this case, the objective is to minimize the disturbance.

The mathematics of diffraction are, in general, extremely complex (Kinsler *et al.*, 1983) and so the present discussion is confined to a qualitative explanation only.

We shall first consider the situation of a 'free field', i.e. one in which the effects of boundaries are negligible throughout the region of interest. At low frequencies (long wavelengths), the microphone is much smaller than the wavelength of the sound. The wave is not disturbed (diffracted) significantly by such a relatively small object. Little energy is scattered by the microphone. The correction for free field measurement is small (Figure 1.16). However, at high frequencies (short wavelengths), the microphone becomes a sizeable obstacle and diffracts significant amounts of energy, causing disturbances to the wave. The reflection of the incident sound wave causes an increase in sound pressure relative to the unobstructed field. This is a maximum when the microphone has an angle of incidence of 0° to the source of the sound as shown in Figure 1.16. The microphone therefore becomes increasingly sensitive as it points towards the source of the sound. Microphones for accurate measurements in a free-field situation are constructed in such a way as to try to remove this increase in sensitivity with frequency to give as near a flat response as possible at 0° incidence.

At even higher frequencies where the sound waves are smaller than the diaphragm dimensions, sections of the diaphragm will be moving in opposition. In the case of the capacitor microphone, this effect causes some regions of the diaphragm to create higher values of capacitance, while others will create lower values than the average. These will tend to interfere and cancel out, therefore reducing sensitivity.

A rather different situation arises when measurements are made in confined spaces, such as the cavity formed in the ear canal between the eardrum and earmould. In this case, the cavity is so small in relation to a wavelength that the pressure at all points is very nearly the same regardless of frequency. The pressure is confined within the cavity and is not permitted to propagate as a travelling wave.

Since the acoustic pressure is the same at all points over the microphone diaphragm, the interference effect does not occur and consequently the output is extended to higher frequencies without degradation in sensitivity.

Many microphones are specifically designed to work in free field or a closed cavity as described above. In summary, care is required in the selection and use of microphones particularly when measuring at high frequencies.

In many situations a diffuse sound field exists where reflections are sufficiently numerous and random that the energy density is uniform. In this case a random incidence microphone is used. It is also possible to use a smaller free field microphone or

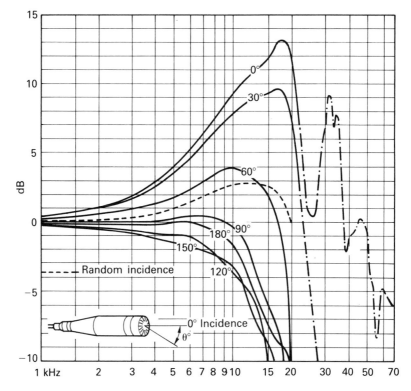

Figure 1.16 Free-field corrections for one-inch microphone cartridge with protecting grid. These are to be added to the electrostatic actuator response curve. (Courtesy of Bruel and Kjaer)

a pressure microphone. Random-incidence correctors are also available for larger free field microphones giving a response equal in all directions, at the expense of sensitivity and bandwidth. A summary of the types of microphone and their use in different sound fields is shown in Figure 1.17.

The electret microphone

The electret is a relative of the capacitor microphone, and is of great importance to audiology since it offers performance that cannot be approached by any other transducer type in subminiature units. Such devices are almost universally used in hearing aids, since they are small (typically 2 mm × 8 mm × 6 mm or less), lightweight (less than 1 g) and require very small amounts of power. Their major advantage is their extreme ruggedness, being resistant to shock, vibration, humidity, and other adverse environments commonly encountered in hearing aids. A schematic diagram of a typical electret microphone is shown in Figure 1.18.

The electret consists of two parallel plates separated by a solid dielectric which is prepolarized. Therefore, an external polarizing supply is not needed. Prepolarization is achieved during dieletric material manufac-

ture where the material is heated beyond its Curie temperature and a high voltage is applied. This aligns the molecules in the material, creating a permanent polarization when the temperature is reduced once more.

The impinging sound wave causes the electret material to be deformed. The resultant voltage appearing across the electret terminals is amplified by an integral preamplifier contained within the case. To maintain the small dimensions, a miniature amplifier using a field effect transistor is used, sometimes constructed on a hybrid microcircuit.

The piezoelectric microphone and earphone

The piezoelectric effect is well known and is exhibited in many materials. Piezoelectric materials are a special set of materials known as electrostrictive substances. In these, an electrical charge is created when the material is deformed. The effect was discovered in 1880 by the Curie brothers, and since then has been exploited in microphones, earphones, underwater and ultrasonic transducers and spark-generating devices.

Materials that are used include quartz (largely superseded due to cost and low sensitivity), ammonium dihydration phosphate (ADP) and Rochelle salt

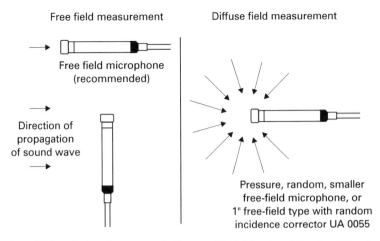

Figure 1.17 Orientation of different microphones types in the sound field. (Courtesy of Bruel and Kjaer)

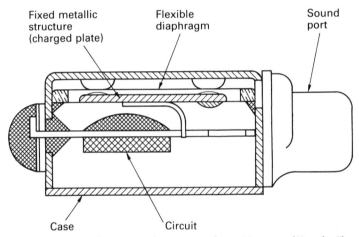

Figure 1.18 Cross-section through a typical miniature electret microphone. (Courtesy of Knowles Electronics)

(which suffer from the disadvantage that they are water soluble), barium titanate and lead zirconate-titanate (PZT) ceramics, which are the most sensitive materials and which are strictly speaking ferroelectric, and more recently piezoelectric plastics such as polyvinylidene fluoride (PVDF).

The piezoelectric effect is reciprocal, i.e. in addition to the effect described above, when an electric charge is applied, the material deforms. It is this property that makes both receivers and transmitters possible with piezoelectric materials.

This type of device has been miniaturized for use in hearing aid microphones and earpieces. Unfortunately, despite their high sensitivity, such devices do not have wide application in precision measurements due to the peaky nature of the frequency response

and temperature sensitivity. In addition, the piezo properties tend to change with ageing giving rise to poor long-term stability.

Piezoelectric materials find greater application in transducers for ultrasonic diagnosis and treatment (MHz region), and in sonar transducers (kHz–MHz). Such devices are capable of generating very high power and detecting small signals with high efficiency and are often formed into arrays to enable narrow beams to be formed to facilitate localization.

Filters and weighting

In addition to the standard flat or 'linear' setting (no filter), which permits sound pressure level (SPL) to be measured, the typical sound level meter may contain filters to enable frequency weighting to be applied to the sound level measurement as described earlier. The number and types of filter depend on the standard to which the instrument was built. The most basic sound level meter would contain at least an 'A' weighting filter (see Figure 1.6). Higher grades of sound level meters contain B, C, D filters and would also have the option to add a bank of external band-pass filters (either octave or one-third octave bandwidth) to permit spectral analysis to take place. The characteristics of these filters are defined within closely specified limits and they operate at standard frequencies (ISO 266, BS 3593). In addition, more specialized filters such as those used to assess infra- and ultrasonic noise or a continuously variable filter, can be substituted for special purposes.

The design of electronic filters is a wide-ranging field, covered comprehensively in many standard text-books and so is not discussed in detail here.

The ideal filter passes all the desired frequencies and rejects all unwanted frequencies completely. The bandwidth of the filter determines the range of frequencies transmitted. In general, it is not possible to achieve complete attenuation in the stopband and zero ripple in the passband and some compromise must be made, as illustrated in Figure 1.19.

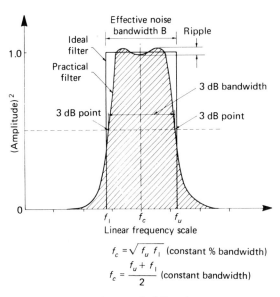

$$f_c = \sqrt{f_u\, f_l} \quad \text{(constant \% bandwidth)}$$

$$f_c = \frac{f_u + f_l}{2} \quad \text{(constant bandwidth)}$$

Figure 1.19 Practical versus ideal filter characteristics. (Courtesy of Bruel and Kjaer)

A good introduction to analogue filter design is given in Horovitz and Hill (1989).

All the previous filters are concerned with analogue signals. It is also possible to construct filters to perform similar operations on digital signals, and in general these have a far greater range of possibilities.

This is beyond the scope of this chapter and the reader is referred to Lynn (1989).

Root mean square (RMS) detector

Amplitude measures were discussed earlier in the chapter, the most widely used being the root mean square (RMS). The RMS detector converts the amplitude of the electrical AC signal derived from the sound wave to a signal proportional to the RMS value. However, not all RMS-to-DC converters perform equally well. Typically, approximations to the ideal conversion are used and this introduces errors. The conversion process is one of the more significant contributors to the precision or otherwise of the sound level meter.

Time weighting/peak detector

In order that averaging of the sound level can be accomplished, the ballistics of the meter can be controlled in many sound level meters. In the majority, fast and slow settings are provided. The fast setting in accordance with IEC 651 has a time constant of 0.125 second, which permits rapidly fluctuating sound pressure levels to be measured, while the slow setting (time constant 1.0 second) smooths out the fluctuations, giving a mean value of sound pressure level without the need for 'eyeball averaging'.

Earlier the problem caused by sounds of short duration being subjectively less loud than a continuous sound of the same sound pressure level was discussed. To enable the meter to display a value closer to the perceived loudness an impulse option is available on some sound level meters. The effect of this on the meter response to various durations of sound is shown in Figure 1.20.

It can be seen that the choice of time constant fast, slow or the use of the impulse setting affects the level and it is clearly very important to ensure that a correct choice is made when monitoring sounds, particularly those of short duration. Finally, it is known that even with the impulse time constant, severe underestimates of the peak amplitude of the impulse can be made. A single very high peak can cause as much hearing damage as continous exposure to a much lower level noise, and therefore an accurate measurement of this type of noise is essential. This measurement limitation is overcome by using a very short time constant (less than 50 μs) in the peak (and peak hold) modes, found on high grade meters.

Other more sophisticated averaging functions exist, in addition to those described above. These are concerned with statistical analysis of the noise level as was briefly described earlier in this chapter. Functions such as L_{50} (the sound level that is exceeded for half of the time), L_{90}, L_{10} and most widely used, L_{eq} (the equivalent continous sound level), are often included in precision integrating sound level meters.

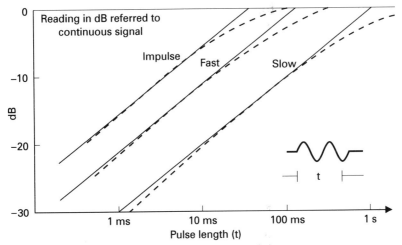

Figure 1.20 Response of time weighting circuit in a sound level meter to tone bursts of varying duration. (Courtesy of Bruel and Kjaer)

Outputs and display

Normally, the sound pressure level is indicated on a display or readout scale of some kind. This may be analogue (i.e. a needle and scale presentation) or digital (numerical presentation). Both have advantages. A digital scale is easier to read precisely, but suffers from the disadvantage that rapid fluctuations are difficult to follow and hard to interpret.

Some sound level meters provide an AC electrical output, corresponding to the sound signal. This can be routed to a tape recorder or other analysis equipment, enhancing the potential of the system considerably since measurements can then be re-examined in more detail at leisure in the laboratory. Also, a DC output signal which is identical to the meter drive signal is often available for driving recorders. Many sound level meters now incorporate a digital output for connection to computers to enable sound level measurements to be stored on the computer for later analysis.

Calibration of sound level meters

In addition to the regular calibration that should be performed on any electroacoustic equipment, it is essential to calibrate the sound level meter 'on site' to allow for any variation due to factors such as temperature, humidity, etc. and to check for damage in transit.

Several methods are available which calibrate the whole instrument in a single operation. In essence, they all involve a precision, calibrated sound source of a portable nature which can be attached to the microphone temporarily. The reading on the meter is then compared with the calibrator value and, if re-

quired, the gain of the meter adjusted to bring it into calibration.

The most popular of the systems are the sound source calibrator and the pistonphone. The sound source calibrator contains a miniature loudspeaker the output level and frequency of which is controlled within fine limits by a built-in electronic circuit. A typical example operates at 1.0 kHz at 94 dB SPL, which corresponds (conveniently) to a sound pressure of 1 Pa. This device permits calibrations to within about ±0.3 dB to be obtained. It is particularly useful for the calibration of A-weighted sound level meters since no correction factor has to be applied. This is because the A weighting is very nearly 0 dB at 1 kHz.

The pistonphone is the most accurate calibrator of this type, permitting accuracies of about ±0.15 dB. The system relies on a pair of opposing pistons being oscillated back and forth within a cavity by means of an eccentric cam on a rotating shaft. The cavity is sealed and contains the microphone. The excursions of the pistons are fixed by the cam dimensions and therefore this provides a simple but reliable precision sound source of exceptional stability. Useful working lives of several decades can be expected from such devices. Quite high sound levels can be produced, and a typical design produces 124 dB SPL at a frequency of about 250 Hz. A barometric correction factor is require to take varying air densitites due to weather and altitude into account. This is determined from a calibrated barometer supplied with the pistonphone. The acoustic signal does contain a high proportion of harmonics which can sometimes lead to problems. Wear of the cams and pistons can cause degradation due to amplitude reduction but, fortunately, these effects are negligible in most cases.

However, it should be noted that both the sound source and pistonphone only calibrate at a single frequency. If the sound level meter lost sensitivity at frequencies other than that tested this would go unnoticed and errors would result.

Standards for sound level meters

Since the sound level meter is the workhorse of acoustics, not surprisingly attention has been focused on the performance that must be attained by these instruments. Many international standards exist. The International Electrotechnical Commission (IEC) Publication 651 (1979) consolidates a number of preceding standards. This divides the performance into several classes, in descending order or sophistication and precision:

Type 0 laboratory reference grade
Type 1 precision grade
Type 2 general field application
Type 3 noise survey application.

The IEC have also published a standard (IEC 804 (1985)) on integrating–averaging sound level meters.

Other noise measuring instruments

In addition to the sound level meter, other noise measuring devices exist. One of the most important of these for routine noise survey and monitoring purposes is the personal sound exposure meter, often called the noise dose meter. This is a small instrument designed to measure personal exposure to noise in industrial situations, e.g. without the need for specialist knowledge of acoustic measurement instrumentation.

The microphone of the device is simply clipped on the lapel or mounted in an alternative position close to the ear, in order to receive approximately the same noise as the wearer's ear. These meters average the noise dose, which takes into account both the sound level and its duration. Occupational safety regulations define a maximum allowable noise exposure for a normal working period. In most countries, 85 dB(A) or 90 dB(A) is the defined equivalent continuous level for an 8-hour day. Higher levels are permitted if a corresponding shorter exposure time occurs. A useful reference is ISO 1999 (1990) which sets out the determination of occupational noise exposure and the estimation of noise-induced hearing impairment. Noise exposure is usually expressed as a percentage of the total allowable dose. In addition, since it is known that exposure to very short, high level impulsive sounds can cause hearing damage, a special peak detection facility is sometimes provided.

Audiometric equipment and calibration

Audiometers

In clinical audiology, pure tone audiometry is still the most frequently used test. The basic elements of the audiometer are shown in Figure 1.21. Earphones are used to test hearing by air conduction and a small vibrator placed over the mastoid to test hearing by bone conduction. The hearing level scale (dBHL) was discussed earlier and all audiometers incorporate a calibration circuit which allows the output sound level to be set at each test frequency so that the sound level control measures in dBHL.

Standards have been produced for both screening and diagnostic audiometers IEC 645–1 (1992). Modern audiometers are very stable in both the level of output and frequency of the test tone. However, faults still occur, particularly in the leads and transducers and it is important to set up a protocol to ensure that errors do not occur in audiometry due to a machine fault.

Practitioners should carry out a daily subjective check of output level and listen for the presence of unwanted sounds which give a false threshold. They should be familiar with their own hearing threshold and have this checked regularly so that they can interpret the results of their daily check accurately.

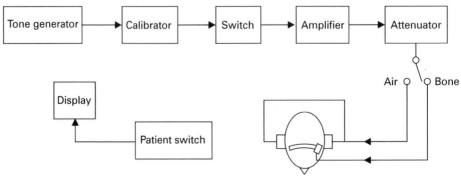

Figure 1.21 Block diagram of a pure tone audiometer

At regular intervals a full laboratory calibration should be carried out. This will be described in the following sections.

The signal presented to the subject by an audiometer can be categorized by its frequency, sound pressure level, and waveform. To obtain reliable audiograms, it is essential that these parameters are controlled. Details of specifications are given in IEC 645 which vary dependent on the type of audiometer. In general, the frequencies must be accurate to within ± 3%, while each harmonic present (with the earphone placed on the acoustic coupler) must be less than 2% of the level attained by the fundamental with the total harmonic less than 2.5%. The attenuator characteristics must be linear, such that the difference between the actual and measured sound levels at adjacent settings (of 5 dB) shall be within ± 1 dB of the difference between the scale readings at the two settings. The time taken for the sound to rise to the test level, and decay when turned off is specified.

Artificial ears and couplers

A number of systems have been evolved to meet the requirements for audiometer calibration. For earphone calibration, an acoustic coupler or artificial ear is used. This consists of a cavity (or cavities) of closely controlled dimensions, containing a microphone. The cavity dimensions are chosen to represent the acoustic characteristics of the ear. The earphone to be calibrated is placed upon the device and the sound pressure level monitored. The type of earphone, the way that it is positioned and the force that is used to keep it in place all affect the result and are all defined in the standard document. The microphone must itself be calibrated to an approved standard (again laid down in the standard) as must the voltmeter used to sense its output.

The older type of acoustic coupler, based on the 6 ml volume NBS 9A coupler (Figure 1.22) (originally defined by the National Bureau of Standards in Washington and defined in IEC 303) has been used for many years but suffers from the disadvantage that is a rather poor representation of the ear, especially at higher frequencies. Because of this, corrections to the reference equivalent threshold sound pressure levels have to be applied to the calibration depending on the type of earphone used (ISO 389 1991). A better representation of the ear overcomes the disadvantage of different reference levels encountered in the 9A coupler and matches the characteristics of the average ear over a wider frequency range. The device is designated the IEC wide-band artificial ear (Figure 1.23) (IEC 318). Different reference equivalent threshold sound pressure levels apply and the levels are defined in BS 2497 (1992), which is equivalent to ISO 389 (1991).

In order that the measurement is not affected by background noise, it is usual to employ a level of about 80 dB hearing level for calibration. However, to measure accurately at levels down to threshold, sophisticated low-noise equipment is required and laboratory noise levels have to be kept low. To overcome this problem, checking of audiometers at low output level is often done by measuring the output voltage and assuming that the transducer (earphone or bone conductor) is linear. In addition to pure tones, most types of audiometers are able to produce masking sounds. The IEC 645 standard for audiometers specifies that the masking levels for narrowband noise be calibrated in effective masking level and that the noise bandwidth be between one-third and one-half of an octave. Where the masking noise is applied by an earphone the reference levels have been standardized in ISO 8798 (1987). The values are given for both one-third and one-half octave masking noise bandwidths.

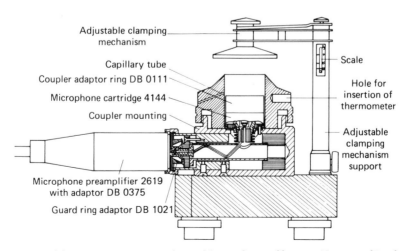

Figure 1.22 Cross-section of the NBS 9A acoustic coupler used for earphone calibration. (Courtesy of Bruel and Kjaer)

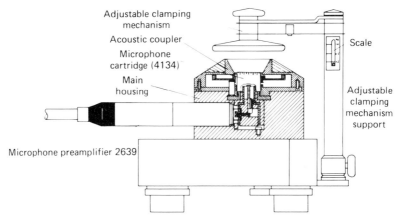

Adjustable clamping mechanism
Acoustic coupler
Microphone cartridge (4134)
Main housing
Scale
Adjustable clamping mechanism support
Microphone preamplifier 2639

Figure 1.23 Cross-section of wideband artificial ear for earphone calibration. (Courtesy of Bruel and Kjaer)

Mechanical coupler (artificial mastoid)

The audiometric reference zero for bone conduction is established with the aid of a mechanical coupler. The first device of this kind was defined in BS 4009, followed by a similar internationally agreed standard (IEC 373 (1990)). The construction is designed to represent the mechanical characteristics of the head in terms of its mass and the compliance of the flesh on the mastoid bone among other factors. A small piezoelectric element is used to sense the vibration induced by the bone vibrator (Figure 1.24). The standard reference equivalent threshold force levels over the frequency range 250 Hz–8 kHz has been defined in ISO 7566 (1987).

Equipment for speech audiometry

Speech audiometry is a useful audiometric test procedure. Unfortunately, because of the long time re-

quired to carry out the test and the poor repeatability it is not widely used in routine clinical audiology. However, with the increasing attention being paid to rehabilitation and the desire to measure the benefits of hearing aids and cochlear implants it is becoming increasingly important in the audiology clinic. The reader is referred to *Speech Audiometry* (Martin, 1987) for an up-to-date description.

In order to carry out speech audiometry, recording equipment is required. This is now a rapidly changing field and the description here will be limited to the use of a standard analogue tape recorder and the use of digital techniques.

Tape recording

Analogue audio (and video) tape recordings encode the signal waveform in the form of a varying permanent magnetic field. Magnetic tape recording has

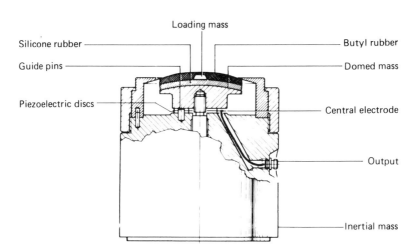

Loading mass
Silicone rubber
Guide pins
Piezoelectric discs
Butyl rubber
Domed mass
Central electrode
Output
Inertial mass

Figure 1.24 Cutaway view of the most important parts of the artificial mastoid. (Courtesy of Bruel and Kjaer)

limitations, particularly in the dynamic range, although noise reduction and compression/expansion techniques such as the 'Dolby' and 'dbx' systems improve performance significantly. The minimum recordable level is dependent on tape quality, and tape speed. Even in the best tapes fluctuations in the magnetic field pattern due to random domain alignment of the magnetic particles on the tape cause the characteristic tape hiss which spreads over the entire audible frequency band.

The maximum recorded level is dependent on the highest magnetic flux that the tape can accommodate before magnetic saturation occurs (the magnetization on the tape does not increase despite increased drive). When the signal level is increased to this level, clipping and harmonic distortion occur. Various schemes are employed to ensure that the saturation level is as high as possible, including the use of a high frequency bias signal. The saturation limit is dependent on the magnetic material, and pure metal tapes offer advantages over ferric oxide and chromium dioxide tapes in this respect. The frequency responses of the different types of tape vary, and this has to be compensated for by the use of different equalization circuits.

A normal analogue tape recorder is capable of achieving a dynamic range of about 50 dB, and noise reduction systems extend this somewhat. The electrical signal is converted to a magnetic field by means of a special electromagnetic transducer. Typically, three electromagnetic tape heads are used, one for recording, one for replay (also called the reproducing head) and one for erasing the tape. Each head consists of a coil wound on a magnetic core which has a minute gap cut in it. The tape passes over the gap, and is magnetized by the strong magnetic flux existing there due to the current in the recording coil. On replay, the magnetic variations on the tape passing over the gap cause a minute current to be generated in the replay head. The erase head is driven by a signal of high frequency, which 'overwrites' the magnetic pattern on the tape. The erase head is always the first that the tape passes over, so that when recording, it may be energized to erase the tape ready for the recording head which follows it. Finally, the replay head may be used to monitor the quality of the recording while it is in progress. Lower-cost tape recorders (and most cassette recorders) sometimes combine the functions of the record and replay head in a single unit. While being satisfactory for many applications, some performance degradation is inevitable since the desirable characteristics of record and replay heads are different and compromises have to be made.

To maintain consistent performance, it is important that the head is not permanently magnetized (since this tends to erase the tape). To maintain performance, they should be demagnetized at regular intervals. Care should be taken during this process to remove tapes from the vicinity as these can be erased by the demagnetizer. Tape heads are quite susceptible to wear since many kilometres of tape pass over the surfaces during their lifetime. This causes an increase in the size of the gap, which impairs performance. Dirty tape often carries minute particles which act in an abrasive manner, and to overcome this very hard materials such as ferrite are commonly used to minimize erosion.

Tape recordings suffer from degradation due to heat and age. In addition, after long storage periods the magnetic field can be transferred from one layer of tape on the spool onto the next. This is known as print-through and causes an echo effect where previous (or future) sections of programme material are heard over quiet passages on the tape. Repeated playing and spooling of the tape can cause the magnetized particles to become detached from the plastic backing layer, causing dropout of the signal. This is shown in a striking way if a pure tone of fixed amplitude is recorded and replayed (such as a calibration tone on a speech audiometry tape). The slightest dropout causes a significant change in the amplitude and this is shown clearly if a meter is used to monitor the replayed signal level.

In summary, although modern analogue tape recorders are reliable, it is important to be aware of the possible deterioration in recorded material. A sensible policy is to retain a master for each tape and use a copy for clinical work replacing it with a new copy at regular intervals.

Digital recording

The recent advent of the compact disc and digital audio tape (DAT) has brought digital recording and its performance capability to the attention of the public. The digital recording system records a numerical representation of the instantaneous amplitude of the waveform. This is done in the form of a binary bit pattern of 1s an 0s. The system is used in compact disc recordings and digital tape recordings. Such systems have considerable advantages over analogue systems. Digital recording is expected to increase in application, eventually rendering analogue recordings obsolete.

The advantages of this system include the reduction of noise to very low levels. The noise limit with digital recording is usually determined by the amplifiers used for the recording microphone and for loudspeaker drive during replay, rather than the recording medium. This is an advance over the analogue system which is generally noise limited by the recording medium. The compact disc, which uses an optical method of retrieving data from the disc, is not susceptible to small amounts of surface dirt on the recording medium since the laser and detector used to reproduce the reflective bit pattern encoded on the disc is designed to use a part of the optical spectrum where grease etc. is relatively transparent.

In the digital system, the difference between the minimum and maximum that can be recorded is determined by the number of different levels (numbers) that can be used to represent the signal amplitude. This also determines the accuracy of reproduction, or resolution. Digitization introduces noise due to the quantization of the signal. Normally, this is arranged to be insignificant by using a large number of quantization levels. At low signal levels quantization noise can become a problem, however. Strangely, one solution (which is adopted in compact disc players) involves adding more low level noise to the recorded signal. This is known as a dither signal.

By the use of suitable error correcting digital encoding, errors due to fairly severe data dropout on the replayed signal can be compensated and near perfect reproduction maintained.

Digital storage using computers

With the low cost of personal computers and interface cards suitable for digitizing analogue signals the use of digital storage of audio signals on computers is becoming more widespread. In addition there are many commercial devices now available for recording studios which enable sound to be digitally stored and edited by linkage to a computer. These developments will enable speech and other audiometric test material to be stored on computer with the potential for a high quality, calibrated sound source.

The limitation with tape recorders that speech material has to be used contiguously will no longer exist as it will be possible to present the stored material in any order.

Speech audiometry calibration

The calibration of speech audiometers which use recorded material is difficult due to the problem of measuring sound pressure levels of speech. The difficulty is complicated by the large amount of different 'standard' speech audiometry material available. In practice, the reference threshold of each word list must be determined from speech audiograms made from groups of normal subjects, a somewhat laborious task. Some of the speech audiometry material is of poor original quality due to the date and method of recording and repeated copying of tapes degrades performance further. Relevant standards in this area are ANSI S3.6, DIN 45626, DIN 45621 and ISO 8253.3.

The move to the use of digitally recorded material should ensure that speech material is of high quality and comparable across centres using it for audiological assessment.

Couplers for insert phones and hearing aids

Two couplers have been defined for the measurement of hearing aids. Both are intended to represent the ear when occluded by an earmould and fitted with either an insert or postaural type earphone. The oldest and most basic is the 2 cc coupler (Figure 1.25) as defined in IEC 126 (1973). This does not represent the response of the occluded ear well, particularly at low and high frequencies and is therefore of limited application. However, because of its simplicity it is still the standard coupler used in commercially available hearing aid test equipment. An improved device, the occluded ear simulator, is defined in IEC 711 (1981) and closely reproduces the physical characteristics of the average human ear (Figure 1.26). This permits the accurate measurement of the performance of insert earphones and postaural hearing aids fitted with tubes. 'In-the-ear' aids can also be measured.

Recent work has shown the importance of measurements *in situ* for hearing aids. The diffraction of sound by the head and body has been found to contribute significantly to the as-worn performance. For this reason, manikins such as the KEMAR have been used together with ear simulators.

It is worth remembering that all the couplers and associated devices describe the average characteristics of a large number of subjects. Individual variations can affect the sound (or vibration) level experienced by the subject. Therefore, different stimuli levels can be generated in different subjects by a single (calibrated) instrument on identical settings. This is one source of audiometric variations, but fortunately is small in most cases. When fitting hearing aids it is now common practice to measure the gain of the aid *in situ* by the use of insertion gain equipment. The problem of having to rely on an average value from coupler measurements is removed. More details of hearing aid measurements are described in Chapter 14, while an extended discussion of audiometric calibration is given in Beagley (1979).

Otoadmittance (acoustic impedance) meters

At the start of the chapter the concept of acoustic impedance was introduced. It was noted that it is normal practice to use the reciprocal measurement of impedance, the admittance, which can be considered to be the sum of its two components conductance and susceptance. Instruments to measure otoadmittance are widely used in audiology to investigate middle ear function. The two main measurements are the variation of admittance with ear canal pressure (tympanometry) and the variation in admittance resulting from an acoustic stimulus (acoustic reflex). These are described in more detail in Chapter 12. A schematic diagram of an impedance meter is shown in Figure 1.27.

A probe is placed in the ear canal forming an airtight seal. The probe contains a sound source, a microphone and a vent through which the air pressure in the ear canal can be altered. The admittance

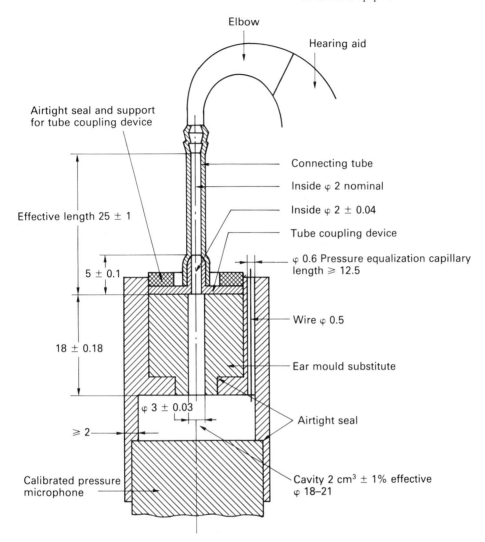

Figure 1.25 Cross-section of a 2 cc coupler to IEC 126

is measured by determining the relationship between the sound power delivered by the sound source and the sound level measured in the ear canal as measured by the microphone. An increase in admittance will reduce the sound level in the ear canal for a fixed sound input power. The air pressure in the ear canal is altered by a pump within the admittance meter.

The specification for acoustic admittance instruments are given in IEC 1027 (1991). In the majority of basic admittance instruments the measurement is made at one frequency, usually at about 220 Hz. At this frequency the admittance is dominated by the elastic components of the middle ear and the ear canal and is usually considered as pure susceptance, the resistive component of the eardrum admittance being negligible. Additionally, at low frequencies the

air in the ear canal and the middle ear can be considered as two separate sources of admittance. The admittance of the air in the ear canal can be measured by decreasing the air pressure until the eardrum becomes taut (about − 3.9 kPa (− 400 mm water) so eliminating the admittance contribution of the middle ear. The admittance of the middle ear is then obtained by subtraction of this value from the total measurement. As was noted at the beginning of the chapter most clinical instruments use equivalent volume as the unit of measurement, corresponding to the volume of a hard walled cavity that has the same acoustic admittance.

The more complex admittance instruments allow both susceptance and conductance to be measured separately and at more than one frequency. These

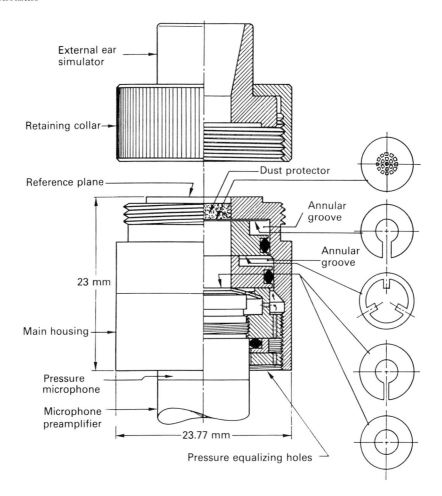

Figure 1.26 Cutaway view of an occluded ear simulator to IEC 711

find application in the diagnosis of such conditions as otoscelerosis and in the measurement of admittance in the neonate. At frequencies higher than that used in the basic instruments it is not possible to disregard the resistive component of the middle ear.

It is possible to carry out daily checks on otoadmittance instruments by the use of test cavities whose volumes cover the range of admittance values found (using units of equivalent volume). In addition, the operator can measure his own tympanogram and reflex thresholds to check whether there is any change which might indicate a fault with the instrument. However, at regular intervals the equipment should be given a full laboratory calibration against the IEC 1027 standard and the manufacturers' specification.

Included in the calibration should be a check of the pressure system against a calibrated pressure meter, a check on admittance values for a range of test cavity sizes and a check on the stimulus generator for acoustic reflex testing using the standards for pure tone audiometers. Many admittance instruments run in an automatic mode only, in particular those instruments used for screening for abnormal middle ear function. This can present a difficulty in that the instrument cannot be adequately controlled to enable comparison of pressure and admittance values with those from calibrated test equipment. One solution to this is to measure the tympanogram of the operator's ear and compare it with that obtained from a diagnostic instrument where an accurate calibration was possible.

Calibration of free-field sound generators

In many audiometric test situations it is desirable to use a stimulus presented in the sound field rather than by earphones. This is particularly the case in

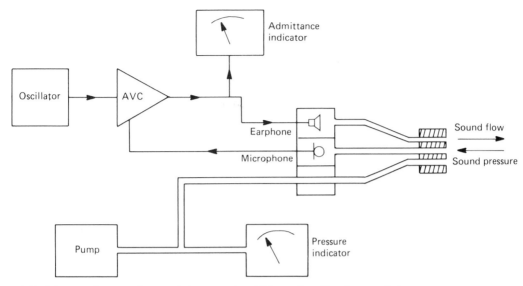

Figure 1.27 Schematic diagram of an otoadmittance meter. AVC = automatic volume control

paediatric audiology where earphones may not be tolerated. However, this presents a problem with calibration as it is more difficult to specify the test conditions. For example, there are many different types of sound generator being used and the geometric relationship to subject and room acoustics can affect the level of sound that reaches the ear under test.

It is common practice to check the sound delivered by a sound-field stimulator by presenting the sound again to a sound level meter. The value obtained is fairly repeatable if the procedure is carried out carefully. The desired aim is to measure a value which relates to the mean threshold in normal subjects to that particular stimulus. However, there are several problems in the use of a sound level meter to achieve this aim.

Sound level meters can only measure down to a level usually dependent on the quality of the microphone employed. Measurement of sound levels close to this limit are subject to error and it is important to be aware of this when making measurements at low sound levels. A typical high quality sound level meter will have a lower limit of about 25 dB(A)SPL for a signal to noise ratio of more than 5 dB whereas a low cost sound level meter, which is the type normally available in an audiology clinic, will have a equivalent lower limit of about 30 dB(A)SPL.

The choice of settings on a low cost sound level meter is usually restricted such that the only sensible option is A weighting with a fast time constant (see earlier in this chapter). The relationship between the recorded level and the level relative to the mean threshold in normal subjects (dBnHL) will depend on the nature of the sound. For example, impulsive noises such as clapping

of hands can have higher dBnHL levels than would be recorded as a dB(A)SPL value with a fast setting. The solution to this is to carry out a study on normally hearing subjects to obtain a reference equivalent threshold sound pressure level for each stimulus used.

To achieve this it will be necessary to carry out the study in a room with adequately low ambient noise levels. This is discussed later under audiometric test environment. The output of the sound generator should be measured under precise conditions, preferably identical to those under which the thresholds of the normal subjects were measured. As with pure tone audiometers the sound measurements will need to be carried out at a high enough attenuator setting to enable an accurate reading on the sound level meter to be obtained. The reference equivalent pressure threshold will then be calculated by taking the difference between this attenuator value and the mean attenuator value, for the threshold of the normal subjects, from the level recorded on the sound level meter. The precision of the attenuator should be checked to ensure an accurate result. A useful standard here is ISO 8253-2.

Electric response audiometry calibration

The stimuli used in electric response audiometry (ERA) vary depending on the type of test being carried out. Click and tone burst stimuli of varying length are the two most common of these (see Chapter 12). At present no international standards exist for these stimuli. The procedure for establishing a reference equivalent threshold sound pressure level (RETSPL) for each stimulus is similar to that described above except that the stimulus sound levels are measured by using a suitable coupler. In the case of earphones the couplers to IEC 303 and IEC 318 referred to earlier are both suitable.

The procedure of establishing the RETSPL for free field and electric response audiometry stimuli is time consuming and it is sensible to exchange information on this between audiology centres to avoid duplication of effort.

The recorded waveform on electric response audiometry equipment is scaled in volts against time. Both of these variables need to be calibrated accurately to ensure that abnormal clinical results are accurately reported. This is beyond the scope of this chapter but users need to ensure that the system is regularly calibrated.

Architectural acoustics and the test environment

Architectural acoustics is the study of sound in enclosures and in particular rooms and auditoria. Sounds radiating from sources in a room will travel until they encounter a wall, ceiling or other boundary. At this point, some of the sound will be reflected back into the room while a proportion will be absorbed by the boundary material. In addition, the remainder of the incident sound will be transmitted through the boundary. A complex sound field is produced as a result of the combination of sound from the sources and the reflected sound. The way in which this sound field grows and decays as a consequence of variations in the sound sources is the principal region of interest in architectural acoustics. In addition, in many applications it is important to consider transmission in some detail to minimize the amount of unwanted sound transmitted into the room from outside sources, and to reduce annoyance caused by noisy activities within a room from disturbing occupants of adjoining rooms.

Growth and decay of sound in a room

The growth and decay of sound in rooms has an important effect on the acoustic environment perceived by the listener. When a source is switched on suddenly, the sound level does not rise abruptly but in a series of steps as the sound arrives from the reflections from the wall, floor and ceiling boundaries and objects within the room. Eventually, an equilibrium is attained where the reflections merge together and the sound amplitude becomes steady when the amount of sound being absorbed by the room is the same as that being radiated.

When the source is switched off, sound continues to be reflected from boundary to boundary, the magnitude decreasing due to absorption with each successive reflection since no boundary is a perfect reflector. This causes a gradual decay of the sound field, called reverberation. The length of time taken for sound

pressure to decay by 60 dB of its original value is known as the reverberation time. The reverberation time has an important effect on room acoustics. It affects the intelligibility of speech, and affects the way music is heard, among many other factors.

Several equations have been derived to express the relationship between the volume of the room, the absorption of the walls and the reverberation time (*RT*). The oldest and best known of these is the Sabine formula, after Sabine (1922) who pioneered the study of auditorium acoustics at the beginning of the twentieth century.

$$RT = \frac{0.161V}{A}$$

Where V is the volume of the room in cubic metres; A is the total absorption of the room in m^2 sabins.

The sabin is the unit of acoustic absorption, corresponding to a surface capable of absorbing the same amount of sound as 1 m^2 of perfectly absorbing material. (This used to be described in terms of an 'open window'.) An alternative unit of absorption is the absorption coefficient which is the ratio of the sound absorbed to the sound incident. Therefore, a perfect absorber has an absorption coefficient of 1 and a perfect reflector 0. The absorption in sabins is therefore simply the product of the area of a surface multiplied by its absorption coefficient. In most rooms, there is a wide variety of surfaces ranging from acoustically 'hard' reflecting ceilings, to good absorbers such as soft furniture (note that all absorbing surfaces must be considered).

The absorption coefficient generally varies with frequency. Therefore, the reverberation time of a room varies depending on the frequency band under consideration. Some typical values of absorption coefficients are given in Table 1.6. Useful tables exist in Rossing (1989), and in Reynolds (1981), among many other sources.

More sophisticated room acoustic models

The geometrical models described above function well in a large number of situations but do not describe the sound field adequately in others. In particular, the formulae given above do not take into account the shape of the room. Practical experience proves that the acoustics of a long corridor are very different from a cubical room, but the simple model would predict the same results for reverberation time in each case. A better method uses wave theory where the boundary conditions set by the sound reflecting surfaces in the enclosure, together with its shape, determine the way in which sound waves propagate inside it.

Unfortunately, the approach is rather mathematical in nature. In the majority of practical cases it is difficult to express the shape of a room in a 'clean' mathematical way and the calculations become in-

Table 1.6 Examples of acoustic absorption coefficients

Material	Frequency (Hz)					
	125	*250*	*500*	*1000*	*2000*	*4000*
Brick	0.03	0.03	0.03	0.04	0.05	0.07
Concrete	0.01	0.01	0.01	0.02	0.02	0.02
Solid wood door	0.1	0.2	0.4	0.52	0.6	0.67
Wood floor	0.15	0.2	0.1	0.1	0.1	0.1
Heavy carpet	0.08	0.24	0.57	0.69	0.71	0.73
Curtains	0.05	0.12	0.15	0.27	0.37	0.5
Acoustic panelling	0.2	0.3	0.75	0.85	0.8	0.4
People in upholstered seats	0.6	0.74	0.88	0.96	0.93	0.85

volved, so this method is generally restricted to simple room shapes. Nevertheless, it provides much insight into the way sound behaves and a qualitative understanding is useful. A full analysis is covered in Reynolds (1981), and in Kinsler *et al.* (1983).

Design of rooms and acoustic defects

There are a number of acoustic defects which impair the properties arising from the size, shape and absorption of the room. Fortunately, these can be alleviated by careful design. A considerable part of architectural acoustics is concerned with the definition of the relevant criteria for rooms for different purposes, since, for example, the desirable acoustic characteristics of a lecture room are quite different to those of an opera house. Whether it is possible actually to achieve all the desirable characteristics once these have been defined is an interesting problem that has only partially been solved.

The basic requirement for any room is that the activity for which it is designed should be heard with adequate loudness. For speech, no perceptible echoes and little reverberation should be present, while for music, sufficient reverberation is a prerequisite. In all cases, it is desirable to exclude external noise (and as a consequence prevent transmission of sound from the inside of the room). After much experimentation, many workers have shown that there is no single optimum reverberation time. The effect of reverberation generally increases the loudness of the received sound. In auditoria used for music, this enhancement can be quite large, doubling the sound level produced by the orchestra.

However, guidelines exist and experience has shown that the reverberation time at about 500 Hz is a good predictor of the intelligibility of speech. Sets of curves of reverberation time for rooms for various purposes have been published in the literature (Kinsler *et al.*, 1983; Rossing, 1989) which give examples based on measurements in rooms that have been judged by listeners to be 'good' (Figure 1.28)

In any room, to maximize intelligibility, there should

be a direct path between the listener and sound source. In large rooms, this dictates that the seating is raked from front to back, as in all good theatres. In addition, if a stage is used, this is sometimes raked in the opposite direction. In large halls, dead spots can arise due to attenuation when sound has to pass over large areas of high absorption, unless precautions are taken.

One technique which has become more popular in the quantification of speech intelligibility in rooms and auditoria is based on the rapid speech transmission index (RASTI) method (IEC 628). In this, a modulated noise source is used to simulate the human voice. A microphone situated at the listener's position is used in conjunction with analysis equipment to calculate various parameters, which are used to express intelligibility.

One of the most blatant of acoustic defects is a distinct echo, which occurs only in relatively large rooms. The echo is a subjectively perceived phenomenon, since the ear requires a gap of at least 0.05 s to distinguish the original sound from the reflection producing the echo. At intervals of less than this, the echo is not audibly distinguishable but merges into and enhances the original sound. This is known as the Haas effect. This is one criterion which can be used to discriminate between an echo (which is a single, distinctive acoustic event occuring at time greater than that quoted after the source sound) from reverberation (which is a multiplicity of indistinguishable echoes). Flutter echo is particularly annoying and occurs when large areas of parallel, low absorption walls are present.

Several experiments have indicated that the initial few arrivals of reverberant sound after the direct sound have an important effect in the listener's perception of reverberation. This indicates that reflecting surfaces in the immediate vicinity of the sound source have to be placed with some care.

Audiometric test environment

Many of the general principles described in the previous section apply to audiometric test rooms. The

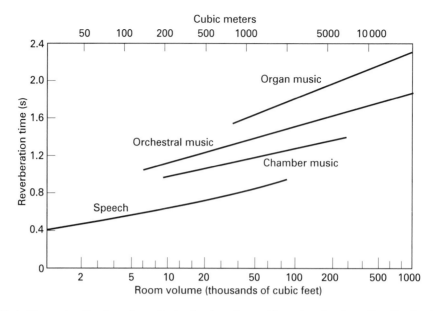

Figure 1.28 Desirable reverberation times for auditoria of various sizes and for various functions (from Rossing, 1989)

environment must be sufficiently quiet for the test signal to be heard and, for free-field tests, enable the sound to be presented at an accurate level without reverberation. Standards have been produced for the maximum permissible ambient noise levels for audiometric test rooms. Two examples are ISO 8253 and ANSI S3.1 (1991). ANSI S3.1 (1991) gives values in both octave and one-third octave bandwidths for 125 to 8000 Hz for two conditions, ears uncovered and ears covered with normal earphones such as the TDH49 type. The ANSI standard specifies maximum levels that will produce negligible masking (≤ 2 dB) of pure tones presented at the reference equivalent threshold sound pressure level as specified in ISO R389. The sound levels required can be difficult to achieve, particularly where the audiometric test room is located in a busy hospital or near to roads with a high traffic density. In many cases it is necessary to use a double sound insulated room, i.e. a room within a room, the inner one of which is mounted on flexible supports and has no rigid structural contact with the outer room. It is very important to carry out a full noise survey and to use these data together with those provided by manufacturers of audiometric test rooms in order to determine whether the desired ambient noise levels will be achieved within the test room.

As well as achieving acceptable ambient noise levels within the test room, it is important to ensure that the room has adequate temperature control, ventilation, lighting and power supply. The additional sound insulation provides very high levels of thermal insulation and it may be necessary to provide cooling within the ventilation system. Most ventilation equipment is too noisy to be used for audiometric test rooms without the addition of silencer ducts. For both temperature and ventilation control careful engineering design procedure is required to ensure that the correct environment will be provided.

Electrophysiological testing has now become routine in clinical audiology. The electrical potentials are of the order of 1–10 microvolts and recordings can be subject to artefacts from electric and magnetic field sources such as power cables, lift motors and fluorescent lights. Artefacts can usually be avoided by location of the test room away from magnetic sources of interference and by the provision of a metal screen lining to the test room which is earthed. The latter will greatly attenuate any electric fields that are present. Finally, care should be taken that no significant electric or magnetic fields are then introduced into the room. For example lighting should be screened or short filament lamps should be used, power cables should be screened or be in screened trunking and the patient should be kept well away from the test equipment.

Appendix 1.1
Selection of standards relevant to audiology

British Standards Institution
2 Park Street,
London, W1

BS 2497: 1992	Specification for standard reference zero for the calibration of pure tone air conduction audiometers (= ISO 389)
BS 2813: 1981 [1990]	Specification for dimensions of plugs for hearing aids (= IEC 90)
BS 3383: 1988	Normal equal-loudness level contours for pure tones under free-field listening conditions (= ISO 226)
BS 3593: 1963 [1993]	Recommendations on preferred frequencies for acoustical measurements (~ ISO 266)
BS 4009: 1991	Specification for artificial mastoids for the calibration of bone vibrators used in hearing aids and audiometers (= IEC 373)
BS 4668: 1971 [1988]	Specification for an acoustic coupler (IEC reference type) for the calibration of earphones used in audiometry (~ IEC 303)
BS 4669: 1971 [1988]	Specification for an artificial ear of the wide band type for the calibration of earphones used in audiometry (~ IEC 318)
BS5108	Sound attenuation of hearing protectors
	Part 1: 1991 Subjective method of measurement (= ISO 4869-1) [+ AMD 7552 which re-numbers this Part as BS EN 24869-1:1993 q.v.]
BS 5330: 1976	Method of estimating the risk of hearing handicap due to noise exposure
BS 5969: 1981 [1989]	Specification for sound level meters [+ AMD 4413 + AMD 5787] (= IEC 651)
BS 6083	Hearing aids
	Parts 0, 1, 2: 1984 [1990]; Part 3: 1991, Part 4: 1981 [1988], Part 5: 1984 [1990]; Parts 6, 7, 8: 1985; Part 9: 1986; Part 10: 1988; Part 11: 1984 [1990] [+ AMDs 6179 to 6184 & 6186 to 6187 to Parts 0, 1, 2, 5, 6, 7, 9, 11 and AMD 6323 to Part 4] (= IEC 118-0 to 118-11)
BS 6111: 1981 [1988]	Specification for reference coupler for the measurement of hearing aids using earphones coupled to the ear by means of ear inserts [+ AMD 6232] (= IEC 126)
BS 6310: 1982	Specification for occluded-ear simulator for the measurement of earphones coupled to the ear by ear inserts [+ AMD 6233] (= IEC 711)
BS 6344	Industrial hearing protectors
	Part 1: 1989 Specification for ear muffs
	Part 2: 1988 Specification for ear plugs
BS 6402: 1983 [1990]	Personal sound exposure meters
BS 6655: 1986 [1993]	Pure tone air conduction threshold audiometry for hearing conservation purposes [+ AMD 7339] (= ISO 6189; = EN 26 189)
BS 6698: 1986	Specification for integrating-averaging sound level meters [+ AMD 6324] (= IEC 804)
BS 6950: 1988	Standard reference zero for the calibration of pure tone bone conduction audiometers [+ AMD 7340] (= ISO 7566)
BS 6951: 1988	Threshold of hearing by air conduction as a function of age and sex for otologically normal persons [+ AMD 7341] (= ISO 7029)
BS 6955	Calibration of vibration and shock pick-ups
	Part 0: 1988 Guide to basic principles (= ISO 5347-0)
BS 7113: 1989	Specification for reference levels for narrow-band masking noise [+ AMD 7342] (= ISO 8798)
BS 7636: 1993	Method for determination of thresholds of hearing using sound field audiometry with pure tone and narrow-band test signals (= ISO 8253-2)

International Standards Organisation
1 rue de Varembe
1211 Geneva 20
Switzerland

ISO 226: 1987   Acoustics – Normal equal loudness level contours
ISO 266: 1975   Acoustics – Preferred frequencies for acoustical measurements
ISO 389: 1991   Acoustics – Standard reference zero for the calibration of pure-tone air
                          conduction audiometers (3rd edn)
ISO 1999: 1990   Acoustics – Determination of occupational noise exposure and estima-
                          tion of noise-induced hearing impairment (2nd edn)
ISO 4869   Acoustics – Hearing protectors
                          4869-1: 1990   Subjective method for the measurement of sound
                                         attenuation
                          TR 4869-3: 1989   Simplified method for the measurement of insertion
                                         loss of ear-muff type for quality inspection purposes
ISO TR 4870: 1991   Acoustics – The construction and calibration of speech intelligibility
                          tests
ISO 6189: 1983 [1988]   Acoustics – Pure tone air conduction threshold audiometry for hearing
                          conservation purposes
ISO 7029: 1984   Acoustics – Threshold of hearing by air conduction as a function of age
                          and sex for otologically normal persons
ISO 8253   Acoustics – Audiometric test methods
                          8253-1: 1989   Basic pure tone air and bone conduction threshold
                                         audiometry
                          8253-2: 1992   Sound field audiometry with pure tone and narrow-
                                         band test signals
ISO 8798: 1987   Acoustics – Reference levels for narrow-band masking noise

International Electrotechnical Commission
3 rue de Varembe,
Geneva,
Switzerland.

IEC 118   Hearing aids
                          118-0: 1993   Measurement of electroacoustical characteristics (2nd
                                         edn)
                          118-1: 1983   Hearing aids with induction pick-up coil input (2nd
                                         edn)
                          118-2: 1983   Hearing aids with automatic gain control circuits (2nd
                                         edn) [+ AMD 1: 1993]
                          118-3: 1983   Hearing aid equipment not entirely worn on the listener
                                         (2nd edn)
                          118-4: 1981   Magnetic field strength in audio-frequency induction
                                         loops for hearing aid purposes
                          118-5: 1983   Nipples for insert earphones
                          118-6: 1984   Characteristics of electrical input circuits for hearing
                                         aids
                          118-7: 1983   Measurements of performance characteristics of hearing
                                         aids for quality inspection for delivery purposes
                          118-8: 1983   Methods of measurement of performance characteristics
                                         of hearing aids under simulated *in situ* working
                                         conditions
                          118-9: 1985   Methods of measurement of characteristics of hearing
                                         aids with bone vibrator output
                          118-10: 1986   Guide to hearing aid standards
                          118-11: 1983   Symbols and other markings on hearing aids and re-
                                         lated equipment
IEC 126: 1973   Reference coupler for the measurement of hearing aids using earphones
                          coupled to the ear by means of ear inserts (2nd edn)

IEC 225: 1966	Octave, half-octave and third-octave band pass filters intended for the analysis of sounds and vibrations
IEC 303: 1970	IEC provisional reference coupler for the calibration of earphones used in audiometry
IEC 318: 1970	An IEC artificial ear of the broadband type for the calibration of earphones used in audiometry
IEC 373: 1990	Mechanical coupler for measurements on bone vibrators (2nd edn)
IEC 645	Audiometers
	645-1: 1992 Pure-tone audiometers (+ Corrigendum: 1992)
IEC 651: 1979	Sound level meters
IEC 711: 1981	Occluded-ear simulator for the measurement of earphones coupled to the ear by ear inserts
IEC 804: 1985	Integrating-averaging sound level meters [+ AMD 1: 1989]
IEC 942: 1988	Sound calibrators
IEC 959: 1990	Provisional head and torso simulator for acoustic measurements on air conduction hearing aids
IEC 1027: 1991	Instruments for the measurement of aural acoustic impedance/admittance

American National Standards,
1430 Broadway,
New York, NY 10018,
USA

ANSI S1.4-1983 (ASA 47)	American National Standard specification for sound level meters
ANSI S1.6-1984 (R 1990)(ASA 53)	American National Standard preferred frequencies, frequency levels, and band numbers for acoustical measurements
ANSI S1.25-1992 (ASA 98)	American National Standard specification for personal noise dosimeters (Revision of ANSI S1.25-1978)
ANSI S1.42-1986 (ASA 64)	American National Standard design response of weighting networks for acoustical measurements
ANSI S3.1-1991 (ASA 99)	American National Standard maximum permissible ambient noise levels for audiometric test rooms
ANSI S3.3-1960 (R 1990)	American National Standard methods for measurement of electroacoustical characteristics of hearing aids
ANSI S3.5-1969 (R 1986)	American National Standard methods for the calculation of the articulation index
ANSI S3.6-1989 (ASA 81)	American National Standard specification for audiometers
ANSI S3.7-1973 (R 1986)	American National Standard method for coupler calibration of earphones
ANSI S3.13-1987 (ASA 74)	American National Standard mechanical coupler for measurement of bone vibrators
ANSI S3.19-1974 (R 1990)(ASA 1)	American National Standard method for the measurement of real-ear protection of hearing protectors and physical attenuation of earmuffs
ANSI S3.21-1978 (R 1986)(ASA 19)	American National Standard method for manual pure-tone threshold audiometry
ANSI S3.22-1987 (ASA 70)	American National Standard specification of hearing aid characteristics
ANSI S3.25-1989 (ASA 80)	American National Standard for an occluded ear simulator
ANSI S3.26-1981 (ASA 41)	American National Standard reference equivalent threshold force levels for audiometric bone vibrators
ANSI S3.35-1985 (R 1990)(ASA 59)	American National Standard method of measurement of performance characteristics of hearing aids under simulated *in situ* working conditions
ANSI S3.36-1985 (R 1990)(ASA 58)	American National Standard specification for a manikin for simulated *in situ* airborne acoustic measurements
ANSI S3.39-1987 (ASA 71)	American National Standard specifications for instruments to measure aural acoustic impedance and admittance (aural acoustic immittance)
ANSI S12.6-1984 (R 1990)(ASA 55)	American National Standard method for the measurement of the real-air attenuation of hearing protectors

References

BEAGLEY, H. A. (1979) *Auditory Investigation – the Scientific and Technological Basis.* Oxford: Clarendon

BENTLEY, J. P. (1988) *Principles of Measurement Systems*, 2nd edn. London: Longman

BURNS, W. (1973) *Noise and Man*, 2nd edn. London: John Murray

HALL, D. E. (1993) *Basic Acoustics.* Krieger

HASSALL, J. R. and ZAVERI, K. (1988) *Acoustic Noise Measurements*, 5th edn. Naenum: Bruel and Kjaer

HOROVITZ, P. and HILL, W. (1989) *The Art of Electronics*, 2nd edn. Cambridge: Cambridge University Press

KAYE, G. W. C. and LABY, T. H. (1986) *Tables of Physical and Chemical Constants.* London: Longman

KINSLER, L. E., FREY, A. R., COPPENS, A. B. and SANDERS, J. Y. (1983) *Fundamentals and Acoustics*, 3rd edn. New York: John Wiley

LYNN, P. A. (1989) *An Introduction to the Analysis and Processing of Signals.* London: Macmillan

MARTIN, M. (1987) *Speech Audiometry.* London: Whurr

RANDALL, R. B. (1987) *Frequency Analysis*, 3rd edn. Copenhagen: Bruel and Kjaer

REYNOLDS, D. D. (1981) *Engineering Principles of Acoustics: Noise and Vibration Control.* Hemel Hempstead: Allyn and Bacon

ROSSING, T. D. (1989) *The Science of Sound.* New York: Addison Wesley

SABINE, W. C. (1922) *Collected Papers on Acoustics*, Boston: Harvard University Press. Reprinted by Dover, New York (1964)

Further reading

ALDRED, J. (1982) *Manual of Sound Recording*, 3rd edn. Hemel Hempstead: Argus Books

BARFORD, N. C. (1985) *Experimental Measurements – Precision, Error, and Truth*, 2nd edn. Wokingham: Addison Wesley

BROCH, J. T. (1980) *Mechanical Vibration and Shock Measurements.* Copenhagen: Bruel and Kjaer

BRUEL and KJAER (1982) Condenser microphones and microphone preamplifiers. In: *Theory and Application Handbook*

BURNS, W. and ROBINSON, D. W. (1970) *Hearing and Noise in Industry.* London: HMSO

COLLOMS, M. (1985) *High Performance Loudspeakers*, 3rd edn. London: Pentech Press Ltd

FAULKNER, L. L. C. (ed.) (1976) *Handbook of Industrial Noise Control.* New York: Industrial Press

GAYFORD, M. L. (1961) *Acoustical Techniques and Transducers.* London: Macdonald and Evans

GAYFORD, M. L. (1970) *Electroacoustics: Microphones, Earphones and Loudspeakers.* London: Newnes-Butterworths

HARRIS, C. M. (1991) *Handbook of Acoustical Measurements and Noise Control.* McGraw

HAUGHTON, P. M. (1980) *Physical Principles of Audiology.* Bristol: Adam Hilger

HINCHCLIFFE, R. and HARRISON, P. (1976) *Scientific Foundations of Otolaryngology.* London: Heinemann

JONES, D. M. and CHAPMAN, A. J. (eds) (1984) *Noise and Society.* Wiley

JONES, M. H. (1985) *A Practical Introduction to Electronic Circuits*, 2nd edn. Cambridge: Cambridge University Press

MORSE, P. M. (1981) *Vibration and Sound.* New York: McGraw Hill

PARKIN, P. H. and HUMPHREYS, H. P. (1979) *Acoustics, Noise and Buildings.* Faber

PETERSON, A. P. G. and GROSS, E. E. (1980) *Handbook of Noise Measurement*, 9th edn. Concord, Mass: General Radio

PORGES, G. (1977) *Applied Acoustics.* London: Arnold

RETTINGER, M. (1988) *Handbook of Architectural Acoustics and Noise Control.* TAB Books

SEDRA, A. S. and SMITH, K. C. (1991) *Microelectronics Circuit.* Philadephia: Saunders College Publishers

TURNER, J. D. and PRESTLOVE, A. J. (1991) *Acoustics for Engineers.* Macmillan

2

Computers in audiology

A. R. D. Thornton

Computers are high speed, unreasoning automata. They do exactly what they are instructed to do, whether it makes sense or not, but they do it very quickly. The hardware of the modern computer represents the end of a long sequence of development of machines which were aids to calculation or calculating devices.

The earliest digital calculating machine was the abacus which initially comprised pebbles placed in grooves made in the sand. In 1642 Blaise Pascal, working in his father's tax office in Rouen, designed and built a mechanical calculator which could perform the operations of addition and subtraction. Some 50 years later, Leibnitz improved Pascal's calculator and incorporated it in a machine which carried out multiplication by repeated addition. This was by no means a successful commercial venture and mechanical calculators were not generally available until the 1880s and even then received no extensive use until the 1920s.

The father of modern computation, Charles Babbage, was born in 1792. He was the first person to design an automatic computer and he laid down the fundamental principles of today's machines. He became involved in a French Government project for the computation of mathematical tables. This was designed to use three or four mathematicians who would decide upon the method of calculation, about seven people who would break down this method to a set of operations that involved only addition and subtraction and about 80 'human computers' who would actually carry out the operations of addition and subtraction. In 1812 Babbage designed his *difference engine* which was intended to replace the 80 'human computers' in the calculation project. He constructed a working model which he demonstrated in 1822 but a complete machine was never finished. He then went on to design his analytical engine

which would be able to perform any type of calculation. The specifications of this machine are essentially the same as those of present day computers. Babbage devoted the rest of his life attempting to perfect the analytical engine which was still unfinished at the time of his death. Nevertheless, it is possible to estimate the timing involved in the operations of the machine. It would have taken about one second for an addition and about one minute for a multiplication.

The first electronic calculator was developed between 1942 and 1946 by Eckert and Mauchly. The machine was known as ENIAC (electronic numerical integrator and calculator) and used some 18 000 valves. The increased speed of electronic operations is reflected in the times for addition (0.2 ms) and for multiplication (28 ms). With so many valves, one was sure to break down after a short interval, reducing the time during which the machine could be used and illustrating the problem of reliability that has been a key factor in the development of the modern computer. ENIAC was not a true computer as it did not have the ability to store a program within the machine.

It was in England, at Cambridge University, that the first machine to use a stored program, EDSAC (electronic delay storage automatic calculator) was built in 1949. In 1951 a similar machine was completed at the University of Pennsylvania and in the same year the Ferranti Mark I became the first commercial system.

Shortly afterwards, computer developments were being carried out at many centres and, as the basic electronic elements became more robust and capable of operating at higher frequencies, so digital computers became more reliable and faster in operation. First generation computers used thermionic valves and were expensive to manufacture and maintain.

Physically they were very large and had a high power consumption requiring special mechanisms for cooling the system.

Second generation machines became possible with the availability of individual transistors in the 1950s. Computers built with these discrete components used low voltages and only small amounts of power.

Third generation systems arrived with the integrated circuit. This was the result of a radical breakthrough in manufacturing techniques which meant that the equivalent of several hundreds of transistors and their interconnecting circuitry could be implemented on a single slice of silicon. This slice was then packaged and connectors added to give the familiar 'chip'. For the first time, a significant change in the hardware of the computer was accompanied by a major effort in the software. A very large amount of work was put into the development of operating systems and time sharing was introduced to cater for the larger and less hardware-oriented users that were coming onto the market.

Fourth generation systems followed and enhanced the work on the integrated circuit. In the early 1970s LSI (large scale integration) chips were developed which contained several thousand transistors per chip and by the mid-1970s VLSI (very large scale integration) chips were capable of containing the whole of the central processing unit on a single chip and was known as a microprocessor. The microprocessor forms the basis of all present day microcomputers. Again, software innovations appeared with this new technology.

Central to this development was the establishment of the IBM PC (personal computer) as an industry standard. This, together with its MS-DOS operating system have been taken up by many manufacturers who have produced machines capable of running the same software. By 1990 there were some 45 million PCs in use.

The present day computers are fourth generation machines but already a great deal of work has gone into the design of fifth generation systems. The concepts involved include input and output systems to deal with speech, images and documents; a knowledge-based problem solving capability; the integration and rationalization of input and output between the various software elements and the improved man-machine interface made possible by artificial intelligence approaches (Moto-Oka, 1983).

The hardware involves elements such as Josephson junction technology in which elements become superconducting when cooled to near absolute zero and parallel processing to increase computational speed. Most current computers have only one processor and by having more processors, or co-processors, the work of the computer can be split between these processors and carried out simultaneously by a technique known as parallel processing. Such an approach is facilitated by arrays of single chip computers known as *transputers*. A modern supercomputer invests heavily in parallel processing and would require less than 3 ns for addition and multiplication operations. However, it is now true to say that, in development costs, it is more expensive to produce software than it is to produce hardware. The changes in circuit elements have also made it possible to build smaller and cheaper machines and over the last decade the real cost of computer power has halved every year.

This increase in computer power has also blurred the distinction between *mainframe, mini- and microcomputers*. The mainframe computer is still a very large machine which costs a great deal of money and is kept in a specially constructed room. Increases in computational power meant that the processing capacity of these computers far exceeded the work load imposed by a single user. *Time-sharing* methods were therefore introduced enabling many people, each with a terminal, to access the computer together. The terminal may be connected from a remote location to the computer via a *modem* which uses a telephone line to transmit and receive data. In this way a modern mainframe can support thousands of users and may have backing store capacity of many billions of numbers and be capable of storing large regional databases and statistics.

The microcomputer requires only a part of a desk top in a normal office and is so cheap that a machine for each user becomes feasible. It will often support only one user although systems of a hundred or so simultaneous users on a network are currently available. It is capable of database storage and analysis for a general practice, a hospital department or, via networking, to provide a records facility for a hospital complex.

Terminology

As in any area of learning, progress can be made only when the terminology has been defined and the relevant jargon understood. In this section, many of the basic elements and concepts of a computer system are introduced and defined and a diagram of a basic computer is shown in Figure 2.1.

Hardware is the term used for the electronic and mechanical parts of the computer system. The *programs* which contain the *instructions* to control the computer operations are known as the *software* of the system. The heart of the hardware of the computer is the *central processing unit* (CPU). This coordinates and controls the activities of all other units. The CPU comprises three elements, the *arithmetic unit*, the *internal memory* and the *program control unit*. The arithmetic unit is where the *logical decisions* and *arithmetic* are carried out in special *registers*. The internal memory is an electronic storage device that

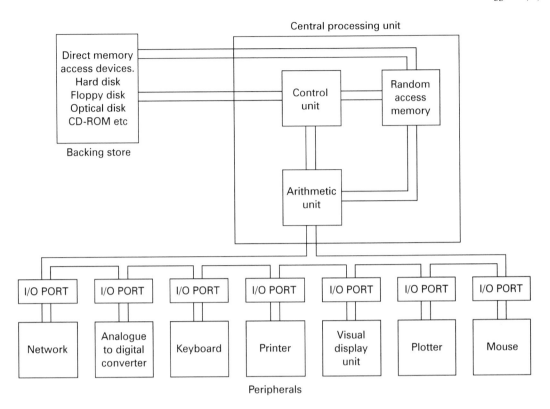

Figure 2.1 Block diagram of the basic elements of a computer

can hold *data* or program *instructions*. Each *location* within memory will hold one *word* which is the basic data unit within the computer. Computer memory may be *volatile* which means that the memory contents are lost when the power is turned off. This is generally referred to as *RAM* or *random access memory*. *ROM* or *read-only memory* is a means of permanent storage of programs. This is *non-volatile memory* that is not destroyed when the power is switched off and hence, unlike the software programs in RAM memory, these permanent programs are referred to as *firmware*. The final part of the central processing unit is the program control unit. This examines each of the individual program instructions in turn, evaluates and interprets the instruction, causes the various transfers of data to be made to or from memory and controls the operation of the arithmetic unit.

Any element of the computer system that is not in the central processing unit is defined as a *peripheral unit*. These include all *input/output* (I/O) devices and *backing store* or *backing memory*. The backing store provides additional storage that is larger in capacity but longer in *access time* than the main computer memory. Computer *disks* and *optical disks* are examples of backing store and programs and data

contained on these devices can be transferred to the internal memory when required.

Input/output devices allow the CPU to communicate with the outside world. These include *mice, digitizing tablets, optical character recognition* or *magnetic ink character recognition* such as the system used on bank cheques. The commonest input device is the *keyboard* of a *visual display unit* (VDU). The majority of output destined for a permanent record will be on some form of *printer*. Both text and graphical output can be sent to the VDU screen and to *plotters* which will produce a *hard copy* output. Input/output devices will be considered in more detail in the next section.

Finally the software used on the machine will be *applications software*, comprising *word processors, spreadsheets, databases* etc, or *system software* comprising *utilities* or *operating system programs*. The utility programs will enable the user to recover deleted programs, search for files, check that the system is working properly together with many other functions. The operating system programs control the system, ensure that data flow in and out is correct and interface the central unit to the peripheral devices. It is this last function that leads to the generic term *DOS* (disk operating system) familiar to PC users.

Operation

Internally, the CPU operates with electronic devices which have two stable states. Switches can be on or off, lamps can be illuminated or not, transistors, or their equivalent within an integrated circuit chip, can act as switches and can be opened or closed. The most suitable arithmetic for such a system is clearly that which is based on two states rather than the normal decimal arithmetic system which has 10 states and so both the data and the program instructions stored within the CPU are represented as binary numbers instead of decimal numbers.

The decimal system has ten digits (0, 1, 2, 3, 4, 5, 6, 7, 8, 9) and the binary system has only two (0, 1) which may be represented electronically as the presence or absence of voltage or as described above. Each digit in a binary number is called a *bit* (short for *Binary digIT*). To represent any number greater than one, several bits must be used. The exact number of bits that are used as a basic 'building block' will vary from one computer to another and examples can be found using 8, 12, 16, 18, 24 and 32 bits. Such a collection of bits is called a *word* and this forms the fundamental unit of the processor memory and arithmetic operations.

The range of values that can be stored in a word will depend upon the word length. An 8 bit word can store 256 values (2^8) which may be interpreted as numbers in the range 0 to 255 or as numbers in the range -128 to 127 where there are 128 negative values (-128 to -1) and 128 positive values (0 to 127). Similarly, a word length of 12 bits can store 4096 values (2^{12}), a 16 bit word can store 65 536 values (2^{16}) and so on. If the range of a single word is not sufficient for the accuracy required then integer values can be represented by two or more words. A different system, again using several words, can further extend the range by using a 'floating point' representation for real numbers. Historically, microprocessors used a word length of 8 bits and this is known as a *byte*. Some systems can process units of 4 bits, that is half a byte, and so a unit of 4 bits is known as a *nibble*.

The binary numbers are stored, manipulated and controlled by the three separate hardware sections of the CPU. The internal memory comprises RAM chips storing the data bits in the equivalent of transistors and the time taken to access one byte can be of the order of 1 ns.

The arithmetic unit (arithmetic logic unit, ALU) contains several special word stores or registers in which the arithmetic operations of addition, subtraction, multiplication and division can be performed. Within most microprocessors the ALU is capable only of addition and subtraction and so multiplication is performed by repeated addition and division by repeated subtraction. There are specialized processors which will do nothing but mathematical operations and carry them out very quickly. These may be added in addition to the main processor chip and are known as arithmetic co-processors. The main processor will pass these arithmetic operations to the co-processor which will then return the result. The most basic of the special registers used for addition and subtraction is called the accumulator or A register and, in most systems, a number passed from a peripheral unit will enter the A register and will then be passed to the memory. If two numbers, stored in memory, are to be added together and the sum stored back in memory then the A register will be cleared, the first number read from memory and added to the A register, the second number added in the same way and finally the value in the A register will be stored back in a memory location.

The control unit within the CPU provides the facilities needed for these operations. It has several registers to enable it to locate addresses in memory, to identify which instruction is to be obeyed and to transfer data between the memory and the arithmetic unit.

In order for the processor to deal with data and to obey program instructions the appropriate binary code must be held in memory. However, memory is relatively expensive and limited in size. Various cheaper forms of mass storage, called backing store, are used to supplement the internal memory.

Various types of cyclic or rotating backing store exist. *Floppy disks* comprise a flexible plastic disk coated with a magnetic material. It is sealed in a square plastic case and 13 cm (5.25 inches) and 9 cm (3.75 inches) diameter disks are the most common at present with the latter now largely replacing the former. The disk is rotated in a drive and a movable magnetic read/write head is moved radially over the disk's surface and data are recorded in tracks on the magnetic material. The amount that can be stored varies between about 100 000 bytes for a minimal configuration of a 13 cm floppy disk to 1 400 000 bytes for a double-sided, high-density 9 cm disk. In order to access a block of data, the worst case would require one revolution of the disk plus the movement time for the read/write head. Floppy disks will commonly have an access time of about 200 ms.

Hard disk systems have been used for a long time and recently these systems have been reduced dramatically in size. They comprise a number of steel disks with magnetic surfaces and information is written to or read from the disk by a series of arms, one for each disk surface. Each arm contains one or several read/write heads and the arms can be positioned across the surface of the disk. Such devices can store between 20 and 2 000 million bytes of information with access times of between 10 and 80 ms. Because of the small distance between the read/write head and the disk surface any dust would ruin the operation of such a system and it is usual for such units to be totally sealed and some contain an inert gas. Thus, although hard disks are more reliable than floppy disks, if there is a fault the user cannot physically access the disk nor replace part of the system. In practice, this disadvantage can be overcome by taking frequent copies of important files from the hard disk to some backup medium such as floppy disks, magnetic tapes or Bernoulli cartridges.

Disks pack binary data onto tracks recorded in the magnetic surface. Track densities range from about 500 to 2000 tracks per inch. *Optical disks*, familiar in the home to all those with compact disk (CD) players, can store 16 000 tracks per inch. Digital data for computers as well as digitized audio signals can be stored on optical disks to produce a CD-ROM of 12 cm (4.75 inches) diameter containing 540 million bytes of data.

The data are written to the disk by a laser beam which creates pits or alters the reflectivity in a reflective surface giving a binary code (reflection of the 'read' laser beam or no reflection) with which to write data. This is an example of *WORM* (*write once, read many* times) technology and is particularly suited to bibliographical databases of which many copies are distributed to libraries. The optical disk has not replaced the magnetic disk because of the difficulties in producing rewritable optical media which would allow the user to store, retrieve and erase files on the optical disk. Examples do exist using dye polymer technology but their general application lies in the future.

Peripheral units such as disk drives generally contain their own subprocessors which allow them to access the memory directly (direct memory access, DMA) without the data having to pass through the main processor. DMA devices can transfer data while the main processor is performing other functions and this feature enables computation to proceed more quickly.

Analogue-to-digital conversion allows for a wide range of versatile peripherals to be connected to the computer. Many devices such as temperature sensors, position sensors for a joystick, systems for measuring heart rate, EEG, ear canal pressure, etc. all have an analogue voltage as their output. An analogue-to-digital converter (ADC) can convert this voltage into a digital representation that can then be fed to the computer. An ADC system therefore provides an interface between the computer and many laboratory measuring devices and also permits manual, analogue input via *graphics tablets* which allow the operator to draw on a surface with an electronic pen whose position is digitized by the table and fed to the computer. There is also a *light pen* which provides the same facility using the surface of the monitor screen directly.

There is similarly a wide range of output devices for the computer. The most common is the visual display unit (VDU) which can range from the domestic television set to an 'intelligent' terminal containing its own microprocessors and memory. These can display characters and graphic output.

Alphanumeric data can also be output by a printer and various types exist. The cheapest form using normal paper is a *dot matrix* printer which has a moving head containing seven or more needles in a vertical line. These are moved forward to hit the ink ribbon and produce marks on the paper in the correct sequence to form each character. Such printers are often capable of graphical output in addition to alphanumeric values. Some very small and cheap printers do not use impact printing at all but have a small dot matrix heating element which moves across heat sensitive paper and hot spots create a colour change on the paper surface. More expensive are *ink jet* printers which spray a fine jet of ink particles which have been electrostatically charged. Deflecting plates set to the appropriate voltages can control the position of these ink particles and give very high speed, quiet printing. Very high quality output can be obtained from a *laser* printer in which a laser beam alters the electrostatic charge on a drum which is then coated with a *toner* and produces a print in he same way as a photocopier. The equivalent speed is variable and depends on the content. Modern systems can output 15 pages of text per minute but, for a page full of graphics, there can be several minutes delay while the data are transferred to the printer memory. Generally, a printer memory of between 1 and 2 million bytes is needed to hold one page of graphics. As even the fastest of printers is still operating very slowly compared to the speed to the CPU, many printers have their own buffer memory so that the CPU can send characters at a high speed to the printer buffer and once the buffer is full the CPU is free to perform other tasks. When the buffer is nearly empty the printer will signal to the CPU that more data are required and the CPU can then send, in a short time, another buffer full of output data.

Direct digital output can be directed through an output port or used to control relays which will operate external devices. An analogue output may be obtained via a digital-to-analogue converter (DAC) enabling a digital computer to be part of an analogue control system by receiving analogue data, converting it and processing it digitally and then outputting an analogue signal back into the system. In this way dedicated microprocessor systems are used to operate automatic record players and washing machines, control the heating of buildings and perform acoustic impedance measurements.

It is possible for many users to run different programs on the same computer by time-sharing. This is based on the fact that the CPU will take approximately 3 ns to perform a simple instruction whereas data coming in from a keyboard will take a minimum time of 100 ms or a factor of 33 million times longer.

The vast disparity between the working rates of the central processor and its peripherals make it possible for the processor, instead of waiting for the next input from a terminal, to service other terminals or to continue with other programs in the intervening period. There are overheads involved in keeping track of which program belongs to which terminal and ensuring that data for each program do not get mixed but, as the time required by the peripheral units is fast compared to human working rates, so far as the user is concerned, all terminals appear to run simultaneously.

The speed at which a processor can work is related to its size and the interconnection distances between the units that make up a computer. The trend towards integrating more and more elements onto a chip continues and this has led to the development of the transputer described earlier.

Languages

In operation, the computer has to implement a series of instructions which is called a program. The operator must first supply the program and there are many different ways in which he can instruct the computer.

The most direct method is to use the binary code which is recognized by the CPU or, for the sake of brevity, to use the equivalent octal or hexadecimal numbers in writing the program and to change these to binary as they are entered in the memory. For example, the code 7000 could mean clear the A register, that is set the A register to 0. Codes 2000 and 3000 could mean 'add' and 'store' respectively. A program to add together two numbers stored in locations 230 and 240 in memory and to place the result of that addition in location 250 could be coded as:

7000 (clear the A register)
2230 (add the contents of location 230)
2240 (add the contents of location 240)
3250 (store the sum in location 250)

This is clearly the most straightforward method as far as the CPU is concerned but it is not an easy task for the programmer. A slightly easier approach is to write the program in a symbolic language or machine code. In this, mnemonics will correspond to the binary arithmetic instructions and labels or tags will correspond to the memory locations. Taking the example defined above the mnemonics CLA (clear A register), ADD (add to the A register) and STO (store the A register) would correspond to the values 7000, 2000 and 3000 respectively. The programmer could also define labels for the locations where the data are stored and the program to add the two numbers stored in locations X and Y and to place the sum in location Z could be written as:

CLA
ADD X
ADD Y
STO Z

Later in the program, the locations would be entered as labels:

X, 3
Y, 2
Z, 0

After the program has been executed the contents of location Z would be equal to 5.

In order to translate this symbolic language into binary code a special program called an assembler is used. The assembler will read the mnemonic symbol, look it up in a table from which it will obtain the binary code, replace the labels by memory address values and thus generate the binary program. Assembler-level or machine code programming gives the programmer direct control over the most basic elements of the computer hardware but can be a laborious and time-consuming means of producing a program.

The next stage of simplification for the programmer is to use a problem-oriented or high level language. In such languages there is a syntax which governs command statements in a standardized form of English and mathematical statements. The example of adding two numbers, given above, would be written as $Z = X + Y$ in such a language. A program to take in two numbers from the keyboard and to print out the sum could be written as:

READ X (read the first number and store it in a variable named X)
READ Y (read the second number and store it in a variable named Y)
S = X + Y (set the variable S equal to the sum)
WRITE S (print out the sum)

While the task has become easier for the programmer, the computer has the difficult job of translating this language to binary code. This is carried out by a special program called a compiler which has to generate one or more words of symbolic code for each statement and to create calls to the correct subroutines. ALGOL (algorithmic language), FORTRAN (formula translation), PASCAL and PL/I are examples of problem orientated high level languages for general and scientific use. The source programs comprise algebraic formulae and standardized but understandable English.

Another form of high level language is provided by interpreters which have all the mathematical and peripheral handling subroutines stored in the main memory and specialized subroutines which translate from the high level language to the binary code as the program is being executed. As its name implies, an interpreter contains routines that will look at the user's program and scan it character by character interpreting the meaning and providing calls to the appropriate subroutines. So far as the operator is concerned there is neither compilation nor assembly, he merely writes a statement in a high level language which can be executed immediately as with a calculator. Alternatively, an ordered series of statements can be written by preceding each line with a number. Again, the program reads in two numbers from the keyboard and prints out their sum, this time in BASIC (*beginners all-purpose symbolic instruction code*) the program is:

```
10 INPUT NUM1
20 INPUT NUM2
30 SUM = NUM1 + NUM2
40 PRINT 'the sum of the two numbers is:' SUM
50 END
```

Each of these languages has advantages and disadvantages which are summarized below.

1 *Symbolic languages* (also known as machine code or assembly-level programming). These allow the programmer the maximum flexibility as he is not committed to fixed subroutines and has control of every peripheral device in the system. In any particular situation the most efficient coding can be achieved and in situations where the program has to operate at the highest possible speed, machine code is the only coding method that can be used. Its disadvantages include the large number of instruction mnemonics that the programmer has to use and the large number of instructions required; it could take several hundred instructions simply to read a non-integer decimal number from the keyboard.

2 *High level languages* (using compilers). These greatly simplify the task of the programmer particularly for complex calculations. The language is only moderately difficult to learn and bears some resemblance to English. However, the final binary program is not optimally coded and is slower in operation than machine code programs. Because the programmer is dependent upon library subroutines and the system is less flexible the efficiency is poor compared to optimal machine code programming. Errors made in the source program may not be discovered until after compilation and so the whole procedure will have to be redone to correct even the simplest errors. However, most errors should be detected by the compiler and high level language programs usually require fewer correction passes than assembler level programs.

3 *High level languages* (interpreters). These simplify the tasks of the programmer even more. Not only are direct statements accepted as well as program lines but the language is normally easier to learn and closer to English. If a mistake is made in the source program it can be corrected and the program rerun immediately without having to go through compilation. One disadvantage is that the program runs more slowly than the compiled languages and machine code programs. Because the program cannot predict the programmer's needs, all subroutines, whether they are needed or not, must be stored in memory thus occupying a large amount of memory space that could otherwise be used by the program. Furthermore, frequently used groups of instructions have to be interpreted every time they are executed whereas a compiler would recode them only once.

Real-time applications

Real-time or on-line computer applications in medicine describe the situation in which the patient is effectively treated as a peripheral device which supplies information of some sort, or as a link between peripheral devices to provide interaction with different parts of the computer system. Many such applications are electrophysiological and signals taken from electrodes attached to a patient are fed to the computer ADC.

Electronystagmographs

Electronystagmographic data may be recorded in this way and the computer program is used to carry out an analysis of the slow phase of the nystagmus. Gentles and Barber (1974) have evaluated the validity of such a procedure by comparing the computer analysis of nine clinical test records with subjective analyses carried out in eight different vestibular laboratories. Various computer techniques for electronystagmographic analysis have been proposed by Herberts *et al.* (1968), Coats and Black (1973) and Allum, Pole and Weiss (1975) and their diagnostic usefulness has been demonstrated. Baloh *et al.* (1976) using such a system, have shown that patients with brain-stem degeneration or with brain-stem compression show impaired pursuit velocity in a smooth tracking task.

Much work has gone into developing computer analysis of electronystagmographic data so that it may be used as a routine test in the clinic. Various detection algorithms and pattern recognition techniques have been used and papers by Hamid, Sayers and Vickery (1979), Vesterhauge *et al.* (1981) and Wortmann, Berg and Haid (1984) trace the progress that has been made in this area. Similar developments have taken place in computer analysis of voluntary eye movements and pursuit tracking performance and different approaches have been described by Wolfe *et al.* (1978), Baloh *et al.* (1980) and Bergenius (1984). More recently, McCullagh and Houston (1990) reported on an algorithm to compute the peripheral nystagmus slow phase velocity. It has been implemented on a commercial microprocessor and shows excellent agreement with user-calculated data. The result of all this work is that many hospitals now use commercially available electronystagmographic analysis systems.

Research into expert systems (see also diagnoses) for vestibular diagnoses is currently being carried out. In 1988 Mira *et al.* described the development of a system called VERTIGO which is used for the detection of peripheral lesions. Gavilan, Gallego and Gavilan (1990) reported on a system called CARRUSEL which attempts to categorize a patient's data into one of 36 diagnoses. A 97% success rate was obtained in relation to expert diagnostic opinion.

Auditory evoked responses

Evoked response measurements play an important role in audiological diagnosis but unlike nystagmographic records, they cannot be recorded directly. This is because the magnitude of the evoked potential is much less than that of other electrical activity which is recorded at the same site. This other activity comprises ongoing EEG, myogenic potentials and electrical noise and as it is larger than the evoked potential it will completely obscure any direct recording. Several computer techniques are available for extracting these low amplitude responses from the background noise; the most common of which is time-domain averaging. This involves improving the signal-to-noise ratio by obtaining the average or sum of a series of responses.

Machine scoring

In addition to obtaining the averaged evoked response, the microcomputer may be used to assess and evaluate the response. By eliminating the operator's subjective decisions about whether a response is present, the evoked response technique can be completely objective. Systems for the automatic estimation of hearing threshold using such techniques have been developed and can provide consistent results which are independent of the experience and consistency of the operator. There have been a number of mathematical response detection and scoring techniques (e.g. Schimmel, Rapin and Cohen, 1974) applied to the slow cortical evoked potential.

Such techniques have also been applied to the auditory brain stem response. Some systems are based on the value of the correlation obtained between the test waveform and a template or 'standard waveform'. The template may be obtained as the mean waveform given by many normally hearing subjects (Elberling, 1979) or the patient may be used as his own control and the template represented by the evoked response obtained at a high stimulation level (Bell, 1979). With either method, the test responses are recorded at various stimulation levels and are correlated with the template. Dependent upon the value of the correlation coefficient a decision is made as to whether a response is present or not.

Other correlation techniques involve calculating the value of the correlation coefficient between two responses obtained at the test stimulation level. Mason and Adams (1984) have reported on such a system which uses a correlation technique together with an estimation of the variability of the background noise. Comparison of subjective and machine scoring of the auditory brain stem response in 75 patients has shown the acceptability of such scoring techniques. Weber and Fletcher (1980) have extended this correlation technique and used two control recordings in addition to the two test runs. More recently methods involving pattern-recognition techniques to detect auditory brain stem response (Bruha, Madhavan and Chong, 1990) and automatically to estimate threshold (Delgado, Ozdamar and Miskiel, 1988) have proved suitable for clinical applications.

Psychoacoustical tests

Computers have been used extensively to control psychoacoustical experiments and this is an example of the patient providing a link between peripheral units as the computer will control the generation of a stimulus and the patient's response will be fed directly back to the computer system. Wood, Wittich and Mahassey (1973) have described a system for computer-controlled automatic audiometry. Both pure-tone and masking stimuli can be generated and the computer was programmed to determine masked as well as unmasked air and bone conduction thresholds. They evaluated the system by comparing the computer results with manually determined thresholds for 20 subjects. High positive correlations between the two measures were obtained ($r = 0.9$) and the maximum difference in the two sets of results was about 5 dB. A similar result was reported by Harris (1979) from his comparison of microprocessor, self-recording and manual audiometry. He found a 4.4 dB maximum difference between manual audiometry and the automatic microprocessor controlled audiometry. The Békésy self-recording instrument gave the most sensitive thresholds but the microprocessor system gave thresholds that were closer to the manual values than those obtained from the self-recording audiometer. Almqvist and Aursnes (1978) have described a fully automated procedure to carry out screening audiometry and threshold measurement. The patient is screened at a preset stimulus level and, if the patient fails the screening test, the computer system will proceed to take the necessary threshold measurements. It has been tested on 82 patients, with ages ranging from 7 to 82 years, and compared with manual audiometry with the conclusion that computer-based audiometry gives a fast and reliable method of screening.

A different approach is described by Meyer-Bisch (1990) with a device called the Audioscan. This can sweep frequencies from 125 Hz to 16 kHz at a fixed level. The starting level, step size and frequency range are selectable. Regions of non-response in the first sweep are retested using secondary, smaller sweeps at higher levels until an audiogram can be obtained. A dedicated computer system is used for control and the procedure will take less than 2 minutes per ear for normally hearing patients but longer times for patients with hearing loss.

A more flexible system has been described by Lutman (1983) which allows a wide range of procedures to be implemented and new test procedures to be configured in a few minutes. A block diagram of the system is shown in Figure 2.2 and the desired flexibility is achieved by providing for various signal sources such as pure-tone oscillators, tape recorders, noise generators, etc. Control files determine the type of test to be done and the control programs have been written in a high level language (FORTRAN) which is relatively device-independent and can be run on different machines. The control files contain the decision rules required in an adaptive test procedure and free the tester from complex manual control. In research applications this will increase the accuracy of test procedures and an additional benefit in the clinic is that the audiologist can concentrate on patient contact rather than the test procedure.

Both the computer-controlled audiometry and the psychoacoustical test system are examples of the microcomputer acting as a controller of peripheral devices that generate the sound signals. Specialized hardware is available as a slot-in card that enables the microcomputer to act as a waveform synthesizer as well as providing the control.

Physical measurements

Commercial microcomputers are available that give a complete hearing aid insertion gain system. Most systems use a 1-mm diameter flexible probe tube which is inserted into the ear canal and measurements are taken first in the open ear canal and second with the hearing aid and earmould in position. The insertion gain may be output as a graph or tabulated and the accuracy and reliability of two such systems has been compared (Thornton *et al.*, 1986). A similar system built around a Hewlett-Packard desk-top computer has been described by Lauridsen and Nielsen (1981) who measured the differences between this real ear insertion gain measurement and that obtained in a 2 cc coupler. They also showed the practical factors involved in using such a system for hearing aid fitting.

Off-line applications

There are many other clinical applications of computers that do not involve a patient being connected to a computer. These include modelling, database systems, word processing and diagnosis. In modelling, the computer may be used as a tool to fit statistical models to data or may be used to process equations that will simulate a physiological system.

Modelling

The auditory brain stem response has been modelled in both the time and frequency domains (Thornton, 1981). The reason for modelling the response was to predict what a patient's response should be in the

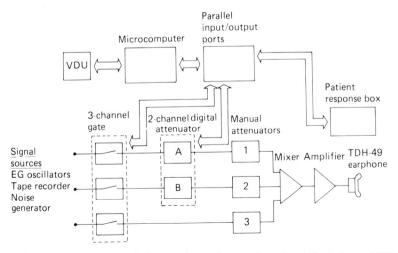

Figure 2.2 Block diagram of a microcomputer-controlled system for psychoacoustic testing. (After Lutman, 1983, by permission)

presence of hearing loss due to end organ or middle ear disorders but with no neurological abnormality. It was possible to test the model by using it to predict the waveforms found in various pathologies and to check these against clinical findings. One such prediction of the model was that, for infiltrating rather than space-occupying lesions, a pathological response could have a larger amplitude than the normal response. While no clinical findings matched this model prediction at the time when it was made, subsequent data have confirmed the model prediction. By this means, a useful addition to the diagnostic criteria used with this test has been made.

An example of statistical modelling may be obtained from epidemiological data. Figure 2.3 shows the prevalence data in the adult population of Great Britain and two mathematical functions have been fitted to these data. Davis (1983) has used a logarithmic model to relate prevalence (PREV) to better ear average hearing loss (HL) that is LOG (PREV) = A + B.HL, where A and B are constants. Thornton (1986), in concentrating on the severe and profound hearing loss end of the distribution, has shown that, over the range of hearing losses shown in Figure 2.3, a Gompertz function provides a slightly better fit to the data. The model is PREV = $a.b^{cHL}$, where a, b and c are constants. The degree to which the fitted mathematical function represents the data may be quantified by calculating the proportion of the variance of the data points that may be explained by the fitted mathematical function. Both models in this case provide a good fit as the percentage of variance accounted for is 99.09% for the log model and 99.91% for the Gompertz function. Curve-fitting procedures such as those illustrated here enable values that lie between measured points to be interpolated and esti-

mates of values that lie beyond the range of measurement to be extrapolated.

Modelling techniques have also been applied to patient management. Smaldino and Traynor (1982) have taken the Goldstein-Stephens (1981) model of audiological rehabilitation and used this as the basis for a computer program. The model is based on three main factors:

1 Communication status which includes auditory and language abilities, visual and manual communication skills and various cognitive factors
2 Associated variables comprising psychological, sociological, vocational and educational factors
3 Related conditions which include mobility, upper limb function and aural pathology.

The model allows all of these data to be combined, their interaction taken into consideration and provides a fast and flexible approach to rehabilitation.

Hearing aid performance has also been modelled by Karzon and Niemoeller (1983) who developed a model for communication hearing aids, implemented on a small desk-top computer. The model can predict output speech and noise levels for any combination of control positions even with the aid driven to saturation. They demonstrated the validity of the model by comparing measured values of hearing aid gain, output noise levels, output speech levels and maximum output levels with corresponding data from the computer model.

More recent work has ranged from modelling the acoustical-neural transduction at the hair cell (Meddis, Hewitt and Shackleton, 1990) to modelling the effects of age on hearing loss (Macrae, 1990).

A whole range of models that can adapt to conditions is now in use. They are known as *adaptive network systems* or *neural networks*. These systems use historical data to model human expertise and are also related to statistical modelling and artificial intelligence techniques. The application areas are extremely wide but include evoked potential recognition (Alpsan and Ozdamar, 1989; Bruha and Madhavan, 1989).

Databases

Research data, patient records, equipment inventories and bibliographic references may be stored on a computer. A database system controls the way in which the data are entered, edited, deleted, stored, accessed, retrieved and output. Related data elements comprise a *record* and a *field* is a subdivision of a record containing the basic unit of information. For example all the data stored about a patient will form the record for that patient. Individual fields within that record may contain the patient's age, sex, name, etc. The simplest form of database is a sequential list of records. Each record may be in a fixed format

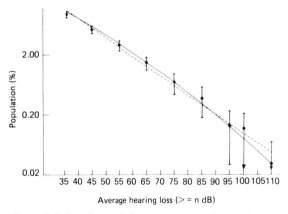

Figure 2.3 Prevalence of a better ear average hearing loss greater than or equal to the value shown on the *x* axis. The average loss is calculated as the mean value of 500, 1000, 2000 and 4000 Hz. Logarithmic (– – – –) and Gompertz (——) curves have been fitted to the data (●) and the vertical bars show the 95% confidence limits

which uses a record length which has been preset and contains spaces for every field whether or not they are used. Alternatively, variable-length records can be created where space is allocated only to the fields that are entered. This has the advantage of more efficient use of file space but has some additional problems in accessing the data.

In order to minimize the amount of incorrect data that is input to the database, various check procedures are used. If the database is built around the patient's serial number or hospital number then, as this is the crucial data element, the database system can require this number to be entered twice and will accept the data only if the number is the same both times. Another example of input checking can be applied to audiometric data where the values should lie between -10 and $+120$ dB and be divisible by 5. If the operator enters a value that does not meet these criteria it will not be accepted by the system.

For clinical records, fast access time is usually necessary and so an indexed database is often used. This involves the use of a unique keyword to define a record. Generally, the keyword will be the patient's hospital number and associated with the keyword will be a pointer which indicates the address in the main data file at which this patient's record can be found. A table containing the keywords and pointers is created when the data are entered and either saved as part of the main data file or as a separate file. Such a system allows fast access because the keyword/pointer table is small enough to be held in the computer memory and so finding a keyword and looking up the associated pointer value takes very little time. The main data file, which is generally too large to maintain in computer memory, may then be accessed and the relevant portion of the file read into memory starting at the address given by the pointer. Clearly, the keyword should be the element that is most commonly used to access the data. Most systems allow multiple keyword indices which are useful but involve a slight speed and storage penalty. In the UK at least two commercially produced audiological database systems are in use. To facilitate computer-based clinical records, an ambitious plan to develop a comprehensive dictionary of standard medical terms is underway. Initially, a clinical thesaurus of 'Read Codes' is being produced by working groups involving over 750 clinicians (West, 1993). The Read Codes are hierarchically organized, alphanumeric codes of up to six characters. The first character defines the broad class, the second the subclass and so on. While these codes and the clinical terms dictionary are being developed within the UK, it is anticipated that they could have a far wider application.

Word processors may be used in conjunction with such databases as most current word processor systems will allow a form letter to be written and then the names and addresses of the recipients accessed from a data file and inserted into individual letters which are output to a printer.

Hearing aid prescription

The task of selecting the electroacoustic characteristics of hearing aids has been made easier by various computer techniques. Seewald, Ross and Spiro (1985) have developed a theoretical computer-assisted approach to the initial selection of amplification characteristics based primarily on audiometric threshold data. These threshold data are entered into the computer together with the desired sensation level for amplified speech as a function of hearing level and frequency, and the desired saturation sound pressure levels as a function of the predicted level of amplified speech. Based on these factors the predicted electroacoustical characteristics of the aid and the target aided sound field thresholds are calculated. Another method has been published by Corell, Ludvigsen and Nielsen (1983) and in clinical trials it was noted that the computer-aided fitting procedure resulted in a greater spread in the types of hearing aid prescribed than had been the case with standard prescription methods. The hearing aid fitting procedure became less dependent on the experience of the technicians fitting the aid and the variable parameters of each aid were utilized to a higher degree than previously. More recently (Jamieson and Raftery, 1989) computers have been programmed to carry out hearing aid prescription, simulation and provide a means of testing the benefit. Recently, programmable hearing aids have become available. The use of computers in programming these hearing aid systems is dealt with in Chapter 14.

Patient interviews

A considerable amount of the available patient contact time in hospitals, clinics and general practitioner's surgeries is used for asking questions of the patient. While the personal interview will remain an important part of medical practice, computer-controlled interviews can obtain a great deal of the necessary information and allow the doctor more time to pursue additional information in the relevant areas of the data provided by the computer. Such computer interviews generally take the following form. On arrival the patient is seated in front of a screen which displays the initial instructions. Usually there are only a few buttons available to the patient to cover the 'yes', 'no', 'don't know' and 'don't understand' conditions. The patient responds by pressing a button and the program follows a branching design in which the next question to be asked depends upon the patient's responses to the previous questions. Checks are made for a repeated failure to respond and for inconsistent answers and the program may be prematurely terminated if these conditions arise. A printout summarizing the interview is then produced which the patient keeps to hand to the doctor when the consultation starts. Experience with such systems suggests that computer interviews can enhance the doctor–patient relationship. Patients are often less anxious about giving the initial history and realize that doctors can focus their skills more effectively when the problems are presented in this way. Milne and Robertson (1979) demonstrated the general acceptance of computer interviews as 73% of the patients found it an interesting experience and less than 12% found it worrying or unpleasant. In 37% of the cases the computer interview contained information that was not elicited by the clinician. Fox, Barber and Bardhan (1979) and Fox, Barber and Malcolm (1982) have reported the successful application of such systems in hospital outpatient clinics. In the audiological domain, the Hearing Measurement Scale (Noble and Atherley, 1970) has been similarly automated and successfully applied in the clinic.

Diagnoses

So far, all of the computer applications described have enabled the clinician to have more information available or to have a larger amount of information available more quickly. The clinician still has to assess all this information in order to draw a diagnostic conclusion. However, computer-aided diagnostic systems can correlate all the information and produce diagnostic options. Rogers, Ryack and Moeller (1979) reviewed the evaluation of 58 diagnostic systems; 40% of these systems showed an accuracy greater than 90% and approximately two-thirds had a diagnostic accuracy of over 80%. More recent developments both in hardware and software have made such systems more 'intelligent' and more widespread. According to the manner in which the diagnostic decision is achieved, they may be classified as probability systems or knowledge-based systems.

Probability systems require tabulated probabilities that relate symptoms to disease. These have to be obtained empirically from many hundreds of case histories. The probabilities are then combined using Bayesian probability theory to give an overall diagnostic conclusion. This method has drawbacks as, in order to reduce the data to a manageable size, an assumption has to be made that the symptoms are independent. However, in specific applications such as De Dombal's (1973) system which is applied to acute abdominal problems, there can be very good diagnostic accuracy. Norris *et al.* (1985) also reported good diagnostic accuracy in neurological diagnosis but some of the errors that can occur with such systems were reported by Szolovits and Pauker (1978) with their application to the diagnosis of left-sided heart disease.

Knowledge-based systems do not suffer from the problems inherent in probability methods. They allow greater flexibility as the patient's symptoms are not required to be forced into particular categories but are allowed to be imprecise and vague. This is clearly a better reflection of the true diagnostic situation and is a major reason for the current interest in knowledge-based systems. As its name implies the systems are created by incorporating decision rules supplied from an expert in a particular area. Although there are technical differences between knowledge-based systems and 'expert systems' both are examples of the artificial intelligence approach. In addition to the decision rule, a level of uncertainty must be associated with each step and this is the main disadvantage of knowledge-based systems because the expert or experts in the field may have great difficulty in associating an exact uncertainty level and a correct weighting for each particular rule. Clearly the greater number of rules in the system the greater will be this problem. Nevertheless, some very good systems have been created. The MYCIN system diagnoses meningitis and blood infections and can recommend drug treatment. It was developed in the mid-seventies by E. Shortcliffe working with the infectious disease group at Stanford University. It is an interactive system and when judged by a panel of experts gave decisions that matched those of the majority of the panel 90% of the time. Currently such approaches are being applied to audiometry (Simler and Ozdamar, 1988) and to audiological diagnosis (Hadzikadic, 1992; Henson-Mack, Chen and Wester, 1992)

Conclusions

The modern computer is a ubiquitous tool and permeates almost every facet of our lives. Computer technology is still advancing rapidly and future medical applications will be more limited by the clinician's or surgeon's reaction to the use of computers than by any technical limitation of computer systems. Relatively few hospitals are without a computer-based patient record system but in the otorhinolaryngological domain, current computer technology has not been fully exploited. An otorhinolaryngological patient record system using a light pen to draw in audiograms or to mark in the position and extent of a tympanic perforation using a graphics screen is well within the capability of today's machines but has not been widely implemented. Computer-controlled patient interviewing and history taking, which has been so successfully applied in the areas of abdominal and back pain, could equally well be used in the otolaryngological clinic. In a National Physical Laboratory survey (Norris *et al.*, 1985) 80% of the patients agreed with the premises that, 'if a computer can ask questions for a doctor, he will spend more time thinking about the patient's answers', and, 'computers make you less nervous than doctors'. The full benefit from computer technology will be obtained in this field only when those involved appreciate both the advantages and limitations of computers and have some knowledge of the kind of problems that are amenable to computer evaluation.

References

ALLUM, J. H. J., POLE, J. R. and WEISS, A. D. (1975) MITNYS. II. A digital program for on-line analysis of nystagmus. *IEEE Transactions in Biomedical Engineering*, DME-22, 196–202

ALMQVIST, B. and AURSNES, J. (1978) Computerised pure tone audiometry. *Scandinavian Audiology*, Suppl. 8, 193–196

ALPSAN, D. and OZDAMAR, O. (1989) A backpropagation network for classifying auditory brainstem evoked potentials: input level biasing, temporal and spectral inputs and learning patterns. *IJCNN: International Joint Conference on Neural Networks*. New York: IEEE TAB Neural Network Committee. p. 605

BALOH, R. W., KUMLEY, W. G., SILLS, A. W., HONRUBIA, V. and KONRAD, H. R. (1976) Quantitative measurement of smooth pursuit eye movements. *Annals of Otology*, 85, 111–119

BALOH, R. W., LANGHOFER, L., HONRUBIA, V. and YEE, R. D. (1980) On-line analysis of eye movements using a digital computer. *Aviation and Environmental Medicine*, 51, 563–567

BELL, I. E. (1979) Audiometric threshold estimation using the brainstem evoked responses. *MSc Thesis*, University of Southampton

BERGENIUS, J. (1984) Computerised analysis of voluntary eye movements. A clinical method for evaluation of smooth pursuit and saccades in otoneurological diagnosis. *Acta Oto-Laryngologica*, 98, 490–500

BRUHA, I. and MADHAVAN, G. P. (1989) Combined syntax-neural net method for pattern recognition of evoked potentials. In: *Computing and Information. Proceedings of the International Conference. ICCI '89*, edited by R. Janicki and W. W. Koczkodaj. Amsterdam: North-Holland. pp. 361–369

BRUHA, I., MADHAVAN, G. P. and CHONG, M. S.-K. (1990) Use of multi-layer perception for recognition of evoked potentials. *International Journal of Pattern Recognition and Artificial Intelligence*, 4, 705–716

COATS, A. C. and BLACK, R. H. (1973) Nystagmus velocity computer. *Transactions of the American Academy of Ophthalmology and Otolaryngology*, 76, 106–108

CORELL, I., LUDVIGSEN, C. and NIELSEN, H. B. (1983) Experiences with computer-aided hearing aid fitting. *Scandinavian Audiology*, 12, 147–150

DAVIS, A. C. (1983) Hearing disorders in the population: first phase findings of the MRC National Study of Hearing. In: *Hearing Science and Hearing Disorders*, edited by M. E. Lutman and M. P. Haggard. London: Academic Press. pp. 35–60

DE DOMBAL, F. T. (1973) Surgical diagnosis assisted by a computer. *Proceedings of the Royal Society*, 184, 433–440

DELGADO, R. E., OZDAMAR, O. and MISKIEL, E. (1988) On-line system for automated auditory evoked response threshold determination. In: *Proceedings of the Annual International Conference of the IEEE Engineering in Medicine and Biology Society*, edited by G. Harris and C. Walker. New York: IEEE. pp. 1472–1473

ELBERLING, C. (1979) Auditory electrophysiology. The use of templates and cross correlation functions in the analysis of brainstem potentials. *Scandinavian Audiology*, 8, 187–190

FOX, J., BARBER, D. C. and BARDHAN, K. D. (1979) Effects of on-line symptom-processing on history-taking and diagnosis. A simulation study. *International Journal of Biomedical Computing*, 10, 151–163

FOX, J., BARBER, D. C. and MALCOLM, A. (1982) Computers in the consulting room. In: *Computers and the General Practitioner*, edited by A. Malcolm and J. Poyser. Oxford: Pergamon Press. pp. 59–78

GAVILAN, C., GALLEGO, J. and GAVILAN, J. (1990) 'Carrusel': an expert system for vestibular diagnosis. *Acta Otolaryngologica*, 110, 161–167

GENTLES, W. and BARBER, H. O. (1974) Human vs. automated techniques in analysis of postcaloric nystagmus. *Canadian Journal of Otolaryngology*, 3, 27–36

GOLDSTEIN, D. P. and STEPHENS, S. D. G. (1981) Audiological rehabilitation: management model 1. *Audiology*, 20, 432–452

HADZIKADIC, M. (1992) Automated design of diagnostic systems. *Artificial Intelligence in Medicine*, 4, 329–342

HAMID, M. A., SAYERS, B. MCA. and VICKERY, J. C. (1979) Implementing a computer-based electro-oculographic analysis system. *Clinical Otolaryngology*, 4, 163–167

HARRIS, D. A. (1979) Microprocessor, self-recording and manual audiometry. *Journal of Auditory Research*, 19, 159–166

HENSON-MACK, K., CHEN, H. -C. and WESTER, D. C. (1992) Integrating probabilistic and rule-based systems for clinical differential diagnosis. *Proceedings. IEEE SOUTHEAST-CON '92*. New York: IEEE. pp. 699–702

HERBERTS, G., ABRAHAMSSON, F., EINARSSON, F., HOFMANN, H. and LINDER, P. (1968) Computer analysis of electronystagmographic data. *Acta Oto-Laryngologica*, 65, 200–208

JAMIESON, D. G. and RAFTERY, E. (1989) A general purpose hearing aid prescription, simulation and testing system. In: *ICASSP-89: 1989 International Conference on Acoustics, Speech and Signal Processing*. New York: IEEE. pp. 1989–1992

KARZON, R. G. and NIEMOELLER, A. F. (1983) A model for predicting hearing aid performance. *Scandinavian Audiology*, 12, 275–284

LAURIDSEN, O. and NIELSEN, H. B. (1981) A new computerised method for hearing aid fitting based on measurements at the ear drum. *Scandinavian Audiology*, 10, 109–113

LUTMAN, M. E. (1983) Microcomputer-controlled psycho-acoustics in clinical audiology. *British Journal of Audiology*, 17, 109–114

MACRAE, J. (1990) An evaluation of methods of predicting the effects of ageing on sensorineural hearing loss. *Australian Journal of Audiology*, 12, 23–32

MCCULLAGH, P. J. and HOUSTON, H. G. (1990) Microcomputer based analysis of nystagmus eye movement. *British Journal of Audiology*, 24, 111–116

MASON, S. M. and ADAMS, W. (1984) An automated microcomputer based electric response audiometry system for machine scoring of auditory evoked potentials. *Clinical Physiology and Physiological Measurement*, 5, 219–222

MEDDIS, R., HEWITT, M. J. and SHACKLETON, T. M. (1990) Implementation details of a computation model of the inner hair cell/auditory nerve synapse. *Journal of the Acoustical Society of America*, 87, 1813–1816

MEYER-BISCH, C. (1990) Audiométrie automatique de dépistage préventif: le balayage fréquentiel asservi (audioscan). Comparison avec les techniques classiques. *Cahiers de notes documentaires*, **139**, 335–345

MILNE, H. and ROBERTSON, J. (1979) The use of a computer in sexual history taking. A pilot study. *British Journal of Sexual Medicine*, **6**, 32–37

MIRA, E., SCHMID. R., ZANOCCO, P., BUIZZA, A., MAGENES, G. and MANFRIN, M. (1988) A computer-based consultation system (expert system) for the classification of dizziness. *Advances in Otorhinolaryngology* **42**, 77–80

MOTO-OKA, T. (ed.) (1983) Challenge for knowledge information processing systems (preliminary report on 5th generation computer systems). In; *Fifth Generation Computer Systems*. Amsterdam: North-Holland Publishing Company. pp. 3–89

NOBLE, W. G. and ATHERLEY, G. R. C. (1970) The hearing measurement scale: a questionnaire for the assessment of auditory disability. *Journal of Auditory Research*, **10**, 229–250

NORRIS, D. E., SKILBECK, C. E., HAYWARD, A. E. and TORPY, D. M. (1985) *Microcomputers in Clinical Practice*. Chichester: John Wiley & Sons Ltd

ROGERS, W., RYACK, B. and MOELLER, G. (1979) Computer-aided medical diagnosis: literature review. *International Journal of Biomedical Computing*, **10**, 267–289

SCHIMMEL, H., RAPIN, I. and COHEN, M. M. (1974) Improving evoked response audiometry with special reference to machine scoring. *Audiology*, **17**, 33–65

SEEWALD, R. C., ROSS, M. and SPIRO, M. K. (1985) Selecting amplification characteristics for young hearing-impaired children. *Ear and Hearing*, **6**, 48–53

SIMLER, D. and OZDAMAR, O. (1988) Experimental expert system for audiometric testing. In: *Proceedings of the Annual International Conference of the IEEE Engineering in Medicine and Biology Society*, edited by G. Harris and C. Walker. New York: IEEE. pp. 1436–1437

SMALDINO, J. and TRAYNOR, R. (1982) Comprehensive evaluation of the older adult for audiological reconditioning. *Ear and Hearing*, **3**, 148–159

SZOLOVITS, P. and PAUKER, S. G. (1978) Categorical and probabilistic reasoning in medical diagnosis. *Artificial Intelligence*, **11**, 115–144

THORNTON, A. R. D. (1981) Computer simulation of auditory brainstem potentials in different pathologies. *Sensus*, **1**, 71–75

THORNTON, A. R. D. (1986) Estimation of the number of patients who might be suitable for cochlear implant and similar procedures. *British Journal of Audiology*, **20**, 221–229

THORNTON, A. R. D., DON, M., MACKENZIE, I. and FARRELL, G. (1986) A comparison of two systems for measuring insertion gain of hearing aids. *IHR Technical Report (Series B)*, **12**

VESTERHAUGE, S., RUNGE, B., MANSSON, A. and ZILSTORFF, K. (1981) Computer analysis of electronystagmographic data. *Clinical Otolaryngology*, **6**, 121–124

WEBER, B. A. and FLETCHER, G. L. (1980) A computerized scoring procedure for auditory brainstem response audiometry. *Ear and Hearing*, **1**, 233–236

WEST, P. (1993) Editorial: the clinical terms project – the development of a computerised clinical language. *Journal of Audiological Medicine*, **2**, ii–iii

WOLFE, J. W., ENGELKEN, J., OLSEN, J. W. and ALLEN, J. P. (1978) Cross-power spectral density analysis of pursuit tracking. Evaluation of central and peripheral pathology. *Annals of Otology*, **87**, 837–844

WOOD, T. J., WITTICH, W. W. and MAHASSEY, R. B. (1973) Computerised pure-tone audiometric procedures. *Journal of Speech and Hearing Research*, **16**, 676–684

WORTMANN, A., BERG, M. and HAID, T. (1984) A new computer analysis of the caloric test. *Acta Oto-Laryngologica Supplementum*, **406**, 174–177

Further reading

CHANDOR, A. with GRAHAM, J. and WILLIAMSON, S. R. (1985) *The Penguin Dictionary of Computers*. London: Penguin Books

COOKE, D., CRAVEN, A. H. and CLARK, G. M. (1983) *Basic Statistical Computing*. London: Edward Arnold

DATE, C. J. (1975) *An Introduction to Database Systems*. Wokingham: Addison-Wesley

EVANS, C. (1983) *The Making of the Micro*. Oxford: Oxford Paperbacks, Wiley

FORD, N. J., FORD, J. M., DENNIS, F. H. and WOODROFFE, M. R. (1991) *Computers and Computer Applications: An introduction for the 1990s*. Chichester: Ellis Horwood Ltd

GRAINGER, J. and HOVER, C. (1981) *The Word Processing Handbook*. London: Drake International

HANSON, O. (1982) *Design of Computer Data Files*. London: Pitman

HUNT, R. and SHELLEY, J. (1988) *Computers and Common Sense*. Hemel Hempstead: Prentice Hall International (UK) Ltd

MALCOLM, A. and POYSER, J. (eds) (1982) *Computers and the General Practitioner*. London: Pergamon

NAIMAN, A. (1983) *Word Processing Buyer's Guide*. Peterborough: BYTE/McGraw-Hill

NORTHERN, J. L. (1986) *The Personal Computer for Speech, Language and Hearing Professionals*. Boston: Little, Brown & Co.

RUSSEL, C. (1993) *Murphy's Laws of DOS*. Almeida: Sybex

3

Epidemiology

Adrian Davis

Scope

The epidemiology of hearing and balance disorders is important for at least three reasons:

1 It shows the scale of need in terms of the prevalence of hearing impairment, disability and handicap
2 It shows those factors that are responsible for the deterioration of hearing and balance
3 It shows how effective hearing services (health and other public services) are at meeting the need.

The epidemiology of hearing disorders should be one of the main inputs into the statement of the public health priorities in terms of hearing health care.

In this chapter the scale of the problem is shown for the UK, where about 8.7m people have a hearing impairment. World-wide the prevalence of hearing impairment is estimated at about 440m people. In the developed world the prevalence of hearing impairment will increase substantially in the next decade or two. The scale of the problem for balance disorders is not known.

The impact of age, occupational group, gender and occupational and other noise exposure on the distribution of hearing thresholds is shown to be frequency specific. Age is the primary risk factor in the population, but the effects of the other demographic variables is systematic. In addition to these, mainly demographic, factors there are significant effects of several other variables on the prevalence of hearing impairment, e.g. the history of childhood ear disease and the family history of hearing impairment. These have not been covered in this chapter to any great extent, but are referred to in Chapters 8 and 10 of this volume.

A major implication of this chapter is that the under provision of hearing health care, regardless of how need is defined and which country is being considered, is a major public health problem that needs considerable effort to find a cost-effective solution.

Introduction

In a previous edition, I outlined several aspects of the epidemiology of hearing disorders (Davis, 1987). This chapter is not a total replacement for that chapter, and relies on that chapter to convey concepts concerning hearing impairment, disability and handicap, the different types of epidemiological evidence and an epidemiological model of hearing disorders. However, it does replace and expand the descriptive epidemiology of hearing impairment and disability, using in particular data from the UK National Study of Hearing (Davis, 1989, 1995). In particular it adds some data from that study and a study in progress concerning reported balance disorders and the associated prevalence of consultation for these disorders.

Over the last 10 years there has been a considerable change in the delivery of health care world-wide. The emphasis has shifted away from provider-based tertiary level care responsive to 'unlimited demand' towards purchaser-based primary level care that tries to adopt a more proactive approach to cost-effective health care in the population. These changes have not been uniformly successful or accepted, particularly when the debate concerns assessing priorities in health care, which may be expressed in a number of ways, e.g. targets, rationing, research initiatives (British Medical Journal, 1993).

The prioritization of health care and the research that is needed to underpin the proper development and implementation of appropriate services for the future is a difficult task. It is a task that is worth doing well, because, even in the developed world, the resources for dealing with the disabilities associated with a rapidly growing elderly population (e.g. mobility, self-care, hearing, vision) are becoming severely limited. This means that the package of health care, for a given cost, has to be optimized against some criteria, e.g. health gain. The inputs into this priority setting are several: political, provider pull, research push, management inertia, lobbying activity on behalf of client groups as well as epidemiology. The epidemiology of hearing impairment and disability should be the main set of information that is required to determine audiological health care needs, the extent to which services that are demanded by individuals, client groups, providers and politicians are relevant to those needs and the health benefit that accrues from the current use of audiogical health care services. Often, the epidemiological data are not available or are ignored and services are developed on the basis of the other factors alone. This leads to services based on prejudice rather than evidence of need met by services that yield benefit to the population. When local epidemiology is not available it may be possible to generalize from data collected elsewhere, always providing that the requisite assumptions are made before so doing. An example of generalization from existing work is shown in this chapter.

In the widest sense, the public health function, in terms of hearing disorders and the stance that a public purchasing authority might take, is to promote and maintain auditory health in the population through preventing and ameliorating the factors that bring about primary and secondary disability. Especially in terms of primary prevention and health education, the public health function is particularly multidisciplinary and multiagency. Considering the public health function the UK government, for example, has suggested that, 'it should ensure that appropriate arrangements are in place to look for (and presumably act on) adverse effects from environmental hazards and sources of pollution' (Public Health, 1994). In terms of auditory health this has considerable implications for possible noise damage to hearing, whether occupational or not, as well as other toxic factors.

In a narrower sense I will concentrate here on three aspects of the public health function viz *who has need*, *what services are asked for or demanded* and finally *what services are actually provided and to what benefit?* The purchasers of auditory health care would like to set targets that specify incremental improvements along the path to providing a 'quality' service. However, to do that there has to be some estimate of the need in the population and how services affect that need. This is often crudely reformulated as: how much can the population benefit for a minimum cost! Clinical guidelines (Grimshaw and Russell, 1993) can often be effective in this context, if developed on the basis of systematic analysis and review

of evidence, rather than prejudice (Chalmers and Haynes, 1994; Clarke and Stewart, 1994; Eysenck, 1994; Knipschild, 1994; Mulrow, 1994; Oxman, 1994) to regulate the quality of the service and ensure a minimum quality service is obtained.

This chapter assumes that the reader appreciates the distinction between hearing impairment (loss of auditory function), disability (impact of that loss on specific tasks, e.g. communication) and handicap (social, economic and psychological impact of the disability on a person, e.g. loss of quality of life). These concepts and their relevance to health care prioritization are covered in various chapters and books (Wood, 1980; Davis, 1983, 1987, 1995; Stephens and Hétu, 1991; Haggard, 1993; Stephens, see Chapter 13). The reader is encouraged to refer to other methods in epidemiology particularly those for assessing evidence from randomized control trials (RCT) which is central to the development of future service developments, e.g. through the Cochrane centres development (Chalmers and Haynes, 1994) and the Health Outcomes Clearing House (Nuffield Institute for Health, 1994).

The three main questions that concern this chapter relate to how we can invest in auditory health care to bring about the greatest gain in the auditory health of the adult population. First, we need to know what the auditory health needs are and how they should be prioritized. We gain this knowledge by assessing the prevalence of hearing impairment and self-reported hearing disability, together with an appreciation of what factors influence the distribution, type and pattern of hearing impairment. Second, we need to know how effective the current services are at meeting the population need; what is the coverage, cost and benefit of those services. Third, we need to know the gaps that exist in our knowledge, the research that is needed and in what priority to underpin the effective development of the auditory health care programme. There are many gaps in our knowledge of the first and second areas, in particular the aetiology, and underlying bases, of adult acquired hearing impairment. Issues relating to access to and the benefits of different types of services, particularly for the over 80s group are poorly understood and will not be covered here in much detail. Tinnitus is an important hearing disorder, with many implications for the organization of audiological and otolaryngological services and is not discussed here but in Chapter 18.

Needs assessment

In order to establish the needs of the population, we have to have a common understanding of what is meant by 'need'. Having tried to establish the concept of 'need', some indicators of 'need' are required if we are to attempt to measure it. Both qualitative and quantitative indicators of need and benefit are relevant here. However, the assessment of need and outcome are usually assigned to the crudest categories, e.g. how many people have a hearing loss and how many have a hearing aid that works. At a gross level this may help to focus on the big task ahead, but it is hardly acceptable when we are assessing the need for cochlear implants or for binaural ITE hearing aids etc. Doyal and Gough (1991) proposed a very useful framework for considering 'need', and it is useful to consider their framework before getting bogged down by the interminable quantification of need and health gain. In particular, they suggested that, after survival has been assured, there is a universal need (that is not culturally relative) for an individual to have an autonomy within their society and to have a say in the organization of that society. In a sense, hearing disability and deafness may interfere with that ability to maintain a critical autonomy within society. Where there is a significant interference then there is obviously a very high priority in trying to assist through rehabilitation and legislation the hearing impaired and deaf to play their full role in society. Where the interference is less significant there is a problem for society in assigning a priority in terms of how much it is prepared to pay for what quality of service for which particular needs/demands/'wants'. It is in this area that there is considerable economic and cultural dependency.

The concepts of need, demand and supply of audiological health services in the population is explored in Figure 3.1, which is adapted from the more general schema proposed by Stevens (1991). Stevens used three circles to denote the three concepts and suggested various ways in which they may or may not overlap depending on the domain of interest. The simplistic model shown in Figure 3.1 has a continuum, represented by a large rectangle, between (1) Need and (2) Demand. This produces three areas, with one central intersection where need and demand are in unison. Obviously the real situation is more complex because need is multidimensional. In this context (Stevens, 1991) need, at the population level (see Davis, 1993a) is functionally defined as the ability to benefit from auditory health care. For general purposes this is a reasonable definition, but it does have as its focus what individual provider units can supply (e.g. cochlear implants, tinnitus counselling, hearing aids, neuro-otology) rather than the problems that people have with communication. It is inherently provider rather than client centred. But this model does have its uses in formulating how current services should change and is an interface between the traditional medical model approach that focuses primarily on demand and tertiary health services and an object-orientated approach that assesses the disabilities and handicaps that people may or will have and meets those needs with a variety of services and resources.

The multidimensionality of need occurs because people may have interacting needs, e.g. they might benefit at the functional level from provision of a hearing aid and from tinnitus counselling. The demand for services may be expressed for one, both or neither of these needs. On the other hand, the demand may be expressed in a completely different context, e.g. for other health services such as visual problems or a medical condition, or the demand may not be expressed by people with the impairment but by the people who interact with them. However, taking one simple audiological health care situation in which a subset of the population has a moderate hearing

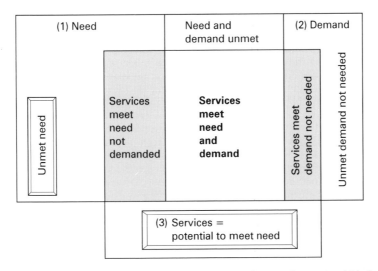

Figure 3.1 The relationship between (1) Need, (2) Demand and (3) Services, showing the way in which they may logically overlap. Each of the seven intersections is labelled and discussed in the text

disability which can be reduced by being trained to use a hearing aid, the model in Figure 3.1 shows seven situations which may occur when a hearing aid service (a subset of the audiological health care service) is provided to meet that need. An eighth situation may be where need is not recognized or demanded, but this is not discussed here (Stevens, 1991).

The extent of need and demand may be arbitrary. Need is constrained on one hand by the availability of benefit from current technology and depends very much on two elements: the ability of a service (e.g. fitting, training and technology) to confer benefit (as demonstrated by reasonable methods such as randomized controlled trials of which there are few examples in audiology); and the cost of realizing that benefit taking into account the change in quality of life that potentially accrues. To take an extreme example, the cost of giving someone with a mild high frequency hearing impairment a substantial improvement in hearing which barely affects major communication tasks may be several times greater than substantially reducing the disability experienced by an individual with a moderate hearing impairment. However, if the livelihood of the first person depends on very good high frequency hearing then the service might be cost-effective. Stevens (1991) addressed these cultural and ethical questions concerning needs assessment that do arise, particularly in a health care system that is socially organized and funded. However, ignoring those elements that relate to the auditory handicap domain for now, it is possible to see that need may be reasonably measured – at least in terms of the size of the problem, its associated severities and types. The surrogate measure of need that I will be using here is the hearing impairment in the population expressed in terms of the better ear averaged (BEA) threshold in the frequency region (0.5, 1, 2 and 4 kHz).

Demand, as discussed above, may be more difficult to assess. Obviously, overwhelmed by demand in certain sectors of health care, some have commented that demand is infinite and that the rectangle of Demand (2) should not be bounded. However, while demand for services that reduce hearing disability are bound to increase as the population of elderly people increases world-wide, there is ample evidence, presented later, that demand is either constrained by services available or restrained! The restraint is exercised by the factors that influence our perception of the services that exist, our perception of hearing disability in old age and indeed of old age itself. Demand is influenced, on the one hand, by the education of people which influences their expectations concerning hearing and hearing aid services but, also, on the other hand, by the education of those in primary care. Demand may also be manipulated by the provider units and the primary care team as well as through skilful use of the media by lobbyists, politicians and providers.

The third rectangle represents the services that have the potential to meet the need in the population. The service overheads, or even surplus services, are shown as in someway neither meeting needs or demands. The simplest objective is to maximize the overlap between need, demand and services and to minimize the surplus services (unless these are construed to be research and development activity needed to meet future needs more effectively and efficiently).

A major question, arising from Figure 3.1, that needs to be answered is the extent of unmet need: What proportion of unmet need is not expressed as a demand and how much would it cost to meet that presently unmet need in a planned manner setting incremental targets for meeting that need? I acknowledge that while the area described as 'Services meet need and demand' shows the overlap between the three concepts, it does not necessarily mean that a successful auditory outcome from hearing aid services has been achieved for all. I will not dwell, in this chapter, on the extent of benefit or its cost-utility.

The two shaded areas of Figure 3.1 are important areas from the public health point of view. In a way, services that meet need not demanded is stretching a point to make an example. A simple case of this area may be cross-referral. So if an elderly person has a hip-replacement and the staff at the hospital realize that there is a hearing problem that could be effectively 'treated' by referral to an otolaryngologist this is a direct expression of this area. However, a more important role of this area is in terms of auditory health education, hearing conservation programmes and hearing screening. In a sense, these are services meeting need and demand because those services may be entrained by society expressing the demand that these services be made available. This depends on our view of demand, whether it is individual or population based. At present there is no great popular demand for these services, because they are relevant for future generations or many years in the future, e.g. when a person has retired or is about to retire. Perceptual discounting occurs for these problems that may be prevented in the future, and are hence not highly valued as ways of spending present resources. Pre-emptive fitting of hearing aids, prior to demand being actively expressed is another example of how service developments can aim to prevent secondary disability (associated with a greater degree of need on all health care services) accruing (Stephens *et al.*, 1990; Davis *et al.*, 1992).

The second shaded area is probably quite small in reality – services that meet demand not needed. In some cases, e.g. occupational compensation schemes, there may be an element of overstated demand, that could be construed as malingering, that wastes services. However, there is a second class of population in this category where the demand is real, but the need lies in another dimension, e.g. mental health or eyesight. This is a very real cost on services and can be minimized by appropriate referral in some cases, but not all.

Depending on the distinct classes of need that we entertain (e.g. mild, unilateral, moderate, severe impairments) it will be possible in this chapter to estimate the extent of unmet need in the UK population, and the cost of meeting some of that need. At present there are no large-scale population studies of how demand is expressed and met as a function of hearing impairment or disability. Boufford (1993), comparing the UK and USA health care systems, suggested that the key difference between the two countries was access to health care: 'The first step in quality health care is access; the ability to get health care when needed'. For the auditory health care system (and presumably other chronic disabling conditions) access depends on many things that have been discussed above concerning demand. At the individual level access is not available until demanded, unless there is some universal screening programme, e.g. health care checks for the over 75s. By this age it may be less beneficial and cost-effective than early intervention. This raises the second problem for auditory health care: how do we define 'when needed' for the majority of people with slowly acquired hearing impairment and disability? The functional answer is, of course, when they would reasonably benefit from intervention. In practice this is difficult to assess because of the knock on advantages of earlier interventions. But as mentioned above, using a very liberal criterion of need a body of evidence suggests that early (mid-life) intervention is acceptable and beneficial (Stephens *et al.*, 1990; Davis *et al.*, 1992).

The following sections try to provide some data on the measurement of need and factors that influence that need and associated demand and uptake of services. The data are specific to the UK, and their generality will be assessed in the light of those factors that influence need. Different aspects of these studies have recently been reported elsewhere (Lutman, Brown and Coles, 1987; Davis, 1989, 1995; Davis, Ostri and Parving, 1991; Browning and Gatehouse, 1992; Davis *et al.*, 1992; Gatehouse and Davis, 1992; Haggard, 1993; Haggard and Gatehouse, 1993; Lutman and Davis, 1994a) as well as in several other publications cited in the previous edition of this chapter. The methodology for that work has been published in detail (Davis, 1989, 1995). Essentially a large random sample of the population in the UK (for the major work reported here the cities Cardiff, Glasgow, Nottingham and Southampton were the primary sampling units, although a smaller national sample replicated the main findings) was contacted and replied to a postal questionnaire. A random subset of 2708 people, aged 18–80 years, had their hearing assessed in good audiological testing conditions. A sample of those who could not attend the clinics for testing were visited at home and no bias was found between attenders and non-attenders.

Other studies should be, but are not, reviewed here in detail. There is reasonable agreement on some aspects of the descriptive epidemiology (Moscicki *et al.*, 1985; US National Center for Health Statistics, 1986; Soucek and Michaels, 1987; Rahko *et al.*, 1988; Gates *et al.*, 1990, 1993; Rosenhall, Pedersen and Svanborg, 1990; Pirila, Jounio-Ervasti and Sorri, 1992; Quarantã and Assenato, 1991; Corso, 1992; Takeda *et al.*, 1992), particularly the age-related aspects, and the under provision of services/demand for hearing aid services. There is still only a small number of studies of hearing impairment using random samples of the population. One of the problems in making comparisons is the lack of uniform data between studies, particularly in the published versions (Davis, 1983, 1993b). The agreement is usually not too problematic for studies that have used the same methods to assess hearing impairment (though few have specified detailed protocols for the audiometry and booths), but can be much greater for less quantitative methods, e.g. reported hearing disability. One area in which there appears to be a discrepancy is between hearing in young people in the UK and in Sweden (Axelsson, Rosenhall and Zachan, 1994). The reasons for this are explored further below.

While a major audiological health care goal (US National Strategic Research Plan, 1989) must be to reduce risk factors that lead to disabling hearing impairments in later life, no great strides have been made in that area (Gates *et al.*, 1993), and factors other than noise and demography only seem to account for a small proportion of hearing impairment in the elderly. These aetiological aspects are covered in Chapters 8 and 10.

The extent and nature of need

Prevalence and distribution of hearing impairment and reported hearing disability

The effect of severity

The prevalence of hearing impairment is the number of people who have a specific degree of hearing impairment at a given time. This can also be expressed as a percentage. The denominator in the percentage has to be made explicit; thus if there are 25 hearing impaired adults in a population of 100 people, of whom there are 50 adults and 50 children, then the population prevalence for adult hearing impairment is 25%, but it is 50% of the adult population. In the following section, I shall be using prevalence to indicate the percentage of adults who have an impairment. In this context I will not be discussing incidence, the number of new cases per given time period (usually a year). Incidence of hearing impairment is discussed further in Davis, Ostri and Parving

(1991) as well as in the previous edition of this chapter (Davis, 1987).

Figure 3.2 shows the broad extent of hearing impairment and reported hearing disability in the UK, in the adult population (aged 18 and over). From this figure we see that almost one in three of UK adults has at least a mild hearing impairment in one ear, with one in five showing a bilateral hearing impairment. One in four people report that they have great difficulty hearing what is said in a background of noise, with one in 10 reporting that they have prolonged spontaneous tinnitus (Coles, Davis and Smith, 1990). At a moderate degree of hearing impairment, in the better ear, there are about 7% of the adult population who are impaired (Davis, 1995, Chapter 8). This represents a substantial number of people in the UK who may have a need for some associated services, i.e. who may benefit from the provision of hearing services. Supplying those services is thus a substantial public health problem, about which there ought to be considerable debate.

For the adult population, aged 18–80 years, Figure 3.3 shows the variation in prevalence of hearing impairment as a function of severity of the hearing impairment and of gender. Davis (1995, Chapter 3) tabulated the prevalence of hearing impairment over a large number of severity criteria for each hearing threshold and each major average of hearing thresholds, for the better and worse ears. In Figure 3.3 the threshold criteria that I have taken is based on the average threshold for the better hearing ear at the frequencies of 0.5, 1, 2 and 4 kHz (BEA). The cut-off for defining the categories of 15+, 25+, 35+ and 45+ dB HL was exactly at those numeric levels. Hence an average of 24.5 was treated as below 25. Rounding up actually adds an extra 0.9%, thus instead of a prevalence of 16.1% of the adult population

having a BEA of 25 dB HL or worse, with rounding it approaches 17%. The prevalences given in Figure 3.3 are already cumulated and should not be added together, because 25+ dB HL already includes 35+ dB HL.

Figure 3.3 shows that there is a difference between males and females, in the expected direction (e.g. Gates *et al.*, 1990) with men having a higher prevalence of hearing impairment. As Davis and Thornton (1990) have pointed out, however, this does not necessarily mean that there are more men than women with hearing impairment, because of the much greater mortality in middle-aged men. The figure shows that the difference exists down to about 45 dB HL where it is very small. However, the major differences are shown for milder hearing impairments at 15+ dB HL and at 25+ dB HL where there is no overlap of the 95% confidence intervals (CI).

The effect of gender

These data give a broad picture of the difference in prevalence of hearing impairment between men and women. Figure 3.4 shows the mean audiograms, with appropriate confidence intervals for the means, for males and females at each of the major age groups used for this study. It is fairly evident from the data shown in this figure that the difference between men and women apparently evolves over time. As this is a cross-sectional study, care has to be taken in attributing change over time. So, there is very little difference between men and women at age 18–30 years. By the age of 31–40 years, there is a significant difference at some high frequencies (3, 4 and 8 kHz) which increases for the decades 41–50, 51–60 and 61–70 years and is still apparent at 71–

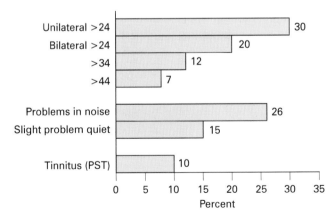

Figure 3.2 The prevalence of hearing impairment at different degrees of severity, hearing disability as shown by finding it 'very difficult' to hear what someone says if there is a background of noise and also by having at least a slight difficulty hearing in quiet. The prevalence of tinnitus that is not only after loud sounds and which lasts for 5 minutes or more (PST, prolonged spontaneous tinnitus) is also shown

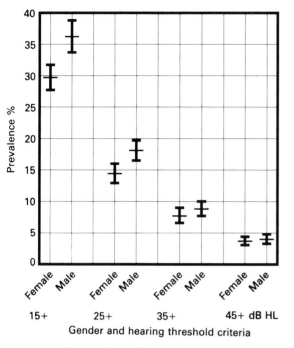

Figure 3.3 The prevalence of hearing impairment with 95% confidence intervals, using the mid-frequency average threshold over 0.5, 1, 2, 4 kHz in the better ear (BEA), at four degrees of severity (15 +, 25 +, 35 +, 45 + dB HL) as a function of gender. (Data from Davis, 1995)

80 years, albeit with greater variation. The 71–80-year-old men actually have slightly better hearing at low frequencies than women in this sample.

It is noticeable from Figure 3.4, that the thresholds at 6 kHz are not necessarily appropriate and must contain almost 10 dB of bias which originates from the ISO standard that was adopted (ISO, 1984). It is also noticeable that the data for the 18–30 year age group deviates systematically from zero dB. This aspect of the data will be mentioned again below and has been extensively examined (Lutman and Davis, 1994a).

The major factor that is associated with the prevalence and distribution of hearing impairment is age (e.g. Davis, 1989). Figures 3.5a and 3.5b shows the variation of prevalence of hearing impairment at two degrees of hearing impairment. Figure 3.5a shows the massive increase in the prevalence of hearing impairments of 25 + dB HL, that in this cross-sectional study, seems to occur at about the age of 51–60 years, where there is no overlap of the confidence intervals at all. This is also reflected in the more severe 45 + dB HL impairments shown in Figure 3.5b. The increase in prevalence of hearing impairments with age is hardly surprising, but its high rate of increase in the over 50s is very large indeed. At 18–30 years the prevalence is 1.8 (1.0–3.2) and 0.2

(0.1–0.6) for 25 + and 45 + dB HL, but by the time of 71–80 years it is 60 (52.9–67.3) and 17.6 (14.3–21.5)% respectively. Data on the over 80s are more difficult to assess, but they have been presented previously (Davis, 1987, 1995) and do indeed continue to show increased prevalence of hearing impairment. A parallel deterioration of hearing is also shown in the worse ear, but with the slope somewhat steeper in the earlier decades.

The effect of age

The extent to which the audiogram changes with age can be assessed from Figure 3.4. However, while the means shown in Figure 3.4 are appropriate for the comparison outlined above, it is often of interest to compare the medians rather than the mean hearing thresholds because of the nature of the distribution of hearing impairment which is not normal but lognormal (Davis, 1987; Bowater *et al.*, 1995). The median thresholds for each decade age group are shown in Figures 3.6a and 3.6b for females and males over better and worse ears. From Figure 3.6 it is evident that there is a much greater effect of age on the high frequencies rather than the low frequencies, but even at the low frequencies there is a substantial variation with age, for both men and women. The effect of age starts to take a differential toll on hearing at above 1 kHz in both genders. The differences between men and women is that the deterioration is more rapid and systematic in men. Note the clear difference even between the 31–40 and the 18–30-year-old males. A second difference is that the slope of the audiogram for hearing between 2 kHz and higher frequencies is more affected in men than in women.

The effect of occupational group

Part of the difference between the genders may emanate from the greater noise exposure of men than women. This is suggested by the way in which the differences between the genders over age are frequency specific. However, not all the difference may be accounted for by the effect of noise exposure, there may be some other reasons such as social class differences and other systemic reasons for the difference. Figure 3.7 shows the prevalence of hearing impairment for three threshold criteria, 25 +, 35 + and 45 + dB HL for BEA as a function of gender and occupational group for adults aged 18–80 years. It is clear from Figure 3.7 that for each gender the prevalence is greater for the manual occupational group. To assess occupational group we ascertained social class, by interview, according to the OPCS Registrar General's Classification of Occupations. This gives six major categories (I, II, IIIN, IIIM, IV and V; or in media terms A, B, C1, C2, D and E) that run from professional occupations (e.g. lawyer) to unskilled occupations. We grouped the first three of these

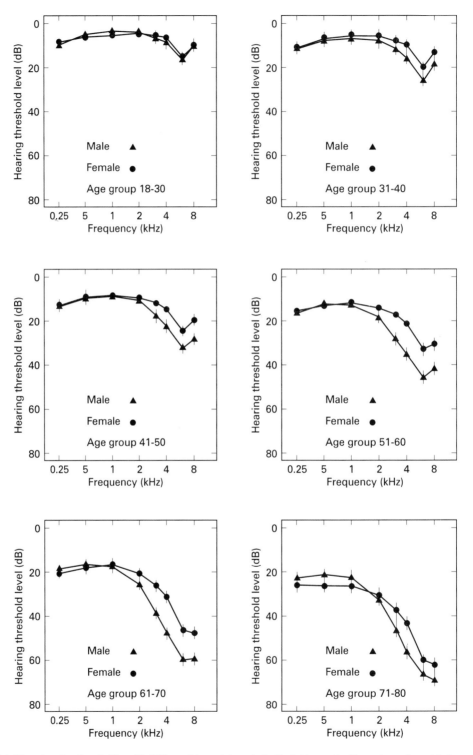

Figure 3.4 Mean hearing thresholds, with 95% confidence intervals, in the better ear for the main audiometric frequencies are shown for each of six age groups as a function of gender. (Data from Davis, 1995)

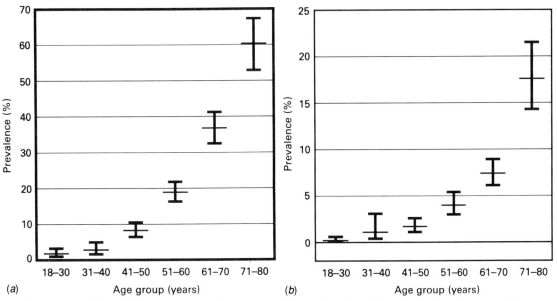

Figure 3.5 (*a*) Prevalence of hearing impairment for BEA 45 + dB HL with 95% confidence intervals as a function of age group. (Data from Davis, 1995.) (*b*) Prevalence of hearing impairment for BEA 45 + dB HL with 95% confidence intervals as a function of age group. (Data from Davis, 1995)

categories together as the non-manual occupational group (N or ABC1) and the remainder as the manual occupational group (M or C2DE).

Figure 3.7 shows that there is a much greater and highly significant effect of occupational group for men than women at the 25 + and 35 + dB HL criteria. At the 45 + dB HL criteria the manual groups for both men and women are significantly greater than the counterparts for the non-manual groups. The right hand portion of Figure 3.7 shows the prevalence of hearing aid possession which will be discussed in more detail below. It does show an interaction between gender and occupational group that is not explained in terms of the prevalence of hearing impairment. Thus while there is no difference in either prevalence of hearing impairment or of hearing aid provision for the non-manual group over gender, there is a significant relative shortfall in the female manual workers.

To look at the difference in pattern of hearing impairment between the occupational groups, as there is an interaction with gender, we need to look at the effect separately in women and men. Figure 3.8 shows the mean hearing thresholds and confidence interval for the females, separated by occupational group. There is a small difference between the occupational groups across all frequencies which is significant in the women aged 18–50 years. For older women the difference is only at the low frequencies.

Figure 3.9 shows for males the same data as Figure 3.8. The difference between the occupational groups is more apparent for the men across all age groups. It does not disappear at higher frequencies. Indeed there is a tendency for considerable overlap at the low frequencies at 60–80 years. This difference between the occupational groups is a major difference and any attempt to isolate risk factors for hearing impairment without taking the occupational group into account will have substantial problems.

It may be that the difference between the occupational groups can be attributed to noise factors alone, but this does not seem to be the case. Lutman and Davis (1994 a,b) have analysed these data extensively to try to reach the roots of the occupational group difference and we have concluded that it is not solely in noise factors. Figure 3.10 shows the difference between the manual occupational group and the non-manual for the 18–30 year age group, for the BEA over the centiles of the BEA distribution. There are bound to be methodological problems here because on the side of good hearing we have only measured down to − 10 dB HL for each frequency. Thus for the low centiles this will tend to underestimate the difference between the groups. There were about 200 people in each occupational group. Figure 3.10 shows the occupational group difference for the whole population (typical population) and for the subset of the population who had negligible noise exposure or any type of conductive hearing impairment (screened or 'otologically normal' population). There is a general increase in the effect of occupational group as the centiles of the distribution are increasing. Thus as hearing worsens the difference

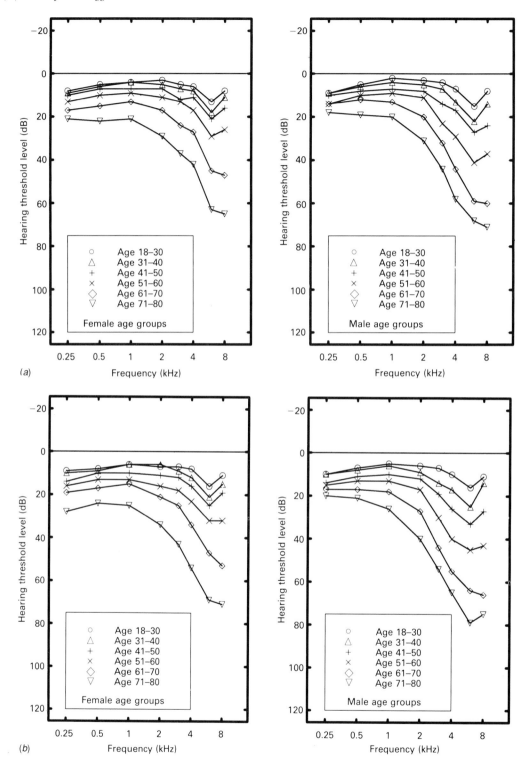

Figure 3.6 (*a*) Median hearing threshold for each of six age groups in the better ear for women (left) and men (right). (Data from Davis, 1995.) (*b*) Median hearing threshold for each of six age groups in the worse ear for women (left) and men (right). (Data from Davis, 1995)

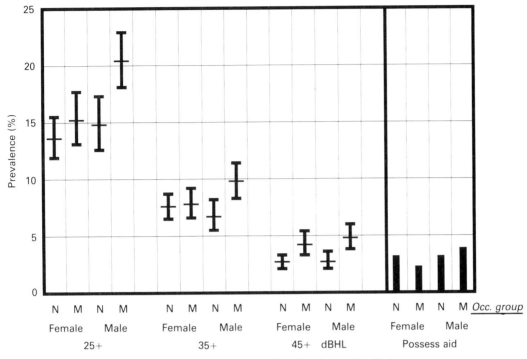

Figure 3.7 The prevalence of hearing impairment, with 95% confidence intervals, for BEA at 25 +, 35 +, 45 + dB HL as a function of gender and occupational group. The prevalence of the possession of a hearing aid is also shown as a function of gender and occupational group. (Occ. group N = non-manual; M = manual)

between the occupational groups increases. This may be an artefact of the methodological problems mentioned above. However, even if it is, the effect of occupational group is of the order 3–5 dB for the screened population and larger for the typical population.

Figures 3.11 and 3.12 show the effect of age on the distribution of hearing impairment for men at the BEA (Figure 3.11) and at 4k Hz in the better ear (Figure 3.12). In each figure seven centiles of the hearing threshold distribution have been estimated and smoothed functions over age have been produced (see Davis, 1995 for the exact estimation procedure). In this set of data only thresholds for people aged 22–78 years have been estimated due to the procedure used. The 5, 10, 25, 50, 75, 90 and 95th centiles have been used together with a mean function (dotted line). The smoothing is necessary because of the small sample in each year of age (2708 overall in 62 age categories) and because of the sampling protocol (Davis, 1989). The data are shown for the screened population and for the typical population, and also for each occupational group.

The first point to note is that the data for 4 kHz show a much greater variation over age than the BEA. The second point is that the asymmetry in the distribution of hearing impairment – shown by the spread in the three upper centiles (75, 90 and 95) compared to the three lower centiles – is much greater for the BEA. In general the asymmetry also increases with (1) age, but is not absent at younger ages, (2) type of population, being greater in the typical population, and (3) occupational group, being much greater in the manual occupational group even for the screened population.

At 4 kHz (Figure 3.12) the modelled thresholds show that the intercept at about 20 years of age is not approaching 0 dB HL in the screened population but is nearer 6–7 dB HL for all occupational groups. This intercept is higher for manual occupational groups.

Figures 3.13 and 3.14 show similar data but for the average threshold in the two ears over the frequencies 0.5, 1, 2 and 3 kHz which has been recommended for evaluation of hearing disability and handicap for medico-legal purposes in the USA (Dobie, 1993). Figure 3.13 shows the distributions for women and Figure 3.14 for men. Similar observations can be made for these data. In particular the distribution of the upper centiles for women in the manual occupational group seems to be highly skewed especially for young age groups. This is true for both screened and typical populations and may reflect the smaller

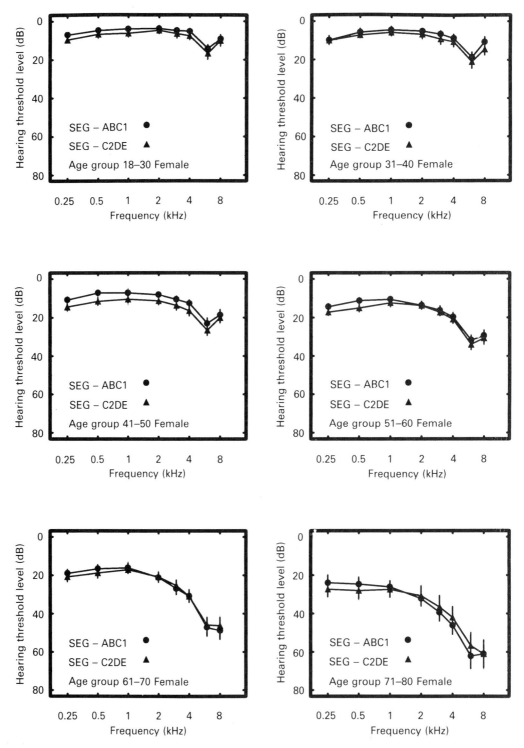

Figure 3.8 The mean threshold, with 95% confidence interval for women as a function of frequency for each age group and occupational group, in the better ear

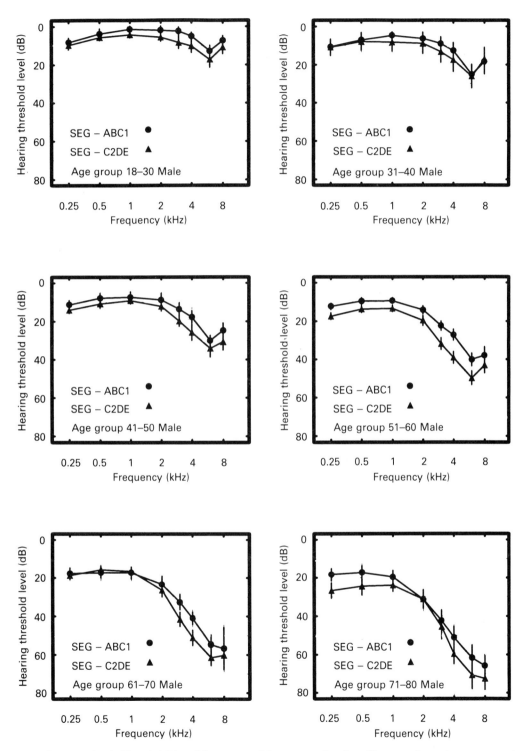

Figure 3.9 The mean threshold, with 95% confidence interval for men as a function of frequency for each age group and occupational group, in the better ear

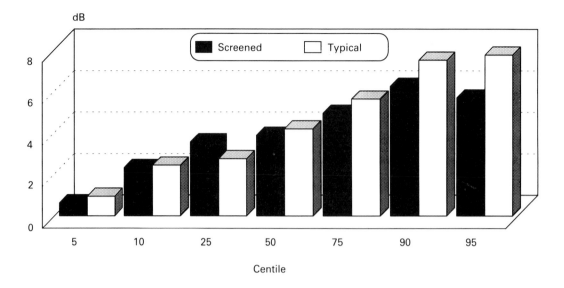

Figure 3.10 The difference between the manual and non-manual occupational groups in BEA as a function of the centile of the distribution in two populations of men (screened, i.e. otologically normal and unscreened, i.e. typical)

number of women at these ages and manual occupational groups who are in the population. For all these models of the impact of age on the different centiles of the hearing threshold distribution for the screened, and otologically normal, population the intercept is always nearer 5 dB than 0 dB HL. If this is correct (Lutman and Davis, 1994a) then it has substantial implications for our understanding of the effect of occupational noise on hearing (ISO, 1984, 1990; King *et al.*, 1992; Dobie, 1993) and, in particular, how we assess the effect of noise exposure and how the apportionment of noise damage for different periods of noise exposure can be viewed (Lutman, 1992).

The effect of occupational noise

We have looked at the effect of age, gender and occupational group on the prevalence of hearing impairment and seen that each has a substantial effect on the prevalence and distribution of hearing thresholds. Both age and gender have frequency specific effects, while occupational group has less of a frequency specific effect than might be hypothesized if it were due to noise alone. Noise immission was rated (NIR) according to a uniform protocol (Davis, 1989; Medical Research Council Institute of Hearing Research, 1985) and the scale of NIR was graded such that an NIR of 0 was < 97 dB(A) NIL, 1 was 97–107, 2 was 107–117, 3 was 117–127 and 4 was > 127 dB(A). The noise immission rating thus represents a five point scale of cumulative lifetime noise exposure. Each value represents a 10 dB range

of NIL values. For example 50 years at Leq of 81–90 dB(A) is equivalent to 97–107 NIL and is an NIR rating of 1. Lutman and Davis (1994b) and Davis, Lutman and Copas (1994) give the most up to date account of how age, gender, occupational group and NIR may affect hearing and there are criticisms of their approach on statistical grounds in Bowater *et al.* (1995). The impact of NIR on the prevalence of hearing impairment was also quantitatively analysed in Davis (1989). Figures 3.15 and 3.16 show the prevalence of BEA at two degrees of hearing impairment (25+ and 35+ dB HL). Combining the NIR groups 2, 3 and 4 the data are shown separately for the genders and occupational groups. Not surprisingly the prevalence of hearing impairment increases with increasing noise immission. This is not related to age, as the mean ages for all groups were surprisingly in agreement to within a few years of age.

Both Figures 3.15 and 3.16 show that the manual occupations had a higher prevalence than the non-manual when there was little noise immission (< 97dB(A)). Figure 3.15 shows that moderate levels of noise immission, NIL 97–107, are associated with raised prevalence of hearing impairment. This is particularly the case for all but the male-manual occupation group which has the lowest increase in prevalence. This may be due to under-reporting of noisy jobs in this group, or the smaller number of people in the other NIRO 1 groups (NIRO = NIR to occupational noise) (147 versus 49 for male non-manual, 84 female manual and 35 female non-manual). The fairly reasonable effect at 25+ dB HL is substantially

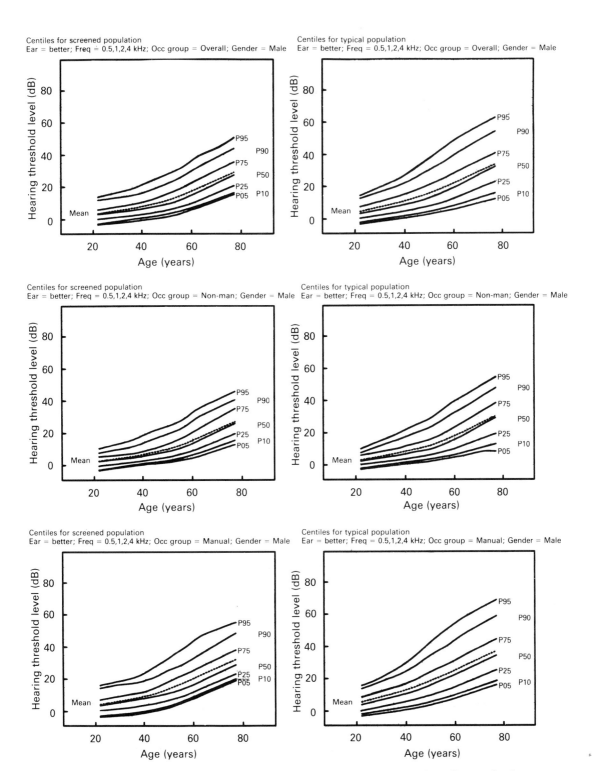

Figure 3.11 Centiles of the distribution of BEA as a function of population, (screened, i.e. otologically normal and unscreened, i.e. typical) as a function of occupational group for men

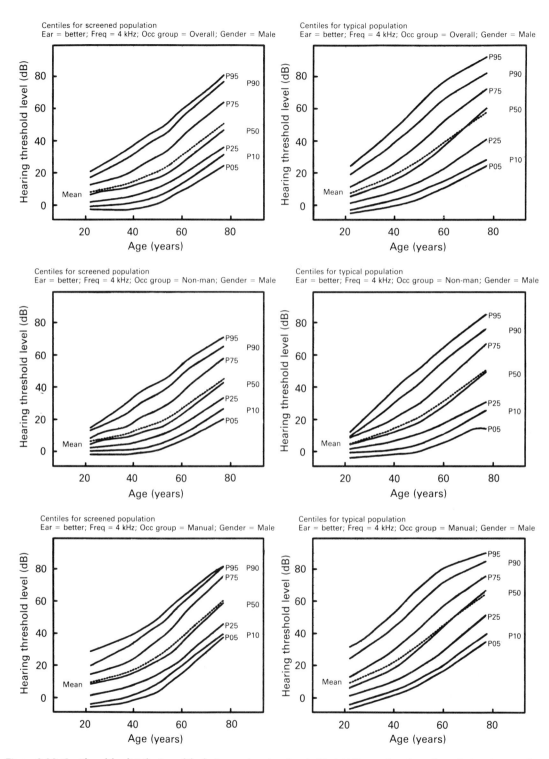

Figure 3.12 Centiles of the distribution of the better ear hearing threshold at 4 kHz as a function of population, (screened, i.e. otologically normal and unscreened, i.e. typical) as a function of occupational group for men

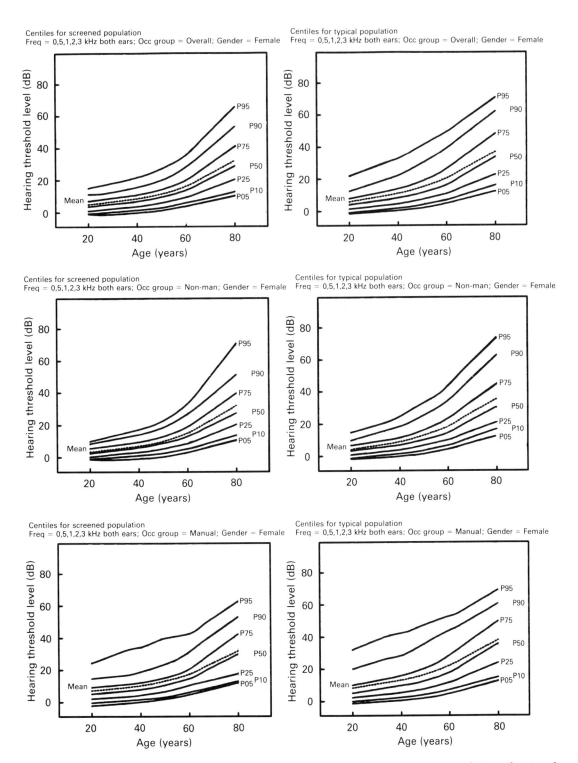

Figure 3.13 Centiles of the distribution of the average threshold for both ears averaged over 0.5, 1, 2, 3 kHz as a function of population, (screened, i.e. otologically normal and unscreened, i.e. typical) as a function of occupational group for females

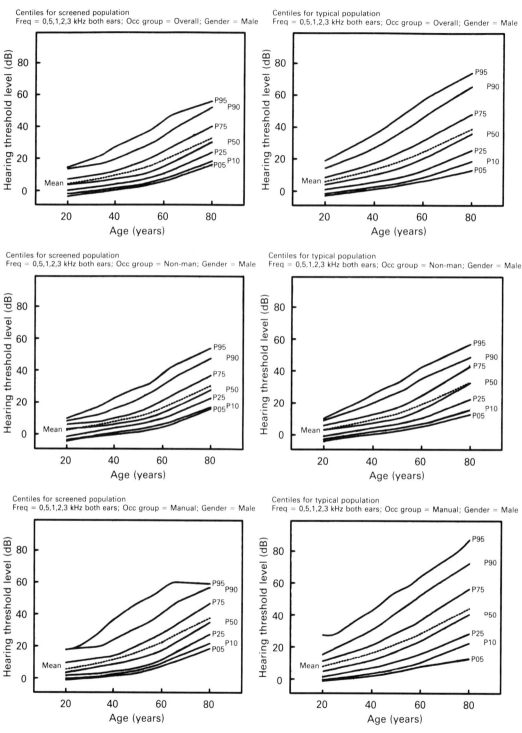

Figure 3.14 Centiles of the distribution of the average threshold for both ears averaged over 0.5, 1, 2, 3 kHz as a function of population, (screened, i.e. otologically normal and unscreened, i.e. typical) as a function of occupational group for males

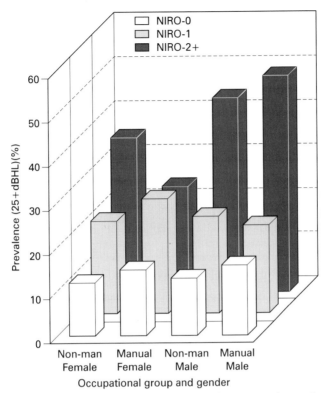

Figure 3.15 The prevalence of BEA 25 + dB HL as a function of gender and occupational group for each of three noise exposure groups (NIRO 0, 1, 2 +)

reduced at 35 + dB HL where the major effect is due to NIRO 2. So the effect of NIRO 1 is quite small on the mean (Davis, Lutman and Copas, 1994; Lutman and Davis, 1994b), but is large on the prevalence of mild hearing impairments becoming much smaller for greater degrees of hearing impairment.

The problems in estimating the parameters in a normal statistical model of the effect of noise and age on hearing impairment are substantial (Lutman and Davis, 1994a; Bowater *et al.*, 1995). Not only does the mean change with NIR, but also the variance and skew of the distribution. However, within certain limits the results obtained within previous models have been robust (Davis, 1995). Another method for examining the effect of NIR is to use a cubic B-spline regression method to fit the age trend to the data from the different levels of NIR. Figure 3.17 shows the results of the fit at 4 kHz, for the four levels of NIR with enough data to use the procedure for the male-manual occupation group alone. This frequency was chosen as it is usually the most sensitive to noise exposure. The associated upper 95% confidence intervals have been derived from the jack-knifed residuals (Hastie and Tibshirani, 1990). The lines shown are the smoothed lines fitted to the estimates derived from the predictions of the

regression equations. The main findings from this analysis are:

1 The intercept at age 20 for NIRO 1 is nearer 5 than 0 dB
2 The mean effect of NIRO 1 was consistent over age, but overlapped the 95% confidence interval for NIRO throughout
3 The effect of NIRO 1 on the mean is probably real, and at its greatest (i.e. 20–30 year age group) is no more than 5–6 dB
4 The effect of NIRO 2 is up to 12 dB, but converges with increasing age to that for NIRO 0 and 1
5 The effect of NIRO 3 + is difficult, well nigh impossible, to measure below about 40 years of age because of the nature of the measure. The effect is a stable 15 dB that decreases in the ages 70–80 years to 0 dB
6 The variability of hearing thresholds for the NIR 3 + condition is very large and hence the wide confidence limits.

These data suggest that the effect of high levels of noise may decrease with age as has been suggested previously (Robinson, 1987; Corso, 1992). However, while the response to moderate levels of noise, NIRO 1, is consistent over age, it is not necessarily the

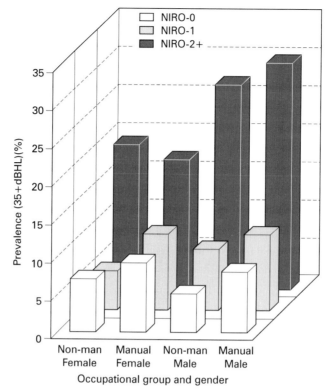

Figure 3.16 The prevalence of BEA 35 + dB HL as a function of gender and occupational group for each of three noise exposure groups (NIRO 0, 1, 2 +)

same as that to greater levels of noise immission. Hence there may be further confounding in the data. It is not surprising that we have difficulty in analysing these data considering the data presenting in Figures 3.15 and 3.16 which show that the effect of moderate levels of noise disappears quite quickly in the tail of hearing impairment.

Leisure noise

Another source of noise exposure that has aroused much media interest in the last 10 years is social or leisure noise (Medical Research Council Institute of Hearing Research, 1985). It has been quite difficult to assess whether leisure noise has a population effect on hearing, because the prevalence of substantial immission akin to that in industry is actually quite small and is restricted very much to those under 40 years and, in the data we have collected, it is only the under 30s that have substantial exposure. Just 5.5% of the 18–30 year age group have leisure noise exposure compared with 11.7% with occupational at the NIL > 97 dB(A) level. This compares to over one-quarter of the adult population having such noise exposure.

Axelsson, Rosenhall and Zachau (1994) reported

that the Swedish young male population who are being conscripted have better hearing than their UK counterparts (not conscripted, but randomly chosen) using a metric of the number of hearing thresholds on either ear that were over 20 dB HL. This yields a metric from 0 to 16 (using both ears). One suggestion might be that social noise exposure may be different between the populations. We cannot test that hypothesis here however, Figure 3.18 shows the prevalence of suitable points on this metric for people aged 18–30 years. This metric is useful because it is sensitive to small problems in hearing. However, it may not be very robust for our needs so has to be interpreted with caution.

Figure 3.18 shows that for up to five thresholds exceeding 20 dB HL there was a noticeable difference between the people who have a social noise NIR (NIRS) of 1 and 0. Figure 3.19 shows the results of an analysis to examine this effect and to take out other effects such as occupational noise and group. As can be seen from Figure 3.19 the increased odds of at least one, or at least two, thresholds exceeding 20 dB HL are increased by a factor of 2.5 to 1 if there has been significant leisure noise exposure.

This should not be surprising. There is no reason

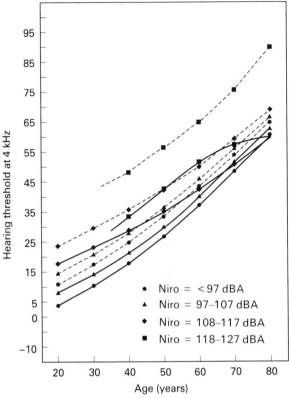

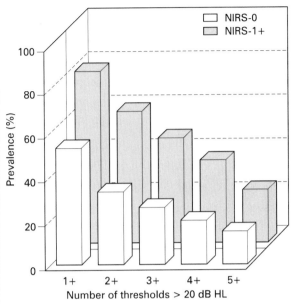

Figure 3.17 The fitted model of hearing impairment at 4 kHz in the better ear as a function of age for each of four occupational noise immission groups (NIRO 0, 1, 2, 3 + corresponding to NIL < 97, 97–107, 108–117, 118–127 dBA). The solid lines give the mean fit using a smoothed spline to fit age to hearing impairment. The dashed lines show the equivalent 95% confidence intervals for the fit shown by the respective solid line. The data are from male, manual occupational group only

Figure 3.18 The prevalence of the number of thresholds for either ear in excess of 20 dB HL as a function of social noise immission rating (NIRS) for the population of young people aged 18–30 years

to believe that leisure noise is any less damaging than occupational noise of similar intensity, duration and pattern of attendance. The problem is that the changes that are seen are obviously smaller in younger people and are confined mostly to young people at present. This is an area where further study, some 10 years since the original fieldwork, may be able to shed light on the present degree of public health hazard due to leisure noise.

Type of hearing impairment

Although 16.1% (15.0–17.3) of the adult population, aged 18–80 years, have a BEA of 25 dB HL or greater, not all of those impairments are due to sensorineural pathologies. Table 3.1 shows the prevalence of hearing impairment that we think is due to conductive

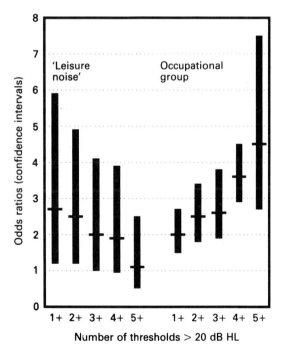

Figure 3.19 The odds ratios (and 95% confidence intervals) for the leisure noise and occupational group parameters as a function of the number of thresholds in excess of 20 dB HL when fitting a general linear model with binomial errors to the prevalence of particular impairment categories

Table 3.1 The prevalence of hearing impairment as a function of type of hearing impairment, ear and severity of hearing impairment for each of three age groups and over all ages

Type of impairment	Ear	Severity (dB HL +)	Prevalence of specified hearing impairment (%)			
			18–40 years	41–60 years	61–80 years	18–80 years
Conductive	Better	25	0.4	3.1	3.8	2.1
Sensorineural hearing loss	Better	25	1.5	10.7	42.0	13.9
Conductive	Worse	25	3.6	9.8	13.4	8.0
Sensorineural hearing loss	Worse	25	3.5	17.4	45.3	17.7
Conductive	Better	45	0.1	1.3	3.1	1.1
Sensorineural hearing loss	Better	45	0.2	1.6	14.3	2.4
Conductive	Worse	45	1.2	5.0	11.3	4.8
Sensorineural hearing loss	Worse	45	0.3	3.0	12.5	4.0

pathologies as opposed to sensorineural. The criterion we have used for this is that for a conductive hearing impairment there should be an air-bone gap of 15 dB or greater over the midfrequencies 0.5, 1 and 2 kHz averaged. Table 3.1 shows the change in each component of prevalence with age, ear and degree of hearing impairment. Using these criteria only 13% of mild or worse impairments have a significant conductive component. However, if the criterion was changed to any frequency showing an air-bone gap of 10 dB or more then this proportion changed to about 28% of the total which amounts to 4.1% impairments with a conductive component – an increase of 2%. Thus the prevalence depends very much on how we define a conductive component to the hearing impairment.

The proportion of conductive pathologies can be seen to change with ear. It accounts for almost one out of three of the impairments at 25 + dB HL in the worse ear, and also with severity of hearing impairment. For impairment of 45 + dB HL conductive impairments in the worse ear account for in excess of 50% of all impairments.

Table 3.1 also shows the massive increase in the prevalence of hearing impairment as a function of age, particularly in the 61–80 year age group. In addition to this big change, the worse ear changes over age for conductive impairments at 45 + dB HL are very large. So the typical person with a 45 + dB HL impairment in the better ear is likely to have a mean hearing impairment of 55 dB HL in the better ear and 64 dB HL in the worse ear, but if the worse ear has a conductive impairment, the worse ear is over 70 dB HL.

The variation of the prevalence of conductive hearing impairments is shown in Figure 3.20 as function of age group, gender and occupational group for the better ear at 25 + dB HL. For all groups bar the male non-manual there is no increase in the prevalence between the 41–60 and 61–80 year age groups. This

is reflected in the first row of Table 3.1. There is no large effect of gender but there is an effect of occupational group, with the older age groups showing an overall difference of 1.5–2.0%, which is almost a 100% increase for the manual occupational group. The effect of age in these data may be due to age alone or they may be cohort effects due to previous medical treatment or other such effects. We cannot distinguish between these hypotheses with these data.

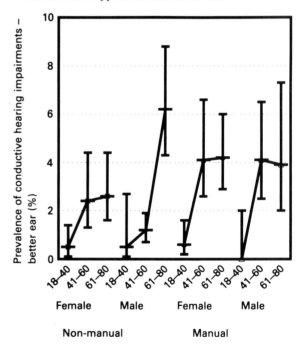

Figure 3.20 The prevalence of conductive hearing impairments (25 + dB HL better ear), with 95% confidence intervals, as a function of age group for gender and occupational groups

Hearing aid provision

Davis (1993b) has presented the prevalence of hearing aid possession in the UK from different samples and over different time periods. There is no evidence in the UK that the prevalence of hearing aid possession and use is going up. Gates *et al.* (1990) reported that in the Framingham cohort (aged 65+ years) there were 10.3% (*n* = 1662) who had worn a hearing aid, one in five of whom had given up. This is close to the UK data, for a sample chosen to match the USA sample for age (i.e. 65 years and over), which was 12.0% (*n* = 7818) who had possessed a hearing aid. A proportion similar to those in the USA study had stopped using them.

Table 3.2 shows the proportion of people who possess a hearing aid as a function of degree of hearing impairment. The population prevalence of each specific severity of hearing impairment on the better ear is shown. Thus there are 4.9% of the population who have BEA in the range 25–29 dB HL; 1.4% of these people possess a hearing aid, representing 2% of the subpopulation of people with a hearing aid. At 35–39 dB HL there are half that number, i.e. 2.4%, of whom only 9.3% possess a hearing aid. It is not until the BEA is >54 dB HL that the proportion

Table 3.2 The prevalence of hearing impairment in each BEA severity category and prevalence of reported hearing aid possession in each degree of hearing impairment. In addition the percentage of those with a hearing aid in each severity category is shown

Degree of impairment (dB HL)	Population prevalence	Percent possess aid	Percent of those with an aid
<25	84.0	0.2	7.0
25–29	4.9	1.4	2.0
30–34	3.0	6.6	6.0
35–39	2.4	9.3	7.0
40–44	1.9	18.6	11.0
45–54	1.8	37.2	21.0
55–64	1.0	57.3	18.0
65+	1.0	88.6	28.0

of people who possess a hearing aid increases above 50%!

The prevalence of hearing aid possession is shown in Figure 3.21 as a function of cumulative severity, gender and occupational group. While we noted earlier in Figure 3.7 that the male manual population had the greatest prevalence of hearing aid possession,

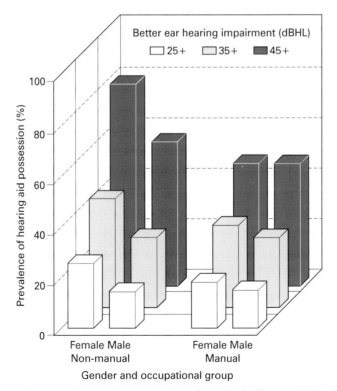

Figure 3.21 The prevalence of hearing aid possession as a function of BEA threshold criteria (25+, 35+, 45+ dB HL) for gender and occupational group

and it seems from Figure 3.7 that the largest preva- lence of hearing aid possession is in this group, it is clear from Figure 3.21 that take-up in this group is lowest. Take up is obviously influenced by degree of impairment as well as gender and occupational group, with the female non-manual group having the highest take-up at all severities.

For England and Wales, we undertook a survey of hearing aid supply in the first six months of 1993 (Davis, Fortnum and Spencer, 1995). This showed an annual rate of prescription of NHS supplied hearing aids of about 577 000 hearing aids, at a cost of £21.8m. About 37% of the hearing aids were given to new users, with the remainder being replacements or repairs. There were approximately 1400 staff in- volved in the provision of hearing aids at an estimated cost of £27.9m. Each hearing aid probably cost the health service of the order of £90, which is about £1 out of £572 spent on health care per head of the population per annum.

In order to improve access to hearing aid services, and supply targets that are set in terms of the severity of hearing impairment and also the ages of those who need a hearing health care service of some sort is a difficult task, and is not likely to be cheap! As we have seen from Table 3.2 and Figure 3.21, there is considerable unmet need. If an overall target was set of improving access so that 5%, rather than 3.2% of people wore a hearing aid (and hopefully found it beneficial) as shown in Table 3.3, then the overall initial cost would be greater than the annual cost of running the whole hearing aid system at about £66m. As two-thirds of the cost of the service is probably spent on replacements and repairs, the run on costs from this initial cost may be as high as £20m per annum, i.e. an increase of 40% per annum in 1993 prices.

The relationship between reported hearing ability and hearing impairment

There are many different ways in which hearing disability can be measured. A behavioural measure

can be made, such as the speech in noise test (SIN) which I reported in the previous edition (Davis and Haggard, 1982; Davis, 1987). This measure of dis- ability was related to BEA, age, gender and tinnitus annoyance. As well as other behaviour measures of disability, self-reported disability questions have been used (e.g. King *et al.*, 1992; Lutman and Robin- son, 1992). Self-report questions and scales (Noble, 1978; Ventry and Weinstein, 1982; Davis, 1995) are useful in assessing aspects of disability. However, disability is multifaceted, and such approaches need to be well validated before using for generic purposes. King *et al.* (1992) proposed a method for assessing disability, based on data from the MRC National Study of Hearing, using a scale of hearing ability where people were asked to rate their hearing from 0 to 100 with relation to how they perceived an abso- lute scale of disability where 100 represented good hearing for a young person. The actual question was:

1 *Imagine that a normal young adult has a hearing ability of 100 and someone who is totally deaf has a hearing ability of 0. We would like you to circle the number that best indicates the state of your own hearing for each ear.*

LEFT EAR	RIGHT EAR
100	100
90	90
80	80
70	70
60	60
50	50
40	40
30	30
20	20
10	10
0	0

Hearing disability is represented in Appendix 2 of their book as a product of the sum of the thresholds over 1, 2 and 3 kHz and the asymmetry between the

Table 3.3 For three age groups, the proportion in each two BEA criteria, the proportion who are aided now and how many people that represents. The aided targets increase by 1, 5 and 10% the proportion aided in each age group. Note that the biggest cost is for the < 71 age group. The costs are calculated in line with the data collected in the first half of 1993, giving about £90 per hearing aid. However, first fittings may be more expensive than the average cost, and hence the costs may be an underestimate

Age group (years)	25 dB HL + (%)	45 dB HL + (%)	Aided now (%)	Number aided (k)	Aided target (%)	Initial cost (£m)
< 71	12.4	2.5	2.2	741	3.2	31
71–80	60.8	18.0	13.7	507	18.7	17
81 +	92.0	65.0	25.6	494	35.6	18
Total	7.8m (people)	2.7m (people)	3.4 (people)	1.7m (people)	5.0	66

ears to the nearest percent. The scientific model and analysis of the data are given in Lutman and Robinson (1992). The idea is a big advance on previous practice in the medico-legal sphere. In the rest of this section, the reciprocity of the relationship between impairment and ability is examined and the data on this question are contrasted with the function relating impairment to an overall measure of disability derived from the IHR Hearing Questionnaire (Lutman, Brown and Coles, 1987; Davis, 1995).

The proposed function (King *et al.*, 1992) has a number of possible limitations as the authors admit. It would be admirable if it were suitable to describe all aspects of hearing abilities. It is more probable that a single measure does not capture the multi-faceted aspects of disability, but is more a surrogate impairment measure. There is nothing wrong with this for the stated purpose (i.e. compensation), but it might be preferable to keep the impairment measure and relate to that (within defined ranges of impairment) without the attendant error in estimating another concept. The rating data are inherently difficult to analyse, because rather than allowing rating between 1 and 100, we used only eleven categories, 0, 10 ... 90, 100, with the top three categories 80, 90 and 100 having over 81% of the data. Thus the scale may be face valid and reliable but it is not really sensitive at the good ability end. In addition there are relatively few people with reported hearing ability less than 40%. Statistically, the disability ratings are non-normal and scarce where most required, however Lutman (personal communication) has collected data from candidates from cochlear implant clinics that would suggest a rating of about 20% ability (80% disability) for people with an average hearing threshold of about 100 dB HL.

Figures 3.22a and b show the reverse relationship to that of King *et al.* (1992) and Lutman and Robinson (1992), i.e. hearing impairment as a function of disability. The data plotted as horizontal lines represent the median and interquartile range of hearing impairment as a function of reported hearing ability, for those people who have a sensorineural impairment with only up to 5 dB asymmetry between the ears. The worse ear is shown because it has more data for the low reported hearing abilities. The solid line represents the fit where auditory ability is being predicted from the averaged hearing threshold at 1, 2 and 3 kHz. The picture given is quite different, as might be expected, and shows that, for a wide range of reported hearing ability (100–60 better ear, and 100–70 better ear), there is very little difference in median hearing level. Figure 3.22b, for the worse ear, shows that there is a clear change and that each change in reported hearing ability is referred to a greater change in hearing impairment. The difference in the two regression functions for the data, depending on which is the dependent variable, cautions us concerning the correct use and interpretation of these data.

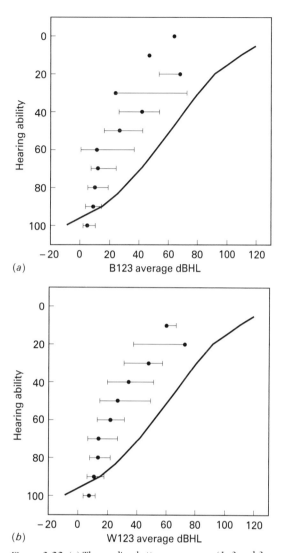

Figure 3.22 (*a*) The median better ear average (1, 2 and 3 kHz), together with the interquartile range, as a function of reported hearing disability for subjects with sensorineural hearing impairment, and interaural thresholds differing by only 5 dB or less. (*b*) The median worse ear average (1, 2 and 3 kHz), together with the interquartile range, as a function of reported hearing disability for subjects with sensorineural hearing impairment, and interaural thresholds differing by only 5 dB or less

Figure 3.23 shows the median of the average better ear threshold (1, 2 and 3 kHz) for those levels of reported hearing ability that had more than five people as a function of type of hearing impairment. For a given level of disability those with a conductive hearing loss had a higher degree of hearing

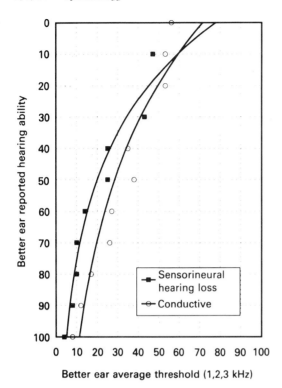

Figure 3.23 The median better ear average hearing thresholds (1, 2 and 3 kHz), together with a fitted exponential curve, as a function of reported hearing disability

impairment than the sensorineural losses, which is fairly sensible in terms of what a conductive loss affects in terms of impairment.

Figure 3.24 shows two aspects of hearing disability. In the left panel it shows the relationship between the data and theory given in King *et al.* (1992) with an analysis I have conducted on the 1703 people in the sample whose better ear had an air-bone gap less than 6 dB. Using a local non-parametric regression function (Hastie and Chambers, 1993), that is more appropriate to these data, the fit given by the solid line was derived and accounts for 18% of the variance in disability. The 95% confidence estimates are derived by a jacknife procedure at nine values of impairment, showing wide intervals at 80 dB and above. The similarity with the fit of Lutman and Robinson (1992), the interrupted line, is very good between 0 and 80 dB, with some divergence thereafter, but the curve definitely asymptotes towards about 80–90%. In the right panel is the result of the similar regression carried out on the overall disability measure (Lutman, Brown and Coles, 1987) derived from the whole disability questionnaire section A, B and C (Davis, 1995). This accounted for 34% of the variance and

gives much better confidence intervals. The major advantage of this measure (a percentage score out of a possible total disability score) is that it has better sensitivity at the low impairment end of the scale, but after 25 dB HL is virtually linear between the two measures. Its disadvantage is that it assumes that each answer has equal intervals between the choices such as 'great difficulty', 'some difficulty', 'easily'.

In summary the data show that:

1 There is similar function for the better and worse ears relating hearing ability to impairment
2 There is a difference between those with conductive and sensorineural pathology in terms of their mapping between disability and impairment
3 There is an expected difference between inferring disability from impairment and the reverse which cautions people not to use the tables in ways they were not intended
4 An appropriate non-parametric analysis of the data corroborates the model of Lutman and Robinson (1992) between 20 and 80 dB HL.

How many people are hearing impaired?

From the data presented here concerning the prevalence of hearing impairment, it may be possible to predict how many people might have a hearing impairment in the UK. In order to make estimates for the UK and for other countries we have to assume that:

1 The risk factors are known and can be accounted for in some way in the estimation
2 That there is cultural independence of the measurement and the risk factors for hearing impairment
3 That mortality is not affected by hearing impairment
4 Co-morbidity is not changing between the sample and the population being estimated.

The main risk factors for hearing impairment have been demonstrated above to be age, gender and occupational group. There is also a part played by noise exposure, exposure to other toxins and possibly the childhood history of otitis media with effusion. The two main risk factors, however, are age and gender. So, if the age and gender specific prevalences of hearing impairment are known they can be convolved with the age/gender population distributions for individual areas, countries or regions. Davis (1995) has done this for the major health and local authority boundaries in the UK. It would seem reasonable that the distribution of risk factors, other than age and gender, might be similar in different parts of the UK, given the corroborating data (Davis, 1989) from a more broadly based sample. To generalize beyond the UK, an assumption of cultural independence has

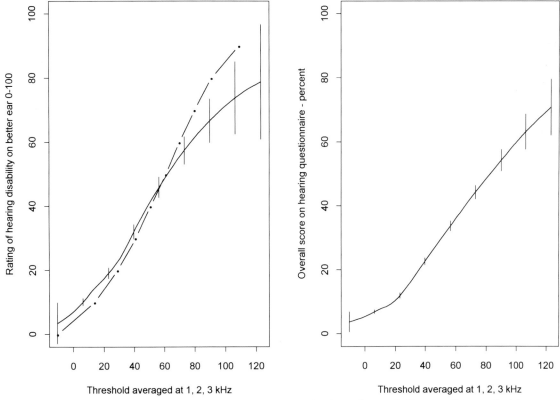

Figure 3.24 The left panel shows the local non-parametric regression for the prediction of self-rating of hearing disability from impairment, with 95% confidence intervals at 9 intervals. This is contrasted with the model of Lutman and Robinson (1992), given in the interrupted lines. The right panel shows the local non-parametric regression for the prediction of an overall self-report of hearing disability from impairment, with 95% confidence intervals at 9 intervals

to be made. This implies, for example, that the incidences of rubella and meningitis are similar and that the treatment effects of antibiotics and other treatments for upper respiratory tract infection and glue ear are not grossly different from one country to another. These assumptions are probably never met. However, the prevalence of the other risk factors may be thought to be lower in the UK than in most other countries and hence the figures are probably lower bound estimates of the true prevalence. On the other hand, there may be some higher co-morbidity and mortality that would reduce the estimates somewhat, particularly in developing countries.

The data on age and gender distributions estimates of all countries (> 500k people) for the period 1950 to 2025 were obtained from the United Nations 1992 revision of population estimates on computer disc. Regions of the world were divided according to the UN codings and the prevalence of hearing impairment was estimated for each region, and for 4 years: 1995, 2005, 2015 and 2025. The data for each region are shown in Tables 3.4, 3.5 and 3.6 and includes:

1 Two countries for comparison; the UK and the USA (Table 3.4)
2 The world divided into more and less developed regions (Table 3.5)
3 The six continents (Table 3.6).

The data concerning hearing impairment were taken in 5-year age bands (18–19, 20–24 ... 70–74, 75–79) for each gender, and the data for the 80 + age band were derived from other studies (see Davis, 1995, Chapter 8).

The columns of Table 3.4 show the total population for the country/region, the adult population and then the estimated number of adults with 25 +, 35 +, 45 +, 65 + and 95 + dB HL using the BEA criterion. All numbers are shown in thousands. Obviously not all degrees of hearing impairment are equally well estimated – particularly those with profound hearing impairments.

Table 3.4 shows that the UN estimate for the whole population of the UK is 58.093 million, and that the estimated number of hearing impaired people using a BEA criterion of 25 + dB HL is 8.759 million. This differs somewhat from estimates I have published elsewhere (Davis, 1993b, 1995; Davis and Fortnum, 1994) because I have used 5-year age bands to estimate prevalences, in these new tables; this probably makes no difference for the estimates for those people under the age of 50 years, but makes quite a bit of difference where the population aged 50–80 years is changing rapidly over time as in some developing countries, and I have used the 1992 revision of the UN World population estimates rather than OPCS data for the UK, and for elsewhere the 1990 UN revision.

From Table 3.4 we can see that in the UK and the USA, while there is a higher prevalence of hearing impairment in men (see above; Gates *et al.*, 1990) there is a larger number of women at each severity. At 25 + dB HL, in 1995, the estimates for women are 6% higher than for men in the UK and 8% in the USA. By 2025 there will be equal numbers or slightly more men. For 45 + dB HL, 1995, there are 41% more women than men in the UK and 39% in the USA, decreasing to 28% and 29% respectively.

The change in the number of hearing impaired people over time is rather different in the USA than in the UK. Estimates for population growth *per se* in the UK are only 3% by the year 2025, compared with 23% growth in the USA. In particular the growth in the over 80s is only 25% in the UK, from 2.248m to 2.816m, compared with a massive 66% growth in the USA, from 7.805m to 12.532m. In the UK therefore I would expect the number of hearing impaired to increase by about 6, 16 and 29% over the next three decades from 8.8m to 11.3m. A similar increase of about 25% should be expected also at 45 + dB HL, with only 10% increase of the profoundly impaired. However in the USA over the same three decades the increase in hearing impaired people is likely to be of the order of 66% at 25 + dB HL and 63% at 45 + dB HL, with the number of profoundly impaired possibly going over a million by 2025.

More than most other countries (apart from some northern European nations and Australia), the increases in the UK and the USA are due to the large numbers of over 80s who are surviving, but who will have some chronic disabilities, the most prevalent of which will be communication. This increase is obvi-

Table 3.4 Population estimates (thousands) of hearing impairment in the UK and the USA as a function of severity, gender and year (derived from UN population estimates)

Region	Year	Gender	Total population	Adult population	Hearing thresholds ≥				
					25 dB	35 dB	45 dB	65 dB	95 dB
UK	1995	Male	28468	21543	4251	2311	1242	401	88
UK	1995	Female	29625	23041	4508	3005	1767	548	92
UK	1995	Overall	58093	44584	8759	5316	3009	949	180
UK	2005	Male	29271	22144	4594	2500	1357	428	83
UK	2005	Female	30092	23314	4687	3122	1833	574	95
UK	2005	Overall	59363	45458	9282	5622	3191	1003	178
UK	2015	Male	29666	22988	5149	2763	1484	469	85
UK	2015	Female	30336	23989	5023	3308	1915	599	101
UK	2015	Overall	60002	46978	10173	6071	3399	1067	187
UK	2025	Male	29801	23485	5693	3150	1678	524	93
UK	2025	Female	30450	24451	5582	3753	2157	675	109
UK	2025	Overall	60251	47937	11275	6903	3834	1199	202
USA	1995	Male	128487	93593	16014	8651	4659	1523	367
USA	1995	Female	134651	101365	17261	11207	6511	1983	326
USA	1995	Overall	263138	194958	33275	19858	11170	3506	693
USA	2005	Male	139999	103082	19000	10199	5571	1789	370
USA	2005	Female	145933	110711	19728	12818	7449	2309	379
USA	2005	Overall	285932	213793	38728	23017	13020	4098	749
USA	2015	Male	149933	113822	23274	12316	6571	2091	410
USA	2015	Female	155688	121258	22777	14608	8343	2609	440
USA	2015	Overall	305621	235080	46051	26923	14914	4700	851
USA	2025	Male	157890	122399	27883	15169	7967	2501	478
USA	2025	Female	164117	130305	27604	18164	10330	3187	527
USA	2025	Overall	322007	252704	55487	33332	18297	5688	1005

Table 3.5 Population estimates (thousands) of hearing impairment in world regions as a function of severity, gender and year (derived from UN population estimates)

Region	Year	Gender	Total population	Adult population	Hearing thresholds ≥ 25 dB	35 dB	45 dB	65 dB	95 dB
World total	1995	Male	2899869	1802725	229004	115563	59984	20319	6167
World total	1995	Female	2859407	1810517	211810	122445	67021	19475	3189
World total	1995	Overall	5759276	3613242	440815	238008	127005	39794	9356
World total	2005	Male	3368611	2165499	294975	149817	77708	25951	7427
World total	2005	Female	3319548	2166846	266746	155554	85122	24794	3988
World total	2005	Overall	6688159	4332344	561541	305371	162830	50745	11415
World total	2015	Male	3829323	2572863	381965	195187	101599	33417	8603
World total	2015	Female	3779643	2573423	335499	197590	107638	31751	5159
World total	2015	Overall	7608966	5146286	717463	392776	209237	65168	13763
World total	2025	Male	4255246	2969748	491434	253737	130699	42239	10257
World total	2025	Female	4217200	2981225	423945	253184	137805	40911	6672
World total	2025	Overall	8472446	5950973	915379	506921	268504	83150	16929
More developed region	1995	Male	604967	445227	77455	40621	21626	7014	1654
More developed region	1995	Female	639209	486670	84086	53737	30807	9436	1592
More developed region	1995	Overall	1244176	931897	161541	94358	52433	16449	3246
More developed region	2005	Male	640313	478550	91592	48526	25638	8128	1713
More developed region	2005	Female	670113	515927	96452	62470	35565	10886	1781
More developed region	2005	Overall	1310426	994476	188044	110996	61204	19014	3495
More developed region	2015	Male	669893	505884	106316	57097	30499	9662	1864
More developed region	2015	Female	696593	540360	107939	70564	40291	12527	2063
More developed region	2015	Overall	1366486	1046244	214255	127661	70790	22189	3927
More developed region	2025	Male	688617	529606	120967	66169	35167	11031	2021
More developed region	2025	Female	714657	563262	121586	80506	46174	14312	2365
More developed region	2025	Overall	1403274	1092868	242553	146675	81341	25343	4386
Less developed region	1995	Male	2294902	1357495	151548	74941	38357	13305	4513
Less developed region	1995	Female	2220198	1323851	127725	68708	36214	10039	1597
Less developed region	1995	Overall	4515100	2681345	279273	143649	74572	23344	6110
Less developed region	2005	Male	2728298	1686951	203204	101292	52069	17824	5714
Less developed region	2005	Female	2649434	1650921	170294	93084	49556	13907	2207
Less developed region	2005	Overall	5377732	3337872	373498	194376	101626	31731	7921
Less developed region	2015	Male	3159431	2066977	275648	138090	71101	23755	6739
Less developed region	2015	Female	3083050	2033065	227559	127024	67347	19223	3096
Less developed region	2015	Overall	6242481	4100041	503207	265114	138447	42979	9836
Less developed region	2025	Male	3566629	2440144	370467	187568	95532	31208	8236
Less developed region	2025	Female	3502542	2417962	302358	172677	91630	26599	4307
Less developed region	2025	Overall	7069171	4858106	672825	360245	187162	57806	12543

ously a very important public health problem that should be tackled via hearing aid and other appropriate services because, in terms of prevention, there are few possibilities, as the generation of people who will be aged 80 in 2025 are already in their 40s, 50s and 60s. A word of caution is needed with regards to the prevalence estimates that rely heavily on the estimates for the over 80s. The data for the over 80s are not aggregated in 5-year age bands as for other age groups, and may not be particularly sensitive to changes in this period. Nor by the nature of things

(e.g. Gatehouse and Davis, 1992) can we expect that the pure tone thresholds obtained from people aged over 80 to be literally the same as those collected for the younger age groups because other psychological factors may enter into the thresholds, e.g. central neurological deficits may appear as perceptual problems. Furthermore, the people from whom these estimates were collected may not be representative of the elderly populations now or in the year 2025. Having exercised this note of caution, the data are still very impressive in terms of the size of the problem

Table 3.6 Population estimates (thousands) of hearing impairment in continental regions as a function of severity, gender and year (derived from UN population estimates)

Region	Year	Gender	Total population	Adult population	Hearing thresholds ≥				
					25 dB	35 dB	45 dB	65 dB	95 dB
Africa	1995	Male	370582	179323	16963	8201	4201	1506	568
Africa	1995	Female	373427	184878	15711	7964	4129	1116	176
Africa	1995	Overall	744009	364202	32674	16165	8330	2622	744
Africa	2005	Male	488830	245123	23067	11175	5756	2065	773
Africa	2005	Female	490995	250916	21305	10832	5650	1522	240
Africa	2005	Overall	979825	496039	44372	22007	11405	3587	1014
Africa	2015	Male	631608	335723	32401	15760	8155	2919	1079
Africa	2015	Female	633142	342238	29407	15105	7907	2150	337
Africa	2015	Overall	1264750	677961	61808	30865	16062	5069	1417
Africa	2025	Male	790504	450833	46780	22851	11761	4150	1478
Africa	2025	Female	792035	458702	41268	21548	11318	3102	492
Africa	2025	Overall	1582539	909535	88048	44399	23079	7252	1970
Asia	1995	Male	1742317	1081725	127497	63279	32306	11074	3606
Asia	1995	Female	1665276	1040973	105937	58031	30696	8590	1374
Asia	1995	Overall	3407593	2122699	233433	121310	63002	19664	4980
Asia	2005	Male	2019456	1311368	169826	85311	43755	14785	4525
Asia	2005	Female	1937474	1266106	139790	78062	41785	11874	1889
Asia	2005	Overall	3956930	2577474	309616	163373	85539	26658	6414
Asia	2015	Male	2270598	1564953	226866	114761	59155	19473	5129
Asia	2015	Female	2190181	1519258	184152	105208	56173	16227	2631
Asia	2015	Overall	4460779	3084211	411017	219969	115329	35699	7760
Asia	2025	Male	2485216	1790326	298497	152872	78058	25142	6135
Asia	2025	Female	2415040	1752716	239858	140200	74947	22041	3574
Asia	2025	Overall	4900256	3543042	538355	293071	153005	47184	9709
Europe	1995	Male	252293	191134	35125	18682	9999	3238	726
Europe	1995	Female	263750	205697	37274	24082	13932	4297	728
Europe	1995	Overall	516043	396831	72399	42764	23932	7535	1454
Europe	2005	Male	260675	199991	40006	21458	11351	3590	735
Europe	2005	Female	270128	212582	41530	27185	15577	4787	782
Europe	2005	Overall	530803	412573	81536	48642	26928	8378	1518
Europe	2015	Male	265929	205444	45142	24426	13071	4119	764
Europe	2015	Female	274017	216702	45447	30039	17302	5390	891
Europe	2015	Overall	539946	422146	90588	54465	30372	9509	1655
Europe	2025	Male	267092	209817	50257	27564	14715	4593	804
Europe	2025	Female	274692	220441	49935	33399	19294	6027	998
Europe	2025	Overall	541784	430258	100192	60963	34009	10620	1803
Latin America	1995	Male	240435	143069	16337	8274	4362	1519	497
Latin America	1995	Female	242042	147278	14851	8212	4431	1253	201
Latin America	1995	Overall	482477	290347	31188	16486	8793	2772	698
Latin America	2005	Male	279727	178896	21898	11106	5851	1995	609
Latin America	2005	Female	282580	184748	19967	11242	6098	1741	278
Latin America	2005	Overall	562307	363645	41866	22347	11949	3736	886
Latin America	2015	Male	316147	214226	29599	15024	7873	2638	736
Latin America	2015	Female	320613	221961	26564	15243	8240	2399	389
Latin America	2015	Overall	636760	436186	56163	30268	16113	5037	1125
Latin America	2025	Male	347449	245657	39179	20124	10405	3382	839
Latin America	2025	Female	354108	255775	35078	20675	11148	3283	535
Latin America	2025	Overall	701557	501432	74257	40799	21553	6665	1374

Table 3.6 *(Continued)*

Region	Year	Gender	Total population	Adult population	Hearing thresholds ≥				
					25 dB	35 dB	45 dB	65 dB	95 dB
Northern America	1995	Male	142596	104075	17789	9597	5163	1688	408
Northern America	1995	Female	149207	112462	10941	12339	7159	2178	358
Northern America	1995	Overall	291803	216537	36830	21936	12322	3867	766
Northern America	2005	Male	155942	115055	21233	11391	6211	1993	413
Northern America	2005	Female	162417	123411	21948	14249	8273	2563	421
Northern America	2005	Overall	318359	238466	43180	25640	14485	4556	833
Northern America	2015	Male	167521	127193	26074	13803	7365	2343	459
Northern America	2015	Female	173917	135473	25481	16351	9341	2921	493
Northern America	2015	Overall	341438	262666	51555	30154	16706	5264	952
Northern America	2025	Male	176770	136985	31287	17035	8953	2811	535
Northern America	2025	Female	183741	145843	30943	20374	11593	3577	591
Northern America	2025	Overall	360511	282828	62230	37409	20547	6388	1126
Oceania	1995	Male	14491	9934	1518	789	415	137	36
Oceania	1995	Female	14300	9982	1417	873	494	147	24
Oceania	1995	Overall	28791	19915	2934	1662	909	284	60
Oceania	2005	Male	16709	11560	1888	991	528	172	42
Oceania	2005	Female	16452	11580	1728	1076	609	185	30
Oceania	2005	Overall	33161	23140	3616	2066	1137	357	72
Oceania	2015	Male	18886	13319	2371	1233	650	209	46
Oceania	2015	Female	18599	13336	2114	1309	735	224	38
Oceania	2015	Overall	37485	26656	4484	2542	1385	433	84
Oceania	2025	Male	20803	15175	2942	1569	821	261	54
Oceania	2025	Female	20539	15223	2667	1690	946	288	47
Oceania	2025	Overall	41342	30398	5609	3259	1767	548	101

in the USA and the UK, the potential for substantial increase in the need for audiological service provision and the sheer size of currently unmet need.

Table 3.5 shows the overall estimates for the world and broken down by more and less developed regions. World-wide there may be at least 441 million people with a hearing impairment at BEA 25 + dB HL, 127 million at 45 + dB HL and 9.3 million profoundly impaired. For the world, there are slightly more men than women with hearing impairment, but in the more developed nations this is reversed as for the UK and USA. If the data can be generalized over countries and time, then the prevalence of hearing impairment is growing at a much faster rate than the population. Over the next three decades world population will increase by maybe 47%, with the number of hearing impaired increasing 107, 111 and 175% at 25 +, 45 + and 95 + dB HL BEA. For the more developed countries the overall increase will be 50% and for less developed 141% at 25 + dB HL BEA. At present, while the more developed world accounts for one in five people it also accounts for about one in three hearing impaired people. In three decades the corresponding percentages will be one in six and one in four. Because the standard of living is increasing

substantially in less developed countries, the rise seen in the number of hearing impaired people is quite large over the next 30 years, but will be substantially greater in the next 50–60 years when the children born in the last 10–20 years will be reaching their 50, 60, 70 and 80th years in far greater numbers than today.

Table 3.6 shows the data derived for different continents; Africa 33 million hearing impaired (BEA 25 + dBHL) increasing to 88 million by 2025, Asia 233 million hearing impaired increasing to 538 million, Europe 72 million hearing impaired increasing to 100 million, Latin America 31 million hearing impaired increasing to 74 million, Northern America 37 million hearing impaired increasing to 62 million and Oceania with 2.9 million hearing impaired increasing to 5.6 million by 2025.

In summary, the scale of the problem has been suggested in different regions of the world. The data are obviously estimates, because there may be factors that are common to different countries and regions that influence the estimates. However, as the main factor that is associated with prevalence is ageing, the estimates given are probably on the low side. It may be that less developed countries have less rigorous occupational noise protection and enforcement than in developed countries and this will tend to inflate the hearing impairments in young and middle-aged men and women employed in the noisy industries.

Other risk factors for hearing impairment

The high priority for finding preventable risk factors of hearing impairment in view of the very large numbers of hearing impaired people is quite understandable (US National Strategic Research Plan, 1989). But most researchers who have looked at possibilities of causal effects, with for instance cardiovascular disease, melanin, diabetes and other systemic diseases, have drawn very little from the relationships that may or may not exist (Davis, 1987; Gates *et al.*, 1990, 1993; Jones and Davis, 1992). This is in part because most of the studies have analysed cross-sectional data and in part because of the confounding of age, noise and social factors with the variables under study. Over a period of several years, I have analysed in great detail over 100 risk factors that were collected in the MRC National Study of Hearing on the 2708 people in the study. Apart from the obvious relationships between hearing impairment and tinnitus, family history of hearing impairment and childhood history of middle ear 'disease', not many of the risk factors were consistent over age groups, ears and genders. The one exception that has come to light in these analyses since the last edition (Davis, 1987) has been the relationship of blood serum bicarbonate with hearing impairment. This relationship is greater in women than in men, is larger in younger people than older, is more consistent at high frequencies and larger in the worse ear. The relationship is that the lower the blood bicarbo-

nate the worse the hearing, and in young people a bicarbonate below 22 mg/mmol increases the odds of a 25 + dB HL BEA impairment by up to 100%.

Figure 3.25 shows the relationship between mean hearing thresholds and the bicarbonate groups low and mid-range, standardized for age, sex and laboratory, for the age range 18–60 years. The audiograms for the two bicarbonate groups at each sex are more or less parallel, indicating an across the board change in audiogram with bicarbonate level, slightly more perhaps at higher frequencies. The difference is about 5 dB in women, which increases with decreasing age, and about 8–10 dB in men. As we did not measure the blood pH, it is difficult to say what, if anything, the decrease in blood bicarbonate is indicating. Blood bicarbonate is one of the main long-term determinants of CSF pressure, and there is some evidence that lower bicarbonate levels are associated with higher CSF pressures which may in turn be associated with altered hearing function (Allen and Habibi, 1962; Beentjes, 1972; Reid *et al.*, 1989). Lower bicarbonate levels, on the one hand, may be associated with chronic respiratory alkalosis or, on the other with metabolic acidosis. It is more likely to be the former rather than the latter in our subjects. This is in turn associated with hypoxia, pulmonary disease, or respiratory stimulation, any one of which might be caused by stress, alcohol intake or pregnancy. Without further data on these it is not possible to investigate this further. The interesting thing to note is that the relationship is not found in the over 60s where low bicarbonate levels are rarer and, if anything, there is an association with raised bicarbonate levels rather than lowered levels. As the relationship is very strong in young women (< 40 years) there may be an association with pregnancy, but unfortunately we did not ask!

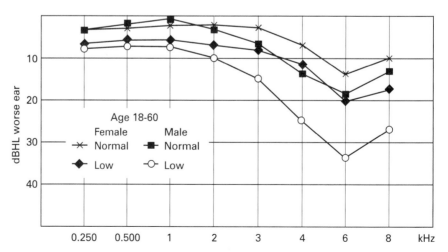

Figure 3.25 The mean hearing threshold levels for adults aged 18–60 years as a function of frequency, gender and bicarbonate group (low and 'normal')

Vestibular dysfunction

Not a great deal is known about the epidemiology of vestibular dysfunction, in terms of balance or dizziness. Using a postal questionnaire with a follow up in the third phase of the National Study of Hearing (NSH), not a great deal of interest was determined apart from the fact that people did find it very difficult to answer questions on balance and dizziness correctly. In the study 40.8% of people overall answered that they had a problem with balance, dizziness or giddiness. The increase with age is shown in Table 3.7, as are the significant differences between the genders and occupational groups. Women showed higher self-reported dizziness than men. The non-manual occupational group also reported more dizziness than the manual occupational group.

Table 3.7 The prevalence of self-reported dizziness as a function of age, gender and occupational group. National Study of Hearing phase 3. $n = 16674$

Age group (years)	Prevalence (%)	Gender/ occupational group	Prevalence (%)
18–30	37.6	Female	46.3
31–40	40.4	Male	34.3
41–50	42.4		
51–60	42.9	Non-manual	42.4
61–70	41.5	Manual	39.1
71–80	42.2		
81 +	47.9		

For the 16674 people who answered this question, 64% did not report tinnitus, and only 29% of these people reported giddiness. However this report of giddiness doubled to 60% for those who had occasional tinnitus and further increased to 65% of that 10% of the adult population who reported prolonged spontaneous tinnitus (PST). In addition, the proportion reporting giddiness, etc. increased from 37.7% of those who reported no problem hearing in quiet to 57.5% of those who had slight difficulty to 60% of those with moderate and 66% of those who had great difficulty (this is using the report on the left ear).

In an investigation conducted in Nottingham (Davis and Lutman, 1994), as part of a study designed to look at hearing in young people, using a postal survey technique that selected households at random, people were asked if they had ever visited a doctor concerning balance or dizziness, or whether they had been referred to a hospital for such a problem. Table 3.8 shows the data from this study in terms of age-group, reported hearing disability in quiet, tinnitus report, and gender. These data are not ideal because we have no information about the 'real' problem. Rather, they are telling something about demand and supply of services in Nottingham and, possibly, in the UK. However, they do all more or less tell the same story. Vestibular problems as manifested by balance and dizziness do increase with age, but not as much as either hearing impairment, disability or tinnitus. There is a higher proportion of women who report vestibular symptoms, and also a

Table 3.8 Consultations concerning balance or dizziness problems as a function of age-group, hearing ability, tinnitus report and gender. Nottingham HIYA study, 1994 ($n = 5474$ adults)

Age	Age group (years)							
	14–20	21–30	31–40	41–50	51–60	61–70	71–80	81 +
Visit family doctor (15.5%)	7.3	8.9	11.4	15.5	18.6	23.3	21.7	31.7
Hospital appointment (5.6%)	1.1	2.6	2.5	5.8	7.3	8.4	9.2	17.7

Reported hearing disability	Better ear reported hearing difficulty in quiet				
	None	Slight	Moderate	Great	Cannot hear
Visit family doctor (15.5%)	12.8	38.5	41.4	66.0	77.8
Hospital appointment (5.6%)	4.1	16.2	19.1	54.2	44.6

Tinnitus	Tinnitus for over 5 minutes		
	None	Some of the time	Most of the time
Visit family doctor (15.5%)	10.9	31.7	41.7
Hospital appointment (5.6%)	3.4	12.1	22.8

Gender	Female	Male
Visit family doctor (15.5%)	19.3	11.3
Hospital appointment (5.6%)	6.6	4.5

higher proportion who have consulted their doctor or been referred to a hospital. The largest association, and one we would have predicted, is that tinnitus report is associated with at least a threefold increase in self-referral and for those with persistent tinnitus it is a sevenfold increase in referral to a 'specialist' hospital service. While the direction of the association is to be expected the size of the association is much bigger than might have been predicted.

For the subset of people in Phase 3 of the NSH who had their hearing assessed, it was possible to estimate the proportion of people who had a low-frequency hearing impairment, prolonged spontaneous tinnitus and 'vestibular problems' as denoted by their questionnaire response. I have defined hearing impairment at low frequency as the averaged threshold at 0.25, 0.5 and 1 kHz and made two criteria at 25 + and 45 + dB HL. Taking our previous definition of hearing impairment defined at the midfrequencies, then 1.6% of people have a BEA of 25 + dB HL with a low-frequency hearing impairment at 25 + dB HL *as well as* tinnitus (PST) *and also* a history of vestibular problems. That is about one in 10 of those with impairment on the better ear. For a 45 + dB HL criterion at both low and midfrequency the prevalence of this set of conditions is 0.6%, i.e. one in five of all impairments at this severity. On the worse ear the respective prevalences were 7.4 and 1.2%.

For these studies there was no vestibular or neuro-otological investigation, so the data are not necessarily valid. However, we can conclude that consultation for vestibular dysfunction is fairly prevalent in adults, but not much is known about its epidemiology, consequences (e.g. a higher prevalence of accidents among this group of people) and health care outcomes. This suggests it should be made a high research priority. About one in 10 people with a hearing impairment in their better ear had low-frequency hearing impairment, tinnitus and some self-reported vestibular symptoms.

Overall summary

At the start of the chapter I discussed the concepts of need, demand and supply, trying to make them pertinent to adult audiology. It was suggested that the key to quality services was access to a broad balance of services that should include prevention, education, screening, assessment and diagnosis, and appropriate technology, e.g. hearing aids and implants, surgery. Decisions on which services should be developed ought to be based on a knowledge of local epidemiology (or the correct application of knowledge to the local community), and on our knowledge concerning the cost and benefits of particular services for the populations and for individuals.

Getting the audiological health care services right

means that there has to be a balance between several things:

1 On the one hand developing new services and on the other 'rationing' of health care
2 The views of the consumers and the interests of the providers
3 Primary and specialist care
4 Auditing the health care process and monitoring appropriate outcomes.

A consideration of the epidemiology of hearing impairment showed the major effect that age has on the whole distribution of hearing impairment, and the important differences that there are between the genders, occupational groups and different degrees of noise immission. A small effect of leisure noise immission was apparent when a strict criterion of 'impaired' hearing was used, i.e. the number of thresholds of 20 + dB HL.

The proportion of people with a conductive impairment does change with age, ear and severity of hearing impairment and there is some evidence of an occupational group effect. The more severe a hearing impairment, the more likely there is to be a conductive impairment. This may have implications for future planning of services targeted at conductive impairments.

The unmet need of the population for help with their hearing disability was shown in terms of the take-up of hearing aids. Although the take-up in the UK has not changed in 15 years, it is a little higher than in a region of the USA (Framingham), but only half of those with moderate-severe impairments possessed a hearing aid, a very small proportion indeed of those who could, do get benefit from properly trained use of a hearing aid(s). The cost of implementing even a small increase in the target for access to hearing aids, to 5% of the whole population would cost more than the £50m budget (1993 prices) for the present hearing aid services.

The relationship of self-reported rating of ability to impairment was shown to be quite different to that of impairment to the same rating. The former was affected by the type of the impairment, with conductive pathologies rating having greater hearing thresholds for a given level of disability. The model of Lutman and Robinson was corroborated by a more appropriate non-parametric analysis of the data over the range 20–80 dB HL, but a more sensitive measure of disability might be needed for investigating those with mild hearing disabilities.

The scale of the public health problem that hearing impairment causes and will cause world-wide has been estimated. These problems are a truly massive burden, that is growing yearly, not because of any increase of the environmental risk factors (although we must be highly aware of those), but because people are healthier and living longer (or are expected to live longer). While on some continents the problem will be tackled with increasing technology, this cannot be the only solution. The majority of the world's hearing impaired in Asia, Africa and Latin America cannot necessarily afford that technology. There is an urgent need for other solutions, that necessarily must be based in the local communities. Such strategies should possibly concentrate on ways of enabling people with communication problems to recognize the problem and learn ways of coping with the effects they have on their everyday activities. The problems of identifying who might best benefit from scarce resources where social health care exists are even more pressing in the less developed countries than in the more developed, and appropriate ear care programmes need to be developed based on a good epidemiology of the local population.

Searching the EMBASE database for references concerning the epidemiology of vestibular disorders or of 'balance' problems did not yield any references over the last 10 years of populations studies of the problems, but there were about 15 articles some of which concern aspects of acoustic neuroma (e.g. Eldridge and Parry, 1992) and Menières syndrome (e.g. Paparella, 1991). The few data available from our studies of hearing impairment, presented here, shows that there is a considerable prevalence of visiting a family doctor for balance or dizziness problems and that this is highly associated with prolonged tinnitus (PST).

Conclusions and priorities for service development

1 There is an urgent need to develop the local epidemiology of hearing impairment and vestibular dysfunction, as outlined above. This should provide the basis for a uniform needs assessment to give:
   a the size of the problem
   b the different types of need in the community
   c the efficacy of current services and their cost-effectiveness.
   A minimum data set providing standardized clear input with agreed definitions pre-coded, with good quality control of the data being entered (this is usually achieved by making sure that those who enter the data have a stake in them being correct) and above all that provides pertinent information will help minimize the problems associated with providing this ongoing epidemiology.
2 Purchasers of auditory health care should increase the role of prevention and education concerning the effects of avoidable hazards (e.g. noise at work, noise in clubs/discos, toxic antibiotics, etc.).
3 Purchasers of auditory health care should increase access to auditory health care, particularly for the pre-retirement group, 50–65 years of age, where intervention is acceptable, beneficial and cost effective.
4 Evidence of the cost-effectiveness of technological innovation should, where possible, be evaluated by randomized control trials.
5 The East Anglian Regional Health Authority (Burton, Jewell and Hadridge, 1993) in the UK have produced a booklet, *Disability and Rehabilitation Services; the example of hearing impairment and deafness*. This is a good example of how a local epidemiology may be attempted/inferred and gives very practical examples of:
   a what the services in a district might be trying to achieve, with a chronic disability such as hearing
   b how that service might be achieved at the primary, secondary and tertiary services
   c how might the service be monitored.
   Obviously the detail of how such a scheme is implemented in each district is going to be different depending on the local context, but it is certain that without a clear statement agreed between purchasers and providers the catalogue and scale of unmet need given in this chapter will not change over the next decades. One thing is sure, the number of people with hearing impairments will not decrease. We need to work now to ensure that the burden of disability and handicap is minimized and that access to good means of communication is not denied to those with hearing impairments.

Priorities for research

The priorities of research can be seen from a number of different perspectives on the basic to applied spectrum. Applied research will obviously vary in its impact depending on the health care system of a particular country. The following are not in any particular order, but encompass a wide range of this spectrum, and have primarily as a focus the health care system in the UK, especially in priorities 1, 5, 6 and 7. The order you put them in will depend on your context and approach to hearing disorders.

1 There is a need for a much more detailed and representative epidemiology of hearing impairment, disability and handicap in the elderly, particularly in those aged over 80. This needs to be population based and to deal with the types of service that are feasible and cost-effective and are not solely technology based. This would enable a better prediction of the size of the problem in the future as well as augment our sparse knowledge about how hearing disability affects quality of life in old age and access to health and social care.

2 The size of the public health hazard associated with high levels of leisure noise, and the extent to which this hazard will lead to disability in future generations need to be assessed. In other words is the damage self-limiting or not.

3 The effect of occupational group on hearing, especially in young adults has no easy explanation. The effect is large (in the context of this age group) and needs to be replicated, and possibly extended to pre-occupational ages. This will help our interpretation of normal hearing and will have clinical and legal ramifications.

4 As mentioned several times above, there is a high priority attached to research that will identify and explain the aetiology of hearing impairment: to see what can modify the effect of age; and to see what other modifiable risk factors may exist and their mechanisms. The findings with respect to aspects such as the effect of bicarbonate levels reported here, blood immunology (Parving *et al.*, 1993), blood viscosity (Gatehouse, Browning and Lowe, 1986) and other factors such as ESR (Jones and Davis, 1992) may be taken as a good place to start. However, it will need a multicentre and disciplinary team to tackle this problem. In addition, it may be that we can harness new imaging technology to take function beyond hearing thresholds and look at changes within the ear in individuals.

5 An understanding of how access to hearing health care is presently controlled and how it might change in a planned way over time is an urgent requirement. Research in this area will need both quantitative and qualitative methodologies to produce advice on what is presently lacking and how change may be achieved in an ordered fashion.

6 The extent to which quality of life in a person with hearing disability is affected by having a hearing aid and the cost-effectiveness of different types of hearing aid need separate population and clinic based research programmes. There is certainly a need to address the issue of the added value that hi-fi or digital hearing aids are purported to supply by conducting large randomized trials of these and other related health technology and training packages that may help acclimatization to specific hearing aids.

7 There is a requirement to provide an epidemiology of vestibular dysfunction on a population basis as has been achieved in the UK for hearing disorders and tinnitus. This should possibly include balance, dizziness, vestibular schwannomas and Menière-like symptoms. The data presented here suggest that these associated problems pose a large burden on the primary and tertiary health care systems in the UK and it is surprising that not much has been accomplished at a population level.

References

ALLEN, G. M. and HABIBI, M. (1962) The effect of increasing the cerebrospinal fluid pressure upon the cochlear microphonic. *Laryngoscope*, **72**, 423–434

AXELSSON, A., ROSENHALL, U. and ZACHAU, G. (1994) Hearing in 18-year-old Swedish males. *Scandinavian Audiology*, **23**, 129–134

BEENTJES, B. I. J. (1972) The cochlear aqueduct and the pressure of the cerebrospinal and endolabyrinthine fluids. *Acta Otolaryngologica*, **73**, 112–120

BRITISH MEDICAL JOURNAL (1993) *Rationing in Action.* London: BMJ

BOUFFORD, M. J. (1993) US and UK health reforms: reflections on quality. *Quality in Health Care*, **2**, 249–252

BOWATER, R., COPAS, J., MACHADO, O. and DAVIS, A. (1995) The log-normal distribution and hearing impairment. *Journal of the Royal Statistical Society* (in press)

BROWNING, G. G. and GATEHOUSE, S. (1992) The prevalence of middle-ear disease in the adult British population. *Clinical Otolaryngology*, **17**, 317–321

BURTON, H., JEWELL, D. and HADRIDGE, A. (1993) *Disability and Rehabilitation Services; the example of hearing impairment and deafness.* Cambridge: East Anglia Health Authority

CHALMERS, I. and HAYNES, B. (1994) Reporting, updating, and correcting systematic reviews of the effects of health care. *British Medical Journal*, **309**, 862–865

CLARKE, M. J. and STEWART, L. A. (1994) Obtaining data from randomised controlled trials: how much do we need for reliable and informative meta-analysis? *British Medical Journal*, **309**, 1007–1010

COLES, R. R. A., SMITH, P. and DAVIS, A. C. (1990) The relationship between noise induced hearing loss and tinnitus and its management. In: *Noise as a Public Health Problem*, edited by B. Berglund and T. Lundvall. Stockholm: Swedish council for building research. pp. 87–112

COLES, R. R. A., DAVIS, A. C. and SMITH, P. (1990) Tinnitus: its epidemiology and management. In: *Proceedings of the 14th Danavox Symposium. Presbyacusis and other Age-related Aspects*, edited by J. H. Jensen. Copenhagen: Stougard Jensen. pp. 377–402

CORSO, J. F. (1992) Support for Corso's hearing loss model relating aging and noise exposure. *Audiology*, **31**, 162–167

DAVIS, A. C. (1983) The epidemiology of hearing disorders. In: *Hearing and Balance in the Elderly* edited by R. Hinchcliffe. Edinburgh: Churchill Livingstone. pp. 1–43

DAVIS, A. C. (1987) Epidemiology of hearing disorders In: *Scott–Browns' Otolaryngology*, 5th edn, edited by A. G. Kerr, Vol 2 *Adult Audiology*, edited by D. Stephens. London: Butterworths. pp. 90–126

DAVIS, A. C. (1989) The prevalence of hearing impairment and reported hearing disability among adults in Great Britain. *International Journal of Epidemiology*, **18**, 911–917

DAVIS, A. C. (1993a) Public health perspective of childhood hearing impairments. In: *Paediatric Audiology 0–5*, edited by B. McCormick. Whurr: London. pp. 1–43

DAVIS, A. C. (1993b) The prevalence of deafness. In: *Deafness*, 5th edn, edited by J. Ballantyne, M. Martin and J. A. M. Martin. London: Whurr. pp. 1–11

DAVIS, A. C. (1995) *Hearing Impairment in Adults.* London: Whurr

DAVIS, A. C. and FORTNUM, H. M. (1994) Estimates of the

number of hearing impaired people in major countries of the world. Paper prepared for ICA meeting, Halifax, July 1994

DAVIS, A. C. and HAGGARD, M. P. (1982) Some implications of audiological measures in the population for binaural aiding strategies. *Scandinavian Audiology*, (suppl. 15, 167–179

DAVIS, A. C. and LUTMAN, M. E. (1994) Hearing in Young Adults Study: Postal Questionnaire data. Work in progress

DAVIS, A. C. and THORNTON, A. R. D. (1990) The impact of age on hearing impairment: some epidemiological evidence. *Proceedings of 14th Danavox Symposium, Presbyacusis and Other Age-related Aspects*, edited by J. H. Jensen, 69–89

DAVIS, A., FORTNUM, H. and SPENCER, H. (1995) Hearing aid provision in the UK. *Paper presented at Second European Conference in Audiology*, Holland, March 1995

DAVIS, A. C., LUTMAN, M. E. and COPAS, J. (1994) Modelling the effect of occupational noise exposure on hearing thresholds in populations: A new statistical approach. In: *Effects of Noise on Hearing; Vth International Symposium*, Gothenburg, Sweden, May 12–14, 1994. (*poster presentation*)

DAVIS, A. C., OSTRI, B. and PARVING, A. (1991) Longitudinal study of hearing. *Acta Otolaryngologica*, Suppl. 482, 103–109

DAVIS, A. C., STEPHENS, S. D. G., RAYMENT, A. and THOMAS, K. (1992) Hearing impairments in middle age: the acceptibility benefit and cost of detection (ABCD). *British Journal of Audiology*, **26**, 1–14

DOBIE, R. A. (1993) *Medical-Legal Evaluation of Hearing Loss*. New York: Van Nostrand Reinhold

DOYAL, L. and GOUGH, I. (1991) *A Theory of Human Need*. Basingstoke: Macmillan Education

ELDRIDGE, R. and PARRY, D. M. (1992) Summary of the vestibular schwannoma consensus development conference, National Institutes of Health, Bethesda, Maryland, December 11–13, 1991. *Otolaryngologic Clinics of North America PY*, **3**, 729–732

EYSENCK, H. (1994) Meta-analysis and its problems. *British Medical Journal*, **309**, 789–792

GATES, G. A., COOPER, J. C. JR, KANNEL, W. B. and MILLER, N. J. (1990) Hearing in the elderly: the Framingham cohort, 1983–1985. *Ear and Hearing*, **4**, 247–256

GATES, G. A., COBB, J. L., D'AGOSTINO, R. B. and WOLF, P. A. (1993) The relation of hearing in the elderly to the presence of cardiovascular disease and cardiovascular risk factors. *Archives of Otolaryngology – Head and Neck Surgery*, **119**, 156–161

GATEHOUSE, S. and DAVIS, A. C. (1992) Clinical pure-tone vs three-inferred forced choice thresholds: effects of hearing level and age. *Audiology*, **31**, 30–44

GATEHOUSE, S., BROWNING, G. G. and LOWE, G. D. O. (1986) Blood viscosity as a factor in hearing impairment. *Lancet*, i, 121–123

GRIMSHAW, J. and RUSSELL, I. T. (1993) Effect of clinical guidelines in medical practice. *Lancet*, ii, 1317–1322

HAGGARD, M. P. (1993) *Research in the Development of Effective Services for Hearing-impaired People*. London: Nuffield Provincial Hospitals Trust

HAGGARD, M. P. and GATEHOUSE, S. (1993) Candidature for hearing aids: justification for the concept and a two-part audiometric criterion. *British Journal of Audiology*, **27**, 303–318

HASTIE, T. and TIBSHIRANI, R. (1990) *Generalised Additive Models*. London: Chapman and Hall

HASTIE, T. J. and CHAMBERS, J. M. (1993) *Statistical Models*. New York: Chapman and Hall

ISO (1984) *ISO 7029 Acoustics – Threshold of Hearing by Air Conduction as a Function of Age and Sex for Otologically Normal Persons*. Geneva: International Organisation for Standardisation,

ISO (1990) *ISO 1999 Acoustics – Determination of Occupational Noise Exposure and of Noise Induced Hearing Impairment*. Geneva: International Organisation for Standardisation,

JONES, N. and DAVIS, A. (1992) Hyperlipidaemia and hearing loss: a true association? *Clinical Otology*, **17**, 463

KING, P. F., COLES, R. R. A., LUTMAN, M. E. and ROBINSON, D. W. (1992) *Assessment of Hearing Disability: Guidelines for Medicolegal Practice*. London: Whurr

KNIPSCHILD, P. (1994) Some examples. *British Medical Journal*, **309**, 719–721

LUTMAN, M. E. (1992) Apportionment of noise-indicated hearing disability and its prognosis in a medicolegal context. A modelling study. *British Journal of Audiology*, **26**, 307–319

LUTMAN, M. E. and DAVIS, A. C. (1994a) The distribution of hearing threshold levels in the general population aged 18–30 years. *Audiology*, **33**, 327–350

LUTMAN, M. E. and DAVIS, A. C. (1994b) Distributions of hearing threshold levels in populations exposed to noise. In: *Noise Induced Hearing Loss*, edited by A. Axelsson, D. Henderson, R. P. Hamernik, R. J. Falvi, P. Helstrom and H. Banchgravik. New York: Thieme Medical Publishers

LUTMAN, M. E. and ROBINSON, D. W. (1992) Disability scales for medicolegal purposes based on self-rating. *British Journal of Audiology*, **26**, 297–306

LUTMAN, M. E., BROWN, E. J. and COLES, R. R. A. (1987) Self-reported disability and handicap in the population in relation to pure-tone threshold, age, sex and type of hearing loss. *British Journal of Audiology*, **21**, 45–58

MEDICAL RESEARCH COUNCIL INSTITUTE OF HEARING RESEARCH (1985) *Damage to Hearing arising from Leisure Noise: a Review of the Literature*. London: HMSO

MOSCICKI, E. K., ELKINS, E. F., BAUM, H. M. and MCNAMARA, P. M. (1985) Hearing loss in the elderly: an epidemiologic study of the Framingham heart study cohort. *Ear and Hearing*, **6**, 184–190

MULROW, C. D. (1994) Rationale for systematic reviews. *British Medical Journal*, **309**, 597–599

NOBLE, W. (1978) *Assessment of Impaired Hearing: a Critique and a New Method*. London: Academic Press

NUFFIELD INSTITUTE FOR HEALTH (1994) *Outcomes Briefing Series*. Leeds: UK Clearing House on Health Outcomes

OXMAN, A. D. (1994) Checklists for review articles. *British Medical Journal*, **309**, 648–651

PAPARELLA, M. M. (1991) Pathogenesis and pathophysiology of Meniere's disease. *Acta Otolaryngologica*, Suppl. 485, 26–35

PARVING, A., HEIN, H. O., SUADICANI, P., OSTRI, B. and GYNTELBERG, F. (1993) Epidemiology of hearing disorders: Some factors affecting hearing. The Copenhagen male study. *Scandinavian Audiology*, **22**, 101–107

PIRILA, T., JOUNIO-ERVASTI, K. and SORRI, M. (1992) Left-right asymmetries in hearing threshold levels in three age groups of a random population. *Audiology*, **31**, 150–161

PUBLIC HEALTH (1994) The public health function (editorial) **108**, 89

QUARANTA, A. and ASSENATO, G. (eds) (1991) Studio epidemiologico dei problemi uditivi netta populazione adulta in Italia. *Audiologica Italiana*, **8**, 257–378

RAHKO, T., KARMA, P., PITKAJARVI, T., NURMINEN, H. and KATAJA, M. (1988) The prevalence of handicapping hearing loss in a middle-aged population in Finland. *Archives of Oto-Rhino-Laryngology*, **245**, 57–59

REID, A., MARCHBANKS, R. J., BATEMAN, D. E., MARTIN, A. M., BRIGHTWELL, A. P. and PICKARD, J. D. (1989) Mean intracranial pressure monitoring by a non-invasive audiological technique: a pilot study. *Journal of Neurology, Neurosurgery and Psychiatry*, **52**, 610–612

ROBINSON, D. W. (1987) Noise exposure and hearing loss: A new look at the experimental data. *Contract Research Report* no. 1/1987. Bootle: Health and Safety Executive

ROSENHALL, U., PEDERSEN, H. and SVANBORG, A. (1990) Presbycusis and noise induced hearing loss. *Ear and Hearing*, **11**, 257–263

SOUCEK, S. and MICHAELS, L. (1987) *Hearing Loss in the Elderly*. London: Springer-Verlag

STEPHENS, S. D. G. and HÉTU, R. (1991) Impairment, disability and handicap in audiology: towards a consensus. *Audiology*, **30**, 185–200

STEPHENS, S. D. G., CALLAGHAN, D. E., HOGAN, S., MEREDITH, R., RAYMENT, A. and DAVIS, A. C. (1990) Hearing disability in people aged 50–65: effectiveness and acceptibility of early rehabilitative intervention. *British Medical Journal*, **300**, 508–511

STEVENS, A. (1991) *Assessing Health Care Needs*. London: NHS Management Executive

TAKEDA, S., MORIOKA, I., MIYASHITA, K., OKUMURA, A., YOSHIDA, Y. and MATSUMOTO, K. (1992) Age variation in the upper limit of hearing. *European Journal of Applied Physiology*, **65**, 403–408

US NATIONAL CENTER FOR HEALTH STATISTICS (1986) Prevalence of selected chronic conditions, United States, 1979–1981. *Vital and Health Statistics, Series 10, no. 155*. OHHS Pub No (PHS) 86–1583. Public Health Service. Washington, DC: US Government Printing Office

US NATIONAL STRATEGIC RESEARCH PLAN (1989) Bethesda: National Institute on Deafness and Other Communication Disorders, National Institutes of Health.

VENTRY, M. and WEINSTEIN, B. (1982) The hearing handicap inventory for the elderly: a new tool. *Ear and Hearing*, **3**, 128–134

WOOD, P. H. N. (1980) The language of disablement: glossary relating to disease and its consequences. *International Rehabilitation Medicine*, **2**, 86–92

4

Otological symptoms and emotional disturbance

S. Jakes

In this chapter the literature on the emotional aspects of disorders of hearing and balance is considered. The major exclusion is developmental, or specifically childhood, aspects of disorders of hearing and balance.

The first section of this chapter deals with some important theoretical issues and it is argued that the role of psychological factors in disease is broader than that often assumed. It is suggested that illness behaviour is not simply determined by disease processes.

The literature review concentrates, to some degree, on the experimental detail of studies cited. When dealing with psychological factors, there are numerous possibilities for complex artefactual influences which may be involved. This is partly because the patients studied may influence the outcome by their apprehension of our purposes (Harre and Secord, 1976). It must be determined how each study was conducted in detail before generalizations can be made.

Psychological factors in medicine

Traditionally, psychological processes have been seen as having only two roles in medical disorders – psychosomatic causes and somatopsychic results. In fact, most attention was paid to psychosomatic processes. Recent work has suggested that psychological processes are involved in a much more far reaching manner. The traditional views of psychosomatic/somatopsychic effect will be briefly characterized, and some deficits with this model of psychological factors in medical disorders are pointed out. Other, possibly more profitable, models are then discussed.

Psychosomatic processes

Since Freud (1895) (and indeed before), psychological processes have been seen as another type of cause of physical symptoms and signs. When an explanation by physical causes could not be found a psychological cause was suggested. It was suggested that this can happen in two ways.

1 Hysterical conversion: symptoms are the result of unconscious conflicts – the symptom serves to satisfy a forbidden wish and does so in a way that symbolically represents that wish.
2 Psychosomatic illness: here the suggestion is that the symptoms have an organic basis but that the causes of the illness are to be sought in psychosocial stressors and the inability of the patient to cope with this stress.

There are many differences between these two supposed processes, for example hysterical symptoms are, in some sense, not real. The concept of hysteria has been subjected to much criticism. Slater (1965) raised several objections to diagnosis of hysteria on logical grounds. He argued that this diagnosis is made on the grounds of exclusion rather than on positive signs – 'all the signs of hysteria are signs of health'. However, demonstrating what is not the case does not give grounds for identification of a syndrome.

With psychosomatic processes there is an organic basis for the symptoms, but the psychological agent is seen as another part of the causal mechanism. This type of psychological explanation has been criticized in a different way. Increasing numbers of diseases have been shown to be related to stress (Steptoe, 1980). Thus the classification of diseases as psychosomatic becomes a matter of degree.

Some authors have criticized the concept of causation by psychological entities or states on the grounds that these are not, logically, the type of state or event which can be included in a scientific analysis of causation of anything. Thus, the behavioural approach to psychology eschewed all mention of psychological states on the grounds that these were unobservable events which could not be objectively verified and, therefore, for all scientific purposes did not exist. However, it is also true of physical science that it makes reference to unobservable processes and events (gravity, atomic structure) which are postulated only on the grounds of their effects. Another problem with this approach is that it implies that everyday accounts of action, are in some way, lacking in validity, e.g. 'I did it because I was bored', makes reference to a causal psychological state.

Over the past 20 years much research has been undertaken looking at the effects of stress on illness and psychiatric disorder. The basic methodology of this 'life change event' research has been to correlate the number of 'life events' during a period (usually between 3 months and 3 years) with subsequent illness rates. Reporting of life events can be undertaken retrospectively, but it is rather better to obtain these estimates prior to the period during which illness rates are recorded. Rahe *et al.* (1974) suggested an optical model to represent the various influences of life events on illness and symptom reporting (Figure 4.1). Life events are represented by light rays of differing intensities. These correspond to the occurrence of life events of differing significance to the individual concerned. Various mediating processes are represented by a series of lenses and filters. The first stage, represented by a filter is the perception of the significance of the event – this is strongly influenced by the past experience of the individual. Next follows ego defences, that is strategies for altering the significance of this perception – this includes, for example denial. This stage is represented as a concave lens diffracting away unpleasant perceptions. The third stage is the conversion of this perceived stress to physiological processes, e.g. increased blood pressure, change in corticosteroid production, etc. (Steptoe, 1980). The fourth stage is the conversion of these psychophysiological processes into organ dysfunctions – this is represented by a colour filter. The

fifth stage, a filter, is coping processes, that is coping with the physiological changes, e.g. by relaxation skills. Finally, these organ dysfunctions may or may not be reported to medical personnel (illness behaviour). This is represented by a convex lens which focuses these light waves at a particular point on the illness rule (see Figure 4.1).

The role of psychological processes postulated by Rahe *et al.* (1974) is rather broader than that characterized above. Five separate stages are postulated, and these do not map easily onto the psychosomatic/somatopsychic model. The effects of stress are mediated by perception of threat, defence against such perceptions, coping with the resultant physiological disturbances and reporting of the consequent organ of dysfunction as illness.

In some ways the most interesting part of this model is the last lens – illness behaviour.

The factors involved here are not linked with causal processes which produce symptoms. It is, therefore, furthest from the traditional model. What counts as an illness for the patient depends on the illness behaviour which the individual has acquired. Waddell *et al.* (1984) described 'inappropriate illness behaviour' by which they seem to mean behaviour which is out of proportion to the symptoms. This seems very much to be another way of calling patients hysterical or at least hystrionic. It is not what the present author means by illness behaviour. Rather one should acknowledge that the process of learning to define a bodily state as a symptom or as requiring medical attention, excusing the individual from normal chores, etc., is subject to a variety of developmental (social and psychological) influences. It rather confuses the issue to talk of such behaviour as being 'appropriate'. Take, for example, tinnitus. What counts as appropriate illness behaviour here? Is it appropriate to be very distressed or totally unmoved? One must recognize that this is a matter of individual differences. Of course, one *can* say which types of illness behaviour are helpful or useful, but this is very different from judging them to be normal or abnormal.

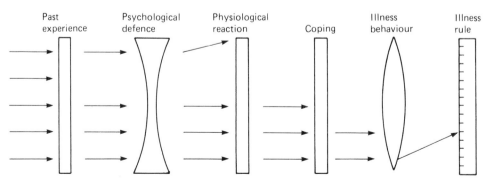

Figure 4.1 Rahe's optical model of life events and illness behaviour

Mechanic (1980) suggested that symptom reporting (i.e. self-definition as ill) is influenced by three main factors.

1 Occurrence of bodily dysfunction
2 General sense of wellbeing
3 Developmental experiences.

Factor 3 is important in that internal monitoring is a learned behaviour, as is presentation of these monitored sensations as illness. Factor 2 is important as general psychological state, and general feelings of wellbeing govern reports of illness (Tessler and Mechanic, 1978; Mechanic, 1980). Patients tend to assess health by overall estimates of feeling good.

Given that presenting symptoms as illness (both to a doctor and to oneself) is not equivalent to having those symptoms, the whole process becomes very complex. Complaining about symptoms is likely to feedback and make symptom monitoring more acute. Self-perception as healthy or unhealthy will, in part, be a self-fulfilling prophecy, and all these behaviours are likely to be susceptible to reward and punishment. (Partly this is what is involved in 'secondary gains', but it should not be seen as applying only to a few, abnormal cases.)

It is hoped that it is clear that these sorts of model lead to different questions to the psychosomatic/somatopsychic model. This is not to say that research conducted into these latter questions is not interesting, indeed, most of this chapter will address these questions. Rather, it is incomplete. This is largely because psychological factors were conceived as alternatives to physical factors. Actually their role is rather different. Although they can serve as efficient causes they are also involved in the presentation of certain physical facts as a problem. If this is true it implies that psychological treatment could be relevant to all illnesses (although this treatment will probably be conducted by the doctor or nurse, not a psychologist).

Most of the work assessing the role of psychological factors in disorders of hearing and balance has looked at one of two questions.

1 Are psychological factors involved in causing the symptoms in some way (psychogenic, psychosomatic)?
2 Does the otological problem result in any psychological (usually emotional) effects?

The degree to which each of these factors has been investigated in each disorder varies a good deal.

Vertigo

A discussion of non-organic vertigo can be found in the fifth edition of this book. Most attention has been paid to the possible involvement of psychological factors in Menière's disease. Typically, the questions which have been addressed have been, 'Are certain types of people more likely to develop Menière's disease than others?' and 'Do stressful events precipitate attacks of Menière's disease?'.

It seems clear that the experience of vertigo is often associated with anxiety or other emotional problems. What is not clear, however, is whether these emotional problems produce (or precipitate) Menière's disease or whether suffering from Menière's disease (and in particular from the associated vertigo) produces or precipitates the emotional difficulties.

Levy and O'Leary (1947) described a 'street neurosis' which can develop in sufferers from this disorder. This involves a fear of venturing out (particularly alone) because of the possibility of a vertiginous attack. Pratt and McKenzie (1958) described 12 patients with 'anxiety states' which they argued had been brought about by a vestibular dysfunction. The emotional problems were obvious but the author's explanation of the organic basis of the disorder, together with head and balance exercises, was a successful treatment.

Fowler and Zeckel (1952, 1953) argued strongly that there is indeed a psychosomatic factor in Menière's disease. They suggested that this effect was mediated through haemorrhage or spasm of the blood vessels in the labyrinth, induced by blood sludging. They reported on 23 patients, whom they divided into five groups on the basis of the type of stress involved in the precipitation of either particular attacks or of the disease itself. They also reported having experimentally induced Menière's attacks in two patients by exposure to emotional stress. In one patient they observed blood sludging of the conjunctiva immediately before the attack occurred.

In a series of papers Hinchliffe examined the psychosomatic hypothesis from several different perspectives. He compared 44 patients with Menière's disease to 20 patients with otosclerosis, attending an audiology clinic (Hinchliffe, 1967a). Twenty-eight of the patients with Menière's disease and two of the patients with otosclerosis claimed that their disease was related to emotional factors. This difference is highly significant ($P < 0.002$).

Twenty-five per cent of the group with Menière's disease had a 'psychosomatic V' type of score on the Minnesota Multiphasic Personality Inventory (MMPI), but none of the otosclerotic group had this pattern. This difference was significant ($P < 0.001$) (Hinchliffe, 1967b).

There was no difference in the number of relatives with psychosomatic diseases reported by the otosclerotic patients and by a control group of hospital employees. The patients with Menière's disease were, however, significantly more likely to have a history of psychosomatic disorder in their families than the controls. Migraine and headache occurred significantly more often in the siblings of the group with Menière's disease. Although the parents of the patients with Menière's disease were twice as likely to have had a psychosomatic disorder this difference was not significant. All the patients with Menière's disease gave a history of migraine and 11 (around 25%) reported cyclical vomiting of childhood.

Finally, Hinchcliffe (1965) examined the severity of the physiological disorder (as indexed by hearing threshold at 250 Hz and duration of the caloric response) as a function of the severity of the psychological disturbance (measured by personality profile on the MMPI). If the psychological disturbance was caused by the vestibular lesion one might expect a positive correlation between these factors. However, a negative correlation was found. The worse the hearing level, or the more abnormal the caloric response, the *less* abnormal the MMPI profile was. However, the number of patients studied was rather small. This series of controlled studies provides at least prima facie evidence that emotional factors may play a role in precipitating the disorder.

One problem with these investigations, however, is that the symptom of vertigo was not controlled. Thus the emotional disturbance on the MMPI could be caused *by* the vertigo rather than the cause *of* the vertigo.

However, it is more difficult to explain away the inverse relationship between physiological dysfunction and emotional disturbance. Hinchcliffe (1967a) suggested that both psychosomatic and somatopsychic processes occur. He suggested that this relationship is probably complicated by a feedback loop. Emotional distress produces vertigo, this in turn produces further anxiety.

Brightwell and Abramson (1975) extended the work on personality in Menière's disease. A group of patients with Menière's disease ($n = 13$) was compared with three control groups. The control groups were vertiginous patients who did not have Menière's disease, patients with otosclerosis, and patients with lymphoma. Subjects completed the Eysenck Personality Inventory (EPI) and the Cornell Medical Index (CMI). The EPI (a personality test) was preferred to the MMPI as it was designed for used in a nonpsychiatric population. Interest focused on the non-Menière's disease vertigo group. However, no significant differences were found between any of the groups except that the non-Menière's disease vertiginous group were more emotionally disturbed on the CMI than the lymphoma group. However, the neuroticism scale (N) (a measure of anxiety) was positively correlated with three measures of severity within the group with Menière's disease. This did not occur in the non-Menière's vertigo group. No such correlation occurred in the other groups. The authors suggested that vertigo cannot be the cause of these correlations and that it may be that anxiety does have a role in influencing the severity of the symptoms. However,

this study is a dis-confirmation of the previous findings of a difference in anxiety level between patients with otosclerosis and those with Menière's disease.

Crary and Wexler's study

An important and carefully conducted study was carried out by Crary and Wexler (1977). This set out to investigate personality factors, the role of life events in precipitating Menière's disease, and the role of stress in the precipitation of Menière's disease attacks. The compared four groups were:

1 Menière's disease (participating in the study)
2 Menière's disease (refused to particpate in the study)
3 Vertiginous (non-Menière's disease group)
4 Non-vertiginous otolaryngological patients.

They followed these patients for a period of 2 years. Subjects participating in the study also kept daily diary records of vertigo attacks and stressful events. Few personality differences were found between the vertiginous groups. Both the male and female Menière's disease patients were, however, distinguished from the respective non-vertiginous controls by more psychosomatic symptoms, more anxiety and higher scores on hypochondriasis, depression and hysteria scales on the MMPI. Crary and Wexler explain this as due to the effects of vertigo.

The Menière's disease group was distinguished by reported higher frequency of tension prior to a vertiginous episode, and by being more likely to have vertiginous attacks when alone. This pattern was not found in the Menière's disease patients who refused to participate in the study.

The relevant percentages of attacks preceded by tension are shown in Table 4.1. It is interesting that in every case the percentage of attacks preceded by tension is lower for men than for women. It seems likely that the men underestimate the number of attacks preceded by tension (given current social mores). For 59% of Menière's attacks in women to be preceded by tension (double the number so reported in the control vertigo group) is strong evidence of a psychosomatic element, (although the authors dismiss this finding). Of course, as this is retrospective self-report this may simply reflect the way these patients view their disease. But as they are no more emotionally disturbed than the non-Menière's vertigo group it is not clear why such perceptions should vary.

Alternatively one could argue that the *participating* Menière's patients were more disposed to look for a psychological explanation (and that was why they agreed to participate).

Subjects reported the number of life events which occurred in the previous 6 months and 6–12 month periods using the life change events questionnaire of

Table 4.1 Percentage of attacks preceded by tension

	Menière's disease group				Non-Menière's disease vertigo	
	Participating in study		Not participating in study			
Men	Women	Men	Women	Men	Women
32	59	7	21	3	26

After Crary and Wexler, 1977

Rahe *et al.* (1974). The authors reported the figures separately for men and women. The combined vertigo group reported more stress than the non-vertigo groups and there was a trend toward the group with Menière's disease reporting more stress than the non-vertigo group (although this was not significant in every case).

The next stage of their investigation involved diaries of stressful events and the occurrence of vertiginous attacks in Menière's disease patients (Table 4.2). They wanted to examine the hypothesis that stress precipitated the vertiginous attacks. They recorded the number of stressful events occurring. Stressful events were not defined for the patients. The number of stressful events pre-and post-vertigo was approximately equal, and the vast majority of vertigo attacks occurred without stress. Crary and Wexler argued that this is evidence against the psychosomatic hypothesis. However, there are several aspects of these data which they did not consider. First, the incidence of stressful events occurring on the day of the vertigo is 6.7 times higher than the incidence of stressful events in the 5 days following the attack and 10.25 times higher than the incidence of stressful events in the preceding 5 days. It seems unlikely that this is due to chance.

Generally Crary and Wexler's study was far more comprehensive than those which had been undertaken previously. In particular the use of prospective diary recordings to assess the role of stress. However, the conclusions they come to (that psychosomatic processes are not involved in Menière's disease) does not seem justified. The personality test results, however, did not corroborate the previous results.

Hinchcliffe (1967c) reported a study which has a bearing on this issue. He used a statistical technique known as numerical taxonomy to identify how many distinct groupings of vertiginous disorder could be identified on the basis of various objective measurements and subjective ratings. These included presence of deafness, fullness in the ears, psychosomatic illness in the family, MMPI profile, caloric test results and the phenomonology of the vertigo.

He excluded any definite medical disorders. Only one cluster was identified. Hinchcliffe concluded that the range of vertiginous disorders were all one disorder, i.e. Menière's disease and form fruste of that disorder. The implication of this study is that the control vertiginous groups may be forms of Menière's disease and, therefore, also psychosomatic.

Recent work

Stephens (1975) using a broad definition of Menière's disease, contrasted a group with Menière's disease (*n* = 164) with a group of idiopathic vertigo sufferers (*n* = 62). He used two personality questionnaires – the Eysenck Personality Inventory (EPI) and the Crown Crisp Experiential Index (CCEI). The EPI was designed for use on a psychiatrically normal population and yields neuroticism (N), extroversion (E) and lie (L) scores. The CCEI yields a variety of measures of psychopathology and has been standardized on a variety of psychiatric and medical populations. Stephens found that the group with Menière's disease was significantly more 'pathological' than the general population on all of the CCEI scales and on N and L.

Table 4.2 Occurrence of stressful events and attacks of vertigo

	Stressful event in the 5 days before vertigo	Stressful events on the day of vertigo	Stress events in 5 days after vertigo	Stressful event with no vertigo	Vertigo with no stressful event
All vertigo days	84	93	76	24	836
Onset of vertigo only	37	76	59	9	330

Adapted from Crary and Wexler

They had a reduced score on E. On comparing the Menière's group with the idiopathic vertigo group he found that the Menière's patients were significantly higher on the obsessionality and depression scales of the CCEI and the N scale of the EPI. In fact, the obsessionality score was higher than the norms for psychiatric patients. The data were reanalysed using the more stringent criteria of Hinchcliffe for the diagnosis of Menière's disease. This made little difference to the results. Furthermore, Stephens replicated Hinchcliffe's finding of an inverse relationship between hearing threshold and anxiety.

These results suggest that patients with Menière's disease do manifest more anxiety than a control vertigo population. However, the severity of the vertigo in the control group is not reported. These results also suggest that, at least psychologically, a distinction exists between idiopathic vertigo and Menière's disease (contra Hinchcliffe, 1967a–c). These results do not agree with Crary and Wexler's findings on personality test scores in Menière's disease patients. It is striking that the group with Menière's disease was higher on the obsessionality scale than the psychiatric patient group.

Hallam and Stephens (1985) examined CCEI scale scores in a series of 62 patients complaining of tinnitus, some of whom also complained of dizziness and/or hearing loss. They compared the following four groups: tinnitus only, tinnitus and dizziness, tinnitus and hearing loss, and tinnitus, dizziness and hearing loss. Testing the equality of the means in these four groups by analysis of variance (ANOVA) they found a significant difference on phobic and somatic anxiety. Hearing loss had no effect on the scores, dizziness being the most important factor.

Hallam and Hinchcliffe (1991) examined the relationship between complaints of dizziness and performance on tests of balance. They found that patients complaining of vertigo did not perform worse on tests of balance than patients attending the same clinic who were not complaining of dizziness. There was also no association between self-rated anxiety and complaint of vertigo. Anxiety did correlate with confidence in balance in those who complained of vertigo, but not in those who did not. It may be that more sensitive measures of dysfunction would have discriminated between the three groups – never experienced dizziness, dizziness main complaint, and dizziness reported but not main complaint. The groups did not differ on postural tests or on self-reported confidence.

It is surprising that postural tests (which are used diagnostically to indicate vestibular problems) did not discriminate between those who had and did not have vertigo. It is unclear why this should be. The relationship between self-confidence and balance could be explained as due to severe dizziness reducing confidence in balance, however, this is not consistent with a difference in correlation between complainers

and non-complainers. It is possible that this is caused by anxiety reducing confidence in balance, rather than the converse.

Stephens and Hallam (1985) and Hallam and Hinchcliffe (1991) both demonstrated a lack of correlation between the complaint of dizziness and clinical tests in patients attending a neuro-otology clinic. Patients attending without complaints of vertigo did as badly on these tests as those complaining of dizziness. Those who had never experienced dizziness were indistinguishable from those who had. These results further applied to balance tests as a series of ordinary tests. One interpretation of these results is that psychological factors are more important in influencing complaints of 'dizziness' than organic factors. It may, however, also reflect error in the balance tests.

Stephens, Hogan and Meredith (1991) studied the relationship of complaints of giddiness and clinical tests of vestibular abnormality in a population who were not attending a clinic for treatment. They surveyed *all* patients, aged between 50 and 65 years registered with two general practices. They found no relationship between the test findings and the complaint of giddiness. The authors suggested that a tendency to complain about symptoms may be partly a psychological tendency, as complaining of dizziness did relate to complaining of hearing loss. The repeated findings of a lack of relationship between complaint of various symptoms and well-established signs of pathology is intriguing and deserves further investigation.

This study has the great advantage of excluding the myriad extraneous factors which lead a person to be referred to a secondary or tertiary neuro-otology clinic (such as persistence). It was also found that those complaining of vertigo did not differ from those not complaining of vertigo on a series of standard balance tests.

Hallam, Prasansuk and Hinchcliffe (1983) administered the Eysenck Personality Questionnaire to patients complaining of all combinations of the symptoms, tinnitus, vertigo and hearing loss. They found that the combination of all three was associated with highest level of neuroticism. Whether this is simply an additive effect or due to anxiety causing Menière's disease is not clear.

Tests of balance were not, however, related to personality scores.

It seems clear that vertiginous patients have elevated scores on various measures of anxiety and depression when compared to the normal population and to non-vertiginous otolaryngological patients. When the symptoms of tinnitus, dizziness and hearing loss are each controlled, dizziness proves to be more important than hearing loss in elevating these scales. It is wrong, of course, to rarefy personality test scores. They consist of a series of self-reports of anxiety, mood, etc. Thus an elevated score can be the result of a disorder as much as the cause.

Little work has been done on the other aspects of

the psychosomatic hypothesis. This is disappointing, as I have argued, that not only does Hinchcliffe's work suggest that Menière's disease has a psychosomatic component, but so do some of Crary and Wexler's data. Hinchcliffe's (1967a) and Stephens' (1975) findings of an inverse relationship between measurable organic impairment and psychopathology is also worth pursuing. It would also be interesting to follow up Fowler and Zeckel's anecdotal report of experimentally induced Menière's attacks. If this could be replicated it would, obviously, be most important.

Grigsby and Johnston (1989) reported two patients with Menière's disease who also experienced feelings of unreality. They suggested that the origins of these sensations of depersonalization are in the dysfunction of the vestibular system and may frequently occur in Menière's syndrome. However, they present no evidence for this suggestion. Fewtrell and O'Connor (1988) suggested that depersonalization and dizziness may be two ways of describing the same perceptual experience or, alternatively, may be two different types of experience (of a very different type), but both describing disturbed self-world relations. The apparent similarities between depersonalization and vertigo (e.g. that on occasion depersonalization will be described as 'dizziness') should not detract from the differences (including the possibility of inducing vertigo by peripheral stimulation of the vestibular system – nothing like this applies to depersonalization).

They argued that 'dizziness names a family of different experiences and many of these experiences may be similar to those of depersonalisation'.

O'Connor, Chambers and Hinchcliffe (1990) administered the rod and frame test (which has been used as a test of dependence on external cues as a perceptual style and also as a personality style) to patients with organic vertigo and to patients with non-organic vertigo. The psychogenic group had less frame-dependent error than the organic group. They also had less frame-dependent error than a normal control group. But this does not achieve significance. The authors suggested that the experience of dizziness in the non-organic group could be produced by these perceptual style differences.

Yardley *et al.* (1992) interviewed vertigo sufferers and reported that they felt stigmatized (often they were perceived as drunk or hypochondriacal). Coping strategies often included social withdrawal and withdrawal from work, and other negative strategies.

The placebo effect in Menière's disease

Evidence of rather a different sort which may implicate psychological factors in Menière's disease comes from the controlled trial of the endolymphatic sac shunt operation by Thomsen *et al.* (1981). They found a strong placebo surgery effect – 77% of patients who had a placebo operation were judged as having had 'good benefit' by the patients and (separately) by doctors (rating blind). Incidence of diary-noted dizziness decreased. This seems to show that a psychological intervention radically affected the symptoms of Menière's disease (although there was no control for this comparison).

What factors influence the illness behaviour related to vestibular problems, although a most interesting question, has not been investigated. However, some work has been conducted on influencing this behaviour in therapy.

Hearing disorders

Most of the work conducted in this area has concerned the emotional effects of hearing loss rather than the emotional causes or precipitants of it. Although a psychological cause for most hearing loss is unlikely, psychological factors are almost certainly involved in illness behaviour or rather complaint behaviour in this area. As evidenced below, the majority of people with hearing loss do not present to a doctor, and a substantial proportion with hearing impairment do not report any hearing loss. That is, they do not define themselves as hearing impaired (even when they are given audiometric test results). This is a most interesting and important area for study.

Psychological causation

Non-organic hearing loss

Psychological causation has been thought to be important in functional hearing loss, non-organic hearing loss or hysterical hearing loss. This is distinguished from deliberate malingering. Psychoanalytic theorists have explained this by reference to unconscious motives. Noble (1978) argued that there is semantic confusion here. When 'non-organic hearing loss' is diagnosed what has been found is not another type of hearing loss; it is the absence of hearing loss, and whatever is wrong with the patient for whom this is true it is not a form of hearing loss. Slater (1965) distinguished the substantive and adjectival use of hysteria. It does not follow from the correct description of symptoms as hysterical that an entity hysteria exists. Applying this to hearing loss would lead to allowing the use of hysterical hearing loss but denying that this was due to an illness or personal characteristic hysteria.

King and Stephens (1992) reported a series of patients complaining of obscure auditory dysfunction (OAD). This is a complaint of hearing loss with a 'normal' audiogram. Twenty patients with obscure auditory dysfunction were compared with 20 controls. Audiometry was conducted up to 10 kHz. Those with obscure auditory dysfunction had a non-significantly higher prevalence of childhood hearing difficulties, they had worse hearing thresholds and higher scores on psychological scales of emotional distress. A history of family concern about health was registered. It seems likely that mild auditory impairments combine with psychological factors to generate a complaint of auditory dysfunction in these patients.

This is an interesting study with regard to obscure auditory dysfunction. However, its importance may lie beyond this group. It seems clear from this study that childhood experience and attitudes acquired toward illness affect the presentation of people with obscure auditory dysfunction. Is this a peculiarity of this group? Are they abnormal psychologically or do the psychological and social factors which cause them to present to a doctor also occur in those with more substantial hearing loss? This study should be taken further to examine this interesting question.

A final area, in which there has been virtually no research, is the possible detrimental effects on hearing of emotional distress. Speech reading (lipreading) is a complex task, involving inference from a variety of cues from lip-movements, context and non-verbal communication. It is also a task which the individual is likely to fail at on at least some occasions. If the speech reading situation becomes a cue for anxiety, then a vicious cycle of anxiety and failure can be set up. This is known as 'performance anxiety'. The anxiety produces the failure which is its object (Masters and Johnson, 1970).

Psychological effects of hearing loss

Much of the work to be reviewed in this section has suffered from an overly narrow psychiatric perspective. Often investigation of the emotional response to hearing loss has been seen as discovering the proportion of patients with a psychiatric illness. Usually this means depression and/or anxiety states. Although this is one way of investigating the emotional impact of hearing loss, it is crude. All adverse emotional states (e.g. mourning) are not psychiatric illnesses. In many ways an adverse emotional reaction to hearing loss is clearly understandable. Construing suffering as a psychiatric illness is likely to lead to confused answers. Adverse emotional consequences are likely to be points on a continuum rather than discrete illnesses or states.

Another feature of some of the literature which relates to this point is the confusion between depression as a mood state and as a psychiatric condition. It is usually a relatively easy matter to assess depression as a mood. We all do it when we say 'I feel very low'. But depressed mood is neither necessary nor sufficient for a psychiatrist to diagnose depression.

There have been two main areas of investigation in this field: the extent and nature of the emotional effects of hearing loss, and the role of hearing loss in precipitating suspiciousness and/or psychosis (paranoia and paraphrenia). One problem with most of this work is that it depends on self-report of emotional consequences.

The psychiatric approach

Early studies

A review of early studies can be found in the fifth edition of this book.

Ramsdell (1962) hypothesized that hearing serves three functions;

1 Symbolic – communication via speech
2 Warning – signals of impending danger, motor horns, threatening cry of animal
3 Background noises associated with various activities going on around us which have no particular informational content.

The most obvious handicap which the hearing impaired suffer is in communication, but Ramsdell argued that the deprivation of background noises was most intimately related to the feelings of depression to which the hearing impaired were prone. This was produced by the feeling of detachment, unreality and isolation that this deprivation produced.

Mahapatra (1974) reasoned that most of the psychological effects of hearing loss would be expected to a far higher degree in patients with a bilateral loss, rather than a unilateral loss. (Ability to perceive speech, for example, is affected to much less an extent with a unilateral loss.) He therefore compared two groups of patients with otosclerosis: those with a hearing loss greater than 40 dB at 250 Hz unilaterally, and those with a hearing loss greater than 40 dB at 250 Hz bilaterally. All the patients were awaiting surgery in an otolaryngological hospital. The two groups were given a psychiatric interview and were compared on the Cornell Index (a questionnaire measuring various personality characteristics related to emotional disturbance). The number of psychosomatic illnesses presented by the patient were also noted. Mahapatra reported that psychiatric illness was more common in the group with bilateral hearing loss ($P < 0.005$), but there was no difference in the number of psychosomatic illnesses in the two groups. Psychiatric illness here largely comprised depressive states, although five of the bilaterally hearing impaired group were diagnosed as paranoid schizophrenics.

The Cornell Index largely corroborated these findings. The bilaterally hearing impaired group obtained higher scores on the following scales: fear, depression, sensitive and suspicious, nervousness and anxiety, neurocirculatory symptoms, hypochondriasis and asthenia. There was a non-significant trend for those who lived alone to receive a diagnosis of psychiatric illness. However, those with a severe hearing impairment were *less* emotionally disturbed than those with moderate hearing impairment. Mahapatra explained this as due to the severely hearing impaired not regarding themselves as part of the hearing world. This might be true if they were prelingually deaf, it seems highly unlikely with otosclerotic patients. Mahapatra postulated that the emotional consequences of hearing impairment are due to sensory deprivation and social isolation. Thomas (1984) has criticized this study suggesting that the inflated Cornell Index scores could have been generated by preoperative stress – this being higher in the bilaterally deaf group because the implications of the operation would have been more far reaching. He also pointed out that 250 Hz lies outside the frequencies considered crucial for speech reception, and is therefore an inappropriate frequency to use. However, preoperative stress ought not to have biased the psychiatric interview (although reliability data ought to have been provided). Although 250 Hz is not the usual frequency for assessing hearing loss, as meaningful differences were found between the groups it seems to have discriminated *some* feature of importance, i.e. it does not seem a completely random categorization. Although it is possible that the differences found are artefactual, as Thomas suggested, the study does provide some evidence of emotional disturbance in the hearing impaired. On the basis of this study, it seems unrelated to severity of loss in any meaningful way.

Recent studies

Thomas and Gilhome Herbst (1980) invited for interview all patients seen for hearing aid fitting at three NHS hearing aid centres between 1975 and 1978. The control group consisted of normally hearing persons matched for age, sex, occupation and geographical location. Patients completed questionnaires which gave information about the perceived effect of their hearing loss on various aspects of their life, their general health and wellbeing; pure tone audiometry was conducted and patients completed the Symptoms of Anxiety and Depression Scale (SAD).

No overall relationship was found between disturbance and pure tone or speech hearing threshold. However, of the 23 respondents who had an average auditory threshold of 70 dB or worse in the better ear together with speech discrimination of 70% or less, wearing a hearing aid, the incidence was significantly higher (12/23). The lack of relationship between psychiatric disturbance and hearing threshold (apart from this group) is to be noted. If hearing impairment produces emotional disturbance, one might well expect increasing levels of hearing impairment to make emotional disturbance more probable. The psychiatrically disturbed group were not differentiated by presence of tinnitus or duration of loss. Both of these factors have previously been thought to

be of importance; tinnitus because it is a potentially stressful stimulus, and duration of hearing loss because it might relate to development of problems by chronic deprivation. Several variables *did* distinguish the psychiatrically disturbed group from the non-disturbed group. Reports of unhappiness at work, changing jobs due to hearing loss, being lonely, having no friends, marriage being affected by hearing loss, feeling near a nervous breakdown and general dissatisfaction with life. Although some of these factors may contribute to the production of emotional disturbance, it seems clear that many quite probably merely reflect that state. The groups were also distinguished by various measures of general health and wellbeing. However, most of the variables which are included here are physical manifestations of anxiety and depression.

Singerman, Riedner and Folstein (1980) examined 174 outpatients at an audiology clinic. Four groups of patients were studied: those with normal hearing, unilateral loss in the speech frequencies, hearing loss outside the speech frequencies, and bilateral hearing loss in the speech frequencies. Patients completed the General Health Questionnaire (GHQ) as a measure of emotional disturbance. This design allows examination of the importance of deprivation of hearing speech. The group with normal hearing had the most abnormal GHQ scores. Of the three groups with hearing loss the bilateral hearing loss group had the highest scores, followed by the group with high or low tone hearing loss. Patients with a unilateral loss were no different from the general population. However, the difference between groups was not significant. This implies that hearing loss outside the speech frequencies (so not affecting conversation) is still associated with emotional disturbance.

The normally hearing group was significantly more likely to have both tinnitus and vertigo. This may explain their raised GHQ scores.

It seems likely that the emotional consequences of hearing loss may in part be mediated by ancillary symptoms. This will be discussed further below. It is worth noting that this factor has been ignored in most previous work.

Gildston and Gildston (1972) examined emotional disturbance in 34 patients with otosclerosis before the restoration of normal hearing by stapedectomy and 3 months later. Patients completed the Guildford-Zimmerman Temperament Survey to assess submissiveness, seclusiveness, emotional lability, depression and suspiciousness. They also completed an optimism scale. Hearing thresholds averaged over the speech frequencies in the better ear were 52.9 dB for pure tone and 54.9 dB for speech reception.

Patients were significantly more disturbed than the general population on four of the seven scales before the operation. Postoperatively they improved on five of the seven scales. Their postoperative scores were not significantly different from the general population scores. The optimism scale also improved. More-over, the few patients whose operations were not successful did not improve on these scales.

Cochlear implants provide another possibility of examining the effect of hearing loss on personality. However, in this case the patients have profound hearing loss. Personality questionnaires have been used pre- and postimplant. McKenna (1986) reviewed this literature. Few changes in personality scores have been found. However, patients who had deviant scores were often not implanted, thus reducing the possibility of improvement.

An important methodological weakness with all of these studies is that self-report questionnaires are open to response-bias. Subjects can deliberately 'fake good' or 'fake bad' or subjects' responses may be influenced unconsciously by the role they are adopt-ing. When a patient adopts the sick role it is quite possible that they will regard adverse mood and poor general wellbeing as expected. This will be true inde-pendently of the actual severity of their symptoms. The use of a lie scale can help to reduce the likelihood of such an interpretation. This has rarely been done.

Gilhome-Herbst and Humphrey (1980) assessed the relationship between hearing impairment and emotional disturbance in an elderly population; 69% of patients aged over 70 years registered with a particular general practice were assessed. Subjects completed the CARE schedule (which yielded a meas-ure of depression), answered various questions about their general hearing and their satisfaction with life and had their hearing tested by pure tone audio-metry. A total of 60% ($n = 98$) was found to have impaired hearing on audiometry (53.5 dB averaged across 1, 2 and 4 kHz). This is far higher than estimates obtained by self-report and, indeed, 27% refused to admit that they had impaired hearing when given the test results. The mean hearing loss in this group was 43.8 dB. Patients were classified as depressed or not depressed. There was a significant relationship between depression and having hearing impairment. However, once again, severity of the hearing loss did *not* relate to the severity of depres-sion, 41% of those with a hearing loss were depressed. It is worth bearing in mind that, therefore 59% were *not* depressed. Thirty patients said their 'hearing loss made them feel different' about themselves (either closed in, frustrated or depressed, or feel inferior). Feeling different was predicted (in order of predictive strength) by onset of hearing loss before retirement, saying that hearing impairment matters, depression, feeling lonely, severity of the hearing loss, saying people get irritable with hearing impaired people and saying people think that the effects of the hearing impairment are absent mindedness.

Self-reports of feeling lonely etc. are problematic as they are conceptually linked to the criterion variable. It is of interest that onset before retirement and severity of loss are predictors. These were predictors

independent of duration of hearing loss. It may well be, as Gilhome-Herbst and Humphrey suggested, that if hearing loss occurs before retirement it is regarded as abnormal and adverse effects attributed to it. If it occurs *after* retirement age it is more likely to be seen as part of normal ageing and, therefore, adverse emotional states are *not* attributed to it. This sort of self-attribution process is one of the crucial problems in dealing with self-report data as if they were physi-cal observations.

Humphrey, Gilhome-Herbst and Faurqi (1981) re-ported further on this survey. Only 29 of the 136 hearing impaired people studied had a hearing aid. These 29 differed from the others in having worse hearing on audiometry, rating themselves as worse at communication, more likely to have tinnitus, and less likely to hear a telephone or radio. There was no difference in sex or class. They were also more likely to be hearing impaired before retirement and to have been hearing impaired longer.

The most obvious explanation of this pattern of differences is that those who had hearing aids had worse hearing. The 27% who refused to admit they had a hearing loss were less impaired, younger, reported less tinnitus and less communication problems. All these factors would seem to make it easier for the patient to deny a hearing impairment, and it may be that, if it is possible, most people would prefer to deny a hearing loss because of the stigma associated with deafness. However, one would not expect someone who *denied* a hearing loss to report difficulties in communication.

Most of the evidence presented seems to suggest that emotional disturbance of more than a transitory nature does occur with hearing loss, and that it is reduced when the hearing loss is cured. It is also clear that not every hearing disabled person is emotionally disturbed. Most attempts to distinguish those who are depressed or anxious from those who are not have been dogged by the problem of criterion-contaminated predictors. It is, however, puzzling that the degree of hearing impair-ment is not a predictor (at least as measured by pure tone audiometry). This raises the possibility that hearing impairment is not causally related to mood disturbance.

A study by Jones, Victor and Vetter (1984) how-ever, complicates this picture somewhat, at least in the elderly. They attempted to interview all patients over 70 years of age registered with a general practice in Wales. They interviewed 657 from a target group of 683. This is a very high response rate (96%) and rather better than those reported by Thomas's group. They used the SAD scale to assess emotional distur-bance, and a semi-structured questionnaire to assess various hearing difficulties. There was reasonably good agreement between the researchers estimate of communication difficulty and by the self-report of the subject. They found that self-assessed hearing diffi-culty related to anxiety and, less strongly, to depres-sion. Probability of emotional disturbance did in-crease with increasing severity of hearing difficulty.

However, other physical disabilities were strongly related to hearing difficulties. The association of reported hearing loss to emotional disturbance was not significant when the effect of physical disability was partialled out. The possibility that associated physical problems could correlate with hearing impairment and be responsible for associated emotional disturbance, at least in the elderly, has not been properly investigated before. This study needs to be replicated using audiometric assessment of hearing. It is also necessary to conduct a longitudinal study. One might follow up persons at retirement age, and investigate the development of emotional disturbance in those who do or do not become hearing disabled.

It has been suggested several times that the categorization of patients into depressed or non-depressed groups (and the identification of clinically depressed individuals) is based on an inappropriate view of emotional disturbance in these patients.

It is also a rather general approach yielding relatively few data on specific and rehabilitation-relevant issues. We still have very little idea about what is likely to predispose a person to develop an adversal emotional reaction to hearing loss. Psychological effects of hearing loss are not restricted to anxiety and depression and they may involve specific changes, e.g. not socializing any more or self-perception as handicapped.

More recent studies

A number of studies have been carried out more recently. Kalayam, Alexopoulous and Young (1991) used a structured interview to evaluate the mental state of subjects over the age of 55 years attending a hearing clinic. They found an association with major depression rather than with paranoid psychoses. However, this may have been partially due to the fact that they had very small numbers of patients with a psychiatric diagnosis, with a very low expectation, therefore, of paranoid psychoses. Knutson and Lansing (1990) investigated the relationship between communication difficulties (measured by a self-report scale) and a variety of measures of emotional difficulties (MMPI, BDI and others), in the profoundly deaf. Communication difficulties correlated with these measures of emotional distress, in particular loneliness and isolation correlated with a scale of hearing problems. The authors concluded that if communication difficulties improved this would reduce psychological distress. This would be worth following up but, of course, the correlation could be due to emotional problems causing people to report worse communication skills, due for example to depression.

Non-psychiatric approaches

Barcham and Stephens (1980) used an open-ended questionnaire to gather information about the effects of hearing loss. Patients were simply asked to list all the problems that they had as a consequence of their hearing loss. The problem most frequently rated as being of most importance was the inability to hear speech. This is important to the assessment of Ramsdell's (1970) hypothesis that it is background sounds which have the greatest emotional effect. The proportion mentioning psychological problems was small – 14% mentioned embarrassment, 6% nervous strain, 5% loneliness, 3% family strain and 2% lack of confidence. Stephens (1980) has argued that open-ended questionnaires minimize the apparent psychological consequences of hearing impairment compared to questionnaire measurement. He argued this may be for one of three possible reasons:

1 The actual incidence of psychological problems is low
2 Few patients recognize these psychological sequelae as a consequence of their hearing impairment
3 The patient may not believe that these problems are relevant to the purposes of the person giving the questionnaire.

It would be interesting to have different professionals (e.g. a medical doctor and a psychologist) administer an open-ended questionnaire to determine whether different types of response are obtained. Another possibility is that patients may well wish to conceal emotional difficulties. A problem with this type of self-report is that patients decide what to report *on* as well as what not to report. However, despite these problems, this study gives us new information. The most commonly reported emotional consequence, embarrassment, has received very little attention in previous work. Depression and suspiciousness are not reported at all.

Patients may also not be able to say if an adverse psychological state is attributable to their hearing loss or not. They simply may not know if their irritability is a consequence of their hearing loss. This type of measure is rather well suited to investigations of illness behaviour. Most of these problems with this scale are actually a part of the data we ought to be investigating. Studies need to be carried out in which the degree and type of hearing impairment, beliefs about hearing, previous experience of illness, family models and more about illness, personality and current stresses are related to the frequency of types of reported problem.

McKenna and Denman (1993) used the repertory grid to assess patients who are being considered for cochlear implantation. They reported the utility of this ideographic method. Patients reported changed self-perception after cochlear implantation. The authors recommended the use of the repertory grid for clinical assessment of hearing-disabled people. It would also be useful to use this tool for research purposes. The great advantage of the 'repertory grid' is that it provides a measure of attitudes towards something which is tailor-made to each individual.

This would produce more detail concerning how the individual's hearing problem functioned in that person's life rather than simple reports of high distress in general, which often is not very illuminating.

Watson, Henggeler and Whelan (1990) found that parents' ratings of the behavioural problems of hearing impaired adolescents are predicted (statistically) by emotional disturbance in the parents and by family stress and family ratings. Parents made both sets of ratings which is an obvious weakness in the design, but the possibility of identifying the mechanism by which distress is occasioned in the hearing impaired is worth pursuing.

One interesting aspect of this study is that the authors attempted to address the question of *how* hearing loss contributes to emotional distress. As emotional disturbance is not universal this is, of course, a most pertinent question, but has not been addressed in most studies. The present author would issue a plea for less time to be spent on atheoretical studies which merely report the association of emotional distress and hearing loss and leave unaddressed the question of *why* this should be.

Experimental studies

An experimental approach which deserves more attention is the examination of non-verbal behaviour in encounters between the hearing and the hearing impaired. Holton (1978) used this technique with prelingually hearing impaired subjects but detected few differences between deaf-deaf, hearing–hearing and hearing–deaf interactions. However, the interactions lasted only 3 minutes and subjects were not informed as to the hearing status of the other person. It would be interesting to know more about non-verbal communication of hearing impaired/hearing interactions of rather longer duration.

Thomas, Lamont and Harris (1982) factor analysed a questionnaire concerning problems experienced at work by the hearing impaired. The four resulting factors were labelled: social relationships at work; loss of status at work; formal work relations; and loss of status/job proficiency. These factors are orthogonal to one another.

Stevens (1982) gave hearing-impaired patients a questionnaire made up of various common statements made by the hearing impaired. He factor analysed this questionnaire and obtained three factors: social isolation; inability to cope; and perceived intolerant attitudes to the deaf. Ability to cope distinguished old from young subjects but not those with hearing aids from those without hearing aids. Conversely, social isolation and perceived intolerant attitudes to the deaf distinguished the aided from the unaided patients, but not the old from the young. The possibility, then, is that self-perception of ability to cope may be refractory to rehabilitation by the provision of a hearing aid but social isolation and perception of intolerant attitudes may respond to this sort of intervention. This could be due to increased and smoother interactions with others. It is interesting that in the studies by Stevens (1982) and by Thomas, Lamont and Harris (1982) social difficulties emerge as a separate factor from other problems. It is obviously very difficult to draw any definite conclusions about different factors of difficulties associated with hearing loss at this stage. This approach, however, potentially offers a much more detailed description of the emotional problems of the hearing impaired. It also allows a whole range of new questions to be asked. For example, what makes people prone to suffer from particular hearing problems or regard certain things as hearing problems.

Stephens, Lewis and Charny (1991) reported data from the Cardiff health survey in which a very large sample was related to various aspects of life-style and attitude about health. They found little relationship. It is not clear why.

Stephens *et al.* (1990) reported the specific complaints about hearing disability made by people who reported hearing problems. From a random sample of 4266, 14.7% indicated that they had a hearing problem. There was a strong relationship with age; 22% complained of having difficulty hearing the television and 20% complained of difficulty in conversation. There was also a large number of other specific complaints. Of patients attending a neuro-otology clinic in London 39% complained of difficulty in conversation and only 4% of difficulty in hearing the television as their main complaint. This may reflect a larger group who do not consider themselves so handicapped as to seek out treatment but who regard themselves as having a minor hearing problem. This study may demonstrate the self-selection on the basis of degree and type of disability and handicap. It would be informative to examine those who present to a clinic with only the complaint of difficulty in hearing the television.

Suspiciousness and/or paranoia

An issue which has attracted a good deal of controversy is the possible role of hearing loss in generating or precipitating suspiciousness and/or paranoid mental states.

Houston and Royse (1954) argued that feelings of inferiority are projected onto the environment and the subsequent ideas of reference are then systematized as delusions.

Several of the early psychiatric reports note clinical impressions of suspiciousness, e.g. Ingalls (1946), Knapp (1948) and Mahapatra (1974).

Several different approaches to examining this hypothesis have been adopted. Some personality questionnaire studies have found elevated scores on scales of suspiciousness. Thomas (1981b) also gave the Eysenck Personality Questionnaire (EPQ) to 88 patients from his hearing aid user sample. The EPQ incorporates a psychoticism (P) scale which purports to be a measure of a personality dimension related to psychosis. The P scale was not elevated in either men or women. However, the N (neuroticism) scale was not elevated either. Thus there was *no* evidence of emotional disturbance in this group. However, the greatest weakness of this study is that the P scale has not been well validated. Groups other than psychotics (e.g. art students) score higher than the psychotics. The content of the items is largely to do with hostility. It is difficult to draw any definite conclusions from these disparate results.

Houston and Royse (1954) set out to examine the hypothesis that hearing loss can produce delusions of persecution. They did this by classifying inpatients in a psychiatric hospital as paranoid or non-paranoid and as deaf and non-deaf. Deaf patients were selected from files and non-deaf patients were randomly selected (but matched for age and sex). Tests of hearing were carried out. Paranoid schizophrenics were twice as likely to be deaf as non-deaf. Although the tests of hearing were crude, this study gave evidence on some important points. Being deaf is associated with receiving a paranoid label if one is a psychiatric patient. There is evidence that difficult interpersonal interactions can lead to relapses in schizophrenia. It would therefore not be particularly surprising if hearing loss, which clearly can interfere with social interaction, could precipitate psychotic states.

Cooper *et al.* (1974) selected two groups of patients – one with affective disorder and the other with paranoid psychosis. Paranoid patients had significantly worse thresholds at four frequencies in the better ear, and there was a trend in the same direction in the worse ear. Social deafness was also significantly more common in the paranoid group.

Kay and Roth (1961) examined the role of hearing loss in paraphrenia. Paraphrenia is a delusional state occurring during old age. Of these patients 40% were found to have hearing disability on interview compared with 7% of patients with affective disorder.

The data at the present time are suggestive of a precipitant relationship between hearing loss and persecutory delusions. It is worth mentioning that it is clear that the vast majority of patients with hearing loss do not have paranoid delusions. What seems possible is that if a person has a psychiatric breakdown hearing loss will tend to produce persecutory delusions. This could well operate because of the ambiguity in hearing that is introduced.

With paraphrenic states it also seems possible that hearing loss may actually precipitate the disorder.

It might be interesting to look at the effect of hearing aid use on outcome. If one could demonstrate an effective hearing aid reduced the incidence or severity of persecutory delusions and/or rate of remission this would be important evidence for a causal role.

Tinnitus

The work that has been conducted on psychological aspects of tinnitus does not fit the same pattern as that reported for other neuro-otological problems. If Menière's disease is a psychosomatic illness then the associated tinnitus is also psychosomatic (at least in those cases where tinnitus occurs only during the attacks). Tinnitus also occurs during attacks of panic or other states of anxiety in some individuals. Clearly in these cases, too, tinnitus can be regarded as psychosomatic. However, apart from these special cases tinnitus has not usually been regarded as psychosomatic. Moreover, it is not clear how one could establish that tinnitus was a hysterical symptom, unless this was by virtue of guilt by association with a non-organic hearing loss.

Fowler and Fowler (1955) argued that emotional strain, although not a cause of tinnitus, was an aggravating factor. They argued for a rather different role of psychological factors in tinnitus. This was that the reduction of emotional threshold led some sufferers to complain about what was actually a trivial symptom.

They recommended procedures designed to reassure the patient that the tinnitus was not indicative of any malignant pathology and to encourage distracting but relaxing activity, and 'Anything which eases the emotional strain, anything which enables the patient to function better in the hearing world, will in the great majority of instances lessen the annoyance from tinnitus, or remove it from consciousness by making it subaudible' (Fowler and Fowler, 1955).

This sort of role for psychological processes is rather different from that discussed for hearing loss and vertigo.

I have argued that these sort of considerations apply to most illnesses. However, there are particular reasons why theorists have argued that there is a psychological component to tinnitus. These reasons will now be discussed.

Loudness of tinnitus

When a tone is adjusted so that it appears to the sufferer to be equally loud as their tinnitus, the result is called a loudness match. This loudness match is usually made using a tone which is similar to tinnitus in pitch. When this procedure has been carried out, the result is usually at most 20 dB above the subject's auditory threshold. Reed (1960), for example, using a binaural matching procedure found that 41% of the tinnitus patients he tested matched their tinnitus to 5 dB SL or less; 95% matched their tinnitus to 30 dB SL or less, and the highest match was 50 dB SL. Other studies have obtained similar results. It was suggested that tinnitus is very soft and complaint about it psychologically determined.

Hazell (1981) has found that loudness matches expressed in dB SPL correlated better with the self-reported loudness of tinnitus than loudness matches expressed in dB SL. He argued that dB SPL therefore better reflected the loudness of the tinnitus, i.e. quite loud. However, Hallam *et al.* (1985) and Jakes *et al.* (1986) found that dB SL expressions of the loudness match correlated better with self-reported loudness than matches expressed in dB HL, both at the tinnitus frequency and at 1 kHz. To complicate matters, these latter workers have also found that converting loudness matches to personal loudness units (PLUs) (Hinchcliffe and Chambers, 1983) yields the highest correlation with self-reported loudness. Personal loudness units are units which express the loudness match relative to an individual loudness function and most comfortable loudness level. This controls for any effect of recruitment as well as other individual differences. Subjects match their most comfortable loudness level at 1 kHz. They then select intensities which correspond to half and twice that loudness. These values are substituted in Scharf and Stevens (1959) loudness function to yield an individual loudness function. The matched loudness is expressed as a proportion of this scale.

However, the important point here for our purposes is that tinnitus is not, as some sufferers claim, 'as loud as a jet engine'. This is important. If tinnitus is not so loud that it *impels* annoyance, the factors which lead to it becoming annoying are of crucial importance.

Most tinnitus patients have tinnitus which is below their most comfortable loudness level (MCLL). That the loudness of tinnitus is less than some workers have believed does not, however, mean that the patients are neurotic. Hallam, Rachman and Hinchcliffe (1984) reported a pilot study in which patients with tinnitus attending a neuro-otology clinic were classified as those who were complaining of their tinnitus and those who were attending the clinic presenting with another symptom but who, incidentally, had tinnitus.

The complainers were compared with the non-complainers on a series of different variables. The self-reported loudness did not distinguish the two groups. Nor did the loudness match at 1 kHz.

Other factors

The existence of people who have tinnitus but who are not presenting with it as a complaint is extremely interesting. Heller and Bergmann (1953) confined a series of normally hearing subjects in a sound proofed room and asked them to report anything that they heard. All subjects reported hearing noises of various sorts. The quality of the noises was similar to the quality of tinnitus (rings, buzzes, hisses). Although these noises were presumably not perceived in ambient noise, this study does demonstrate that some degree of tinnitus is normal.

Epidemiological work demonstrates that awareness of tinnitus, (lasting for more than 5 minutes and not due to noise) is very common (15% of the general population) (OPCS 1983); 2% report tinnitus which is always present. An important finding of this work is that 2% of the population said that tinnitus bothered them 'a good bit' or 'quite a lot'. Thus the majority of tinnitus sufferers did not find it very annoying. Although there is a relationship between being bothered by tinnitus and how frequently it occurs, this does *not* hold for those whose tinnitus is present for an hour or more, once a week or more (i.e. those whose tinnitus occurs to a clinically significant degree). About one-third of people who have tinnitus continuously, for an hour or more every day, or an hour or more once a week or more found it bothered them 'a great deal' or 'quite a lot'. The proportion is invariable across these three groups. So it seems unlikely that being bothered by tinnitus is determined by simple sensory qualities of the noise or frequency of occurrence.

Because of these sort of findings, Hallam, Rachman and Hinchcliffe (1984) have proposed that habituation to tinnitus should be regarded as the norm and continued annoyance should be regarded as a failure of this habituation process (see below). Of particular relevance here is the series of experiments by Glass and Singer (1972). They demonstrated that the physiological response to annoying noise decreased with continued presentation. Although the noise they used was of a much greater loudness than that of tinnitus, it seems likely that the same process ought to occur.

Hallam, Rachman and Hinchcliffe (1984) proposed an important model of tinnitus-related distress. It is based on the observation that most people who have tinnitus do not complain about it. They postulated that the normal course of events is for a person who develops tinnitus to adapt to it. They argued that what needs to be explained is why people do not adapt. Complaining about tinnitus is a failure of adaptation. They further argued that the process of adaptation is a special case of habituation. The response to a stimulus which is repeatedly presented, and which has no significance for the subject is a decrement in response. The response to a novel stimulus is to orient to it. That is to turn towards the apparent origin of the stimulus, to become alert and for other activity to be halted. This is the orienting reflex. With repeated presentation this behaviour declines. The subjective experience is of ceasing to be aware of a novel stimulus as it continues to occur providing that the stimulus is without significance.

Hallam and his colleagues argued that the usual

course of events is for the sufferer to habituate to tinnitus, in a manner analogous to that by which the orienting response habituates to a novel sound.

Possible causes of non-habituation include unspecified differences at a neural level, any factor which renders the tinnitus meaningful. By this is meant any factor (belief or attitude) which gives the tinnitus any significance for the sufferer. These factors include the belief that the tinnitus is the symptom of a serious medical or psychological disorder, or an indication that one is getting old, but also more general beliefs such that it is possible to treat tinnitus. Ellis (1962) believed that all neurotic suffering is born of demanding that oneself or the world must be other than what they are. In this case the beliefs that one *must* have perfect health or that it is *unfair* if one suffers from tinnitus also render the tinnitus meaningful. The belief that tinnitus is a problem recursively also renders tinnitus meaningful and hence, according to the above theory, noticeable and a problem.

Time, medical reassurance and any factors which potentiate to adaptation are postulated by Hallam and colleagues to be therapeutic.

This model of tinnitus complaint-behaviour has been very important in the development of a broadened understanding of the patient with tinnitus. It also gives a rationale for many of the psychological therapies for tinnitus (which often appeared to have simply been transplanted from work with people with anxiety problems). If it is possible to reduce the level of tension or anxiety and encourage a goal of coping (to replace the maladaptive attitude that a cure must be found) then the normal process of habituation will be allowed to occur. This model focuses the attention on the processes which make the experience of tinnitus into a complaint, and as such it seems both to fit with the known epidemiological facts and is consistent with attempts to alleviate the distress of tinnitus. For example why should a masking noise from a masker be helpful to someone with tinnitus? Maskers can be helpful when the masking noise is very similar to the tinnitus sound and perceived as louder than the tinnitus sound. Surely the explanation here is that the masker is helpful simply because it is *not* the tinnitus and possibly because the sufferer knows that it can be switched off. This therapeutic process is unclear if the aim is simply to change the quality or intensity of the noise.

One ambiguity with the habituation model is whether the process being addressed is the simple process of habituation of the orienting reflex or whether a more general process of adaptation to noise. If habituation of the orienting reflex (or of attention to the noise) is meant to be the *sole* explanation it is not clear why the time factor involved is so different. An individual will habituate to a neutral stimulus over a short series of presentations, but tinnitus is adapted to over a period of months or years. It could be argued that this is because an

attitudinal change needs to take place for the habituation to happen and this is probably correct. But the process of this attitudinal adaptation is then the most important part of the process and this is not a peripheral phenomenon such as habituation to a tone. Another problem with the habituation model of tinnitus annoyance is that it is really a model of tinnitus awareness. But many sufferers report the awareness of tinnitus without reporting being annoyed by it.

The factors which generate annoyance from the perception of tinnitus are far more central than the habituation model allows for. It seems possible that it is attitudinal factors which generate annoyance and distress from tinnitus. These attitudes and beliefs do not merely serve to make tinnitus a salient stimulus (although they *do* do this), they serve to render it a problem.

Some people report having always had tinnitus, not having been bothered by it until they realized it was abnormal.

Finally, the habituation model (or adaptation model) needs to be understood in the context of the general life situation of the sufferer. Clearly if the person has many other disavowed problems, tinnitus can become a non-threatening explanation or if health seems too difficult for the sufferer it can provide an alternative, more acceptable role in life. It is crucial to assess the person's difficulties in context and not merely the one *presented* difficulty.

Carlsson and Erlandsson (1991) carried out a purported test of Hallam and colleagues' habituation theory of tinnitus tolerance. They took two groups of people who reported tinnitus. One group was highly distressed by their tinnitus while the second was not bothered by it. They compared the rate of habituation of the orienting response to a repetitive tinnitus-like sound. They found no difference in rate of habituation in either group. Both groups demonstrated significant habituation. They claimed it is unlikely that differences in orienting reflex habituation susceptibility could explain the difference between the two groups. They suggested that this evidence is not consistent with the habituation theory of tinnitus tolerance. But, of course, that theory never maintained that simple differences in rate of habituation in general explained the difference between those who tolerate tinnitus and those who cannot. Rather it argued that *other factors* prevent habituation occurring, e.g. beliefs and attitudes about tinnitus. In so far as these beliefs and attitudes are tinnitus-specific no general habituation factor would be predicted. It does, however, rule out the more general factors, e.g. personality, mood, level of anxiety that Hallam and colleagues postulated might be involved.

A study by Webb and Warren (1967) examined adaptation to noise in experiments over several months. Explosive charges were detonated over a small town 20 times a day in a barrage balloon. The authors surveyed the population and recorded how annoyed the residents were by noise in the area. The proportion who were annoyed dropped from 51% to 20%. This then is evidence that tolerance develops.

Tinnitus is more likely to be annoying on this hypothesis if factors exist which retard habituation to it. Penner (1983) found that although the minimal masking level of tinnitus was only weakly correlated with self-reported annoyance, and the increase in intensity of masker necessary to keep the tinnitus inaudible was unrelated to annoyance, the rate of change of the intensity of noise necessary to keep the tinnitus inaudible was quite strongly related to annoyance. It seems likely that this demasking process would render tinnitus more noticeable in varying ambient noise. This might well make habituation to tinnitus difficult.

Facets of complaint about tinnitus

Hinchcliffe and King (1992) in a recent review of the literature on the medico-legal aspects of tinnitus concluded that: 'The probability that tinnitus is a source of complaint and the probability that it will be associated with a particular degree, or pattern of distress appears to be primarily related to the psychological characteristics of the individual, the stresses to which he or she has been exposed, and the circumstances surrounding the onset of the tinnitus'. Does this imply that people who complain about tinnitus suffer from a psychiatric illness?

McKenna, Hallam and Hinchcliffe (1991) used a structured interview conducted by a clinical psychologist to assess the need for psychological help in 120 consecutive patients with tinnitus attending a tertiary referral clinic. Forty-two per cent of patients were assessed as being in need of psychological help and 86% of these accepted the offer of help. They were assessing need for *psychological* help not whether the client had a psychiatric illness.

Lewis, Stephens and Huws (1992) reported five case histories in which tinnitus patients committed suicide and one in which a suicidal tinnitus patient was murdered by his son. These were all patients attending a particular tinnitus clinic in Wales. Most of the patients were male, were socially isolated and working class. In all but one case there was a clear history of major psychiatric disorder. Tinnitus tended to be of recent onset, left sided and pulsatile. It seems possible that the tinnitus was purely incidental to the patient's suicide, but a larger series would be very interesting. To what degree is this the 'tip of the psychiatric iceberg?'. This question has been explicitly examined in a challenging series of studies by Katon and colleagues.

Sullivan *et al.* (1988) used a structured psychiatric interview and various questionnaire methods of rating psychological distress to compare patients with troublesome tinnitus, those with a hearing loss and a normal control group. They found that the tinnitus patients had a higher incidence of major depression than control subjects both currently and throughout their life. The authors argued that the association of tinnitus with affective disorder may be explained by complaint about tinnitus merely being a symptom of depression. This interesting argument raises a number of important questions. However, it should be noted that a higher current prevalence or lifetime prevalence of depression in tinnitus patients is not evidence that tinnitus is merely secondary to depression. Clearly, unless it is established that the tinnitus *followed* the depression it could equally be that the tinnitus caused the depression. Obviously it could be the case that this occurred in people vulnerable to that state. The assumption that major depression is an illness or not susceptible to environmental causation is at least debatable. It does seem that Sullivan and his colleagues make such an assumption.

Harrop-Griffiths *et al.* (1987) studied the first 21 patients attending a newly established tinnitus clinic. All patients suffered from severe tinnitus. They used a structured psychiatric interview to classify the patients in terms of psychiatric diagnosis. They compared these tinnitus patients to 14 control patients attending an otolaryngology clinic because of hearing loss. The tinnitus patients had a significantly greater prevalence of major depression. Sixty two per cent of tinnitus patients had been depressed at some point in their lives and 46% were currently depressed. The corresponding figures for the hearing loss controls were 21% and 7%. However, depression as a psychiatric category shades into misery as a human category. That is to say a concordance between tinnitus and depression cannot be considered to be a concordance of two independent entities (unlike influenza and gout, for example). Furthermore, the first 21 patients of an otolaryngological clinic are unlikely to be representative of tinnitus patients attending clinics nor people who experience tinnitus. Tinnitus patients who were currently depressed scored as more distressed than tinnitus patients who were not currently depressed, on the SCL-90. However, this merely shows that the SCL-90 is higher in people who are depressed.

Kirsch, Blanchard and Parnes (1989) compared tinnitus sufferers whom they classified as high copers to those whom they classified as low copers. They found that patients who were low in coping ability scored higher on measures of psychological distress than those classified as high in coping ability. Low copers were similar to chronic pain patients.

Dimensions of distress

Wilson *et al.* (1991) reported a questionnaire designed to assess the psychological distress associated with tinnitus, the Tinnitus Reaction Questionnaire (TRQ). They achieved good test-retest reliability. They extracted four factors which they named general distress, interference, severity and avoidance. The TRQ scales correlated with depression and anxiety but not with neuroticism. This questionnaire, using a different set of questionnaire items replicated the finding of Hallam and colleagues, that emotional distress, the intrusiveness of tinnitus and the severity of tinnitus load on separate orthogonal factors. Of course, the statistical independence of these factors is imposed on the data by the statistical tools used. However, if distress were determined by the intensity of tinnitus it would be unlikely to load on a factor independent of distress. Another interesting finding in this study is the association with depression. It has been suggested that tinnitus becomes problematic in those suffering from depression on other grounds (see above).

Hallam, Jakes and Hinchcliffe (1988) developed a tinnitus effects questionnaire which they factor analysed. This analysis produced three main dimensions of complaint. The authors labelled these dimensions emotional distress, auditory perceptual difficulties and sleep disturbance. These factors were statistically independent of each other. Insomnia and problems related to hearing were also identified in a previous study by these authors, with a different questionnaire.

These studies demonstrate that the way in which people are bothered by tinnitus varies and that different complaints are not strongly associated. Although lack of correlation can be simply due to a high degree of error, the extraction of different factors suggests this is not the case.

Kirk *et al.* (1990) reported the development of a tinnitus handicap questionnaire. They factor analysed a 27-item questionnaire. They obtained three common factors which they named physical, emotional and social consequences of tinnitus, hearing ability, and patients' view of tinnitus. None of these factors correlated with the loudness match. The consequences of tinnitus correlated at only $r = 0.56$ with subjective loudness reports. These findings broadly confirm the major findings of Jakes and colleagues (see below).

Tyler and Baker (1983) used an open-ended questionnaire to investigate different types of problems that tinnitus sufferers report. Responses were obtained from a tinnitus self-help group. They classified these problems on an ad hoc basis. The resulting categories were: effects on hearing, effects on life style, effects on general health, and emotional problems. There was a significant negative correlation between the number of problems reported and the duration of the tinnitus ($P = 0.029$). This implies that the passage of time (even in those who attend a tinnitus group and therefore presumably define themselves as having a problem), may reduce the overall number of problems that tinnitus causes.

Jakes *et al.* (1985) reported a factor analytical study of various complaints made about tinnitus, together with audiometric data, and certain information about reported symptoms. They used a varimax rotation, thus the resultant factors are orthogonal to one another, i.e. the different factors are not correlated. The tinnitus-complaint factors they obtained in order of extraction, were intrusiveness of the tinnitus, distress due to the tinnitus, insomnia and effect on passive listening activities. Audiometric indices of tinnitus intensity loaded separately. Hearing difficulties and vestibular symptoms were separate factors, and did not relate to problems with tinnitus. There is some degree of agreement between this study and the ad hoc categories of Tyler and Baker. It is not clear what predisposes a person to complain in these various different ways about tinnitus.

It is also unclear at this stage to what extent different dimensions of complaint reflect differential occurrence of different problems, or merely report of these problems.

In our latest factor analysis (Hallam, Jakes and Hincliffe, 1986) we included a series of unhelpful thoughts, beliefs and attitudes along with reports of particular difficulties. To a large extent these thoughts (e.g. 'It will be dreadful if this noise never stops' or 'It's unfair that I should suffer from this tinnitus') loaded on the emotional distress factor, but several smaller attitudinal factors were also found. These were labelled hopelessness, ability to ignore the noises and irrelevance of psychological factors. These were, of course, orthogonal factors. It seems possible, then, that many, but not all, of these sorts of belief are associated with emotional distress. Some of our recent therapeutic work has aimed at altering these beliefs in order to try to reduce emotional disturbance. To a large extent the factors which lead to differential complaints about tinnitus, (and indeed to complain about it at all) are unknown. Possible interactions with personality, noise sensitivity, previous illness experiences, religious convictions and practices and marital status are virtually unexplored. This is a profitable and important area for more research.

Psychological therapies for tinnitus

No attempt will be made here comprehensively to review psychological therapies. What counts as a psychological therapy is not easy to determine. The existence of the placebo effect gives drug treatment and indeed surgery (see Thomson *et al.*, 1983) a psychological component. Patients expect certain results, and feel optimistic or pessimistic. Suggestion and motivational factors serve to change personal habits, and so affect the physical condition in this way. However, they also affect illness behaviour – interpretation of physical disturbance as symptoms alter – as does the appraisal of the affect of symptoms.

Psychological therapy can have two basic aims for tinnitus sufferers: to abolish tinnitus or change its sensory qualities (e.g. make it quieter), or to reduce the adverse effects of the tinnitus on the person (e.g. reduce how annoying the tinnitus is, or the disruption it causes to sleep). A third aim, to help psychological problems causally unrelated to tinnitus to improve the ability to cope with the noise, will not be considered. Although this approach is indubitably valuable, it is not tinnitus-specific, and will thus be omitted. Hallam and Jakes (1985) reported a single case study in which treatment of psychological problems (other than the response to tinnitus) selectively reduced the distress due to tinnitus more than the loudness of the tinnitus.

Possible mechanisms by which various psychological therapies might reduce the loudness of tinnitus or abolish it altogether are unclear.

Hypnosis

Hypnotherapy has been used on occasions. A variety of different suggestions has been made during hypnosis. Sometimes patients visualize a dial and it is suggested that as the dial is turned down the tinnitus will become quieter. Another approach is to suggest relaxation to the subject despite tinnitus. Marlowe (1973) reported the successful use of a mixture of these techniques on three patients.

Marks, Karl and Onisphorou (1985) used a cross-over design to evaluate three types of hypnotic intervention. These were induction of hypnotic state alone, ego boosting during hypnosis, and suggestions of active suppression of the tinnitus. Each treatment was given for 2 weekly sessions with 3 weeks between treatments. Patients rated the loudness and unpleasantness of the tinnitus on visual analogue scales; loudness matching was also conducted. Five of the 14 patients found that the induction of hypnosis was helpful, making tinnitus more tolerable. One of the 14 found the active suppression helpful. No differences in loudness matching were found. Although no placebo condition was used it is moderately encouraging that some patients found the hypnotic induction helpful. Attias *et al.* (1990) treated tinnitus by self-hypnosis and two other conditions (waiting list or presenting a brief stimulus to the tinnitus ear). They reported the disappearance of tinnitus in 73% of the self-hypnosis group during the treatment sessions and significant improvement following treatment. This study, conducted on army personnel, is notable in the remarkable effects of the treatment on the perception of tinnitus. The most likely explanation is that the peculiar circumstances of being on active service increased dissimulation or suggestibility.

Biofeedback

House (1978) used biofeedback with 41 tinnitus patients to teach relaxation. This was intended to influence the tinnitus. Patients kept daily tinnitus charts recording how loud the tinnitus was. Thirty-three of the 41 patients showed improvement on the diaries. At one year post-treatment seven patients reported they were 'much improved' or 'very much improved', 16 'slightly improved' and 18 'no change'. House reported that many patients became less aggravated by understanding the role of tension in precipitating tinnitus. No control condition was used so it is hard to evaluate the outcome.

Borton, Moor and Clark (1981) reported using electromyographic (EMG) feedback from the frontalis muscle using an experimental single subject reversal design. Although EMG activity responded to treatment, there was no improvement in ratings of tinnitus loudness, annoyance or loudness match levels.

Grossan (1976) used biofeedback with 51 patients; 40 of the patients reported some therapeutic improvement at the end of a short course. It seems improvement was measured simply by report. No control condition was used.

Haralambous *et al.* (1987) compared biofeedback with neutral instruction to biofeedback with counterdemand exercises. They found no significant difference, or indeed any effect in either group.

As biofeedback is used simply to induce relaxation, an alternative approach has been simply to train tinnitus patients in progressive muscle relaxation.

Relaxation training

Ireland *et al.* (1985) gave relaxation training to 30 tinnitus patients. Pre-, post- and mid-treatment assessments of self-reported tinnitus loudness/insomnia were made. Mood was assessed pre- and post-treatment, as was the loudness match. Relaxation training was compared with a waiting list control. No significant differences were found, except for the Beck Depression Inventory scores which were lower after treatment. No assessment of annoyance *about* tinnitus was made.

Scott *et al.* (1985) used relaxation training combined with certain cognitive techniques in the treatment of tinnitus patients. Treatment involved 10 hourly sessions of learning progressive muscle relaxation, conditioned relaxation and quick relaxation. It also involved 'perceptual restructuring', i.e. training of distraction using exercises to relocate attention. Patients imagined a scene which was associated with tinnitus being particularly troublesome and, when the patient's attention was directed to the tinnitus, quick relaxation was introduced. Visualization of a pleasant scene then followed. Finally, this procedure was used in difficult real-life situations. A waiting list group served as a control. Dependent variables were daily diaries of tinnitus loudness and discomfort from the tinnitus. They also rated depression and irritability for the whole day. Loudness matching (dB HL) or a tone pitch matched to the tinnitus was also undertaken. Significant improvements were found in diary-rated loudness, discomfort and in depression. No significant change in the matched loudness of tinnitus was found.

Jakes *et al.* (1986) investigated relaxation training only and combined with a cognitive technique distraction training. Every patient was also assessed during a pre-therapy period during which a booklet was provided which gave information about the role of attitudes, thoughts and beliefs in maintaining attention to tinnitus and distress about tinnitus. The dependent variables were factor-scores from a tinnitus questionnaire – distress, auditory perceptual difficulties and insomnia, a check list of interference with a number of activities and diary records of loudness and annoyance of tinnitus. These measures were made before and after the pre-treatment period as well as after therapy. The Crown Crisp Experiential Index was administered at the beginning of the orientation phase and after therapy. Auditory perceptual difficulties did not change during therapy, and the diary-rated loudness decreased only slowly (this decrease achieved significance by the end of treatment). Most other variables decreased constantly during orientation and therapy phases. However, the annoyance of tinnitus decreased faster once treatment began than during the orientation phase.

Taking the studies of Jakes *et al.* (1986) and Scott *et al.* (1985) together, it seems that relaxation training is more effective than a waiting list control and that distraction training adds little or nothing to simple relaxation. Self-rated annoyance seems to respond to therapy before self-rated loudness.

Not only did Ireland *et al.* (1985) find no significant difference between waiting list and relaxation groups but no change across time was found in either therapy group. That is, failure to demonstrate a difference was *not* due to a control group who also improved. How is the difference between Ireland and her colleagues' study and the other studies mentioned above to be explained? The most obvious difference between their procedure and that used in the other relaxation studies is that in both other studies relaxation training was incorporated into a more general cognitive approach. The utility of applied relaxation for many different problems (including tinnitus) has been reported by several authors. This may suggest that it is worth trying to understand a common mechanism of treatment.

Lindberg *et al.* (1987) followed up 20 patients with tinnitus 9 months after behavioural treatment. They found that the self-reported discomfort caused by tinnitus was still reduced after this period of time. However, the loudness of tinnitus and associated depression and irritation did not remain reduced. This finding (a selective effect of psychological therapy on the *distress* associated with tinnitus) is replicated in many of the studies reported above. As it seems unlikely that psychological treatment would affect the intensity of the tinnitus, this selective effect could be argued to be evidence of a genuine response rather than simply a response given by the therapist. Unfortunately, there is no control group for this follow-up period.

Kirsch, Blanchard and Parnes (1987) treated six tinnitus sufferers using relaxation training and biofeedback. Ratings made by the patients of the effect of their tinnitus on them improved. However, there was much less change in the daily diary ratings. Unfortunately, although the authors claimed that their patients were treated because their lives were 'significantly affected' by their tinnitus the average diary ratings *pre*-treatment indicate tinnitus was a 'slight problem'. It may be that this indicates that their diary scale was in some way not sensitive or that the subjects did not complete them correctly. It could be that tinnitus was severely troublesome but, intermittently so, so that the effects are obscured by averaging. However, why Jakes *et al.* (1986), using a similar treatment *did* find improvement in diary ratings of the annoyance of tinnitus is obscure. Possibly all that can be said is that if similar results do not come from different centres replication must be called for. One possibility which seems important to address is that disparate results may be due to different subject populations. More description of the patients included in the studies is to be encouraged (e.g. Do the clients have major problems in other areas of their life? Is there any possibility of secondary gain?). Alternatively if the lack of effect when tinnitus is measured in this way is accurate, this lack of correspondence requires further investigation.

Cognitive psychotherapy

Cognitive techniques have been reported by several authors. By cognitive techniques is meant any procedure which seeks to help the sufferers by manipulation of thoughts, beliefs, attitudes or imagery.

Sweetow (1985) has used cognitive therapy which concentrated on altering the beliefs and attitudes of the patients in groups. This focuses on demonstrating to patients that they engage in a series of cognitive distortions (e.g. over generalization 'Tinnitus bothers me all the time'). The patient's reaction to the tinnitus is taken as the focus of treatment.

Although no formal results are reported Sweetow claimed that they have found this more effective than tinnitus maskers and biofeedback.

Jakes *et al.* (1993) randomly allocated patients to five treatment conditions: group cognitive therapy, group cognitive therapy plus the provision of a tinnitus masker, a tinnitus masker, a placebo masker, and waiting list control group. Only patients who received cognitive therapy were improved at 3-month follow up. These patients were improved in that the distress occasioned by tinnitus had reduced.

Loumidis, Hallam and Cadge (1991) tested the hypothesis (derived from the studies reported by Jakes and Hallam above) that the provision of a booklet which gave information about tinnitus and which explained a coping model of tinnitus would reduce distress by itself. They gave such a booklet to a random sample of patients presenting with a main complaint of tinnitus. There was no difference between patients who were given the booklet and those who were not. They gave the TEQ to both groups at their second appointment. This study rules out one explanation of the decrease in distress in the previous studies. It is unclear why there was a decrease in emotional distress prior to treatment. The authors suggested that possible explanations include the expectation of treatment or that the effects were the result of prior medical reassurance (not given in the study). Clearly this requires further investigation.

Conclusion

Most of the research in this area has been conducted within the psychosomatic/somatopsychic paradigm. Although these questions are valid and interesting they leave out many psychosocial factors of the utmost importance. These have to do, broadly, with what has been described as illness behaviour, the process whereby bodily occurrences are defined as medical symptoms, and the medical symptoms (so defined) are considered sufficiently troublesome to be presented to a doctor. Illness behaviour also incorporates various coping strategies, so that the degree to which the problems are compensated or decompensated is also involved.

These can seem like side issues if one understands medicine as diagnosis and removal of the cause of the illness. 'Whatever the patients thinks *we* know if it's an illness or not'. However, in the field of rehabilitation these issues are crucial (see Stephens, Hallam and Jakes (1986) for an application to tinnitus). If we continue to see them as 'obvious' side issues we are ignoring a large area of study which might help us to help our patients. After all converting a decompensated symptom to a compensated one must be worthwhile. It may be necessary to understand how patients end up complaining of a symptom in order to do this.

One important way in which these issues could be examined is demonstrated by some of the more recent work examining tinnitus patients. In particular the developing work using cognitive therapy has important theoretical implications. If it can be demonstrated that illness behaviour can be affected by direct manipulation of the way in which the signs and symptoms are construed then this is experimental evidence that these processes exist and are of importance (Jakes *et al.*, 1985; Scott *et al.*, 1985; Sweetow, 1985). Such psychological interventions also have the added advantage that they are clearly needed on clinical grounds. There is a high level of distress associated with chronic neuro-otological problems to

which there is no medical solution. Psychological intervention is a positive alternative which seems most promising. The techniques which are being developed with tinnitus patients seems to be equally applicable to hearing impairment and vertigo. It is hoped that psychologists will take on the challenge of making this application.

References

ATTIAS, T., SHEMESH, Z., SHAHAM, C. and SHAHAR, A. (1990) Efficacy of self-hypnosis for tinnitus relief. *Scandinavian Audiology*, **19**, 245–249

BARCHAM, L. J. and STEPHENS, S. D. G. (1980) The use of an open-ended problems questionnaire in auditory rehabilitation. *British Journal of Audiology*, **14**, 49–58

BORTON, T., MOOR, W. and CLARK, S. (1981) Electromyographic feedback for tinnitus aurium. *Journal of Speech and Hearing Disorders*, **46**, 39–45

BRIGHTWELL, D. R. and ABRAMSON, N. (1975) Personality characteristics in patients with vertigo. *Archives of Otolaryngology*, **101**, 364–366

CARLSSON, S. and ERLANDSSON, S. (1991) Habituation and tinnitus: an experimental study. *Journal of Psychosomatic Research*, **35**, 509–514

COOPER, A. F., CURRY, A. R., KAY, D. W. K., GARSIDE, R. F. and ROTH, M. (1974) Hearing loss in paranoid and affective psychoses of the elderly. *Lancet*, ii, 851–854

CRARY, W. G. and WEXLER, M. (1977) Meniere's disease: a psychosomatic disorder? *Psychological Reports*, **41**, 604–645

ELLIS, A. (1962) *Reason and Emotion in Psychotherapy.* New York: Lyle Stuart

FEWTRELL, W. and O'CONNOR, K. P. (1988) Dizziness and depersonalisation. *Advances in Behaviour Research and Therapy*, **10**, 201–218

FOWLER, E. P. and FOWLER, E. P. JR (1955) Somatopsychic and psychosomatic factors in tinnitus, deafness and vertigo. *Annals of Otology, Rhinology and Laryngology*, **64**, 29–37

FOWLER, E. P. JR and ZECKEL, A. (1952) Psychosomatic aspects of Meniere's disease. *Journal of the American Medical Association*. **148**, 1265–1268

FOWLER, E. P. JR and ZECKEL, A. (1953) Psychophysiological factors in Meniere's disease. *Psychosomatic Medicine*, **15**, 127–129

FREUD, S. (1895) On the grounds for detaching a particular syndrome from neurasthenia under the description of 'anxiety neurosis'. In the *Standard Edition*, III, London: Hogarth

GILDSTON, H. and GILDSTON, P. (1972) Personality changes associated with surgically corrected hypoacusis. *Audiology*, **11**, 354–367

GILHOME HERBST, K. and HUMPHREY, C. (1980) Hearing impairment and mental state in the elderly living at home. *British Medical Journal*, **281**, 903–905

GLASS, D. C. and SINGER, J. E. (1972) *Urban Stress*, New York: Academic Press

GRIGSBY, J. P. and JOHNSTON, C. L. (1989) Depersonalisation, vertigo and Menieres disease. *Psychological Reports*, **64**, 527–534

GROSSAN, M. (1976) Treatment of subjective tinnitus with bio-feedback. *Ear Nose and Throat Journal*, **55**, 314–318

HALLAM, R. S. and HINCHCLIFFE, R. (1991) Emotional stability: its relationship to confidence in maintaining balance. *Journal of Psychosomatic Research*, **35**, 421–430

HALLAM, R. S. and JAKES, S. C. (1985) Tinnitus: differential effects of therapy in a single case. *Behaviour Research and Therapy*, **23**, 691–694

HALLAM, R. S. and STEPHENS, S. D. G. (1985) Vestibular disorders and emotional distress. *Journal of Psychosomatic Research*, **29**, 408–413

HALLAM, R., JAKES, S. and HINCHCLIFFE, R. (1988) Cognitive variables in tinnitus annoyance. *British Journal of Clinical Psychology*, **27**, 213–222

HALLAM, R. S., PRASANSUK, S. and HINCHCLIFFE, R. (1983) Neuroticism and the number of complaints of ENT outpatients in London and Bangkok. *Personality and Individual Differences*, **4**, 689–691

HALLAM, R. S., RACHMAN, S. and HINCHCLIFFE, R. (1984) Psychological aspects of tinnitus. In: *Contributions to Medical Psychology*, Vol. 3, edited by S. Rachman. Oxford: Pergamon Press. pp. 31–54

HALLAM, R. S., JAKES, S. C., CHAMBERS, C. and HINCHCLIFFE, R. (1985) A comparison of different methods for assessing the 'intensity' of tinnitus. *Acta Otolaryngologica*, **99**, 501–508

HARALAMBOUS, G., WILSON, P., PLATT-HEPWORTH, S. and TOMKIN, J. (1987) EMG biofeedback in the treatment of tinnitus: an experimental evaluation. *Behaviour Research and Therapy*, **25**, 49–55

HARRE, R. and SECORD, P. (1976) *The Explanation of Social Behaviour*. Oxford: Basil Blackwell

HARROP-GRIFFITHS, J., KATON, W., DOBIE, R., SAKAI, G. and RUSSO, J. (1987) Chronic tinnitus: association with psychiatric diagnosis. *Journal of Psychosomatic Research*, **31**, 613–621

HAZELL, J. (ed.) (1981) Measurement of tinnitus in humans. In: *Tinnitus*. Ciba Foundation, London: Pitman Books Ltd

HELLER, M. F. and BERGMANN, M. (1953) Tinnitus aurium in normally hearing persons, *Annals of Otology*, **62**, 73

HINCHCLIFFE, R. (1965) *A Psychophysiological Investigation into Vertigo*. Unpublished PhD thesis. University of London

HINCHCLIFFE, R. (1967a) Emotion as a precipitating factor in Meniere's disease. *Journal of Laryngology and Otology*, **81**, 471–475

HINCHCLIFFE, R. (1967b) An attempt to classify the primary vertigos. *Journal of Laryngology and Otology*, **81**, 849–859

HINCHCLIFFE, R. (1967c) Personal and family medical history in Meniere's disease. *Journal of Laryngology and Otology*, **81**, 661–668

HINCHCLIFFE, R. and CHAMBERS, C. (1983) Loudness of tinnitus: an approach to measurement. *Advances in Oto-Rhino-Laryngology*, **29**, 163–173

HINCHCLIFFE, R. and KING, P. (1992) Medicolegal aspects of tinnitus. I: medicolegal position and current state of knowledge. *Journal of Audiological Medicine*, **1**, 38–52

HOLTON, S. A. (1978) Not so different: spatial and distancing behaviour of deaf adults. *American Annals of the Deaf*, December, 920–924

HOUSE, J. W. (1978) Treatment of severe tinnitus with biofeedback training. *Laryngoscope*, **88**, 406–412

HOUSTON, F. and ROYSE, A. B. (1954) Relationship between deafness and psychiatric illness. *Journal of Mental Science*, **100**, 990–993

HUMPHREY, C., GILHOME HERBST, H. and FAURQI, S. (1981) Some characteristics of the hearing-impaired elderly who do not present themselves for rehabilitation. *British Journal of Audiology*, **15**, 25–30

INGALLS, G. S. (1946) Some psychiatric observations on patients with hearing defect. *Occupational Therapy and Rehabilitation*, **25**, 62–66

IRELAND, C. E., WILSON, P. H., TONKIN, J. P. and PLATT-HEPWORTH, S. (1985) An evaluation of relaxation training in the treatment of tinnitus. *Behaviour Research and Therapy*, **23**, 423–430

JAKES, S. C., HALLAM, R. S., CHAMBERS, C. and HINCHCLIFFE, R. (1985) A factor analytical study of tinnitus complaint behaviour. *Audiology*, **24**, 195–206

JAKES, S. C., HALLAM, R. S., CHAMBERS, C. and HINCHCLIFFE, R. (1986) Matched and self-reported loudness of tinnitus: methods and sources of error. *Audiology*, **25**, 92–100

JAKES, S., HALLAM, R. S., MCKENNA, L. and HINCHCLIFFE, R. (1993) Group cognitive therapy for medical patients. An application to tinnitus. *Cognitive Therapy and Research*, **16**, 67–82

JAKES, S. C., HALLAM, R. S., RACHMAN, S. and HINCHCLIFFE, R. (1986) The effects of relaxation training and distraction on chronic tinnitus sufferers. *Behaviour Research and Therapy*, **24**, 497–507

JONES, D. LA., VICTOR, C. A. and VETTER, N. J. (1984) Hearing difficulty and its psychological implications for the elderly. *Journal of Epidemiology and Community Health*, **38**, 75–78

KALAYAM, B., ALEXOPOULOUS, G., MERRELL, H. and YOUNG, R. (1991) Patterns of hearing loss and psychiatric morbidity in elderly patients attending a hearing clinic. *International Journal of Geriatric Psychiatry*, **6**, 131–136

KAY, D. W. K. and ROTH, M. (1961) Environmental and hereditary factors in the schizophrenias of old age ('late paraphrenia') and their bearing on the general problem of causation in schizophrenia. *Journal of Mental Science*, **107**, 649–686

KING, K. and STEPHENS, D. (1992) Auditory and psychological factors in auditory disability with normal hearing. *Scandinavian Audiology*, **21**, 109–114

KIRK, F., TYLER, R., RUSSELL, D. and JORDAN, H. (1990) The psychometric properties of a tinnitus handicap questionnaire. *Ear and Hearing*, **11**, 434–445

KIRSCH, C. A., BLANCHARD, E. B. and PARNES, S. (1987) A multiple baseline evaluation of the treatment of subjective tinnitus with relaxation training and biofeedback. *Biofeedback and Self Regulation*, **12**, 295–312

KIRSCH, C., BLANCHARD, E. and PARNES, S. (1989) Psychological characteristics of individuals high and low in their ability to cope with tinnitus. *Psychosomatic Medicine*, **51**, 209–217

KNAPP, P. H. (1948) Emotional aspects of hearing loss. *Psychosomatic Medicine*, **10**, 203–222

KNUTTSON, J. and LANSING, C. (1990) The relationships between communication problems and psychological difficulties in persons with profound acquired hearing loss. *Journal of Speech and Hearing Disorders*, **55**, 656–664

LEVY, I and O'LEARY, J. L. (1947) Incidence of vertigo in neurologic conditions. *Transactions of the American Otologic Society*, **35**, 329–347

LEWIS, J., STEPHENS, D. and HUWS, D. (1992) Suicide in tinnitus patients. *Journal of Audiological Medicine*, **1**, 30–37

LINDBERG, P., SCOTT, B., MELIN, L. and LYTTKENS, L. (1987) Long term effects of psychological treatment of tinnitus. *Scandinavian Audiology*, **16**, 167–172

LOUMIDIS, K. S., HALLAM, R. S. and CADGE, B. (1991) The

effect of written reassuring information on out-patients complaining of tinnitus. *British Journal of Audiology*, **25**, 105–109

MCKENNA, L. (1986) The psychological assessment of cochlear implant patients. *British Journal of Audiology*, **20**, 29–34

MCKENNA, L. and DENMAN, C. (1993) Repertory grid technique in the assessment of cochlear-implant patients. *Journal of Audiological Medicine*, **2**, 75–84

MCKENNA, L., HALLAM, R. S. and HINCHCLIFFE, R. (1991) The prevalence of psychological disturbance in neuro-otology patients. *Clinical Otolaryngology*, **16**, 452–456

MAHAPATRA, S. B. (1974) Deafness and mental health: psychiatric and psychosomatic illness in the deaf. *Acta Psychiatrica Scandinavica*, **50**, 596–611

MARKS, N. J., KARL, H. and ONISPHOROU, C. (1985) A controlled trial of hypnotherapy in tinnitus. *Clinical Otolaryngology*, **10**, 43–46

MARLOWE, F. I. (1973) Effective treatment of tinnitus through hypnotherapy. *American Journal of Clinical Hypnosis*, **15**, 162–165

MASTERS, W. and JOHNSON, V. (1970) *Human Sexual Inadequacy*. New York: Little, Brown and Co

MECHANIC, D. (1980) The experience and reporting of common physical complaints. *Journal of Health and Social Behaviour*, **21**, 146–155

NOBLE, W. (1978) *Assessment of Hearing Impairment*. New York: Academic Press

O'CONNOR, K., HINCHCLIFFE, R. and CHAMBERS, C. (1989) Dizziness and perceptual style. *Psychotherapy and Psychosomatics*, **51**, 169–174

OFFICE OF POPULATION CENSUSES AND SURVEYS (1983) *The Prevalence of Tinnitus 1981*. General Household Survey. London: OPCS

PENNER, M. J. (1983) The annoyance of tinnitus and the noise required to mask it. *Journal of Speech and Hearing Research*, **26**, 73–76

PRATT, R. T. C. and MCKENZIE, W. (1958) Anxiety states following vestibular disorders. *Lancet*, ii, 347–349

RAHE, R., FLOISTAD, I., BERGAN, T., RINGDAL, R., GERHARDT, R., GUNDERSON, E. *et al.* (1974) A model for life changes and illness research. *Archives of General Psychiatry*, **31**, 172–177

RAMSDELL, D. A. (1970) The psychology of the hard of hearing and the deafened adult. In: *Hearing and Deafness*, edited by H. Davis and S. R. Silverman. New York: Holt, Richard and Winston. pp. 499–510

REED, G. (1960) An audiometric study of two hundred cases of subjective tinnitus. *Archives of Otolaryngology*, **71**, 94–104

SCHARF, B. and STEVENS, J. (1959) The form of loudness function near threshold. *Proceedings of 3rd International Congress of Accoustics*, Stuttgart. Amsterdam: Elsevier

SCOTT, B., LINDBERG, P., LYTTKENS, L. and MELIN, L. (1985) Psychological treatment of tinnitus. An experimental group study. *Scandinavian Audiology*, **14**, 223–230

SINGERMAN, B., RIEDNER, E. and FOLSTEIN, M. (1980) Emotional disturbance in hearing clinic patients. *British Journal of Psychiatry*, **137**, 58–62

SLATER, E. (1965) Diagnosis of hysteria. *British Medical Journal*, **1**, 1395–1399

STEPHENS, D., LEWIS, P. and CHARNY, M. (1990) Are attitude and lifestyle important health factors in the hearing disabled elderly? In: *Presbyacusis and Other Age Related Aspects. Proceedings of the 14th Danavox Symposium*, edited by J. H. Jensen. Copenhagen: Danavox. pp. 239–252

STEPHENS, S. D. G. (1975) Personality tests in Meniere's disorder. *Journal of Laryngology and Otology*, **89**, 479–490

STEPHENS, S. D. G. (1980) Evaluating the problems of the hearing impaired. *Audiology*, **19**, 205–220

STEPHENS, S. D. G. and HALLAM, R. S. (1985) The Crown-Crisp experiential index in patients complaining of tinnitus. *British Journal of Audiology*, **19**, 151–158

STEPHENS, S. D. G., HALLAM, R. S. and JAKES, S. C. (1986) Tinnitus: a management model: 2 *Clinical Otolaryngology*, **11**, 227–238

STEPHENS, S. D. G., HOGAN, S. and MEREDITH. R. (1991) The desynchrony between complaints and signs of vestibular disorders. *Acta Otolaryngologica*, **111**, 188–192

STEPHENS, S. D. G., LEWIS. P. A., CHARNY, M. C., FARROW, S. C. and FRANCIS. M. (1990) Characteristics of self-reported hearing problems in a community survey. *Audiology*, **29**, 93–100

STEPTOE. P. (1980) Stress and medical disorders. In: *Contributions to Medical Psychology*, II, edited by S. Rachman, Oxford: Pergamon Press. pp. 139–158

STEVENS, J. J. (1982) Some psychological problems of acquired deafness. *British Journal of Psychiatry*, **140**, 453–456

SULLIVAN, M., KATON, W., DOBIE, R., SATAI, C., RUSSO, J. and HARROP-GRIFFITHS, J. (1988) Disabling tinnitus: association with affective disorder. *General Hospital Psychiatry*, **10**, 285–291

SWEETOW, R. W. (1985) Cognitive behavioural modification in tinnitus management. *Hearing Instruments*, **35**, 14–52

TESSLER, R. and MECHANIC, D. (1978) Psychological distress and perceived health state. *Journal of Health and Social Behaviour*, **19**, 254–262

THOMAS, A. J. (1981a) Acquired deafness and mental health. *British Journal of Medical Psychology*, **54**, 219–229

THOMAS, A. J. (1981b) The effect of severe hearing loss on personality. *IRCS Medical Science*, **9**, 941–942

THOMAS, A. J. (1984) *Acquired Hearing Loss: Psychological and Psychosocial Implications*. London: Academic Press

THOMAS, A. and GILHOME-HERBST, K. (1980) Social and psychological implications of acquired deafness for adults of employment age. *British Journal of Audiology*, **14**, 76–85

THOMAS, A., LAMONT, M. and HARRIS, M. (1982) Problems encountered at work by people with severe acquired hearing loss. *British Journal of Audiology*, **16**, 39–43

THOMSEN, J., BRETLAU, P., TOS, M. and JOHNSEN, N. J. (1981) Placebo effect in surgery for Meniere's disease. *Archives of Otolaryngology*, **107**, 271–277

THOMSEN, J., BRETLAU, P., TOS, M. and JOHNSEN, N. J. (1983) Meniere's disease: a 3 year follow-up of patients in a double-blind placebo-controlled study on endolymphatic sac shunt surgery. *Advances in Oto-rhino-Laryngology*, **30**, 350–354

TYLER, R. S. and BAKER, L. J. (1983) Difficulties experienced by tinnitus sufferers. *Journal of Speech and Hearing Disorders*, **48**, 150–154

WADDELL, G., BIRCHER, M., FINLAYSON, D. and MAIN, C. J. (1984) Symptoms and signs: physical disease or illness behaviour? *British Medical Journal*, **289**, 739–741

WATSON, S., HENGGELER, S. and WHELAN, J. P. (1990) Family functioning and the social adaptation of hearing-impaired youths. *Journal of Abnormal Child Psychology*, **18**, 143–163

WEBB, D. R. B. and WARREN, C. H. E. (1967) An investigation into the effects of bangs on the subjective reaction of a community. *Journal of Sound and Vibration*, **6**, 375

WILSON, P., HENRY J., BOWEN, M. and HARALAMBOUS, G. (1991) Tinnitus reaction questionnaire: psychometric properties of a measure of distress associated with tinnitus. *Journal of Speech and Hearing Research*, **34**, 197–201

YARDLEY, L., TODD, W., LACOUDRAYE-HARTER, M. and INGHAM, R. (1992) Psychosocial consequences of recurrent vertigo. *Psychology and Health*, **6**, 85–96

5

Clinical tests of hearing and balance

I. R. C. Swan

Clinical tests of hearing

Prior to the introduction of pure-tone audiometry into clinical practice in the 1940s, clinical tests were the only means of assessing hearing. Most tests employed either the human voice or tuning forks, though various other instruments and ingeniously devised tools were also used. Nowadays, hearing is usually assessed by pure-tone audiometry but this is not always readily available. Even when it is available, reliable results require, among other things, a competent technician and a cooperative patient. Few otologists will invariably rely upon audiometric thresholds without confirming that they are compatible with their own clinical assessment.

There are three main aims in clinical assessment of hearing:

1 Estimation of threshold
2 Differentiation of conductive and sensorineural impairment
3 Identification of non-organic hearing loss.

Estimation of threshold

Clinical voice tests

Voice tests are probably the oldest test used to assess hearing. The human voice has a wide intensity range, but only three intensities should be used clinically in order to provide a degree of standardization: a whispered voice, a conversational voice, and a loud voice.

A whispered voice is usually described as a forced whisper – the loudest whisper that the clinician can produce. Traditionally it was held that the clinician should exhale normally prior to making the forced whisper, though it seems unlikely that such a whisper

will be significantly different from one made without exhaling. The important limiting factor is that the vocal cords should be abducted throughout. A conversational voice represents the intensity used by the clinician when conversing normally in a quiet room. A loud voice is as loud a shout as the clinician can comfortably produce.

The clinician should take care to stand to one side of the patient so that visual clues are excluded. Stimuli should be simple so that they are readily understood by all patients. Suitable stimuli are combinations of three numerals (e.g. 6–1–4). The patient is asked to repeat whatever she hears. A positive test result is when the patient is able to repeat correctly more than 50% of the stimuli presented.

Tests are commonly carried out at distances of 60 cm (2 feet) and 15 cm (6 inches) from the patient's ear. Sixty centimetres (two feet) represents arm's length from the non-test ear as it is essential to mask the non-test ear during all testing (see below). Hearing may be assessed by forced whisper at greater distances; a normally hearing individual will easily hear a whispered voice at 10 m.

The author's voice levels at each intensity for 10 test items were recorded on each of 4 days to assess his own consistency (Table 5.1). The intensity of voice used in these three categories by different clinicians will vary, but an individual clinician should maintain his or her own consistency. The clinician should also be aware of the tendency to raise the voice as the distance from the patient increases, i.e. the voice used at 60 cm (2 feet) tends to be louder than that used at 15 cm (6 inches) unless care is taken to avoid this (King, 1953). Table 5.2 shows the equivalent pure-tone audiometric thresholds for a range of voice test thresholds in a prospective study of 101 patients tested by two otologists (Swan, 1984). The whispered voice test at 60 cm (2 feet) can detect

Table 5.1 Voice levels of the author at each intensity and distance

Voice	Mean (dBA)	Standard deviation
WV (2 ft)	51	3
WV (6 in)	54	3
CV (2 ft)	73	8
CV (6 in)	76	8
LV (2 ft)	92	7

Swan, 1984
WV = whispered voice; CV = conversational voice; LV = loud voice.

Table 5.2 Comparison of voice test thresholds with pure-tone audiometric thresholds (mean of 0.5, 1, 2 and 4 kHz) in 101 patients

Voice test threshold	10th centile	Mean (dB HL)	90th centile
WV (2 ft)		12	25
WV (6 in)	22	34	45
CV (2 ft)	40	48	60
CV (6 in)	48	56	62
LV (2 ft)	67	76	87

Swan, 1984
WV = whispered voice; CV = conversational voice; LV = loud voice.

a speech-frequency hearing impairment greater than 30 dB with a sensitivity of 96% and a specificity of 91% (Browning, Swan and Chew, 1989). These data provide a rough guide to interpretation of voice tests, but are no substitute for the experience gained by a clinician comparing his or her own voice test results with pure-tone audiometric thresholds.

Masking for voice tests

Shaw (1974) quantified the effect of location of a sound source on the amount of sound energy arriving at the tympanic membrane. The difference in the sound energy arriving at the tympanic membrane of the test and non-test ears is commonly known as the head shadow effect (Table 5.3). When using voice tests, the sound source is usually at an azimuth of 90° and the attenuation of sound at the non-test ear is small, so it is essential to mask the non-test ear. This can be achieved by tragal rubbing or the use of a Bárány noise box.

Tragal rubbing requires occlusion of the external auditory meatus by fingertip pressure on the tragus. The clinician's finger is then gently rotated thus producing a broad band noise in the patient's external

Table 5.3 The difference in the sound pressure level at each tympanic membrane with a sound source at 90° azimuth

Frequency (kHz)	0.25	0.5	1	2	3	4	6	8
Attenuation (dB)	4	6	7	9	12	13	21	18

Data adapted from Shaw, 1974

ear. The masking noise thus produced is sufficient to attenuate speech by about 60 dB (range of attenuation 45–75 dB) (Swan, 1989). This is adequate to mask a whispered or conversational voice in the contralateral ear (Swan, 1989). Tragal rubbing has the major advantage that there is no cross-masking of the other ear because the noise is confined within the external auditory canal.

The Bárány noise box is a traditional method of masking the non-test ear which produces broad band noise in the region of 100 dB(A). As the sound levels recorded at the contralateral external auditory meatus are over 60 dB(A) (Swan, 1989), the Bárány noise box is not a suitable instrument for masking the non-test ear while using a whispered voice as there will be over-masking of the test ear. The use of the Bárány noise box in clinical voice testing should be restricted to occasions on which it is necessary to use a loud voice as a stimulus.

Other methods of masking the non-test ear have been described in the past, such as rubbing tissue paper over the external ear. The efficacy of such methods is difficult to assess as there are many variables, such as the type of paper used. These other methods are rarely used.

Limitation of voice tests

Clinical voice tests are not a substitute for pure-tone audiometry. They are, however, an essential tool for the otologist to check unreliable audiometry (Browning, Swan and Chew, 1989) and especially unreliable patients (see Non-organic hearing loss below). They are also frequently used in testing those patients unable to comply with pure-tone audiometry, for example the very young, the mentally handicapped and the very old.

Other methods

Finger-snapping or finger-friction tests are of minimal value in assessing hearing thresholds as the stimulus cannot be standardized. Lever pocket watch tests have been made obsolete by the widespread use of quartz watches. An account of these and other historical tests is given by Hinchcliffe (1987).

Differentiation of conductive and sensorineural impairment

A careful history will usually lead the clinician to suspect either a conductive or a sensorineural hearing impairment. Associated symptoms of otorrhoea or otalgia usually indicate a conductive impairment while the complaint of difficulty making out what is said despite hearing the spoken voice is suggestive of a sensorineural impairment. If otoscopy reveals significant pathology in the external or middle ear then there will be a conductive component to the hearing impairment. The clinician must remember however that many impairments are mixed, i.e. have a conductive and a sensorineural component.

Tuning fork tests

Tuning fork tests were the traditional method of differentiating conductive from sensorineural impairments prior to the advent of pure-tone audiometry. Numerous tests have been described in the past and these tests are usually named after their inventors who were mostly 19th century physicians. Only those few tests which are still in use in modern audiological practice will be described. An account of the early history of tuning fork tests is given by Ng and Jackler (1993). Sheehy, Gardner and Hambley (1971) provide a description of other rarely used tests. Hinchcliffe (1987) gives a comprehensive historical account of tuning fork tests.

Tuning fork tests should be carried out in a reasonably quiet room as excessive ambient noise may significantly influence the results. The most commonly used tuning forks are those tuned to 256 or 512 Hz. Though the 256 Hz fork produces more overtones than the 512 Hz fork (Samuel and Eitelberg, 1989), it has been shown in clinical practice to be more sensitive in detecting air-bone gaps than the 512 Hz fork (Stankiewicz and Mowry, 1979; Doyle, Anderson and Pijl, 1984; Browning and Swan, 1988).

The fork should not be struck on a hard surface as this may produce overtones which may give a false result and, in addition, the fork may be damaged (Samuel and Eitelberg, 1989). It should be struck gently on the elbow or knee or on a hard rubber pad. Striking the fork about two-thirds of the way along the tines will minimize distortion products.

Before carrying out any tuning fork test, it is important to assess the overall severity of the hearing impairment by voice testing, as ignorance of the patient's hearing thresholds may lead to misinterpretation of tuning fork test results.

Rinne test

The Rinne tuning fork test was described in detail by Heinrich Rinne in 1855 though Huizing (1975)

noted that Polansky (1842) had earlier described the principles of the test. There are two main variations of the test: the loudness comparison method and the threshold comparison method.

The loudness comparison method is the more commonly used method. The fork is struck and held with the tines either parallel to or perpendicular to the axis of the external auditory canal (Samuel and Eitelberg, 1989) and the tips of the tines approximately 2.5 cm from the external auditory meatus (Figure 5.1a). The clinician should confirm that the patient

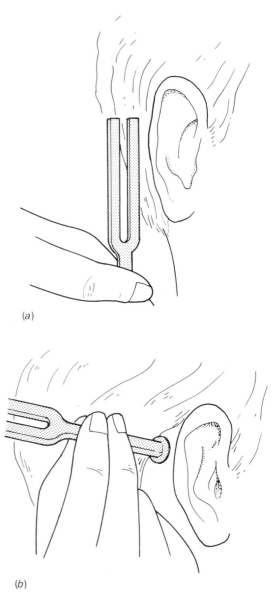

(a)

(b)

Figure 5.1 Placement of the tuning fork in the Rinne test (*a*) for air conduction and (*b*) bone conduction

can hear the fork 'in front of the ear'. The fork is then immediately transferred so that the base of the fork is pressed firmly against the bone overlying the mastoid. The preferred site is the flat area of non-hair bearing skin immediately posterior and superior to the external auditory canal (Figure 5.1b). Placing the fork over the tip of the mastoid process will give false results because an insufficient area of the base of the fork will be in contact with the bone. Care should be taken to ensure that the pinna does not lie against the tines of the fork. Counter pressure should be applied to the opposite side of the head with the clinician's free hand. The clinician should confirm that the patient can hear the fork 'behind the ear' and should ask the patient to judge whether the tone sounds louder in front of or behind the ear.

In an ear with a normal conduction mechanism (i.e. normal hearing or a sensorineural hearing loss), the air conduction tone should be louder than the bone conduction tone. This is described as a positive test result though there is less scope for misunderstanding if the result is described as air conduction better than bone conduction. When bone conduction is louder than air conduction, the result may be referred to as Rinne negative and this indicates a significant conductive component to the hearing loss. If air conduction and bone conduction are equal, this should also indicate a conductive hearing loss, though it may simply indicate indecision on the part of the patient. The clinician should be aware of the 'false Rinne negative' which can occur when there is a severe sensorineural hearing loss in the test ear. In this case the bone conduction stimulus will be heard in the non-test ear and therefore will be louder than air conduction. This situation can usually be identified using the Weber test (see below). Indeed, if clinical voice testing has indicated a unilateral hearing loss, the Weber test should precede the Rinne test.

In the threshold comparison method the fork is pressed against the bone over the mastoid. The patient is asked to raise her hand if she hears the tone and to keep her hand raised until the tone disappears. When the patient indicates that she can no longer hear the tone, the fork is immediately placed outside the external auditory meatus. If there is no conductive component to the hearing impairment, the patient should be able to hear the tone again, thus giving a positive result. This method is not so commonly used because it takes longer and is more likely to be influenced by ambient noise levels. It has also been shown to be less sensitive than the loudness comparison method (Browning and Swan, 1989).

Masking of the non-test ear is sometimes advocated. This is not to be recommended, however, as it introduces further sources of error. If tragal rubbing is used (see above) the clinician is unsure whether adequate masking is being provided. If a Bárány box is used then it is likely that excessive masking will be provided which will overmask the test ear (Swan, 1989). In addition, the use of either form of masking is likely to alter the counter-pressure the clinician applies to the opposite side of the head; the loudness of the sound heard by bone conduction is highly dependent on the pressure with which the fork is held against the bone.

The Rinne tuning fork test merely gives a guide as to the presence of a significant conductive component to the hearing loss. Used as a test for detecting conductive hearing loss, the Rinne test has a high specificity but a low sensitivity (Crowley and Kaufman, 1966; Wilson and Woods, 1975; Stankiewicz and Mowry, 1979; Capper, Slack and Maw, 1987; Browning and Swan, 1988). All of these authors showed that the sensitivity of the Rinne test did not reach 90% until the air-bone gap exceeded 30 dB, though the specificity of the test exceeded 95% in that the test very rarely showed bone conduction to be better than air conduction in the absence of an air-bone gap greater than 10 dB. Thus small airbone gaps (up to about 30 dB) will frequently not be detected by the Rinne test, while a Rinne negative result is a reliable indicator of the presence of a conductive hearing impairment. It is reported that the crossover point at which the Rinne test is likely to become negative is at an air-bone gap of around 18 dB (Sheehy, Gardner and Hambley, 1971; Golabek and Stephens, 1979; Capper, Slack and Maw, 1987). This merely indicates the point at which the Rinne test will be negative 50% of the time; the patient's response will be variable with an air-bone gap around this level.

Weber test

The test is named after Ernst Weber who described the lateralization of bone-conducted sound to an occluded ear (1834) though, according to Huizing (1973), Schmalz (1846) first described the clinical application of the test. The aim of the Weber test is to detect the better hearing cochlea. A tuning fork (usually 512 or 256 Hz) is struck and placed on the midline of the patient's head. The commonly used sites are forehead, bridge of the nose, vertex and upper incisors. Of these, the bridge of the nose is to be preferred as the skin between fork and bone is thinnest here; the vertex can only be used in bald patients while the upper incisors should not be used because of the risk of cross-infection. The patient is asked whether the sound is heard better in one ear or equally in both ears (often described as being in the middle of the head). In a normally hearing patient the tone is heard centrally, otherwise the tone should be heard on the side of the better-hearing cochlea, except when there is a conductive component to the hearing impairment. In this case, if cochlear function is symmetrical, the tone should appear louder on the side of the conductive impairment or, if there is a bilateral conductive impairment, on the side with the larger conductive component. The reasons for this are complex.

Unfortunately, the results of the Weber test do not always agree with the results of pure-tone audiometry (Stankiewicz and Mowry, 1979; Capper, Slack and Maw, 1987) and 'wrong' results may be found in up to 25% of patients with unilateral hearing impairment. In cases of bilateral hearing impairment, it is difficult to predict on theoretical grounds in which ear the patient should hear the tone louder; interpretation in practice is impossible and the Weber test should be reserved for cases of unilateral hearing impairment.

Bing test

The Bing test (Bing, 1891) is based on the principle that occlusion of the external auditory meatus will make bone-conducted sounds appear louder in ears with a normal conduction mechanism. This phenomenon was first described by Wheatstone (1827). A vibrating tuning fork is applied to the bone overlying the mastoid as in the Rinne test (see above). As with the Rinne test, there are two methods: threshold comparison and loudness comparison. In the threshold comparison method, the patient is asked to raise his hand for as long as he can hear the tone. When the patient indicates that he can no longer hear the tone, the examiner occludes the patient's external auditory meatus by fingertip pressure on the tragus. If the patient can once again hear the tone, this indicates that the conduction mechanism is functioning. In the loudness comparison method, the meatus is alternately left patent and occluded and the patient is asked to judge whether the tone is louder with the ear occluded or patent.

Many otologists have recommended the use of the Bing test to detect conductive hearing impairment (e.g. Csovanyos, 1961; Sheehy, Gardner and Hambley, 1971). It has been found to be more sensitive than the Rinne test in selected groups of patients and normal subjects. Golabek and Stephens (1979) reported a crossover point from positive to negative at an air-bone gap of 9 dB. When evaluated on unselected groups of patients, however, the Bing test has been found to be less reliable than the Rinne test (Stankiewicz and Mowry, 1979; Swan and Browning, 1989) and to identify conductive impairments only slightly better than chance (Wilson and Woods, 1975). It is likely that the discrepancy in opinion arises because many patients find the test difficult to do. In addition, errors arise because of the difficulty the clinician experiences in applying a constant pressure with the base of the tuning fork when he or she has to use the other hand to occlude the meatus. The Bing test is not sufficiently reliable to be of significant clinical value.

Role of tuning fork tests

Tuning fork tests are not a substitute for correctly performed pure-tone audiometry with full masking and should certainly never be used as an excuse for omitting assessment of bone conduction thresholds. They are a useful tool for alerting the clinician to a possible inaccuracy in pure-tone audiometry. In this role they are particularly important for the otologist, to whom the presence or absence of a conductive hearing loss is of utmost importance. The clinician must remember, however, that tuning fork tests tend to overlook small conductive components and thus they should not be relied upon when making clinical decisions.

Identification of non-organic hearing loss

The most important factor in detection of non-organic hearing loss is clinical suspicion. Clinical suspicion will automatically be raised in any patient where there is a question of compensation for either noise exposure or injury. The alert clinician will always consider whether the results of hearing assessment, both clinical and audiometric, are compatible with the general behaviour of the patient. The patient's ability to hear should be observed from the initial greeting to final departure. Many patients who exaggerate their hearing loss can be identified by their general behaviour. Most severely hearing-impaired patients will sit down in the obvious chair regardless of whether they have heard the clinician's invitation to do so; only those with non-organic hearing loss will decline to sit down when invited to do so on the pretext of not having heard the invitation. It is most unusual for the genuinely hearing-impaired patient to sit forward on his seat, cup his hand behind his ear and stare intently at the clinician's lips. It is surprising how often normal conversation can be achieved with a patient with non-organic hearing loss yet, when the clinician carries out voice tests, the patient can only hear a loud voice 15 cm (6 inches) from his ear. Some better trained patients can be caught off guard by social pleasantries if the clinician leads them to believe that the consultation is over and escorts them out of the consulting room.

Most of these patients have some degree of hearing impairment but exaggerate their thresholds. It is important to compare carefully the clinician's clinical impression based on general observation of communication ability with more formal assessment of hearing by voice tests. Further indications of exaggerated thresholds will be found at audiometry.

Only a small proportion of cases of non-organic hearing loss are unilateral. These can be identified by Erhard's loud voice test (1872) which makes use of the patient's lack of knowledge of acoustics and physiology. During voice testing, the 'good' ear should be tested first to establish normal thresholds. When testing the 'deaf' ear, the good ear should be masked by simple tragal occlusion. This should not be confused with tragal rubbing (see above) as simple occlusion of the external auditory meatus by tragal pressure will attenuate sound by less than 30 dB so the patient should still be able to hear a loud voice presented to the 'deaf' ear. The patient will be unaware of this and will deny hearing the stimulus.

Stenger test

The Stenger test is nowadays rarely used as a tuning fork test but is used as a pure-tone audiometric test. The aim of the Stenger test is to detect patients who feign a unilateral hearing loss (Stenger, 1900). The test is based upon the phenomenon that if pure tones of the same frequency but different intensities are presented simultaneously to each ear, the patient will only be aware of the louder stimulus. In the tuning fork test, two tuning forks of the same frequency are presented simultaneously to both ears of the patient. The fork presented to the 'deaf' ear is held close to the ear while the other fork is held some distance from the good ear. In a genuine unilateral hearing loss, the patient will hear the fork in the good ear. In a feigned loss, the patient will only be aware of the fork in the 'deaf' ear and therefore will deny hearing the fork. The great problem with the tuning fork test is judging the relatively intensity of the two forks so the test is better performed using a pure-tone audiometer where the relative intensities of the stimuli are known.

Identification of diplacusis

Diplacusis is the perception of an additional or different tone to that which is presented to the patient. Binaural diplacusis is more commonly encountered than monaural diplacusis. In binaural diplacusis the same tone is perceived differently in each ear by the patient. This phenomenon was reported by several 19th century physicians and is most commonly found in Menière's disorder. Jones and Pracy (1971) demonstrated differences of up to 37% between tones matched to give the same pitch perception in each ear. The point at which the travelling wave reaches its maximum amplitude in the basilar membrane is governed in part by the stiffness of the basilar membrane at different points along its length. In endolymphatic hydrops the stiffness of the basilar membrane is increased and this presumably leads to the altered pitch perception. This phenomenon has, however, been reported in other conditions such as noise-induced temporary threshold shift (Elliott, Sheposh and Frazier, 1964; Brandt, 1967). The explanation for the phenomenon in these cases is not known. In the 19th century, the phenomenon was detected by presenting the same tuning fork to each ear and noting that the patient perceived the tones differently. This method is still used as a quick clinical test. However, accurate detection and quantification of binaural diplacusis is better obtained nowadays by pure-tone audiometric pitch matching. The presence or absence of diplacusis is rarely of diagnostic significance.

In monaural diplacusis, when a pure-tone is presented to one ear, the patient reports hearing an additional second tone in that ear. This is a rare phenomenon and the cause is uncertain.

Clinical tests of balance

Few clinicians find the diagnosis of the cause of dizziness easy because the clinician can rarely identify pathology, either visually or by imaging, and the control of equilibrium depends on a complex interaction between different systems. In the great majority of cases the diagnosis is made on the basis of a thorough history and clinical examination. The aim of this chapter is to guide the clinician in localizing the abnormality; the conditions causing dizziness are described elsewhere (Chapter 17).

History

The clinician should first determine precisely what the patient means by dizziness by encouraging the patient to describe the sensation and any accompanying symptoms. Dizziness can usually be assigned to one of the three following types:

1 Vertigo
2 Unsteadiness
3 Light-headedness.

Vertigo is defined as an illusion of movement of the subject or of his surroundings. Commonly there is a feeling of rotation or spinning but some patients merely complain of falling to one side. The symptom arises because of imbalance between the tonic signals arising from each vestibular system. Abnormalities may lie anywhere within the system, that is in the labyrinth, the VIIIth nerve, or the vestibular nuclei. It occurs in episodes of variable duration, usually with a sudden onset. There are associated symptoms of nausea and sometimes vomiting.

Unsteadiness is a sensation of being off-balance and usually only occurs while walking. This may be caused by abnormalities of the cerebellum or the proprioceptive system. There may be associated symptoms of incoordination and occasionally of weakness or numbness of the limbs.

Light-headedness describes a presyncopal state. The patient becomes pale and perspires; visual upset may occur, most commonly described as flashing lights; there may be palpitations. The signs of light-headedness can usually be seen by a companion and the episode may culminate in syncope. The attacks usually last for a few minutes and are rapidly relieved by sitting down or, preferably, lying down. They are caused by diffuse cerebral ischaemia and the aetiology should usually be sought in the cardiovascular system.

Psychogenic causes must always be considered. These may be the sole cause of symptoms, e.g. dizziness precipitated by fear of heights, but more commonly patients present with a psychogenic overlay to a mild peripheral vertigo. In this case, a careful history will elucidate the psychogenic overlay which can usually be managed by explaining the organic symptoms and reassuring the patient of their simple nature.

Other aetiological factors should also be sought. Dizziness is a side effect of many drugs and a careful drug history is essential in any dizzy patient. It may be a manifestation of a systemic condition (e.g. diabetes, anaemia). The clinician should enquire regarding precipitating factors, e.g. head injury.

Examination

The aim of examination in a patient with imbalance is to look for signs which will localize the abnormality. Clinical examination should include: the vestibular system; cerebellar and proprioceptive function; other structures possibly affected by the pathology, i.e the cranial nerves; and other systems which might affect the balance control systems, principally the cardiovascular system. The following should be examined in all patients with imbalance:

Otoscopic examination and hearing assessment
Eye movements
Stance and gait
Coordination
Positional tests
Other cranial nerves.

Eye movements

The range of eye movements should be tested by asking the patient to follow the clinician's finger. This tests the function of cranial nerves III, IV and VI. It also tests the smooth pursuit function of the vestibulo-ocular reflex (VOR) though other factors may affect smooth pursuit. Nystagmus is the abnormality most commonly sought but other abnormalities may also be identified.

Nystagmus is an involuntary rhythmic to and fro movement of the eyes. It can be divided into three main types: physiological nystagmus, peripheral vestibular nystagmus and central nystagmus; other rare types also occur.

Physiological nystagmus

Physiological nystagmus occurs in normal individuals on extreme lateral gaze and is due to fatigue of the ocular muscles. Sometimes the term is also applied to the nystagmus induced by moving objects, for example when looking out of a moving vehicle at rapidly passing telegraph poles, though this form of nystagmus is more properly called optokinetic nystagmus.

Peripheral vestibular nystagmus

Nystagmus is the only objective sign of vestibular system disorder. Its presence or absence should be sought with the patient looking directly ahead, looking to either side and looking up and down. The eyes should not deviate more than 30° from the resting position as nystagmus occurs in normal individuals on extreme lateral gaze.

In peripheral vestibular nystagmus, there is a slow drift of the eyes followed by a rapid flick back to the original position. The slow drift is the abnormal phase caused by faulty input to the vestibulo-ocular reflex while the rapid flick is the brain's restoration of the correct position. The direction of the nystagmus is conventionally named after the direction of the fast phase. Peripheral vestibular nystagmus is caused by a lesion in the labyrinth or vestibular nerve. It most commonly occurs in the horizontal plane though it may also be rotatory, but not vertical. The severity of the nystagmus may be classified in three degrees: first degree nystagmus occurs when the eyes are deviated in the direction of the fast phase; second degree nystagmus occurs when the eyes are central; third degree nystagmus occurs when the eyes are deviated away from the direction of the fast phase.

Spontaneous vestibular nystagmus may be unmasked by the removal of visual fixation. This can readily be achieved in the clinic by using Frenzel's glasses (Frenzel, 1925). These are goggles fitted with thick bi-convex lenses (+ 20 dioptres) which prevent the patient from focusing on anything (Figure 5.2).

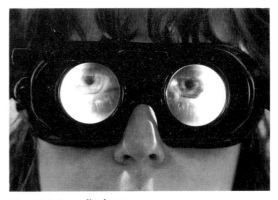

Figure 5.2 Frenzel's glasses

Two small bulbs inside the goggles allow the eyes to be illuminated and the observer has a magnified view of the eyes. Lifting the front of the glasses allows the patient to focus on the surroundings and the clinician to observe the effect of visual fixation. They are not as effective in removing visual fixation as observing eye movements electrically in complete darkness.

In peripheral lesions nystagmus is never present in the absence of dizziness and the eye movements are always conjugate. The fast phase will usually be in the same direction regardless of eye position. The nystagmus will always be more marked when the eyes are deviated in the direction of the fast phase (i.e. first degree nystagmus will be more marked than second degree nystagmus which will be more marked than third degree nystagmus). Visual fixation will suppress or abolish the nystagmus.

Nystagmus may be induced by positional tests or by caloric stimulation (see below). It can be more accurately assessed by electro-oculography (more commonly, though inappropriately, referred to as electronystagmography (ENG)) (Chapter 18).

Central nystagmus

Various characteristics of nystagmus can differentiate between peripheral and central lesions. Central disorders may cause vertical nystagmus as well as horizontal or rotatory nystagmus. The nystagmus may be present in the absence of imbalance. The direction of nystagmus may change and the nystagmus may be most marked with the eyes in a position other than looking in the direction of the fast phase. Sometimes there is dissociated eye movement. The nystagmus may be unaffected or even enhanced by visual fixation.

Other types of nystagmus

The eye movements do not have the rhythmic slow and fast phase characteristics of vestibular nystagmus, but may be equal in both directions or grossly irregular. They are not associated with imbalance. The most common causes are congenital and ocular (e.g. coalminer's nystagmus due to macular degeneration).

Other disorders of eye movement

Oscillopsia describes an inability to maintain eye position during head movement. The patient most commonly complains of difficulty focusing while walking. The symptom may be reproduced in the clinic by rapid side to side or up and down movement of the head. It is caused by bilateral vestibular failure or generalized cerebellar disease. It is sometimes associated with a downbeat nystagmus which occurs on

looking straight ahead and may be enhanced by looking to the side.

Abnormalities of slow pursuit and saccadic (rapid) eye movement can also be identified in the clinic. Slow pursuit can be assessed by asking the patient to follow the examiner's finger which is moved very slowly across his field of vision. Jerkiness of eye movement in one direction indicates cerebellar disease on that side; jerkiness in both directions indicates bilateral cerebellar disease. Saccadic movement can be tested by asking the patient to fixate on an object in front of his eyes and then to look rapidly at another object held to one side. In cerebellar disease, the eyes may overshoot and several small adjusting movements may be necessary to focus on the second target.

Stance and gait

The assessment of stance and gait should commence when the patient walks into the consulting room. Patients with cerebellar disease have a characteristic reeling gait and tend to stagger to the side of the lesion. Those with proprioceptive loss walk with a broad gait and may be observed to take high steps to avoid hitting their feet on the ground. If a patient can stand on one leg with the eyes closed, the balance is essentially normal and it is not necessary to carry out other tests of stance and gait.

The traditional test of stance is Romberg's test which was originally described by Romberg in 1846. Rogers (1980) described the original test and discussed its interpretation. The patient is asked to stand erect and is then asked to close his eyes. It is important to reassure the patient that the clinician will support him if he loses his balance. With posterior column disease the patient will not sway significantly with eyes open, but will sway progressively and fall over on closing his eyes. This is described as a positive Romberg's test and may also be found in bilateral complete vestibular failure. In cerebellar disease, the patient is likely to be unsteady with eyes open but eye closure will not worsen this. With unilateral labyrinthine disease, there will be no significant sway, except in the acute phase when the patient will tend to fall to the side of the lesion with eyes open and will be worse with eyes closed. Hysterical patients have exaggerated truncal movements on eye closure and tend to fall over but usually recover at the last moment.

Some clinicians find a sharpened Romberg test of value (Fregly, 1974). The patient stands with one foot behind the other, heel to toe. Normal subjects should be able to maintain this stance for at least 30 seconds while Fregly claims that patients with unilateral or bilateral vestibular impairment can rarely manage this.

The stepping test has been described by Unterberger (1938), Fukuda (1959) and others. The patient stands with hands clasped together and arms outstretched in front and is asked to mark time on the spot with eyes closed. In unilateral vestibular lesions, the patient will rotate to the side of the lesion. The test should continue for at least 30 seconds. Rotation of up to 30° is considered normal (Fukuda, 1959).

The patient's ability to walk in a straight line should be assessed by asking them to walk with one foot in front of the other. Cerebellar lesions may cause a variety of abnormalities. The patient should be able to carry out the test adequately with a labyrinthine lesion unless this is acute when they will veer to the side of the lesion. The test can be repeated with eyes closed. Patients with posterior column disease or bilateral vestibular failure will then find it impossible, as will those patients with acute unilateral labyrinthine disease. Patients with unilateral chronic labyrinthine disease will veer to the side of the lesion. Hysterical patients will deviate to both sides, more so with eyes closed, but again will not fall.

Coordination

Three aspects of limb coordination are tested:

1 The ability to carry out repeated opposite movements
2 The ability to carry out rapid fine movements
3 The ability to coordinate the movement of the whole limb.

Repeated opposite movements are tested by asking the patient to place the palm of one hand on top of the opposite hand. He is then asked to supinate the first hand then pronate it again and keep repeating this procedure. The opposite hand is then tested. Clumsiness in performing this test on one side indicates a lesion affecting the ipsilateral cerebellar hemisphere (dysdiadochokinesia).

Rapid fine movements are assessed by asking the patient to touch the tip of each finger in turn, from the index finger to the little finger, with the tip of the thumb of the same hand and then to return along the row of fingers. This action is then repeated with the other hand. Minor differences between the two hands may occur due to handedness. Marked slowness or inaccuracy of placement indicates cerebellar disease.

The finger–nose test assesses the movement of the whole arm. The patient is asked to touch the tip of his index finger against the tip of the examiner's index finger which is held in front of the patient. The patient then moves his index finger to the tip of his nose and back to the examiner's finger. The examiner then moves her finger slowly from side to side while the patient continues moving his finger from the examiner's finger to his nose and back again. In

labyrinthine disease the patient may overshoot to either side of the examiner's finger (past pointing), but more commonly the test will be normal. In cerebellar disease the patient will usually overshoot to the side of the lesion or the patient's finger may fall short of its target (dysmetria). The test can then be repeated with the examiner's finger stationary in front of the patient and the patient's eyes closed. With cerebellar disease, the patient's performance should not change on closing the eyes; proprioceptive problems affecting the upper limbs will cause significantly poorer performance in the absence of vision; with labyrinthine disease the test will be normal.

Positional tests

These tests look for nystagmus in different positions of the head. There are three factors which may cause nystagmus:

1 The position of the head with respect to gravity
2 The position of the head in relation to the neck
3 Movement of the head.

The traditional positional test, as described by Dix and Hallpike (1952), may induce nystagmus in any of these three ways as it involves elements of each. The test is carried out by sitting the patient on a couch so that when she lies down the head will hang over the end (Figure 5.3). The examiner stands to one side, grasps the patient's head, turns it 45° to the side and instructs the patient to look between the examiner's eyes. The examiner then quickly lies the patient down holding the head 30° below the horizontal. The patient should continue to look between the examiner's eyes while he watches closely for nystagmus. The patient should report any dizziness. As the onset of nystagmus may be delayed, the position should be maintained for at least 20 seconds. The patient is then returned to the sitting position, while still looking between the examiner's eyes. If any nystagmus is provoked, the test should be repeated. The test is then carried out with the patient's head to the other side. In labyrinthine lesions the nystagmus will be associated with vertigo and is usually rotatory with the upper pole of the eye rotating to the downmost ear. There is usually a latent interval and the nystagmus fatigues on repeated testing and is present to one side only. In positional nystagmus of central origin there is no latent interval, the nystagmus varies in type and does not fatigue; it may be present on both sides and there may be no associated vertigo. It should be remembered that alcohol produces a central type of positional nystagmus, even several hours after ingestion.

The effect of neck movement should be examined by full rotation to either side, lateral flexion, flexion and extension and the patient asked whether any dizziness is provoked.

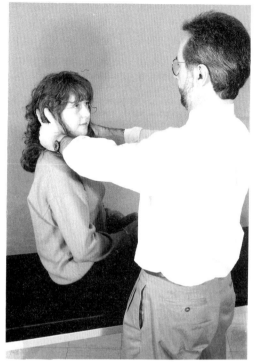

(a)

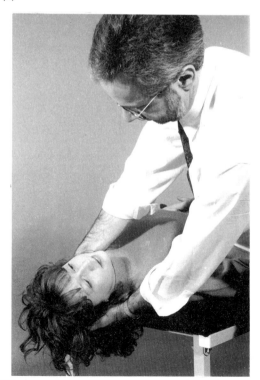

(b)

Figure 5.3 The Hallpike positional test

Caloric testing

Caloric stimulation of the lateral semicircular canal is best carried out with electro-oculographic (ENG) monitoring. However, it can also be carried out in the clinic using cold water at a temperature of 20–25°C. Ice cold water is sometimes suggested but this is most unpleasant for the patient and induces a marked vertiginous response in the normal labyrinth and consequent nausea. The test should be carried out with the patient lying supine on a couch and the head elevated at an angle of 30°. In this head position, the lateral semicircular canal is vertical. The duration of any evoked nystagmus can be timed with a stopwatch. Accurate comparison of the two sides is not possible unless the water temperature is thermostatically controlled, in which case it would seem more appropriate to use electro-oculographic (ENG) monitoring as well. Frenzel's glasses can be placed on the patient prior to commencing the test. The glasses can then be closed when the nystagmus disappears to assess the effect of removal of visual fixation.

The response to caloric stimulation can also be measured by using the phenomenon of oculogyral illusion (Arroyo and Hinchcliffe, 1977). This term describes the sensation, caused by the caloric response, that a particular point in space is moving. The test is carried out in a darkened room with a small light on the ceiling above the patient. The patient is asked to state whether or not the light appears to move and, if it does so, its direction of movement. He is then told to state when the light stops moving. The time interval is measured and used to compare ears. This method is said to have the advantage that the examiner does not have to detect the nystagmus herself.

Clinical caloric tests performed as described without electro-oculographic (ENG) monitoring provide a very crude comparison of vestibular function and can only detect gross unilateral vestibular dysfunction.

Other cranial nerves

The IIIrd, IVth and VIth nerves will have been tested while examining eye movements. Particular attention should be paid to cranial nerves V, VII and IX to XII.

Patients will usually volunteer any loss of sensation in the area of the Vth (trigeminal) nerve on the face. Traditionally, otolaryngologists assessed Vth nerve function by testing the corneal reflex; absence of the reflex was regarded as a strong indicator of a large cerebellopontine angle tumour, most commonly a vestibular schwannoma. However, this test is difficult to perform and interpret and risks damage to the patient's cornea. Unreliable results can be obtained by the patient seeing the approach of the stimulus. As the absence of the corneal reflex is a rare finding in vestibular schwannomas, routine testing of the corneal reflex cannot be recommended. Trigeminal sensation is readily assessed by inquiring about facial sensory loss. The motor function can be assessed by asking the patient to open the mouth fully; if there is a weakness, the chin will deviate to the paretic side.

Function of the VIIth (facial) nerve is assessed by testing the muscles of facial expression.

The IXth (glossopharyngeal) nerve provides pharyngeal sensation and is tested by the gag reflex. However, this is an unpleasant test to experience and can usually be omitted as pharyngeal sensation is rarely abnormal in the absence of other lower cranial nerve palsies.

Unilateral Xth (vagal) nerve lesions are usually readily apparent because of voice problems. The simplest test is to inspect palatal movement; in a unilateral vagal lesion, the uvula deviates to the normal side.

The XIth (accessory) nerve is tested by placing the clinician's hand on the patient's forehead and asking the patient to push forward while the clinician observes or palpates the sternomastoid muscles to compare their contraction. It may also be assessed by asking the patient to shrug the shoulders against resistance though this method can be affected by arthritic problems in the neck and shoulder.

The XIIth (hypoglossal) nerve is assessed by inspecting the tongue at rest in the mouth for evidence of atrophy or fibrillation. In a unilateral hypoglossal weakness, the tongue will deviate to the paralysed side on protrusion.

Other examination

In all dizzy patients, some consideration should be given to the cardiovascular system. If the patient complains of lightheadedness related to changes in posture, it is appropriate to measure lying and standing blood pressure. The pulse should be examined for evidence of arrhythmias. The carotid arteries should be auscultated for bruits. Clinical signs of anaemia should be sought.

Patients with recurrent vague dizziness, particularly young women, should be asked to hyperventilate to see if this reproduces their symptoms.

Conclusions

The examination of the dizzy patient can, with practice, be carried out very rapidly. Differentiation of normal and abnormal is often difficult and requires much experience of examining normal function.

References

ARROYO, J. A. and HINCHCLIFFE, R. (1977) Caloric test with oculogyral illusion as response. *Journal of Laryngology and Otology*, **91**, 309–321

BING, A. (1891) Ein neuer Stimmgabelversuch. *Wiener medizinische Blatt*, **14**, 637–638

BRANDT, J. F. (1967) Frequency discrimination following exposure to noise. *Journal of the Acoustical Society of America*, **41**, 448–457

BROWNING, G. G. and SWAN, I. R. C. (1988) Sensitivity and specificity of the Rinne tuning fork test. *British Medical Journal*, **297**, 1381–1382

BROWNING, G. G., SWAN, I. R. C. and CHEW, K. K. (1989) Clinical role of informal tests of hearing. *Journal of Laryngology and Otology*, **103**, 7–11

CAPPER, J. W. R., SLACK, R. W. T. and MAW, A. R. (1987) Tuning fork tests in children (an evaluation of their usefulness). *Journal of Laryngology and Otology*, **101**, 780–783

CROWLEY, H. and KAUFMAN, R. S. (1966) The Rinne tuning fork test. *Archives of Otolaryngology*, **84**, 406–408

CSOVANYOS, L. (1961) The Bing test in the diagnosis of deafness. *Laryngoscope*, **71**, 1548–1560

DIX, M. R. and HALLPIKE, C. S. (1952) Pathology, symptomatology and diagnosis of certain disorders of the vestibular system. *Proceedings of the Royal Society of Medicine*, **45**, 341–354

DOYLE, P. J., ANDERSON, D. W. and PIJL, S. (1984) The tuning fork – an essential instrument in otologic practice. *Journal of Otolaryngology*, **13**, 83–86

ELLIOTT, D. N., SHEPOSH, J. and FRAZIER, L. (1964) Effect of monaural fatigue upon pitch matching and discrimination. *Journal of the Acoustical Society of America*, **36**, 752–756

ERHARD, J. (1872) Das Gehörorgan als Object der Kriegsheilkunde. *Deutsche Militararztl Zeitschrift*, 157–159

FREGLY, A. R. (1974) *Handbook of Sensory Physiology, vol 6*, edited by H. H. Kornhuber. Springer Verlag

FRENZEL, H. (1925) Untersuchungsmethodik der Vestibularisstörung. *Klinische Wochienschrift*, **4**, 138–142

FUKUDA, T. (1959) The stepping test. *Acta Otolaryngologica*, **50**, 95–108

GOLABEK, W. and STEPHENS, S. D. G. (1979) Some tuning fork tests revisited. *Clinical Otolaryngology*, **4**, 421–430

HINCHCLIFFE, R. (1987) The clinical examination of aural function. In: *Scott-Brown's Otolaryngology*, 5th edn, Vol. 2, edited by S. D. G. Stephens. London: Butterworths. pp. 203–243

HUIZING, E. H. (1973) The early descriptions of the so-called tuning fork tests of Weber and Rinne. I. The 'Weber Test' and its first description by Schmalz. *Journal for Oto-Rhino-Laryngology and its Borderlands*, **35**, 278–282

HUIZING, E. H. (1975) The early descriptions of the so-called tuning fork tests of Weber, Rinne, Schwabach and Bing. II. The 'Rinne Test' and its first description by Polansky. *Journal for Oto-Rhino-Laryngology and its Borderlands*, **37**, 88–91

JONES, R. O. and PRACY, R. (1971) An investigation of pitch discrimination in the normal and abnormal hearing adult. *Journal of Laryngology and Otology*, **85**, 795–802

KING, P. F. (1953) Some imperfections of the free-field voice tests. *Journal of Laryngology and Otology*, **67**, 358–364

NG, M. and JACKLER, R. K. (1993) Early history of tuning-fork tests. *American Journal of Otology*, **14**, 100–105

POLANSKY, P. (1842) *Grundriss zu einer Lehre von den Ohrenkrankenheiten*. Vienna.

RINNE, H. A. (1855) Beiträge zur Physiologie des menschlichen Ohres. *Vjschr. prakt. Heilkunde. Med. Fak. Prag.*, **12**, 71–123

ROGERS, J. H. (1980) Romberg and his test. *Journal of Laryngology and Otology*, **94**, 1401–1404

ROMBERG, M. H. (1846) *Lehrbuch der Nerven Krankenheiten des Menschen*. Berlin: A. Dunker

SAMUEL, J. and EITELBERG, E. (1989) Tuning forks: the problem of striking. *Journal of Laryngology and Otology*, **103**, 1–6

SCHMALZ, E. (1846) *Erfahrungen über die Krankenheiten des Gehörs und ihre Heilung*. Leipzig: Teubner

SHAW, E. A. G. (1974) Transformation of sound pressure level from the free field to the eardrum in the horizontal plane. *Journal of the Acoustical Society of America*, **56**, 1848–1861

SHEEHY, J. L., GARDNER, G. and HAMBLEY, W. M. (1971) Tuning fork tests in modern otology. *Archives of Otolaryngology*, **94**, 132–138

STANKIEWICZ, J. A. and MOWRY, H. J. (1979) Clinical accuracy of tuning fork tests. *Laryngoscope*, **89**, 1956–1963

STENGER, S. (1900) Ein Versuch zue objectiven Festellung einseitiger Taubheit bzw. Schwerhörigkeit mittelst Stimmgabeln. *Archiv für Ohrenheilkunde*, **50**, 197–198

SWAN, I. R. C. (1984) Clinical aspects of hearing aid provision. *MD Thesis*. University of Glasgow, Scotland.

SWAN, I. R. C. (1989) Clinical masking with tragal rubbing and the Bárány noise box. *Clinical Otolaryngology*, **14**, 535–537

SWAN, I. R. C. and BROWNING, G. G. (1989) The Bing test in the detection of conductive hearing impairment. *Clinical Otolaryngology*, **14**, 539–548

UNTERBERGER, S. (1938) Neue objective registrierbare Vestibularis-Drehreaktion, erhalten durch Treten auf der Stelle. Der 'Tretversuch'. *Archiv für Ohren-, Nasen- und Kehlkopfheilkunde*, **145**, 478

WEBER, E. H. (1834) De pulsu, resoptione, auditu et tactu. In: *De utilitate cochleae in organo auditus*, Chap. VI. Leipzig: pp. 25–44

WHEATSTONE, C. (1827) Experiments in audition. *Quarterly Journal of Scientific Literature and Arts*, 57–72

WILSON, W. R. and WOODS, L. A. (1975) Accuracy of the Bing and Rinne tuning fork tests. *Archives of Otolaryngology*, **101**, 81–85

6

Pharmacological treatment of hearing and balance disorders

Gary J. McKee

This chapter examines the scientific basis and rationale for the practice of drug therapy in treatment of hearing and balance disorders. We have entered an age where proof of efficacy of drug therapy is important and the accepted management of hearing and balance disorder is constantly being questioned and reappraised. Drug therapy is discussed in sections covering the symptom or disease which is the major indication. Two aspects are discussed: a review of the literature is presented to justify use of each drug, and relevant pharmacology is summarized.

The prescription of medical therapy by the otolaryngologist or audiological physician, should be influenced by evidence from clinical trials. An attempt is made to evaluate the efficacy of each drug prior to an account of its pharmacology. There is a large number of drugs still in use for management of specific hearing and balance disorders which have little or no proof of efficacy. These drugs have been listed and briefly discussed at the end of each section.

The chapter has been structured into three sections covering the pharmacotherapy for:

- Wax
- Symptoms of inner ear disease
- Inner ear disease resulting from local or systemic pathology.

Pharmacotherapy for removal of wax

Patients presenting with wax impacted in the external auditory canal are regularly seen in otolaryngology and audiological medicine clinics. Over the years many organic solvents and solutions have been used to treat impacted wax. An ideal cerumenolytic would be a preparation which dissolves impacted wax and facilitates transport from the ear canal without any chemical irritation. The ideal drug has not been developed and even the optimal frequency of administration of available agents is controversial. The choice of available agents to treat impaction of wax is wide. Some preparations clear wax by softening the wax to facilitate removal while others both soften and dissolve wax.

Commonly prescribed ceruminolytics

- Chlorobutal-paradichlorobenzene-turpentine oil (Cerumol)
- Arachis oil-almond oil-rectified camphor oil (Earex)
- Docusate sodium (Waxsol)
- Sodium bicarbonate 10%
- Distilled water

Softening agents

Many preparations have been shown to soften and lubricate impacted wax to facilitate removal by syringing, with wax hook or suction. Organic solvents appear best suited for this purpose. This group includes: olive oil; almond oil; Cerumol (paradichlorobenzene 2%, chlorobutal 5%, oil of terebinth (turpentine) 5%); Earex (arachis oil 33.3%, almond oil 33.3%, rectified camphor oil 33.3%). Agents which are incorporated into cerumenolytic preparations include choline salicylate for analgesic and anti-inflammatory activity; polyoxypropylene glycol as a cerumen softener and glycerin as an emollient. Some organic solvents can cause irritation of the meatal skin but this is unlikely with simpler remedies.

Results

Fraser (1970) reported a controlled trial of wax solvents *in vitro* and *in vivo* in a geriatric population. The following solvents were compared with sodium bicarbonate BPC ear drops: olive oil, Cerumol, Waxsol, dioctyl ear capsules and Xerumenex. The capacity to facilitate syringing *in vivo* and to disintegrate wax *in vitro* were assessed. Cerumol alone was significantly more effective than sodium bicarbonate at facilitating syringing. Olive oil and Waxsol eased syringing more than sodium bicarbonate but not significantly so. The four oil-based preparations, (Cerumol, olive oil, dioctyl capsules and Xerumenex) softened and lubricated the surface of the wax but did not disperse it. Two water-based preparations, Waxsol and sodium bicarbonate, caused complete disintegration of wax.

Audax and Cerumol have similar effects in softening and reducing the amount of wax (Dummer, Sutherland and Murray, 1992). A study based on ease of syringing suggested that Audax was superior to Earex but syringing was still required for most subjects with each preparation (Lyndon *et al.*, 1992).

Dissolving agents

There is evidence that aqueous solutions may dissolve and liquefy ear wax in addition to acting as softening agents. Aqueous solutions such as distilled water, Waxsol (docusate sodium 0.5% in a water-miscible base) and 5–10% sodium bicarbonate solution have been shown to liquefy wax during *in-vitro* studies. This property is important in prophylaxis against build-up of wax, unblocking of grommets and clearance of wax in children or uncooperative patients. Non-aqueous preparations cause little disintegration of the wax within the ear canal (Bellini, Terry and Lewis, 1989).

Results

Bellini and colleagues found that docusate sodium preparations (Waxsol and stores own brand) proved most effective *in vitro* at disintegrating human cerumen over a 2-hour period (Bellini, Terry and Lewis, 1989). Docusate sodium (dioctyl sodium sulphosuccinate) is also used as a faecal softener and stimulant laxative. Many proprietary preparations contain docusate 0.5–5% as an ingredient. It is surprising that distilled water was as effective as docusate sodium in this study. Chen and Caparosa (1991) advocated that docusate sodium be warmed to body temperature prior to use. They advised the use of docusate sodium drops once a month in patients who have repeated extractions of impacted wax. In a clinical consultation, an application of drops for 10 minutes will help

soften hard wax and facilitate a difficult removal by instrument or lavage.

This assessment is not accepted by many authors who feel that sodium bicarbonate is superior to docusate sodium. Robinson and Hawke (1989) stated that 10% sodium bicarbonate solution is the cerumenolytic of choice as it caused marked swelling of cerumen *in vitro*, particularly at higher temperatures. Sodium bicarbonate solution was advocated as an adjunct to syringing or suction clearance in cases of impaction. They recommended that drops should be instilled twice daily for 2 days prior to syringing or 2 hours prior to suction clearance. In young children or uncooperative patients, sodium bicarbonate ear drops may be used twice daily for 1 week to facilitate wax disintegration.

Pharmacotherapy for symptoms resulting from inner ear disease

Otolaryngologists and audiological physicians commonly meet patients who require treatment for symptoms of inner ear disease of unknown aetiology. Pharmacotherapy can be used to provide excellent relief from vertigo, equivocal improvement of hearing loss but regrettably little or no relief for tinnitus sufferers. Elderly patients with imbalance pose a particular problem and a subsection is devoted to the management of this problem.

Sudden hearing loss

Idiopathic sudden hearing loss can be usefully defined as a sensorineural hearing loss exceeding 30 dB occurring in at least three contiguous frequencies in less than 3 days (Wilson, 1986). It is an alarming experience for the patients who often require hospital admission and investigation to exclude serious causes. During admission, there is often real or imagined pressure on the clinician to 'do something for the patient'.

Treatment of sudden hearing loss is controversial. Natural remission without treatment occurs in over half of these patients. Mattox and Simmons (1977) reported that 16 of 28 cases (57%) had good or complete resolution of hearing loss with restriction of physical activity alone. This rate of 'spontaneous' remission is frequently misreported as 65% by workers in the field. A rate of 65% remission has been mistakenly used as a standard against which medical treatments of sudden hearing loss have been compared. Few controlled clinical trials have shown any medical therapy to exceed this rate by a significant margin. There is doubt therefore, that medical therapy alters the rate of spontaneous remission. The highest rates of remission are observed in patients with a mid-or-low-frequency loss or those where therapy has been commenced within 1–2 weeks. These factors may be more significant than the particular drug combination chosen for treatment.

Pharmacotherapy itself has associated risks (Anderson and Meyerhoff, 1983). This may explain why some authors prefer not to use pharmacotherapy for sudden hearing loss (Cowan and Chow, 1988). Drugs which have some evidence of beneficial effect in sudden hearing loss are listed below.

Glucocorticoids

Glucocorticoids will be referred to as 'steroids' throughout this chapter as this term, though inaccurate, is used in most clinical trials of treatment. Wilson, Byl and Laird (1980) reported the only controlled study which showed a beneficial effect from steroids in treatment of sudden hearing loss. It was a double-blind study with oral steroid, placebo, and refusal of treatment in 119 patients. Patients with mid-frequency hearing loss recovered best, regardless of therapy. Those with profound hearing loss in excess of 90 dB at all frequencies had a disappointing recovery rate of 24% with steroids. Patients with audiograms between these two configurations, 14 of 18 (78%) had partial or complete recovery in the steroid group, but this occurred in only eight of 21 (38%) in the placebo group (Table 6.1). Delay prior to treatment and the characteristics of the audiogram heavily influenced the outcome of treatment. Moskowitz, Lee and Smith (1984) reported an uncontrolled study of 27 patients treated with steroids against nine patients treated by rest and restriction of salt, alcohol and tobacco. Eighty-nine per cent of those treated with steroid recovered 50% or more of their hearing loss compared with 49% of the untreated group.

Other trials have failed to show a treatment benefit from steroids (Huang *et al.*, 1989).

Pharmacology

The mechanism of action of steroids in sudden hearing loss is not established but it is likely that suppression of the immune response is involved. Glucocorticosteroids are used to suppress inflammation, allergy, and immune responses (Kimberley, 1991). Prednisolone acts by entering the cell and binding reversibly to a specific cytoplasmic receptor. The steroid–receptor complex undergoes a reaction which enables it to enter the nucleus where it regulates transcription of specific gene sequences and thus protein synthesis. The alteration of protein synthesis modifies the function and behaviour of cells.

Glucocorticoids have a profound anti-inflammatory effect. The formation of prostaglandins, leukotrienes and platelet activating factor is inhibited. Glucocorticoids also have immunosuppressive effects. They inhibit complement, migration inhibition factor, T and B lymphocyte function and decrease circulating macrophages and lymphocytes (Williams and Yarwood, 1990). When used to treat sudden hearing loss, they are administered as a high initial daily dose, reduced gradually over a 7–10 day period.

Carbogen

Carbogen is a safe treatment with some evidence that it may restore sudden hearing loss. Fisch (1983) reported a randomized controlled study of 1–2 weeks' treatment with carbogen or active control (papaverine and low molecular weight dextran) in 46 patients. No difference in hearing improvement was observed

Table 6.1 Summary of favourable controlled studies of drug treatments of sudden hearing loss

Authors	Subjects	Success rate			Control	Side effects
		Drug	*Relief*	*Effect*		
Wilson, Byl and Laird (1980)	33	Steroid	Mid-frequency Mild–severe Profound	4/4 14/18 2/11	Double-blind controlled	None
	34	Placebo	Mid-frequency Mild–severe Profound	1/1 8/21 2/12		
	52	No-treatment	Mid-frequency Mild–severe Profound	6/6 17/35 4/11		
Fisch (1983)	29	Carbogen	30 dB improvement		Active control	None listed
	17	Dextran/ papaverine	16 dB improvement			

at 5 days but the carbogen group had significantly better hearing at 1 year follow up. Fisch concluded that carbogen did not cure sudden hearing loss, rather it improved the likelihood of spontaneous recovery (see Table 6.1). It is conceivable that the 5-day period of bed-rest necessary to undertake carbogen treatment is more beneficial than the treatment itself.

Pharmacology

Carbogen produces an increase in oxygen tension within the labyrinthine fluids (Nagahara, Fisch and Yagi, 1983). The mixture of 95% oxygen and 5% carbon dioxide produces maximal perilymphatic oxygenation with minimal side effects. However, the gas mixture is not thought to have a direct effect on cochlear vasculature (Kallinen *et al.*, 1991). Perilymphatic oxygen tension depends on both the partial pressure of carbon dioxide in serum and the oxygen saturation. Subjects breathing *room air* enriched with 5% carbon dioxide experience marked vascular effects resulting from constriction of the systemic arterial tree, respiratory acidosis, activation of the sympathetic nervous system and hypertension. Carbogen is usually administered by inhalation for 30 minute periods every hour throughout the day for 5 days.

Histamine receptor agonist

There is some evidence from an uncontrolled trial that betahistine (a histamine receptor agonist) may have a useful treatment effect. The pharmacology of betahistine is discussed later in the section on vertigo. Betahistine has been incorporated into multi-drug regimens used to treat sudden hearing loss. Khanijow and Raman (1988) in an uncontrolled trial reported good improvement in eight of 11 (73%) patients treated with bed rest, steroids, histamine receptor agonists and plasma expanders. Betahistine, 8 mg three times a day, was recommended in this study but this dose may be doubled.

Drugs with no evidence of effect in sudden hearing loss

Over the years, many drugs, or combinations of drugs have been used for treatment of sudden hearing loss. These drugs have subsequently been subjected to controlled trials. Drugs with little or no supporting evidence are discussed below.

Anticoagulants

Anticoagulants have been used to treat sudden hearing loss. Donaldson (1979) reported an uncontrolled study in which 16 of 23 patients (70%) seen within 1 week of hearing loss made a good or complete recovery after treatment with 6500 international units of heparin infused three times daily for 5 days. The author felt that 70% recovery was of the order expected through natural remission and that heparin was ineffective for treatment of sudden hearing loss. This is an excellent success rate but the study was uncontrolled and all patients were recruited early in the disease when remission rates are highest. A controlled study of the effectiveness of heparin as a treatment of sudden hearing loss would be necessary to determine its usefulness.

Other forms of anticoagulant therapy have been tried. In a double-blind study. Shiraishi, Kubo and Matsunaga (1991) reported recovery of hearing after sudden hearing loss in 57% of 82 patients given defibrinogenation treatment but in only 39% of 86 patients treated with steroid therapy. Batroxobin (a derivative of snake venom) was used to cleave fibrinogen into fibrinmonomer and FDP (fibrin degradation products) which were then excreted into the urine. Batroxobin can reduce blood viscosity to approximately 20% of the control value. The success rate claimed for defibrinogenation therapy is comparable to that expected with natural remission. The poor results from steroid therapy in this study should be noted.

Thymoxamine

Thymoxamine (Opilon) is an α-adrenoreceptor blocking agent with a primary action causing relaxation of smooth muscle in peripheral arteriolar vessel walls leading to systemic vasodilatation. It is indicated for treatment of Raynaud's disease. It has also been included in polypharmacy therapy for sudden hearing loss, presumably to augment perilymphatic oxygenation caused by carbogen. Intestinal absorption of thymoxamine is very poor. Large oral doses are required to cause increased skin blood flow. Side effects include flushing, headache and dizziness. No recent studies have been reported on the efficacy of the drug and further studies are required to assess the value of thymoxamine as a treatment for sudden hearing loss.

Plasma expanders

A number of drugs which reduce blood viscosity are in use for the treatment of sudden hearing loss. These include hydroxyethylstarch (HES), pentoxifylline and Dextran-40. Controlled trials have failed to show convincing treatment effects except that plasma expanders may possibly have a useful effect in polycythaemic patients.

Results

Probst *et al.* (1992) reported a double-blind trial of Dextran-40 with pentoxifylline, saline infusion with pentoxifylline, and saline infusion with placebo medication in 184 patients with sudden hearing loss. No treatment benefit from dextran or pentoxifylline in sudden hearing loss or acute acoustic trauma was discerned. Kronenberg *et al.* (1992) reported no treatment effect from low-molecular-weight Dextran and intravenous procaine (local anaesthetic with vasodilator properties) in sudden hearing loss. The combination of procaine and Dextran was not superior to placebo. Desloovere, Lorz and Klima (1989) reported a double-blind trial of HES and pentoxifylline in 150 patients. There was no benefit from treatment overall. Approximately 50% of patients who received either treatment or placebo (saline infusion) recovered hearing. There was a slight treatment advantage to patients with hypertension or haemoglobin > 14 mg/dl (2.17 mmol/l).

Zaytoun, Schuknecht and Farmer (1983) reported a case where renal failure and death complicated treatment of sudden deafness with Rheomacrodex, a low molecular weight dextran. This unfortunate result raises major concerns about the the advisability of using drugs with known serious side effects when other safer forms of treatment are available.

Pharmacology

HES, like Dextran-40, is a glycopolysaccharide derivative which acts as a potent plasma expander and haemodiluting agent. It increases the cardiac output and decreases blood viscosity. Pentoxifylline is a drug which affects red cell rigidity causing red cells to become more malleable and thus permitting them to pass more easily through capillaries.

Radiological contrast media

Emmett and Shea (1979) stimulated interest in the possible therapeutic effect of radiological contrast media in treatment of sudden hearing loss. Huang *et al.* (1989) concluded that neither hypaque (diatrizoate meglumine) nor steroids resulted in better recovery rates than that which occurs with natural remission. The rate of recovery was heavily influenced by the initial audiometric picture but not by any medical treatments.

Calcium antagonists

Mann, Beck and Beck (1986) reported an uncontrolled study of 50 patients on the effect of oral nifedipine and intravenous naftidrofuryl given concomitantly with vitamin A, vitamin E and zinc. The drugs had no useful effect on hearing loss.

Diuretic vitamins

Diuretic-vitamin preparations do not seem to help recovery of hearing after sudden hearing loss. Kon-

ishi, Nakai and Yamane (1991) carried out an uncontrolled study of the value of infusions of frusemide, and vitamins B_{12}, B_1, thioctic acid, pantothenic acid and betamethasone 4 mg for sudden hearing loss. Overall, 56% of 453 patients treated with frusemide-vitamin therapy improved compared with 55% of 140 given conventional treatment.

Coenzyme Q_{10}

Sato (1988) stated that coenzyme Q_{10} is a widely reported treatment of sudden hearing loss in the Japanese literature. Coenzyme Q_{10} is a co-factor in metabolic reactions. Unfortunately, the paper does not clearly state the outcome of the treatment.

Chronic sensorineural deafness

There is currently no place for pharmacotherapy in the treatment of long-standing sensorineural deafness but research into the field continues. Yohimbine is an α_2-adrenoreceptor antagonist. It has been shown to increase noradrenalin in the brain affecting attention, anxiety and libido levels. Yohimbine encourages sexual behaviour in mice. In humans, the resulting rise in noradrenalin levels has been shown to improve the signal-noise ratios of sensory systems, including the auditory system.

Hughes *et al.* (1988) reported a double-blind crossover controlled trial of 14 sensorineurally impaired subjects with a single dose of 10 mg yohimbine and placebo. Auditory brain stem response latencies III–V were shortened (improved) by yohimbine but there was no evidence of improved speech intelligibility in background noise. Adverse effects reported were flushing, nausea, sweating, nervousness, dizziness, salivation and a metallic taste.

Tinnitus

Tinnitus is best managed by developing a positive attitude in the patient towards his or her tinnitus. Belief that the tinnitus will improve with time facilitates the process of habituation to the noise. A large number of drug therapies has been tried for tinnitus. Most drugs cause side effects and few produce beneficial effects superior to that obtained with placebo. At present, only a small minority of patients with tinnitus obtain benefit from pharmacotherapy (Sirimanna and Stephens, 1992). Some drugs are helpful in specific clinical situations:

- Sedatives and hypnotics – in carefully selected patients with high anxiety levels
- Tricyclic antidepressants – in some patients who suffer from depression and sleep disturbance
- Treatment of systemic and specific diseases –

such as anaemia (iron supplements), hypertension (antihypertensives) or Menière's disorder.

The major problem with drug therapy in tinnitus is that the beneficial effects of the drugs are short lived and the patient is again faced with his or her tinnitus. Temporary relief from tinnitus is likely to delay habituation by the patient. In many cases a short-term therapeutic response is achieved only with high drug levels at which side effects are common.

Drugs with a probable beneficial effect in tinnitus

Murai *et al.* (1992) published a comprehensive review of drug therapy for tinnitus. Controlled studies have demonstrated that some drugs have a useful action against tinnitus. As yet none of these drugs has entered mainstream medical practice. As tinnitus is likely to have many causes, it is unlikely that a single drug will be developed which will be effective in all cases.

Lignocaine

Intravenous lignocaine has been shown in many controlled trials to abolish tinnitus temporarily (e.g. Martin and Colman, 1978; Isreal *et al.*, 1982). Unfortunately this property cannot be utilized for the benefit of tinnitus sufferers as the drug cannot be administered orally. Laffree, Vermeij and Hulshof (1989) found no effect from transporting lignocaine through the tympanic membrane by iontophoresis. Coles, Thompson and O'Donoghue (1992) delivered lignocaine to five patients via intratympanic injection. These patients obtained no lasting benefit and suf-

fered violent vertigo for several hours after injection. The authors felt that this mode of treatment was ineffective and poorly accepted.

Pharmacology

Local anaesthetic drugs cause a reversible block of electrical conduction along nerve fibres. Molecules penetrate the axon in a non-ionized form. Once inside, ionized molecules form and these block sodium channels to prevent the generation of action potentials. Intravenous infusion is the only practical method of administration because of the short half-life and the first-pass effect of the liver. Treatment with lignocaine is impractical as a treatment for tinnitus except in selected cases. Side effects such as unsteadiness, slurring of speech and dizziness are common. All members of this group of drugs can cause cardiac arrhythmias. Oral analogues such as tocainide, mexiletine and flecainide do not seem to have the same activity against tinnitus.

Oxazepam and clonazepam

At first glance, oxazepam and clonazepam would appear promising drugs for the treatment of tinnitus, with initial success rates of over 50%. Lechtenberg and Shulman (1984) reported a controlled study comparing the effect of antihistamine (active control) with various benzodiazepines. Twelve of 23 (52%) patients given oxazepam and 18 of 26 patients (69%) given clonazepam reported improvement. The active control reduced tinnitus in only four of 37 patients. Surprisingly, no treatment effect was seen with diazepam or flurazepam (Table 6.2).

Table 6.2 Summary of controlled trials showing treatment effects on tinnitus

Authors	Subjects	Success rate			Control	Side effects
		Relief (%)	Lignocaine	Placebo		
Martin and Colman (1980)	32	0	7/32	28/32	Double-blind	None listed
		25–75	11/32	3/32	cross-over	
		100	14/32	1/32		
Isreal *et al.* (1982)	26	Worse	4/26	1/26	Double-blind	Numbness
		No change	0/26	21/26	Cross-over	Dizziness
		Better	22/26	4/26		Tingling

Benzodiazepines
Lechtenberg and Shulman (1984). Single-blind trial with side effects of sedation, nausea and vomiting

Medication	Patients	Improved	< 50%	50–80%	> 80%	Worse	No change
Antihistamine	37	4	1	1	2	3	30
Oxazepam	23	12	4	1	7	0	11
Clonazepam	26	18	6	8	4	0	8

NB: Diazepam was shown to have no beneficial effect

Pharmacology

Clonazepam is a potent anticonvulsant with additional anxiolytic, hypnotic and muscle relaxant actions. These actions of drugs from the benzodiazepine group are thought to be caused by the enhancement of GABA-mediated inhibition in the central nervous system. The effect on the central nervous system is extensive as around 30–50% of synapses in the brain are believed to be GABA-ergic. Benzodiazepines have low toxicity but it is now realized that chronic treatment may cause cognitive impairment, tolerance and dependence. In addition, clonazepam may impair ability to drive and operate machinery and oxazepam, which is a short-acting hypnotic, carries a high risk of withdrawal symptoms after long-term use. The risks of dependence would be high with prolonged courses of benzodiazepines. Because of their addictive nature benzodiazepines should be reserved for situations where there is a clear short-term objective for treatment.

Drugs with possible beneficial effects

Eperisone hydrochloride

Kitano *et al.* (1987) reported a study of the effect of a muscle relaxant, eperisone hydrochloride, combined with vitamin B_{12} and sulpiride compared with the placebo effect of vitamin B_{12} and sulpiride. Tinnitus was significantly reduced in 65 of 164 patients (39%) receiving eperisone but in only eight of 54 patients (15%) receiving placebo. A controlled study of the efficacy of eperisone, which is not available in the UK, would be of interest.

Glutamic acid

McIlwain (1987) in an uncontrolled study found seven of 21 patients (33%) claiming improvement in tinnitus but adequate follow up was not possible. No side effects were observed. Ehrenberger and Brix (1987) reported the unspecified beneficial effect of glutamic acid diethylester and glutamic acid in more than 100 patients. The long-term follow up was not stated and treatment relapses appeared common.

Pharmacology

Amino acids are used as transmitters in fast point-to-point neural circuits in the central nervous system. Glutamate is the main central excitatory transmitter and is present within the auditory pathways. It depolarizes neurons by triggering an increase in membrane Na^+ conductance. Glutamic acid diethylester (GDEE) is an antagonist to glutamic acid (Glu) and both must be given as an infusion. In overdose glutamate can lead to serious neurotoxicity within the central nervous system.

Aspirin

Aspirin has an ototoxic effect on hair cells and produces tinnitus in high doses. Penner (1989) reported a single case where aspirin appeared to abolish tinnitus caused by spontaneous otoacoustic emissions. It was suggested that in this case, cochlear mechanical tinnitus (loud otoacoustic emissions perceived as tinnitus) was suppressed by aspirin. Further research is required into this fascinating area. Within the vascular system, aspirin acts by inhibiting the synthesis of thromboxane-A_2 which is a powerful inducer of platelet aggregation.

Drugs where trials suggest no beneficial effect on tinnitus

Antidepressants

Tricyclic antidepressants are used in the treatment of depressed or suicidal patients complaining of tinnitus. The high rates of response observed within this patient group seem to be due to a combination of placebo effect and reduced levels of depression. There is no evidence of a direct treatment effect on tinnitus. Two controlled studies by Mihail *et al.* (1988) and Dobie *et al.* (1993) found that trimipramine and nortriptyline, respectively did not directly affect perception of tinnitus. Both studies showed that placebo effects were large and that benefit was more likely to be reported by depressed patients. The absence of treatment effect and the frequency of side effects such as dry mouth indicates that tricyclics should only be used in carefully selected cases. The advice of a psychiatrist should be sought prior to commencing treatment. There is little experience in treatment of tinnitus with other groups of antidepressant drugs.

Pharmacology

Tricyclics act by blocking the reuptake of noradrenalin into the presynaptic nerve ending. They resemble the phenothiazines in structure and have similar blocking actions at cholinergic muscarinic receptors, α-adrenoreceptors and histamine receptors. These actions often result in side effects such as dry mouth, blurred vision, constipation, urinary retention, tachycardia and postural hypotension. Within the ear, anticholinergic effects can lead to decreased production of endolymph and reduced inhibition of the afferent fibres to the organ of Corti and olivocochlear bundle. Other adverse effects may occur including sedation, and a range of dangerous cardiac, haematopoietic and endocrine-metabolic effects. This family of drugs is toxic in overdose.

Oral administration of local anaesthetic derivatives

There is evidence that tocainide, mexiletine and flecainide have no effect on tinnitus. Controlled studies have found that tocainide (Hulshof and Vermeij, 1984 a,b; Blayney *et al.*, 1985), mexiletine (McCormick and Thomas, 1981) and flecainide (Harker *et al.*, 1987; Fortnum and Coles, 1991) did not lead to a reduction of tinnitus. These drugs have pro-arrhythmic actions which are clinically important. They are best avoided in tinnitus.

Anticonvulsants

Anticonvulsants such as carbamazepine or amino-oxyacetic acid (similar to vigabatrin) are ineffective against tinnitus in controlled trials. Hulshof and Vermeij (1985) found that carbamazepine 150 mg three times a day was less effective than placebo. Guth *et al.* (1990) reported that 14 of 66 patients (21%) taking carbamazepine 75 mg four times a day for 1 week, showed a subjective decrease in tinnitus. The majority of these patients (71%) developed side effects. Reed *et al.* (1985) found no treatment benefit from amino-oxyacetic acid over placebo.

Barbiturates

Barbiturates have a depressant action throughout the central nervous system, but with particular affinity for the reticular activating system which is concerned with state of arousal. Marks, Onisiphorou and Trounce (1981) reported that a single dose of sodium amylobarbitone 120 mg did not alter the loudness or frequency of tinnitus.

Calcium antagonists

Hulshof and Vermeij (1986) reported that flunarizine was ineffective against tinnitus in a double-blind study.

Nicotinamide (vasodilator)

Nicotinamide is a B complex vitamin which is thought to cause vasodilatation by reducing the release of adrenalin at sympathetic nerve endings within vascular smooth muscle. Hulshof and Vermeij (1987) reported a controlled trial of the administration of 70 mg nicotinamide three times a day for 30 days on tinnitus. Side effects were common and nicotinamide was found to have a similar effect to placebo.

Xanthines

Xanthines are phosphodiesterase inhibitors which block the breakdown of cyclic AMP within the cell. They have inotropic, diuretic and bronchodilator actions and cause a pro-arrhythmic effect. Pentoxifylline is a member of the xanthine group which acts to decrease blood viscosity. This is achieved by increasing the red cell deformability and reducing platelet aggregation. Salama, Bhatia and Robb (1989) re-

ported a single-blind controlled trial where oxypentifylline 400 mg three times a day was administered for 6 weeks. No useful effect on tinnitus was observed.

Ginkgo biloba extract

Coles (1988) reported an uncontrolled pilot study using 40 mg *Ginkgo biloba* extract three times a day for 12 weeks. Only four of 21 patients had an improvement in tinnitus. The mechanism of action was unknown but side effects were common and included tiredness, headache, depression, nausea and palpitations. It was concluded that *Ginkgo biloba* had no useful therapeutic effect.

Adrenalin

Willatt *et al.* (1987) found in a controlled double-blind study that tinnitus relief after iontophoresis of the tympanic membrane with 4% lignocaine and 1:2000 adrenalin was no better than that obtained by placebo.

Zinc

Paaske *et al.* (1991) reported the effect of 100 mg zinc sulphate three times daily for 8 weeks on 48 patients with tinnitus. They observed that zinc deficiency was rare and did not demonstrate any beneficial effect from zinc on tinnitus.

Vertigo

Drug therapy for vertigo is mainly directed towards relief of symptoms rather than the modifying the underlying aetiological process. The choice of drug therapy is dictated by the clinical picture rather than the aetiology with the exception of Menière's disease.

Animal studies

The study of vestibular function and the effect of drugs in vestibular pathology is instructive but the findings must be applied to humans with caution. Pyykkö *et al.* (1988) and Flohr, Abeln and Luneburg (1985) reported the effects of drug administration in frogs after vestibular compensation for unilateral labyrinthectomy (Table 6.3). Equilibrium was said to have decompensated, when there was reappearance of functional defects typical of an acute vestibular lesion. Decompensation occurred after receiving the following drugs: nicotine, GABA-agonists (benzodiazepines), parasympathetomimetics (carbachol and cholinesterase inhibitors), sympathomimetics and alcohol. Some drugs caused overcompensation with the appearance of functional defects opposite to those observed with the original lesion. These drugs included cholinolytics such as hyoscine and atropine, GABA-antagonists and β-blockers. Sedatives such as

Table 6.3 Drugs and effects after compensation for labyrinthectomy in frogs

Effect	Drugs which cause effect
Decompensation	Nicotine, carbachol, cholinesterase inhibitors, GABA-agonists, sympathomimetics, alcohol
Overcompensation	Hyoscine, atropine, GABA-antagonists, β-blockers
Slowed compensation	Alcohol, benzodiazepines, neuroleptics, narcotics
Accelerated compensation	Caffeine, amphetamine, ACTH

alcohol, benzodiazepines, neuroleptics and narcotics slowed vestibular compensation; excitant drugs including caffeine, amphetamine and ACTH accelerated the compensation by the central vestibular pathways.

Peppard (1986) observed that vestibular compensation in cats was accelerated when vestibular sensory imbalance was not suppressed during the acute phase of injury. Stimulant or antiemetic drugs were also found to accelerate compensation. This observation suggested that the perception of vestibular imbalance is the stimulus for the adaptive mechanism. Overall, drug therapy to reduce vegetative symptoms was felt to be helpful by facilitating mobilization.

Classification of vertigo

In humans, it is convenient to categorize causes of vertigo as peripheral or central. Most presentations of peripheral vertigo respond to oral medications. The exception to this rule are patients with acute vestibular failure. Destruction of the labyrinth frequently causes severe disorder with acute vertigo accompanied by vegetative symptoms. Severe incapacitation of the patient may result, demanding supportive measures and parenteral drug therapy. In most other disorders where vertigo arises from peripheral vestibular disease, there is no requirement for such intensive management. Central vertigo is variable in presentation and treatment is also symptomatic.

Classification from a pharmacotherapeutic perspective

Peripheral vertigo
● Destructive lesion:
  a acute phase
  b compensation phase
● Episodic vertigo
Central vertigo

Peripheral vestibular disorders

Destructive lesions

In the acute stage after vestibular failure, the patient experiences intensely unpleasant symptoms. As time passes over weeks and months, the central nervous system compensates for the loss of input from the affected labyrinth. This process allows the patient to re-establish balance for most postures and movements.

Acute phase after destructive lesions

Normal balance is maintained in part by the vestibular nuclei through their control over vestibulospinal and vestibulo-ocular reflexes. When the function of one labyrinth is reduced, the central nervous system fails to receive a reciprocally balanced input. In the early stages, this unnatural pattern of input arouses vegetative symptoms at rest, such as nausea and vomiting as well as vertigo and ataxia. These symptoms can be controlled by pharmacotherapy.

Pharmacotherapy

Drugs can effectively suppress both vestibular and vegetative symptoms during the acute stage of a complete vestibular lesion. The choice and timing of therapeutic intervention is dependent on the severity of the clinical condition. It has been argued that suppression of vestibular symptoms might prolong recovery by retarding or preventing the natural habituation process (Zee, 1985). However, in practice it is necessary to suppress the vegetative symptoms to commence rehabilitation.

Vestibular symptoms

Vestibular symptoms such as vertigo are controlled by calcium-blockers, phenothiazines, benzodiazepines or combinations of these three groups of drugs. In addition, there is one study which suggests that steroids may also have a role in the treatment of acute vestibular failure (Ariyasu *et al.*, 1990).

Calcium antagonists

Flunarizine is not generally available within the UK but it is widely used to treat certigo and has been extensively studied in Europe and elsewhere. Cinnarizine (Sturgeon) is a closely related compound which is available in the UK. Flunarizine has been shown to reduce nystagmus induced by rotation (Lee, Watson and Boothby, 1986). Cullen, Hall and Allen (1989) showed that cinnarizine had a similar effect. Comparative studies seem to suggest that flunarizine is more potent than cinnarizine (Wouters, Amery and Towse, 1983).

Pharmacology

Calcium antagonists act by blocking the ready influx of calcium, which is required for contraction, into cardiac and smooth muscle cells (Kazda, Knorr and Towart, 1983). This group of drugs is anti-vasoconstrictive causing a reduction in peripheral resistance and a slight negative inotropic effect. Each drug from the group has an individual pattern of affinity for various arteries. Both cinnarizine and flunarizine (a difluorinated derivative) have been shown to increase cerebral blood flow. Flunarizine causes vascular relaxation in the basilar artery at 1/100 the concentration required to induce a similar effect in the coronary vessels. There is also evidence of a direct effect of calcium antagonists on the vestibular system. Sterkers *et al.* (1988) suggested that interference with the Ca^{++} messenger system may influence mechano-electrical transduction of energy within vestibular hair cells. Calcium ions may also modulate the secretion of endolymph. Finally, cinnarizine may increase blood flow by preventing calcium entry into ischaemic erythrocytes, thereby preserving flexibility in the microcirculation. Side effects of calcium antagonists include drowsiness, headache, nausea, insomnia, dry mouth, rash and gastric pain.

Phenothiazines

Prochlorperazine (Stemetil) is a neuroleptic which suppresses acute vertigo, associated distress, nausea and vomiting. All neuroleptics are antagonists to dopamine receptors. They also have muscarinic receptor and α-adrenoreceptor blocking actions and therefore cause autonomic side effects including postural hypotension, dry mouth and constipation. The chemical class dictates which peripheral side effects are predominant. Prochlorperazine is in the piperazine group which has less sedative and anticholinergic effects but more pronounced extrapyramidal effects. This drug causes less drowsiness and dry mouth than chlorpromazine but is more likely to cause movement disorders such as acute dystonia particularly in the elderly and children.

Benzodiazepines

Diazepam is thought to act by the enhancement of GABA-mediated inhibition in the central nervous system. It is a GABA-agonist. In the acute phase of vestibular failure, potentiating the effect from inhibitory cerebellar GABA-ergic neurons on the vestibular nuclei may be important. Ishikawa and Igarashi (1984) studied the effect of diazepam on vestibular compensation in monkeys. They noted that ataxia was alleviated, spontaneous nystagmus was prolonged and significantly, that the period of compensation was not prolonged in animals receiving benzodiazepines.

Steroids

Ariyasu *et al.* (1990) reported the beneficial effect of methylprednisolone in a double-blind crossover trial of 20 patients with acute onset of vestibular vertigo. A course of methylprednisolone reducing from 32 mg to 0 after 8 days was given orally. Eighty per cent of patients felt prednisolone controlled vertigo more effectively than placebo (Table 6.4). Steroids were claimed to be an effective treatment for vestibular failure irrespective of the aetiology. The mode of action was not suggested but presumably it involves accelerated compensation by the central nervous system. Steroid-induced effects on mood and local anti-inflammatory action may also be factors.

Vegetative symptoms

Vegetative symptoms are controlled with antiemetic drugs. As with vestibular symptoms, there is also some evidence that steroids have a beneficial effect.

Antiemetics

Metoclopramide is a dopamine antagonist and it produces an antinausea/antiemetic action by blocking central dopamine receptors in the chemoreceptor trigger zone of the brain stem. Metoclopramide acts locally to alter upper gut motility and can lead to adverse reactions including extrapyramidal movement disorders similar to those of phenothiazines. Cyclizine is a phenothiazine with prominent antihistamine activity which acts centrally to suppress emesis and cause sedation. It has adverse reactions including antimuscarinic effects (dry mouth, blurred vision etc.).

Ondansetron (Zofran) is a serotonin type 3 receptor antagonist which exerts a potent antiemetic effect by blocking neurotransmission by serotonin within the gut and brain stem. The major indication is treatment of nausea and vomiting resulting from cytotoxic chemotherapy (Markham and Sorkin, 1993). However, it has also been used successfully to reduce postoperative nausea and vomiting (Haigh *et al.*, 1993). The drug is safe with minor side effects such as constipation and headache. It may become a useful alternative therapy for patients who are not controlled by conventional antiemetic treatment.

Compensation phase after vestibular failure

Rectifying the neurological mismatch which occurs after acute vestibular failure and the restoration of balance requires neural modifications within the cen-

Table 6.4 Summary of studies which used drugs to treat vestibular symptoms

Authors	Drug	Subjects	Success			Control	Side effects
			Good/v.good	*Poor/none*			
Destructive lesion							
Ariyasu *et al.*	Methylprednisolone	10	9/10	1/10		Double blind	
(1990)	Placebo	10	3/10	7/10		crossover	
Episodic vertigo							
			Cure	*Better*	*No change*		
Elbaz (1988)	Flunarizine + placebo	58	35/58	18/58	5/58	Double-blind	Gastrointestinal tract disorder, sleepiness
	Betahistine + placebo	48	19/48	11/48	18/48		
			Better	*No difference*	*Worse*		
Oosterveld	Betahistine	24	19/24	1/24	4/24	Double-blind	None
(1984)	Placebo	24	4/24		20/24	crossover	

tral nervous system. These processes require reorganization of sensory input into the vestibular nuclei to permit correction of vestibular dysmetria. Exposure of the central pathways to conflicting sensory information is necessary to signal the need for and direction of adaptive change. When neural adaptation has occurred, the patient is said to have compensated.

Pharmacotherapy should be discontinued when nausea has settled and balance has been restored with the head stationary. This stage is reached after a period of approximately 1 week for most patients. Thereafter, mobilization should be actively encouraged. Imbalance experienced during movement will speed the habituation process. Ideally, formal vestibular exercise programmes may be followed to acquire dynamic vestibular balance (head and body moving). Indeed vestibular habituation training has long been used to speed compensation (Cawthorne, 1945; Cooksey, 1945). In practice, the return of the patient to their former lifestyle substitutes for habituation training in the majority of cases.

The role of drugs during the compensatory phase is unclear. Animal experiments suggest that they are best avoided but many uncontrolled studies have suggested that symptomatic relief does not slow compensation significantly.

Episodic vertigo

The place of pharmacotherapy is not clearly established for patients with episodic vertigo from whatever cause. Pharmacotherapy often produces frustrating results despite the frequency with which it is prescribed. In the long term, most patients with episodic vertigo tend to remit due to compensation within the central nervous system. As pharmacotherapy may influence compensation, it would seem best to avoid it where possible. Drugs should be reserved for patients with marked distress or in whom impaired function interferes with lifestyle or employment.

Drugs may be employed symptomatically and prophylactically. Phenothiazines, calcium antagonists and antihistamines can be used to relieve vertigo and imbalance. The prophylactic properties of betahistine (histamine receptor agonist) in patients with episodic vertigo is not proven but despite the lack of evidence, the drug is widely prescribed for this purpose by specialists and general practitioners alike.

Prochlorperazine

The sublabial preparation (Buccastem) is an appropriate means of delivering the drug in the treatment of episodic vertigo. This formulation avoids the side effects encountered during oral maintenance therapy. There is no evidence of a prophylactic effect in episodic vertigo. Buccastem is not helpful in situations such as postural hypotension, where the duration of vertigo is shorter than the onset of action.

Calcium antagonists

Flunarizine has been shown to alleviate episodic vertigo in a number of double-blind trials. Oosterveld (1982) found that 10 mg flunarizine had a significant effect on vertigo. Elbaz (1988) compared flunarizine and betahistine in peripheral vestibular lesions and vertebrobasilar insufficiency. Flunarizine was significantly better, giving relief of vertigo in 60% of patients compared with 40% of patients taking betahistine (see Table 6.4). It is necessary for clinicians to be circumspect with all drug trials for episodic vertigo. Difficulty occurs with construction of reliable drug trials because of a tendency toward natural remission and large placebo effects.

Antihistamines and anticholinergics

Sedation is an important side effect which prevents the use of H_1-receptor blocking drugs (antihistamines) and anticholinergic drugs in treatment of episodic vertigo. Hyoscine and dimenhydrinate have no sustained benefit in chronic diseases such as Menière's disorder, vestibular neuronitis or benign paroxysmal positional vertigo (Wennmo *et al.*, 1987).

Newer selective H_1-receptor blocking drugs such as astemizole (Hismanal) have also been shown to possess an antivertiginous effect. Jackson and Turner (1987) reported the benefit of astemizole in patients with prolonged vertigo or dizziness combined with spontaneous or positional nystagmus. Twenty-eight of 38 patients (74%) given 5–20 mg of astemizole had symptomatic relief and reduced nystagmus. No results from a placebo group were reported.

Pharmacology

Astemizole is an H_1-receptor blocker with a long half-life. It does not cause antimuscarinic effects (drowsiness and psychomotor impairment) because of a limited ability to cross the blood–brain barrier. Sedation with other antihistamines such as dimenhydrinate results from blockade of histaminergic neurons in the mid-brain reticular formation and posterior mamillary bodies which control states of wakefulness and sleep. As with a related compound, terfenadine, ventricular arrhythmias have followed excessive dosage and care is required in liver impairment.

Betahistine

The place of betahistine as a prophylactic agent for episodic vertigo is unresolved but has important clinical and financial implications. It is widely prescribed within the UK for many causes of episodic vertigo despite the fact that it is only indicated for treatment of Menière's disorder. Some studies suggest that betahistine acts as a prophylactic by reducing the frequency of vertiginous attacks (Fischer, 1991). Evidence from double-blind crossover trials appear to support this conclusion. Oosterveld (1984) reported a trial on patients with peripheral vertigo for more than 2 months which showed betahistine to be superior to placebo. Nineteen of 24 patients reported a decrease in the incidence and severity of vertigo and less nausea and vomiting during the betahistine period of treatment compared with four who preferred placebo (see Table 6.4). Deering *et al.* (1986) reported a study of 88 patients in general practice with two or more episodes of vertigo of unknown origin during the preceding 3-month period. The frequency and

duration of attacks of vertigo during treatment were compared for 3 month courses of 24 mg betahistine three times daily or 30 mg cinnarizine three times daily. Significantly fewer and shorter attacks of vertigo occurred with betahistine therapy. However, patients did not express a preference for it over cinnarizine.

No firm conclusions can be drawn from these studies as the inclusion criteria were not specified. The role, if any, of betahistine in the treatment of episodic vertigo has still to be defined. The influence of the drug on vestibular compensation also needs to be evaluated.

Pharmacology

Betahistamine dihydrochloride is an histamine analogue which is thought to cause capillary vasodilatation in the cerebral circulation and stria vascularis of the cochlea. Betahistine may also act centrally on histaminergic synapses in the mid-brain reticular formation which regulates the state of arousal. It is associated with few side effects but can cause gastrointestinal upset and drowsiness.

Vestibular inadequacy

There is little place for drug therapy in the unfortunate group of patients with chronic vestibular inadequacy. Provision of walking sticks or walking frames is the primary mode of treatment.

Central lesions

Central vertigo commonly arises from cardiovascular disease, musculoskeletal degeneration of the spine, toxic effects from drugs, demyelinating diseases and intracranial masses. Treatment of imbalance arising from central nervous system pathology is symptomatic but appropriate medical or surgical management of the disease can be curative, for example drainage of a cerebellar abscess.

Imbalance in the elderly

Imbalance is a common symptom in the elderly. It may lead to many complaints from patients, ranging from frequent falls or loss of confidence in walking, to fear of going out and total immobility. There is impairment of balance mechanisms and increased body sway with advancing age. This explains the predisposition to balance disorders in the elderly population. However, a variety of disease processes must also be involved. The sense of imbalance is aggravated by functional impairments and disease of several other body systems. The multitude of factors which can contribute to imbalance in the elderly are listed below.

Factors contributing to imbalance in the elderly

- Visual impairment
- Bedrest and lack of regular walking
- Falls and fear of further falls
- Drugs
- Debility
- Neurological disease
- Carotid/vertebral disease
- Cardiovascular diseases
- Mental impairment

Treatment of imbalance in the elderly is best achieved by determining then avoiding the cause. It is usually advisable to apply the principle of avoidance and/or withdrawal of any unnecessary drug therapy. The latter is particularly important as many elderly patients are receiving multiple drugs on repeat prescriptions while their requirements decrease with advancing age.

Determining the cause of imbalance

Clinical evaluation may determine the cause of imbalance to be of purely an otogenic, cardiovascular, neurological, metabolic or haematological origin. Alternatively, the patient may have vague symptoms distinguishable from classical presentations of disease. Light-headedness is such a symptom and is common in patients with multiple sensory deficiencies. Elderly patients often suffer from cervical spondylosis and multiple minor sensory impairments such as visual loss and peripheral neuropathy. These patients often complain of imbalance in the absence of an identifiable cause. When the cause of the dizziness is established, appropriate treatment may be prescribed. Non-specific dizziness is not a serious problem. Often all the patient needs is reassurance and possibly the provision of a walking stick.

Avoidance or withdrawal of drugs

Avoidance of those drugs which predispose to imbalance is especially helpful including sedatives, antihypertensives and diuretics.

Wild, Nayak and Isaacs (1980) found evidence of association between falling and the consumption of the following drugs: antihypertensives, hypnotics, sedatives, alcohol and antidepressants. These drugs presumably slow neural conduction within the central nervous system and impair the accuracy of corrective movements. Hypnotics continue to act for a longer time in old people. Antidepressant drugs such as imipramine and amitriptyline may be associated with falls as a consequence of their postural hypotensive effects.

Postural hypotension

Dizziness resulting from postural change is a major problem in the elderly. Postural hypotension occurs in patients who have defective postural vasomotor reflexes: it is common in diabetics, in patients receiving antihypertensive drugs or in cases where diuretic therapy has caused sodium and fluid depletion. Treatment consists of advice to the patient on standing up slowly and to raising the bed head to improve autonomic tone. Medications should be reviewed and drugs such as diuretics and sedatives discontinued if possible. Fludrocortisone (a mineralocorticoid) 100 μg daily may be helpful for controlling the condition. Fludrocortisone causes retention of fluid which will correct fluid depletion in the elderly but peripheral oedema and congestive heart failure can complicate treatment. Postural dizziness, without detectable change in blood pressure on standing, is much more common than clinically proven postural hypotension. It may also be improved by withdrawal of drugs.

Pharmacotherapy for inner ear disease resulting from local or systemic pathology

Pharmacotherapy is the principal mode of treatment used in the management of many disorders of the inner ear. Motion sickness arising from excessive stimulation of the labyrinth and disorders caused by infection, hydrops and autoimmune ear disease respond to pharmacotherapy to a greater or lesser degree.

Motion sickness

Tolerance (vestibular compensation) to continuous motion in normal subjects occurs over a period of days. Motion sickness can occur during this time, and is due to excessive and changing neural input from the labyrinths. A wide variety of other factors predispose an individual to motion sickness; these include previous experience, reading, warm environment, a full stomach and powerful odours.

Motion sickness is easier to prevent than cure. Estimation of the likely duration of exposure will influence the choice of drug for prophylaxis. Hyoscine (scopolamine) and cyclizine have a short duration of action but the former may cause confusion in the elderly. Meclozine and promethazine have long half-lives and are suitable for prolonged journeys. These drugs may cause drowsiness and should not be combined with alcohol or used where a long car drive is necessary. Most of these drugs are antihistamines with anticholinergic properties.

When sickness occurs, difficulties with administration of drugs arise. Motion sickness inhibits gastric motility, making the oral route ineffective for medication. The transdermal and intramuscular routes are effective alternatives.

Hyoscine

Acetylcholine is the neurotransmitter released from postganglionic nerve terminals. The effects of stimulating acetylcholine at these sites is reproduced by administration of the toxin muscarine. Muscarinic effects include: constriction of the pupil, accommodation for near vision, profuse watery salivation, bronchiolar constriction, bronchosecretion, hypotension (due to bradycardia and vasodilatation), increase in gut motility and secretion, contraction of the urinary bladder and sweating. Hyoscine (scopolamine) is a natural alkaloid which *blocks* acetylcholine at postganglionic nerve terminals and acts centrally to cause an antiemetic effect, sedation, drowsiness and amnesia. Pyykkö, Schälen and Jantti (1985) showed a beneficial effect on motion induced vertigo and nausea with transdermal patches containing hyoscine. These are useful when short periods of nausea are anticipated and they avoid the problems which arise with oral administration when sickness occurs.

Antihistamines

Promethazine (Phenergan) is a phenothiazine derivative which is widely used for its antihistaminic properties. It is sedating and has anticholinergic side effects but is probably the drug of choice for intramuscular use because of a longer duration of action than hyoscine and a high level of effectiveness. Wood *et al.* (1992) measured the amount of increased head movement before onset of sickness with various antimotion drugs. Hyoscine was superior to promethazine and had a duration of action of 4 hours compared with 12 hours for promethazine. The effect of both drugs was significantly enhanced by adrenalin (epinephrine).

Flunarizine is a calcium antagonist which is an effective treatment for motion sickness. It causes less central depressive side effects which characterize treatment with antihistamines and anticholinergics. The mode of action in motion sickness may be due to antihistaminic and antidopaminergic effects rather than calcium antagonism (Rascol, Clanet and Montastruc, 1989).

Phenytoin and other anticonvulsant drugs such as carbamazepine have been shown to increase the tolerance to motion stress without adverse effects such as blurred vision, dry mouth or sedation (Chelen *et al.*, 1990). A trial of the effect of 1–1.4 g of phenytoin administered in five divided doses over a 20-hour period prior to challenge with severe rotational stimulation demonstrated significant benefit. A single daily dose of phenytoin was suggested as being most effective. Light-headedness is a frequent side effect (Chelen *et al.*, 1993).

Otosyphilis

Hearing and balance disorders are most common in late congenital and late acquired syphilis. Hearing loss in both forms tends to be sudden, partially asymmetrical, fluctuating and often accompanied by tinnitus and episodic vertigo. Severe sensorineural hearing loss, usually bilateral, is the usual outcome of untreated syphilitic labyrinthitis. Primary syphilis is treated with 600 000 international units of procaine penicillin daily for a 10-day course. Recovery of hearing and/or vestibular function in early otosyphilis is excellent. In contrast, pharmacotherapy for late congenital and acquired otosyphilis is often prolonged and less successful. Late otosyphilis is best treated with antibiotics and steroids.

Antibiotics

Smyth (1968) postulated that the treponeme in late syphilis is in a more dormant state with division times of up to 90 days. Accordingly treponemocidal levels must be maintained for prolonged periods. Ampicillin has been successfully used in the treatment of otosyphilis and has the advantage that it may be administered orally. The penicillins produce their bactericidal effect by preventing the cross-linkage between the linear peptidoglycan polymer chains which are important structural elements of the cell wall. Adams *et al.* (1983) found that ampicillin (1.5 g four times daily for 4 weeks) in combination with prednisolone (10 mg three times daily for 10 days), gradually reduced over a subsequent 10-day period, preserved the hearing in about half the cases they followed up over 5–14 years. In those patients who failed to respond to ampicillin and steroid, regular injections of ACTH over *many years* has resulted in the maintenance of hearing in the majority of cases. Amoxycillin has been shown to produce treponemicidal levels in the CSF using 6 g combined with 2 g probenicid daily (Faber *et al.*, 1983).

Penicillin is also effective when combined with steroids. Dobbin and Perkins (1983) gave 10 million units penicillin G intravenously daily for 2 weeks then intramuscular injections on alternate weeks for 10 weeks. Concomitant steroids were given for a 1-month period but a lasting response was observed in only two out of 13 patients. This poor outcome may have been due to the fact that steroids were not continued over the long term. If the patient is allergic to penicillin, doxycycline (a tetracycline) can be administered as 300 mg daily for 21 days to treat late syphilis. Cephaloridine 1 g twice daily intramuscularly for 21 days or erythromycin 500 mg orally four times a day for 21 days have also been recommended (Dunlop, 1985).

Steroids

Most studies show hearing improvement in 35–50% of late congenital and acquired syphilitics with combined antibiotic and steroid treatment. Darmstadt and Harris (1989) reviewed the literature and suggested that prednisolone 40–60 mg/day for 2 weeks was the minimum treatment. The possible mechanisms of action are non-specific reduction of vasculitis or suppression of the immune response to antigens released on lysis of spirochaetes. The side effects of treatment include the Jarisch-Herxheimer reaction (JHR), penicillin allergy and steroid toxicity and these are fully described in the relevant chapter. Relative contraindications for steroid therapy include duodenal ulceration, diabetes mellitus, hypertension, tuberculosis, pregnancy, glaucoma and psychiatric illness. The features of Cushing's syndrome may develop in cases of prolonged steroid therapy.

Menière's disorder

The AAO-HNS guidelines (Pearson and Brackmann, 1985) state that reporting of clinical results for treatment of Menière's disorder will only be valid if evaluated 2 years after initiation of therapy, whether medical or surgical. No controlled drug trial adheres to the guidelines although some reports on aminoglycoside administration during surgery have a 2-year follow up. Short-term trials with no information on the relapse rate after termination of the trial are unhelpful in this chronic relapsing disease which may last decades.

Acute attack

Drug therapy is used to manage acute attacks of Menière's disorder. In severe cases, bed rest and correction of fluid and electrolyte imbalance may be necessary. The control of vertigo and vomiting is discussed above. Gejrot (1976) reported successful control of attacks with infusion of lignocaine. The risk of serious adverse effects limits the usefulness of this form of treatment.

Prophylaxis

Medical treatment of Menière's disorder has many aspects. Psychological support, pharmacotherapy and dietary modification are frequently used to assist patients. The role of drugs in long-term treatment of Menière's disorder is controversial. Evidence is mounting that drug therapy in Menière's disorder only produces symptomatic relief, rather than influencing the disease process as was previously supposed.

Histamine-receptor agonist

The unproven hypothesis that Menière's disorder results from ischaemia of the stria vascularis has been used as a justification for the use of capillary vasodilators. Histamine is a natural vasodilator which causes flushing. It is rarely used because of the disadvantages of a narrow therapeutic range and of being ineffective when administered orally. Betahistine is a synthetic analogue of histamine (Fischer, 1991). The reduction in vertigo observed with betahistine in drug trials does not seem to continue after discontinuation of therapy. Two double-blind crossover trials of betahistine provide evidence of short-term control of vertigo in Menière's disorder by betahistine (Frew and Menon, 1976; Wilmott and Menon, 1976). Both studies were small and of insufficient duration (36 and 24 weeks respectively). Fraysse *et al.* (1991) compared the efficacy and safety of betahistine and flunarizine in 55 patients with probable Menière's disorder in a double-blind study. Betahistine was superior to flunarizine in terms of reduction in severity, duration and number of vertiginous attacks and in other vestibular and cochlear symptoms. Side effects were significantly fewer with betahistine. This result is at odds with the results of the study by Elbaz (1988). Bertrand (1982) reported a long-term evaluation of betahistine treatment in Menière's disorder. In this study of 60 patients treated for 12–14 years; 13 were symptom free at death or follow up, 36 required continuous treatment to avoid relapse and 11 were failures and had revision surgery.

Betahistine appears to offer limited prophylaxis against attacks during therapy but does not modify the disease process (Oosterveld, 1984; Deering *et al.*, 1986).

Drugs with possible prophylactic value in Menière's disorder

Diuretics

There is no convincing evidence that thiazide diuretics are effective in Menière's disorder. Early reports by Klockhoff and Lindblom (1967) and Klockhoff, Lindblom and Stahle (1974) claimed to show a significant reduction in attacks of vertigo from a double-blind controlled trial of hydrochlorthiazide and a long-term study of chlorthalidone respectively. Ruckenstein, Rutka and Hawke (1991) reviewed the study and observed that 15 of 26 (58%) had less vertigo with hydrochlorthiazide compared with 14 of 26 (54%) given placebo. In a second paper by Klockhoff, Lindblom and Stahle (1974), 26 of 34 of patients (76%) treated for 7 years had a reduction in the frequency and intensity of vertiginous episodes. This figure falls within the 60–80% range of success which has been reported for most treatment modalities in use for Menière's disorder (McKee *et al.*, 1991). Thiazide diuretics induce a diuresis by blocking sodium reabsorption in the proximal portion of the distal tubule of the nephron. Their clinical effect on the inner ear is unknown.

Controlled trials suggest that other types of diuretics have no treatment benefit in Menière's disorder. Van Deelan and Huizing (1986) reported that hydrochlorthiazide and triamterine were ineffective in a double-blind trial of 33 patients. Preference for diuretic was expressed by only half of the treatment group. Acetazolamide is a carbonic anhydrase inhibitor that causes a diuresis by decreasing sodium–hydrogen exchange in the renal tubule. Brookes and Booth (1984) found that acetazolamide did not reduce symptoms and was associated with side effects in 46% of patients. Corvera and Corvera (1989) in a retrospective review found that long-term treatment with chlorthalidone or acetazolamide did not prevent deterioration of hearing in Menière's disorder.

Salt

Salt can be used to destroy the cochleovestibular neuroepithelium of the affected ear in Menière's disorder. Colletti, Fiorino and Sittoni (1989) described inserting salt crystals into the vestibule after stapedectomy. Vertiginous episodes were controlled in all 21 patients over a follow-up period of 32–81 months. This procedure is associated with hearing loss from what is in essence a chemical labyrinthectomy.

Lignocaine and steroid

Itoh and Sakata (1991) compared the use of lignocaine and dexamethasone or dexamethasone alone injected into the tympanic cavity in Menière's disorder and labyrinthine vertigo. Success rates of 79–84% were reported in large groups of patients but no follow-up period was specified in this open trial. Coles, Thompson and O'Donoghue (1992) found a similar method used to treat tinnitus was ineffective and unpleasant for patients.

Immunotherapy

Derebery and Valenzuela (1992) proposed that desensitization to inhalant allergens and elimination of foods allergens from the diet was a useful treatment in patients with Menière's disorder and evidence of allergy on skin or RAST (radio-allergosorbent) testing. Fifty-six of 90 (62%) patients had improvement in symptoms but one patient had a severe reaction requiring adrenalin. This adverse effect raises major concerns about the risk of treatment with immunotherapy in a disease with no proven allergic basis.

Ototoxic vestibular ablation

Aminoglycosides

Aminoglycosides exert their bacteriocidal effect by inhibiting protein synthesis. Non-functional proteins are synthesized by the bacterium which leads to cell death. One of the most important side effects of aminoglycosides is ototoxicity. The antibiotic accumulates in perilymph and leads to hair cell death. The ototoxic effects of streptomycin and gentamicin are predominantly vestibulotoxic but cochleotoxicity occurs at higher doses. Neuroepithelium within the cristae then the utricle and finally the saccule are affected by increasing dose. Systemic and local administration of these drugs have been used to attempt therapeutic ablation of vestibular function in incapacitating Menière's disorder where useful residual hearing is present.

Systemic administration

Intramuscular titration of streptomycin is a therapeutic option in patients with disabling vertigo from bilateral disease or disease in the only hearing ear. Schuknecht (1957) established the standard indications and treatment regimen for systemic streptomycin therapy. Silverstein *et al.* (1984) reported the use of streptomycin sulphate 1 g twice daily for 2–3 weeks to a maximum dose of 18–54 g in six patients. All patients were relieved of vertigo with preservation of hearing but all had profound ataxia and oscillopsia. Controlled trials have not been performed. Langman, Kemink and Graham (1990) administered 5–50 g in 19 patients. Good control of vertigo was achieved in 16 of 19 but permanent post-treatment dysequilibrium occurred in 47%. It would seem that the patient is at significant risk of having worse symptoms after this form of treatment.

Local administration

Patients with unilateral disease and serviceable hearing present most frequently to the clinician. It is desirable to use a mode of treatment which cures vertigo but conserves hearing in these patients. Local vestibulotoxic injury can be harnessed successfully to ablate vestibular function in the target ear. There are two principal methods of delivery in use. The first method involves delivery of aminoglycoside into the middle ear cleft by intratympanic injection or via a catheter delivery device. The second method involves perfusion with aminoglycoside solution or insertion of a dried flake of aminoglycoside into the labyrinth via a fenestration of the lateral semicircular canal. Chemical ablation of a diseased labyrinth offers good control of vertigo in Menière's disorder but carries a considerable risk of sensorineural hearing loss. Table 6.5 summarizes the results of local administration of aminoglycoside in Menière's disorder.

Results

Schmidt, Beck and Lange (1980) reported 37 of 40 patients (93%) free from vertigo after application of gentamicin through a polyethylene tube placed through the eardrum. Patients were claimed to have excellent relief from tinnitus and fullness, although 15% had hearing loss. Nedzelski *et al.* (1992) used a

Table 6.5 Results of local administration of aminoglycoside in Ménière's disorder

Authors	Number	Mean dose and drug	Delivery	Vertigo control (%)	Hearing loss (%)	Follow up
Schmidt, Beck and Lange (1980)	40	144 mg Gent	Tube to ME	93	15	2–6 years
Laitakari (1990)	20	48 mg Gent	Tube to ME	60	45	1–6 years
Nedzelski *et al.* (1992)	20	208 mg Gent	Tube to ME	90	15	2 years
Møller *et al.* (1989)	15	200 mg Gent	Inject to ME	93	33	1–6 years
Odkvist (1988)	29	130 mg Gent	Inject to ME	97	31	1–9 years
Shea (1989)	12	150 μg Strep	Perfused SCC	92	25	?
Amedee, Morris and Risey (1991)	8	125 μg Strep	Flake in SCC	65	50	2.2 years
Monsell and Shelton (1992)	47	Streptomycin	Perfused SCC	83	68	10 months

Gent = gentamicin; Strep = streptomycin; ME = middle ear; SCC = semicircular canal

similar delivery method for daily injection of gentamicin in 20 patients. Eighteen of 20 (90%) were free from vertigo, hearing deteriorated in 15% and no change was observed in tinnitus. Møller *et al.* (1988) reported 14 of 15 patients (93%) free from vertigo after treatment with 3–11 daily intratympanic injections of 30 mg gentamicin. Odkvist (1988) reported 28 of 29 (97%) were free from vertigo after treatment. Approximately one-third of patients suffered increased hearing loss but many reported alleviation of tinnitus and fullness in the ear. Laitakari (1990) reported 60% control of vertigo and 45% hearing loss in 20 patients after delivering gentamicin through a polyethylene tube into the middle ear. He felt that the technique was less useful than previously stated.

Aminoglycosides may also be administered via fenestration of the lateral semicircular canal. Shea (1989) described perfusing a 1 ml solution of 150 μg streptomycin sulphate and 20 mg methyl prednisolone in Ringer lactate. Surgery was accompanied by a single intramuscular injection of 1 g streptomycin sulphate. Vertigo was controlled in 11 of 12 patients (92%) but no follow-up period was specified. Amedee, Norris and Risey (1991) inserted a dried flake of 125 or 250 μg streptomycin powder into the lateral semicircular canal in 15 patients with intractable Ménière's disorder. The 250 μg dose was abandoned because of unacceptable sensorineural hearing loss. Successful control of vertigo was achieved in 65% with the 125 μg flake but sensorineural hearing loss was observed in four of eight patients. Early results from the Labyrinthotomy Streptomycin Infusion (LSI) Multicenter Study Group are discouraging (Monsell and Shelton, 1992). This group reported the outcome on 47 cases and concluded that LSI was associated with severe postoperative hearing loss (57%), and revision surgery (failure) was required in 17% of patients. Kerr (1995) described an additional opening into the labyrinth, into the posterior semicircular canal. In a 3-year follow up of 11 patients he controlled the vertigo in 91% with hearing preservation in 45%.

Hearing loss frequently complicates topical aminoglycoside therapy in Ménière's disorder. This suggests that dosages used may be unnecessarily high. Magnusson and Padoan (1991) observed that following intratympanic instillation of gentamicin, vertigo and nystagmus occurred 3–5 days after treatment was stopped. They suggested that gentamicin treatment should not be continued until symptoms of ototoxic effects on the cochlea were apparent as is the present practice. They argued that extremely low-dose treatment produced sufficient loss of vestibular function with less risk of affecting the hearing level.

Autoimmune inner ear disease

Autoimmune inner ear disease is a concept proposed by McCabe (1979). It is thought to result from targeting of inner ear type 2 collagen by the host's immune system (Cruz *et al.*, 1990; Harris and Sharp, 1990). The disease is uncommon and presents as progressive bilateral sensorineural deafness responsive to treatment with immunosuppression. Episodic vertigo similar to that of Ménière's disorder may accompany auditory symptoms.

Diagnosis is made if a response is observed to a 3-week trial of treatment with immunosuppression (McCabe, 1989). Clearly it is not ideal to diagnose the disease in this way and some workers are sceptical about the existence of autoimmune inner ear disease. Response to treatment is defined as an improvement in pure-tone thresholds of 15 dB at three sound frequencies or of 20% speech discrimination scores. Treatment consists of combination therapy with cyclophosphamide and prednisolone for a period of 3 months. The dose of cyclophosphamide is 2 mg/kg twice daily and that of prednisolone is 30 mg on alternate days. Prednisolone is continued for a further 2 weeks then tailed off over 2 weeks. The treatment regimen can be repeated up to eight times for a total of 2 years.

Luetje (1989) suggested that plasmapheresis may be effective as an alternative or adjunctive therapy in autoimmune inner ear disease. The role of plasmapheresis remains to be clarified.

Cyclophosphamide

Cyclophosphamide is an alkylating agent which reacts with bases in the DNA strand and prevents cell division by cross-linking the two strands of the double helix. It is metabolized in the liver to form active metabolites. One metabolite, acrolein, occasionally causes a serious complication, haemorrhagic cystitis. Cyclophosphamide can cause profound neutropenia. The drug should be stopped if the white cell count falls below $4000 \times 10^6/l$ and recommenced when the white cell count exceeds this figure.

Vertebrobasilar insufficiency

The classification of patients with posterior cerebral circulation disease requires a combination of clinical observation and vertebral angiography (Caplan, 1981). Because of attendant risk, angiography is seldom undertaken except when there is probable ischaemic disease. The clinical syndrome resulting from vertebrobasilar insufficiency is therefore not a diagnosis. The use of the term vertebrobasilar insufficiency is usually inaccurate if it has been applied to patients with unclassified vertigo associated with vascular risk factors and cervical arthritis. These criteria are not relevant to the diagnosis of vertebrobasilar insufficiency.

Diagnosis requires a history of several transient ischaemic attacks causing at least two and preferably three of the following symptoms: vertigo, drop attacks, diplopia, bulbar symptoms, hemianopia, and occipital headache: vertigo alone is insufficient. In the rare true case of vertebrobasilar insufficiency, vascular stenosis or embolism from intimal plaques may be displayed by angiography. Kessler *et al.* (1991) studied 35 patients with Doppler-sonograpy and found evidence of reduced carbon dioxide dependent reactivity of the basilar artery in patients with vertebrobasilar insufficiency. The basilar artery was found not to dilate as fully in this group of patients where carbon dioxide tension in arterial blood was elevated. The significance of this observation is unknown.

Results

Hofferberth (1986) reported a number of double-blind crossover trials in patients with true vertebrobasilar insufficiency. Flunarizine and nimodipine 40 mg three times a day for 4 weeks were found to reduce dizziness significantly. Nimodipine is a calcium antagonist which is used to relieve vascular spasm after subarachnoid haemorrhage. There are no trials of cinnarizine in vertebrobasilar insufficiency although theoretically it should be helpful. Aspirin 75 mg daily may be a useful treatment of true vertebrobasilar insufficiency. Its major action would be to reduce the risk of stroke rather than relief of imbalance.

Wegener's granulomatosis

Wegener's granulomatosis is a systemic granulomatous disease which frequently presents with ear or nasal manifestations. Sensorineural hearing loss and serous otitis media are common features of the disease (Kempf, 1989). Sensorineural hearing loss is potentially reversible with immunosuppressive therapy. It is advisable to seek the opinion of an experienced physician to exclude renal or pulmonary lesions in patients with otolaryngological manifestations of Wegener's disease.

Therapy with cyclophosphamide 100–200 mg and prednisolone 50–60 mg daily in an adult male is recommended. Azothioprine 250 mg may be substituted for cyclophosphamide. Kornblut, Wolff and Fauci (1982) recommended continued medication for about 1 year *after* clinical remission of the disease. There is growing evidence for the efficacy of co-trimoxazole (sulfamethoxazole-trimethoprim) in Wegener's granulomatosis (DeRemee, McDonald and Weiland, 1985). Co-trimoxazole is an antimicrobial drug that inhibits nucleic acid synthesis by blocking purine and pyrimidine nucleotide synthesis. It is thought to have an immunosuppressive action in Wegener's disease. It is significant that azothioprine is converted into the antimetabolite mercaptopurine within the body. This compound also impairs the synthesis of purine nucleotides but the mechanisms involved are not clear. McRae and Buchanan (1993) reviewed the beneficial effect of co-trimoxazole 480 mg twice daily for 2–8 week courses. Co-trimoxazole seems to allow the early reduction of the dose of immunosuppressive therapy. It has also been used over the long term to maintain remission as a substitute for immunosuppressive therapy.

Systemic autoimmune diseases causing deafness

Several systemic autoimmune diseases cause deafness. These conditions are rare and are treated with a variable degree of success by immunosuppressive drugs. Disease states include: Behçet's disease, Cogan's syndrome, polyarteritis nodosa, temporal arteritis and Takayasu's disease.

Behçet's disease

Behçet's disease is thought to be an autoimmune vasculitic disease producing a classical triad of oral, genital and ocular lesions. Hearing loss has been demonstrated in 80% of sufferers (Elidan *et al.*, 1991). These authors reported the beneficial effect of cyclosporin A in a randomized double-blind trial compared with conventional therapy (prednisolone and chlorambucil) in 35 patients. Five of 20 (25%) Behçet's patients treated with cyclosporin A had significantly improved hearing thresholds after treatment.

Pharmacology

Cyclosporin A is a metabolite of soil fungi which is a potent immunosuppressant used to prevent the rejection of heart and kidney transplants. Side effects are common and include paraesthesia, gingival hypertrophy, fatigue and gastrointestinal discomfort. It is nephrotoxic and hepatotoxic. Serum creatinine and liver function must be monitored closely.

Cogan's syndrome

Cogan's syndrome is a rare systemic autoimmune disease with prominent ophthalmological and vestibulocochlear manifestations (Wilder-Smith and Roelcke, 1990). Sensorineural hearing loss, vertigo and tinnitus are present in almost all patients. Reports suggest that associated sensorineural hearing loss is reversible only if treatment is commenced early. Vollertsen *et al.* (1986) reviewed the subject. Eleven of 19 patients (58%) in the literature with mild to moderate hearing loss had improvement in their hearing within 1 week of commencing treatment. They proposed an initial regimen of 1–1.5 mg/kg of prednisolone daily, gradually reducing depending on clinical response. Steroids were discontinued if there was no response after 2 weeks of treatment.

Polyarteritis nodosa

Hearing loss is a rare feature of polyarteritis nodosa. Two case reports suggest that hearing loss is potentially reversible with immunosuppression and/or corticosteroid therapy (Wolf *et al.*, 1987; Vathenen, Skinner and Shale, 1988).

Temporal arteritis

Hearing loss is an extremely rare presenting feature of temporal arteritis. One case report indicated that hearing loss reversed with 2 weeks of steroid therapy (Kramer, Nesher and Sonnenblick, 1988).

Takayasu's disease

Hearing loss is a recognized feature of Takayasu's disease which mainly affects large arteries in middle-aged females. Kunihiro *et al.* (1990) reported five cases of this rare disease who had sensorineural

hearing loss, all of whom were responsive to steroid therapy.

Hormonal disturbance

There is a widespread belief that correction of metabolic disturbance in conditions such as hypothyroidism and diabetes mellitus will reverse hearing loss. There is no conclusive evidence that this is the case (Parving, 1991). Hearing thresholds were measured in 15 hypothyroid patients before and after 32–46 months of thyroxine therapy. No improvement in hearing levels was observed.

Similarly there is no proof that treatment modifies sensorineural hearing loss in diabetes. Insulin-dependent diabetics with short- and long-term disease and matched controls have similar hearing thresholds and speech discrimination scores. Long-term insulin-dependent diabetics have evidence of encephalopathy which may impair central auditory processing. Impairment of functions within the central auditory pathway may create a hearing disability which is not apparent with basic audiometric testing.

References

ADAMS, D. A., KERR, A. G., SMYTH, G. D. L. and CINNAMOND, M. J. (1983) Congenital syphilitic deafness – a further review. *Journal of Laryngology and Otology*, **97**, 399–404

AMEDEE, R. G., NORRIS, C. H. and RISEY, J. A. (1991) Selective chemical vestibulectomy: preliminary results with human application. *Otolaryngology – Head and Neck Surgery*, **105**, 107–112

ANDERSON, R. G. and MEYERHOFF, W. L. (1983) Sudden sensorineural hearing loss. *Otolaryngologic Clinics of North America*, **16**, 189–195

ARIYASU, L., BYL, F. M., SPRAGUE, M. S. and ADOUR, K. K. (1990) The beneficial effect of methylprednisolone in acute vestibular vertigo. *Archives of Otolaryngology – Head and Neck Surgery*, **116**, 700–703

BELLINI, M. J., TERRY, R. M. and LEWIS, F. A. (1989) An evaluation of common cerumenolytic agents: an in-vitro study. *Clinical Otolaryngology*, **14**, 23–25

BERTRAND, R. A. (1982) Long-term evaluation of the treatment of Meniere's disease with betahistine HCL. *Advances in Oto-Rhino-Laryngology*, **28**, 104–110

BLAYNEY, A. W., PHILLIPS, M. S., GUY, A. M. and COLMAN, B. H. (1985) A sequential double blind cross-over trial of tocainide hydrochloride in tinnitus. *Clinical Otolaryngology*, **10**, 97–101

BROOKES, G. B. and BOOTH, J. B. (1984) Oral acetazolamide in Meniere's disease. *Journal of Laryngology and Otology*, **98**, 1087–1095

CAPLAN, L. R. (1981) Vertebrobasilar disease: time for a new strategy. *Stroke*, **12**, 111–114

CAWTHORNE, T. (1945) Vestibular injuries. *Proceedings of the Royal Society of Medicine*, **39**, 270–273

CHELEN, W., KABRISKY, M., HATSELL, C., MORALES, R., FIX, E. and SCOTT, M. (1990) Use of phenytoin in the prevention of motion sickness. *Aviation, Space, and Environmental Medicine*, **61**, 1022–1025

CHELEN, W., AHMED, N., KABRISKY, M. and RODGERS, S. (1993) Computerized task battery assessment of cognitive and performance effects of acute phenytoin motion sickness therapy. *Aviation, Space, and Environmental Medicine*, **64**, 201–205

CHEN, D. A. and CAPAROSA, R. J. (1991) A nonprescription cerumenolytic. *American Journal of Otology*, **12**, 475–476

COLES, R. (1988) Trial of an abstract of Ginkgo biloba (EGB) for tinnitus and hearing loss. *Clinical Otolaryngology*, **13**, 501–502

COLES, R. R. A., THOMPSON, A. C. and O'DONOGHUE, G. M. (1992) Intra-tympanic injections in the treatment of tinnitus. *Clinical Otolaryngology*, **17**, 240–242

COLLETTI, V., FIORINO, F. G. and SITTONI, V. (1989) NaCl deposition in the vestibule: a simple, safe, and effective method of cochleovestibular deafferentation. *American Journal of Otology*, **10**, 451–455

COOKSEY, F. S., (1945) Rehabilitation in vestibular injuries. *Proceedings of the Royal Society of Medicine*, **39**, 273–278

CORVERA, J. and CORVERA, G. (1989) Long-term effect of acetazolamide and chlorthalidone on the hearing loss of Meniere's disease. *American Journal of Otology*, **10**, 142–145

COWAN, P. F. and CHOW. J. M. (1988) Sudden sensorineural hearing loss. *American Family Physician*, **37**, 207–210

CRUZ, O. L. M., MINITI, A., COSSERMELLI, W. and OLIVEIRA, R. M. (1990) Autoimmune sensorineural hearing loss: a preliminary experimental study. *American Journal of Otology*, **11**, 342–346

CULLEN, J. R., HALL, S. J. and ALLEN, R. H. (1989) Effect of betahistine dihydrochloride compared with cinnarizine on induced vestibular nystagmus. *Clinical Otolaryngology*, **14**, 485–487

DARMSTADT, G. L. and HARRIS, J. P. (1989) Luetic hearing loss: clinical presentation, diagnosis and treatment. *American Journal of Otolaryngology*, **10**, 410–421

DEERING, R. B., PRESCOTT, P., SIMMONS, R. L. and DOWNEY, L. J. (1986) A double-blind crossover study comparing betahistine and cinnarizine in the treatment of recurrent vertigo in patients in general practice. *Current Medical Research and Opinion*, **10**, 209–214

DEREBERY, M. J. and VALENZUELA, S. (1992) Meniere's syndrome and allergy. *Otolaryngologic Clinics of North America*, **25**, 213–224

DEREMEE, R. A., MCDONALD, T. J. and WEILAND, L. H. (1985) Wegener's granulomatosis: observations on treatment with antimicrobial agents. *Mayo Clinic Proceedings*, **60**, 27–32

DESLOOVERE, C., LORZ, M. and KLIMA, A. (1989) Sudden sensorineural hearing loss influence of hemodynamical and hemorheological factors on spontaneous recovery and therapy results. *Acta Oto-Rhino-Laryngologica Belgica*, **43**, 31–37

DOBBIN, J. M. and PERKINS, J. H. (1983) Otosyphilis and hearing loss: response to penicillin and steroid therapy. *Laryngoscope*, **93**, 1540–1543

DOBIE, R. A., SAKAI, C. S., SULLIVAN, M. D., KATON, W. J. and RUSSO, J. (1993) Antidepressant treatment of tinnitus patients: report of a randomised clinical trial and clinical prediction of benefit. *American Journal of Otology*, **14**, 18–23

DONALDSON, J. A. (1979) Heparin therapy for sudden sensorineural hearing loss. *Archives of Otolaryngology*, **105**, 351–352

DUMMER, D. S., SUTHERLAND, I. A. and MURRAY, J. A. (1992) A single-blind, randomized study to compare the efficacy of two ear drop preparations (Audax and Cerumol) in the softening of ear wax. *Current Medical Research and Opinion*, **13**, 26–30

DUNLOP, E. M. C. (1985) Survival of treponemes after treatment: comments, clinical conclusions, and recommendations. *Genitourinary Medicine*, **61**, 293–301

EHRENBERGER, K. and BRIX, R. (1987) Tinnitus treatment: intravenous administration of glutamate and its antagonist glutamic acid diethylester. In: *Proceedings of the Third International Tinnitus Seminar, Munster, 1987*, edited by H. Feldmann. Karlsruhe: Harsch Verlag. pp. 331–334

ELBAZ, P. (1988) Flunarizine and betahistine. Two different therapeutic approaches in vertigo compared in a double-blind study. *Acta Otolaryngologica*, Suppl. **460**, 143–148

ELIDAN, J., LEVI, H., COHEN, E. and BENEZRA, D. (1991) Effect of cyclosporine A on the hearing loss in Behçet's disease. *Annals of Otology, Rhinology and Laryngology*, **100**, 464–468

EMMETT, J. R. and SHEA, J. J. (1979) Diatrizoate meglumine (Hypaque) treatment for sudden hearing loss. *Laryngoscope*, **89**, 1229–1238

FABER, W. R., BOS, J. D., RIETRA, P. J. G. M., FASS, H. and VAN EIJK, R. V. W. (1983) Treponemicidal levels of amoxicillin in cerebrospinal fluid after oral administration. *Sexually Transmitted Diseases*, **10**, 148–150

FISCH, U. (1983) Management of sudden deafness. *Otolaryngology Head and Neck Surgery*, **91**, 3–8

FISCHER, A. J. E. M. (1991) Histamine in the treatment of vertigo. *Acta Otolaryngologica*, Suppl. **479**, 24–28

FLOHR, H., ABELN, W. and LUNEBURG, U. (1985) Neurotransmitter and neuromodulator systems involved in vestibular compensation. In: *Adaptive Mechanisms in Gaze Control: Facts and Theories*, edited by A. Berthoz and G. Melville Jones. Amsterdam: Elsevier Science Publishers. pp. 269–277

FORTNUM, H. M. and COLES, R. R. A. (1991) Trial of flecainide acetate in the management of tinnitus. *Clinical Otolaryngology*, **16**, 93–96

FRAYSSE, B., BEBEAR, J.-P., DUBREUIL, C., BERGES, C. and DAUMAN, R. (1991) Betahistine dihydrochloride versus flunarizine. A double-blind study on recurrent vertigo with and without cochlear syndrome typical of Meniere's disease. *Acta Otolaryngologica*, Suppl. **490**, 1–10

FRAZER, J. G. (1970) The efficacy of wax solvents: *in vitro* studies and a clinical trial. *Journal of Laryngology and Otology*, **84**, 1055–1064

FREW, I. J. C. and MENON, G. N. (1976) Betahistine hydrochloride in Meniere's disease. *Postgraduate Medical Journal*, **52**, 501–503

GEJROT, T (1976) Intravenous xylocaine in the treatment of attacks of Meniere's disease. *Acta Otolaryngologica*, **82**, 301–302

GUTH, P. S., RISEY, J., BRINER, W., BLAIR, P., REED, H. T., BRYANT, G. et al. (1990) Evaluation of amino-oxyacetic acid as a palliative in tinnitus. *Annals of Otology, Rhinology and Laryngology*, **99**, 74–79

HAIGH, C. G., KAPLAN, L. A., DURHAM, J. M., DUPREYON, J. P., HARMER, M. and KENNY, G. N. (1993) Nausea and vomiting after gynaecological surgery: a meta-analysis of factors affecting their incidence. *British Journal of Anaesthesia*, **71**, 517–522

HARKER, L. A., TYLER, R. S., FREDELL, P. A., KUK, F., SELLERS, J.

A., FOX, T. L. *et al.* (1987) Evaluation of flecainide acetate (Tambocor) as a treatment for tinnitus. In: *Proceedings of the Third International Tinnitus Seminar*, Munster, 1987, edited by H. Feldmann. Karlsruhe: Harsch Verlag. pp. 322–325

HARRIS, J. P. and SHARP, P. A. (1990) Inner ear autoantibodies in patients with rapidly progressive sensorineural hearing loss. *Laryngoscope*, **100**, 516–524

HOFFERBERTH, B. (1986) Calcium entry blockers in the treatment of vertebrobasilar insufficiency. *European Neurology*, **25**, (Suppl. 1), 80–85

HUANG, T-S., CHAN, S-T., HO, T-L., SU J-L. and LEE, F-P. (1989) Hypaque and steroids in the treatment of sudden sensorineural hearing loss. *Clinical Otolaryngology*, **14**, 45–51

HUGHES, E. C., GOTT, P. S., WEINSTEIN, R. C. and BINGGELI, R. (1988) Noradrenergic cerebral stimulation of sensorineural impaired subjects: Yohimbine effects on speech intelligibility and the auditory brain response. *American Journal of Otology*, **9**, 122–126

HULSHOF, J. H. and VERMEIJ, P. (1984a) The effect of intravenous Lidocaine and several different doses oral tocainide HC1 on tinnitus. *Acta Otolaryngologica*, **98**, 231–238

HULSHOF, J. H. and VERMEIJ, P. (1984b) The effect of several doses of oral tocainide HC1 on tinnitus: a dose finding study. *Journal of Laryngology and Otology*, **9**, 257–258

HULSHOF, J. H. and VERMEIJ, P. (1985) The value of carbamazepine in the treatment of tinnitus. *Journal of Otorhinolaryngology and Related Specialties*, **47**, 262–266

HULSHOF, J. H. and VERMEIJ, P. (1986) The value of flunarizine in the treatment of tinnitus. *Journal of Otorhinolaryngology and Related Specialties*, **48**, 33–36

HULSHOF, J. H. and VERMEIJ, P. (1987) The effect of nicotinamide on tinnitus: a double-blind controlled study. *Clinical Otolaryngology*, **12**, 211–214

ISHIKAWA, K. and IGARASHI, M. (1984) Effect of diazepam on vestibular compensation in squirrel monkeys. *Archives of Otolaryngology*, **240**, 49–54

ISREAL, J. M., CONNELLY, J. S., MCTIGUE, S. T., BRUMMETT, R. E. and BROWN, J. (1982) Lidocaine in the treatment of tinnitus aurium. *Archives of Otolaryngology*, **108**, 471–473

ITOH, A. and SAKATA, E. (1991) Treatment of vestibular disorders. *Acta Otolaryngologica*, Suppl. 481, 617–623

JACKSON, R. T. and TURNER, J. S. (1987) Astemizole: its use in the treatment of patients with chronic vertigo. *Archives of Otolaryngology – Head and Neck Surgery*, **113**, 536–542

KALLINEN, J., DIDIER, A., MILLER, J. M., NUTALL, A. and GRENMAN, R. (1991) The effect of CO_2 and O_2 gas mixtures on laser Doppler measured cochlear and skin blood flow in guinea pigs. *Hearing Research*, **55**, 255–262

KAZDA, S., KNORR, A. and TOWART, R. (1983) Common properties and differences between various calcium antagonists. *Progress in Pharmacology*, **5**, 83–116

KEMPF, H.-G. (1989) Ear involvement in Wegener's granulomatosis. *Clinical Otolaryngology*, **14**, 451–456

KERR, A. G. (1995) Streptomycin perfusion of the labyrinth. *Proceedings of the Irish Otolaryngological Society* (in press)

KESSLER, C., VON MARAVIC, M., ALBRECHT, D. M., VON MARAVIC, C., MULLER, M., SCHMIDT, P. *et al.* (1991) Doppler CO_2 test in patients with vertebrobasilar ischemia. *Acta Neurologica Scandinavica*, **84**, 519–522

KHANIJOW, V.K. and RAMAN, R. (1988) Idiopathic sudden sensorineural deafness – an approach to the problem. *Singapore Medical Journal*, **29**, 76–77

KIMBERLEY, R.P. (1991) Mechanisms of action, dosage schedules, and side effects of steroid therapy. *Current Opinion in Rheumatology*, **3**, 373–379

KITANO, H., KITAHARA, M., UCHIDA, K. and KITAJIMA, K. (1987) Treatment of tinnitus with muscle relaxant. In: *Proceedings of the Third International Tinnitus Seminar*, Munster, 1987, edited by H. Feldmann. Karlsruhe.' Harsch Verlag. pp. 326–330

KLOCKHOFF, I. and LINDBLOM, U. (1967) Meniere's disease and hydrochlorthiazide (Dichlotride) – a critical analysis of symptoms and therapeutic effects. *Acta Otolaryngologica*, **63**, 347–365

KLOCKHOFF, I., LINDBLOM, U. and STAHLE, J. (1974) Diuretic treatment of Meniere disease: long-term results with chlorthalidone. *Archives of Otolaryngology*, **100**, 262–265

KONISHI, K., NAKAI, Y. and YAMANE. H. (1991) The efficacy of lasix-vitamin therapy (L-V therapy) for sudden deafness and other sensorineural hearing loss. *Acta Otolaryngologica*, Suppl. 486, 78–91

KORNBLUT, A. D., WOLFF, S. M. and FAUCI, A. S. (1982) Ear disease in patients with Wegener's granulomatosis. *Laryngoscope*, **92**, 713–717

KRAMER, M. R., NESHER, G. and SONNENBLICK, M. (1988) Steroid-responsive hearing loss in temporal arteritis. *Journal of Laryngology and Otology*, **102**, 524–525

KRONENBERG, J., ALMAGOR, M., BENDET, E. and KUSHNIR, D. (1992) Vasoactive therapy versus placebo in the treatment of sudden hearing loss: a double-blind clinical study. *Laryngoscope*, **102**, 65–68

KUNIHIRO, T., KANZAKI, J., O-UCHI, T. and YOSHIDA, A. (1990) Steroid-responsive sensorineural hearing loss associated with aortitis syndrome. *Journal of Otlaryngology and Related Specialties*, **52**, 86–95

LAFFREE, J. B., VERMEIJ, P. and HULSHOF, J. H. (1989) The effect of iontophoresis of lignocaine in the treatment of tinnitus. *Clinical Otolaryngology*, **14**, 401–404

LAITAKARI, K. (1990) Intratympanic gentamycin in severe Meniere's disease. *Clinical Otolaryngology*, **15**, 545–548

LANGMAN, A. W., KEMINK, J. L. and GRAHAM, M. D. (1990) Titration streptomycin therapy for bilateral Meniere's disease. Follow-up report. *Annals of Otology, Rhinology and Laryngology*, **99**, 923–926

LECHTENBERG, R. and SHULMAN, A. (1984) Benzodiazepines in the treatment of tinnitus. *Journal of Laryngology and Otology*, (Suppl.) **98**, 271–276

LEE, J. A., WATSON, L. A. and BOOTHBY, G. (1986) Calcium antagonists in the prevention of motion sickness. *Aviation, Space, and Environmental Medicine*, **57**, 45–48.

LUETJE, C. M. (1989) Theoretical and practical implications for plasmapheresis in autoimmune inner ear disease. *Laryngoscope*, **99**, 1137–1146

LYNDON, S., ROY, P., GRILLAGE, M. G. and MILLER, A. J. (1992) A comparison of the efficacy of two ear drop preparations ('Audax' and 'Earex') in the softening and removal of impacted ear wax. *Current Medical Research and Opinion*, **13**, 21–25

MCCABE, B. F. (1979) Autoimmune sensorineural hearing loss. *Annals of Otology, Rhinology and Laryngology*, **88**, 585–589

MCCABE, B. F. (1989) Autoimmune inner ear disease: therapy. *American Journal of Otology*, **10**, 196–197

MCCORMICK, M. S., and THOMAS, J. N. (1981) Mexiletine in the relief of tinnitus: a report on a sequential double-blind crossover trial. *Clinical Otolaryngology*, **6**, 255–258

MCILWAIN, J. C. (1987) Glutamic acid in the treatment of

tinnitus. *Journal of Laryngology and Otology*, **101**, 552–554

MCKEE, G. J., KERR, A. G., TONER, J. G. and SMYTH, G. D. L. (1991) Surgical control of vertigo in Meniere's disease. *Clinical Otolaryngology*, **16**, 216–227

MCRAE, D. and BUCHANAN, G. (1993) Long-term sulfamethoxazole-trimethoprim in Wegener's granulomatosis. *Archives of Otolaryngology – Head and Neck Surgery*, **119**, 103–105

MAGNUSSON, M. and PADOAN, S. (1991) Delayed onset of ototoxic effects of gentamicin in treatment of Meniere's disease. Rationale for extremely low dose therapy. *Acta Otolaryngologica*, **111**, 671–676

MANN, W., BECK, C. and BECK, CHL. (1986) Calcium antagonists in the treatment of sudden deafness. *Archives of Otorhinolaryngology*, **243**, 170–173

MARKHAM, A. and SORKIN, E. M. (1993) Ondansetron. An update of its therapeutic use in chemotherapy-induced and postoperative nausea and vomiting. *Drugs*, **45**, 931–952

MARKS, N. J., ONISIPHOROU, C. and TROUNCE, J. R. (1981) The effect of single doses of amylobarbitone sodium and carbamazepine in tinnitus. *Journal of Laryngology and Otology*, **95**, 941–945

MARTIN, F. W. and COLMAN, B. H. (1980) Tinnitus: a double-blind crossover controlled trial to evaluate the use of lignocaine. *Clinical Otolaryngology*, **5**, 3–11

MATTOX, D. E. and SIMMONS, F. B. (1977) Natural history of sudden sensorineural hearing loss. *Annals of Otology, Rhinology and Laryngology*, **86**, 463–480

MIHAIL, R. C., CROWLEY, J. M., WALDEN B. E., FISHBURNE, J., REINWALL, J. E. and ZAJTCHUK, J. T. (1988) The tricyclic trimipramine in the treatment of subjective tinnitus. *Annals of Otology, Rhinology and Laryngology*, **97**, 120–123

MOLLER, C., ÖDKVIST, L. M., THELL, J., LARSBY, B. and HYDEN, D. (1988) Vestibular and audiological functions in gentamicin-treated Meniere's disease. *American Journal of Otology*, **9**, 383–391

MONSELL, E. M. and SHELTON, C. (1992) Labyrinthotomy with streptomycin infusion: early results of a multicenter study. *American Journal of Otology*, **13**, 416–422; discussion 422–425

MOSKOWITZ, D., LEE, K. J. and SMITH, H. W. (1984) Steroid use in idiopathic sudden sensorineural hearing loss. *Laryngoscope*, **94**, 664–666

MURAI, K., TYLER, R. S., HARKER, L. A. and STOUFFER, J. L. (1992) Review of pharmacologic treatment of tinnitus. *American Journal of Otology*, **13**, 454–464

NAGAHARA, K., FISCH, U. and YAGI, N. (1983) Perilymph oxygenation in sudden and progressive sensorineural hearing loss. *Acta Otolaryngologica*, **96**, 57–68

NEDZELSKI, J. M., SCHESSEL, D. A., BRYCE, G. E. and PFLEIDERER, A. G. (1992) Chemical labyrinthectomy: local application of gentamicin for the treatment of unilateral Meniere's disease. *American Journal of Otology*, **13**, 18–22

ODKVIST, L. M. (1988) Middle ear ototoxic treatment for inner ear disease. *Acta Otolaryngologica*, Suppl. 457, 83–86

OOSTERVELD, W. J. (1982) Flunarizine in vertigo. A double-blind placebo-controlled cross-over evaluation of a constant dose schedule. *Oto-Rhino-Laryngology*, **44**, 72–80

OOSTERVELD, W. J. (1984) Betahistine dihydrochloride in the treatment of vertigo of peripheral vestibular origin: a double-blind placebo-controlled study. *Journal of Laryngology and Otology*, **98**, 37–41

PAASKE, P. B., PEDERSEN, C. B., KJEMS, G. and SAM, I. L. K. (1991) Zinc in the management of tinnitus: placebo-controlled trial. *Annals of Otology, Rhinology and Laryngology*, **100**, 647–649

PARVING, A. (1991) Hearing problems and hormonal disturbances in the elderly. *Acta Otolaryngologica*, Suppl. 476, 44–53

PEARSON, B. W. and BRACKMANN, D. E. (1985) Committee on hearing and equilibrium guidelines for reporting treatment results in Meniere's disease. *Otolaryngology – Head and Neck Surgery*, **93**, 579–581

PENNER, M. J. (1989) Aspirin abolishes tinnitus caused by spontaneous otoacoustic emissions. A case study. *Archives of Otolaryngology – Head and Neck Surgery*, **115**, 871–875

PEPPARD, S. B. (1986) Effect of drug therapy on compensation from vestibular injury. *Laryngoscope*, **96**, 878–898

PROBST, R., TSCHOPP, K., LUDIN, E., KELLERHALS, B., PODVINEC, M. and PFALTZ, C. R. (1992) A randomised, double-blind, placebo-controlled study of dextran/pentoxifylline medication in acute acoustic trauma and sudden hearing loss. *Acta Otolaryngologica*, **112**, 435–443

PYYKKÖ, I., SCHALÉN, L. and JÄNTTI, V. (1985) Transdermally administered scopolamine vs. dimenhydrate. 1. Effect on nausea and vertigo in experimentally induced motion sickness. *Acta Otolaryngologica*, **99**, 588–596

PYYKKÖ, I., MAGNUSSON, M., SCHALÉN, L. and ENBOM, H. (1988) Pharmacological treatment of vertigo. *Acta Otolaryngologica*, Suppl. 455, 77–81

RASCOL, O., CLANET, M. and MONTASTRUC, J. L. (1989) Calcium antagonists and the vestibular system: a critical review of flunarizine as an antivertigo drug. *Fundamentals of Clinical Pharmacology*, **3**, 79s–87s

REED, H. T., MELTZER, J., CREWS, P., NORRIS, C. H., QUINE, D. B. and GUTH, P. S. (1985) Amino-oxyacetic acid as a palliative in tinnitus. *Archives of Otolaryngology – Head and Neck Surgery*, **111**, 803–805

ROBINSON, A. C. and HAWKE, M. (1989) The efficacy of ceruminolytics: everything old is new again. *Journal of Otolaryngology*, **18**, 263–267

RUCKENSTEIN, M. J., RUTKA, J.A. and HAWKE, M. (1991) The treatment of Meniere's disease: Torok revisited. *Laryngoscope*, **101**, 211–218

SALAMA, N. Y., BHATIA, P. and ROBB, P. J. (1989) Efficacy of oral oxpentifylline in the management of idiopathic tinnitus. *Journal of Otolaryngology and Related Specialties*, **51**, 300–304

SATO, K. (1988) Pharmacokinetics of Coenzyme Q_{10} in recovery of acute sensorineural hearing loss due to hypoxia. *Acta Otolaryngologica*, Suppl. 458, 95–102

SCHMIDT, C. L., BECK, C. and LANGE, G. (1981) Intratympanic application of gentamycin for treatment of Meniere's disease. In: *Proceedings of the Sixth Shambaugh International Workshop on Otomicrosurgery*, Chicago 1980, edited by G. E. Shambaugh and J. J. Shea. Huntsville, Alabama: Strode Publishers, pp. 291–294

SCHUKNECHT, H. F. (1957) Ablation therapy in the management of Meniere's disease. *Acta Otolaryngologica*, Suppl. 132, 1–42

SHEA, J. J. (1989) Perfusion of the inner ear with streptomycin. *American Journal of Otology*, **10**, 150–155

SHIRAISHI, T., KUBO, T. and MATSUNAGA, T. (1991) Chronological study of recovery of sudden deafness treated with defibrinogenation and steroid therapies. *Acta Otolaryngologica*, **111**, 867–871

SILVERSTEIN, H., HYMAN, S. M., FELDBAUM, J. and SILVERSTEIN D. (1984) Use of streptomycin sulfate in the treatment of Meniere's disease. *Otolaryngology – Head and Neck Surgery*, **92**, 229–232

SIRIMANNA, T. and STEPHENS, D. (1992) Coping with tinnitus. *Practitioner*, **236**, 821–826

SMYTH, J. L. (1968) Spirochetes in late seronegative syphilis, despite penicillin therapy. *Medical Times*, **96**, 611–623

STERKERS, O., BERNARD, C., FERRARY, E., SZIKLAI, I., TRAN BA HUY, P. and AMIEL, C. (1988) Possible role of Ca ions in the vestibular system. *Acta Otolaryngologica*, Suppl. 460, 28–32

VAN DEELAN, G. W. and HUIZING, E. H. (1986) The use of a diuretic (Dyazide) in the treatment of Meniere's disease. *Journal of Otolaryngology and Related Specialities*, **48**, 287–292

VATHENEN, A. S., SKINNER, D. W. and SHALE, D. J. (1988) Treatment response with bilateral mixed deafness and facial palsy in polyarteritis nodosa. *American Journal of Medicine*, **84**, 1081–1082

VOLLERTSEN, R. S., MCDONALD, T. J., YOUNGE, B. R., BANKS, P. M., STANSON, A. W. and ILSTRUP, D. M. (1986) Cogan's syndrome: 18 cases and a review of the literature. *Mayo Clinic Proceedings*, **61**, 344–361

WENNMO, C., BERGENIUS, J., HENRIKSSON, N. G., HYDEN, D., ENBOM, H., MAGNUSSON, M. *et al.* (1987) Transdermal scopolamine and vertigo of peripheral vestibular origin. In: *The Vestibular System. Neurophysiologic and Clinical Research*, edited by M. D. Graham and J. L. Kemik. New York: Raven Press. pp. 607–611

WILD, D., NAYAK, U. S. L. and ISAACS, B. (1980) How dangerous are falls in old people at home? *British Medical Journal*, **282**, 266–268

WILDER-SMITH, E. and ROELCKE, U. (1990) Cogan's syndrome. *Journal of Clinical Neuro-Ophthalmology*, **10**, 261–263, editorial comment 264–265

WILATT, D. J., O'SULLIVAN, G., STONEY, P. J., JACKSON, S. R., PRITCHARD, J. and MCCORMICK, M. S. (1987) A sequential double blind crossover trial of iontophoresis. In: *Proceedings of the Third International Tinnitus Seminar*, Munster, 1987, edited by H. Feldmann. Karlsruhe: Harsch Verlag. pp. 316–319

WILLIAMS, T. J. and YARWOOD, H. (1990) Effect of glucocorticosteroids on microvascular permeability. *American Review of Respiratory Disease*, **141**, S39–S43

WILMOT, T. J. and MENON, G. N. (1976) Betahistine in Meniere's disease. *Journal of Laryngology and Otology*, **90**, 833–840

WILSON, W. R. (1986) Sudden sensorineural hearing loss. In: *Otolaryngology: Head and Neck Surgery*, edited by C. W. Cummings. St Louis: C. V. Mosby. pp. 3219–3224

WILSON, W. R., BYL, F. M. and LAIRD, N. (1980) The efficacy of steroids in the treatment of idiopathic sudden hearing loss – a double-blind clinical study. *Archives of Otolaryngology*, **106**, 772–776

WOLF, M., KRONENBERG, J., ENGELBERG, S. and LEVENTON, G. (1987) Rapidly progressive hearing loss as a symptom of polyarteritis nodosa. *American Journal of Otolaryngology*, **8**, 105–108

WOOD, C. D., STEWART, J. J., WOOD, M. J. and MIMS, M. (1992) Effectiveness and duration of intramuscular antimotion sickness medications. *Journal of Clinical Pharmacology*, **32**, 1008–1012

WOUTERS, D. V. M., AMERY, W. and TOWSE, G. (1983) Flunarizine in the treatment of vertigo. *Journal of Laryngology and Otology*, **97**, 697–704

ZAYTOUN, G. M., SCHUKNECHT, H. S. and FARMER, H. S. (1983) Fatality following the use of low molecular weight dextan in the treatment of sudden deafness. *Advances in Oto-Rhino-Laryngology*, **31**, 240–246

ZEE, D. S. (1985) Perspectives on the pharmacotherapy of vertigo. *Archives of Otolaryngology*, **111**, 609–612

7

Legal and ethical matters

Ronald Hinchcliffe and Susan Bellman

At the outset one should distinguish a number of concepts or domains, e.g. ethics, jurisprudence, justice, law, moral philosophy, morality, mores, philosophy and, last but not least, sociology.

Philosophy can be considered to be the critical evaluation of assumptions and arguments, investigating the ultimate nature of knowledge and existence. Moral philosophy is then defined as the philosophical enquiry about norms, values, right and wrong, good and bad and what ought and ought not to be done (Raphael, 1981). Gillon (1986) equated ethics with moral philosophy. And as Dias (1970) pointed out, ethical evaluation cannot be kept apart from sociology; social problems are grounded in ethical evaluation.

Law, morality, mores and religion make up what Allott (1980) referred to as normative systems. These can be interpreted as culturally-based behavioural control systems. *Law* is what is made in a political society to be imposed on its citizens in order to regulate their behaviour in that society. *Religion* purports to be an account of reality, of what is and why it is there, as well as being a set of rituals, practices and prescriptions. A moral system is a set of precepts for right living, which may or may not be associated with belief in and about the supernatural implied by religion. *Mores* refers to the habitual practices, conventions and etiquette of a society.

Jurisprudence is the science of law and of legal systems but, as Dias (1970) pointed out, it is more concerned with *thought* about law rather than with *knowledge* of law. *Justice* implies fairness, impartiality.

The development of the law is shaped by logic, history, custom and utility, as well as by the accepted standards of right conduct (Cardozo, 1921).

Philosophy, ethics, science, logic, laws and the concept of justice all had their roots in ancient Greece. It is therefore useful to consider the historical perspective of this subject.

Historical

In his *Conjectures and Refutations*, Popper (1981) pointed out that science had its beginnings in ancient Greece when the Greek philosophers invented a new tradition, i.e. that of critically discussing myths when they were retold. Thus knowledge progresses by guesses and tentative solutions to our problems, i.e. by conjectures. These conjectures are controlled by criticism, i.e. by refutations. Conjectures may survive these tests but they can never be positively justified; they can be established neither as definitely true nor even as probable. But all this brings us nearer to the truth. One can then trace Popper's falsifiability concept of scientific methodology through Robert Grosseteste's (an English scholar c. 1168–1253) *Principle of Falsification*, i.e. that a hypothesis should be rejected if experience proves that its conclusions are false. We shall return to this concept later in discussing legal logic.

In his *Early Greek Law*, Gagarin (1986) traced the emergence of law from the eighth to the sixth centuries BC, i.e. from the oral culture of Homer and Hesiod to the written codes of law in most city states. As a result of his studies, Gagarin proposed a three-stage model for the development of law in society. The first, i.e. *pre-legal*, stage is where the society has no recognised, viz. formal and public, procedures for peacefully settling disputes[1] between its members. The second, i.e. *proto-legal*, stage is where a society possesses legal procedures, i.e. ways of going about resolving disputes, but no legal rules, i.e. no corpus of substantive law. The arrival of the latter, i.e. the third, *legal*, stage had to await the development of a written language.

[1] Thus we see here the prime function of law as a dispute-resolving system (see later) in society

Table of Cases

Table of Cases – *Continued*

Law – comparative

A study of the law of the various countries of the world (e.g. David and Jauffret–Spinosi, 1992) indicated that there are broadly two superfamilies of legal systems, i.e. the European and the Afro-Asian group. There are three broad families within the European grouping, i.e. the Romano-Germanic, the Socialist and the Common Law family.

Romano-Germanic law, which dominates Western Europe, is characterized by codification. Socialist law is derived from, and subordinate to, Marxist-Leninist doctrine. The Common Law is a uniquely English derivation. Following the end of the Roman occupation in 430 AD, England saw invasions by a number of tribes (Angles, Jutes, Saxons and Vikings) from northwestern Europe over the next six centuries. Each brought with them their own *customary law*. It was William the Conqueror's arrival from Normandy

in 1066 AD which resulted in defining what these various customary laws had in common. Hence the designation of this collated law as the 'Common Law'. This was completed about 1250 AD. Interestingly, any customary law in what are now the European states from where the invaders originated, has long since disappeared or been codified. (This is not entirely true since the general law in France on civil liability (*responsabilité délictuelle*) has never been codified.) Despite the occupation lasting for four centuries, Roman law had no lasting impact on the law of England. (It may well be said that the *Corpus Iuris Civilis* of Justinian was not completed until 534 AD, but this had incorporated the law of 13 centuries.) Similarly, the Roman occupation of Wales (Agricola completed the conquest of Wales in 78 AD) over essentially the same time span had no lasting impact on the law of Wales, the *Law of Hywel Dda* (Jenkins, 1986). However, the Law of Hywel Dda was replaced by the laws of England when Wales was politically assimilated to England under the Act of Union of 1535. By contrast, basic Scottish law survived the political union with England in 1707 (although James VI of Scotland had succeeded Elizabeth I of England in 1603). The survival of Scotland's distinct and independent system of jurisprudence (Black, 1993) was largely due to the publication of Viscount Stair's *Institutions of the Law of Scotland* in 1681. Paradoxically, although the Romans advanced only so far as the Forth-Clyde isthmus (Antonine Wall) and occupied that part of Scotland for a relatively brief period, Scottish Law owes much to Roman law. This stems from the links that independent Scotland had with continental Europe in the mediaeval ages. There is no evidence that the laws and customs of the non-Aryan, pre-Celtic inhabitants of the British Isles, the Picts, survived the assimilation of these peoples by the Scots.

It should thus be clear that the law of England and Wales is neither the law of the UK nor that of Great Britain because Northern Ireland, Scotland, the Channel Islands and the Isle of Man are not ruled by 'English law'. Éire has been enacting its own statutes since the Dáil Éireann (National Parliament) came into being in 1921. But because of the long association with England, and notwithstanding the prior existence in the mediaeval ages of an Irish Parliament, the Irish legal system (Byrne and McCutcheon, 1989) is broadly similar to that of England and Wales, with a common law/doctrine of precedence dominating.

Many developing countries have sought to modernize their legal systems by bringing in European jurists to codify the *mélange* of their various laws. For example, the many laws of Ethiopia, i.e. religious (Christian and Islamic), traditional (Amharic and Pagan) and European, were reduced to a single, uniform system, the 1960 Ethiopian Civil Code. This codification was a 'high intellectual achievement', but a dismal failure in practice (Allott, 1980).

Classification

If the reader expects to find a classification of English law similar to Simpson's (1945) classification of the mammalia, or a classification based upon the Sokal and Sneath's (1963) principles of numerical taxonomy, he will be disappointed. Nevertheless, classifications exist, such as into *adjectival* law and *substantive* law, corresponding roughly to methodology and systematic or descriptive knowledge. But, particularly since the law of England and Wales is amorphous, one talks about the *sources* of law, or of *areas* of law.

Currently, the main *sources* of English law are the common law, legislation, and EC Law (Steiner, 1994). Note that the term European Union (EU), introduced in Article A of the Maastricht Treaty on European

Union (TEU), is not strictly applicable to matters of law relating to the European Community (EC) Treaty, the amended EEC Treaty.

Areas of law constitute practical operating regions for lawyers. They comprise, e.g. Charities (Picarda, 1994), Company Law (Mayson, French and Ryan, 1994), Computer Law (Reed, 1993), Environmental Health Law (McManus, 1994), Family Law (Black and Bridge, 1994), Information Technology (Lloyd, 1993), Intellectual Property Rights (Bainbridge, 1994), Land Law (MacKenzie and Phillips, 1994), Medical Law (Kennedy and Grubb, 1994), Personal Injuries Litigation (Goldrein and de Haas, 1994) and Road Traffic Law (McMahon, 1994).

The English Common Law

As well as being uncoded, the Common Law system is characterized by two other features, i.e. by the method of acquisition of evidence (adversarial, as opposed to inquisitorial), and the practice of *judicial precedent* (see later). It is the latter which gives rise to what is termed *case law*. There are now some 400 000 *case reports* contained in 1000 volumes of law reports. Kennedy and Grubb's (1994) text on medical law cites well over 1000 case reports. But compare this with the two million medical articles published annually in some 20 000 journals.

The common law doctrine of abiding by precedent is known as *stare decisis* (short for *stare decisis et non quieta movere*). Thus for civil cases, the hierarchy of authority is House of Lords > Court of Appeal (Civil Division) > High Court of Justice > County Courts. It is thus a vertical, and not a horizontal, authority. Moreover, in 1966, the House of Lords declared that it would not be bound by its own decisions (*Practice Statement*). Thus the judgments of primary interest are those of the latest House of Lords and Court of Appeal decisions relevant to the matter in question. Yet these may be ones which are universally ignored by medical men. For example, in *Robinson v. British Rail Engineering*, the Court of Appeal disposed of hearing disability/loss of amenity assessments based upon pure tone audiograms in no uncertain terms. Yet professionals in the area of hearing disorders continue to produce disability/handicap assessments using such methods. Hearing disability is a multifactorial value of which hearing impairment is only one factor (Williams, 1992). It is so much easier (at least for adults) to ask a plaintiff, 'What difficulties do you have?' That is what the courts require. Moreover, such an approach is more consistent with clinical practice.

Important House of Lords judgments have been confirmations of the *Bolam test* (see below) on at least three occasions (and therefore well established by precedent), i.e. in *Whitehouse v. Jordan* [1981] re treatment, in *Maynard v. West Midlands Regional Health Authority* [1984] re diagnosis, and in *Sidaway v. Bethlem Royal Hospital Governors* [1985] re informed consent. But it could well be that the Bolam test will not survive into the twenty-first century (Brennan, 1995).

The doctrine of *stare decisis* must be distinguished from that of *res judicata*, i.e. a matter which has been adjudicated on. *Res judicata* means that the final judgment on a dispute between two parties may not be disputed subsequently by those *parties*.

The only thing in a judge's decision binding as an authority upon a subsequent judge is the principle upon which the case was decided (*Osborne to Rowlett* 1880). This principle on which a case is decided is known as the *ratio decidendi*. The acertainment of the *ratio decidendi* of a case depends upon a process of abstraction from the totality of facts that occurred in it. The higher the abstraction, the wider the *ratio decidendi* (Williams, 1982b).

Dias (1970) contended that the rigidity of *stare decisis* is largely mythical and judges have considerable latitude in evading unwelcome authorities. In the first place, a judge may lower the level of generality of a precedent when stating its facts and, in so doing, distinguish one case from another. Thus judges have much discretion in the handling of precedent. Moreover, as Stuttard (1969) pointed out, there is no test which can be applied to show which part of a previous case constituted the *ratio decidendi*. Anything which is not part of the *ratio decidendi* and which is not part of the facts of a case is referred to as *obiter dicta* (things said by the way). Consequently, the common law has the capacity to develop and to progress. As Lord Evershed said, the ancient rules of the English common law have the characteristic that in general they can never be said to be final and limited by definition, but have the capacity of adaptation in accordance with the changing circumstances of succeeding ages (*Haley v London Electricity Board* 1965).

Equity

Equity was a peculiar development of the Middle Ages which sought to modify the rigidity of the common law by proceeding on flexible principles of 'good conscience'. However, equity was a system that was known to the Greeks. Aristotle distinguished between Justice (see later) and Equity, arguing that the law is necessarily generalizing and often harsh in application to the individual case. Equity mitigates and corrects its harshness by considering the individual case (Friedmann, 1949).

Statute law – legislation
In general

The dominance of the common law is not to say that there is no legislation (making of laws by the legisla-

ture – Parliament) in the English legal system. This is the principal function of Parliament. About 70 statutes (Acts of Parliament) are produced each year, although one-fifth are consolidating Acts. In addition to these statutes, there is also *subordinate legislation*. More than 2000 *statutory instruments*, the commonest form of subordinate legislation, are issued each year. Parliament is omnipotent; it can make and unmake laws to an unlimited extent.

The unprecedented development of legislation in the nineteenth century owed much to the concepts and reforming zeal of Bentham (1789) who has subsequently been considered as one of the greatest analytical jurists of all time (Friedmann, 1949). In his theory of legislation, Bentham defined the main function of law as being to provide subsistence, to aim at abundance, to encourage equality, and to maintain security. From these concepts there emerges the increasing social legislation which reached its peak in the middle of the twentieth century.

As Dias (1970) pointed out, there is now universal recognition that deliberate law making is indispensable to the efficient regulation of the modern state. The most important consequence of judicial acceptance of the supremacy of Parliament is the doctrine that no court can challenge the validity of an Act. In *Ex parte Canon Selwyn* (1872), Cockburn C. J. said, 'There is no judicial body in the country by which the validity of an Act of Parliament could be questioned'. In *Cheney v Conn* [1968] the judge (Ungoed-Thomas) said, 'What the statute itself enacts cannot be unlawful, because what the statute says and provides is itself the law, and the highest form of law that is known to this country . . . and it is not for the court to say that (it) . . . is illegal'. In *Pickin v British Railways Board* [1974], Lord Morris of Borth-y-Gest said, 'In the courts there may be an argument as to the correct interpretation of the enactment: there must be none as to whether it should be in the Statute book at all'.

This contrasts with the position in some other countries where a higher court can declare statutes as 'unconstitutional' and therefore inoperative. However, with Britain having joined the European Economic Community (now termed the European Union), the doctrine of unlimited supremacy of Parliament may have to be modified. This may well be the only legal safeguard for the possibility, envisaged by Dicey (1905), that Parliament could, if it wished, enact a law ordering all blue-eyed babies to be killed.

In *Ellen Street Estates v Ministry of Health* [1934] Lord Justice Maugham said that the one thing that Parliament could not do is bind its successors. This reflects the doctrine of *implied repeal*, i.e. the appearance of a new Act of Parliament implies that any preceding Act, or parts of such Acts, that could conflict with the new legislation are automatically repealed. Over 300 years ago, it was held that Parliament was entitled to ignore any provisions in an earlier Act purporting to prevent that Act from being repealed (*Godden v Hales*).

In respect of Acts of Parliament, the role of judges is limited to interpreting them. As Miers and Page (1990) pointed out, judicial interpretation in practice will hinge primarily, if not exclusively on the purpose of the enactment, as indicated in *Maunsell v Olins, Stock v Frank Jones (Tipton) Ltd, Hanlon v Law Society* and *Ealing London Borough Council v Race Relations Board*. This 'purposive' approach goes back to what has been termed 'the celebrated formulations' in *Heydon's* case in 1584. Most recently, Lord Justice Glidewell in the Court of Appeal has ruled that there is nothing in the 1992 Social Security and Contributions Act to suggest that a disabled person was entitled only to an allowance for the maintenance of life. The disability allowance is there to enable people to live full lives. The Department of Social Security had appealed against a decision by the Social Security Commissioner to allow the claim of a young congenitally deaf woman for an interpreter (News Item, 1995a). It thus follows that decisions based upon an application of an Act and its interpretation by the courts are all important; the actual provision of the Act is less important.

Statute law may impose certain limitations on the common law. In particular, the Limitation Act 1939 stated that actions founded on tort shall not be brought after the expiration of a certain duration (6 years) from the date on which the cause of action accrued. The Law Reform (Limitation of Actions) Act 1954 reduced this period to 3 years in connection with actions for damages for negligence, nuisance, or breach of statutory duty where personal injury was concerned. The time commences on the date on which the cause of action accrues. Thus, an injustice might have arisen in a case where an injury was inflicted in a way that could become discoverable only after a lapse of time. Such a manner is, of course, characteristic of many occupational disorders, noise-induced hearing loss being an example *par excellence*. This injustice was removed by the Limitation Act 1963. This Act enables the plaintiff to bring a claim even though the 3-year limit is past, provided that he neither knew about the injury, nor ought to have known about it, and provided that he brings the claim within 1 year of his knowing about it.

David and Jauffret-Spinosi (1992) view legislation as a secondary source only of English law, a series of errata and addenda to the main body of the law which is formed by the decisions of the courts.

More specifically

About 100 statutes are relevant to medical law (Jones and Morris, 1992; Kennedy and Grubb, 1994) aside from a number of others which are relevant to habili-

tation and rehabilitation. Over the past 5 years we have seen the Human Organ Transplants Act 1989, the Children Act 1989, the Access to Health Records Act 1990, the National Health Service and Community Care Act 1990, the Human Fertilisation and Embryology Act 1990, the Social Security Act 1993 and the Education Act 1993.

The Human Organ Transplants Act 1989 prohibits commercial dealings in human organs and restricts transplants to persons who are genetically related. The Children Act 1989 (Bridge, Bridge and Luke, 1989) came into force on 14 October 1991. It brought the law relating to children and families into one piece of legislation. In seeking to redefine the balance between securing the safety of children and the responsibility and rights of parents to bring up children witin their own families, the act adopts as its guiding principle the welfare of the child. The Access to Health Records Act 1990 is mentioned later. The National Health Service and Community Care Act 1990 provides for NHS contracts and NHS Trusts. The Human Fertilisation and Embryology Act 1990 governs experimentation with embryos and gametes (Morgan and Lee, 1991). The Social Security Act 1993 essentially amended the Social Security Act 1986. Part III of the Education Act 1993, which implements proposals made in the Department of Education Consultative paper 'Special Educational Needs and Access to the System', makes provision for children with special educational needs. For the purposes of the Act, a child has a 'special educational need' if he has a learning difficulty which calls for special educational provision to be made for him. Section 156 (2) considers a child to have a 'learning difficulty' if he has a significantly greater *difficulty in learning* than the majority of his age, or he has a *disability* which either prevents or hinders him from making use of educational facilities of a kind generally provided for children of his age in schools within the area of the local educational authority.

The only statute which could be considered as specific to our field is the Hearing Aid Council Act 1968 together with the Hearing Aid Council (Extension) Act 1975 and the Hearing Aid Council (Amendment) Act 1989. For the purpose of the 1968 Act, a body termed the 'Hearing Aid Council' was set up. The Council has the function of securing adequate standards of competence and conduct among persons engaged in dispensing hearing aids in the private sector. It also advises on methods for improving training facilities for hearing aid dispensers. Section (3) requires the Council to draw up both standards of competence and codes of practice for dispensers. Section 1(6) provides for the Council to receive complaints from members of the public and to investigate such complaints. Section 2 requires the Council to establish a register of dispensers of hearing aids. A person may be registered if, prior to the commencement of the Act, he had acted as a dispenser of hearing aids for a period of at least 6 months in the 2 years prior to the Act, or he satisfies the standards of competence laid down by the Council. The Council was also empowered by s5(1) to set up a committee termed the 'Investigating Committee' to investigate disciplinary cases. The function of the Investigating Committee was to decide whether a disciplinary case (a case being investigated) ought to be referred to the Disciplinary Committee. If a person is judged by the Disciplinary Committee to have been guilty of serious misconduct in connection with the dispensing of hearing aids, the Committee may direct his name to be erased from the register. Section 14 of the Act defined a 'dispenser of hearing aids' as 'an individual who conducts or seeks to conduct oral negotiations with a view to effecting the supply of a hearing aid, whether by him or another, to or for the use of a person with impaired hearing'. A 'hearing aid' was defined as 'an instrument intended for use by a person suffering from impaired hearing to assist that person to hear better but does not include any instrument or device designed for use by connecting conductors of electricity to equipment or apparatus provided for the purpose of affording means of telephonic communication'.

The purpose of the Hearing Aid Council (Extension) Act was to extend the Act to Northern Ireland. The main purpose of the Hearing Aid Council (Amendment) Act was to amend the composition of the Hearing Aid Council and make provision to further secure adequate standards of conduct and regulation for private hearing aid dispensers.

EC law

In the case of *Costa v ENEL* [1964], the European Court of Justice (ECJ) ruled *inter alia*,

> 'The transfer by the States from their domestic legal system to the Community legal system of the rights and obligations arising under the Treaty carries with it a permanent limitation of their sovereign rights, against which a subsequent unilateral act incompatible with the concept of the Community cannot prevail'.

Thus the European Court of Justice (ECJ) showed that EC provisions which do not specifically mention individuals may still create rights for them. Moreover, the ECJ indicated that the logic of EC law gives it supremacy over the domestic laws of its member states.

As Allen, Thompson and Walsh (1994) pointed out, the pre-eminence of EC law was brought home most forcefully in a decision regarding fishing rights and the Merchant Shipping Act 1988. In July 1991 the House of Lords ruled, following a judgment to the same effect by the EC court (the European Court of Justice), that where national law contravenes EC law, Britain was bound by the terms of the 1972 European Communities Act to repeal or amend the law accordingly (*R v The Secretary of State for Transport, ex p. Factortame*). In relation to EC law parliamentary sovereignty is already a dead letter.

Law – methodological matters

This covers what the lawyers would refer to as *adjectival law*.

Legal procedures in Britain

General

In practice, litigation and prosecutions are no more conducted with scrupulous regard to, say, Sime's (1994) *Practical Approach to Civil Procedure* and Blackstone's (1994) *Criminal Practice* than are wars with regard to the Geneva Convention. A departure from the strict pattern may be referred to euphemistically as 'stage management'. 'Ambushes' are referred to openly (Letters to the Editor, 1995). Surrogate actors may be in place. One action showed parallels to the trial set up in John Le Carré's *The Spy who came in from the Cold* to protect Comrade Mundt. It is these and other problems that Lord Woolf (1995) has in mind in his plans for a sweeping shake up of our civil law system which has become too adversarial with the rules of court 'too often ignored by the parties and not enforced by the court'. Medical examiners will welcome the recommendation that there will be no oral evidence from expert witnesses but, with hearings limited to 3 hours, reports will need to be much more detailed than at present to diminish the risk of misinterpretations (News Item, 1995b).

Specific

The Royal Commission on Criminal Justice recommended the provision of interpreting services for deaf and hard-of-hearing people within the criminal justice system. However, as Grear (1993) pointed out, there is the need to provide adequate funds to ensure defendants have access to qualified interpreters while in police stations, which are usually the point of entry into the system. It is at this stage that clear and accurate communication is of paramount importance.

Adversarial vs. inquisitorial systems

As Eggleston (1983) pointed out, unlike the continental (*inquisitorial*) system of trials the English system based upon the Common Law is an *adversary* (or *adversarial*, or *accusatorial*) system.

Under the continental system, the witnesses are examined before the trial, and their evidence recorded and placed on file. The judge takes an active part, questioning the parties. For example, under German law, the *Grundsatz der freien richterlichen Beweiswürdigung* (principle of the unfettered consideration of the evidence) means that there are no legal rules compelling the judge to consider evidence in any particular way and saying what emphasis, if any, should be put on any particular piece of evidence (Foster, 1993).

Under the *adversarial system*, the parties (not the judge) decide what documents and evidence they should lay before the court. In a civil case, the judge cannot himself call a witness but must rest content with what the parties provide (*Jones v National Coal Board*). As Cohen (1977) pointed out, if the overriding aim of the court were to discover the full truth about the relevant past, the trier of fact (the judge) would need to have general powers to summon his own witnesses and the right to use his own information that is not before the court. And this is what an adversarial, as distinct from an inquisitorial, system does not permit. The adversarial system sees the judge as an arbiter in a contest of proof-strength rather than a research worker in the science of the past. Thus, under an adversarial system, parties oppose each other, much as boxers do, with the judge as umpire to see that the parties obey the rules (Du Plessis, 1992). The system is thus similar to trial by battle, a Norman (not Anglo-Saxon) institution. The parties, or their champions (now the Counsel in English courts), each armed with a leather shield and a staff, fought each other until one side gave in, or until nightfall (in which case the Plaintiff was considered to have lost). Trial by battle was not abolished in England until 1819 (Curzon, 1968).

Evidence, proof, probability and logic

Evidence

> 'While seeming to leave no stone unturned in its quest, deploying a panoply of procedures which have no true equivalent in inquisitorial systems, the English law of evidence nonetheless applies a number of rules which an outside observer could be forgiven for thinking had been designed for the express purpose of preventing the Court from getting at the truth' (Reynolds, 1994).

In one common law action for alleged occupational noise damage to the hearing, the Plaintiff's lawyers had retained a senior member of a national prestigious centre who was in effect held *incomunicado* in court, not being allowed to give evidence, while the work of his centre was being attacked.

Medical records

Confidential information communicated to medical practitioners is not protected by privilege (*Garner v Garner* 1920). However, a witness may refuse to produce a document or give evidence until ordered by the court to do so. In any claim for damages for personal injury, the court has the power under ss.31 and 32 of the Administration of Justice Act 1970 to order the disclosure and production of documents. Section 31 relates to legal proceedings which are contemplated; s32 relates to legal proceedings which have been commenced. It entitles either party to the action to apply for an order for the production of relevant documents in the possession of a third person who is not a party to the action. Documents which may be the subject of an order under either section include medical correspondence, records, reports and X-rays. As a result of three decisions in the Court of Appeal in the early 1970s, it had become the practice in applications under both ss.31 and 32 for medical records to be disclosed only to a medical expert nominated by the applicant, and not to the applicant himself or to his solicitors. In the case of *McIvor v Southern Health and Social Services Board* 1978, a hospital submitted that the consequences of not confining production of hospital records to the medical advisers of the applicant would in some cases be so dire that Parliament must have intended to confer on the courts a power so to do. The hospital's appeal to the House of Lords was dismissed. The House of Lords held that the Act meant what it said. However, the medical protection societies strongly advise their members to consult with them before complying with any request for the disclosure of records. It does not follow that every application from solicitors for the disclosure of records in the possession of a doctor must automatically be complied with, for the applicant has to satisfy the court on affidavit that there are grounds for making an order (Annual Report and Accounts, 1978). In practice, disclosure is now becoming less of a problem in relation to medical negligence claims.

Medical reports and evidence

Reports

It has been held, both by the courts and by doctors (e.g. Morrison, 1993) that an expert medical report is meant for the impartial assistance of the court and not simply to buttress one party's case. (One medical examiner went so far as to say in his report that he wished to represent the plaintiff in court.) Consequently, a doctor is right in refusing to amend a report at the behest of the solicitor requesting it (Medicolegal, 1979). However, Sir Joseph Molony QC (1966) has asked, 'What is the authority for this proposition (that the expert witness owes a duty solely to the court)? The only duty of an expert witness that I know of is to answer the questions they are asked truthfully and in accordance with their knowledge of the facts, combined with their experience and understanding of the subject. A supplementary duty, I would say, is not to allow to pass any apparent misunderstanding of their evidence which the Court or either advocate may entertain'.

Nevertheless, concern has been expressed regarding the manner in which expert evidence comes to be organized by lawyers. Comments have been made both in the Court of Appeal and in the House of Lords. In a House of Lords' judgment, Lord Wilberforce said that, 'while some degree of consultation between experts and legal advisers was entirely proper it was necessary that expert evidence presented to the Court should be, and should be seen to be, the independent product of the expert, uninfluenced as to form or content by the exigencies of litigation. To the extent that it was not, the evidence was likely to be not only incorrect but self-defeating (*Whitehouse v Jordan and Another* 1980). However, Bartlett (1994b) wrote:

'This incautious dictum has caused confusion as to counsel's role. In practice, it is impossible to comply with it and at the same time properly prepare a case for trial. It is the *duty* of the lawyers conducting litigation to ensure that the experts' reports are suitable both in form and content for the needs of the litigation. To the extent that a report is *not* influenced in form and content by the needs of the litigation, it is likely to hinder the due administration of justice and to result in costs being wasted'.

It could therefore well be that some examiners are placed in an invidious position. Moreover, such a concept could well explain observations that some examiners take a different line in court than they would at a medical or scientific meeting.

The Code of Conduct for the Bar (para. 607.3) states that a barrister must not rehearse, practise or coach a witness in relation to his evidence or the way in which he should give it. There is of course nothing to stop him delegating the task to someone else.

What should a report include? 'If the expert's opinion is to carry proper weight he must show that he has already taken account of all facts which might tend to weaken his stated conclusions on the issues with which his report is concerned' (Bartlett, 1944a). Thus, for example:

a In connection with thalidomide claims, the medical examiner should point to the similarity of the clinical picture to the Holt–Oram syndrome; some of the 430 British thalidomide victims are now going back to court to seek greater compensation because they are alarmed over their financial future; one of the original claimants has fathered a daughter with similar limb abnormalities (News Item, 1993a).

b In connection with 6 kHz audiometric notches, the examiner should point out, *inter alia*, that the first Medical Research Council hearing survey encountered earphone calibration difficulties at 6 kHz (Hinchcliffe, 1959). An apparent deviation at 6 kHz from the reference hearing level of Royal Naval recruits (Knight and Coles, 1960) was subsequently shown to be due to a calibration problem (Knight, 1966). Pressure of the audiometer earphone on the soft structures of the ear can also produce spurious results in attempts to measure the hearing threshold level. This is particularly so at 6 kHz where a 70 dB spurious notch may be produced (Coles, 1967). Screening audiometry of teenagers shows a number with discrete audiometric dips, most commonly at 6 kHz (Axelsson *et al.*, 1981). The National Physical Laboratory has said that the standard reference zero for the calibration of pure tone air conduction audiometers is set at too low a level by 8 dB (Robinson, Shipton and Hinchcliffe, 1981). The Medical Research Council's Institute of Hearing Research is saying that it is set too low by 9 dB (Lutman and Davis, 1994). Finally, patients who have hearing impairment only at very high frequencies ($\geqslant 6$ kHz) do not report speech communication problems (Dobie, 1993).

c In connection with auditory damage claims where the hearing threshold level is within the range of normality but there are complaints of hearing difficulties, the examiner should draw attention to the King–Kopetzky syndrome (or its local appellation) (Hinchcliffe, 1992); he should distinguish this from Merluzzi and Hinchcliffe (1973) thresholds, and bear in mind the clinical condition of labelling (Haynes *et al.*, 1978).

Handling quantitative data

As Martin (1979) pointed out, an expert, when giving evidence in court must state the reasons for his opinions, how they were reached and by what criteria his conclusions can be tested. At least three methods (descriptive, numerical, graphical), together with variations of these methods, have been suggested to us on how an expert witness should explain quantitative data to the court. Decisions need to be made before entry to the court, otherwise hesitancy in making a choice can be misinterpreted. Perhaps the solution is to use all three. Incorporation of explanations of the principal data sets in use onto a template which is employed for word-processor based reports would then be seen to be advantageous. This approach also has the advantage that all the expert's evidence is set out ready for the Court of Appeal if necessary.

Some courts may have difficulty in appreciating that quantitative models of, for example, hearing threshold levels, are statistical regression equations so that they do not have the precision of, say, geometrical equations such as that which describes the area of a rectangle as the product of its length and breadth, i.e. $A = l \times b$. This is but one of the many problems that the expert witness may encounter in using quantitative methods in his evidence (Hinchcliffe, 1994a).

It would be natural to believe that any medical examiner would accept an equation or formula if it fitted their data. Such is not the case. One may need to go through some formal reasoning such as:

- Has the equation been derived by a reputable scientific institution using an acceptable method of scientific analysis?
- Is there any reason to question the experimental design that produced the data?
- Is the equation or formula scientifically plausible?
- Does the equation or formula fit the data in question?
- Is there any reason to believe that the law of parsimony has been repealed?
- Is there any reason to doubt Tarski's concept that truth is conformity with the facts?

There are a number of numerical expressions which describe the hearing threshold level in terms of a number of components, e.g. ageing, gender, socioeconomic factors, noise exposure. With litigation in the field of audition being pursued within the range of normal hearing, factors which may be of no significance in the management of the individual, now assume significance in medico-legal practice. The existence of each of these factors, whether it be the one associated with ageing (Willott, 1991), gender (Jerger *et al.*, 1993), socioeconomic level (Hinchcliffe, 1994b) or noise (Sataloff and Sataloff, 1993) has been known for over half a century.

It is almost certain that these factors are multifactorial in nature. For example, in addition to the general and specific socioeconomic factors mentioned previously, Evans (1994) reported that low social status produces long-term elevation of blood glucocorticoid levels which increase low density lipoproteins, a risk factor for heart attacks. But the origin of this and other socioeconomic influences on health in adult life goes back to childhood (Kaplan and Salonen, 1990; Patel *et al.*, 1994) and even fetal life (Barker, 1990). Herrnstein and Murray (1994) go even further back to assert that the genome is the major factor determining socioeconomic level. Doctors tend to marry lawyers, lawyers, doctors, and factory workers, factory workers. It is therefore unlikely that assigning a woman the same socioeconomic grading as her partner, as in the National Study of Hearing, would incur a significant error. It is also unlikely that any sudden change in socioeconomic level, whether it be a manual worker coming up on the football pools or a Lloyds' name losing all that he has, would be associated with a change in hearing threshold level. Nevertheless, with increasing gender reassignments associated with the increasing incidence of gender dysphoria, there is a need to know what, if any, auditory consequences are associated with such an event. There are practical medico-legal implications. For example, what gender factor should a medical examiner use in assessing a hearing claim of an ex-Regimental Sergeant Major? Moreover, there could well be long-term changes in the magnitude and pattern of these various factors. There could well be secular changes in both the socioeconomic factor and the gender factor over this period of time. The social attributes of gender have been changing, whether in relation to occupational preferences or smoking or other habits. Human semen quality has declined substantially over the past 50 years (Skakkebaek, Giwercman and de Kretser, 1994). It is therefore incumbent on medical examiners in looking at hearing threshold levels to consider what birth cohort populations are available for comparison. If it is confirmed that subfecundity is an occupational risk for welders (Bonde, 1993), should a modified gender constant be used in the hearing regression expressions when such workers are litigating in respect of their hearing?

Given the magnitude of these various factors, it would not be possible to determine clinically the magnitude that a factor contributed to an individual's hearing level.

But, when all is said and done there may still be difference between different examiners. As Montaigne concluded in Chapter XXXVII of his *Essais*:

> '*Et ne fut jamais au Monde deux opinions pareilles, non plus que deux poils ou deux grains. Leur plus universelle qualité, c'est la diversité.*' (There never was in the world two opinions alike, no more than two hairs or two grains; the most universal quality is diversity.)

Evidence in court

It is for the court to determine whether or not it wishes to accept an expert's opinion, or which of conflicting opinions, if any, it prefers. The court is not bound to accept any opinion, even if undisputed. According to s.1 of the Perjury Act, if any person lawfully sworn as a witness or as an interpreter in a judicial case wilfully makes a statement material in that proceeding which that person knows to be false or does not believe to be true, that person shall be guilty of perjury. However, aside from the possibility of evidence being contaminated by deliberate false statements, witnesses have vaying degrees of defective memory, including genuine false memories. Experimental studies have demonstrated that individuals may assert with complete confidence that they remember things that have not happened (Roediger, 1994).

There is a curious notion among some medical men that they must, as well as presenting their expert evidence, also dwell on the rights and wrongs of a legal case. As Martin (1979) pointed out, a witness, however distinguished, cannot assume the mantle of a judge; he does not relieve the court of its responsibility for the judicial decision. Lord President Cooper has clearly distinguished between the separate roles of the expert and of the court (*David v Edinburgh Magistrates* 1953).

Use of quotations

There appears to be an increasing tendency by all the actors in a court scenario to make use of quotations to embellish their observations. As a former Master of the Rolls (Denning, 1986) indicated, such actions received their *imprimatur* from the Roman poet, Horace, who lived in the century before Christ. In his *De Arte Poetica* we read:

> *'Inceptis gravibus plerumque et magna professis*
> *Purpureus, late qui splendeat, unus et alter*
> *Adsuitur pannus'* [2]

Where there are actions relating to alleged damages in the millibel range, an appropriate quotation might well be: 'Take care of the pence, for the pounds will take care of themselves'. A saying that the Earl of Chesterfield (Stanhope, 1747) attributed to a one time Secretary of the Treasury, William Lowndes (1652–1724). But, with alleged damages of such a magnitude, the ageing, gender and socioeconomic factors remain insignificant no longer.

Alexander Pope's

> *'Be not the first by whom the New are try'd,*
> *Nor yet the last to lay the Old aside.'*
>   (*Essay on Criticism*, line 335)

provides a commendable guideline for irreversible interventions, e.g. surgical management. However, applying the quotation to, for example, the Medical Research Council's Institute of Hearing Research's model of auditory threshold (Lutman and Spencer, 1991) could well result from failure to appreciate that problems known to be associated with the measurement of hearing at 6 kHz particularly have been recognized for over 30 years (Hinchcliffe, 1959), that the existence of a socioeconomic factor (or factors) has been known for more than half a century (Hinchcliffe, 1994b), that the relevance of what is now

known as Leijon's (1992) quantization error has been appreciated for over 30 years (e.g. by Knight and Coles, 1960), that the non-dichotomous nature of the screening process has been recognized for over 10 years (Robinson, Shipton and Hinchcliffe, 1979) and that occupational noise *may* not be as damaging as some reports would indicate has been known for over 40 years (Wheeler and Dickson, 1952), but that the ageing of hearing has not changed in the UK over a period of 30 years (Hinchcliffe, 1993).

In such cases, a more appropriate quotation from Pope would therefore be from his *Windsor Forest* (line 13):

> *'Not Chaos-like together crush'd and bruis'd,*
> *But as the world, harmoniously confus'd:*
> *Where Order in Variety we see,*
> *And where, tho' all things differ, all agree.'*

Undoubtedly the best 'purple patch' to apply to the MRC model and its detractors would be one from Molière's *Le Médecin Malgré Lui*, 1666. Sganarelle, who symbolizes the pseudo-doctor in the literature of Molière, says, '*Oui, cela était autrefois ainsi; mais nous avons changé tout cela, et nous faisons maintenant la médecine d'une methode toute nouvelle*'. (Yes, it used to be so but we have changed all that. Everything's quite different in medicine nowadays.) Sganarelle was alluding to the post-mortem finding of transposition of the viscera in a condemned criminal (reported in the *Gazette* of 17 December 1650). Thus, just as Sganarelle was being cynical about there being more than one internal structural model of man, so current Sganarelles have difficulty in comprehending that there could be more than one model of man's hearing.

Much of the difficulty that some people have in accepting that there could be more than one quantitative model of hearing is that there exists a precise mathematical formula. The numerical models used in medico-legal reports are statistical, and not mathematical, models, i.e. they are not formulae to give precise predictions of expected hearing threshold levels (Hinchcliffe, 1994a).

Often when a medical examiner's opinion runs counter to another's he will take refuge in the clinical experience resulting from seeing several thousand similar cases. One is reminded of an eminent philosopher's comments (Popper, 1981) on 'clinical observations'.

> 'The Freudian analysts emphasised that their theories were constantly verified by their "clinical observations". As for Adler, I was much impressed by a personal experience. Once, in 1919, I reported to him [3] a case which to me did not seem

[2] 'When you are covering, as with a garment, some weighty or important matter, you should sew on one or two purple patches so as to attract the attention of those who are unfamiliar with it.'

[3] During the time that he lived in Vienna, Popper helped Adler with his social work among the working-class young.

particularly Adlerian, but which he found no difficulty in analysing in terms of his theory of inferiority feelings, although he had not even seen the child. Slightly shocked, I asked him how he could be so sure. "Because of my thousandfold experience", he replied; whereupon I could not help saying: "And with this new case, I suppose, your experience has become a thousand-and-onefold".'

Like the law, medicine and science are in a state of continual evolution. This was well summarized by Montaigne (1580) who died 400 years ago:

'*Les arts et les sciences ne sont pas coulés dans un moule mais formés et perfectionnés par degrés, par de fréquents maniements et polissages, comme les ourses lèchent patiemment leurs petits pour les éveiller au monde.*' (Arts and sciences are not cast in a mould, but are formed and perfected by degrees, by frequent handling and polishing, as bears patiently lick their cubs into form.)

Role of the expert witness in the legal process

Jones (1994) has examined the role of the expert witness in the legal process. She concluded that the effect of the harnessing of science to law has been the concealment of the way in which scientific evidence is constructed. She argued that the legal profession and the judiciary perceived the growing professionalism of scientists as a threat to the dominance of the law as the principal method of dispute resolution, and responded by developing various types of control strategies.

Standard of proof

What is referred to as the *standard of proof* in English law civil cases is that of the balance of probabilities (*Cooper v Slade* 1858).

'In civil cases the case must be proved by a *preponderance of probability*, but there may be degrees of probability within that standard. The degree depends on the subject matter. A civil court, when considering a charge of fraud, will naturally require for itself a higher degree of probability than that which it would require when asking if negligence is established' (*Bater v Bater* per Denning L.J.).

In criminal cases the standard of proof

'need not reach certainty, but it must carry a high degree of probability. Proof beyond a reasonable doubt does not mean proof beyond the shadow of a doubt. The law would fail to protect the community if it admitted fanciful possibilities

to deflect the course of justice. If the evidence is so strong against a man as to leave only a remote possibility in his favour, which can be dismissed with the sentence "of course it is possible but not in the least probable" the case is proved beyond reasonable doubt, but nothing short of that will suffice' (*Miller v Minister of Pensions per* Denning L.J.).

In French law there is the expression '*bénéfice du doute*', to give someone the benefit of the doubt. In his final submission, Edgar Demange, Counsel for Dreyfus (see section on Law – systematic), addressed the court: '*Ce doute me suffit; ce doute, c'est un acquittement!*' (Alas! it was not).

The English distinctions between different degrees of proof have not gone unquestioned by the judiciary. Lord Goddard said that he had difficulty in understanding how there are or can be two standards (*R v Hepworth and Fearnley*). One British Judge, Hilbery J. said 'If a thing is proved, it is proved, but I am not entitled to that view'.

Probability

Bertrand Russell is purported to have said, 'Probability is the most important concept in modern science, especially as nobody has the slightest notion what it means' (Bell, 1945).

Historically, the concept of 'probability' goes back to the *probabilitas* of Aristotle which referred to the degree of conviction, and it is in this sense that it is used in medicine and in jurisprudence (Schneider, 1983). In that sense it must be a very personal concept.

Jeremy Bentham (1825) considered that the doctrine of chances, i.e. Pascal's mathematical calculus of probability, inapplicable to the measurement of probative force. Current case law is as expressed in *Re J S* (*a minor*),

'The concept of "probability" in the legal sense is certainly different from the mathematical concept; indeed it is rare to find a situation in which the two usages co-exist although, when they do, the mathematical probability has to be taken into the assessment of probability in the legal sense and given its appropriate weights'.

It would thus appear that the term 'probability' is used differently in law, medicine and science.

Medical examiners frequently refer to 'the balance of probabilities'. What probabilities are they balancing? And in respect of causation, disability, handicap, explanation of symptoms? Not infrequently, when the phrase is used, one is reminded of John Gay's *The Painter who Pleased Nobody and Everybody*:

'*Lest men suspect your tale untrue,
Keep probability in view.*'

Mechanism of proof

There are two distinct schools regarding what is considered to be the mechanism of legal proof. There is the Pascalian probability concept of a former Chancellor of Monash University (Eggleston, 1983) and the Baconian probability concept of a former President of the British Society for the Philosophy of Science (Cohen, 1977). The latter approach, being an experimental, 'gradually dissecting' analysis, is more akin to how both clinicians and scientists approach these problems. However, one should distinguish between *probability* and *degree of corroboration* (Popper, 1934).

Legal logic

The logic adopted by judges in handling evidence has been studied by Williams (1982a). He concluded that judicial argument can often be translated into intuitionistic inductive logic. This would be consistent with the view that courts use Baconian concepts in the approach to proof since Bacon is frequently identified as the promulgator of the inductive method. It can, nevertheless, be traced back to Aristotle. Although supported by John Stuart Mill, the fallacy of the inductive method was demonstrated first by Hume and then by Popper (1981). Bacon also erred in other matters. For example, he opposed Copernicus' heliocentric concept on the grounds that it, 'needlessly did violence to our senses'. In the courts, *non sequiturs* (e.g. in *Williams, Hunter and McPoland v. Robinson Willey Ltd*) may have been attributable to the use of inductive logic.

There is a strong belief that many judges decide what their decision will be, then back-track from there, but produce what may appear to be a forward looking argument. There is also the uncertainty of the extent that both judges and juries seek spiritual guidance before coming to a decision; British judges are physically backed by the logo *Dieu et mon droit*; juries have been reported to use Ouija boards (Slapper, 1994).

Alternative systems of dispute resolution (ADR)

In recent times there has been, for a variety of reasons, an increasing dissatisfaction with litigation as a means of resolving disputes. Systems of dispute resolution other than litigation have therefore been developed and implemented (Mackie, 1991; Brown and Marriott, 1993).

'Compared to modern business, civil courts have changed very little ... Alternative dispute resolution gives lawyers an opportunity to use new processes, encourages a problem-solving attitude and an openness to compromise' (Coulson, 1989).

But, in the historical introduction to this chapter, we referred to Gagarin's idea of law developing first as a dispute-resolving system in society. Arbitration (διαιτηδια) was recognized by the Greeks. Thus the dispute-resolving processes now being established and implemented are not new to society. They have existed since the earliest times, antedating litigation. Indeed in the pre-literate societies which still exist there is no alternative to the 'alternative' systems of dispute resolution. One is also reminded of the *Essais de Michel de Montaigne* over 400 years ago:

En voilà qui, pour tout juge, emploient en leurs causes le premier passant qui voyage le long de leurs montagnes. Et ces autres élisent le jour du marché quelqu'un d'entre eux, qui sur-le-champ décide tous leurs procès. Quel danger y aurait-il que les plus sages vidassent ainsi les nôtres, selon les occurences et à l'oeil, sans obligation d'exemple et de conséquence? A chaque pied son soulier.' (Some have no judges, but take the first traveller to pass through their mountains to decide their disputes for them; and others, on their market day, elect one of their own number to decide their disputes at once. What risks would there be if the wisest amongst us were to settle our disputes in the same way, according to circumstances and at sight, without being bound by precedents and consequences. For every foot its own shoe.) (A parallel account is given by Guillaume Bouchet de Brocourt in his *Sérées* which appeared about the same time.)

ADR is not restricted to the field of civil justice. It is now being used as an adjunct to the administration of justice in the criminal field in Britain, Germany and North America. In the USA, the applications are referred to as VORPS (Victim Offender Reconciliation Programs) and in Britain as *reparation schemes* (Marshall, 1984; Marshall and Merry, 1990). Meeting the offender was the most commonly identified reason for the victim (if he survives!) being satisfied with the process (Coates and Gehm, 1985).

Although there are indications of a changing attitude in the new CIS (Commonwealth of Independent States), and in the old USSR arbitration had no role where disputes betwen individual citizens were concerned. 'In the USSR, citizens do not make use of arbitral jurisdictions because they have complete confidence in the people's courts' (Kudrjavcev, 1956). In contrast to the negligible role of private arbitration in Russia, public arbitration (between state organizations) is the rule. Around half a million disputes were settled when this activity was at its peak.

Law – systematic (substantive)
Private (civil)

Tort and delict

The *law of torts* (Hepple and Matthews, 1991; Jones, 1994) was a creation of the common law and it was evolved from the principle of providing a remedy for an unjustifiable injury done by one person to another. A tort is a civil wrong. As pointed out by Lord Denning, the province of tort is to allocate responsibility for injurious conduct. In the context of this chapter, the three most important torts are nuisance, negligence, and trespass to person.

As Atiyah (1970) pointed out, the concept of *fault* dominates the existing compensation systems. Although it has virtually no place in personal insurance compensation or in the social security system, it underlies almost the entire law of torts. The concept of the fault principle derives much from the writers on tort, particularly Sir John Salmond, at the beginning of this century. Salmond strove to reduce the whole law of torts to a set of moral principles around the concept of fault. But compensation payable bears no relation to the degree of fault.

Those legal systems which belong to the Romano–Germanic group have a substantial input from Roman Law. The *law of delict* is based upon the second of the three precepts of Ulpian: *Juris praecepta sunt haec: honeste vivere, alterum non laedere, suum cuique tribuere.* (The maxima of the law are these: to live honestly, to harm no one, and to give everyone his due.) Both Scottish law and South African law derive from Roman–Dutch law. Consequently in both these legal systems the law of delict governs civil legal wrongs, although in Scotland it is referred to as the law of reparation. Although under Roman law a delict could be public (termed a crime in modern legal systems) or private. The latter covers what under English law is termed the law of tort. Delict has shown considerable evolution since Roman times when it was essentially legalized vengeance. Delict has now been defined as an unlawful act which violates the subjective right(s) of a legal subject (Du Plessis, 1992).

Nuisance

A nuisance has been defined as:

> 'an inconvenience materially interfering with the ordinary comfort, physically, of human existence, not merely according to elegant or dainty modes of living, but according to plain and sober and simple notions among the English People' (*Walter v Selfe* 1851).

A nuisance is thus an unlawful interference with a person's use or enjoyment of land, or of some right over or in connection with it. As Mr Justice Cusack

(1969) pointed out, English land law has for many centuries laid stress upon the entitlement of lawful occupiers to what is termed 'quiet enjoyment', meaning that they are to be protected against unjustifiable interference from outsiders. In modern times this ancient expression has been found to have a new and literal significance. Quiet enjoyment is increasingly menaced by intrusive noise.

That air-borne noise may constitute a nuisance was first established in 1867 in the case of *Crump v Lambert*. That structure-borne noise may constitute a nuisance was established in the case of *Hoare and Company v McAlpine* in 1923. In *Vanderpant v Mayfair Hotel Co* 1930 it was made clear that intrusive noise need not be injurious to health. What matters is whether or not it interferes with ordinary comfort.

In contrast to the statute law on noise, it is no defence for the defendant to show that he has taken all reasonable steps and care to prevent the noise (*Rushmer v Polsue and Alfieri Limited* 1906). The judgment in this case was expressly approved by the House of Lords on appeal. Lord Loreburn stated that, 'It would be no answer to say that the steam hammer is of the most modern improved pattern and is reasonably worked'. This principle was upheld in the case of *Halsey v Esso Petroleum Company Limited* 1961. The plaintiff was granted both damages for loss caused by acid smuts from the defendant's depot and injunctions to restrain the making of noise at night and the emission of pungent smells at any time. The action was also of note because in evidence the plaintiff brought noise level measurements to court.

A landlord may be liable if he has authorized the creation of a nuisance expressly or by implication. Thus a landlord has been held liable for his tenant's blasting operations because he had let the property for that specific purpose (*Harris v James* 1876).

Gunfire, especially when malicious, can be a cause for nuisance. A fox farmer was granted an injunction restraining his neighbour from firing guns so as to frighten the foxes during the breeding season (*Hollywood Silver Fox Farm v Emmett* 1936). Noises other than those due to gunfire or machinery can also constitute a nuisance. In the case of *Tinkler v Aylesbury Dairy Co. Limited* 1988, it was held that noise resulting from moving milk churns when being loaded interfered with the personal comfort of the nearby residents and thereby constituted a common-law nuisance. Noise from carts and shouts from their drivers during the night, so that they made the plaintiff unable to sleep, also constituted a common-law nuisance (*Bartlett v Marshall* 1896). Noisy animals can constitute a common-law nuisance. As well as the case of *Leeman v Montagu* 1936, there was, more recently, the case of *Harrison v Metropolitan Police* 1972. In the latter case, the plaintiff obtained an injunction with respect to the howling and barking of dogs kept in a police station compound. These noises had disturbed his sleep and made it difficult for him to work in his study even when he wore earplugs and had installed both double glazing in the bedroom and internal shutters. 'Corky', a noisy cockerel, became a *cause célèbre* in a North Devon village (News Item, 1994a).

Malice may be a factor in an action for noise nuisance. In the case of *Christie v Davey* 1983, a music teacher was granted an injunction restraining ·a neighbour from knocking on the party wall and otherwise creating a noise to interfere with professional teaching.

However, *temporary noise*, e.g. that due to the demolition of a building, may not, if the operation is reasonably conducted and all proper reasonable steps taken to ensure that no undue inconvenience is caused to neighbours, form a basis for a successful action for nuisance at common law (*Andreae v Selfridge* 1938). Nevertheless, a teacher in New Zealand was successful in claiming damages in the New Zealand Supreme Court because nearby construction noise forced him to shout and this caused him to develop a tumour on the vocal folds (News Item, 1969).

At common law, *prescriptive right* is a defence in an action for nuisance. This arises after 20 years. However, the time begins only when the act in fact becomes a nuisance. Thus it was held that the defendant had no prescriptive right in a case where he had used the machinery for more than 20 years but the vibrations caused by it became a nuisance only when the plaintiff, a physician, put up a consulting room at the end of his garden near the noise (*Sturges v Bridgman* 1879). This decision thus also upheld the principle, established in the case of *Bliss v Hall* 1838, that it is no defence to show that the plaintiff came to the nuisance.

The Noise and Statutory Nuisance Act 1993 principally amends the Control of Pollution Act 1974 and the Environmental Protection Act 1990 and makes new provision relating to the operation of loudspeakers in streets and roads and to audible intruder alarms.

Negligence

In general

Negligence is a failure to provide against reasonably foreseeable hazards. Indeed the concept of foreseeability is an essential element in all cases of nuisance and of negligence [Privy Council in the *Wagon Mound* case (*Overseas Tankship (UK) Limited v Miller Steamship Co.* 1967 – *Wagon Mound No. 2*, so-called because it refers to the ship SS *Wagon Mound*.)]. However, as Munkman (1985) pointed out,

'negligence as the criterion of liability involves the further test of reasonable foreseeability, which has been shown up as vague, capricious and subjective when applied to anything more complex than bow and arrows, or horses and carts'.

Some learned judges are able to foresee very little; others, by taking a complex succession of events step by step, are able to foresee almost anything.

The same court can reach opposite results on two cases based on the same happening. In the *Wagon Mound* case, different plaintiffs took action on the same occurrence. The lower court in one case held that a particular event was not reasonably foreseeable, while, in the second case, another lower court held that the same event might have been foreseeable.

In British courts, the concept of foreseeability is usually interpreted in the sense given to it by Lord Oaksey in the case of *Bolton v Stone* 1951 (the plaintiff was injured by a cricket ball hit over a fence onto a road; it was held that the cricket club was not liable as the possibility of injury was so slight). The reasonable man does not take precautions against everything which he can foresee, but only against those things which he can foresee are reasonably likely to happen.

In an action for negligence, the plaintiff must prove that the defendant was under a duty of care to him, that there was a breach of such duty, and that, as a direct consequence, the plaintiff suffered damage. Thus, the essential prerequisites have been given as the four Ds: duty of care, dereliction of duty, damage, and directness.

In practice, there is usually no doubt about the existence of the duty of care and it is then assumed to exist. However, in the case of *Donoghue (or M'Alister) v Stevenson*, Lord Atkin formulated the general concept that, 'you must take reasonable care to avoid acts or omissions which you can reasonably foresee will be likely to injure your neighbour'. He then defined 'neighbours' as 'persons so closely and directly affected by my act that I ought reasonably to have them in contemplation as being affected when I am directing my mind to the acts or omissions which are called in question'. Thus there will be a 'duty' situation wherever the relationship of the parties is such that the likelihood that the plaintiff would be affected by the defendant's conduct ought reasonably to have been contemplated by the defendant.

Prior to Lord Atkin's unifying concept in *Donoghue (or M'Alister) v Stevenson*, negligence cases belonged to one or other category. Since then the law of negligence has undergone considerable development, coming full circle with the 1990 judgment in *Caparo Industries plc v Dickman*. Once more we are back to categories. Giving a House of Lords judgment in this case, Lord Bridge said,

'What emerges is that, in addition to the foreseeability of damage, necessary ingredients in any situation giving rise to a duty of care are that there should exist between the party owing the duty and the party to whom it is owed a relationship characterised by the law as one of "proximity" or "neighbourhood" and that the situation should be one in which the court considers it fair, just and reasonable that the law should impose a duty of a given scope on the one party for the benefit of the other . . . It is preferable in my view, that the law should develop novel categories of negligence incrementally and by analogy with established categories, rather than by a massive extension of a prima facie duty of care restrained only by indefinable "considerations" which ought to be negative, or to reduce or limit the scope of the duty or the class of person to whom it is owed'.

This is the present position of the law of negligence.

Defences available in an action for negligence are, apart from denying the alleged negligence, that:

1 It was an inevitable accident (mishap)
2 The negligence was that of someone else
3 The risk was assumed by the plaintiff (*volenti non fit injuria*)
4 There was contributory negligence by the plaintiff.

It is a defence to an action in tort that the defendant neither intended to injure the plaintiff nor could have avoided doing so by the use of reasonable care.

Until 1945, *contributory negligence* was a complete defence to an action in tort. However, in that year, the Law Reform (Contributory Negligence) Act was enacted. Section 1 of that Act states that,

'Where any person suffers damage as the result partly of his own fault and partly the fault of any other person, a claim in respect of that damage shall not be defeated by reason of the fault of the person suffering the damage, but the damages recoverable in respect thereof shall be reduced to such an extent as the court thinks just and equitable having regard to the claimant's share in the responsibility for the damage'.

In two decisions (*Parnell v Shields*, 1973 and *Salmon v Newland and others*, 1983) 20% was deducted from damages awarded as the result of road accidents in which the plaintiff was not wearing a seat belt.

Associated with the concept of contributory negligence is the doctrine of 'hypothetical causation'. A steel erector had died following a fall from a tower. Although on the day in question no safety belts were available, it was held, from the evidence given, that the deceased would not have worn one. The plaintiff's act of omission may therefore constitute a *novus actus interveniens*.

Medical negligence

Medical negligence (Dingwall, Fenn and Quam, 1990; Powers and Harris, 1990) is the one area of law which has the greatest impact on medical practice. As Lord Bridge (1990) pointed out, the growth in litigation in this field is attributable to two principal causes: first, the greater awareness of patients of their legal rights and a greater willingness to enforce them; secondly, the ever increasing sophistication of medical procedures. It is ironic but inevitable that the further medical science advances the more the medical profession lays itself open to attack in respect of mistakes which can occur in the highly complex and delicate procedures necessary for effective treatment.

Yet a medical man cannot decline to go along with current developments. A physician in the UK undertakes 'to keep myself informed of advances in Medicine'. It is also implicit in *Bolam* (see below) that the professional man has an obligation to keep up to date in the exercise in his particular skill. However, he is not negligent if harm could have been avoided by using equipment commonly available in another country but rare in the UK (*Whiteford v Hunter*). Moreover, he is not expected to implement the findings of reports which have appeared only within the past 6 months (*Crawford v Board of Governors of Charing Cross Hospital*).

A trainee is expected, legally, to demonstrate the same standard of care as someone who has completed training. This applies equally to learning to drive a car (*Nettleship v Weston* 1971) and to learning to care medically for premature babies (*Wilsher v Essex Area Health Authority* 1988). However, there have been conflicting interpretations of the judgments in the last case. Finch (1986) claimed that the headline of The Times Law Report on this case 'Doctor's Inexperience no Defence to Negligence' is not supported by the full original transcript of the judgment. An inexperienced senior house officer was acquitted by all three Court of Appeal judges. However, the decision qualified significantly the ability of inexperienced doctors. Finch argued that it is misinterpretations such as these that give rise to medical misconceptions of legal responsibility. These have two results. First, defensive medicine is practised. This is not defensiveness, it is defensivism, which is the enemy both of doctors and of patients. Secondly, a cry goes up for a new type of compensation independent of the need to prove fault. Havard (1986) drew our attention to the views expressed by the dissenting judge (the Vice-Chancellor) in the above case:

'Should the authority be liable if it demonstrated that due to the financial stringency under which it operated it could not afford to fill the post with those with the necessary experience? However, the law should not be distorted by making findings of personal fault against individual doctors who were, in truth, not at fault, in order to avoid such questions . . . the courts would not do society a favour by distorting the existing law so as to conceal the real social questions which arises.'

It is normal for the plaintiff to establish that the defendant's negligence had caused him injury. However, the onus is on the defendant if the principle of *res ipsa loquitur* (things speak for themselves) operates. For example, a patient went into hospital with two stiff fingers (due to Dupytren's contracture) and came out with four. In reversing the decision of the trial court, Lord Denning held it to be a case of *res ipsa loquitur* (*Cassidy v Minister of Health* 1951). Two conditions are required before this doctrine will apply. First, the event which caused the damage must have rested within the control of the defendant. Second, the mere occurrence of the event itself implies that the defendant has been negligent. One would also presume that this doctrine would be applied to cases of permanent complete facial palsy following a stapedectomy. For example, a plaintiff underwent this operation and the stapes was replaced with a politef piston. The only unusual feature encountered at operation was a greater than usual amount of posterior meatal wall which had to be drilled before the stapes and foramen ovale were exposed. The patient developed a complete ipsilateral facial palsy 48 hours after the operation. A subsequent exploration showed that the facial nerve had been damaged in the horizontal portion of a facial nerve canal, at which site there was a dehiscence. The claim for damages was settled for £10 000 (Annual Report and Accounts, 1978).

Actions for medical negligence allow for a 'chain of causation'. Thus failure in the treatment of the infected finger of a pregnant woman was held to be the cause of a voice disorder. The chain of causation here was via a septicaemia and subsequent damage to the cranial nerves.

An action cannot be pursued if the ultimate outcome has not been influenced by the doctor's negligence. For example a patient developed loss of hearing and of balance 24 hours after the onset of an illness which in retrospect was considered to have been meningitis. The patient had been examined within 6 hours of the onset of his illness by his general practitioner, who, on the basis of the contemporary records, made a not unreasonable diagnosis of gastroenteritis. The doctor prescribed antibiotics but ignored requests for further visits despite a deterioration in the patient's condition which was associated with the loss of hearing and balance. It was held that the outcome would have been no different had the doctor visited the patient as requested. In the *Wilsher v Essex Area Health Authority* case mentioned above, the House of Lords decided that it had not been established on the balance of probabilities that negligence on the part of the junior doctor was primarily responsible for the damage (blindness).

In respect of medical practice, Lord Denning has said that a doctor was not to be held to be negligent simply because something went wrong. He was liable only when he fell below the standard of care of a reasonably competent practitioner in his field so much that his conduct might be deserving of censure or be inexcusable (*Cole v Hucks* 1968). However, this holds only when the *mishap* cannot be avoided by any such precaution as a reasonable man may be expected to take. Risks are inherent in most medical and surgical procedures but a practitioner must not take 'an unwarranted and unnecessary risk'. The 'broken needle' cases best illustrate the law relating to medical mishaps. When the needle of a hypodermic syringe breaks off during a diagnostic or therapeutic procedure, the plaintiff must produce evidence of negligence as such. The evidence may be that the needle was not the appropriate one for the particular injection or that it was inserted wrongly.

In a Court of Appeal decision, Lord Denning said that:

'if medical men were to be found liable whenever they did not effect a cure – or whenever anything untoward happens – it would do a great disservice not only to the profession itself but to society at large. Heed should be taken of what had happened in the United States. There ''medical malpractice'' cases were very worrying, especially as they were tried by juries who had sympathy for the patient and none for the doctor – who was insured – and damages were colossal. Experienced practitioners refused to treat patients for fear of being accused of negligence. In the interest of all we must avoid such consequences. The courts must say firmly that, in a professional man, an error of judgment was not negligent' (*Whitehouse v Jordan and Another* 1979).

However, the case went to the House of Lords where disagreement was expressed with this statement. Their Lordships nevertheless upheld the Court of Appeal's decision in reversing the trial judge's finding. In concurring with Lord Wilberforce, Lord Fraser stated that Lord Denning must have meant to say that an error of judgment 'is not necessarily negligent'. Another Law Lord, Lord Edmund–Davies, concluded by saying:

'doctors and surgeons fell into no special legal category, and, to avoid any future disputation of a similar kind, his Lordship would have it accepted that the true doctrine was enunciated – and by no means for the first time – by Mr Justice McNair in *Bolam v Friern Hospital Management Committee* 1957. In that case, McNair J. in directing the jury, enunciated what has become to be known as the *Bolam test*: "The test is the standard of the ordinary skilled man exercising and professing to have that special skill. A man need not possess the highest expert skill at the risk of being found negligent . . ." A doctor is not guilty of negligence if he has acted in accordance with a practice accepted as proper by a responsible body of medical men skilled in that particular art. In words applied by the Privy Council in *Chin Keow v Government of Malaysia* 1967: "When you get a situation which involves the use of some special skill or competence, then the test as to whether there has been negligence or not is not the test of the man on the top of a Clapham omnibus, because he has not got this special skill. The test is the standard of the ordinary skilled man exercising and professing that special skill." If a surgeon failed to measure up to that standard in any respect ("clinical judgment" or otherwise) he had been negligent and should be so judged' (*Whitehouse v Jordan and Another* 1980).

In comparison, a jeweller, when piercing ears, must exercise the degree of care appropriate to jewellers, and not aural surgeons (*Philips v William Whiteley*).

Mistakes must be differentiated from mishaps. As a general rule in the law of torts, a mistake is no defence. However, the law has taken a different view in respect of medical mistakes. A mistake in diagnosis has been construed as an 'error of judgment'.

Thus, in an action for damages brought by a widow in respect of the misdiagnosis of her late husband's chest pain, the judge ruled that the case was one of mistake and not of negligence because the doctor had examined the case carefully for an hour. However, failing to make a correct diagnosis must be differentiated from failure to examine a patient adequately. The latter may amount to negligence. Failure to use a stethoscope in a casualty department to diagnose fractured ribs in an intoxicated injured patient has been held to be negligent. Failure to request a radiological examination in possible bony disorders or injuries would probably be held to be negligent. But, surprisingly, failure to employ an endoscope which would have diagnosed a rare condition may not amount to negligence. If a doctor does not feel competent to diagnose a particular case, he may be held negligent for failing to refer the case to the appropriate specialist. Although, in cases concerning surgical treatment, the question of negligence hinges on what other competent practitioners would, or would not, have done, so often the principle of *res ipsa loquitur* (see above) is applied. This principle would hold where the wrong operation was performed or the wrong side was operated on. Lord Goddard held that the principle applied in 'swab cases' also (*Mahon v Osborn* 1939).

If a patient dies as a result of gross negligence by a doctor then a criminal charge (manslaughter) would arise (see later).

In the Court of Appeal, Lord Denning said that the *hospital authorities* are responsible for all of their staff (*Roe v Ministry of Health* 1954). In January 1990, Health Authorities accepted full vicarious liability for the negligent (but not other) actions of their medical staff, the so-called Crown indemnity. In *Bull v Devon AHA* [1993] the Court of Appeal, in the course of holding the health authority liable in negligence, accepted that the authority owed the plaintiff and her son a duty of care directly.

Viewed globally, the central concern of law in the various countries of the world is to give 'due and consistent protection to the patients' rights', with the sole and significant exceptions of the countries of the British Isles (Giesen, 1988a).

SYRINGING CASES

A perforated ear drum following aural syringing in a 50-year-old man resulted in otorrhoea which, in turn, resulted in inability to go swimming or take a shower, resulting in an expensive holiday to the Canary Islands being ruined. The doctor who syringed the ear recorded that 'unfortunately, the nozzle of the syringe slipped during the procedure and the external auditory canal was lacerated'. The case was settled out of court for £4222. This sum covered a 'profound sensorineural hearing loss' on the affected side as well as surgical fees for a myringoplasty and legal fees (Annual Report and Accounts, 1978).

In another case of a perforated ear drum following syringing, the plaintiff was reported to have suffered a 'permanent 40-dB hearing loss and tinnitus' (*James v SKF [UK]* 1977).

In a third case of ear-drum perforation following syringing, subsequent treatment (repeated myringoplasties) by a consultant was considered to have made things worse rather than better. 'There was a 50 per cent hearing loss in the affected ear with vestibular function significantly diminished.' The claim was settled after negotiation by payment of damages of £8000 and costs of £810 (Annual Report and Accounts, 1979).

However, not all claims in respect of ear-drum perforation due to syringing have been successful. An 18-year-old youth attended for a medical examination at a recruiting centre. Impacted wax in both ears required syringing. The youth denied any previous ear trouble. Syringing was successful in clearing the wax from one ear but,

> 'the third and last effort to eliminate the wax from the other ear proved so painful that the doctor desisted, instilled more oil into the ear and told the young man to return a week later . . . the boy reported at the examination centre a week later

with a piece of lint over his ear on which there was some brownish-yellow discharge . . . He had had some bleeding from the ear during the evening of the day when it had been syringed . . . On examination, the ear was found to be cleared of debris and there was a small perforation in the tympanum. The papers were submitted to two experienced otologists, both of whom were of the opinion that it is impossible to perforate a healthy ear drum by syringing.' In view of this evidence, the judge gave a judgment for the doctor with costs (Taylor, 1971).

OTOTOXIC DRUGS

The law of negligence affords some protection for a patient against the adverse effects of therapeutic substances or procedures. The doctor, the hospital, or the pharmaceutical manufacturer could be liable. Injury sustained as a result of being given a drug could be considered an aspect of product liability. Decisions in a given case would be based on *Donoghue v Stevenson* 1932 which has been referred to earlier. The plaintiff in that case had drunk ginger beer from an opaque bottle which was subsequently found to contain a decomposed snail. The plaintiff, who became ill, was unable to sue under the law of contract because another person had purchased the bottle. The law of contract may also not be applicable for other reasons. For example, in *Pfizer v Ministry of Health* 1965, the House of Lords ruled that the supply of drugs under the NHS scheme was not a contract, even when a prescription charge had been levied. The patient has a statutory right to demand the drug; the hospital has the statutory obligation to supply it.

The case of *Watson v Buckley* 1940 showed that a plaintiff may sue (successfully) the distributors of an unsafe pharmaceutical product, in that case a hair dye. But in the UK there has not yet been a successful court action against a pharmaceutical company in respect of adverse side effects of one of of its products. Out of court settlements have been reached without any admission of liability.

Much of the legal interest in the adverse effect of drugs centres on thalidomide, $\alpha - (N - phthalimido)$-glutarimide. This was a psychotropic drug which was discovered in 1954, first marketed in West Germany in 1956 and in the UK in 1958. An ataxic polyneuritis was soon observed as an adverse effect. Wiedemann (1961) reported congenital abnormalities in cases where the mothers had taken the drug in the early stages of pregnancy. In the same year, the drug was withdrawn from the market. During the 5-year period that it was on the market, thalidomide probably produced 10 000 defective children, about 400 in the UK. The congenital abnormality was characterized by phocomelia, microtia and, frequently, defec-

tive hearing. Legal proceedings began in 1962 but the case was never fully litigated. Instead, there were a series of settlements, beginning in 1968 and ending 10 years later (News Item, 1978). Nevertheless, as Teff and Munroe (1976) pointed out, the thalidomide catastrophe has had many repercussions and a profound influence on the law. It provoked an extensive assessment by the Law Commission on the Problem of Liability for Antenatal Injury. This culminated in the Report on Injuries to Unborn Children 1974. Based upon the Law Commission's recommendations, the Congenital Disabilities (Civil Liability) Act 1976 provided for the unborn child to sue for negligence. At the time of the thalidomide catastrophe, doubts were expressed as to whether or not a right of action existed with regard to antenatal injury. This was exemplified by a decision in 1884 in the USA in which it was held that a child was part of its mother and had no independent legal personality (*Dietrich v Northampton* 1884). However, a British judge involved in the thalidomide settlements held that the mother had a right of action and was entitled to damages for 'grievous shock at seeing her child born deformed'.

The likelihood of a thalidomide claim succeeding also hinges as it does in occupational noise-induced hearing loss cases, on the general state of medical and scientific knowledge at the time in question. The time in question was between 1956 and 1958 when the drug was being developed. The likelihood of success of a claim would also hinge on whether or not the pharmaceutical company could be held to have discharged their duty of care. At the time in question, teratogenicity tests were not part of standard screening procedures for new drugs. Risks which ought reasonably to have been known must be interpreted in the light of medical knowledge and experience prevailing at the time (*Roe v Ministry of Health* 1954).

As Teff and Munroe (1976) pointed out, public reaction to the thalidomide tragedy created an atmosphere in which both the medical profession and the pharmaceutical industry were prepared to accept controls. The result was the Medicines Act 1968. This Act provided for the legal control of various aspects of the advertising, manufacture, labelling, distribution, and use of medicines.

The 1968 Act also provided for the establishment of the Medicines Commission Licences for new products. Certificates to subject these to clinical trials must be obtained from the Commission's Committee on Safety of Medicines. The Committee also monitors adverse reactions to drugs already in use. As a result the hazards of practolol, 4-(2-hydroxy-3-isopropylaminopropoxy) acetanilide, were detected and their frequency assessed. The drug, which is a β-adrenergic blocker, was used for the treatment of angina pectoris, cardiac dysrhythmias, and hypertension. It produces an oculomucocutaneous disorder (Felix, Ive and Dahl, 1974), which is sometimes associated with tinnitus and/or impairment of hearing (Wright, 1975). The hearing disorder may be conductive or sensorineural. Various audiometric patterns occur, including one that is similar to that of noise-induced hearing loss (McNab Jones *et al.*, 1977).

An Australian case mentioned by Lockhart (1980) is cited as an example of the duty of a doctor to use competent assistants. The plaintiff, who had been surfing, attended hospital complaining of 'a thundering noise in the ear'. After examination of the plaintiff's ear in the casualty department, a resident doctor asked a student nurse to provide the plaintiff with some glycerol and phenol ear drops. The nurse misunderstood and the plaintiff was given what was essentially pure phenol. As a result 'a part of his ear drum was destroyed, and his hearing was permanently impaired'. The judge said that:

'the real cause of the error was the giving of instructions in terms which were not as specific as they should have been to a pupil nurse who was not competent to take them. The doctor should not have given her instructions, or he should, before giving her the instructions, have satisfied himself that she was competent to take them and knew what was intended' (*Henson v The Board of Management of the Perth Hospital and Another* 1938).

Actions relating to the adverse effects of ototoxic drugs frequently allege medical negligence in respect of dosage. Even 10-fold errors in dosage have occurred. Fortunately an isolated single high dose of some drugs, e.g. gentamicin, is usually rapidly cleared from the body in individuals with normal renal function, so that no permanent damage occurs.

But antibiotics not usually considered ototoxic have been the basis of negligence actions where overdosage is concerned. One $2\frac{1}{2}$-year-old child who developed permanent hearing impairment after pneumococcal meningitis was awarded £102 000 damages because the judge decided that the deafness had been contributed to by an intrathecal injection by mistake of 300 000 units instead of 10 000 units of penicillin (Annual Report and Accounts, 1986). The judgment was reversed on appeal. The President of the appeal court said it was 'wholly improper for a judge to neglect the principle of doing justice between the parties and of fairness to both parties by going further and giving a decision in favour of one party upon a ground of his own devising . . .' In a unanimous decision in May 1988, the House of Lords dismissed an appeal by the plaintiff, finding that the deafness was caused by the meningitis and that there was no causal connection between the deafness and the overdose (*Kay v Ayrshire & Arran Health Board*, 1987).

A woman who had been admitted to hospital suffering from boils was prescribed a course of streptomy-cin. The day after the last injection, symptoms of damage to the vestibulocochlear nerve developed and the plaintiff was left with the loss of her sense of balance. The claim for negligence was based upon the fact that a total of 30 injections had been ordered by the house surgeon but 34 injections had been given. The judge considered that it was the last injection which had caused the damage. The defendants were therefore liable (*Smith v Brighton and Lewes Hospital Management Committee* 1958).

Another woman, after a holiday in Taiwan and in Australia, developed first, a middle ear infection and then a subacute bacterially negative endocarditis. She was prescribed a 19-day course of benzylpenicillin in conjunction with gentamicin. Almost immediately after the end of the treatment she had symptoms of vestibular labyrinthine damage. The plaintiff's case was that there had been no monitoring of gentamicin blood levels in the last week of the treatment. However, the judge accepted the views of the expert witnesses called on behalf of the defendants. They gave evidence to the effect that the defendants' doctors treated the patient in a manner which conformed to a proper standard of medical treatment. Consequently, the defendants' doctors could not be held to be negligent (*Vernon v Bloomsbury Health Authority* 1986). Having regard to the judgment in the previous case, one wonders whether another judge at another time in another place would have come to the same decision. Unfortunately, the plaintiff could not afford to go to the Court of Appeal.

AURAL SURGERY

In a claim for damages arising out of an unsuccessful stapedectomy, the plaintiff claimed that he had not carefully read the consent form and was under the impression that it signified authority only for a general anaesthetic and an examination. The plaintiff was employed as a claims manager by an insurance company where careful scrutiny of forms and their small print is all important. Not surprisingly, therefore, the judge completely rejected the plaintiff's evidence.

NOSE AND THROAT SURGERY

A family doctor, working in the otolaryngological department of a general hospital performed a nasal polypectomy on an elderly man. Later in the day the man became unconscious and was transferred to an intensive care unit. The condition deteriorated and he died on the seventh postoperative day. Post-mortem examination revealed a 5 mm by 20 mm defect in the cribriform plate with damage to the right anterior cerebral artery. The case was settled out of court (Annual Report and Accounts, 1983).

A young girl developed postoperative brain damage after tonsillectomy and adenoidectomy as a day case in South Africa (Annual Report and Accounts,

1990). The claim was settled for a 'considerable sum' since:

- The amount of anaesthetic agents administered were somewhat greater than normally given for a day case
- The anaesthetist had allowed the child to return to the ward too soon
- There were no records of the postoperative care.

NEW MEDICAL OR SURGICAL PROCEDURES

The institution of an experimental therapeutic procedure can be particularly hazardous – legally for the doctor as well as medically for the patient. The law governing the institution of new (experimental) treatments of patients was established over 200 years ago (*Slater v Baker and Stapleton* 1767). In that case, the plaintiff sued the then Head Surgeon (Mr Baker) of St Bartholomew's Hospital. Mr Baker had refractured the plaintiff's healed leg so that it could go through the 'operation of extension using a heavy steel invention with fearsome teeth'. On appeal, the Chief Baron held that:

> 'although the Defendants in general may be as skilful in their respective professions as any two gentlemen in England, yet the Court cannot help saying that, in this particular case, they have acted ignorantly and unskilfully contrary to the known rules and usage of surgeons'.

The law applicable to actions for negligence in respect of a new therapeutic procedure was systematized in a Scottish case (*Hunter v Hanley*) by Lord President Clyde in 1955. Three facts must be established. First, that there does exist a normal, usual practice. Second, that the defendant had not adopted the practice. Third, that the course of management adopted was one that no professional of ordinary skill would have taken if he/she had been acting with ordinary care.

A defence of *volenti non fit injuria* in medical cases of actions for negligence can only be made if consent – informed consent – has been freely given. Any medical or surgical procedure, including the simplest diagnostic examination which is conducted without the patient's consent (expressed or implied) is a trespass to person (see later). For minor diagnostic and therapeutic procedures, consent is usually implied. It is argued that, when a patient presents to a doctor seeking treatment, he/she has clearly implied consent to a physical examination and, at least, some minor therapeutic procedure. Sitting down in the examination chair or lying down on a couch may be taken as tacit consent. In other cases, written consent should be obtained. If an emergency operation is necessary to save a patient's life and consent cannot be obtained, the principle of 'agency of necessity' is invoked.

In some experimental therapeutic procedures, actions for negligence have hinged, not on whether or not an unusual course of action was adopted, but on whether or not informed consent had been really given. In a case where a facial paralysis developed after an operation involving the insertion of an electronic device in the para-aural tissues to treat deafness, the judge held that there was inadequate warning of all the risks involved.

However, in non-experimental therapeutic procedures, the courts will admit to the necessity for 'therapeutic misrepresentation'. In an action for negligence arising from damage to the recurrent laryngeal nerve during a thyroidectomy, the trial judge said:

> 'on the evening before the operation, the surgeon told the plaintiff that there was no risk to her voice, when he knew that there was some slight risk, but he did that for her own good because it was of vital importance that she would not worry. He told a lie, but he did it because in the circumstances it was justifiable. The law does not condemn the doctor when he only does what a wise doctor so placed would do' (*Hatcher v Black* 1954).

Similarly, a surgeon advising a patient on the risks of undergoing a major operation was under a duty to inform the patient according to the practice adopted by substantial body of medical practitioners competent in a particular field, but not under an absolute duty of full disclosure (*Hills v Potter and Another* 1983). The case concerned a woman who underwent an operation to relieve torticollis. Subsequent to the operation she was paralysed from the neck downwards.

PAEDIATRIC NEGLIGENCE CASES IN GENERAL

The approach to paediatric cases in respect of negligence claims is different to that in adult cases. Figures 7.1 and 7.2 illustrate the ambit of paediatric negligence cases.

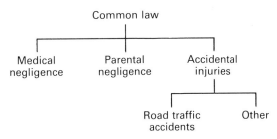

Figure 7.1 Common law aspects of paediatric practice

With adults there is usually an assumption of normal function of a structure, e.g. the ear, prior to the alleged damage. At least it is possible to take a

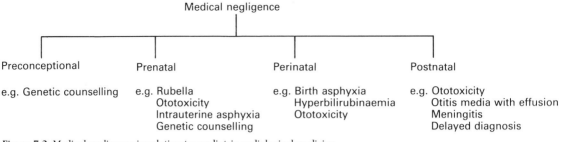

Figure 7.2 Medical negligence in relation to paediatric audiological medicine

history and review the previous medical records. With children there is rarely reliable proof of normal aural function prior to the alleged damage, particularly when the damage is said to have occurred very early in life, e.g. prior to the aquisition of language. Not only is the time of the injury difficult to ascertain in many cases in children, but even the existence or extent of any abnormality can be difficult to assess. In young children, there are problems in establishing frequency specific thresholds of hearing prior to the age of 3–4 years (5–6 years for masked thresholds). This means that, in practice, an auditory abnormality is often identified for the first time some months or even years after the alleged injury. This can lead to difficulties in demonstrating a definite causal link between the disability and the alleged negligent act. This difficulty is further compounded by the difficulty even in non-litigating cases in ascertaining a cause for a hearing loss in a child. Even today, following full investigation, the cause of a hearing problem remains 'unknown' in a substantial proportion of the children with congenital or early onset hearing loss. The likelihood of a hearing loss following the alleged negligent act (if proven) then has to be compared with the general risk of hearing loss within the appropriate population (Table 7.1). The occurrence of hearing loss as part of a genetic syndrome finds relevance in cases of alleged negligence in respect of genetic counselling. Causation is also clear in congenital rubella, where faulty management may have led to an absence of appropriate counselling and the birth of a handicapped child.

Although there can be no 'wrongful life' claims in UK jurisdictions (see below), a parent can sue for the extra care needed to bring up such a child.

Funding of litigation has been a greater hurdle for child plaintiffs than adult plaintiffs. However, children have recently been allowed to claim legal aid in their own right. Cases are now being pursued in the UK that might earlier have been dropped for lack of funding. This means that many more cases relate to alleged negligence many years previously. This in turn can pose problems in obtaining adequate records. A lack of appropriate investigations at the relevant times may be a significant contributory

Table 7.1 Incidence of hearing loss (moderate or greater) of varying causation in children

General population	1 : 1000
Genetic causation	1 : 2000
Autosomal dominant	1 : 2
Autosomal recessive	1 : 4
Rubella	
< 13 weeks	1 : 1.25
13–20 weeks	1 : 2
21–35 weeks	1 : 5
Cytomegalovirus	
Any loss	1 : 7
Significant loss	1 : 17
Preterm/low birthweight	
Any loss	1 : 10–1 : 20
Severe loss	1 : 50–1 : 100
Severe asphyxia	1 : 12–1 : 25
Hyperbilirubinaemia	1 : 12–1 : 25
Meningitis	
Pneumococcal	
Any loss	1 : 2.5
Severe loss	1 : 7
Meningococcal	1 : 8–1 : 10
Haemophilus influenzae	1 : 10–1 : 17
Congenital loss of unknown causation	1 : 3000

factor in failing to establish clear links between the alleged negligent act and the current disability.

The level of damages awarded in paediatric cases is frequently much greater than in adult cases, not only because of the much greater consequences of, for example, aural and neurological impairment on a child's development and future, but also because pre- and perinatal injuries, in particular, often lead to multiple handicaps.

There is a dominating psychological need of the parents of handicapped children to identify the cause of their child's problem. The expectation that one's own child should be normal is widespread, one might almost say, universal. Affected parents experience feelings of guilt, even though unwarranted. There is an understandable need to assign blame, preferably away from themselves.

WRONGFUL CONCEPTION, BIRTH AND LIFE

'Wrongful conception', 'wrongful birth' and 'wrongful life' claims are topics of considerable interest.

'Wrongful conception' claims, i.e. negligence leading to birth of a healthy child, relate to either negligent contraceptive advice or treatment, or a failed abortion carried out under section 1(1)(a) of the 1967 Abortion Act to prevent the birth of a child who would be healthy. As Kennedy and Grubb (1994) pointed out, sterilization is quite commonly practised outside the NHS. Thus actions under this heading usually arise in contract.

'Wrongful birth' claims are claims brought by the parents of a child who has been born disabled as a result of negligence before birth. Thus this action arises out of the same circumstances as a 'wrongful life' claim.

A 'wrongful life' claim is one brought by a disabled child complaining of negligent actions prior to its birth which result in its birth. As Stolker (1994) pointed out, the child-plaintiff argues: 'You, the doctor, ought to have given my mother the opportunity of having me aborted. My life is not worth living; I would prefer no life to the life I have'. Obviously, the child is not interested in the remedy of the cost of suicide, but in the wish to live out the rest of her life without cares, at least financially. Hepple and Matthews (1991) pointed out that the Pearson Commission agreed with the Law Commission that there should be no cause of action for damages for 'wrongful life'. In *McKay v Essex Area Health Authority* [1982] the Court of Appeal accepted that s. 1(2)b of the 1976 Congenital Disabilities (Civil Liability) Act achieved that goal.

PRECAUTIONS

The Medical Protection Society offers the following recommendations to doctors for a successful defence in negligence cases:

1 Keep clear and accurate records
2 Report early to the Society any incident which might give rise to a possible claim, setting out full details of the incident while it is fresh in the memory and giving the names and addresses of anyone else who witnessed the incident.
3 Seek the advice of the Society before replying to a letter of complaint which might lead to an allegation of negligence or breach of terms of service or an accusation of professional misconduct
4 Reply promptly to letters from the Society or its solicitors requesting comments or instructions
5 Keep the Society informed of any change of address, so that letters do not go astray. If a principal witness goes overseas without leaving a forward-ing address and cannot be traced when a trial is imminent, the defence is embarrassed (Annual Report and Accounts, 1978).

Occupational

As mentioned later, a number of occupational diseases may attract compensation under the tort system. The doctor with a particular interest in certain of these diseases may therefore find himself being asked to examine and prepare a report on one or other of them.

OCCUPATIONAL AND NOISE-INDUCED HEARING LOSS (ONIHL)

Occupational noise-induced hearing loss (Prescribed disease A10) is the negligence case *par excellence* with which the medical examiner is involved.

The *evidence presented by clinicians*, collectively (including at least 10 specialists with a particular interest and considerable experience in the matter) and individually (British Association of Otorhinolaryngologists – Head and Neck Surgeons and British Medical Association), to the Industrial Injuries Advisory Council enquiring as to whether or not there are degrees of hearing loss due to noise which satisfy the conditions for prescription under the National Insurance (Industrial Injuries) Act, was that, 'apart from a characteristic pattern on the audiogram showing typically the greatest loss at the 4000 Hz frequency, there are no signs or symptoms which are specific to noise-induced deafness' (Report by the Industrial Injuries Advisory Council, 1973). Or, as some of our Canadian colleagues have put it,

> 'There are no unique characteristics of NIHL which differentiate it absolutely from other causes of cochlear dysfunction, although traditionally it is believed that it produces a bilateral symmetrical sensorineural hearing loss, worse in the higher frequencies, typically with a notch at or about 4 kHz, with some recovery above this frequency' (Alberti, Symons and Hyde, 1979).

Although specialists, individually and collectively, have described the symptomatology of ONIHL, and the results of the special investigations (specifically, audiometry), as 'non-specific', clearly this is a relative term. Afflicted individuals do not present with a gnawing pain in the left knee, blurred vision or difficulty in walking. The complaint is one of hearing difficulty, which is of insidious onset and which, the individual may or may not claim, is progressive. Moreover, it is not an affliction of one particular ear, is not of sudden onset, and does not fluctuate.

The diagnostic difficulty was perhaps best summarized by the lecturer at the Medico-Legal Society on the 14th February 1974 who said:

> 'Diagnosis of noise deafness is difficult. There is

nothing positive about it; it is done by exclusion of other factors. There has to be an audiogram which fits the diagnosis to ensure that it is not obviously due to something else, that there is not deafness due to congenital causes, head injury, ear disease or a number of other things. But by the time you have severe noise exposure, particularly the kind in the occupational cover that we are considering, and the man has something approaching the right kind of deafness – that is to say, he has a correct history and there is nothing else competing for the diagnosis, then there is a very strong presumption of noise-induced hearing loss' (Coles, 1975).

Diagnosis has become even more difficult in the 20 years that have followed that appraisal. We are encountering much less the cases with 'severe noise exposure, particularly the kind in the occupational cover that we are considering'. Nowadays we are encountering alleged minimal damage (a better term than 'minimal loss' since many of the cases would not meet the criteria for having a hearing loss) cases. Indeed this is very puzzling since many of these cases would meet the Medical Research Council's Institute of Hearing Research's criteria for the diagnosis of obscure auditory dysfunction (OAD) (Saunders and Haggard, 1989). ONIHL is not a cause of OAD (Hinchcliffe, 1992). The distinction between OAD and ONIHL is important because the management of OAD (Saunders, Haggard and Field, 1989) is distinct from that of ONIHL (Harrowven, Greener and Stephens, 1987).

Since the clinical picture of occupational noise-induced hearing loss is non-specific, the *role of the medical examiner* is first to examine the audiogram of a claimant to see whether it is genuine or spurious, and, if genuine, whether or not:

- The hearing threshold levels (HTLs) are what one might expect to find for an individual of the same age, same gender and same socioeconomic group. Up-to-date data for the UK (Davis, 1992, 1995) are now available to make such a meaningful comparison. There is, of course, no reason why a given individual should be at *one particular point* on the distribution curve of such HTLs.
- The audiometric pattern is that of occupational noise-induced hearing loss or otherwise (e.g. as the Medical Research Council confirmed (Lutman and Spencer, 1991) notching at 4 kHz is a feature of individuals who have been exposed to hazardous occupational noise levels, notching at 6 kHz is a feature of those who have not been so exposed).

Should the level of hearing and/or the audiometric pattern point to the possibility of the hearing having been damaged by occupational noise then the medical examiner's clinical and audiometric expertise comes into play to confirm whether or not this is so. There is now a wealth of clinical and audiometric knowledge on hearing and its disorders. There is also a plethora of formulae and data sets with which to analyse a Claimant's audiograms to see whether or not the latter are compatible with the alleged negligent hazardous occupational noise exposure. For example, in the UK, there are those of the Health and Safety Executive (Robinson, 1988; Robinson, Lawton and Rice, 1994), the Medical Research Council (Lutman and Spencer, 1991; Lutman, Davis and Spencer, 1993) and the National Physical Laboratory (Robinson and Shipton, 1977).

The problem of using ISO 7029 (identical with data base A of ISO 1999: 1990) as the *yardstick* is that the values therein represent essentially the age-shifted thresholds of a 'highly screened' population re a selected group of well-motivated young British adults (Dadson, 1949; Dadson and King, 1952; Wheeler and Dickson, 1952), meticulously examined and selected[4] and the hearing measured under strictly controlled laboratory conditions with a precision unmatched in any other study[5]. The *modal* values were then used to define the reference zero for the first British standard which related to the hearing of young, healthy ears (BS 2497: 1954). Unfortunately, this first British standard was entitled 'The Normal Threshold of Hearing . . .' so it could easily be inferred that every threshold of hearing which did not conform to that, i.e practically everybody, was abnormal. Subsequent British Standards omitted the word 'normal'. None of the American or the International Standards for the calibration of audiometers included the word 'normal' in their titles. There are also internal inconsistencies (specifically regarding what exactly the thresholds are relative to) in ISO 7029 which are now being resolved by the appropriate committee.

The problem of using the data base B in ISO 1999 is that it refers to an *unscreened* population. Specifically, it is that derived from the USPHS National Health Survey 1960/62. The data would therefore have included not only ageing effects but also some nosoacusis as well as effects of occupational and non-occupational noise exposure.

There is, of course, no dichotomy between highly screened and unscreened (Robinson, Shipton and

---

[4] Test subjects were excluded not only if there was evidence for outer or middle ear disorder, i.e. they were *tympanologically* abnormal, but also if there was evidence for inner ear disorder, as indicated by inability to hear a forced whisper at a distance of 20 feet (6.1 m), i.e. they were *labyrinthologically* abnormal also. In fact only in these British studies could the subjects be considered to be truly clinically *otologically* normal.

[5] The scientists used a special audiometer which moved in 2 dB steps, in contrast to the manual audiometers which are almost invariably used by clinicians, epidemiologists and medical examiners (movement in 5 dB steps).

Hinchcliffe, 1979). What the medical examiner requires for medico-legal work is a data base (or formula) which is appropriate to the population that he is sampling, and to his method of examination and level of rejection. In general, medical examiners test a claimant's hearing with manual pure-tone audiometry. Although they pay lip service to the 'clinical examination', there is no evidence that, by and large, they do more than check the ears with an otoscope to ensure that there is no obstructing wax and that the eardrums are intact. There is seldom a clinical examination of the internal ear, despite the numerous clinical tests available (Hinchcliffe, 1987). In such cases, the ears should never be reported as being 'clinically otologically' normal. At the most, they can say that the ears are *tympanologically* (or perhaps, *pre-labyrinthologically* in lieu of tympanologically since this term would encompass the external ear also (bear in mind that the term 'labyrinth' is a synonym for the internal ear)) normal. But an examiner will not infrequently designate a Plaintiff's ears as being 'clinically normal' when the eardrums are scarred, the term 'clinically abnormal' being reserved for gross middle ear disease. Having regard to the structural change/functional deficit correlation for middle ear disease, the typical examiner's level of rejection could well correspond to that of the Medical Research Council's formula for ageing/noise effects (Lutman and Spencer, 1991), where, 'Only ears free from any material conductive hearing impairment (air-bone gap averaged over the frequencies 0.5, 1 and 2 kHz < 15 dB) were included in the analysis'.

There have also been allegations that the Medical Research Council data were contaminated with the effects of hazardous occupational noise exposure so that the ageing/noise formula may underestimate the effect of occupational noise. However, the Institute of Hearing Research used staff specially trained to administer an in-depth interview and compile a noise immission rating (NIR) according to a protocol devised by an audiological scientist and an audiological physician with extensive experience with this type of work. Had the MRC's non-noise exposed threshold data been contaminated with noise damage they would have shown a different ageing shift than that shown by the first MRC Survey and ISO 7029. This is not the case. The MRC's age/noise formula, ISO 7029 and the results for the first MRC Hearing Survey are entirely consistent with one another in respect of the ageing component (Hinchcliffe, 1993).

The statistical method used to analyse the National Study of Hearing data has also been criticized. But the method used, i.e. generalized linear interactive modelling (GLIM), is a highly respected method for the analysis of complex biological, medical and sociological data (McCullagh and Nelder, 1983; Healy, 1988; Aitkin *et al.*, 1989) and has the backing of the Economic and Social Research Council and the Royal Statistical Society. The technique was introduced in 1972 (Nelder and Wedderburn, 1972) and so was not available for either the first Medical Research Council Survey of Hearing or the Medical Research Council/National Physical Laboratory Survey of Hearing and Noise in Industry.

The final question is, 'Does the MRC formula work?' The formula fitted the data for the three Plaintiffs in a recent common law action (*Williams, Hunter and McPoland v Robinson Willey* 1992) for occupational noise-induced damage to the hearing. The formula was consistent with the gender, age, socioeconomic group, hearing threshold levels and noise exposure data for the group. Medical examiners using the formula should be explicit in their report about the reasons for the formula's validity; that they are endeavouring to compare like with like since this is what it is all about. The MRC has now published the results for the National Study of Hearing in tabular form (Davis, 1992). The latter are the best data to use initially by a medical examiner in the UK in order to see whether or not the hearing threshold levels are consistent with the Plaintiff's gender, age and socioeconomic group without having the need to postulate that some additional factor has been operating, whether occupational noise, head injury or ototoxic drugs. The examiner should, however, indicate the level of any drug, noise, or traumatic induced component in the measured hearing threshold levels. One cannot assume [6] that if this is at a *de minimis* (short for *de minimis non curat lex* (the law does not concern itself with trifles)) level medically, it will also be at a *de minimis* level so far as the lawyers are concerned.

HYPERBARISM

Hyperbarism (decompression sickness) (McCallum, 1987; Macmillan, 1988), which is prescribed occupational disease A3, sometimes presents with otoneurological (specifically, brain stem) symptoms.

NASAL CARCINOMA

Adenocarcinoma of the nasal cavity and sinuses which is a particular risk for woodworkers in the furniture industry (Acheson *et al.*, 1968; Hadfield, 1970) is prescribed occupational disease D6. Squamous cell carcinoma in nickel workers (Barton, 1977; Alderson, 1986) is prescribed occupational disease C22.

MUCOUS MEMBRANE DISEASE

Mucous membrane disease is now receiving increasing attention from personal injuries lawyers. This is prescribed occupational disease D4 (Inflammation or ulceration of the mucous membranes of the upper

---

[6] As one might if the hearing thresholds conformed essentially to what one might expect having regard to the gender, age and socioeconomic group for the general population, otherwise one might risk being accused of being dismissive.

respiratory passages or mouth produced by dust, liquid or vapour). Negligence claims are now being pursued outside the industrial arena. Are local authorities, landlords or central government negligent if individuals develop one or other upper respiratory tract inflammatory or allergic disease due to environmental pollution?

STRESS

The appearance of a report on stress in doctors (Caplan, 1994) 2 weeks prior to an announcement (News Item, 1994b) that a county council was liable to a social worker for job-induced stress should pave the way to claims by doctors.

Negligence in preparing reports for lawyers

Actions against doctors for negligence may arise not only in relation to their management of patients but also in their management of lawyers. A consultant in charge of a casualty department of a London teaching hospital was asked by solicitors to prepare a report on their client who had been examined there after a fall. Without looking at the X-rays or the radiologist's report, the consultant prepared a report on the basis of the casualty officer's notes which reported superficial bruising only. On this basis the solicitors settled the claim for a few hundred pounds. A medical reappraisal prompted by persistence of pain showed that the solicitor's client had sustained a fracture. This would have attracted greater damages. A claim against the consultant for negligence in the preparation of his report was settled out of court (Annual Report and Accounts, 1986).

Trespass

Trespass to the person is any direct, intentional interference with an individual without lawful justification. Trespass to person encompasses both assault (the threat or attempt to use force against another person) and battery (the actual application of force). Unlike the law of negligence, the plaintiff need not prove that the defendant was negligent or had a duty of care to him. He need only prove that the act was harmful to him. He must, however, establish an intention. Where the battery does not amount to a serious crime, a defence of *volenti* can be maintained, as in the law of negligence.

Thus the question of whether or not there has been a trespass to person in medical practice hinges on whether or not *consent* has been given.

Adults

It is not a battery to make a medical examination of a patient who consents to it. But a battery does take place if a person is examined against his or her own will (*Latter v Braddell and Sutcliffe* 1881). However, Lord Justice Winn's Committee on Personal Injuries

Litigation concluded (Cmnd 3691, 1968, para. 312) that it:

> 'entertained no doubt that every claimant for personal injuries must be bound to submit himself to medical examination of a reasonable character which is reasonably required, subject, of course, to proper safeguards and to the claimant's right to object to any particular doctor'.

Nevertheless, Mr Justice Lawson condemned the procedure whereby a person could be compelled to submit a medical examination by indirectly staying proceedings as not being conducive to respect for the administration of justice (*Baugh v Delta Water Fittings* 1971). Mr Justice Lawson pointed out that a requirement to submit to a medical examination could be justified only where Parliament had specifically authorized it. Compulsory medical examinations are required by various statutes, e.g. of school children under the Education Act 1944. Even then, the examination can only be done after the requisite notice has been served on the parent.

The Court of Appeal has held that:

> 'if a Defendant in a personal injuries case made a reasonable request for the Plaintiff to be medically examined by a doctor whom the Defendant had chosen then the Plaintiff should accede to such a request unless he had reasonable ground for objecting to that particular doctor and was prepared to disclose his reason to the Court' (*Starr v National Coal Board* 1977).

In giving judgment in this case, the judge said that:

> 'the Defendant is not to be regarded as making an unreasonable request merely because he wishes to have the Plaintiff examined by a doctor unacceptable to the Plaintiff ... it can only be the interests of justice that could require one or other of the parties to have to accept an infringement of a fundamental human right cherished by the common law. The Plaintiff can only be compelled, albeit indirectly, to an infringement of his personal liberty if justice requires it. Similarly, the Defendant can only be compelled to forego the Expert Witness of his choice if justice requires it.'

A particular forensic audiological case over 15 years ago concerned attempts to impose constraints on the nature and extent of the medical examination to be conducted by an expert witness. The plaintiff alleged that he was suffering from impaired hearing as a result of exposure to an occupational noise hazard. He had a partial hearing loss on one side, a total hearing loss on the other side, and he also suffered from tinnitus and recurrent episodes of vertigo. The defendant's expert witness proposed to conduct a medical examination that would have included tomography of the internal acoustic meatus, caloric tests and transtympanic electrocochleography. The patient refused to submit to the examinations and the defendant applied to stay the proceedings. The application first came before a registrar who was also furnished with an affidavit sworn by the expert witness for the plaintiff. The affidavit stated, among other things, that the radiological examination would 'involve considerable radiation dosage to the brain and eyes . . .'.

'My experience is that the caloric test is frightening to some patients, causes giddiness to most, nausea to many and vomiting to a few.'

Transtympanic electrocochleography 'is somewhat unpleasant and frightening for many patients. It is not without danger; very occasionally it has punctured the inner ear membranes and damaged the ear; or caused infection.'

The registrar accepted these statements and concluded that it would not be appropriate to grant a stay as asked by the defendant. However, he did say, in referring to the X-ray examination: 'it seems to me that this is an infringement of his (the Plaintiff's) liberty which, if it were the only test proposed, and subject to it not involving the Plaintiff in more than the safe dosage limit of X-rays, the Plaintiff could be obliged to accept.'

The defendant appealed and the case was heard by Mr Justice Webster on July 22 1980. The judge refused to choose between the conflicting evidence produced by two expert witnesses.

'For the reasons for the decisions I have already reached it has not been necessary for me to determine any factual conflict between the evidence of the Plaintiffs and the Defendants. All it is for me to determine is a reasonableness of the Defendants' request as reasonably seen by them and the reasonableness of the Plaintiff's objection as seen by him, and then to compare the weight of the reasonableness of the request with the reasonableness of the objection. For that purpose it does not seem to me (at any rate, in this case) to be necessary to involve such conflicts as there are between the various deponents, and I accordingly dismiss that application' (*Prescott v Bulldog Tools Limited* 1981).

In an interlocutory action, Mr Justice Mais ordered an action to be stayed unless the plaintiffs submitted to caloric testing and polytomography. Liberty to apply for electrocochleography was also provided (*Bird v Cadbury Schweppes Overseas Ltd* 1981, *Pearson v Cadbury Schweppes Overseas Ltd* 1981).

In a subsequent interlocutory action (*Holt v British Aerospace* 1983), the plaintiff's solicitors had endeav-oured to constrain the medical examination which two medical examiners instructed by the defendants had proposed to conduct. It was a case of alleged noise-induced hearing loss. The case was heard before the district registrar who ruled, 'so long as the Defendants choose a professional man with obviously good qualifications, then it seems to me that he should be given the right to make the decision (regarding which tests to do)'. The Registrar distinguished this case from the one of *Prescott v Bulldog Tools* 1981 on the grounds that in Holt 'nothing is really known about the Plaintiff's deafness'.

Investigations as to the cause of, for example, a hearing impairment are clearly of benefit to the individual, as well as helpful in medico-legal issues of causation. Adult plaintiffs are as likely as other members of the population to have conditions such as vestibular schwannomas, treponemal infections, hypothyroidism and other treatable causes of their problems. Investigations may be more important in paediatric cases to clarify the medical diagnosis, since there is frequently no useful pre-injury data as a basis for comparison. For example an 8-year-old child had a unilateral dead ear, allegedly following a road traffic accident at the age of 6 years. There was said to have been a normal sweep test on school audiometry at the age of 5 years. Because of the relatively mild trauma which was associated with the accident, one needed to rule out, for example, a developmental anomaly, such as a dilated vestibular aqueduct, which could have explained the total loss of hearing after a minimal injury. A CT scan of the petrous temporal bones showed that instead of a radiologically normal cochlea on the affected side, the child had only a primitive otocyst; the child could never have had any hearing in that ear.

It is within the discretion of a judge to admit the evidence derived from a specimen of blood that has been unlawfully obtained (*R v Trump* 1979).

Surgical operations which are technically successful may amount to a trespass if consent has not been obtained. 'A doctor who operates without consent of his patient is, save in cases of emergency or mental disability, guilty of the civil wrong of trespass to the person; he is also guilty of the criminal offence of assault,' (*Sidaway v Board of Governors of the Bethlem Royal Hospital* [1985] *per* Scarman LJ). In *Mohr v Williams* (1905) the plaintiff consented to an ear specialist operating on a diseased right ear. When the plaintiff was anaesthetized the defendant decided that the condition of the right ear did not warrant operation but the condition of the left ear warranted operation. He immediately operated on that left ear, and did so skillfully and successfully. An action for battery succeeded.

In an English case (*Chatterton v Gerson and Another* 1980), the plaintiff claimed that consent to a therapeutic procedure, which was associated with complications, was vitiated by a lack of explanation of what the procedure entailed and its implications. Consequently, the plaintiff had given no real consent. The procedure was therefore a trespass to her person. There was no claim that the doctor had been negligent. The judge said that the duty of a doctor was to explain what he intended to do, and its implications, in the way that a careful and responsible doctor in similar circumstances would have done. His Lordship was satisfied that the doctor had told the plaintiff what the procedure (an intrathecal phenol injection for pain relief) was all about. The plaintiff's consent was not vitiated by any lack of information. The judge also said that it would be very much against the interests of justice if actions which were really based on a failure by the doctor to perform his duty adequately to inform were pleaded in trespass. The action therefore failed.

Children

Following the House of Lords decision in *Gillick v West Norfolk and Wisbech AHA* [1985], a child below the age of 16 years may be given medical advice and treatment without parental agreement, provided that the child has achieved sufficient maturity to understand fully what is proposed. However, in *Re R* [1991] Lord Donaldson, in a Court of Appeal decision, said that the right to consent which a competent child had did not include the right to veto treatment. Treatment could proceed on the consent of the parents or those in *loco parentis*.

Informed consent

Strictly speaking this topic is not part of negligence since a particular medical or surgical procedure has not been done negligently so the patient cannot bring an action for negligence against the doctor. Nor can there be a question of trespass if consent has been obtained. What is in issue is whether or not the patient has been adequately apprised of the risks attendant on the procedure. They are then in a better position to make an informed decision on whether or not to undergo the procedure. It can thus be argued that, although the doctor has not been negligent in carrying out the procedure, he has been negligent in not apprising the patient of the attendant risks.

Faden, Beauchamp and King (1986) approached the matter of informed consent from a historical perspective, reasoning from a background of both moral philosophy and law. The ethical principle that each person has a right to self-determination finds its expression in law through the concept of consent.

'The aphorism "informed consent" has entered the language as being synonymous with valid consent. This is not so. It gives only a partial view. The requirement that consent be informed is only one, albeit a very important, ingredient of valid consent' (Kennedy and Grubb, 1994).

A London Queen's Counsel has said,

'I do not like the phrase "informed consent". It implies that one can only consent to a course of action if one understands its implications, which is neither true nor sense ... I as a patient would prefer doctors to think not so much of "consent" as something to be obtained before treating a patient as of "counselling", a process involving both parties ... it implies that there is one clear legal doctrine of "informed consent". This is not the case. In the United States of America there are many varieties of the doctrine ... and the law ... is still evolving in the United Kingdom' (Whitfield, 1990).

Other English legal perspectives have been presented by Brazier (1987), Hare (1988) and Eekelaar (1989). A broad assessment has been provided by Appelbaum, Lidz and Meisel (1987).

Otolaryngological perspectives of informed consent have been given by Bailey (1988) from the USA, and Smith (1988) from England. The medical experience is that patients who take legal action are more likely to be those who think that inadequate time has been spent in explaining either the proposed treatment or its alleged failure (Morrison, 1993). As Dawes and his colleagues (Dawes, O'Keefe and Adcock 1992; Dawes and Davison, 1994) pointed out, patients now want to be told more about their condition and its proposed treatment. These authors demonstrated that use of a structured interview changes patient's attitudes towards informed consent. Such a procedure made them feel that they had been more involved in the decision-making process, i.e. an approach which was consistent with Whitfield's concept. Such changes in patient attitude are consistent with changes world-wide, i.e. a change from paternalism to shared decision-making (Giesen, 1988b).

One should distinguish the 'informed consent' concept in the UK from that in North America. The concept emerged first in the USA in *Canterbury v Spence*. The judgment in this case should be compared with that in *Sidaway v Bethlem Royal Hospital Governors* in the UK and *Reibl v Hughes* in Canada. *Sidaway* uses the Bolam test (see above), i.e. 'the doctor knows best' approach. *Canterbury* and *Reibl* use a more objective approach, i.e. what the reasonable patient would want to know regarding the probability of various complications arising.

An Australian judge has said, extrajudicially, that 'the fact that a patient gave an informed consent will not prevent him from suing; a warm relationship with a competent and caring physician will' (Kirby, 1983).

To summarize, informed consent involves more

than the disclosure of risks. Informed consent also depends on the discussion and consideration of alternative courses of action (Lee, 1986). In practice most actions concerned with informed consent are brought in negligence on the basis that part of the duty of care is to secure valid consent to what is proposed. The plaintiff has to prove (a) the information that he was given was inadequate, and (b) he would not have consented had he been properly informed. The plaintiff often fails on (b).

Contract

The law of contract (Guest, 1994) is that branch of the law which determines whether a promise is binding and, if it is, what are the consequences of breaking it (Smith, 1992). The characteristic feature of a contractual obligation (contract) is that it is not imposed by law but is voluntarily undertaken by one or more parties to a contract. A promise which is not contained in a deed is binding only if given 'for consideration', i.e. the promisor must have asked for and have received something in return for his promise. A purely gratuitous promise cannot be enforced by the law unless it is made in a deed.

Actions for 'wrongful conception' (see above) usually arise in contract. This is because the cause for action has arisen from, for example, a sterilization operation done outside the NHS.

Public

Constitutional

Constitutional law may be defined as that body of the law which regulates the structure of the principal organs of government and their relationship to each other and to the citizen (Wade and Bradley, 1994). The UK is one of the three countries in the world which is said not to have a written constitution. It would be more correct to say that it does not have a *codified* constitution. Over a quarter of a century ago, Lord Bolingbroke wrote, 'By constitution we mean . . . that assemblage of laws, institutions and customs . . . that compose the general system according to which the community hath agreed to be governed' (Allen, Thompson and Walsh, 1994). As Harden and Lewis (1986) pointed out,

> '"the British constitution" and "the rule of law" are the two powerful concepts which embody the idea that British people live under a system of open, accountable, democratic government. In practice this is not the case.'

Éire has a constitution which, in its original form, came into operation on 6 December 1922 although constitutional links with the UK were not severed finally until the Republic of Ireland Act 1948 came into operation on 18 April 1949.

Administrative

A formal definition of administrative law is that it is that branch of public law concerned with the composition, procedures, powers, duties, rights and liabilities of the various organs of government which are engaged in administering public policies (Wade and Bradley, 1994). In the matter of the Health Service this is dealt with in Sweet and Maxwell's Encyclopedia of Health Services and Medical Law (Davies and Jacob, 1987).

Criminal

> 'Criminal law is a subject of great complexity which students find both fascinating and frustrating. The complexity is in large part caused by the uncertainty created by judges in courts at all levels, who fail to understand or adhere to fundamental principles. As a result the subject is both challenging and potentially frustrating' (Allen, 1994).

As Harpwood and Alldridge (1989) pointed out, the criminal law (Murphy, 1994) exists to protect various interests, e.g. those of life, limb and property. Unlike most jurisdictions, England and Wales has no criminal code, but from very early times Parliament has created criminal offences (Smith and Hogan, 1993). A crime may be defined as an act (or omission or a state of affairs) which contravenes the law and which may be followed by prosecution in criminal proceedings with the attendant consequences, following conviction, of punishment (Allen, 1994).

The majority of significant offences in criminal law require proof of either intention or recklessness. The result is that the prosecution can secure a conviction for an offence without going so far as proving that the defendant intended to commit it, recklessness being sufficient. Central to the concept of recklessness is the fact that the defendant is being punished for taking an unjustifiable risk. Clearly one needs to distinguish between those risks which have a social utility, and those which do not (Molan, 1994).

In the matter of unlawful homicide, the crimes include murder, manslaughter, causing death by reckless driving and infanticide.

In *R v Hancock and Shankland* [1986], the leading case on the *mens rea* for murder, the House of Lords reaffirmed that the prosecution has to establish that the defendant intended to kill or do grievous bodily harm, but Lord Scarman said that a defendant cannot be assumed to foresee a consequence simply because it was a natural result of his actions.

Murder has occurred in the NHS. In 1993, a children's nurse was convicted of killing four children and injuring nine more (Dyer, 1993). A disturbing feature about the case was that the relevant Consultant Paediatricians were subsequently penalized (Appleyard, 1994). This despite the fact that Nottingham's Professor of Paediatrics who was consulted in the police investigation considered in retrospect that, except in one case, there was no definite evidence to raise a question of foul play.

Manslaughter can be classified as either *voluntary* or *involuntary*. With the former offence the *malice aforethought* required for a murder charge can be established, but there are conditions (provocation, diminished responsibility, suicide pacts) which require a murder conviction to be reduced to one of manslaughter. With the latter offence, no *malice aforethought* can be established. Nevertheless, a degree of fault/negligence is required in excess of that required in a civil action for negligence. A *high degree of negligence* was considered to be the required level by Lord Atkin in *Andrews v DPP* 1937. The Court of Appeal has held that an unlawful act causing the death of another cannot, simply because it is an unlawful act, render a manslaughter verdict inevitable. For such a verdict, the unlawful act must be such that all sober and reasonable people must inevitably recognize it must subject the other person to the risk of some harm resulting therefrom, albeit not serious harm (*R v Church* 1966).

In the 1980s and the 1990s, *reckless manslaughter* and *killing by gross negligence* emerged as two distinct heads of involuntary manslaughter. The former emerged as a result of the House of Lords decision in *R v Seymour* 1983. The defendant had crushed the victim fatally in an attempt to move her car out of the way with his truck.

It is more correct to say that *killing by gross negligence* re-emerged since there appears to have been such a case at the beginning of the 19th century. In *R v Williamson* 1807, the defendant, an accoucheur, as a result of a misdiagnosis, inflicted on the patient such terrible injuries that she died. Lord Ellenborough said,

> 'To substantiate that charge [of manslaughter] the prisoner must have been guilty of criminal misconduct, arising either from the grossest ignorance or the most criminal inattention'.

As Smith and Hogan (1993) pointed out,

> 'the word "criminal" in any attempt to define a crime is perhaps not the most helpful, but it is plain that Lord Ellenborough meant to indicate to the jury a high degree of negligence'.

Seventy years ago, a family doctor who undertook a domiciliary delivery, removed part of the uterus in the belief that it was the placenta. The conviction was quashed on appeal because the Chief Justice held

that, in order to establish criminal liability the accused would have to have shown such disregard for the life and safety of others that it would amount to a crime against the State and conduct deserving punishment (*R v Bateman* 1925). Two years ago, in *R v Prentice and Others* 1993, the Court of Appeal quashed a manslaughter conviction arising out of the treatment of a 16-year-old leukaemic patient on the grounds that the appropriate test was not 'recklessness' but 'gross negligence'. In 'motor manslaughter' a 'recklessness' test was appropriate but it was inappropriate in manslaughter trials where death is caused by breach of duty of care. The Court redefined, in the context of breach of duty of care, what had come to be known as the *Bateman* test for gross negligence. Killing by gross negligence involves proof of the existence of the duty, breach of the duty causing death, and gross negligence. Gross negligence can take a number of forms: (1) indifference to an obvious risk of injury to health, (2) foreseeing the risk and deciding to run it; (3) appreciating the risk, intending to avoid it, but displaying a high degree of negligence in adopting avoidance techniques; and (4) failure to advert to a serious risk that goes beyond 'mere inadvertence' and which the defendant should have adverted to because of the duty he was under.

Compensation and punishment

Compensation

General

In one way or another, an individual may receive compensation for loss of property or money, or for personal injuries or disease which has occurred. Personal injuries or disease may attract compensation under the tort system (or under delict), under the criminal injuries compensation scheme, under social security legislation, under contract law or under personal insurance schemes (Atiyah, 1970).

Under the tort system, compensation (termed *damages*) is based upon what is termed *loss of amenity*. To some degree this can be equated with loss of quality of life. If the medical examiner has difficulty in assessing this so does the lawyer, including the judge.

Lord Devlin said, in respect of compensation for loss of amenity:

> 'Limbs and faculties cannot be turned into cash as property can. If it were not that the objective element has already been given a place in the assessment by authorities, I should question whether it should be there at all. I think that deprivation should be measured mainly if not wholly by the sense of loss' (*H. West and Son Ltd and another v Shephard* 1963).

But when the case came to the House of Lords, their Lordships thought otherwise. Compensation should be on a more 'objective' assessment of the loss, e.g. loss of a limb; deprivation of life's pleasures; inability to pursue hobbies (*H. West and Son Ltd and another v Shephard* 1964). In a prior case, Diplock L. J. had argued for basing assessments on loss of happiness (*Wise v Kaye* 1962).

A continually up-dated compendium, Kemp and Kemp (Kemp, 1994), based on court decisions, informs lawyers what a limb, a finger or a loss of hearing is worth.

A general approach to the problem of compensation has been presented by Stapleton (1986). She argued that there are serious distortions underlying the modern debate on compensation for personal injuries because it focuses on the victims of traumatic accidents. Alternative forms of support for the disabled are suggested.

A recent development in the USA considers loss of enjoyment and satisfaction of life using a statistico-economic approach which places a monetary value on the whole life of an individual above and beyond his value as a wage earner or productive member of society (Manning, 1993). Hedonic (Greek ηδονη, strict translation: 'sensual pleasure', but perhaps this is what it should be) damages are already recognized in about half the jurisdictions in the USA. This legal concept can be traced back through Bentham to Aristotle. The chief good for Aristotle was ευδαιμνια (eudaemonia, happiness or, more correctly, prosperity).

So should we not consider the enjoyment of life in terms that are expressed, say, by modern Greek poets? For example, by the 1963 Nobel Laureate George Seferis' ΔΙΑΛΕΙΜΜΑ (*Interlude of Joy*).

And should the yardstick for happiness be that of Catullus?

> *quis me uno uiuit felicior, aut magis hac re*
> *optandum in uita dicere quis poterit?*
> (*Who in the world lives happier than I? Or who can say*
> *What's more to be prayed for in life than this*).

'No-fault' compensation

Clinical service

As previously pointed out, the current system in the UK for compensating for the adverse consequences of medical intervention depends on an assessment of negligence. And so often this ends up in a litigation process under the tort system. But, as Simanowitz (1993a) pointed out, this is damaging to the parties and indeed to the practice of medicine. The tort system has been widely criticized as being expensive, inefficient and unfair. The 1990/1991 cost of compensating victims of medical accidents under this tort system was £52.3 m (Fenn, Hermans and Dingwall, 1994). Many proposals have been put forward not merely for altering the tort system but even for its total abolition (Maclean, 1989). Consequently, as Lewis (1988) said, it has often been said that a system of compensation for medical and other injuries that does not depend upon proof of fault, but merely requires proof of injury having been sustained as a result of treatment, would be of great benefit to the community. Such systems are in operation in Denmark, New Zealand and Sweden. Both the British Medical Association (1983) and the Royal College of Physicians of London (1990) are in favour of some form of 'no-fault' system.

Having discussed the present British position on product liability in respect of drugs, Diamond and Laurence (1985) concluded that a no-fault scheme for drug-induced injury in particular is desirable, workable and need not cost so much as to render serious discussion on implementation a waste of time. Such a scheme would obviate unsuccessful plaintiffs being encumbered by crippling financial costs. For example, the plaintiff in *Vernon v Bloomsbury Health Authority* 1986 will have to sell the family home to pay not only her own lawyer's bills but also the defendants' costs, which have been awarded against her. However, a 'no-fault' system introduced into the UK could well cost four times that of the current system (Fenn, Herman and Dingwall, 1994).

A 'development risks' defence operates under the Consumer Protection Act 1987. Thus a pharmaceutical company would not be liable under the Act if an adverse reaction was unknown before a drug was marketed.

The problem for the *future* regarding providing for the adverse consequences of medical intervention is one of forecasting accuracy at provider level. Too high a guess and current patient care will suffer; too low a guess and future patient care will suffer (Fenn, Herman and Dingwall, 1994).

Simanowitz (1993b) has pointed out that accountability has proved to be of far greater importance to victims of medical accidents than compensation. From the victim's point of view, accountability means that something is done to ensure that those responsible are required to give an account of themselves, that an explanation is given to the victim or the family, and that steps are taken to try to avoid a similar accident happening again. Indeed the majority of patients who approach AVMA (Action for Victims of Medical Accidents) come with distress, bewilderment and anger generated by a feeling of helplessness.

AVMA/ACHCEW (Association of Community Health Councils in England and Wales) have proposed the formation of a statutory body, A Health Standards Inspectorate, i.e. similar to the Danish system. The main thrust of the inspectorate would be to improve and maintain standards in health care.

This Inspectorate would be the sole point of entry for any complaint from a patient of whatever nature. A major advantage of this proposal is that it would not require the prior demolition of the whole system (Simanowitz, 1993a).

Clinical research

Bodies such as the Royal College of Physicians have influenced local research ethics committees towards 'no-fault' compensation when research subjects have suffered untoward effects. Harvey and Chadwick (1992) maintain that such an approach does not embrace the concept of the autonomy of the individual. They therefore consider it more desirable to inform research subjects what compensation arrangements are available rather than for ethics committees to make no-fault compensation a general requirement before ethical approval is given.

Punishment

As Allen (1994) pointed out, the idea which has gained ascendancy in recent years is that of 'just deserts', based upon the philosophical concepts of Kant. A person who commits a crime has gained an unfair advantage over other members of society. Punishment cancels out the advantage, particularly when the court orders confiscation, restitution or compensation.

Justice

The Athenians were preoccupied with the problem of *justice* (δικη), as shown in the poems of Hesiod and of Solon and the theoretical formulations of Aristotle. Diverging from his mentor, Bentham, John Stuart Mill (1863) linked justice with general utility.

The judicial oath does not enjoin a judge simply to do justice, nor simply to apply law; it requires him to do justice according to law. In most cases the judge has an instinctive sense of justice born of vast knowledge and experience of the law. Even with precedent and statute, there is room for much judicial discretion (Dias, 1970). MacGormick and Birks (1986) have explored the patterns of thought peculiar to lawyers and the forces which influence the concepts, methods and preoccupation's of the legal mind.

Although lawyers chide doctors and scientists on their inconsistency, there is considerable interjudicial variability. This is manifest in judgments delivered by the Court of Appeal, the House of Lords or the Privy Council; so often there is a dissenting judgment. As Pope would have it in *An Essay on Criticism* (line 9):

'Tis with our Judgments as our Watches, none
Go just alike, yet each believes his own.

As Cohen (1977) pointed out, the advancement of truth in the long run is not necessarily the same as the dispensation of justice in each individual case.

There are reports that judges are becoming ruder, undoubtedly reflecting that they also are not immune from the stresses which are afflicting other professionals. On one occasion, after a judge had been offensive to a doctor in court, the doctor's professional insurance society made a strongly worded formal protest to the Lord Chancellor. In the fullness of time, the Society received a reply signed personally by the Lord Chancellor. *Inter alia*, the Lord Chancellor said, 'Having investigated the facts now very fully, I am satisfied that (the doctor) was treated without the courtesy that is called for in judicial proceedings and the Judge has asked me to convey his personal apologies, to which I add my own'.

Demands for justice arise from the existence of *injustice*. Alexandre Dumas' *Le Comte de Monte–Cristo* was published exactly 150 years ago. The novel, in which the hero, Edmond Dantès, dedicated his life for vengeance, epitomized personal injustice. The Dreyfus affair (Zola, 1898; Bredin, 1983) and the Seznec affair (Langlois, 1992) have brought home to the French not only the realities of personal injustice, but its persistence over the past 100 years. The recent saga of the Birmingham Six, the Guildford Four, the Maguire Seven and the Tottenham Three have brought home to the British that personal injustice is not confined to foreign countries with different legal systems. As Walker and Starmer (1993) pointed out, each of these events has highlighted serious failures in the English *criminal justice* system which have contributed to miscarriages of justice. Among the many disturbing features are the obtaining of confessions by unacceptable means; the fabrication of evidence; the failure to disclose evidence adverse to the prosecution and the inadequacy of appeal and reference-back systems. Failures in the English *civil justice* system have been relatively unexplored, or, should we say, unpublicized. They undoubtedly exist. There are similar parallels. And is it so much different from that in other parts of the world where deficiencies in the legal system are portrayed in, e.g. Tawfik Al–Hakim's (1989) savage satirical *Maze of Justice*.

Ethical aspects
In general

Having equated ethics with moral philosophy Gillon (1986) immediately sought to distinguish philosophical *medical ethics* from what might be called traditional medical ethics, that is the long and honourable tradition in which doctors have established and promulgated among themselves rules and codes of behaviour considered to be morally binding. The purpose of philosophical medical ethics is to make medico-moral decision-making a more thoughtful and intellectually rigorous exercise. Its ultimate purpose is to construct and defend comprehensive and moral theory for medical practice based on universal principles applying to all and capable of justifying particular lines of conduct in individual cases. In a series of articles he then proceeded to conduct such an analysis. A prominent issue concerns: 'What are rights?' The answer to this question immediately elicits the fact that there are two major types of ethical theory. One type is based on rights and duties (so-called 'deontological theories of ethics', from the Greek word for duty; much religious moral theory is deontological). The other is based on the consequences of actions (consequentialist theories of, for example utilitarianism).

Professional medical ethics

As Dunstan (1981) pointed out, the ethics of medicine are as old as the profession itself. In Western civilization history goes back to the Hippocratic tradition. The foundations for modern medical ethical standards in Britain are derived from the code of Professional Conduct produced by Thomas Percival in Manchester over 200 years ago (1789). His proposals, *Medical Ethics or a Code of Institutes and Precepts adapted to the Professional Conduct of Physicians and Surgeons* were published in 1803 (British Medical Association, 1984). The British Medical Association's Handbook pointed out that, while other European countries' ethical systems have been codified and incorporated in national civil and criminal law, the UK has proceeded along a different path. The General Medical Council, whose powers derive from the Medical Acts and which is responsible to the Privy Council, has enforced professional standards on the basis of guidance rather than through a codified system. The General Medical Council's (1991) booklet *Professional Conduct and Discipline: Fitness to Practice*, should be consulted regarding the broad aspects of etiquette, professional discipline and the law.

Doctor–patient relationship

Dunstan (1986) argued that the basis of the doctor–patient relationship is trust and confidence. The patient had to be given sufficient information so that consent to treatment could be grounded in trust. The patient did not need to understand everything that the doctor said to him, but he did have to trust him. But how does this mesh with *medical audit* (Frostick, Redford and Wallace, 1995), the collection and use of information allegedly for effective resource management and improved patient care? How does one measure and quantify 'trust' or 'confidence'?

Research on human subjects

Pappworth (1978) pointed out that there are basically two ethical problems in respect of medical research. First, is there valid consent? And in this context, consent to an action which is basically wrong cannot change it into a rightful one. Second, do the ends justify the means? To these two basic problems, one should add a third problem: Is the confidentiality of the required data safeguarded?

As pointed out by the Council for International Organisations of Medical Sciences (1982), the generalized application of the experimental scientific method by medical research is a product of the present century. Consideration is required in developed and developing countries alike as to whether prevailing legal provisions and administrative arrangements ensure that the rights and welfare of subjects involved in research are adequately considered and protected in conformity with the ethical principles prescribed in the Declaration of Helsinki by the Eighteenth World Medical Assembly 1964, as revised by the Twenty-ninth World Medical Assembly, Tokyo, 1975.

In Britain, the concept of *local ethical research committees* developed with a recommendation of the Royal College of Physicians in the late 1960s that clinical research investigations should be subject to ethical review. Subsequently, the Royal College of Physicians (1984) produced *Guidelines on the Practice of Ethics Committees on Medical Research*. In 1991, the Department of Health produced its own guidelines, *Local research ethics committees*. These guidelines attempt to provide detailed guidance on how the principles and the declarations of the World Medical Assembly should be applied to individual research proposals. The College of Physicians' guidelines make it clear that research ethical committees should concern themselves, not only with experimental research but also with non-experimental research, e.g. use of case records. They also indicate that there should be a mandatory review of *all* research projects affecting human subjects, including fetal material and the recently dead, in an institution. In the case of adverse decisions, the Committee is empowered, *at the request of an investigator*, to appoint referees by mutual agreement or, in the case of special difficulty, to ask the appropriate Royal College to appoint referees, who will consider the views of both the investigator and the ethics committee in the presence of both. Local ethical research committees have no direct sanctions but, in the event of their discovering that their advice is not heeded or that clinical investigations are being conducted without reference to them, then they should report the facts to the body that set them up. The Department of Health Guidelines have been critically reviewed by Moodie and Marshall (1992).

Julia Neuberger's (1992) review of local ethical research committees emphasized the need to monitor research projects. She emphasized spot checks on on-going research to ensure that it is being conducted in accordance with whatever was approved by the ethical committee.

The routine treatment of an individual patient, using a procedure which has not yet been validated by an experimental comparative study, and which is not part of a research project, is in effect an uncontrolled experiment of a sample size of one and where the study is frequently not replicated; i.e. the antithesis of a good experimental comparative study.

The Scientific Affairs Board of the British Psychological Society (1978) enumerated 12 ethical principles which should govern research on human subjects.

Particular groups, for example children (Nicholson, 1986) and healthy volunteers (Royal College of Physicians, 1986) have been the subject of special studies. The first study stemmed from the fact that, in the UK, four sets of guidelines for medical research in children had been produced. The four proposals were in conflict. Some children's rights activists argue that children should never be used for research. But, how can the health of children be improved without the possibility of doing research on children? A Working Group of the Institute of Medical Ethics has sought to resolve these conflicts. Among other things, the Report of the Royal College of Physicians recommended that there should be no financial inducement or any coercion that might persuade a volunteer to take part in a study against his better judgment.

The French approach to setting up ethical standards for experimental comparative studies is well set out by Arpaillange, Dion and Mathé (1985).

In the case of an investigator wishing to experiment on himself, particularly when he is conducting research in his own field of expertise, it could not be argued that there was no informed consent nor could there ever be a charge of breach of confidence. However, it could be argued that the subject was in a dependent relationship with the investigator. But perhaps the investigator could take refuge in the right to privacy as defined by a judge (Cooley) towards the end of the last century of the right to be let alone. Or take refuge in the right to decide what is to be done with one's body.

Confidentiality

Confidentiality and the use of medical records for research has been discussed by Knox (1986). Hippocrates was the first to set out the confidential basis of medical practice. However, he said nothing about the conflict between the needs for confidentiality and the communication of data for research. The EC considered the matter (Commission of the European Communities, 1984). Two principal points emerged. First, modern reformulations of the Hippocratic Oath, such as the Declaration of Geneva, assert a joint concern for the good of man as an individual and for the corporate benefit of mankind. In a competitive world, the two principles sometimes come into conflict. Second, appeals to broader principles, e.g. contractual agreements, property rights and the right to privacy, do not solve the dilemma. The rules of personal contract demand secrecy, but the integrity of the society that sanctions and supports such contracts, demands a broader view. The EC study concluded that there was no formal solution to the dilemma. A positive statement of all legitimate uses, including for research, to which medical records might be put, was preferred. It was considered that any strictly enforced legislation on confidentiality would almost always be harmful in one way or another. Consequently, they recommended a code of practice. This would provide a set of interpretable rules which could be applied in day-to-day decisions.

Confidentiality can be considered as one aspect of the right to privacy. Specifically, it can be considered the right to the privacy of personal information. Over 20 years ago, the Younger Committee on Privacy concluded that the main concern about what is termed 'invasions of privacy' involves the treatment of personal information. The Committee considered that, in medicine, the question of privacy was a matter for ethics and not for legislation. As a result of information which the Medical Research Council submitted to the Younger Committee, the MRC published a Code of Practice on 'Responsibility in the Use of Medical Information for Research'. The Council accepted that medical information about identified patients could be made available for medical research without the patients' explicit consent. However, all medical information that could be related to an identified individual should be treated as confidential and should be communicated only to medical research workers who are engaged in investigations in the interests of the health of the community. Even then, the MRC expressed great fears that confidentiality would break down with the increasing use of computers. At the same time, as a result of the active discussion in Parliament on privacy, the British Psychological Society's Standing Committee on test Standards produced an interim report a quarter of a century ago which was then subsequently amended in respect of the section on 'Relevant Information'. The amended section read:

> 'How much personal information should be sought from an individual, even by those who have good reason for doing so, is a difficult question which faces psychologists. Almost any information will, in certain circumstances, be relevant but the use of some information is controlled by law. The decisions of psychologists would be ex-

pected not to contravene the Universal Declaration of Human Rights adopted by the United Nations General Assembly 1948.'

The desire to protect computerized data resulted in the Data Protection Act 1984. As Elbra (1986) pointed out, the eight principles, which are the keystone of the legislation, state that data must be:

1 Obtained fairly and lawfully
2 Held only for registered lawful purposes
3 Not used or disclosed except as registered
4 Adequate, relevant and not excessive
5 Accurate and, where necessary, up to date
6 Not kept longer than necessary
7 Available to the individual concerned
8 Kept secure.

The Act was primarily introduced to enable the UK to confirm with an EC directive and thus allow British companies to continue to transfer computerized information across national boundaries. Some lobbyists saw it as a means for the introduction of 'freedom of information' but they have been disappointed by the narrowness of the Act (Anon, 1986).

As Black (1984) pointed out, there is something of an anomaly in more concern being focused on protection of data held in mechanically processed systems than on the much larger amount of information held in manual records.

Baldry *et al.* (1986) and Bird and Walji (1986) argued cogently for giving patients access to their own medical records. The Data Protection Act 1984 gave patients the right to access electronically stored health records. The Access to Health Records Act 1990 complemented this right for manually stored records.

Reflections
Towards the attobel

In the field of hearing, litigation has now entered the millibel domain (but whether either medical examiners or lawyers are aware of this is uncertain). But this can be considered merely as an application of the philosophy that 'every decibel counts'. And if 'every decibel', why not 'every attobel (10^{-18} bels)' and why not every frequency? If negligent damage to even a single hair of an individual may attract damages, why not a single hair on a single hair cell? The answers to these questions will depend on where the courts will draw the line at *de minimis* (see above). Nevertheless, medical examiners will need to be aware of the relevance and importance of such clinical conditions as the King-Kopetzky syndrome (Hinchcliffe, 1992) and labelling (Haynes *et al.*, 1978) and bear in mind the experience of clinicians, that those who have elevated hearing threshold levels for fre-

quencies of around 6 kHz and above do not report problems in auditory communication (Dobie, 1993).

Beyond Homo sapiens

A recent series of cases in the English courts has shown that the law can no longer be accused of being speciest. One man was charged with leaving a South American sucking loach at 'home alone', although a veterinarian had said that the fish appeared to be in good condition. Another man who left his pet zebra tarantula spider without food and water for at least 9 days was fined £50 (News Item, 1993b). (But zoologists say that these animals feed only monthly.) A third man had neglected his pet stick insects. But all this is consistent not only with age-old religious beliefs but with current developments in molecular biology. In the third century BC, Buddhists set up hospitals in India both for man and for other animals; to Buddhists all animals are sacrosanct. At the molecular level there is so little difference between the various species. Body shape is the one thing which we see as distinguishing us from other animals and other animals from one another. Yet nearly identical molecular mechanisms define body shape in all animals. An interrelated group of genes, the *HOM* genes in invertebrates and the *Hox* genes in vertebrates govern similar aspects of body design. One can use some human and mouse *Hox* genes to guide development of the *Drosophila* (fruit fly) embryo (Zhao, Lazzarini and Pick, 1993; McGinnis and Kuziora, 1994). Moreover, according to Margulis' (1981) theory, we, like all eukaryotic cellular organisms, are biologically eclectic. Our mitochondria are the lineal descendants, like the cells which contain them, of bacteria which were incorporated into these cells perhaps two billion years ago.

Codification

The opinion of perhaps the greatest comparative jurists of this century regarding the English legal system is of interest:

> *'Les juristes du continent européen étaient élevés dans le culte de la loi et pénétrés d'admiration pour les codes. Il leur paraissait étrange, et presque inconvenant, de voir un pays hautement civilisé, le plus grand pays commerçant du monde, rejeter la formule de la codification et demeurer attaché à une formule à leurs yeux périmée, voyant dans la jurisprudence la source fondamentale du droit.* (European continental jurists have been educated to the superiority of legislation and are filled with admiration for codes. For them it was strange, almost unseemly, that a highly civilized country and the greatest trading

nation on earth should reject codification and remain attached to the philosophy, outdated in their eyes, that decided cases are the fundamental source of law.) (David et Jauffret-Spinosi, 1992).

It is difficult to reconcile the resistance to codification of the law in England, when one considers what has actually been possible. In 1932, the British codified the law of torts for use in the then Crown Colony of Cyprus. This was then copied as the Civil Wrongs Ordinance of 1944 for use in what was then Palestine (Tedeschi, 1969). Following the Declaration of Independence of 14 May 1948, this codified law of torts was incorporated into Israeli law. A Hebrew version of the law was, however, published according to the Law and Administration Ordinance of 19 May 1948. Similarly, the Israeli Penal Code of 1977 is the substantially unchanged Criminal Code Ordinance of 1936. This in turn had originated in an Australian (Queensland Criminal Code of 1899) codification of what was essentially the English criminal law (Abrams, 1972). However, as Bin-Nun (1992) pointed out, the binding force of the English *stare decisis* was never unreservedly recognized by Israeli judges. The official link with English law was finally abolished by the Law and Administration (Amendment No. 14) Ordinance 1972. Nevertheless, 'quotations from English sources are still part of well-founded court decisions'. Moreover, according to the Basic Law: Judicature, a given 'court is bound by a higher court's decisions, whereas the Supreme Court is free in its considerations and not bound even by its own decisions'.

Towards an inquisitorial system

The adversarial system is not well suited to a scientific analysis of specialized evidence (Donnelly, 1994). But what makes the common law/adversarial system unacceptable to doctors and scientists is its divisive nature. One can, for example, contrast the divisive nature of current tort litigation with the cohesive effect of gathering medical and scientific evidence in the 1960s relative to the proposed legislation to designate noise-induced hearing loss as a prescribed occupational disease.

More radical legal changes

Not only the English legal system is under attack. The legal systems of advanced capitalist states in general are subject to criticism from both right and left shades of political opinion. The former see these systems as the domain in which legitimate public power is improperly challenged by both individuals and groups and communal values are destroyed. The latter reject the abstraction, conservatism and formal-ism of these systems. In *The End of Law?*, O'Hagan (1984) addressed these issues. He proposed a politico-legal model which combines John Stuart Mill's (1863) libertarian pluralism with Karl Marx' egalitarianism but rejects the Marxist myth of the withering away of the state and of the law. For Mill the most important condition for attaining a free society is that there should be a minimum of interference by the state in the citizen's organization of his or her own life. Mill advocated diversity of life styles, of different experiments in living. But O'Hagan goes beyond Mill to argue that, 'a system of rights can be understood and defended as a solution to the problem posed by a particular stage of social evolution, which is to find a form of autonomous, non-manipulated social intercourse for citizens of a technologically advanced state'.

Towards ADR

But, in the area which most concerns the doctor, i.e. cases involving negligence in health care services or in industry, one would forsee in the more immediate future an escape from the traditional judicial system of dispute resolution (tort system). As Lord Mustill (1995) has pointed out, dispute resolution needs to be performed harmoniously and humanely. ADR offers a better and faster method than the present tort system for medical negligence cases (Chapman, 1994). The Chartered Institute of Arbitrators' (1993) scheme involves, initially, mediation, which is non-adversarial. If this is unsuccessful then the dispute would proceed to arbitration with at least one medically qualified arbitrator. A technically qualified arbitrator removes much of the need for expert evidence, but, where it is needed, he is able to guard against misinterpretations.

Conclusions

As pointed out at the beginning of this chapter, ethics and the law are influenced by accepted standards of right conduct. Ethics and the law will reflect changes in these standards.

As a Past President of the Royal College of Physicians has indicated, the three principal medico-legal problems confronting doctors now, and increasingly in the future, are:

- The definition of the legal boundaries within which clinicians are able to practise their profession; acceptance that medical authoritarianism is being replaced increasingly by a greater demand by patients to be involved in the decision-making process
- The legal aspects of regulating resources within a health service; but *triage* has long been recognized as a feature of military medicine

- Medical complaints; the questions of professional accountability, liability and litigation (Hoffenberg, 1989).

The 'new' discipline of socio-legal studies hopes to provide the solution to these problems by beginning from, and returning to, the practical circumstances of doctors and other health care workers (Dingwall, 1989). It is perhaps only the name 'socio-legal' that is new since one can trace a sociological interpretation of the law back through the Harvard jurist Roscoe Pound (1943/4), who saw the aim of modern law as being one of 'social engineering', to Bentham and Ihering. Following an intensive study of Roman law (published as *Der Geist des römischen Rechts* (The Spirit of Roman Law)), Ihering (1873) incorporated Bentham's utilitarianism concepts into a major work, *Der Zweck im Recht* (The Law as a means to an End). His thesis, now generally accepted (but common sense), is that the law needs to reconcile individual and community interests. Consequently Ihering has been described as the 'father of modern sociological jurisprudence'.

In the future, many cases which are currently dealt with under the tort system will be settled under one or other scheme of ADR, particularly medical negligence cases.

References

ABRAMS, N. (1972) Interpreting the Criminal Code Ordinance 1936 – the untapped well. *Israel Law Review*, **7**, 29–32

ACHESON, E. D., COWDELL, R. H., HADFIELD, E. and MACBETH, R. G. (1968) Nasal cancer in woodworkers in the furniture industry. *British Medical Journal*, **2**, 587–591

AITKIN, M., ANDERSON, D., FRANCIS, B. and HINDE, J. (1989) *Statistical Modelling in GLIM*. Oxford: Oxford University Press

ALBERTI, P. W., SYMONS, F. and HYDE, M. L. (1979) Occupational hearing loss: the significance of asymmetrical hearing thresholds. *Acta Otolaryngologica*, **87**, 255–263

ALDERSON, M. R. (1986) *Occupational Cancer*. London: Butterworths

AL-HAKIM, T. (1989) *Maze of Justice*. Translated by Abba Eban. London: Saqi

ALLEN, M. J. (1994) *Textbook on Criminal Law*. London: Blackstone

ALLEN, M. J., THOMPSON, B. and WALSH, B. (1994) *Cases and Materials on Constitutional and Administrative Law*. London: Blackstone

ALLOTT, A. (1980) *The Limits of Law*. London: Butterworths

ANNUAL REPORT AND ACCOUNTS (1978) London: The Medical Protection Society Limited

ANNUAL REPORT AND ACCOUNTS (1979) London: The Medical Protection Society Limited

ANNUAL REPORT AND ACCOUNTS (1983) London: The Medical Protection Society Limited. p. 25

ANNUAL REPORT AND ACCOUNTS (1986) London: The Medical Protection Society Limited. pp. 41, 44

ANNUAL REPORT AND ACCOUNTS (1987) London: The Medical Protection Society Limited. p. 32

ANNUAL REPORT AND ACCOUNTS (1990) London: The Medical Protection Society Limited. p. 29

ANON (1986) Spotlight on the data protection act. *British Medical Association News Review*, **12**, 36

APPELBAUM, P. S., LIDZ, C. W. and MEISEL, A. (1987) *Informed Consent: Legal Theory and Clinical Practice*. Oxford: OUP

APPLEYARD, W. J. (1994) Murder in the NHS. *British Medical Journal*, **308**, 287–288

ARPAILLANGE, P., DION, S. and MATHÉ, G. (1985) Proposal for ethical standards in therapeutic trials. *British Medical Journal*, **291**, 887–889

ATIYAH, P. S. (1970) *Accidents, Compensation and the Law*. London: Weidenfeld and Nicolson.

AXELSSON, A., JERSON, T., LINDBERG, U. and LINDGREN, F. (1981) Early noise-induced hearing loss in teenage boys. *Scandinavian Audiology*, **10**, 91–96

BAILEY, B. J. (1988) What is informed consent? In: *Dilemmas in Otorhinolaryngology*, edited by D. F. N. Harrison. London: Churchill Livingstone. pp. 1–14

BAINBRIDGE, D. I. (1994) *Intellectual Property* 2nd edn. London: Pitman

BALDRY, M., CHEELE, C., FISHER, B., GILLITT, M. and HEWITT, B. (1986) Giving patients their own records in general practice: experience of patients and staff. *British Medical Journal*, **292**, 596

BARKER, D. J. P. (1990) The fetal and infant origins of adult disease. *British Medical Journal*, **301**, 1111

BARTLETT, A. (1994a) The preparation of experts' reports. *Arbitration*, **60**, 94

BARTLETT, A. (1994b) The preparation of experts' reports. *Arbitration*, **60**, 222

BARTON, R. T. (1977) Nickel carcinogenesis of the respiratory tract. *Journal of Otolaryngology*, **6**, 412–422

BELL, E. T. (1945) *The Development of Mathematics*. New York: McGraw-Hill. p. 587

BENTHAM, J. (1789) *Introduction to the Principles of Morals and Legislation*. London: Payne

BENTHAM, J. (1825) *Treatise on Judicial Evidence*. London: Payne. p. 41

BIN-NUN, A. (1992) *The Law of the State of Israel*. Jerusalem: Rubin Mass

BIRD, A. P. and WALJI, M. T. I. (1986) Our patients have access to their medical records. *British Medical Journal*, **292**, 595

BLACK, D. (1984) Iconoclastic ethics. *Journal of Medical Ethics*, **10**, 179–182

BLACK, J. and BRIDGE, J. (1994) *A Practical Approach to Family Law*. London: Blackstone

BLACK, R. (ed) (1993) *Laws of Scotland: Stair Memorial Encyclopaedia*. London: Butterworths

BLACKSTONE'S CRIMINAL PRACTICE. (1994) London: Blackstone

BONDE, J. P. E. (1993) The risk of male subfecundity attributable to welding of metals: studies of semen quality, infertility, adverse pregnancy outcome and childhood malignancy. *International Journal of Andrology*, **16**, 1–29

BRAHAMS, D. (1993) Doctors and manslaughter. *Lancet*, i, 1404

BRAZIER, M. (1987) *Medicine, Patients and the Law*. London: Penguin

BREDIN, J.-D. (1983) *L'Affaire*. Paris: Julliard

BRENNAN, D. (1995) The Bolam test and medical negligence – a valedictory assessment for the twentieth century. *Medico-Legal Journal*. (in press)

BRIDGE, LORD (1990) Foreword. In: *Medical Negligence*, edited by M. Powers and N. Harris. London: Butterworths

BRIDGE, J., BRIDGE, S. and LUKE, S. (1989) *The Children Act 1989*. London: Blackstone

BRITISH MEDICAL ASSOCIATION (1983) *Report of the Working Party on No-Fault Compensation for Medical Injury*. London: British Medical Association

BRITISH MEDICAL ASSOCIATION (1984) *The Handbook of Medical Ethics*. London: British Medical Association

BROWN, H. and MARRIOTT, A. (1993) *ADR Principles and Practice*. London: Sweet and Maxwell

BYRNE, R. and MCCUTCHEON, P. (1989) *The Irish Legal System*. London: Butterworths

CAPLAN, R. P. (1994) Stress, anxiety, and depression in hospital consultants, general practitioners, and senior health service managers. *British Medical Journal*, **309**, 1261

CARDOZO, B. N. (1921) *The Nature of the Judicial Process*. New Haven, Connecticut: Yale University Press

CHAPMAN, M. (1994) Medico-legal reports. *Journal of the Royal Society of Medicine*, **87**, 186

CHARTERED INSTITUTE OF ARBITRATORS (1993) *The Med-Arb Scheme. Proposal for a Mediation and Arbitration Scheme for Medical Negligence Cases in the NHS*. London: The Chartered Institute of Arbitrators

COATES, R. and GEHM, J. (1985) *Victim Meets Offender: an Evaluation of Victim Offender Reconciliation Programs*. Cited by Umbreit (1988)

COHEN, L. J. (1977) *The Probable and the Provable*. Oxford: Clarendon

COLES, R. R. A. (1967) External meatus closure by audiometer earphone. *Journal of Speech and Hearing Disorders*, **32**, 296–297

COLES, R. R. A. (1975) Medico-legal aspects of noise hazards to hearing. *Medico-Legal Journal*, **43**, 3–19

COMMISSION OF THE EUROPEAN COMMUNITIES (1984) *The Confidentiality of Medical Records*. Report EUR 9471 EN

COMMITTEE ON PERSONAL INJURIES LITIGATION (WINN COMMITTEE) (1968) *Report Cmnd 3691*. London: HMSO

COULSON, R. (1989) The lawyer's role in dispute management. *Dispute Resolution*. American Bar Association Standing Committee on Dispute Resolution. Issue 25

COUNCIL FOR INTERNATIONAL ORGANISATIONS OF MEDICAL SCIENCES (1982) *Human Experimentation and Medical Ethics*. Geneva: CIOMS

CURZON, L. B. (1968) *English Legal History*. London: Macdonald and Evans

CUSACK, R. (1969) Foreword. In: *The Law on Noise*. London: Noise Abatement Society

DADSON, R. S. (1949) Standardization of audiometers. *Acta Otolaryngologica Supplementum*, **90**, 59

DADSON, R. S. and KING, J. H. (1952) A determination of the normal threshold of hearing and its relation to the standardization of audiometers. *Journal of Laryngology and Otology*, **66**, 366–378

DAVID, R. and JAUFFRET-SPINOSI, C. (1992) *Les Grands Systèmes de Droit Contemporains*. Paris: Dalloz

DAVIES, J. V. and JACOB, J. (1987) *Encyclopedia of Health Services and Medical Law*. London: Sweet and Maxwell

DAVIS, A. (1992) *The Distribution of Hearing Thresholds in GB: 1980–86*. IHR Internal Report: Series A Number 10. Volume 2. Nottingham: MRC Institute of Hearing Research

DAVIS, A. (1995) *Hearing in Adults*. London: Whurr

DAWES, P. J. D., O'KEEFE, L. and ADCOCK, S. (1992) Informed consent: the assesment of two-structured interview approaches compared to the current approach. *Journal of Laryngology and Otology*, **106**, 420–424

DAWES, P. J. D. and DAVISON, P. (1994) Informed consent: what do patients want to know? *Journal of the Royal Society of Medicine*, **87**, 149–152

DENNING, A. T. (1986) *Leaves from my Library*. London: Butterworths. p. vi

DEPARTMENT OF HEALTH (1991) *Local Research Ethics Committees*. HSG(91)5. London: DoH

DIAMOND, A. L. and LAURENCE, D. R. (1985) Product liability in respect of drugs. *British Medical Journal*, **290**, 365–368

DIAS, R. W. M. (1970) *Jurisprudence*. London: Butterworths

DICEY, A. V. (1905) *Lectures on the Relation between Law and Public Opinion in the 19th century*. London: Macmillan

DINGWALL, R. (1989) *Socio-Legal Aspects of Medical Practice*. London: Royal College of Physicians

DINGWALL, R., FENN, P. and QUAM, L. (1990) *Medical Negligence: a Review and Bibliography*. Oxford: Centre for Socio-Legal Studies

DOBIE, R. A. (1993) *Medical-Legal Evaluation of Hearing Loss*. New York: Van Nostrand and Reinhold

DONNELLY, P. (1994) The prosecutor's fallacy. *Royal Statistical Society News*, number 1, **22**, 1–2

DUMAS, A. (1845) *Le Comte de Monte Cristo*. Republished 1984. Paris: Livre de Poche

DUNSTAN, G. R. (1981) In: *Dictionary of Medical Ethics*, edited by A. S. Duncan, G. R. Dunstan and R. B. Welbourn. London: Darton, Longman & Todd

DUNSTAN, G. R. (1986) Report on junior members forum. *British Medical Journal*, **292**, 1028

DU PLESSIS, L. M. (1992) *Inleiding tot die Reg*. Kaapstad: Juta

DYER, C. (1993) Medico-legal. *British Medical Journal*, **306**, 1431–1432

EEKELAAR, J. (1989) Consent to treatment: legal and empirical questions. In: *Socio-legal Aspects of Medical Practice*, edited by R. Dingwall. London: Royal College of Physicians of London. pp. 21–26

EGGLESTON, R. (1983) *Evidence, Proof and Probability*. London: Weidenfeld and Nicolson

ELBRA, A. (1986) Living with the Data Protection Act. *Linkup*, April–June, p. 59

EVANS, R. (1994) *Proceedings of British Association for Advancement of Science*, September

FADEN, R. R., BEAUCHAMP, T. L. and KING, N. M. P. (1986) *A History and Theory of Informed Consent*. Oxford: Oxford University Press

FELIX, R. H., IVE, F. A. and DAHL, M. G. C. (1974) Cutaneous and ocular reactions to practolol. *British Medical Journal*, **iv**, 321–324

FENN, P., HERMANS, D. and DINGWALL, R. (1994) Estimating the cost of compensating victims of medical negligence. *British Medical Journal*, **309**, 389–391

FINCH, J. (1986) Letter to the editor. *The Times*, September 18th, p. 15

FORD, R. (1993) *The Times*, 25th February

FOSTER, N. (1993) *German Law and Legal System*. London: Blackstone

FRIEDMANN, W. (1949) *Legal Theory*. London: Stevens

FROSTICK, S. P., RADFORD, P. J. and WALLACE, W. A. (1995) *Medical Audit*. Cambridge: Cambridge University Press

GAGARIN, M. (1986) *Early Greek Law*. Berkeley, CA: University of California Press

GAY, J.(early 18th c) *The Painter who Pleased Nobody and*

Everybody. Quoted by J. Bartlett (1955) *Familiar Quotations*. 13th edn. Boston: Little, Brown and Co. p. 308

GENERAL MEDICAL COUNCIL (1991) *Professional Conduct and Discipline: Fitness to Practise*. London: General Medical Council

GIESEN, D. (1988a) *International Medical Law*. Tübingen: JCB Mohr

GIESEN, D. (1988b) From paternalism to self-determination to shared decision-making. *Acta Juridica (Cape Town)*, pp. 107–127

GILLON, R. (1986) *Philosophical Medical ethics*. London: Wiley

GOLDREIN, I. S. and DE HAAS, M. R. (1994) *Butterworths Personal Injury Litigation Service (Looseleaf)*. London: Butterworths

GREAR, J. (1993) Letter to the Editor. *The Times*, 15th July

GROSSETESTE, R. (c 1230) Commentaries on the *Physics and Posterior Analytics of Aristotle*. Quoted by C. L. Parkinson (1985) *Breakthroughs*. London: Mansell. p. 4

GUEST, A. G. (ed) (1994) *Chitty on Contracts*. London: Sweet and Maxwell

HADFIELD, E. H. (1970) A study of adenocarcinoma of the paranasal sinuses in woodworkers in the furniture industry. *Annals of the Royal College of Surgeons of England*, **461**, 301–319

HARDEN, I. and LEWIS, N. (1986) *The Noble Lie: The British Constitution and the Rule of Law*. London: Hutchinson

HARE, D. J. (1988) What is informed consent? In: *Dilemmas in Otorhinolaryngology*, edited by D. F. N. Harrison. London: Churchill Livingstone. pp. 21–24

HARPWOOD, V. and ALLDRIDGE, P. (1989) *GCSE Law*. London: Blackstone

HARROWVEN, R. G. C., GREENER, J. D. F. and STEPHENS, S. D. G. (1987) A double blind cross-over study of high-frequency emphasis hearing aids in individuals with noise-induced hearing loss. *British Journal of Audiology*, **21**, 209–219

HARVEY, I. and CHADWICK, R. (1992) Compensation for harm: the implications for medical research. *Sociology, Science and Medicine*, **34**, 399–402

HAVARD, J. (1986) Where should responsibility lie? *British Medical Association News Review*, **12**, 5

HAYNES, R. B., SACKETT, D. L., TAYLOR, D. W., GIBSON, E. S. and JOHNSON, E. L. (1978) Increased absenteeism from work after detection and labeling of hypertensive patients. *New England Journal of Medicine*, **299**, 741–744

HEALY, M. J. R. (1988) *GLIM An Introduction*. Oxford: Oxford University Press

HEPPLE, B. A. and MATTHEWS, M. H. (1991) *Tort: Cases and Materials*. London: Butterworths

HERRNSTEIN, R. and MURRAY, C. (1994) *The Bell Curve*. New York: Free Press

HINCHCLIFFE, R. (1959) The threshold of hearing of a random sample rural population. *Acta Otolaryngologica*, **50**, 411–422

HINCHCLIFFE, R. (1987) *The Clinical Examination of Aural Function*. In: *Scott-Brown's Otolaryngology*, 5th edn, edited by A. G. Kerr, vol. 2, *Adult Audiology*, edited by D. Stephens. London: Butterworths. pp. 558–576

HINCHCLIFFE, R. (1992) King–Kopetzky syndrome: an auditory stress disorder? *Journal of Audiological Medicine*, **1**, 89–98

HINCHCLIFFE, R. (1993) Hypoacousies et bourdonnements: une perspective globale. *Revue de Laryngologie*, **114**, 93–102

HINCHCLIFFE, R. (1994a) Quantitative methods re expert testimony. *Proceedings of 10th World Congress on Medical Law, Jerusalem*. Ramat Gan, Israel: Steir

HINCHCLIFFE, R. (1994b) A socio-economic factor for hearing? *Journal of Audiological Medicine*, **3**, 107–112

HOFFENBERG, R. (1989) Foreword. In: *Socio-Legal Aspects of Medical Practice*, edited by R. Dingwall. London: Royal College of Physicians

IHERING, G. (1873) *Der Zweck im Recht*. Reprinted as *Law as a Means to an End*. London: Modern Legal Philosophy Series

JENKINS, D. (1986) *The Law of Hywel Dda*. Llandysul, Dyfed: Gomer

JERGER, J., CHMIEL, R., STACH, B. and SPRETNJAK, M. (1993) Gender affects audiometric shape in presbyacusis. *Journal of the American Academy of Audiology*, **4**, 42–49

JONES, M. A. (1994) *Textbook on Torts*. London: Blackstone

JONES, M. A. and MORRIS, A. E. (1992) *Blackstone's Statutes on Medical Law*. London: Blackstone

KAPLAN, G. A. and SALONEN, J. T. (1990) Socioeconomic conditions in childhood and ischaemic heart disease. *British Medical Journal*, **301**, 1121–1123

KEMP, D. (1994) *Kemp and Kemp – The Quantum of Damages*. London: Sweet and Maxwell

KENNEDY, I. and GRUBB, A. (1994) *Medical Law: Text with Materials*. London: Butterworths

KIRBY, M. (1983) *Reform the Law: Essays on the Renewal of the Australian Legal System*. Melbourne: OUP

KNIGHT, J. J. (1966) Normal hearing threshold determined by manual and self-recording techniques. *Journal of the Acoustical Society of America*, **39**, 1184–1185

KNIGHT, J. J. and COLES, R. R. A. (1960) Determination of the hearing threshold levels of naval recruits in terms of British and American standards. *Journal of the Acoustical Society of America*, **32**, 800–804

KNOX, E. G. (1986) Confidentiality and the use of medical records for research. *Journal of the Royal College of Physicians of London*, **20**, 234

KUDRJAVCEV, P. I. (1956) *Juridiceskij slovar*. Quoted by David and Jauffret–Spinosi, 1992

LANGLOIS, D. (1992) *L'Affaire Seznec*. Paris: Plon

LEE, S. (1986) *Law and Morals*. Oxford: OUP

LEIJON, A. (1992) Quantization error in clinical pure-tone audiometry. *Scandinavian Audiology*, **21**, 103–108

LETTERS TO THE EDITOR (1995) Eliminating 'ambushes' in court. *The Times*, 23rd May, p. 17

LEWIS, C. J. (1988) *Medical Negligence: A Plaintiff's Guide*. London: Cass

LLOYD, I. (1993) *Information Technology and the Law*. London: Butterworths

LOCKHART, M. R. (1980) Medical malpractice in Australia. In: *Medical Practice*, edited by J. Leahy Taylor. Bristol: John Wright

LUTMAN, M. E. and DAVIS, A. C. (1994) The distribution of hearing threshold levels in the general population aged 18–30 years. *Audiology*, **33**, 327–350

LUTMAN, M. E. and SPENCER, H. S. (1991) Occupational noise and demographic factors in hearing. *Acta Otolaryngologica*, Suppl. 476, 74–84

LUTMAN, M. E., DAVIS, A. and SPENCER, H. S. (1993) Interpreting NIHL by comparison of noise exposed subjects with appropriate controls. In: *Noise and Man '93 – Proceedings of the 6th International Conference on Noise as a Public Health Problem*, Nice 5–9 July, Volume 3, Actes INRETS No. 34. edited by M. Vallet. Arcueil: Institut Nationale de Recherche sur les Transports et leur Sécurité, Service Publications

MCCALLUM, R. I. (1987) Increased barometric pressure. In: *Hunters Diseases of Occupations*, edited by P. A. B. Raffle, W. R. Lee, R. I. McCallum and R. Murray. London: Hodder and Stoughton. pp. 523–547

MACCORMICK, N. and BIRKS, P. (1986) *The Legal Mind*. Oxford: Oxford University Press

MCCULLAGH, P. and NELDER, J. A. (1983) *Generalised Linear Models*. London: Chapman and Hall

MACKIE, K. J. (ed) (1991) *A Handbook of Dispute Resolution: ADR in Action*. London: Sweet and Maxwell. p. 104

MCGINNIS, W. and KUZIORA, M. (1994) The molecular architects of body design. *Scientific American*, **36**, 270

MACKENZIE, J.-A. and PHILLIPS, M. (1994) *A Practical Approach to Land Law*. London: Blackstone

MACLEAN, M. (1989) Alternatives to litigation: no-fault or effective social security? In: *Socio-legal Aspects of Medical Practice*, edited by R. Dingwall. London: Royal College of Physicians of London. pp. 37–42

MCMAHON, R. (1994) *A Practical Approach to Road Traffic Law*. London: Blackstone

MACMILLAN, A. J. F. (1988) Decompression sickness. In: *Aviation Medicine*, edited by J. Ernsting and P. King. London: Butterworths. pp. 19–26

MCMANUS, F. (1994) *Environmental Health Law*. London: Blackstone

MCNAB JONES, R. F., HAMMOND, V. T., WRIGHT, D. and BALLANTYNE, J. C. (1977) Practolol and deafness. *Journal of Laryngology and Otology*, **91**, 963–973

MANNING, S. (1993) Hedonic damages. *Journal of the Medical Defence Union*, **3**, 50

MARGULIS, L. (1981) *Symbiosis in Cell Evolution*. San Francisco: Freeman

MARSHALL, T. F. (1984) *Reparation, Conciliation and Mediation*. Paper 27. London: Home Office Research and Planning Unit

MARSHALL, T. F. and MERRY, S. (1990) *Crime and Accountability*. London: HMSO

MARTIN, C. R. A. (1979) *Law Relating to Medical Practice*. Tunbridge Wells: Pitman Medical

MAYSON, S., FRENCH, D. and RYAN, C. (1994) *Company Law*. London: Blackstone

MEDICOLEGAL (1979) Medical reports not to the lawyers' liking. *British Medical Journal*, ii, 1376

MERLUZZI, F. and HINCHCLIFFE, R. (1973) Threshold of subjective auditory handicap. *Audiology*, **12**, 65–69

MIERS, D. R. and PAGE, A. C. (1990) *Legislation*. London: Sweet and Maxwell. p. 170

MILL, J. S. (1863) *Utilitarianism*. Republished 1962 edited by M. Warnock. Glasgow: Fontana

MOLAN, M. T. (1994) *Criminal Law Textbook*. London: HLT Publications

MOLIERE, J. B. P. (1966) *Le Médecin Malgré Lui*. Act II, sc. 4, line 730. Republished 1984, edited by F. Angué. Paris: Bordas

MOLONY, J. (1966) Letter to the Editor of *The Times*. Quoted by Chapman, 1994

MONTAIGNE, M. E. DE (1580) *Essais 2: De La Ressemblance des Enfants aux Pères*. Chapitre XXXVII. Reprinted (1972) Paris: Librairie Générale Française

MOODIE, P. C. E. and MARSHALL, T. (1992) Guidelines for local research ethics committees. *British Medical Journal*, **304**, 1293–1295

MORGAN, D. and LEE, R. G. (1991) *The Human Fertilisation and Embryology Act 1990*. London: Blackstone

MORRISON, M. C. T. (1993) Medico-legal Reports. *Journal of the Royal Society of Medicine*, **86**, 247

MUNKMAN, J. (1985) *Employer's Liability at Common Law*. London: Butterworths

MURPHY, P. (ed) (1994) *Blackstone's Criminal Practice*. London: Blackstone

MUSTILL LORD (1995) Closing Speech at 'Entitlement to NHS Treatment: The Resolution of Disputes.' Conference at Royal Society of Medicine, 14 June

NELDER, J. A. and WEDDERBURN, R. W. M. (1972) Generalised linear models. *Journal of the Royal Statistical Society A*, **135**, 378–384

NEUBERGER, J. (1992) *Ethics and Health Care: the Role of Research Ethics Committees in the United Kingdom*. London: King's Fund Institute

NEWS ITEM (1969) *The Times*, 4th September

NEWS ITEM (1978) *The Times*, 4th August

NEWS ITEM (1993a) *Guardian*, 6th August

NEWS ITEM (1993b) *The Times*, 14th May, p. 3

NEWS ITEM (1994a) Torturer Corky brought to book. *The Guardian*, 18th August, p. 1

NEWS ITEM (1994b) Stress case paves way for damages claims. *British Medical Journal*, **309**, 1391

NEWS ITEM (1995a) Deaf woman wins court battle over 'social life' benefit. *The Times*, 16th June. p. 4

NEWS ITEM (1995b) Fast trials plan in civil law shake-up. *The Times*, 16th June. p. 1

NICHOLSON, R. H. (ed.) (1986) *Medical Research with Children*. Oxford: Oxford University Press

O'HAGAN, T. (1984) *The End of Law?* Oxford: Blackwell

PAINTER, A. A. and HARVEY, B. W. (1994) *Butterworth's Law of Food and Drugs*. London: Butterworths

PAPPWORTH, M. (1978) Medical ethical committees: a review of their functions. *World Medicine*, **13**, 199–201

PATEL, P., MENDALL, M. A., KHULUSI, S., NORTHFIELD, T.C. and STRACHAN, D.P. (1994) *Helicobacter pylori* infection in childhood: risk factors and effect on growth. *British Medical Journal*, **309**, 1119–1123

PEARSON, H. and MILLER, C. (1990) *Commercial Exploitation of Intellectual Property*. London: Blackstone

PICARDA, H. A. P. (1994) *The Law and Practice Relating to Charities*. London: Butterworths

POPE, A. (c 1709) *An Essay on Criticism*. Republished 1992, In: *The Poems of Alexander Pope*, edited by J. Butt. London: Routledge. p. 144 and 145

POPE, A. (1713) *Windsor-Forest*. Republished 1992, In: *The Poems of Alexander Pope*, edited by J. Butt. London: Routledge. p. 195

POPPER, K. (1934) *Logik der Forschung*. Vienna. Translated as *The Logic of Scientific Discovery* (1983) London: Hutchinson

POPPER, K. (1981) *Conjectures and Refutations*, 4th edn. London: Routledge and Kegan Paul

POUND, R. (1943/4) *A Survey of Social Interests* 57 Harvard Law Review 1, Cambridge, Mass, USA

POWERS, M. and HARRIS, N. (1990) *Medical Negligence*. London: Butterworths

RAPHAEL, D. D. (1981) *Moral Philosophy*. Oxford: Oxford University Press

REED, C. (1993) *Computer Law*. London: Blackstone

REPORT BY THE INDUSTRIAL INJURIES ADVISORY COUNCIL (1973) In accordance with Section 62 of the National Insurance (Industrial Injuries) Act 1965 on the question whether there are degrees of hearing loss due to noise which satisfy the conditions for prescription under the Act. Cmnd. 5461. London: HMSO. para 31

REYNOLDS, K. (1994) Getting at the truth in arbitration –

admissibility, confidentiality and compulsion. *Arbitration*, **60**, 24–29

ROBINSON, D. W. (1988) *Tables for the Estimation of Hearing Impairment due to Noise for Otologically Normal Persons and for a Typical Unscreened Population, as a function of Age and Duration of Exposure.* London: HSE Contract Research Report No. 2/1988. Health and Safety Executive

ROBINSON, D. W. and SHIPTON, M. S. (1977) *Tables for the Estimation of Noise-induced Hearing Loss. NPL Acoustics Report Ac 61 (2nd.)* Teddington: National Physical Laboratory

ROBINSON, D. W., LAWTON, B. W. and RICE, C. G. (1994) *Occupational Hearing Loss from Low-level Noise.* HSE Contract Research Report No. 68/1994. London: Health and Safety Executive

ROBINSON, D. W., SHIPTON, M. S. and HINCHCLIFFE, R. (1979) *Normal Hearing Threshold and its Dependence on Clinical Rejection Criteria.* Teddington: NPL Acoustics Report Ac 89

ROBINSON, D. W., SHIPTON, M. S. and HINCHCLIFFE, R. (1981) A verification and critique of International Standards. *Audiology*, **20**, 409–431

ROEDIGER, R. (1994) Rembering events that never happened. *Psychologist*, **7**, 257

ROYAL COLLEGE OF PHYSICIANS OF LONDON (1984) *Guidelines on the Practice of Ethics Committees in Medical Research.* London: Royal College of Physicians of London

ROYAL COLLEGE OF PHYSICIANS OF LONDON (1986) Research of healthy volunteers. A report of the Royal College of Physicians. *Journal of the Royal College of Physicians*, **20**, 243–257

ROYAL COLLEGE OF PHYSICIANS OF LONDON (1990) *Compensation for Adverse Consequences of Medical Intervention.* London: Royal College of Physicians

SATALOFF, R. T. and SATALOFF, J. (1993) *Occupational Hearing Loss.* New York: Dekker

SAUNDERS, G. H. and HAGGARD, M. P. (1989) The clinical assessment of obscure auditory dysfunction – 1. Auditory and psychological factors. *Ear and Hearing*, **10**, 200–208

SAUNDERS, G. H., HAGGARD, M. P. and FIELD, D. (1989) Clinical diagnosis and management of obscure auditory dysfunction (OAD). *British Journal of Audiology*, **23**, 358

SCHNEIDER, I. H. (1983) In: *Dictionary of the History of Science*, edited by W. F. Bynum, E. J. Browne and R. Porter. London: Macmillan. p. 338

SCIENTIFIC AFFAIRS BOARD (1978) Ethical principles for research with human subjects. *Bulletin of the British Psychological Society*, **31**, 48–49

SEFERIS, G. (1965) ΔΙΑΛΕΙΜΜΑ ΧΑΡΑΣ (Interlude of joy). In: *Collected Poems* Athens: Ikaros. Republished 1982, In: *Collected Poems* edited by E. Keeley and P. Sherrard. London: Anvil. p. 228

SIMANOWITZ, A. (1993a) Alternative dispute resolution. *AVMA Medical and Legal Journal*, **4**, 1

SIMANOWITZ, A. (1993b) Accountability. In: *Medical Accidents*, edited by C. Vincent, M. Ennis and R. J. Audley. Oxford: OUP. ch. 14

SIME, S. (1994) *A Practical Approach to Civil Procedure.* London: Blackstone

SIMPSON, G. G. (1945) The Principles of Classification and a Classification of Mammals. *Bulletin of the Museum of Natural History*, vol. 85, New York

SKAKKEBAEK, N. E., GIWERCMAN, A. and DE KRETSER, D. (1994) Pathogenesis and management of male infertility. *Lancet*, i, 1473–1479

SLAPPER, G. (1994) The dangers of spiritual guidance. *The Times.* 25 October, p. 37

SMITH, C. W. (1988) What is informed consent? In: *Dilemmas in Otorhinolaryngology*, edited by D. F. N. Harrison. London: Churchill Livingstone. pp. 15–20

SMITH, J. C. (1992) *Smith and Thomas: A Casebook on Contract.* London: Sweet and Maxwell

SMITH, J. C. and HOGAN, B. (1993) *Criminal Law: Cases and Materials.* London: Butterworths

SOKAL, R. R. and SNEATH, P. H. A. (1963) *Principles of Numerical Taxonomy.* San Francisco: Freeman

STAIR VISCOUNT (1681) *Institutions of the Law of Scotland.* Quoted by Black, 1993

STANHOPE, P. D. (1747) *Letters*, November 6th

STAPLETON, J. (1986) *Disease and the Compensation Debate.* Oxford: Oxford University Press

STEINER, J. (1994) *Textbook on EC Law.* London: Blackstone

STEPHENS, S. D. G. and RENDELL, R. J. (1988) Auditory disability with normal hearing. *Audiologia*, **4**, 233–238

STOLKER, C. J. J. M. (1994) Wrongful Life: The Limits of Liability and Beyond. *International and Comparative Law Quarterly*, **43**, 521–536

STUTTARD, A. R. D. (1969) *English Law Notebook.* London: Butterworths

TAYLOR, J. L. (1971) *The Doctor and Negligence.* Tunbridge Wells: Pitman Medical. p. 110

TEDESCHI, G. (ed) (1969) *The Law of Civil Wrongs, General Part.* Jerusalem: Rubin Mass, (Hebrew)

TEFF, H. and MUNROE, C. R. (1976) *Thalidomide: The Legal Aftermath.* Farnborough, Hants: Saxon House

UMBREIT, M. S. (1988) Mediation of victim offender conflict. *Journal of Dispute Resolution*, **2**, 85–105

WADE, E. C. S. and BRADLEY, A. W. (1994) *Constitutional and Administrative Law.* London: Longman

WALKER, C. and STARMER, K. (1993) *Justice in Error.* London: Blackstone

WHEELER, L. J. and DICKSON, E. D. D. (1952) The determination of the threshold of hearing. *Journal of Laryngology and Otology*, **66**, 379–395

WHITFIELD, A. (1990) Informed consent: does the doctrine benefit patients in the United Kingdom? In: *Medicine and the Law*, edited by D. Brahams. London: Royal College of Physicians of London. pp. 1–10

WIEDEMANN, H. R. (1961) Hinweis auf eine derzeitige Haufung hypo- und aplasticher Fehlildungen des Gliedmassen. *Medizinische Welt*, **37**, 1863–1866

WILLIAMS, A. G. P. (1982a) *Applicable Inductive Logic.* London: Edsall

WILLIAMS, G. (1982b) *Learning the Law.* London: Stevens

WILLIAMS, R. G. (1992) The evaluation of hearing impairment. *Journal of Audiological Medicine*, **1**, 156–160

WILLOTT, J. F. (1991) *Aging and the Auditory System.* San Diego, California: Singular Publishing. p. 246

WOOLF LORD (1995) *Access to Justice.* Interim Report to the Lord Chancellor on the Civil Justice System in England and Wales. Quoted by Leading Article in *The Times* 19th June. p. 21

WRIGHT, P. (1975) Untoward effects associated with practolol administration: oculomucocutaneous syndrome. *British Medical Journal*, i, 595–598

ZHAO, J. J., LAZZARINI, R. A. and PICK, L. (1993) *Genes and Development*, no. 3. **71**, 343–354

ZOLA, E. (1898) J'accuse. *L'Aurore.* 13th January

Glossary of terms and abbreviations

AAHL age-associated hearing loss

acoustic trauma the permanent loss of hearing that immediately follows a brief exposure to a very intense noise, e.g. gunfire.

ADN abbreviation for auditory disability with normal hearing (syn OAD; King-Kopetzky syndrome)

ARHL abbreviation for age-related hearing loss (synonymous with AAHL)

audiogram a chart which portrays in graphic form the results of audiometry

audiology that part of human knowledge and endeavour (educational, medical and scientific) concerned with hearing and its disorders (a word which is sometimes used incorrectly as a synonym for audiometry)

audiometry the measurement of hearing using electroacoustic equipment

BAAP British Association of Audiological Physicians (the association concerned with advancing the interests of those medical specialists who are concerned with disorders of balance and auditory communication)

BAO–HNS British Association of Otorhinolaryngologists – Head and Neck Surgeons (the association concerned with advancing the interests of British ear, nose and throat specialists)

BS 2497 the British Standard Specification for the Standard reference zero for the calibration of pure tone air conduction audiometers (currently BS 2497: 1992; equivalent to ISO 389 1991) [note that the term 'normal' which appeared in the title of the first British Standard, i.e. BS 2497: 1954, was subsequently deleted]. The original samples (Royal Air Force; National Physical Laboratory) on which the standard was based provided *modal* values for a *clinically otologically normal* population.

BS 5330: 1976 specifies a relationship between noise exposure and the expected incidence of hearing handicap (now referred to as a 'hearing disability'). The hearing of a person is deemed to be impaired sufficiently to cause a handicap if the arithmetic average of the hearing threshold levels, of the two ears combined, is equal to or greater than 30 dB (re BS 2497). 'Since this standard is based upon statistical data it cannot be expected to provide an accurate assessment of hearing handicap in individual persons.'

BS 6951 the British Standard Specification for the Threshold of Hearing by air conduction as a function of age and sex for otologically (this cannot be so since the data reflect the effects of ageing (as the standard intends)) normal persons (currently BS 6951: 1988; equivalent to ISO 7029-1984).

BSA British Society of Audiology (the British multidisciplinary national society of doctors, engineers, scientists and other professionals who are interested in hearing and its disorders).

CERA abbreviation for cortical electrical response audiometry (sometimes written just ERA).

clinical picture the constellation of symptoms and physical signs, i.e. ignoring the contribution of special tests (e.g. X-rays, blood tests, audiometry), which either characterizes a disorder or characterizes a particular individual's disorder. (Clinical picture thus relates to the use of zero-level or low-level technology)

clinician a health care professional (medical, scientific or surgical) concerned with the clinical investigation and management of *individuals* seeking help.

dB abbreviation for decibel

deafness total hearing loss

decibel the unit used for expressing the physical magnitude of sounds.

disability 'In the context of health experience, a disability is any restriction or lack (resulting from an impairment) of ability to perform an activity in the manner or within the range considered normal for a human being . . . Disability represents a departure from the norm in terms of performance of the individual, as opposed to that of the organ or mechanism . . . To say that someone *has a disability* is to preserve neutrality . . . However, . . . to say that someone is *disabled* . . . is to risk being dismissive.' International Classification of Impairments, Disabilities, and Handicaps: A manual of classification relating to the consequences of disease (1980) World Health Organization. Geneva. As regards hearing, it would cover everyday use, as in the ability to converse under different conditions.

expected value (or 'expectation'): an expression used in statistical work to indicate the *mean* that would occur among some group on the basis of a given hypothesis (Hill, A. B. and Hill, I. D. (1991) *Bradford Hill's Principles of Medical Statistics*. Edward Arnold. London. p. 66.). For example, we might look at the mean HTLs of a *group* of noise-exposed (or not exposed) Plaintiffs to see whether this matches the MRC ageing/noise model of hearing.

handicap 'In the context of health experience, a handicap is a disadvantage for a given individual, resulting from an impairment or a disability, that limits or prevents the fulfilment of a role that is normal (depending on age, sex, and social and cultural factors) for that individual . . . It is thus a social phenomenon, representing the social and environmental consequences for the individual stemming from the presence of impairments and disabilities.' International Classification of Impairments, Disabilities, and Handicaps: A manual of classification relating to the consequences of disease (1980) World Health Organization. Geneva, p. 29. As regards hearing, it covers the non-auditory consequences of hearing impairment, e.g. economic, psychological, social. (These are difficult concepts. Even ISO 1999: 1990 confuses 'handicap' and 'disability' (p. 3).)

hearing level (HL) for a specified frequency of pure-tone and testing system, the sound pressure level (essentially the physical magnitude of the sound in the case of air conduction audiometers) or vibratory force level (essentially the physical magnitude of vibration in the case of bone conduction audiometers) of the tone relative to that of a reference zero (as defined by an International or National Standard). It is the dial setting of an audiometer if the instrument has been properly calibrated. Expressed in decibels, i.e. as dB HL.

hearing loss an impairment of hearing that exceeds a criterial level; no units, but may be qualified, in terms of severity, as mild, severe etc.

hearing threshold level (HTL) for a particular ear, and a given frequency and test system, it is an individual's threshold of hearing (i.e. the quietest sound that he can hear) as determined in a stated manner and expressed by the system's indicated hearing level value. Expressed in decibels, i.e. as dB HTL.

hearing threshold shift the change in the threshold of hearing for a given frequency (or group of frequencies) over a particular period of time; expressed in decibels.

hertz unit of frequency (formerly cycles per second)

HL abbreviation for hearing level

HTL abbreviation for hearing threshold level

Hz abbreviation for hertz

IAPA International Association of Physicians in Audiology (the international association of medical men and women whose particular interest is the investigation and care of individuals with disorders of hearing and/or of balance)

IHR Institute of Hearing Research (the MRC unit for research on hearing; epidemiology forms a strong component in its research programme)

ILO Institute of Laryngology and Otology, University College, London University (the principal UK postgraduate medical school for teaching and research in ear, nose and throat diseases and disorders of hearing)

impairment 'In the context of health experience, an impairment is any loss or abnormality of psychological, physiological, or anatomical structure or function . . . Thus the term is more inclusive than "disorder", e.g. the loss of a leg is an impairment but not a disorder.' International Classification of Impairments, Disabilities, and Handicaps: A manual of classification relating to the consequences of disease (1980) World Health Organization. Geneva. Assessments of hearing in individual ears relate to impairment. A 1991 Editorial in *Audiology* (the journal of the International Society of Audiology) pointed out that there is a continuum of hearing tests ranging from simple pure-tone audiometry to the more complex tests of speech recognition in noise. (Stephens, D. and Hétu, R. (1991) Impairment, disability and handicap: towards a consensus. *Audiology*, 30, 185–200)

ISA International Society of Audiology (the international multidisciplinary society concerned with disseminating knowledge of hearing and its disorders)

ISO 1999: 1990 International Standard for the determination of occupational noise exposure and estimation of noise-induced hearing impairment. (not yet endorsed by UK)

ISVR Institute of Sound and Vibration Research, University of Southampton (a prestigious centre for research into the effects of sound and vibration, including the effects on man)

labelling all the consequences, medical and social, which occur when an individual is informed, rightly or wrongly, that he has some disease or other body abnormality. (Haynes, R. B., Sackett, D. L., Taylor, D. W., Gibson, E. S. and Johnson, E. L. (1978) *New England Journal of Medicine*, 299, 741–744).

mean the arithmetic mean (colloquially termed the 'average') is the sum of all the observations divided by the number of observations. In hearing surveys, 'the difference between "mean" and "median" hearing level can be significant . . . The mean, however, . . . gives a better description of the sample when supplemented with stand-

ard deviations. Mean HTLs are indeed particularly sensitive to clinical rejection criteria.' (Robinson, D. W., Shipton, M. S. and Hinchcliffe, R. (1979) *NPL Report Ac 89*.)

median this is essentially the middle point when a series of measurements is ranked in ascending order.

mode the most frequently occurring value in a distribution.

MRC Medical Research Council (the main UK Government agency for the promotion of medical and related biological research)

normal threshold of hearing 'A term which should be avoided because of its medical and medicolegal implications.' (Davis, H. and Silverman, S. R. (1978) *Hearing and Deafness*. New York: Holt, Rinehart and Winston. p. 540.) There is no single normal threshold of hearing; there are indeed a number of normal thresholds of normal hearing.

nosoacusis hearing loss due to all factors other than ageing, industrial and non-industrial noise exposure. (Ward, W. D. (1977) '*Effects of Noise Exposure on Auditory Sensitivity*'. In: *Handbook of Physiology*, vol. 9: *Reaction to Environmental Agents*, edited by D. H. K., Lee. Bethesda: American Physiological Society. pp. 1–15.)

NPL National Physical Laboratory (the main UK Government physics laboratory)

NSH National Study of Hearing (the principal epidemiological programme of IHR)

OAD abbreviation for obscure auditory dysfunction (syn ADN)

ONIHL abbreviation for occupational noise-induced hearing loss

otological relating to the ear; this organ has three component structures, i.e. the outer ear, the middle ear and the inner ear, or labyrinth, and the last named is divided into the auditory labyrinth, or cochlea, and the vestibular labyrinth; an ear should not be termed 'clinically otologically normal' unless tests for the functional integrity of all the structural components of the ear have been shown to be normal; so often an ear is referred to as being 'otologically' normal when the examiner has screened only for middle ear disorders, i.e. the designation should be '*tympanologically* normal'. Hence the difficulty of reconciling these clinical concepts with the definition of 'otological' given by ISO 7029 (BS 6951).

PTA abbreviation for pure-tone audiogram

range of normal hearing the scatter of actual determinations of hearing sensitivity of normal-hearing persons with respect to age and gender. Sometimes, the limit is taken arbitrarily as two standard deviations from the mean, sometimes as the 95th centile.

socioacusis non-industrial noise-induced threshold shifts. (Glorig, A. (1958) *Noise and Your Ear*. New York: Grune and Stratton.)

tinnitus a sensation of sound which is not associated with any external acoustic, electrical or mechanical stimulus.

tympanological: relating to the middle ear.

8

The prevention of hearing and balance disorders

Katherine Harrop-Griffiths

Disorders of hearing and of balance are common problems which may affect people of all ages world-wide and may lead to marked disability and handicap. Various specific preventive measures are possible and can be effectively adopted in order to reduce both the incidence and the results of pathology.

Epidemiology

'The principal scientific basis for preventive audiology is epidemiological audiology. Not only does epidemiology provide the clues to the factors which are important in the causation of auditory disorders, but it also provides the means for monitoring the effectiveness of preventive audiological measures' (Hinchcliffe, 1975). In addition, epidemiological studies provide information about the size and extent of the problem, thereby enabling forward planning for provision of prevention and care.

It is only for those conditions in which the aetiology and pathogenesis of the condition are fully understood that we can hope to effect adequate and effective preventive measures. In some cases a direct cause may be obvious; in others the precipitating factor or factors may not be so clear-cut; there may be a multifactorial cause or a delay between causation and presentation. Hence the need for detailed epidemiological studies to unravel these enigmas.

Hearing loss

The size of the problem

Precise figures are impossible to obtain, but it is estimated that more than 200 million people, or approximately 4% of the world's population, have a degree of hearing impairment sufficient to interfere with normal life (Alberti, Kapur and Prasansuk, 1993), while 5 million or more are thought to be profoundly deaf (Holborrow, 1985) (see also Chapter 3). Two-thirds of the hearing-impaired population live in underprivileged countries. Alberti (Alberti, Kapur and Prasansuk, 1993) has pointed out the potential increase in the percentage with ageing populations, while Wilson (1990) predicted a doubling of the elderly population in North America in the next 50 years. Other developed countries will have similar statistics.

From the above figures it can be seen that hearing impairment is a significant world-wide problem.

International preventive initiatives

Several preventive programmes have been initiated both nationally and internationally. On the international level the World Health Organization (WHO) has been particularly active in identifying the need for preventive strategies, establishing programmes of prevention and supporting their management, especially in developing countries.

Following the eradication of smallpox in the late 1970s, the WHO adopted the optimistic slogan 'Health for All by the Year 2000' in order to establish an impetus for preventive medicine. In 1988 they declared their aim of global eradication of poliomyelitis by 2000, while Europe and the USA hoped to eradicate measles, mumps and rubella by 2010, with the Caribbean having stated a similar aim by 2005.

The Expanded Immunisation Programme introduced in the early 1980s (WHO) has contributed significantly to the establishment of effective vaccination programmes world-wide. In order to encourage vaccine development, the Children's Vaccine Initiative was launched in 1990, with the aim of encouraging the development of vaccines which require fewer doses in order to establish lasting immunity at a younger age, can be stored without refrigeration and are cheaper than existing vaccines (Begg, 1993).

IMPACT (International Initiative against Avoidable Disablement) was launched in 1981 (Wilson, 1988) and, in 1986, the WHO established the Programme of Prevention of Deafness and Hearing Impairment (PDH), the focus of which was to 'prevent and control the major avoidable causes of deafness and hearing impairment and make basic ear care available as an integral part of primary health care to populations in greatest need'. Attention was also to be given to standardizing data collection, national planning of services, training of personnel, the development of inexpensive diagnostic and amplification services and to education (Alberti, Kapur and Prasansuk, 1993).

'Hearing International' came into being in 1992 as a global project aimed at promoting 'the prevention and management of hearing impairment and deafness world-wide'. The founding agencies were the International Society of Audiology (ISA) and the International Federation of Otological Societies (IFOS). The project aims to collaborate with other agencies including the WHO (Suzuki, 1993). Under this project a number of otological centres have been established both in developing and developed countries, and quarterly newsletters are aimed at facilitating communication between professionals in order to improve ear care world-wide.

Cost of prevention

For any planned preventive measure, consideration has to be given to the limited resources of the community concerned. Prevention of illness or disability makes moral sense, but may not always make economic sense. The saving to society, as a result of prevention, should outweigh the cost of that prevention. Therefore, for preventive audiology to be effective, it must be aimed at disorders of hearing and balance which are relatively common, of a severity to cause significant disability and handicap, and which are potentially avoidable by simple or straightforward measures involving minimal financial cost.

A further consideration is the delay in achieving obvious financial results. Rehabilitation is expensive and, especially for a child, the time-lag between expenditure and the obvious financial benefit to society of an independent wage-earner (as opposed to a dependent adult) exceeds the terms of office of most governments, a fact of possible significance in developing countries.

Public health considerations

Developing countries

Preventive measures appropriate to developed countries, such as the USA and Europe, are not applicable to the deprived areas of the world where basics such as standards of housing, sanitation, nutrition and general education are often inadequate. Money is scarce and civil war not uncommon, depriving the populace of finances as well as stability. Distances between medical centres are enormous and transportation limited, making the movement of medical supplies and personnel difficult. Medical resources are often inadequate, with a dearth of trained people and facilities. Electricity is frequently absent and refrigeration of vaccines may be a major problem. However, energy and finances spent on primary prevention, such as avoidance of infectious diseases, improved antenatal, obstetric and neonatal care, prompt treatment of common infections and training of primary health care workers is immensely valuable and probably cost-effective when compared to the cost of treatment. Improving the health education of village dispensers, teachers and other community leaders in the early recognition of health problems does much to supplement and extend primary health care, while the need for training of medical personnel at all levels is a priority.

Developed countries

Many of the problems facing the poorer countries are not issues for the developed countries where good nutrition, adequate housing, basic education and good health-care are commonplace. There still remain many hazards where preventive action is needed: control of industrial pollution, overcrowding and social deprivation in inner cities, unemployment, poverty, drug and alcohol abuse and smoking. While many problems are the concerns of public health officials and politicians, there is much that the individual can do by altering behaviour to reduce the risk of contracting disease or suffering injury. Health education, both in schools and in the media, is essential to provide information and motivation for individual to adopt healthy life-styles.

Balance disorders

Balance disorders are complex. Normal balance requires the central integration of neural input from the vestibular system, vision, superficial sensation and proprioceptors in the spinal column and limbs. Pathology affecting one or more of these sensory systems, or the central processing of information, can result in a feeling of unsteadiness, instability or dizziness. Because of this complex mechanism of control, balance disorders are difficult to define and measure. Whereas pathology of the labyrinthine end-organ can often be associated with cochlear pathology, this is not always the case. However, preventive measures applicable to cochlear pathology can also result in reduction of vestibular pathology, particularly those arising from genetic or infective causes.

Where the vestibular system is known to be affected by a particular surdogenic insult this will be discussed below but, for the most part, there are few specific primary preventive measures. Nor is screening for vestibular pathology worthwhile, because although labyrinthine dysfunction is common, it may produce no disability. Conversely, balance disorders may be associated with normal peripheral vestibular function. There is, however, a number of tertiary preventive measures which have impact and these will be discussed later.

Tinnitus

This is a common problem causing moderate to severe annoyance for approximately 8% of people in the UK (Coles, 1987). The basic cause of tinnitus is understood to be pathology of the auditory system, although damage may be minimal and not give rise to a measurable hearing impairment. Surdogenic insults of all kinds may lead to tinnitus and therefore the primary preventive measures outlined below are effective. Secondary prevention plays no part in this complaint because, by its very nature, it only gives rise to disability when it is brought to conscious awareness. Tertiary prevention is applicable, as is briefly discussed later in this chapter, but covered in more detail in Chapter 13.

Classification

There are three levels of prevention:

Primary prevention: prevention of pathology by reduction in the causative factors leading to that pathology.

Secondary prevention: prevention or limitation of disability and handicap in those individuals with impairment, by screening for affected individuals prior to clinical presentation and, when possible, providing treatment to prevent progression of pathology and impairment.

Tertiary prevention: prevention or limitation of handicap by early management of disability.

These are illustrated in Figure 8.1, with a subclassification in Table 8.1.

Table 8.1 Subclassification of the three levels of prevention

1 Primary prevention

Genetic
Infective
Traumatic
   noise
   physical trauma
   barotrauma
Ototoxic and vestibulotoxic drugs
Perinatal factors
Environmental and socioeconomic factors

2 Secondary prevention

Screening
Treatment

3 Tertiary prevention

Specific to hearing disorders
Specific to balance disorders

Primary prevention

The impact of a variety of primary preventive strategies, both specific and general, over the last century has been considerable. Effective prevention of some categories of audiological disease has been the result of improved public health and education, as well as an increased understanding of disease pathogenesis in general and the effects of surdogenic insults in particular. As a consequence, the aetiological profile of the hearing-impaired community in developed countries has altered markedly in recent decades. The incidence of chronic suppurative otitis media has fallen, as has congenital rubella syndrome and rhesus incompatibility, but there still remains the need for a wider application of preventive knowledge. The need for further research into causative factors of hearing and balance disorders is unquestioned. Prevention of disease in poorer countries lags markedly behind and much needs to be done to improve health provision and uptake of preventive care.

Genetic hearing loss

It is recognized that a significant proportion of hearing disorders have a genetic basis. There have been numerous studies into the aetiology of childhood hearing disorders in recent years. Although actual figures vary according to the population studied, the degree of hearing loss and the depth of investigation, findings have been fairly consistent in developed countries: about 45% of cases can be attributed to identifiable genetic causes, 30–35% to acquired causes and 20–25% to unknown causes, of which most are

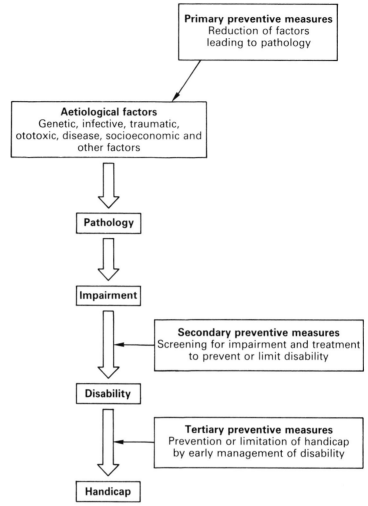

Figure 8.1 The three levels of prevention

likely to be genetic (Cremers, Van Rijn and Hageman, 1989).

Of the acquired hearing losses, evidence is accumulating to support a genetic predisposition to various ototoxic insults. Patients with brown eyes have been shown to have a greater tendency to hearing impairment as a result of cis-platinum therapy, the presumption being that the drug is bound to melanin in the stria vascularis (Barr–Hamilton, Matheson and Keay, 1992), whereas brown eyes, again due to a greater concentration of melanin, are protective when noise exposure is considered (Hood, Poole and Freedman, 1976; Carter, 1980). A familial tendency to ototoxic damage with streptomycin has been described and Higashi (1989) and Hu *et al.* (1991) attributed this tendency to mitochondrial inheritance. Barr (1982) suggested a genetic susceptibility to congenital ru-

bella infection. There are also well-recognized familial tendencies to the development of 'presbyacusis' and otitis media. Thus genetic predisposition could explain the variable effect of surdogenic insult between individuals and within families.

There are two facets to the issue of prevention with reference to genetic hearing loss: there is the question of prevention for an individual and his family; and there is the wider question of prevention within the community as a whole.

Prevention within the community

Consanguinity

Probably the most important factor when one considers prevention within the community is the question of consanguineous marriages. It is evident that consanguineous matings increase the expression of recessive genetic characteristics and, in societies such as isolated communities, where consanguineous matings are common there can be a high incidence of hearing loss. For example, Kloepfer, Laguaite and McLaurin (1966) described a high incidence of Usher's syndrome in the Arcadian population of Louisiana where, by virtue of religious and geographic isolation, there was marked inbreeding. Similar clusters of other recessively inherited conditions have been described and Vanniasegaram, Tungland and Bellman (1993) recently showed a high incidence of deafness occurring in a Bengali community in East London where, for cultural reasons, marriages between cousins are relatively common.

Avoidance of consanguinity in these tight-knit communities would obviously be a useful preventive factor. In a recent paper from Israel (Feinmesser, Tell and Levi, 1990) it was noted that a decrease in the prevalence of congenital hearing impairment was related to a decrease in the rate of consanguinity among parents. Improvements in education, both secular and religious, regarding the risks involved, together with the increasing population mobility and ethnic interbreeding should decrease the incidence of consanguineous marriages and go some way to preventing deafness (Holborrow, 1985).

Assortive mating

The assortive mating of deaf with deaf individuals can increase the risk of expression of recessive characteristics. Improved amplification has led to increased integration of the hearing-impaired, both in educational settings and in the work-place. This advance may lead to fewer assortive matings and although a relatively minor factor, may play some role in prevention.

Prevention for the individual

Fundamental to offering preventive advice to the individual and his family is an accurate diagnosis of the cause of hearing impairment. The importance of this cannot be underestimated. The diagnosis enables the doctor to provide an explanation to the patient and his family, and this information can itself aid acceptance and understanding of the sensory impairment. In addition, knowledge of the pathogenesis enables the audiologist to advise on prognosis for the individual, and it opens the way for effective but non-directive genetic counselling. Furthermore, diagnostic labels advance our knowledge and understanding of the heterogeneity of the hearing impaired population which, in turn, will enhance our preventive capabilities.

The diagnosis of a genetic hearing loss is based on the following factors:

A detailed family history

A positive family history of the same kind of hearing loss may indicate the pattern of inheritance, i.e. autosomal dominant, autosomal recessive, X-linked or mitochondrial. Such a pattern may only be apparent in a large family, particularly with recessive inheritance, and in these days of reduced family size a definite pattern may not emerge. However, the lack of such does not exclude an inherited cause. In fact, Taylor *et al.* (1975) suggested that those children in whom, after full investigation, the cause of the hearing loss is unknown should be considered as having a genetically determined hearing loss, either recessively inherited or a new mutation. This point is controversial, but certainly a genetic cause is a distinct possibility in these children.

For more details on the genetics of hearing disorders please refer to Chapter 3 in Volume 6.

Syndromic markers

The recognition by the clinician, after examination and investigation, of other markers constituting a syndromic condition aids diagnosis, e.g. the white forelock or heterochromia iridis of Waardenberg's syndrome, or the widened QT interval on ECG of Jervell Lange–Nielsen syndrome. These markers are numerous and diverse and can be subtle. Knowledge of their importance to the eventual diagnosis is an essential element of training for those managing the hearing impaired.

Absence of acquired cause of hearing impairment

The history of definite surdogenic insult suggests the diagnosis of an acquired hearing loss as opposed to a genetic defect. However, the existence of a multifactorial aetiology must also be borne in mind, and the presence of a risk factor such as neonatal hypoxia or hyperbilirubinaemia must be considered critically; a mother's history and recorded medical facts may not agree.

Identification of carriers

Evidence of carrier status in other members of the family, particularly the obligate carriers, may clarify a diagnosis of a genetic condition. In those conditions with variable expressivity, such as Waardenberg's syndrome and Treacher Collins syndrome, other markers of the syndrome can be apparent in members of the family, e.g. areas of pigmentation or abnormal facial features. A minor degree of hearing impairment may be detected on routine pure tone audiogram of family members. The presence of abnormalities leading to recognition of carriers is variably reported, and several papers suggested that it may be possible to identify carriers of Usher's syndrome and Alport's syndrome by observing notches or dips in either Békésy audiogram (Anderson and Wedenberg, 1968) or the Audioscan (Meredith *et al.*, 1992) or hearing loss in very high frequency audiometry, above 12 kHz.

Examination of family members for evidence of carrier status should form part of the investigation of the newly diagnosed hearing-impaired child where the aetiology is in doubt.

Gene mapping

Advances in gene mapping and in the identification of mutations responsible for the various hearing disorders have been a feature of recent research. Work has been largely based on families displaying inherited deafness, but comparative studies using mice have also been valuable in contributing to our understanding of some forms of genetic deafness. Not only does this work demonstrate something of the complexity of genetic coding for normal hearing mechanisms and the heterogeneity of disorders which may present with the same phenotypic pattern but it also enables detection of the exact fault in the amino acid sequence in the strand of DNA which is responsible for hearing loss in particular disorders. Furthermore, this knowledge could help detection of carrier status and it is felt by some possibly to point the way for substitution therapy and gene transfer therapy (Snow, 1992).

Genetic counselling

Once the genetic nature of the hearing loss is established or suspected, the individual and his family can and should be offered genetic counselling.

The role of the genetic counsellor is to inform the family of the risks to unborn children of inheriting the condition leading to hearing impairment. The service is of most value when directed at parents who already have one hearing-impaired child and wish to continue procreation, or for young couples, with a family history of hearing loss, about to start a family of their own. It enables a couple to decide whether to embark upon subsequent pregnancies aware of the risks.

Although it is important to determine the exact nature of the inheritance pattern to be able to predict risk accurately, in the absence of such information an empirical risk can be offered which may be altered when more information is available.

Early prenatal diagnosis of major abnormalities allows parents the opportunity to elect for termination of the pregnancy. Chorionic villus sampling, amniocentesis and detailed ultrasound scans are methods enabling prenatal diagnosis of chromosomal abnormalities, e.g. Down's syndrome, recognized familial genetic disease, e.g. muscular dystrophy, or major developmental anomalies, e.g. anencephaly, spina bifida. However, the ethical considerations of offering a termination for non-life-threatening conditions, such as hearing loss, are complex and beyond the scope of this chapter. Nevertheless, prenatal diagnosis and termination of affected fetuses offers a means of prevention of hearing loss which can occur as part of another more disabling condition.

With X-linked conditions, such as muscular dystrophy, there is now an opportunity to decide the sex of the unborn child using sperm separation techniques prior to artificial insemination (Johnson *et al.*, 1993). Again, it is ethically debatable whether the method should be applied to X-linked hearing impairment.

Gene therapy

This new advance in the treatment of conditions with a genetic basis is in its infancy and its ultimate role in the prevention of hearing loss can only be guessed. It is a technique which may have value in conditions where a defective gene leads to an absence of an essential substance, and where it is possible to treat before damage is done. Work in the treatment of children with cystic fibrosis is in progress.

Ethics of genetic counselling

The offer of genetic counselling must be treated with the utmost sensitivity. Most families where hearing loss has a dominant mode of transmission, such as in Waardenburg's syndrome, may be fully aware of the likely expression of the condition and some look on genetic counselling as superfluous to requirements or even as interference. There are others who are too stunned by the birth of their deaf child to accept counselling because of the feeling of 'blame' which may be attached to one partner, or the mother may be pregnant with another child and reluctant to consider the possibility of a second hearing-impaired child. Most hearing-impaired children (particularly the profoundly deaf) are the product of hearing parents who view the challenge of bringing up a deaf child as something to be avoided, and many will voluntarily limit their family even without counselling. But it must not be presumed that all couples seeking advice wish to avoid having a deaf child. Some deaf couples actively wish for a deaf child who will use the same method of communication, namely signing, and be part of the same culture.

Although genetic counselling plays a significant role in the primary prevention of hearing impairment, the aim of the service is not to eradicate deafness. This is probably an unachievable aim and, in some people's eyes, an incorrect one. It serves merely as an information-giving service where the individual is as fully informed as possible about the risks and is made aware of the options they have over treatment or prevention. It should give an opportunity to make a balanced decision as to whether to continue procreation or not, but the ultimate decision lies with the individual.

There are considerable ethical concerns about the question of primary prevention, particularly of genetic deafness. Although hearing individuals believe deafness to be a handicap, many deaf individuals do not see deafness as a disease or abnormality; they see it as a social and cultural variation, the only handicap being the lack of acceptance from hearing society. They belong to a group with a rich language and distinct culture and have pride in this culture. They may perceive research into preventive measures as an attempt to decimate their culture because of the inherent assumption in the term prevention that deafness is to be avoided and is therefore bad. Sensitivity has to be displayed by those investigating the subject of prevention of genetic variation (Grundfast and Rosen, 1992).

Infective hearing loss

A number of infectious diseases are known to cause hearing loss and it is in this particular field that primary prevention is particularly effective. Improvements in housing, sanitation and education over the last century has led to a remarkable reduction in the prevalence of infectious diseases; treatment with antibiotics has also been effective as have the immunization programmes of recent years. The number of people affected in developed countries has fallen dramatically but more needs to be done, particularly in developing countries where infectious diseases are still a major cause of mortality and morbidity, with hearing loss being a significant sequel.

Consideration of specific infective causes is usually temporal viz prenatal and postnatal, because of the differing impact of the timing of hearing loss. However, it is perhaps of greater value to discuss these infections according to the methods of prevention we have at our disposal, with the understanding that some categories, e.g. meningitis, may command more than one major preventive measure. This is illustrated in Table 8.2.

Prevention by immunization

The principle of vaccination is exposure of the individual, either by injection or oral administration, to antigenic material sufficient to cause an immune reaction without overt disease. This immune reaction is then protective against the pathogenic organism. The vaccine used can be live, attenuated (non-pathogenic) organisms, e.g. mumps, rubella and measles, inactivated organisms, e.g. pertussis, or immunizing components of the organism, e.g. part of a virus, or the bacterial capsular polysaccharides, e.g. *Haemophilus influenzae* B vaccine, or toxoids, e.g. tetanus and diphtheria vaccines.

Mumps, rubella and measles are all viral infections which are effectively prevented by vaccination with live, attenuated virus. As man is the only source and reservoir of these viral pathogens, elimination by an effective immunization programme is a possibility. Recent introduction of a single vaccine against these three infections (the MMR vaccine) provides the opportunity to eradicate at a reasonable cost. In the UK, MMR vaccination was introduced in 1987 and is offered to infants of 12–15 months of age. The same vaccine is offered to previously unimmunized children at school entry. Efficacy is reliant on a high uptake of vaccine within the community (at least 95%). In order to achieve this in the USA certificates of vaccination are required at school entry. In the UK there is a financial incentive for general practitioners to achieve high vaccination rates.

As the result of a study (Brobby, 1988) into the aetiological factors leading to deafness in tropical countries, Brobby in 1989 predicted a 50% reduction in the incidence of prelingual deafness in the Third World with effective immunization against 'measles, meningitis, mumps, tetanus and rubella'.

Rubella

Rubella (German measles) is caused by an RNA virus of the togavirus group. It is spread by droplets and is highly communicable, to the extent that immunity at child-bearing age, prior to the introduction of vaccination, was 85–90%. It is a mild febrile illness, usually without sequelae, in children and young adults but it is the teratogenic effect of maternal rubella infection during early pregnancy which has prompted attempts at eradication. Major epidemics occur every 6–9 years and there appears to be variation in teratogenicity with different mutations of the virus. The relationship of epidemics to the subsequent birth of affected infants led to the realization of the effects of rubella. Gregg (1941) described the association of rubella infection in pregnancy with a number of congenital defects and Swan *et al.* (1943) described sensorineural hearing loss as one of the sequelae.

Table 8.2 Methods of prevention

1 *Prevention by immunization*

   a Rubella
   b Measles
   c Mumps
   d Meningitis

2 *Prevention by early treatment*

   a Meningitis
   b Syphilis
   c Toxoplasmosis
   d Lyme disease

3 *Prevention by avoidance and education*

   a Sexually transmitted diseases
   b Toxoplasmosis
   c Cytomegalovirus
   d Lyme disease

4 *Prevention by vector eradication*

   a Lassa fever

The virus produces a generalized chronic infection of the embryo or fetus with inhibition of cell multiplication, leading to deranged and delayed organogenesis. The extent of damage is dependent on the gestational age, with earlier infection causing greater damage than later illness. Infection between the 8th and 10th weeks can result in up to 90% of infants being affected with the congenital rubella syndrome: cataracts, sensorineural deafness, cognitive handicap, cardiac lesions, poor intrauterine growth and inflammatory lesions of the brain, liver, lungs and bone marrow. The risk of congenital rubella syndrome is about 10–20% at 16 weeks and thereafter declines. Sensorineural hearing loss, however, has been described as occurring alone, or with pigmentary retinopathy as the only accompanying sequel, in the middle or even the last trimester of pregnancy. Martin in the EEC survey of 1979 (Martin, 1982a) reported rubella to be the causative factor in 16% of children with losses of 50 dBHL average or greater.

The isolation of the virus in 1962 led to diagnostic laboratory tests for rubella, and the subsequent development and introduction of an effective vaccine in 1972 has done much to reduce the incidence of congenital rubella syndrome. Initially the vaccine was offered in the UK to girls of 10–14 years of age and to women of child-bearing age. The aim of the policy was to increase the incidence of immunity in pregnant women and this aim was achieved; immunity was 85–90% in 1970 prior to the vaccination programme and 97–98% in 1987. The incidence of congenital rubella syndrome decreased, but there re-

mained a pool of rubella with continuing risk of infection. In 1988, in the UK, a new vaccination policy was introduced following other countries such as the USA and Finland that had already found the use of combined MMR vaccine effective. This policy is aimed at reducing the circulation of rubella within the community thus reducing (and eventually eliminating) the risk of infection. MMR vaccine was introduced for children of both sexes aged 12–15 months of age. Immunity is achieved after one injection in 90% or more, and should be life-long, although cases of congenital rubella syndrome have been reported in previously immunized mothers (Keith, 1991).

It is an accepted part of antenatal care in the UK to establish rubella immunity status for every pregnancy regardless of previous test results. Non-immune women are offered vaccination after the birth of the child, although the vaccine itself is not considered to be teratogenic. The definitive diagnosis of rubella infection is made serologically and evidence of infection during pregnancy is an indication for offering termination. Treatment with immunoglobulin does not prevent infection but may possibly reduce risk to the fetus and is recommended if termination is unacceptable.

The current vaccination programme has led to a dramatic reduction in the number of rubella cases (a notifiable disease since 1988) in the UK. In 1991 there were only 15 serologically-confirmed cases of rubella in pregnant women reported to the CDSC (Communicable Diseases Surveillance Centre) compared with 164 in 1987. Termination of pregnancy for rubella infection has shown a similar trend; 738 in 1972 and 10 in 1992 (HMSO, 1992). Similar effects of vaccination have been reported in the USA and other countries. Clearly, effective vaccination programmes have a significant preventive effect and adoption of similar immunization policies by developing countries is required.

Measles

Measles is a particularly contagious disease caused by an RNA virus of the paramyxovirus group. It is one of the exanthematous illnesses of childhood with epidemics occurring every 2–3 years. A mixed hearing loss is one of the more common sequelae. Complication rates are high; in the UK, otitis media occurs as a complication in 5–9% of cases and pneumonia in 1–6%. Measles encephalitis is an uncommon but serious complication, occurring in approximately 0.1% of cases and is associated with a mortality rate of 15% with a further 25–35% developing permanent neurological sequelae such as sensorineural hearing loss (HMSO, 1992; Orenstein, Markowitz and Hinman, 1992). Another rare complication (one in every 100 000 cases) is subacute sclerosing panencephalitis. A 0.1–0.2% death rate overall has been quoted for the USA but the complication rate is much higher in developing countries where the death rate can reach 20%, with a complication rate of over 80% in some series (Clements *et al.*, 1992). Factors predisposing to complications include young age, over-crowding, malnutrition and coincident infections. Brobby (1988) ascribed as many as one-third of acquired cases of hearing impairment in Ghana to measles.

Measles has been a notifiable disease since 1940 in the UK and, prior to the introduction of vaccine in 1968, approximately 95% of the urban population had been infected by the age of 15 years. Prior to 1968, cases of measles varied between 160 000 and 800 000 per annum but widespread vaccination led to a reduction to between 50 000 and 180 000 cases per annum in the 1970s. MMR vaccination (see above) was introduced in 1987 for infants of 12–15 months, leading to reporting of only 9985 cases in 1991 with no deaths among children during 1990 and 1991. In developing countries, because of a high rate of complications during the first year of life, the vaccine is given at 9 months of age. Although vaccination rates of over 90% are being achieved in developed countries, vaccination programmes in developing countries are hampered by limited finances and personnel.

Mumps

Mumps is an infective illness, characterized by parotid swelling, which is caused by an RNA virus of the myxovirus group. Spread is by direct contact or droplets and about one-third of cases are subclinical. Complications include oophoritis, orchitis, pancreatitis, meningitis, encephalitis and sensorineural hearing loss. Meningeal signs are seen in about 15% of cases, while encephalitis occurs in approximately 0.5% of cases and carries a 1.4% death rate. Sensorineural hearing loss is reported as occurring in 0.5–5.0 cases per 100 000 cases of mumps (Stehr–Green and Cochi, 1992). The loss is generally unilateral and often total, although bilateral losses have been described. In the UK, mumps has been a notifiable disease since 1988 following the introduction of the MMR vaccine. Prior to vaccination, hospital admissions for mumps were around 1200 per year with an estimated average of approximately 6.5 cases of mumps/100 000 population. Since vaccination there were only 2924 cases in total notified in 1991 (an average of <1 case/ 100 000 population) (HMSO, 1992). In the USA vaccination has been available since 1967 and in routine use since 1977. The result has been a dramatic reduction in the number of cases reported, from 185 691 in 1967 to 4866 in 1988 (Stehr–Green and Cochi, 1992).

Meningitis

Meningitis is the most common cause of severe acquired deafness in childhood, accounting for up to 90% of such acquired impairments in the UK. Incidence figures generally vary between 6 and 10% of the hearing-impaired population, although Davis, in 1993, stated an incidence of 18% among profoundly deaf children with 12% among the severely hearing impaired and 3% of those with moderate losses. Fortnum (1992) quoted reports giving figures between 3.5 and 37.2% of those surviving meningitis having some degree of hearing impairment. Immunization against some organisms which cause meningitis, is available.

Haemophilus meningitis

Haemophilus influenzae is a Gram-negative coccobacillus and a major cause of infections in man. Invasive disease is associated with a high rate of morbidity and mortality and is caused by the encapsulated strains of the bacteria of which six types (a–f) are known to be pathogenic to man (Drugs and Therapeutics Bulletin, 1993). Over 99% of invasive infections are due to type b (Hib); and affect 34 per 100 000 children per year, i.e. one in 600 children will develop illness due to Hib before the age of 5 years. Sixty per cent of these cases are meningitis, 15% epiglottitis, and 10% septicaemia. *H. influenzae* is responsible for 45% of all cases of meningitis. The mortality rate from meningitis is 4–5% with 11–30% developing permanent neurological sequelae such as sensorineural hearing loss. The disease has a high incidence between the ages of 3 months and 4 years, with a peak at 10–11 months of age. There had been an increase in cases in the 1980s in the UK from 869 cases reported in 1983 to 1259 cases reported in 1989 (HMSO, 1992). The non-encapsulated strains are associated with respiratory tract infections including otitis media.

Vaccines against *H. influenzae* were first introduced in the 1970s but were ineffective in very young children. Recent developments, whereby the capsular component, polyribosylribitol phosphate, is conjugated with either tetanus or diphtheria toxoids, have increased their immunogenicity particularly in the very young. An immunization programme was introduced in October 1992 in the UK whereby Hib vaccine is given to infants as part of their primary immunization from the age of 2 months. The vaccine has previously been used in both the USA and Finland and found to be very effective in reducing the incidence of invasive disease. Early reports indicate a marked reduction in cases of haemophilus meningitis in the UK since immunization.

Meningococcal meningitis

Meningococcal meningitis accounts for up to 50% of cases of deafness occurring as a result of meningitis, although it causes only 15–25% of cases of bacterial meningitis. *Neisseria meningitidis* or the meningococcus is a Gram-negative diplococcus which gives rise to both meningitis and also meningococcal septicaemia, which can occur alone or in association. Asymptomatic nasopharyngeal carriage rates are around 10% (4–25%: Klein, Heyderman and Levin, 1993) and spread is by droplets or direct contact from carriers or individuals incubating the disease. The bacteria can be classified into antigenically different groups, of which A, B, C, Y and W135 are the most common. Group B organisms are the major cause of disease in the UK, but group C organisms can be responsible for institutional outbreaks. In other parts of the world the risks of contracting meningococcal disease are relatively high with groups A and C causing many major epidemics. The aptly named 'meningitis belt' of Africa, lying between 15° and 5° North, being one such place.

The course of the disease can vary between being rapidly fatal within hours of the first symptoms to a more insidious and mildly progressive illness. The maximum incidence is in infants and small children, with another peak of occurrence in teenagers and young adults. Mortality is quoted as being 10%; 1–4% of cases suffer bilateral profound sensorineural hearing loss.

Vaccines are available against groups A, C, Y and W135 and are used to combat small outbreaks as well as more widespread epidemics. There is no vaccine available for group B meningococcus, and instead, prophylaxis (oral rifampicin) for contacts of a confirmed case is recommended, with vaccination only if the illness is caused by group C (or rarely group A) bacteria. In the epidemic areas mass vaccination is considered to be of value, although reports suggest that seroconversion in children is low (Klein, Heyderman and Levin, 1993) and long-term protection is poor (Ceesay *et al.*, 1993).

There is a need for more research into long-term effective vaccines against all strains of the disease.

Pneumococcal meningitis

There is no effective vaccine against pneumococcal meningitis, although vaccines have been developed to combat other pneumococcal diseases.

Streptococcus pneumoniae is an encapsulated Gram-positive coccus. There are about 84 recognized strains of which 23 types cause 90% of cases. Infections with pneumococcus are relatively common and carry a high mortality and morbidity rate. The pneumococcus is responsible for about one-fifth of the cases of bacterial meningitis, with a mortality rate of 50%, and with 25% or more of survivors having residual neurological problems of which sensorineural hearing loss is common. The vaccine currently available is against the 23 commonly pathogenic capsular types of pneumococcus and is reported as being 60–70% effective in preventing pneumococcal pneumonia. Consequently, it is of particular value postsplenectomy. Its efficacy in children is reduced, particularly in those under 2 years of age, and it does not prevent otitis media nor exacerbations of chronic bronchitis. As these primary infections lead on to pneumococcal meningitis this vaccine therefore has little value as a preventive agent against meningitis. Research is continuing into vaccines against this disease.

Prevention by early treatment

Meningitis

There is evidence that prompt treatment of meningitis reduces the morbidity and mortality of this infection. Klein, Heyderman and Levin (1993) recommended penicillin as the first-line treatment of choice for meningitis, although third generation cephalosporins have an improved spectrum of activity because of emerging resistance to penicillin among the bacteria concerned (Nathavitharana and Tarlow, 1993). It is recommended practice to initiate treatment at home, with parenteral penicillin, on clinical suspicion of meningitis prior to urgent transfer to hospital (Cartwright *et al.*, 1992; Strang and Pugh, 1992). However, as some authorities believe hearing loss occurs early in the illness, the efficacy of early treatment in the prevention of deafness is questioned (Fortnum, 1992). Cremers, Van Rijn and Hageman (1989) stated that since the widespread use of antibiotics the death rate for meningitis had fallen by 50%.

The use of steroids, in particular dexamethasone, is recommended as an adjunct to antibiotic therapy in some cases of meningitis. Administration has been shown to reduce mortality and also to reduce the incidence of hearing loss and other neurological deficits following infection with *Haemophilus influenzae* and also pneumococcus (Odio *et al.*, 1991). There is no evidence of benefit with meningococcal disease.

Syphilis

Syphilis is a sexually transmitted disease known from earliest times. It is spread by direct mucosal contact or by inoculation (e.g. needle-sharing). The causative organism is the spirochaete, *Treponema pallidum*, which is sensitive to penicillin. Adequate treatment of syphilis in its primary stage of the chancre, prevents further pathology, but once the disease has entered its tertiary stage, sensorineural hearing loss can develop as a result of involvement of the cochlea. Reports on treatment at this stage have been variable. It is generally felt that antibiotic treatment will slow down progression but may not improve the hearing loss. However, Gleich, Linstrom and Kimmelman in 1992, reported improvements in symptomatology among about one-quarter of patients treated with penicillin and steroids. They concluded that the earlier treatment is started the better the results are likely to be.

Congenital syphilis is also associated with a progressive sensorineural hearing loss, but antenatal diagnosis and treatment can prevent fetal infection. Therefore, preventive strategies include routine antenatal serological monitoring.

Toxoplasmosis

Toxoplasmosis is an infection caused by the protozoan *Toxoplasma gondii*. Transplacental colonization can occur, resulting in a generalized infection of the fetus with sensorineural hearing loss as a possible sequel. Toxoplasma is carried by domestic cats and dogs and is present in their excrement. There is a marked variation in incidence between countries with a high incidence in the tropics and undeveloped areas. Although rates of infection are low in the UK, they are significantly higher in the USA. The world-wide figures show 0.1–1% of pregnant women become infected and in 40% of these cases the child is also infected (Stray–Pedersen, 1993).

Most pregnant women who become infected are asymptomatic, although symptoms of a mild 'flu-like illness with lymphadenopathy are sometimes noticed. The risk of congenital infection increases with advancing gestation, from 20% in the first trimester up to 65% in the third (Bakht and Gentry, 1992). Most infected infants are asymptomatic at birth, but up to 85% develop sequelae including chorioretinitis, sensorineural hearing loss ('educationally significant in 10–15%', McGee *et al.*, 1992) and cognitive impairment.

Early recognition and treatment is effective in reducing placental colonization by 60% or more. Diagnosis is made serologically either by routine antenatal screening or following overt illness. Confirmation of infection in the fetus is obtained from an umbilical cord blood sample, or by serial ultrasound scans to identify abnormalities suggestive of infection, e.g. enlarged cerebral ventricles, intracranial calcifications, ascites, hepatomegaly and increased placental thickness (Bakht and Gentry, 1992). The drugs of choice are pyrimethamine and sulphadiazine. Pyrimethamine is contraindicated in the first trimester, in which circumstance spiramycin is the initial medication of choice with a change to pyrimethamine and sulphadiazine when infection of the fetus is confirmed.

Prompt antibiotic treatment reduces the risk of fetal infection and also modifies established infection. For the child with evidence of congenital infection, treatment during the first year of life improves the prognosis. McGee *et al.* (1992) reported no sensorineural hearing loss in 30 treated children.

Although treatment is effective in reducing disease transmission, prevention of infection by avoidance must also be practised (see below).

Lyme disease

This is a tick-borne infection caused by the spirochaete *Borrelia burgdorferi*. It is prevalent in many areas of the world, e.g. North America, Europe, China and parts of Russia. Transmission is by *Ixodes dammini* ticks which feed on deer, sheep and other large mammals, including humans. The other hosts for the larval and nymph stages of the tick are small rodents which harbour the spirochaete. The illness is not dissimilar to syphilis and gives rise to multiple skin lesions, arthritis, myocarditis, aseptic meningitis and cranial or peripheral polyneuritis. Sensorineural hearing loss and vertigo have been described. Early treatment prevents progression of pathology. Even delayed treatment may lead to improvement in symptoms of vertigo and in hearing thresholds (Hanner, Rosenhall and Kaijser, 1988).

Prevention by avoidance and education

Sexually transmitted disease

Marked changes in sociosexual behaviour in recent years have affected the epidemiology of sexually transmitted diseases. The 1960s heralded increased promiscuity, particularly among young adults, and the 1970s brought the public acceptance of homosexuality. Both these changes in attitude have affected the prevalence of venereal disease. In addition, drug abuse and addiction has led to an increase in needle-sharing for parenteral administration as well as the exchange of sex for drugs or for money to buy drugs. As a result of these changes the incidence of gonorrhoea and herpes increased in the 1960s and 1970s, while that of syphilis and AIDS rose during the 1980s.

Acquired immune deficiency syndrome (AIDS) is a sexually transmitted disease which has been reported to be associated with sensorineural hearing loss, vertigo and tinnitus as well as middle ear pathology (Rarey, 1990; Birchall *et al.*, 1992). In the 1980s, AIDS was prevalent in the homosexual population but the adoption of 'safe sex' has led to a decrease in incidence among this group in the 1990s, along with a concomitant decrease in the incidence of syphilis. Adoption of the policy of 'safe sex' demonstrates the effectiveness of education as a means of prevention: the routine use of the condom and a reduction in casual sex has been effective in avoiding spread of infection. Thus the explosion in cases originally predicted has not occurred. Heterosexual transmission has not halted, however, both in the developed world, and most particularly the developing world where AIDS is a major cause of morbidity and premature death.

Herpes simplex virus type 2 (HSV-2) is associated with genital herpes and is prevalent, with 10–20% of adults having positive serology (Andersen, 1992). Of concern is the effect of perinatal infection which can give rise to a severe multisystem disease, of which hearing impairment is a known complication. Infection is acquired through direct contact with herpetic lesions in the birth canal or secretions, or through nosocomial spread by hospital personnel. Prevention is by performing Caesarian section when the mother is known to have active herpetic lesions at the time of delivery. Nosocomial spread can be prevented by proper ward hygiene.

Although most sexually transmitted diseases can be effectively treated there is, as yet, no cure for herpes nor for AIDS, and so avoidance is the only preventive measure. Education begins with the young at school but the message must be spread by all methods of communication to the entire population on a world-wide basis.

Toxoplasmosis

Infection by *Toxoplasma gondii* is by ingestion of oocysts present in contaminated soil or food, ingestion of undercooked meat containing cysts and transplacentally. A campaign in the USA informing pregnant women of the risks to the unborn child of toxoplasmosis and giving practical advice on avoidance, is gaining widespread acceptance (Bakht and Gentry, 1992). The incidence of toxoplasma infection in the UK is not high but there is a need for similar information to be available to the public.

Cytomegalovirus

Human cytomegalovirus (HCMV or CMV) is a herpes virus which is widespread and causes a generally mild illness. Most adults possess antibodies. However, infection of the developing fetus can cause severe life-threatening disease. Approximately 10% of infected neonates have symptomatic infections characterized by petechial rash, jaundice, hepatosplenomegaly, chorioretinitis, thrombocytopenia or anaemia (Bale, 1992). The mortality rate is approximately 30%. Survivors frequently have neurological sequelae, e.g.

visual loss, hearing loss, and intellectual disability. Asymptomatic infants are also at risk of developing sensorineural hearing loss and other neurological sequelae. Accurate figures for cytomegalovirus as a cause of hearing impairment are not known, as the diagnosis of infection must be made within the first few weeks of life, prior to presentation with hearing impairment. Positive serology later in the first year of life may indicate acquired infection which is a mild illness and is not associated with hearing impairment.

Studies world-wide indicate that 0.5–3.0% of infants excrete cytomegalovirus in their urine at birth. The virus is excreted in milk, urine, saliva, blood, tears, semen or cervical secretions and transmission is by direct contact. At present there is no effective vaccination, although research is progressing. Prevention is by good hygienic practice: washing of hands, disposing of soiled articles such as nappies, and the use of condoms to reduce sexual transmission.

Lyme disease

There are a number of steps recommended to reduce the risks of acquiring Lyme disease: if possible avoid tick-infested areas, keep legs and feet well-covered, use insect repellents on exposed skin and frequently inspect and remove ticks on clothing or skin when in high-risk areas.

Prevention by vector control

Lassa fever

Lassa fever is an acute febrile illness which is endemic in West Africa. It is caused by an arenavirus carried by the rodent *Mastomys natalensis*, a small rat-like animal. The virus is excreted in the animal's urine, but person-to-person transmission can also occur. Mortality is high (approximately 16% in hospitalized cases; Monath and Johnson, 1992) and sudden sensorineural hearing loss is a known complication (White, 1972; Cummins *et al.*, 1990; Cummins, 1992).

Preventive measures against Lassa fever must include control of the rodent population in endemic areas, as well as research into effective vaccination.

Traumatic hearing loss

Noise

That noise leads to cochlear damage is well documented and is covered in detail in Chapter 11. The prevention of noise-induced hearing loss is an important topic, particularly in the industrialized world where noisy machinery has increasingly become part of every-day life.

Present EU (European Union) legislation regarding the permissible noise exposure in the workplace is designed to give protection to those employed in noisy industry. The implementation of this act is a most important preventive measure. Although legislation on noise is now uniform throughout the EU, developing countries often lack the financial reserves to implement preventive measures, which include reduction of noise emission where possible, acoustic screening of noisy areas, the wearing of effective ear-defenders and limitation of noise exposure as well as continuing education of the work-force and employers.

Physical trauma

Trauma to the ear or otic capsule can give rise to both vestibular and auditory impairment. Most trauma is preventable.

Noise occurring as a result of leisure pursuits is another area of concern.

Iatrogenic

Inexpert syringing and attempts at removal of foreign bodies from the ear canal are common causes of trauma and are prevented by adequate training of doctors and nurses. Trauma during ear surgery leading to hearing impairment or vestibular damage is reduced with training and experience and it is well recognized that surgeons in training have a higher incidence of complications than experienced surgeons. This has been illustrated with regard to stapedectomy where the incidence of 'dead ear' is lower in those surgeons with the greatest experience and expertise. This supports the need for adequate training and supervision of young surgeons and for increasing specialization (otologists among otolargyngological surgeons) with centralization of certain procedures which are infrequently performed, such as stapedectomy. Also supported is the need for peer review, or audit, of clinical practice and continuing education of consultants, both of which needs are currently being addressed in the UK.

Radiation

Therapeutic radiation to the head and neck, particularly for tumours of the parotid gland or nasopharynx, can include the ear and eustachian tube within the radiation field. Effects include middle ear effusion as a result of oedema of the nasopharynx and also sensorineural hearing loss. The sensorineural hearing loss tends to be high frequency and can occur as a late complication. Prevention includes the careful choice of radiation fields in order to limit or avoid exposure of the cochlea (Schot *et al.*, 1992).

Car accidents

The introduction of legislation regarding the wearing of seat belts in the UK has led to a marked decrease in the number of trauma cases as a result of road traffic accidents. This is particularly so with regard to head and chest injuries. Legislation on wearing helmets while riding a motorcycle has had similar effects. As a result helmets are now popular wear for cyclists of all ages, skateboarders, rollerskaters, cricketers and anyone participating in sports where there is an increased risk of head injury. The spin-off from this growing market has led to more effective protection – light-weight, comfortable, and even fashionable, headwear.

Head restraints are another preventive measure and have succeeded in lowering the incidence of whiplash injury, which is a common cause of vertigo and imbalance, probably as a result of disruption of the normal cervical proprioceptive input into the vestibular system. Other safety systems in cars have led to a reduced risk of impact (e.g. anti-locking brakes), greater shock absorption (e.g. crumple zones) and protection (e.g. air bags) from the effects of impact. These have all had an indirect preventive effect on ear trauma by reducing the incidence of head injury.

One can also regard public education and enforced legislation on drink-driving and speeding as preventive measures.

Childhood accidents

In recent years an increased regard for safety in children's playgrounds has been noticeable; the introduction of dense rubberized tiles or of a thick layer of pieces of tree bark to replace hard tarmac is aimed at reducing injury. Stair gates, straps and reins serve a similar preventive function. Equipment is designed to provide fun while limiting danger and the many safety devices available today go some way towards prevention of head injury and thus also ear trauma.

Barotrauma

The effect of variation in atmospheric pressure, or dysbarisms, on the ear is well recognized and documented. Barotrauma occurring as the result of exposure to reduced pressure, first reported following a balloon descent in the late eighteenth century, is an important factor in aviation medicine. However, it is in the field of underwater diving and hyperbaric pressure changes that barotrauma assumes major significance. In recent years, advanced technology has resulted in an increase in the availability and sophistication of diving equipment, which has enabled extended exploration of the seabed, particularly for fuel resources, and has also led to increased popularity of scuba (self-contained underwater breathing apparatus) diving as a sport. Concomitant to the increase in diving has been an increase in the incidence of diving-related injuries and an enhanced understanding of the mechanism of such injuries (Talmi, Finkelstein and Zohar, 1991).

Mechanism

Middle ear barotrauma

Middle ear barotrauma occurs as a result of failure of equalization of air pressure within the middle ear compared to external air pressure. This occurs as a result of poor eustachian tube function. On descent, the comparatively low pressure within the middle ear can lead to otalgia, congestion, and a haemorrhagic effusion with an associated conductive hearing loss and sometimes symptoms of tinnitus and vertigo. The symptoms usually resolve completely.

Middle ear barotrauma is the most common cause of morbidity among divers and pressure workers and can occur with dives as shallow as 2.3 metres. Inherent eustachian tube dysfunction will precipitate the problem, as will failure of pressure equalization by the diver on descent due to inexperience or very rapid descent. Atmospheric pressure increases rapidly over a short distance underwater, necessitating divers to perform frequent Valsalva techniques to maintain equalization; failure to do this leads to 'locking' of the eustachian tube orifice by the greatly increased pressure in the postnasal space. Voluntary opening of the eustachian tube is prevented and pathology results. Middle ear barotrauma also occurs after air travel when it is usually associated with an upper respiratory tract infection, or in the case of children, with poor eustachian tube function.

Inner ear barotrauma

Inner ear barotrauma was first described as a different entity from middle ear barotrauma by MacFie in 1964, although previous reports of permanent sensorineural hearing loss associated with middle ear barotrauma were probably as a result of inner ear barotrauma. The mechanism is similar: the diver uses a forced Valsalva manoeuvre in an attempt to equalize middle ear pressure and the resultant violent increase in pressure causes pathology by either of two proposed routes:

1 *Implosive route* – if the manoeuvre opens the eustachian tube there is massive increase in pressure in the middle ear cavity with either rupture of the round window membrane or disruption of the stapes footplate.
2 *Explosive route* – if the eustachian tube remains

closed the resultant increase in intracranial pressure can be transmitted along a patent cochlear duct or along the internal auditory meatus causing disruption of the round window, the stapes footplate, or even intracochlear membranes.

With either the implosive or explosive mechanism the resultant perilymphatic leak or intracochlear membrane damage gives rise to sensorineural hearing loss and vertigo (Goodhill, 1971).

Decompression sickness

Decompression sickness is another mechanism responsible for sensorineural hearing loss in divers. This occurs when dissolved gas (usually nitrogen) comes out of solution on a diving ascent forming bubbles in soft tissues or blood vessels leading to a variety of symptomatology dependent on the site of pathology, including:

• The major joints leading to pain and sometimes bone necrosis (the bends)
• The spinal cord leading to paraplegia
• The brain stem and inner ear precipitating vertigo and imbalance (the staggers)
• The cochlea and auditory pathways with resultant sensorineural hearing loss
• The pulmonary vasculature leading to respiratory difficulty (the chokes).

Prevention

Air travel

As a significant reduction of ambient pressure occurs even within the pressurized cabins of commercial aircraft, preventive measures are important for all travellers. These include avoidance of air travel during and immediately after upper respiratory tract infections. Most airlines insist on this for their staff but passengers are frequently unaware of the risks taken when travelling even with a mild cold or catarrh. Sucking sweets or sipping drinks facilitate pressure equalization through frequent swallowing and should be encouraged during ascent and descent, particularly for children. The use of topical nasal decongestants, e.g. ephedrine, can be of value.

Diving

Training for divers must include instruction on equalizing pressure within the middle ear. They should not be allowed to dive when unable to equalize pressure in their ears for whatever reason and, if at any stage in a dive, difficulty is experienced the dive should be abandoned. Following middle ear or inner ear barotrauma the advice given regarding further diving is dependent on the precipitating cause, persistent eustachian tube dysfunction being a contraindication. Avoidance of diving is usually recommended to those suffering inner ear barotrauma but a recent report showed that damage does not necessarily recur on subsequent dives and recommended that total abstinence may not be necessary (Parell and Becker, 1993). All patients with middle ear and inner ear barotrauma should be reinstructed on techniques for optimizing eustachian tube function prior to further diving.

Decompression sickness (Caisson disease) following a deep dive is well recognized and international tables exist recommending safe decompression times related to the time and depth of the dive. Flying following a dive should also be discouraged until sufficient time has elapsed for full elimination of nitrogen from soft tissues, which can take several days.

Ototoxic and vestibulotoxic agents

The fact that some drugs and chemicals have ototoxic properties has been known for some considerable time. Evidence exists of the ototoxic effects of mercurial poisoning as far back as the 15th or 16th century BC. Recent research has led to increased knowledge and recognition of a number of toxic agents in use either as therapeutic agents, or in industry. This knowledge, in turn, can be used to prevent or limit exposure and so reduce the damage.

Industry

A number of chemical agents occurring widely in industry as commercial products, waste products or contaminants are recognized as having ototoxic and vestibulotoxic effects. Trichloroethylene, carbon disulphide, toluene, arsenic, mercury, lead and manganese are recognized for their ototoxic properties and xylene, styrene, hexane, butyl nitrate and tin have also been implicated, although evidence is less conclusive for ototoxic damage (Rybak, 1992). There are reports of synergism between the chemicals and noise exposure and also between different chemical substances in the same work-place.

Mercury is well recognized as giving rise to disequilibrium due to effect on the sensory cells, nerve fibres and central brain stem and cerebellar connections. Both lead and manganese are also reported as giving rise to vestibular symptoms as well as hearing loss. Industrial solvents, such as xylene, styrene, trichloroethylene and methylchloroform can give rise to symptoms of fatigue and dizziness, while nystagmus has been demonstrated in studies (Odkvist *et al.*, 1979).

Rybak, in 1992, outlined the evidence of toxicity, citing reported cases in humans and animal evidence, and called for further research. Certainly increased knowledge is essential, but of greater import is the acceptance of the need for tight controls in minimizing exposure to these and other toxic substances, both for the industrial worker and the general public. Minamata disease, a severe neurological disorder resulting from ingestion of fish and shellfish contaminated by mercurial waste effluent from a chemical manufacturing plant in Minamata, Japan in 1953, resulted in many cases of death and of severe disability, and is an illustration of the need for stringent control in pollution world-wide. Legislation, in this respect, is essential, but education to enhance public awareness of the dangers of pollution is equally important.

Abuse

Solvent and drug abuse is reported to be increasing, particularly among the young, and a number of the abused substances (e.g. toluene) are associated with reports of sensorineural hearing loss. Although the incidence is thought to be low, it nevertheless is a preventable problem. Alcohol is well known to cause balance problems; the effects of acute alcoholic intake inducing acute vertigo ('the whirlies'), vomiting and imbalance is a common phenomenon. Alcohol also has a chronic effect on the cerebellum and brain stem leading to poor coordination which, in turn, affects balance.

The increasing abuse of both alcohol and drugs has a multifactorial basis – social, financial, psychological, etc. Preventive measures include improved education in schools and at home in order to increase public awareness, coupled with legislation to penalize those abusing or supplying drugs.

Therapeutic agents

Drug-induced dizziness is very common and has been reported with almost every drug. There is, however, a limited number of drugs where the symptom is a common side effect and in many cases is not unexpected, as in antihypertensives, diuretics, sedatives, tranquillizers and analgesics (Ballantyne and Ajodhia, 1984). In the elderly, multiple drug prescriptions combined with multisensory dizziness can be debilitating and a reappraisal and rationalization of medication is a potent method of management.

In the past both arsenic and mercury have been used as therapeutic agents but, because of toxicity and the emergence of more effective, safer treatment since the 1930s, their use has ceased.

The aminoglycosides are well known for their effects on hearing and balance. Streptomycin was the first developed and was used to treat tuberculosis from 1945. It was seen as a therapeutic breakthrough but the debilitating vestibulotoxic effect was fairly soon evident with both Berg (1949) and Causse (1949) reporting on the pathological changes in the vestibular sensory epithelium. Sensitivity to streptomycin has a familial basis (see above).

The later aminoglycosides are also ototoxic but vary in their effect, some affecting the cochlear hair cells more than the vestibular, e.g. dihydrostreptomycin, neomycin and kanamycin, while others are more vestibulotoxic, e.g. gentamicin, tobramycin and amikacin (Ballantyne and Ajodhia, 1984).

The toxic effects of aminoglycosides are permanent and can continue to have effect after cessation of treatment, due to retention within the perilymph and hair cells. The ototoxic effect is related to serum levels of the drug and there are well established 'safe' levels where therapeutic activity is sufficient and the toxic effects minimal. The dose of aminoglycoside is dependent on renal function and needs to be reduced in cases of renal insufficiency and also in premature babies. Potentiation of the ototoxic effect occurs with the concurrent use of other ototoxic agents such as loop diuretics and also by concurrent exposure to noise (Pye and Collins, 1991). Prevention is afforded by avoidance where possible and by close monitoring of serum levels, both pre-dose and post-dose with appropriate adjustment of dose where indicated.

In developed countries prevention of these ototoxic effects of the aminoglycosides is effectively practised. However, in developing countries there is an increased and unmonitored use of the drugs; not only is tuberculosis still endemic and streptomycin the treatment of choice (Brobby, 1989) but, in addition, these and other antibiotics are available for 'over-the-counter' purchase. There also exists the belief among the populace that parenterally administered drugs are superior in action to oral preparations, and also that antibiotics are 'cure-alls', which has led to misuse of these inexpensive drugs in the Third World with a resultant increase in cases of ototoxicity (Alberti, 1993, personal communication), to the extent that ototoxicity is one of the common causes of childhood deafness in China (Hu *et al.*, 1991). In these areas the need for limiting availability of these drugs and for education into their side effects is urgent.

The safety of aminoglycosides in ear drops has been questioned and limitation of their use, particularly in dry ears with a defect or absence of the tympanic membrane, is recommended.

Cis-platinum

Cis-platinum (cis-dichlorodiammineplatinum II; C-DDP) is an antineoplastic drug which is used as a chemotherapeutic agent for a wide variety of neoplasms in both adults and children. It is known to be ototoxic and to produce a permanent, dose-related, high frequency sensorineural hearing loss. Its effect is said to be enhanced in those patients with brown eyes (because of increased binding to melanin), in those having bolus injections, in those who have undergone cranial irradiation and in children. The reported incidence of hearing loss varies considerably:

in adults the range quoted is 25–86% and in children 84–100% (Pasic and Dobie, 1991). The frequencies affected are 4 kHz and above and losses are often asymptomatic.

Weatherly *et al.* (1991) stressed the need for audiological monitoring before treatment and at regular intervals during a course of treatment particularly after a cumulative dose of 360 mg/m^2. Altering the therapeutic regimen, in the light of hearing loss, is a decision for the oncologist and the patient, but must be made in the knowledge of the effects of progression of the hearing loss.

Teratogenic drugs

Probably the best known and most potent teratogenic drug is thalidomide. This was widely available between 1959 and 1962 and prescribed to pregnant women to counteract the nausea of early pregnancy. It was an effective antiemetic but produced a well-defined pattern of skeletal deformities, affecting mainly the limbs and face, including the ear – external, middle and also the inner ear (Takemori, Tanaka and Sizuli, 1976). In animal experiments the drug has been shown to be almost invariably teratogenic when taken even on a single day during the susceptible period, from the 35th to the 50th day after the last menstrual period (Lenz and Knapp, 1962). The drug was banned when the effects were known and litigation against the drug company pursued. However, the drug has recently been shown to be effective in treatment of leprosy, other skin conditions and AIDS. In particular, the use in South America has grown over recent years with the result that deformities among children as a result of ingestion has increased markedly. Where there is no alternative to this treatment it is essential that the public are made aware of the dangers of the drug so that contraception or therapeutic abortion can be offered. Thus again, education of medical and lay personnel is a vital preventive step.

Many other drugs, e.g. chloroquine, tetracycline, antifungal agents, antineoplastic drugs are known to have teratogenic effects and their use in pregnancy is contraindicated. Since the 1960s research into the effects on the embryo of drugs taken during gestation has been carefully conducted and the results publicized. However, the prescribing of drugs during pregnancy should ideally be limited, using only drugs with a proven record where possible. In addition, prior to prescribing known teratogenic agents, it is encumbent upon the medical practitioner to advise the patient appropriately.

Perinatal factors

There are several preventable factors which pose recognized risks to auditory function during the perinatal period. These factors include hypoxia, hyperbilirubinaemia, neonatal meningitis, aminoglycoside toxicity and noise. Disorders of balance are also common sequelae either because of damage specifically to the vestibular system, as in meningitis, or because of related motor problems, e.g. cerebral palsy, as a result of neurological insult.

Prematurity exposes the infant to an enhanced risk of problems because of the increased likelihood of the above factors occurring alone or together. Advances in knowledge and technology have enabled the survival of increased numbers of very premature babies (28–30 weeks' gestation) with good prognoses. The limits of infant viability are falling and successful resuscitation of 25-week fetuses is not uncommon. Extreme prematurity carries with it increased risk (up to 50% of survivors) of neurological sequelae. The cost of neonatal intensive care is very high and the wisdom of resuscitation of extremely premature infants is actively questioned.

Hypoxia

Hypoxia or asphyxia during the perinatal period is thought to be a major causative factor in developmental problems in the neonate. But, although a history of hypoxia, or anoxia, is commonly elicited for hearing impaired infants, and McCormick and Davis (1994 personal communication) have suggested a definite association between recurrent apnoeic attacks and sensorineural hearing loss, it is now generally considered more likely to be one of a number of risk factors, the combination of which leads to damage. Good antenatal care and obstetric practice minimize the incidence of hypoxia at delivery. These preventive elements, while commonly available in developed countries, are lacking in poor areas.

Hyperbilirubinaemia

Markedly elevated levels of unconjugated bilirubin in the neonate are associated with kernicterus, a neurological syndrome resulting from the deposition of unconjugated bilirubin in the corpus striatum, midbrain and brain-stem nuclei. Clinical manifestations include choreoathetoid cerebral palsy, severe high frequency sensorineural hearing loss and cognitive delay. Common causes of hyperbilirubinaemia include haemolytic disease of the newborn and prematurity. In both cases, liver metabolism (conjugation of bilirubin) is insufficient to cope with demand and the elevated unconjugated bilirubin exceeds the blood–brain barrier limit. Haemolytic disease of the newborn occurs as a result of Rhesus, or occasionally ABO group, incompatibility when the formation of bilirubin as a result of red cell haemolysis is high. In premature infants the primary problem is an immature liver with a slow rate of conjugation coupled with a lower serum threshold for brain damage from un-conjugated bilirubin. In addition, breakdown of red cells may be high as a consequence of concurrent infections.

Reduction in morbidity by prevention of hyperbilirubinaemia has been successful in developed countries over the last 20 years. The preventive measures taken include:

Antenatal care which includes identification of 'at-risk' pregnancies and monitoring of antibody levels through pregnancy in these mothers in order to effect early delivery of affected fetuses.

Monitoring of serum bilirubin levels on all infants with the early introduction of ultraviolet phototherapy or exchange transfusion when indicated.

Exchange transfusion which was introduced in the late 1960s is effective in rapidly reducing unconjugated bilirubin levels and intrauterine exchange transfusion is now practised for severely affected fetuses. The Committee on Fetus and Newborn (1982) recommended the serum bilirubin levels, as a function of the infant's birthweight, at which exchange transfusion is indicated.

Phototherapy using ultraviolet light was introduced as a treatment in the 1970s as it reduces levels of unconjugated bilirubin by breaking down the pigment. By well-timed use the need for exchange transfusion can often be obviated.

Anti-D immunization, which has been available since the early 1970s, is given to all Rhesus-negative mothers before delivery or after the birth of a Rhesus-positive child, and also after all abortions, in order to reduce the formation of Rhesus antibodies. It is the effect of the anti-D antibodies, produced by the mother, on the fetal red cells which results in haemolysis and jaundice.

These preventive steps have been effective in reducing the incidence of kernicterus in developed countries such that it is now a rare occurrence.

Hypothyroidism

Hypothyroidism is a major cause of hearing impairment world-wide, probably accounting for at least 50 000 hearing-impaired infants born each year (Wilson, 1988). The problem is particularly prevalent in those regions of the world where endemic goitre is common, such as the sub-Himalayan regions of the Indian subcontinent, parts of Africa and Latin America. The regular use of iodized salt with further supplementation during pregnancy by iodized oil can prevent deafness due to hypothyroidism. Although the cost of such measures is minimal, iodine supplies are thought to be limited (Wilson, 1990).

Environmental and socioeconomic factors

Improvements in environmental factors and education are among the most potent means of prevention which we have at our disposal. This is particularly evident when one considers middle ear disease which is the most common cause of hearing impairment world-wide.

Socioeconomic factors

It is well recognized that the incidence of chronic suppurative otitis media in children and adults in developed countries has fallen markedly this century. This has coincided with improvement in housing, sanitation, diet and public health. The advent of antibiotics in post-war years has helped fuel the decline in the severity of the problem, as have improved surgical techniques in dealing with early stages of chronic suppurative otitis media. The incidence of the disease still remains high in deprived areas, both in developing and in developed countries, and much needs to be done to reduce morbidity from middle ear disease by attention to socioeconomic factors and improving the general health of the populace.

Education

Education of the public as to the value of diet, hygiene and health surveillance has been shown to be effective. In developed countries baby clinics and antenatal clinics are now accepted as valuable by the general public, and immunization programmes are routine. The result has been a marked reduction in perinatal and infant mortality in recent decades. Infant screening and school health checks are considered part of normal care and, more recently, there is increasing awareness of the value of health screening in the older age groups – 'well-women clinics', cervical smears and breast screening. Prevention of noise-induced hearing loss is part of our legislation as is the wearing of seat-belts. Secondary school children are counselled about healthy life-styles, personal hygiene, safe sex, and the dangers of smoking and drugs.

Recent changes in health education have gone beyond thought of prevention of infectious diseases and survival; current emphasis is on improved lifestyle with maintenance of good health. The value of good hearing and balance is not as apparent as other modalities of health such as heart disease and cancer and more needs to be done to increase public awareness of audiological health.

Prevention programmes in developing countries are still in their infancy, delayed by financial, cultural and educational barriers. Prevention of hearing impairment must be seen as part of the overall process to improve health by improving the socioeconomic status of these areas. Education is fundamental to this process – education of those responsible for provision of care, be it ministerial or practical, and education of the public in the need for uptake.

Smoking

Cigarette smoking is a major cause of morbidity and mortality. In spite of anti-smoking promotions, limitation of advertisements and high taxation, people continue to smoke and young people continue to experiment. Exposure to environmental tobacco smoke has been reported as being associated with an increased incidence of otitis media with effusion and acute otitis media in children (Kraemer *et al.*, 1983; Lyons, 1992; Stenstrom, Bernand and Ben–Simhon, 1993). Association of smoking and sudden hearing loss has not been proven (Matschke, 1991), although the vascular disease associated with smoking is thought to contribute to hearing impairment in old age.

Diet

The importance of a good balanced diet has long been recognized for its role in increased resistance to infection and disease. Education in the UK has resulted in enhanced nutritional status over the last century with consequent improvements in health. Increasing research in recent years continues to supplement our knowledge about diet and its role in disease, to the association of saturated lipids, cholesterol and sugars in the diet with atherosclerosis. Certain aspects of diet therefore have obvious roles in the prevention of ear disease; improved general health has reduced middle ear problems, and reducing the prevalence of atherosclerosis and hyperlipidaemia may lower the incidence or severity of presbyacusis, tinnitus or sudden hearing loss, and also of balance disorders occurring as a result of cerebral ischaemia.

Education as to the advantages of breast-feeding has had partial success in developed countries but, in many areas, it remains a social stigma indicating poverty. Its value in prevention of middle ear disease is in the improved immunity and nutritional status of the infant in early months as well as the modification of the allergic response to milk protein in atopic children.

The association of manioc or cassava, a cereal which forms part of the staple diet in areas of West Africa, with a neuropathy, among the symptoms of which is sensorineural hearing loss and ataxia, illustrates a possible preventive step by adaptation of diet in these areas. Cassava contains cyanide in the form of linamarin and the symptoms of disease are the results of chronic cyanide poisoning (Osuntokun, Monekosso and Wilson, 1969; Hinchliffe, 1983).

Allergy

Nasal allergy is now accepted as one of the aetiological factors in the pathogenesis of otitis media with effusion and, as a consequence of this, also acute otitis media and chronic suppurative otitis media. Treatment using either topical steroid or sodium cromoglycate in combination with allergen avoidance advice to parents of children with otitis media with effusion has been found to be of significant value in treatment and prevention of recurrence of symptoms (Scadding *et al.*, 1993). This advice includes steps to reduce contact with house-dust mite and animal dander, treatment of damp and mould in the house and also avoidance of smoking in the house. Breast-feeding and the avoidance of cows'-milk proteins in the early months of life reduces the allergic response to milk which may be a factor in some children with otitis media with effusion.

Stress

Psychological stress is a potent causative agent of ill health. The vasoconstriction resulting from the adrenergic stress reaction is thought to contribute to the pathogenesis of stress-related illness such as peptic ulceration, migraine and Menière's disease, while the increased efferent tone seen in stressed individuals may explain the association with tinnitus. Dizziness is also perpetuated by stress, leading to poor compensation following peripheral vestibular disturbance.

Modern life in the western world is fast-moving and stressful. The need for stress-management as part of everyday office life is becoming accepted, and the active pursuance of leisure pursuits encouraged. Of infinitely greater value would be education of our young school children on how to cope with stress and how to relax; the old maxim of 'all work and no play makes Jack a dull boy' perhaps should read 'all work and no play makes Jack (and Jill) ill.'

Secondary prevention

This level of prevention encompasses both screening and treatment.

Screening

Screening for disease or impairment forms the basis of secondary prevention programmes, where the aim is to identify the individual at risk at an early stage in order to institute treatment and thus prevent or limit disability and handicap.

Definition

The definition of the term 'to screen' is 'to select, eliminate or sift'. In the words of Northern and Downs (1984), 'The process (of screening) is one of applying to a large number of individuals certain rapid, simple measures that will identify those individuals with a high probability of disorders in the function tested'.

Principles

For a screening procedure to be acceptable a number of criteria must be met:

1 Within the population to be screened the prevalence of the disease is frequent enough, or serious enough, to make mass screening a cost-effective proposition.
2 The disease or condition is amenable to treatment which will improve the expected outcome.
3 Facilities and resources for treatment of the identified individual are readily available.
4 Screening must be cost-effective. The benefits of early identification and intervention must outweigh the costs of screening.
5 A screening protocol must be practically feasible and acceptable to the community; both the members of the public and the medical profession involved.
6 A screening test must exist which will reliably and effectively differentiate between affected and non-affected individuals.

Hearing loss is a condition which lends itself well to the practice of screening, therefore considering these criteria in relation to hearing loss:

1 Hearing loss occurs frequently. The incidence of significant (> 50 dBHL average in the better hearing ear) congenital or perinatal hearing loss is 0.9 to 2/1000 live births and the incidence of hearing loss at school age is 2–4% (Bellman, 1987). Although hearing loss is not a life-threatening condition, delay in appropriate treatment is detrimental to a child's development. The prevalence of hearing loss in the elderly population is high (see below) and it is one of the major causes of disability in the elderly.
2 Hearing impairment is eminently amenable to treatment. Both medical and surgical treatment is valuable in the management of middle ear disease and, although there are limited means of preventing progression of sensorineural hearing loss, rehabilitation is effective in reducing disability and handicap particularly when instituted early.
3 It is unethical to screen for hearing loss, obtain early identification of hearing impairment and then not have the means to offer treatment. Facilities and resources, both medical and educational, sufficient to cater for those individuals identified, must exist prior to the introduction of screening programmes. This is of particular importance in developing countries where enthusiasm to develop screening may lead to overloading of existing limited rehabilitative resources – establishing tertiary prevention must precede secondary prevention.
4 Screening is costly, as is rehabilitation, but the earlier identification of a hearing-impaired individual leads to earlier rehabilitation and improved communication skills. Communication skills are crucial to the individual's independence and his ability to lead an economically productive life. The comparison of an individual dependent on the state compared with one independent and paying

taxes has to make economic sense. The cost-effectiveness of screening for hearing disorders has to be viewed over a long time-span. Of equal importance, but more difficult to quantify, is quality of life for the individual and his family.

5 The screening protocol has to offer benefits which outweigh the inconvenience and problems with screening both for the patient and the professional. In the UK screening of hearing in children is conducted within the school, facilitating coverage. Testing of babies and infants forms part of regular developmental tests which are now accepted as routine as a result of public education. Although the methods and periodicity of testing is under constant reappraisal, nevertheless, the present system is considered of value. Older age groups need more convincing that the benefits are greater than the inconvenience.

6 The screening test must be inexpensive, safe (non-invasive), reliable, sensitive, specific, easy and quick to perform. The disease must be identifiable; pass or fail criteria should be definite and easily differentiated; the population must be accessible. We are fortunate in the tools we have available for screening of hearing impairment, e.g. auditory brain stem responses, transient evoked otoacoustic emissions, distraction testing, pure tone audiogram. These tests are effective and valid but none is perfect and there is continued debate as to the relative merits of each for each particular screen.

Paediatric screening

Hearing impairment can have a marked deleterious effect on the emotional, social and educational development of the child. This can be reduced or avoided by early detection and intervention. Early intervention has been shown to be of value in the development of speech and language. Markides (1986) reported better intelligibility of speech of congenitally hearing-impaired children aided before 6 months of age and Ramkalawan and Davis (1992) likewise found significant correlation between some measures of language, particularly vocabulary and quality of interaction, with the age of intervention.

Screening for hearing loss was introduced for infants of 7–9 months of age in 1938, but the age of detection of significant losses remains unacceptably high (Martin, 1982b; Newton, 1985; Parving, 1991; Watkin, 1991; Davis and Wood, 1992), although a recent paper reported the median age of referral to three well-supported audiological centres to be 12 months of age (Davis, 1993).

Recent advances in technology have made screening for significant hearing impairment in the neonatal period a practicality, and the prospect of reducing the age of detection below 6 months a reality for a high proportion of the congenitally hearing-impaired infants in developed countries.

Neonatal screening

Identifying a hearing-impaired child in the neonatal period allows the earliest possible diagnosis and habilitation. Screening prior to discharge enhances accessibility but, with early discharge policies, time may be at a premium. Testing is relatively expensive in terms of technical time and equipment, depending on the technique used. Facilities for follow up of the test failures must be readily available so that delay is not incurred at this point. Three testing techniques are available: transient evoked otoacoustic emissions, auditory brain-stem responses and the auditory response cradle (or Crib-o-gram). For discussion on the relative merits of each I refer you to Chapter 6 in Volume 6.

The majority of centres performing neonatal screening identify an 'at risk' group, (Table 8.3) usually comprising those babies with a positive family history and those receiving care on the neonatal intensive care unit (NICU). Because of the significantly increased risk of hearing loss in the NICU group, estimated to be approximately 10.2 times that of the non-NICU population (Davis and Wood, 1992), screening of this restricted population is more cost-effective than universal screening, and more easily achieved. However, a recent report from Rhode Island (White, Vohr and Behrens, 1993) demonstrated the practical feasibility of universal screening using transient evoked otoacoustic emissions.

Table 8.3 At risk criteria – Joint Committee on Infant Hearing (1991)

1 Family history of congenital or delayed onset childhood sensorineural hearing loss
2 Congenital infections – toxoplasmosis, syphilis, rubella, cytomegalovirus, herpes
3 Craniofacial abnormalities
4 Birthweight < 1500 g
5 Hyperbilirubinaemia at a level exceeding indication for exchange transfusion
6 Ototoxic medication
7 Bacterial meningitis
8 Severe respiratory depression at birth
9 Prolonged mechanical ventilation for 10 or more days
10 Stigmata or other findings associated with a syndrome
· known to include sensorineural hearing loss (e.g. Waardenburg's or Usher's syndromes)

The 'at risk' criteria (Table 8.3) apply to approximately 7–9% of live births (Bellman, 1987) and of these 2.5–5% have been reported as having a moderate to severe hearing loss (Horsford–Dunn *et al.*, 1987; Joint Committee on Infant Hearing, 1991). Screening on the basis of the 'at risk' criteria will identify 50–70% of the hearing impaired population.

The adoption of a neonatal screening programme does not obviate the need for further screening or surveillance to identify those with moderate, acquired, progressive or late onset hearing impairment, whether sensorineural or conductive.

Infants, preschool and school screens

Screening of children at 7–9 months of age by the health visitor distraction test was initially adopted to detect those with significant sensorineural hearing losses. Current practice viz. neonatal screening combined with increased awareness among child health doctors and health visitors of 'at risk' criteria, as well as improved education of new mothers using information leaflets, has reduced the numbers of those with significant congenital sensorineural hearing loss identified by this route. Nevertheless, the test has value in the identification of those with hearing impairment sufficient to interfere with the normal acquisition of language, either as a result of middle ear disease, or because of moderate, progressive or late onset sensorineural losses. Its use has been criticized in recent years and the results of policies to abandon health visitor distraction test in favour of neonatal screening of at risk babies and surveillance in Berkshire (Scanlon and Bamford, 1990) and Wandsworth are awaited with interest.

Surveillance of language acquisition in the preschool and young school child is advocated as a screen for hearing as well as other communication disorders. The use of a sweep audiogram during the first year at school (British Association of Audiological Physicians, 1989) identifies late onset losses, unilateral losses and persistent middle ear problems, all of which may result in a hearing deficit which constitutes an educational disability.

Elderly

Hearing impairment is much more prevalent in the elderly; at least 90% of those with a hearing loss of 45 dBHL average (over 500 Hz to 4 kHz) in the better hearing ear are over 52 years of age, while approximately 35% of those aged over 50 years have at least a mild hearing loss in their better ear (Davis, 1987). Results of a recent questionnaire conducted in South Wales (Stephens *et al.*, 1990) found the prevalence of hearing disability among 50–65 year olds in two villages to be about 50%, whereas ownership of a hearing aid ran at 7% of the group.

The onset of hearing loss is usually insidious and is often temporally associated with deteriorating vision and mobility. Hearing impairment can lead to frustration, depression and confusion. It affects relationships with family and friends and can result in isolation and dependency. Many believe it to be an inevitable consequence of ageing while some deny its existence because of the social stigma attached to hearing impairment. In general, help is sought late after significant handicap is evident and frequently the patient is too old and set in their ways to be able to take optimal advantage of rehabilitation.

Most patients being fitted for the first time with hearing aids are in their late 60s or early 70s and report problems in hearing for 10–20 years prior to presentation (Stephens *et al.*, 1991). The need for screening for hearing impairment in the older age group is highlighted by a number of authors (Davis, 1987; John, Davies and Stephens, 1989; Weinstein, 1989; Sangster, Gerace and Seewald, 1991; Stephens *et al.*, 1991). The value of a simple questionnaire (Institute of Hearing Research questionnaire) and the forced whisper test as simple inexpensive screening tests for general practice was reported by John, Davies and Stephens (1989). Stephens *et al.* (1991) illustrated the value of a screening programme in the pre-retirement group (50–65 years) using simpler questionnaires to identify those with disability (Stephens *et al.*, 1990). Both papers demonstrated a marked increase in the take up and use of hearing aids with early identification. This can therefore be regarded in some ways as tertiary prevention.

While recent general practitioner contract changes in the UK have encouraged interest in preventive care for the elderly (Tulloch, 1991), there is a need to establish screening for hearing impairment prior to retirement in order to facilitate rehabilitation and to reduce the stigma of hearing loss.

Handicapped

Hearing impairment exacerbates the degree of handicap in those who have an additional problem, particularly visual or intellectual disability. Early recognition of remediable disability, such as hearing loss facilitates rehabilitation and care. In particular those with Down's syndrome are accepted as being at risk of an unrecognized hearing loss because of the high incidence of middle ear disease and also of progressive sensorineural hearing loss which develops in their third decade (Davies, 1988). Screening for hearing impairment should constitute part of regular assessments for intellectually disabled individuals of all ages and in all children with visual impairment. However, because of the difficulty in testing these individuals, these particular 'screens' should be undertaken formally by experienced audiologists in tertiary centres rather than in the community.

Industrial workers

Compensation for cases of noise-induced hearing loss as a result of noise exposure at work has led to routine monitoring of workers' hearing in order to detect early signs of damage and, by reducing exposure, to minimize hearing impairment. Pure-tone audiometry is commonly used, although the method has been criticized (Alberti, 1987). It is time-consuming, inaccurate because of the noisy testing environment, subjective and the learning effect of repeated testing may prejudice early identification of hearing loss

(Hinchcliffe, 1979). Otoacoustic emissions have recently been suggested for screening in this particular field; they are objective, quick, stable, less reliant on a quiet environment and are sensitive to subtle changes in cochlear function which precede audiometric changes (Kemp, 1988; Probst, Harris and Hauser, 1993).

Screening of hearing for industrial workers is becoming accepted preventive practice in the developed world; adoption by developing countries will necessarily follow legislation on noise exposure (see above).

Disorders of balance

Screening for balance disorders is generally inappropriate as vestibular pathology does not necessarily indicate disability nor handicap. Furthermore, disability may not be associated with a measurable impairment. Posturography is probably the only technique which could lend itself to the role of a screening tool in order to predict those liable to fall and may be of some value in a population at risk, such as the elderly. Even then the cost-effectiveness of screening is in doubt.

Treatment

Identification of impairment by screening facilitates prompt treatment to limit the extent of pathology. Certainly, in conditions where the surdogenic insult is recognized early, as in noise-induced hearing loss and cis-platinum treatment, cessation of exposure will limit impairment. In Refsum's disease modification of diet will halt progression of the hearing loss. However, in most cases of sensorineural hearing loss, treatment has a limited effect on impairment, rehabilitation being the treatment of choice.

Middle ear disease, however, is eminently amenable to treatment, and early effective management will prevent progression to chronic suppurative otitis media and subsequent cholesteatoma and sensorineural hearing loss (Alberti, Kapur and Prasansuk, 1993). Chronic middle ear disease is no longer common in the Western world, but is a major cause of morbidity in poorer countries where it is the most prevalent ear disease. In some dry, dusty areas, 90% of children have discharging ears (Holborrow, 1985) and Lundborg (1987) estimated that 4–5% of the population in developing countries is in need of ear surgery. Wilson, in 1988, stated that 5.6% of school-age Burmese children had hearing impairment sufficient to interfere with education and that 80% of these cases were due to otitis media. In 1985 there were reportedly 30–40 otolaryngological doctors to 1 million population in industrialized countries, whereas in Africa there was less than one otolaryngological doctor to 1 million population.

Primary ear care is dependent on early identification by village community workers. Simple first line treatment with antibiotics, aural toilet and ear drops should be readily available and would prevent much chronic disease. Surgical intervention can do much to minimize disability from chronically infected ears and limit the consequent hearing impairment and other sequelae. The establishment of mobile surgical teams in developing countries extends surgical care to the provincial poor and promotes awareness among the public of middle ear disease and its treatment. The success of such teams has been demonstrated in Thailand; the limitation being a shortage of trained personnel as well as finances (Alberti, Kapur and Prasansuk, 1993).

Tertiary prevention

Tertiary prevention is the management of disability in order that handicap may be minimized or prevented. Disability can be defined as the loss or reduction of functional ability of the individual as a result of impairment, and in the context of this chapter, impairment occurs as the consequence of pathology of the auditory or vestibular systems.

The term 'handicap' refers to the adverse effects on the lifestyle of the individual occurring as a consequence of the disability. Handicap, therefore, encompasses effects on social, emotional, educational or occupational aspects of life.

Rehabilitation is the provision of tertiary preventive care. The term implies the restoration, as far as possible, of impaired function, presupposing previously normal function (Stephens, 1987). The term is also used to refer to management for those individuals born with hearing disorders as similar methodology is involved, although the term 'habilitation' may be more appropriate.

Tertiary prevention is a reactive management system which is orientated towards the individual needs of the patient. Management is based on the problems faced by the individual in real-life rather than physiological measurements, such as audiograms or bithermal calorics. A multidisciplinary approach is ideal in order to deliver appropriate and effective assistance in the various different areas of difficulty experienced by the patient. The different components of the rehabilitative process are illustrated by the Goldstein and Stephens model (1981) which is discussed in detail in Chapter 13. A similar multidisciplinary problem-solving approach is appropriate to both paediatric audiological habilitation and vestibular rehabilitation. For more details on these three different fields of rehabilitation you are referred to the appropriate chapters in this volume and in Volume 6.

Tertiary prevention specific to hearing disorders

Provision of appropriate amplification is a main feature of rehabilitation of the hearing impaired and recent advances in technology have extended the options available, enabling more people to benefit from improved amplification. The scope of hearing aids is enormous, the limiting factor being cost. It is not just the cost of provision of hearing aids, but also of well-fitting ear moulds, and the cost of maintenance of equipment (including batteries, which deteriorate rapidly in humid tropical conditions) and training, both for the patient and the provider, which limits the use of amplification in the developing countries. The need to provide inexpensive hearing aids, preferably financed by the state, has been highlighted by Prasansuk (Alberti, Kapur and Prasansuk, 1993). Wilson (1988) recommended the development of solar-powered battery packs.

Other aspects of auditory rehabilitation, e.g. assistive listening devices, communication training including sign language, hearing tactics, vocational training, psychological support, etc. are important as part of an integrated programme incorporating a multidisciplinary approach and tailored to the particular needs of the individual. There is need for similar programmes in the Third World, necessarily modified according to the environment. Of particular importance is the education and support of the family of the hearing-impaired child or adult in order that they can understand the particular and special needs of their family member. The value of the primary care team in delivering education and advice of this sort in poorer countries cannot be underestimated. Holborrow, in 1985, writing about tertiary prevention in tropical countries, stressed the need for early, simple and repeated advice, and for support and education of parents and sibling-mothers (where the older child takes charge of the baby while the mother works) in order to maximize residual hearing and establish communication with a hearing-impaired child.

Tinnitus

Prompt and effective management of tinnitus prevents handicap. A history, examination and audiological tests, with reassurance, discussion and explanation, combined with advice about the value of relaxation and tuition in the rudiments of cognitive therapy are potent but simple psychological tools, the use of which aids rehabilitation enormously. General management includes appropriate use of hearing aids and masking devices with continuing support from a multidisciplinary rehabilitation team. For further information on tinnitus you are referred to Chapter 18.

Education of the general public

Acceptance and understanding of the needs of those with hearing impairment is an important part of prevention. Advances in amplification and educational techniques have enabled integration of hearing-impaired children into mainstream schools and into the work place, but there remain many misconceptions about the ability and the communication needs of the deaf and partially-hearing, leading to unfounded discrimination. This discrimination is particularly evident in poorer countries where the deaf are often denied education and independence. Acceptance of those with disabilities as valuable members of society is a prerequisite for effective rehabilitation.

Tertiary prevention specific to vestibular disorders

Balance disorders lead to limitation of mobility for a significant number of people, mainly the elderly, but often remain unrecognized and untreated. There is a need for greater awareness among professionals of the handicap caused by balance disorders and also of the value of rehabilitation. Rehabilitation follows similar methodology as audiological rehabilitation and the problem-based, multidisciplinary approach is covered in detail in Chapter 22.

General care of the elderly

The elderly are particularly prone to disorders of balance for a number of reasons; age-dependent degenerative changes such as cerebrovascular disease, cardiovascular disease, visual problems and reduced proprioception as a result of arthritic conditions, a multiplicity of drugs and psychological factors result in the so-called multisensory dizziness of old age. Essential to effective management is the investigation and identification of treatable causes, regardless of age.

Prevention of falls in this age group is an important aspect of care. Regular visits to the optician and appropriate spectacles are essential. Chiropody, well-fitting low-heeled shoes, the use of a stick, frame or shopping trolley will maintain mobility. Handrails and grips, non-slippery floors, appropriately arranged furniture are of value in the home, while general practitioners can do much to rationalize drug treatment. Effective social support to enable the elderly to remain in familiar surroundings can prevent confusion and disorientation. Falls are a frequent reason for hospital admission among the elderly, but simple preventive steps can reduce morbidity significantly, and in some cases also mortality.

Conclusion

Preventive strategies are numerous and diverse. The above discussion attempts to illustrate the concept of preventive medicine as applied to hearing and balance disorders but, by its very nature, this discussion cannot be exhaustive. As knowledge advances our preventive ability will increase, but as provision of health care is an expensive commodity, financial resources are a limiting factor world-wide. Health education is a fundamental issue in prevention. It is very much dependent on improved standards of general education in developing countries. In developed countries there remains a need to combat behavioural aberrations, such as drug abuse, smoking, drinking etc., which continue to threaten public health endeavours. Much has already been achieved by preventive strategies in both the developed and developing worlds but still more needs to be done.

References

ALBERTI, P. W. (1987) *Noise and the Ear*. In: *Scott-Brown's Otolaryngology*, 5th edn, edited by A. G. Kerr, vol. 2 *Adult Audiology*, edited by D. Stephens. London: Butterworths. pp. 594–641

ALBERTI, P. W., KAPUR, Y. P. and PRASANSUK, S. (1993) Prevention of deafness and hearing impairment. *World Health Forum*, **14**, 1–12

ANDERSEN, R. D. (1992) Herpes simplex virus. In: *Maxcy–Rosenau–Last Public Health and Preventive Medicine*, edited by J. H. Last and R. B. Wallace. London: Prentice-Hall International UK. pp. 142–144

ANDERSON, H. and WEDENBERG, E. (1968) Audiometric identification of normal hearing carriers of genes for deafness. *Acta Otolaryngologica*, **65**, 535–554

BAKHT, F. R. and GENTRY, L. O. (1992) Toxoplasmosis in pregnancy: an emerging concern for family physicians. *American Family Physician*, **45**, 1683–1690

BALLANTYNE, J. C. and AJODHIA J. M. (1984) Iatrogenic dizziness. In: *Vertigo*, edited by M. Dix and Hood. Chichester: John Wiley & Sons Ltd. pp. 217–248

BALE, J. F. (1992) Cytomegalovirus infections. *Maxcy–Rosenau–Last Public Health and Preventive Medicine*, edited by J. H. Last and R. B. Wallace. London: Prentice-Hall International UK. pp. 144–145

BARR, B. (1982) Teratogenic hearing loss. *Audiology*, **21**, 111–127

BARR-HAMILTON, R. M., MATHESON, L. M. and KEAY D. G. (19) Ototoxicity of cis-platinum and its relationship to eye colour. *Journal of Laryngology and Otology*, **105**, 7–11

BEGG, N. T. (1993) Vaccination: the next ten years (Editorial). *British Journal of Hospital Medicine*, **49**, 83–84

BELLMAN, S. C. (1987) Hearing disorders in children. *British Medical Bulletin*, **43**, 966–982

BERG, K. (1949) The toxic effect of streptomycin on the eighth cranial nerve. *Annals of Otology, Rhinology and Laryngology*, **58**, 448–456

BIRCHALL, M. A., WIGHT, R. G., FRENCH, P. D., COCKBAIN, Z. and SMITH, S. J. M. (1992) Auditory function in patients infected with the human immunodeficiency virus. *Clinical Otolaryngology*, **17**, 117–121

BRITISH ASSOCIATION OF AUDIOLOGICAL PHYSICIANS (1989) *Paediatric Audiological Medicine*. Policy document of the British Association of Audiological Physicians, edited by S. Bellman and S. Snashall. Wembley: Adept Press Ltd

BROBBY, G. W. (1988) Causes of congenital and acquired total sensorineural hearing loss in Ghanaian children. *Tropical Doctor*, **18**, 30–32

BROBBY, G. W. (1989) Personal view: strategy for prevention of deafness in the Third World. *Tropical Doctor*, **19**, 152–154

CARTER, N. L. (1980) Eye colour and susceptibility to noise-induced permanent threshold shift. *Audiology*, **19**, 86–93

CARTWRIGHT, K., REILLY, S., WHITE, D. and STUART, J. (1992) Early treatment with parenteral penicillin in meningococcal disease. *British Medical Journal*, **305**, 143–147

CAUSSE, R. (1949) Action toxique vestibulaire et cochleaire de la streptomycine du point de vue experimental. *Annales d'Otolaryngologie (Paris)*, **66**, 518–538

CEESAY, S. J., ALLEN, S. J., MENON, A., TODD, J. E., CHAM, K., CARLONE, G. M. *et al.* (1993) Decline in meningococcal antibody levels in African children 5 years after vaccination and the lack of effect of booster vaccination. *Journal of Infectious Diseases*, **167**, 1212–1216

CLEMENTS, C. J., STRASSBURG, M., CUTTS, F. T. and TOREL C. (1992) The epidemiology of measles. *World Health Statistics Quarterly*, **45**, 285–289

COLES, R. R. A. (1987) Tinnitus and its management. In: *Scott-Brown's Otolaryngology*, 5th edn, edited by A. G. Kerr, Vol. 2 *Adult Audiology*, edited by D. Stephens. London: Butterworths. pp. 368–414

CREMERS, C. W. R. J., VAN RIJN, P. M. and HAGEMAN M. J. (1989) Prevention of serious hearing impairment or deafness in the young child. *Journal of the Royal Society of Medicine*, **82**, 484–487

CUMMINS, D., MCCORMICK, J. B., BENNETT, D., SAMBA, J. A., FARRAR, B., MACHIN, S. J. *et al.* (1990) Acute sensorineural deafness in lassa fever. *Journal of the American Medical Association*, **264**, 2093–2096

CUMMINS, D. (1992) Rats, fever and sudden deafness in Sierra Leone. *Tropical Doctor*, **22**, 83–84

DAVIES, B. (1988) Auditory disorders in Down's syndrome. *Scandinavian Audiology*, Suppl 30, 65–68

DAVIS, A. C. (1987) Epidemiology of hearing disorders. In: *Scott-Brown's Otolaryngology*, 5th edn edited by A. G. Kerr, Vol. 2, *Adult Audiology* edited by D. Stephens. London: Butterworths. pp. 90–126

DAVIS, A. (1993) A public health perspective on childhood hearing impairment. In: *Paediatric Audiology 0–5 years*, edited by B. McCormick. London: Whurr. pp. 1–41

DAVIS, A. and WOOD, S. (1992) The epidemiology of childhood hearing impairment: factors relevant to planning of services. *British Journal of Audiology*, **26**, 77–90

DRUGS AND THERAPEUTICS BULLETIN (1993) *Haemophilus influenzae* B immunisation. **31**, 1–2

FEINMESSER, M., TELL, L. and LEVI, H. (1990) Decline in the prevalence of childhood deafness in the Jewish Community: ethnic and genetic aspects. *Journal of Laryngology*, **104**, 675–677

FORTNUM, H. M. (1992) Hearing impairment after bacterial meningitis. *Archives of Diseases of Childhood*, **67**, 1128–1133

GLEICH, L. L., LINSTROM, C. J. and KIMMELMAN, C. P. (1992) Otosyphilis: a diagnostic and therapeutic dilemma. *Laryngoscope*, **102**, 1255–1259

GOLDSTEIN, D. P. and STEPHENS, S. D. G. (1981) Audiological rehabilitation: management model I. *Audiology*, **20**, 432–452

GOODHILL, V. (1971) Sudden deafness and round window rupture. *Laryngoscope*, **81**, 1462–1474

GREGG, N. M. (1941) Congenital cataract following German measles in the mother. *Transactions of the Ophthalmological Society of Australia*, **3**, 35–45

GRUNDFAST, K. M. and ROSEN, J. (1992) Ethical and cultural considerations in research on hereditary deafness. *Otolaryngologic Clinics of North America*, **25**, 973–978

HANNER, P., ROSENHALL, U. and KAIJSER, B. (1988) Borrelia infection in patients with vertigo and sensorineural hearing loss. *Scandinavian Audiology*, Suppl. 30, 201–203

HIGASHI, K. (1989) Unique inheritance of streptomycin-induced deafness. *Clinical Genetics*, **35**, 433–436

HINCHCLIFFE, R. (1975) Prevention of disorders of hearing. *Proceedings of the Seminar of the Commonwealth Society for the Deaf*. London: Commonwealth Foundation Occasional Paper, 34 pp. 95–103

HINCHCLIFFE, R. (1979) Epidemiology of hearing. In: *Auditory Investigation: the Scientific and Technological Basis*, edited by H. A. Beagley. Oxford: Clarendon Press. pp. 552–595

HINCHCLIFFE, R. (ed.) (1983) Epidemiology of balance disorders in the elderly. *Hearing and Balance in the Elderly*. Edinburgh: Churchill Livingstone. pp. 227–250

HMSO (1992) Immunisation against infectious diseases. London: HMSO

HOLBORROW, C. (1985) Prevention of deafness in rural tropical areas. *Tropical Doctor*, **15**, 39–41

HOOD, J. D., POOLE, J. P. and FREEDMAN, L. (1976) The influence of eye colour upon temporary threshold shift. *Audiology*, **15**, 449–464

HORSFORD-DUNN, H., JOHNSON, S., SIMMONS, F. B., MALACHOWSKI, N. and LOW, K. (1987) Infant hearing screening: program implementation and validation. *Ear and Hearing*, **8**, 12–20

HU, D. N., QUI, W. Q., WU, B. T., FANG, L. Z., ZHOU, F., GU, Y. P. *et al.* (1991) Genetic aspects of antibiotic induced deafness: mitochondrial inheritance. *Journal Medical Genetics*, **28**, 79–83

JOHN, G., DAVIES, E. and STEPHENS, D. (1989) Predicting who will use a hearing aid. *Practitioner*, **233**, 1291–1294

JOHNSON, L. A., WELCH, G. R., KEYVANFAR, K., DORFMANN, A., FUGGER, E. F. and SCHULMAN, J. D. (1993) Gender preselection in humans? Flow cytometric separation of X and Y spermatozoa for the prevention of X-linked diseases. *Human Reproduction*, **8**, 1733–1739

JOINT COMMITTEE ON INFANT HEARING (1991) *1990 Position Statement.* ASHA, **33** (Suppl. 5), 3–6

KEITH, C. G. (1991) Congenital rubella infection from reinfection of previously immunised mothers. *Australian and New Zealand Journal of Ophthalmology*, **19**, 291–293

KEMP, D. T. (1988) Development in cochlear mechanics and techniques for non-invasive evaluation. *Advances in Audiology*, **5**, 27–45

KLEIN, N. J., HEYDERMAN, R. S. and LEVIN, M. (1993) Management of meningococcal infections. *British Journal of Hospital Medicine*, **50**, 42–49

KLOEPFER, H. W., LAGUAITE, J. K. and MCLAURIN, J. W. (1966) The hereditary syndrome of congenital deafness and retinitis pigmentosa. *Laryngoscope*, **76**, 850–862

KRAEMER, M. J., RICHARDSON, M. A., WEISS, N. S., FURUKAWA, C. T., SHAPIRO, G. G., PIERSON, W. E. *et al.* (1983) Risk factors for persistent middle ear effusions. *Journal of the American Medical Association*, **249**, 1022–1025

LENZ, W. and KNAPP, K. (1962) Die Thalidomide-embryopathie. *Deutsche Medizinische Wochenschrift*, **87**, 2132–2142

LUNDBORG, T. (1987) Clinical rehabilitation of the deaf. *Advances in Oto-Rhino-Laryngology*, **37**, 158–161

LYONS, R. A. (1992) Passive smoking and hearing loss in infants. *Irish Medical Journal*, **85**, 111–112

MACFIE, D. D. (1964) ENT problems of diving. *Medical Services Journal, Canada*, **20**, 845–861

MCGEE, T., WOLTERS, C., STEIN, L., KRAUS, N., JOHNSON, D., BOYER, K. et al. (1992) Absence of sensorineural hearing loss in treated infants and children with congenital toxoplasmosis. *Otolaryngology – Head and Neck Surgery*, **106**, 75–80

MARKIDES, A. (1986) Age at fitting of hearing aids and speech intelligibility. *British Journal of Audiology*, **20**, 165–167

MARTIN, J. A. M. (1982a) Aetiological factors relating to childhood deafness in the European community. *Audiology*, **21**, 149–158

MARTIN, J. A. M. (1982b) Diagnosis and communicative ability in deaf children in the European Community. *Audiology*, **21**, 185–196

MATSCHKE, R. G. (1991) Smoking habits in patients with sudden hearing loss. *Acta Otolaryngologica*, Suppl. 476, 69–73

MEREDITH, R., STEPHENS, D., MEYER–BISCH, C., REARDON, W. and SIRIMANNA, T. (1992) Audiometric detection of carriers of Usher's syndrome type II. *Journal of Audiological Medicine*, **1**, 11–19

MONATH, T. P. and JOHNSON, K. M. (1992) Diseases transmitted primarily by arthropod vectors – Viral infections. In: *Maxcy-Rosenau-Last Public Health and Preventive Medicine* edited by J. M. Wallace and R. B. Wallace. London: Prentice-Hall International UK. pp. 213–231

NATHAVITHARANA, K. A. and TARLOW, M. J. (1993) Current trends in the management of bacterial meningitis. *British Journal of Hospital Medicine*, **50**, 403–407

NEWTON, V. (1985) Aetiology of bilateral sensorineural hearing loss in children. *Journal of Laryngology and Otology*, Suppl. 10, 1–57

NORTHERN, J. L. and DOWNS, M. P. (1984) Identification audiometry with children. In: *Hearing in Children*, 3rd edn. Baltimore: Williams & Wilkins. pp. 223–267

NORTHERN, J. L. and DOWNS, M. P. (1991) Medical aspects of hearing loss. *Hearing in Children*, 4th edn. Baltimore: Williams & Wilkins, pp. 51–102

ODIO, C. M., FAINGEZIGHT, I., PARIS, M., NASSAR, M., BALTODANO, A., ROGERS, J. *et al.* (1991) The beneficial effects of early dexamethasone administration in infants and children with bacterial meningitis. *New England Journal of Medicine*, **324**, 1525–1531

ODKVIST, L. M., LARSBY, B., THAM, R. and ASCHAN, G. (1979) Influence of industrial solvents on the vestibular system. *Advances in Oto-Rhino-Laryngology*, **25**, 167–172

ORENSTEIN, W. A., MARKOWITZ, L. E. and HINMAN, A. R. (1992) Measles. In: *Maxcy-Rosenau-Last Public Health and Preventive Medicine*, edited by J. M. Last and R. B. Wallace. London: Prentice-Hall International UK. pp. 65–98

OSUNTOKUN, B. O., MONEKOSSO, G. L. and WILSON, J. (1969) Relationship of a degenerative tropical neuropathy to diet. Report of a field survey. *British Medical Journal*, **1**, 547–550

PARELL, G. J. and BECKER, G. D. (1993) Inner ear barotrauma in scuba divers. A long-term follow-up after continued diving. *Archives of Otolaryngology – Head and Neck Surgery*, **119**, 455–457

PARVING, A. (1991) Detection of the infant with congenital/early acquired hearing disability. *Acta Otolaryngologica* Suppl. 482, 111–116

PASIC, T. R. and DOBIE, R. A. (1991) Cis-platinum ototoxicity in children. *Laryngoscope*, **101**, 985–991

PROBST, R., HARRIS, F. P. and HAUSER, R. (1993) Clinical monitoring using otoacoustic emissions. *British Journal of Audiology*, **27**, 85–90

PYE, A. and COLLINS, P. (1991) Interaction between sound and gentamicin; immediate threshold and stereociliary changes. *British Journal of Audiology*, **25**, 381–390

RAMKALAWAN, T. W. and DAVIS, A. C. (1992) The effects of hearing loss and age of intervention on some language metrics in young hearing-impaired children. *British Journal of Audiology*, **26**, 97–107

RAREY, K. E. (1990) Otologic pathophysiology in patients with human immunodeficiency virus. *American Journal of Otolaryngology*, **11** 366–369

RYBAK, L. P. (1992) Hearing: the effects of chemicals. *Otolaryngology – Head and Neck Surgery*, **106**, 677–686

SANGSTER, J. F., GERACE, T. M. and SEEWALD, R. C. (1991) Hearing loss in elderly patients in a family practice. *Canadian Medical Association Journal*, **144**, 981–998

SCADDING, G., MARTIN, J. A. M., ALLES, R., HAWK, L. and DARBY, Y. (1993) Glue ear guidelines (comment). *Lancet*, i, 57

SCANLON, P. E. and BAMFORD, J. M. (1990) Early identification of hearing loss: screening and surveillance methods. *Archives of Diseases of Childhood*, **65**, 479–485

SCHOT, L. J., HILGERS, F. J., KEUS, R. B., SCHOUWENBURG, P. F. and DRESCHLER, W. A. (1992) Late effects of radiotherapy on hearing. *European Archives of Otorhinolaryngology*, **249**, 305–308

SNOW, J. B. (1992) Foreword. *Otolaryngological Clinics of North America*, **25**, xv–xvi

STEHR-GREEN, P. A. and COCHI, S. L. (1992) Mumps. In: *Maxcy-Rosenau-Last Public Health and Preventive Medicine*, edited by J. M. Last and R. B. Wallace. London: Prentice-Hall International UK. pp. 68–70

STENSTROM, R., BERNARD, P. A. M. and BEN-SIMHON H. (1993) Exposure to environmental tobacco smoke as a risk factor for recurrent acute otitis media in children under the age of five years. *International Journal of Pediatric Otorhinolaryngology*, **27**, 127–136

STEPHENS, S. D. G. (1987) Audiological rehabilitation. In: *Scott–Brown's Otolaryngology*, 5th edn, edited by A. G. Kerr, Vol. 2, *Adult Audiology*, edited by D. Stephens. London: Butterworths. pp. 446–480

STEPHENS, S. D. G., CALLAGHAN, D. E., HOGAN, S., MEREDITH, R., RAYMENT, A. and DAVIS, A. C. (1990) Hearing disability in people aged 50–65: effectiveness and acceptability or rehabilitative intervention. *British Medical Journal*, **300**, 508–511

STEPHENS, S. D. G., MEREDITH, R., CALLAGHAN, D. E., HOGAN, S. and RAYMENT, A. (1991) Early intervention and rehabilita-

tion: factors influencing outcome. *Acta Otolaryngologica* Suppl. 476, 221–225

STRAY-PEDERSEN, B. (1993) Toxoplasmosis in pregnancy. *Baillieres Clinical Obstetrics and Gynaecology*, **7**, 107–137

STRANG, R. J. and PUGH, E. J. (1992) Meningococcal infections: reducing the case fatality rate by giving penicillin before admission to hospital. *British Medical Journal*, **305**, 141–143

SUZUKI, J.-I. (1993) Editorial: Hearing International: the birth of a new agency. *Journal of Audiological Medicine*, **2**, ii–iii

SWAN, C., TOSTEVIN, A. L., MOORE, B., MAYO, H. and BARHAM BLACK, G. H. (1943) Congenital defects in infants following infectious diseases during pregnancy. *Medical Journal of Australia*, **2**, 201–210

TAKEMORI, S., TANAKA, Y. and SUZULI, J. I. (1976) Thalidomide anomalies of the ear. *Archives of Otolaryngology*, **102**, 425–427

TALMI, Y. P., FINKELSTEIN, Y. and ZOHAR, Y. (1991) Barotrauma-induced hearing loss. *Scandinavian Audiology*, **20**, 1–9

TAYLOR, I. G., HINE, W. D., BRASIER, V. J., CHIVERALLS, K. and MORRIS, T. (1975) A study of the causes of hearing loss in a population of children with special reference to genetic factors. *Journal of Laryngology and Otology*, **89**, 899–914

TULLOCH, A. J. (1991) Preventive care of elderly people: how good is our training? *British Journal of General Practice*, **41**, 354–355

VANNIASEGARAM, I., TUNGLAND, O. P. and BELLMAN, S. (1993) A 5-year review of children with deafness in a multiethnic community. *Journal of Audiological Medicine*, **2**, 9–19

WATKIN, P. M. (1991) The age of identification of childhood deafness – Improvements since the 1970s. *Public Health*, **105**, 303–312

WEATHERLY, R. A., OWENS, J. J., CATLIN, F. I. and MAHONEY, D. H. (1991) Cis-platinum ototoxicity in children. *Laryngoscope*, **101**, 917–924

WEINSTEIN, B. E. (1989) Geriatric hearing loss: myths, realities, resources for physicians. *Geriatrics*, **44**, 42–60

WHITE, H. A. (1972) Lassa fever – a study of 23 hospital cases. *Transactions of the Royal Society for Tropical Medicine and Hygiene*, **66**, 390–398

WHITE, K. R., VOHR, B. R. and BEHRENS, T. R. (1993) Universal newborn hearing screening using transient evoked otoacoustic emissions: results of the Rhode Island hearing assessment project. *Seminars in Hearing*, **14**, 18–29

WILSON, J. (1988) Deafness in developing countries – Approaches to a global programme of prevention. *Scandinavian Audiology*, Suppl. 28, 37–58

WILSON, J. (1990) Hearing impairment in developing countries. *Journal of Otolaryngology*, **19**, 368–371

9

Hearing overview

Dafydd Stephens

Within this volume we have grouped together the chapters specifically about hearing disorders rather than intermingling them with general topics and with balance disorders. In this way they cover a wide range of components, but components which, in the clinic, need to be brought together as an integrated whole. This is essential for the clinician faced with a patient complaining of hearing difficulties.

Clinical history (anamnesis)

The first role of the clinician is to determine the patient's primary problem which may or may not be identical to that specified in the referral letter. The initial history taking will then concentrate on that problem, be it hearing disability, tinnitus, otalgia, vertigo, ataxia or any other related complaints. Thus the clinician will determine the duration of any hearing loss, whether one or both ears is affected, its onset sudden or gradual and its subsequent progress. He will want to know whether the loss is steady or fluctuant, whether it is associated with distortion or phonophobia, whether the individual hears better in the quiet or noise and whether he has difficulty in localization. These questions will be of relevance both from an aetiological diagnostic standpoint and from the standpoint of planning therapy. Indeed, throughout the anamnesis, matters which can influence both the aetiological decision and the management decisions are intertwined, and this needs to be borne in mind when taking the history. We must, however, concentrate on questions which are *relevant* to either or both of these needs. A useful question to the patient is, 'What do you think is the cause of your hearing loss?'. This can sometimes give useful diagnostic cues and also insight into the patient's personality and attitudes.

Apart from the main symptom, patients will need to be asked next for relevant related symptoms which can contribute both to the diagnosis and to the management of the hearing problems (e.g. see Chapter 13). The most closely related to hearing loss will be tinnitus and indeed Davis, Coles and their colleagues (see Chapters 3 and 18) have shown that the level of hearing at the high frequencies is the best predictor of tinnitus. In Chapter 18 Coles has discussed the relevant questions to be asked about tinnitus.

Other specific areas the clinician should cover include the sensation of pressure in the ear, important for some inner ear conditions as well as external and middle ear problems, otalgia, otorrhoea, and previous surgery to the ears, as well as ear problems experienced as a child.

In patients with suspected sensorineural hearing loss, questioning about balance problems is also essential and is discussed in Chapter 19.

Where the clinician moves now depends much on his orientation and the age and type of patient. It is important to consider factors which might have influenced the patient's hearing. In those with long-standing hearing loss there may be a history of head injury, noise – including occupational, social and gunfire (see Chapter 11) – together with past and present ototoxic medication. These need to be addressed initially almost in a screening manner, leading on to pursuing further details where relevant. Other important areas are relevant family history, which generally requires careful probing questions, together with aspects of the individual's general health. This last should focus on serious illnesses which may result in hearing problems, e.g. mumps, measles, meningitis and cardiovascular disorders.

In elderly patients it is also important to ask about other conditions associated with cerebrovascular disease such as speech disorders, swallowing difficulties, tremors, paraesthesiae, and also visual problems. The last may be aetiologically relevant, but will also have an important bearing on the rehabilitative management.

In individuals with hearing problems dating back to childhood, a history of birth and pregnancy and relevant milestones may give useful further information.

Moving on to questions of specific relevance to the management of the patient, the most important questions to ask are, 'What are the problems which you have because of your hearing loss?' and 'What made you do something about it now?'.

As mentioned in Chapter 13, the former can be usefully addressed in a form sent to the patient with his appointment letter, but this will need to be discussed further during the clinical interview.

Finally, it is important to be aware of the patient's social situation, whether he lives alone, with a partner or family or in an institution, and also what rehabilitative help he has had in the past. This should cover hearing aids, environmental aids (assistive listening devices) and communication training/skills, together with social service and employment training support where relevant.

Clinical examination

Clinical examination begins as soon as the patient walks into the clinic or consulting room and is complemented by observations made by the clinician while taking the patient's history. Swan in Chapter 5 has highlighted the importance of this in non-organic hearing loss, but careful observation may also highlight neurological and metabolic abnormalities such as tremors, proptosis, exophthalmos, together with pre-auricular or neck pits indicative of branchio-oto-renal syndrome or asymmetry of the individual's facies. Pinna abnormalities may also be apparent at this stage.

Furthermore, during the history-taking the clinician will be able to form a good opinion of any speech abnormalities which may reflect on the hearing loss and also have implications for the rehabilitative management.

Examination of the ears to determine the state of the external canal and tympanic membrane is the most central part of this examination, together with tuning fork tests. These have been discussed in Chapter 5. A combination of the Weber, Rinne and Bing tests together with testing for diplacusis binauralis can be performed very rapidly and provide useful diagnostic information. Carefully performed they avoid the pitfall of incorrect diagnoses arising from inaccurate audiometry, although inevitably they cannot provide as much information as careful audiometry.

Speech tests of hearing have a similarly confirma-

tory role and may either be performed at fixed distances as outlined by Swan or at variable distances. It is important for each clinician to calibrate themselves against careful audiometry and to be aware of the difficulties which may arise in different levels of ambient noise. From a rehabilitative standpoint, such speech tests can give the clinician useful information about the differences between the two ears which can influence any decisions about which ear to aid.

Other aspects of the clinical examination will depend very much on the specific patient. In patients with pulsatile or clicking tinnitus, auscultation, both of the ear (Figure 9.1) and of the neck, will be indicated (in pulsatile tinnitus) together with simultaneous observation of any movements of the soft palate (clicking tinnitus). Meatal occlusion giving rise to an increase in tinnitus loudness usually points to cochlear tinnitus, and emphasizes the need for the use of non-occluding earmoulds. Pressure on the vessels of the neck can provide other valuable information in vascular tinnitus.

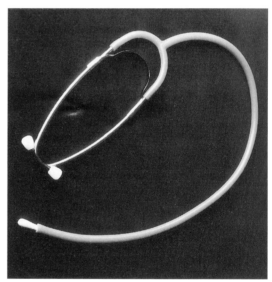

Figure 9.1 Stethoscope modified for aural auscultation by K. S. Sirimanna

If examination of the tympanic membrane indicates middle ear abnormalities then a full otolaryngological examination will be indicated, particularly with unilateral problems of recent onset, when examination of the postnasal space is essential. It may be necessary in such cases to proceed to fibreoptic endoscopy.

Many patients with problems arising from the cochlea or cochlear nerve may also have vestibular problems and, in these cases, examination for nystagmus and clinical tests of balance such as Unterberger's test will be indicated. This is particularly true in the case of unilateral sensorineural hearing losses.

More general physical examination for vascular and thyroid abnormalities, fundoscopy, testing of gait and other clinical tests will be indicated in certain patients according to their anamnesis and general clinical appearance.

Examination of the cranial nerves is essential in those with unilateral hearing loss or tinnitus and when complaints of specific problems are indicated. It may also be indicated by a general observation of the facies indicating abnormalities.

Finally, as part of the clinical examination it may be relevant to check the individual's visual acuity if they are going to be very dependent on speech reading (lip reading) to complement their limited auditory input. This may be also the time to check their speech reading ability with a simple test of speech reading as outlined in Chapter 13, particularly in the case of those individuals with severe communicative problems.

Audiometric investigations

Determination of the patient's threshold of hearing by pure tone audiometry is the most basic and universal audiometric test. This can be performed by air and bone conduction, although under certain circumstances the latter may be truncated or omitted altogether. If bone conduction is performed, adequate masking is essential, as discussed by Lutman in Chapter 12.

While the most common audiometric threshold measure is manual audiometry, semiautomatic techniques which cover the full frequency range in detail, such as Békésy audiometry or Audioscan may give more useful information in certain cases, particularly when there may be sudden irregularities of the audiogram or if the individual's hearing is clinically normal.

While manual pure tone audiometry is being performed, two short tests may be added which can provide useful diagnostic information, namely a Stenger test to confirm asymmetries and a modified Carhart test of abnormal adaptation. The latter can be performed at 20 dB SL at 4 kHz for 30 s and can provide a useful pointer towards neural abnormalities, leading on to further investigations if abnormal (Stephens and Hinchcliffe, 1968).

After pure tone audiometry, the most important single test procedure is otoadmittance testing giving information on admittance, middle ear pressure, eustachian tube dysfunction, the stapedial reflex arc and acoustic reflex decay. This is discussed at length in Chapter 12.

Speech audiometry has little relevance for diagnosis but may give useful information to support rehabilitative management decisions (Chapter 13).

The next most important investigation is the auditory brain stem response (ABR) which is the most sensitive audiometric measure of cochlear nerve dysfunction and also gives valuable information in the investigation of central auditory dysfunction (see Chapters 12 and 17). It does not generally have good frequency specificity and for medicolegal purposes the best evoked response measure is the slow vertex response (ERA).

Other evoked response measures and a variety of behavioural measures may be useful in the investigation of central auditory function and are discussed in Chapter 17.

Finally, in Chapter 18, Coles discusses the various measures of tinnitus which may be used. Enthusiasm for the value of these has waned, but they still have an important role in the therapeutic investigation of the patient with disturbing tinnitus. A small proportion of such patients has abnormal spontaneous otoacoustic emissions. The role of evoked otoacoustic emissions in anything other than screening remains to be defined and is considered by Lutman in Chapter 12.

Imaging and pathological investigations

Imaging of the ear, particularly with MRI and CT scanning has several roles in the hearing impaired patient. It features in the definition of possible cochlear nerve neoplasia (particularly the vestibular schwannoma/acoustic neuroma) where MRI scanning with gadolinium enhancement is the 'gold standard', giving optimum results, although there have been a few cases in which there have been false positive results.

CT scanning still has an important role in examination of the cochlea for congenital abnormalities, to examine the vestibular aqueduct, to seek evidence of cochlear otosclerosis and to define the patency of the cochlear turns in potential candidates for cochlear implants. In patients with pulsatile tinnitus, CT scanning may be used to test for glomus jugulare tumours, and MRI angiography is developing an important role in this field.

The decision as to which haematological and biochemical investigations, if any, should be performed in patients presenting with hearing problems is one which depends very much on the clinician involved. It will also depend much on the age and general health of the patient concerned and the extent to which he has been investigated by his primary physician and/or other physicians.

Many indications will come from a careful anamnesis and examination of the patient, and a number of investigations may be indicated when there are no obvious causes for the loss. A variety of possible aetiological factors is discussed in Chapter 10. In general, the approach is to screen for major systemic conditions rather then to adopt a blunderbuss approach.

However, particularly in young individuals with

a progressive hearing loss, it is important to exclude preventable or stoppable causes of progressive hearing loss. Thus an approach of using basic haematological indices (haemoglobin, white blood cell count, platelets), screening for autoimmune disorders (ESR, immunoglobulins, complement, autoantibody screen), general metabolic measures (lipids, glucose, liver function tests, urea and electrolytes, thyroid function tests) including an appropriate measure of blood viscosity, together with treponemal serology is advocated by many clinicians. In acute auditory failure (sudden deafness) virological antibody measures, particularly for mumps, measles and herpes zoster, should be added. The role of antibody tests for *Borrelia* and HIV remains more controversial. In addition the relevance of abnormal bicarbonate measures, reported by Davis in Chapter 3, needs further clarification.

Patient treatment

Most hearing loss is not amenable to treatment and, for the large majority of patients, the main relevance of aetiological investigation is to help them to come to terms with the permanency of their hearing loss. A small proportion of hearing impaired patients (e.g. those with otosclerosis, some cases of otitis media, osteogenesis imperfecta) may have improved hearing from middle ear surgery and are discussed in Volume 3. In others, such as vestibular schwannoma, surgery is usually destructive of hearing but may save the patient from a life-threatening condition. In yet others (e.g. Menière's disorder), surgery may provide relief from other disabling symptoms.

Pharmacological approaches to a variety of conditions are discussed by McKee in Chapter 6 and are generally more orientated towards prevention of the progression of the condition than towards achieving an improvement in hearing. This is true whether the condition is infectious (e.g. syphilis), autoimmune or idiopathic (e.g. Menière's disorder). In most of these, early intervention may result in an improvement of the hearing (secondary prevention, see Chapter 8), but once the condition is established, usually the best that can generally be expected is arrest of the progress of the condition and possibly some relief of the related aural symptoms.

Rehabilitation

For most patients with hearing loss the only effective management is rehabilitative. The various aspects of this are pulled together in Chapter 13. This covers the non-instrumental as well as the instrumental aspects of the process; some of the specifically psychological aspects of that process are also addressed by Jakes in Chapter 4. Certainly such psychological factors play an important role in determining whether the patient accepts the permanency and irreversibility of his condition and is hence prepared to make the effort necessary to obtain optimum benefit from the rehabilitative process.

Instrumental intervention, using hearing aids, tactile aids and cochlear implants, has a unique role within the rehabilitative process, although without non-instrumental support maximal benefit cannot be achieved from these. (These types of intervention are discussed in Chapters 14, 15 and 16.) The need for additional support stems in part from the stigma associated with use of any instrumentation and also the fact that such instruments are rarely able to 'correct' hearing loss in the same way as spectacles in a myopic individual.

The level of hearing loss at which hearing aids can be fitted should depend on the individual and his disability rather than on any strict audiometric criterion. The level at which cochlear implants or tactile aids could be considered will broadly depend on the clinical judgement that the individual is likely to obtain more benefit from them than from hearing aids. In patients with good speech discrimination, the choice of hearing aids is clear; in those with no measurable hearing the choice of implant or tactile aid is also clear. However, again there is a grey area between these two which will depend in part on the state of current technology (both of improving hearing aids as well as of improving cochlear implants) and also on the clinician's judgement, the patient's wishes and, inevitably, certain socioeconomic factors.

The choice between implants and tactile aids is again a multifactorial decision based on the patient's feelings, the respective potential benefits of the two and also on the health status of the patient. Patients with severe cardiovascular, respiratory and other disorders may not be fit for a 3-hour non-life-saving surgical procedure involved in a cochlear implant, however audiologically appropriate it may be. Others with inadequate cochlear nerve fibres may present a problem and in many cases again the experience of the physician or surgeon is critical in making the appropriate decision.

Reference

STEPHENS, S. D. G. and HINCHCLIFFE, R. (1968) Studies on temporary threshold drift. *International Audiology*, 7, 267–279

10

Causes of hearing disorders

Lam Hoe Yeoh

There can be few practitioners of audiological medicine and otolaryngology who have not experienced the feeling of helplessness occasioned by watching the inevitable progression of sensorineural hearing loss in an adult patient. For this type of deafness to be alleviated or prevented the cause must be understood if there is to be any chance of treatment which is anything other than empirical. Our ignorance is such that practitioners will often avoid a fruitless search for a cause. This approach is short-sighted as investigation does occasionally reveal treatable pathology, with *Borrelia* infection and autoimmune disease being two examples. More importantly, it is only by constantly attempting to understand the pathological basis of deafness that the possibility of effective treatment for such a patient can be realized. The hearing system is like any other and subject to the same groups of disorders, so that we can apply basic pathological categories such as congenital, infection, inflammation, vascular, metabolic, trauma, degenerative and neoplastic. There are of course some disorders such as vasculitis which fall into more than one category. When attempting to ascertain the cause of deafness the history may often be sufficient to indicate the cause, e.g. noise exposure, but sometimes exhaustive investigation is required, and each case should be considered on its own merits. For some it is essential to establish the cause quickly if hearing is to be preserved, e.g. autoimmune disease, and infections such as syphilis. For others it is important to detect associated impairment such as retinitis pigmentosa or renal dysfunction.

The causes of deafness given below cannot be exhaustive but are representative of the types of disorder that should be considered when faced with an adult patient whose hearing is deteriorating. For some disorders the effect upon hearing is debatable, e.g. myxoedema and diabetes, and in these cases the clinician has to weigh the probabilities of attributing the hearing impairment to the disorder. Genetic disorders can present in adult life and the associated abnormalities may not be apparent in the course of an otolaryngological examination. It is important to discover any genetic defect as there are implications for other members of the family. With an ageing population a label of degenerative deafness or presbyacusis can be used indiscriminately to the detriment of appropriate medical care and the advancement of our understanding of the pathology of deafness.

Causes of hearing loss

Hereditary

Autosomal dominant: early onset degenerative hearing loss; otosclerosis
Autosomal recessive: difficult to identify and uncommon, unless syndromal
Syndromal: includes Alport's, Usher's, Pendred's, Waardenburg's, Crouzon (all may have late expression); neurodegenerative disorders, e.g. osteogenesis imperfecta; craniometaphyseal dysplasia; hereditary sensory neuropathy (HSN-I); Charcot-Marie-Tooth; facioscapulohumeral muscular dystrophy; Paget's disease; neurofibromatosis 2
Inherited metabolic: Refsum's disease; mucopolysaccharidoses
X-linked
Mitochondrial

Infections

Viral: including acquired immunodeficiency syndrome (AIDS); Ramsay Hunt syndrome

Microbial: syphilis; meningitis; Lyme disease; post-chronic suppurative otitis media
Fungal

Ischaemia

Ischaemic heart disease
Macrovascular disorders: including arteriovenous malformations, ectasia, aberrant vessels
Strokes
Hypertension
Vasculitis
Coagulopathies: hereditary coagulation disorders, sickle cell anaemia, blood viscosity

Inflammation

Autoimmune hearing loss: rheumatoid arthritis, Cogan's syndrome, systemic lupus erythematosus, Takayasu's disease, IgA nephropathy, Behçet's syndrome, polyarteritis nodosa (PAN)
Demyelination

Neoplastic

Primary and secondary lesions
Vestibular schwannoma (acoustic neuroma)
Leukaemia

Metabolic and endocrine disorders

Diabetes mellitus
Thyroid dysfunction
Hyperlipoproteinaemia
Renal failure
Hyperuricaemia
Other disorders

Trauma and toxicity

Head injury
Barotrauma

Radiotherapy
Ototoxicity
Acoustic trauma

Degenerative

Age-related hearing impairment ('presbyacusis')

Miscellaneous

Ménière's syndrome
Bell's palsy
Sarcoidosis
Obscure auditory dysfunction

Sudden sensorineural hearing loss

Hereditary

The various genetic causes of hearing loss are shown in Table 10.1.

Chromosomal disorders associated with sensorineural hearing loss include Down's syndrome (trisomy 21), trisomy 18, trisomy 13 and deletion of the long arm of chromosome 18. The hearing impairment with these disorders is predominantly from childhood.

Autosomal dominant hearing loss in isolation

This condition is difficult to identify and diagnosis may be based on exclusion. The major cause of late-onset hearing loss is genetic (Konigsmark and Gorlin, 1976). This may either be single gene mutations, or polygenic control with several gene loci influencing the auditory system (Steel and Bock, 1985). It is thought that the latter is more likely. Genetic hearing loss may be autosomal dominant, autosomal recessive or X-linked. Autosomal recessive hearing loss in

Table 10.1 Genetic causes of hearing loss in adults

	Syndromal	*Non-syndromal*
Autosomal dominant	Craniometaphyseal syndrome; Waardenburg's type II; osteogenesis imperfecta; hereditary sensory neuropathy (HSN-I); Charcot-Marie-Tooth disease; facioscapulohumeral muscular dystrophy; ataxia with hearing loss; neurofibromatosis 2	Late-onset hearing loss; otosclerosis.
Autosomal recessive	Late-onset hearing loss; Friedreich's ataxia; Refsum's disease, mucopolysaccharidoses	Late onset hearing loss
X-linked dominant	Alport's syndrome	Late onset hearing loss
X-linked recessive	Mixed hearing loss associated with fixation of stapedial footplate; X-linked hypophosphataemic rickets; ocular albinism	(Late onset hearing loss)
Mitochondrial	MELAS; MERRF	Familial streptomycin ototoxicity

isolation is uncommon, often appearing as part of a syndromal picture. Over 60 types of hereditary deafness exist in man, most of which have defects in hearing and other systems, but in 10 conditions, deafness appears to be the only known manifestation of the genetic defect (Konigsmark, Mengel and Berlin, 1971).

Dominant progressive early onset sensorineural hearing loss in childhood or early adult life often occurs with high frequency hearing loss and preservation of hearing below 2000 Hz. Hearing loss is progressive affecting the middle frequencies. Huizing, van Bolhuis and Odenthal (1966) found severe loss only in subjects over 45 years of age. A similar progressive loss was reported by Teig (1968).

Konigsmark, Mengel and Berlin (1971) described early onset or congenital low frequency sensorineural hearing loss at 500 and 1000 Hz, with progressive deterioration of the high frequencies above 4000 Hz in middle decades. Hearing at 2000 Hz and 4000 Hz was better preserved. After the fourth decade all frequencies were likely to be affected. This may result in patients presenting in middle age with a low and high frequency hearing loss or a loss affecting all frequencies from their fifth decade onwards. Inheritance is autosomal dominant, with normal vestibular function. The site of lesion was suggested to be the cochlea at the apical turn of the organ of Corti, or in the related spiral ganglion fibres.

Dominant mid-frequency sensorineural hearing loss may develop in childhood and progress to involve all frequencies in adulthood, although low and high frequencies are preserved in early years. Variable expression of the gene occurs.

Dominant high frequency progressive deafness presents with an abrupt loss, lower frequencies being affected with progressive age.

Khetarpal *et al.* (1991) reported on five temporal bone findings from three patients from two kindreds with adult onset autosomal dominant progressive sensorineural hearing loss. They observed deposits of polymucosaccharide ground substance in the spiral ligament, limbus and spiral lamina of the cochlea and the macula and cristae. Based on a subsequent report on the temporal bones of the above, Khetarpal (1993) suggested that autosomal dominant sensorineural hearing loss was classifiable into cochlear and cochleovestibular subtypes.

Otosclerosis

Otosclerosis is an autosomal dominant condition with variable penetrance. The reader is invited to refer to Chapter 14 in Volume 3 for further information regarding this condition. Characteristic audiological features include a conductive hearing loss, a midfrequency U-shaped sensorineural hearing loss, a notch at 2000 Hz for bone conduction thresholds, and the on-off effect of the acoustic reflex (the abnormal negative impedance seen at the beginning and end of reflex measurements in early otosclerosis). Debruyne (1992) reported this effect in 40 patients with sensorineural hearing loss, including eight with symptoms suggestive of endolymphatic hydrops. He proposed that the effect was due either to the effects of otosclerotic foci in the cochlea, or from increased pressure on the footplate. Forquer and Sheehy (1981) found this effect present in 42% of subjects with cochlear otosclerosis. The reliability of tympanometric findings in the diagnosis of this condition is uncertain due to the overlap in the results between normal subjects and those with otosclerosis, although testing with a probe tone of 660 Hz has been reported to give abnormal results in approximately two-thirds of such patients.

Causse *et al.* (1989) suggested that otosclerosis arises from the release of enzymes from the otosclerotic foci which damage the inner ear and result in deposition of new bone in the oval window niche. The release was thought to be an autoimmune process.

Hearing loss in the adult may arise in addition from audiometric dips which extend in adult life; early onset degenerative hearing loss may also be associated with the branchio-oto-renal.

Hearing loss associated with syndromes

Several syndromes have an association with sensorineural hearing loss, although most of these, including Alport's, Usher's, Pendred's, and Waardenburg's, present in childhood. However, hearing loss may develop in the second decade onwards. Some conditions are listed below.

Alport's syndrome

Alport's syndrome is a predominantly X-linked dominant, variably expressed disorder more common in males, although autosomal forms have also been described. It is caused by mutations in a collagen chain gene (COL4A5) located in the Xq22 region (Tryggvason *et al.*, 1993). The mutations, including single base mutations, large deletions and other rearrangements, are sufficient to cause structural and functional defects in the type IV collagen molecule. The syndrome consists of sensorineural hearing loss associated with hereditary nephritis, the latter manifesting at an earlier age, usually as recurrent haematuria in the first or second decade, ending in renal failure by the third decade in men (Glassock and Brenner, 1987). Deafness develops later, and is variable in frequency and intensity, although the high frequencies are more likely to be involved earlier on. Other signs include cataract, spherophakia, anterior or posterior lenticonus, myopia or scotomata in 10% (Konigsmark and Gorlin, 1976). Clinical hearing loss occurs in 45% of subjects and is described as slowly progressive and asymmetrical (Arnold, 1984). Temporal bone data include stria vascularis degeneration, loss of cochlear neurons, atrophy of the spiral ligaments and non-specific basophilic substance deposition in the stria. It has been suggested (Myers and Tyler, 1972) that as many as five variants of this condition occur: renal disease with organ of Corti damage, renal disease with spiral ganglion loss, renal disease and deafness with no histological inner ear lesion, renal disease with normal hearing and deafness without renal disease. However, the variants may be due to poor diagnostic criteria in the identification of the disorder, rather than specific variations. Following transplantation the condition does not recur. Improvement in hearing threshold levels after transplantation was reported by McDonald *et al.* (1978) in one out of six patients with stabilization of hearing loss in the remainder.

Edwards *et al.* (1989) reported a new syndrome of autosomal recessive nephropathy, deafness and hyperparathyroidism distinct from Alport's syndrome, in which five out of six siblings of parents who were first cousins had sensorineural hearing loss, with no haematuria.

Craniometaphyseal dysplasia

Craniometaphyseal dysplasia, an autosomal dominant disorder of enchondral bone formation, presents with conductive hearing loss arising from bony annulus deformity, fixation of the malleus head, and thickened ossicles on temporal bone examination. Sensorineural hearing loss may arise because of heredodegenerative involvement, cochlear involvement, encroachment of the internal auditory canal, or obliteration of the foramen (Morgan, Aldren and Hoare, 1990).

Waardenburg's syndrome type II

Waardenburg's syndrome type II is an autosomal dominant genetic disorder with moderate progressive bilateral sensorineural hearing loss in more than half of such subjects. This may be missed in childhood, without dystopia canthorum or typical facial features of type I subjects, and present with a progressive hearing loss (Hildesheimer *et al.*, 1989).

Osteogenesis imperfecta

Osteogenesis imperfecta, inherited predominantly as an autosomal dominant condition is a congenital disorder presenting with easily fractured bones, blue sclerae, laxity of joints and deafness, usually in the second or third decade, due to mutations in type I collagen fibres. Such mutations may either have reduced production of normal collagen or defective collagen production (Byers, Wallis and Willing, 1991). Classification, based on the clinical features, is into four distinct subtypes, with hearing loss being common in osteogenesis imperfecta types I and III, and less frequently in type IV (Sillence, Senn and Danks, 1979). Osteogenesis imperfecta type II is usually lethal in the perinatal period. Pedersen (1985) found conductive hearing loss which became mixed by the third and fourth decade. Stewart and O'Reilly (1989) in a study on 56 patients concurred, with conductive hearing loss noted initially in the second and third decades. Approximately one-quarter of the subjects had a purely sensorineural hearing loss. In a review of 15 stapes from patients with osteogenesis imperfecta tarda, Pedersen (1985) noted two causes of stapedial fixation. One had a focus which resembled, histologically, early active otosclerosis, while in other cases fixation was due to diffuse structural alteration. Stapes with localized foci resembling otosclerosis have different biochemical and histochemical findings from otosclerotic stapes, and are not thought to be otosclerotic.

Hereditary sensory neuropathy

Hereditary sensory neuropathy (HSN-I) is another autosomal dominant condition with an unknown metabolic defect resulting in sensory neuropathy distal to the wrist and knee, often leading to involuntary mutilation of hands and feet. Sensorineural deafness has been observed in some families with this disorder (Asbury, 1987).

Hearing loss is very infrequently reported in *peroneal muscular dystrophy* (Charcot-Marie-Tooth disease), an autosomal dominant condition with atrophy of anterior tibial and calf muscles ('stork legs').

Facioscapulohumeral muscular dystrophy

Facioscapulohumeral muscular dystrophy is an autosomal dominant condition affecting males and females equally, usually starting in the third to fourth decades. The abnormal gene is located on chromosome 4. High frequency hearing loss has been reported by Meyerson, Lewis and Ill (1984). Brouwer *et al.* (1991) reviewed 11 publications which had shown subjects to have retinal abnormalities, mental retardation and bilateral high frequency sensorineural hearing loss which was progressive in some cases. They did not see this in their study of 56 subjects compared with 72 normal family members and suggested that expression of the hearing loss was variable possibly due to genetic heterogeneity, a pleiotropic effect of a single gene or involvement of tightly linked genes.

Friedreich's ataxia

Friedreich's ataxia is characterized by degeneration of the spinocerebellar tracts and of ascending and descending tracts of the spinal column. This is usually an autosomal recessive condition although it may be dominantly inherited. Presentation starts in childhood affecting the lower limbs and spreading proximally. Nystagmus may be present. Survival into adulthood is rare. Ell, Prasher and Rudge (1984) found a mild to moderate sensorineural hearing loss in nine of 10 patients. Abnormalities on auditory brain-stem responses usually affect wave IV which may be more prominent than wave V.

Other conditions

Hearing impairment has also been reported in *oculopharyngeal dystrophy with progressive external ophthalmoplegia* (Walton, 1977). Rare autosomal dominant endocrine-neuroectodermal syndromes involving sensorineural hearing loss in adults with alopecia, hypogonadism, mental retardation and diabetes mellitus have also been described (Oerter *et al.*, 1992).

Ataxia, epilepsy, and myoclonus, thought to represent an autosomal dominant disorder, have been associated with a high frequency sensorineural hearing loss (May and White, 1968). In addition, Konigsmark and Gorlin (1976) noted the association between ataxia with pes cavus and adult-onset sensorineural hearing loss, ataxia with hyperuricaemia, renal insufficiency and deafness in the third decade, and ataxia with cataract, nystagmus, psychosis and/or dementia and sensorineural deafness, with hearing impairment presenting in the third decade after onset of ocular findings.

In addition to the condition reported by May and White in 1968, Yih *et al.* (1993) have reported an association between spastic paraplegia with epilepsy, mental retardation and hearing impairment in a family.

Neurofibromatosis 2, another autosomal dominant disorder, is discussed in this chapter under the heading for Neoplastic lesions.

Inherited metabolic losses

Refsum's disease

Also known as phytanic acid storage disease, or heredopathia atactica polyneuritiformis, Refsum's disease is an autosomal recessive inborn error of metabolism manifesting in the first or second decade of life. It is a demyelinating process, due to a defect in α-oxidation of β-methylated fatty acids, presenting with night blindness or polyneuropathy, with cerebellar ataxia and cardiac abnormalities being later features. Cochlear hearing loss is present in up to 80% of

cases, from the second decade onwards. Hallpike (1967) found collapse of Reissner's membrane, disorganization of the organ of Corti and degeneration of stria vascularis. Treatment with a low phytanate diet and plasmapheresis therapy may arrest hearing deterioration (Djupesland, Flottorp and Refsum, 1983).

The mucopolysaccharidoses

The mucopolysaccharidoses are inherited disorders of mucopolysaccharide metabolism with defective activity of genetically determined pathways of lysosomal degradation. The resulting build-up of intracellular acid mucopolysaccharides leads to characteristic skeletal and clinical changes. Some are also associated with deafness, usually conductive or mixed (Konigsmark and Gorlin, 1976). Most of these conditions result in death by the second decade. Inheritance is autosomal recessive with the exception of Hunter's.

Hurler syndrome (MPS I–H) is the classical prototype with features of growth failure, marked mental retardation, corneal clouding, progressive lack of joint mobility, and coarsening of facial features. A progressive conductive hearing loss is reported. *Scheie syndrome* (MPS I–S) is an allelic form of Hurler syndrome, with normal intelligence; 10–20% have a mixed loss in middle age. *Hunter syndrome* (MPS II) presents in two forms – mild (type A) and severe (type B). Approximately 50% have a mixed hearing loss. *Sanfilippo syndrome* (MPS III) has a less significant picture than Hurler syndrome with death by the second decade. *Morquio syndrome* (MPS IV) subjects have normal intelligence, normal facies, disproportionately long extremities and growth failure. Most have a mixed hearing impairment. *Maroteaux-Lamy syndrome* (MPS VI) patients have a severe Hurler-like appearance with normal intelligence. The mild form appears around the age of 6 years and survival into adulthood is common while in the severe form death occurs usually in adolescence. One-quarter of these patients have a mainly conductive hearing loss from recurrent otitis media.

There is a possible correlation between mucolipidoses and sphingolipidoses with hearing impairment (Konigsmark and Gorlin, 1976).

Sex-linked sensorineural hearing loss

X-linked non-syndromal hearing loss is reported to be genetically heterogeneous, with at least two gene loci on the X-chromosome (Reardon *et al.*, 1992) presenting with diverse clinical patterns. Reardon *et al.* (1992) found different audiometric configurations in their study of seven pedigrees, and concluded that audiological parameters did not reflect genetic differences in this form of deafness.

Pelletier and Tanguay (1975) reported a family with X-linked recessive hearing loss occurring around adolescence which was progressive, resulting in a bilateral flat moderate sensorineural hearing loss.

X-linked hypophosphataemic rickets

X-linked hypophosphataemic rickets (the commonest form of all genetically determined osteomalacias) is due to a dominant defect in cellular transport in the renal tubule and may cause a low frequency cochlear hearing loss. O'Malley *et al.* (1988) suggested that this was due to a hydropic pattern from stria vascularis metabolism alteration or from occlusion of the endolymphatic duct or sac. Davies, Kane and Valentine (1984) reported cochlear hearing loss in 76% of subjects with X-linked hypophosphataemic (vitamin D-resistant) osteomalacia.

Ocular albinism

Ocular albinism has also been reported in a family with seven males having high frequency sensorineural hearing loss, horizontal nystagmus and blue irides. The hearing loss developed in the fifth decade, differentiating this X-linked condition from autosomal dominant oculocutaneous albinism with congenital hearing loss (Winship, Gericke and Beighton, 1984).

Turner's syndrome

Turner's syndrome, first described more than 50 years ago, is classically associated with a 45XO monotype, with the clinical features resulting from loss of material from the short arm of the X chromosome. Twenty per cent of Turner's syndrome patients are mosaic with some cells in these women having a normal 46XX constitution. Classically presenting with short stature, typical facial features and a short webbed neck, as well as auricular deformity, the prevalence is one in 5000 of the female population. Watkin (1989) found 83% of a small sample with a history of middle ear disorder, with sensorineural hearing loss in 20% developing after the age of 8 years. He also observed a midfrequency cochlear loss in another 20% of his sample. Sylven *et al.* (1991) in their study of 49 subjects found a mild sensorineural hearing loss in 61% of them. The loss was similar for both 45XO subjects and for mosaic Turner's patients.

Mitochondrial myopathies with hearing loss

MELAS syndrome

MELAS (mitochondrial encephalomyopathy, lactic acidosis and recurrent cerebral insults resembling strokes) syndrome is one of several such syndromes having diverse clinical features, but all affecting mitochondrial function. The pathological picture in all of them shows ragged red fibres on muscle biopsy. Cortical blindness and seizures have also been described. Mosewich *et al.* (1993) reported on a family with a female predilection towards progressive bilateral sensorineural hearing loss.

Kearns-Sayre syndrome

Kearns-Sayre syndrome, another mitochondrial myopathy, has a triad of progressive external ophthalmoplegia, retinal degeneration, and heart block or cerebellar syndrome. Ohkoshi *et al.* (1989) reported the presence of bilateral moderate sensorineural hearing loss in a subject with the triad of symptoms.

MERRF syndrome

Hearing loss is a common feature in MERRF syndrome, another mitochondrial condition, with myoclonic epilepsy, ragged red fibres, dementia and ataxia (Mendell and Griggs, 1987).

Infections
Viral infections
Spumaretrovirus

Pyykko *et al.* (1994) reported on the incidence of human spumaretrovirus (HSRV) in patients with sudden sensorineural hearing loss. The human spumaretrovirus is a recently characterized retrovirus which resembles other exogenous retroviruses in causing neurodegenerative diseases. Four subjects out of 30 presenting with sudden sensorineural hearing loss were found to have raised titres to human spumaretrovirus, with two having bilateral hearing loss. The pattern was mainly flat. Of the six ears affected, thresholds recovered in four, and deteriorated in two. The recovery period varied from hours to months. One patient had a fluctuating loss and it was postulated that reactivated human spumaretrovirus infection was responsible.

Lassa fever

Cummins *et al.* (1990) found an incidence of sensorineural hearing loss in 29% of confirmed cases of Lassa fever, noting an eightfold increase in the titre of anti-Lassa IgG in 26 of 32 subjects with varying degrees of hearing loss. Recovery was partial or complete in more than 50% of subjects. Liao, Byl and Adour (1992), using audiometric criteria from the earlier study, assessed 222 patients with sudden hearing loss. They suggested that similarities between the distribution of the severity of the loss, and the percentage and extent of hearing improvement, between Lassa fever patients and their subjects supported the theory that viral infection played a major role in sudden hearing loss.

It was believed by Cummins *et al.* (1990) that an antigen-antibody immunological reaction to various viruses was the basis for hearing loss in susceptible patients. The improvement in hearing threshold levels to steroid therapy, as reported by some authors (Wilson, Byl and Laird, 1980) might support this. Veltri *et al.* (1981) found seroconversion in two-thirds of subjects with sudden hearing loss, with multiple seroconversions seen in half of the subjects with positive seroconversion. The most common seroconversion occurred with influenza B and rubeola virus.

Acquired immune deficiency syndrome (AIDS)

AIDS is an epidemic of the current century with a multitude of presentations which at present has no cure. Identification of the HIV virus dates back to a blood sample from Zaire in 1959. The 5-year mortality in the USA varies between 90% and 100% with an infected population between 1 and 1.5 million (Sorvino and Lucente, 1992). The HIV virus is a retrovirus with a tropism for T-helper lymphocytes, as well as a neurotropic tendency. Infection is spread via sexual contact, contaminated blood and blood products, use of contaminated needles by drug addicts, and transplacentally.

An increasing number of patients has been reported with otological symptoms from AIDS, while reports have also noted the correlation between AIDS and syphilis. Sensorineural hearing loss in AIDS may be due to infection with other viruses, e.g. cytomegalovirus, hepatitis B, herpes simplex or with *Treponema pallidum* (Smith and Canalis, 1989; Veltri *et al.*, 1981). Mishell and Appelbaum (1990) have reported Ramsay Hunt syndrome presenting in a subject with an AIDS-related complex.

Birchall *et al.* (1992) found abnormalities on pure-tone audiometry in 39% of a small sample of patients with neurologically asymptomatic, syphilis-negative, HIV infection, with five of the 18 subjects having increased latencies of waves III and V on auditory brain-stem response audiometry. They suggested that auditory brain-stem response audiometry might be a sensitive predictor of central nervous system degeneration in HIV infection. Recently, subjects presenting with sudden sensorineural hearing loss have been reported (Real, Thomas and Gerwin, 1987; Timon and Walsh, 1989). Schinella, Breda and Hammerschlag (1987) reported a man with a sloping sensorineural hearing loss in one ear and a mixed mild to profound loss in the other, secondary to *Pneumocystis carinii* presenting as an otic polyp, with antibody to the human immunodeficiency virus (HIV). Sandler *et al.* (1990) reported a similar case and reviewed previous cases, concluding that extrapulmonary manifestation of *P. carinii* was becoming increas-

ingly common in patients with HIV, presenting with external ear polyps and middle ear disease, without concomitant pulmonary disease.

Johns, Tierney and Felsenstein (1987) noted an increased number of HIV patients developing neurosyphilis, contrary to the recent trend. They reported on four cases in a year, one with a severe bilateral sensorineural hearing loss which improved after treatment for syphilis. Smith and Canalis (1989) reported on five patients with HIV infections who presented with otosyphilis. It was suggested that infection with HIV modified the natural history of syphilis by increasing the propensity for development of neurosyphilis, reducing the latency period and increasing the manifestation of syphilis through the severe defects of cell-mediated immunity. The mode of action was postulated to be through the reduction of immunological response to treponemal infection.

Michaels, Soucek and Liang (1994) found cytomegalovirus in 24% of 49 temporal bones from subjects with AIDS, with a 20% incidence of otitis media.

Ramsay Hunt syndrome

This condition, first reported in 1907, has a triad of facial palsy, hearing loss and auricular herpes infection. The virus may be herpes zoster or herpes simplex. The incidence of deafness in this condition ranges from 24% of 122 patients (Wayman *et al.*, 1990) to 69% of 32 patients (Devriese, 1968). Hyperacusis is a more common presentation while the presence of vertigo is associated with a poorer prognosis. The incidence of the latter is variable due to differing criteria for patient selection, with Abramovich and Prasher (1986) reporting its presence in 11 of 13 patients, while Devriese (1968) reported vestibular symptoms in 23 of 32. The site of lesion may be both cochlear and retrocochlear, as well as involvement of the vestibular nerve and facial nerve by lymphocytic or round cell infiltration (Blackley, Friedmann and Wright, 1967; Abramovich and Prasher, 1986). Yagi, Yamaguchi and Nonaka (1988), in addition to sensorineural hearing loss, found abnormal results on positional and positioning tests and on caloric testing in more than 50% of such patients, and nystagmus in all their subjects.

Microbial infections

Syphilis

Otosyphilis is more common in late acquired syphilis and in congenital syphilis. Varying presentation patterns have been observed, including sudden hearing loss, although it had been previously suggested that the typical finding is consistent with a Menière's syndrome pattern. Infection by *Treponema pallidum* is becoming more common in the USA, and there are increasing numbers of patients with AIDS and syphilis (Johns, Tierney and Felsenstein, 1987). Estimates of the prevalence of otosyphilis among otological patients is around 0.6% as reported by Darmstadt and Harris (1989) who reviewed the literature relating to luetic hearing loss and found that sensorineural hearing loss had been reported in primary, secondary and late acquired syphilis. Steckelberg and McDonald (1984) reviewed 79 cases of syphilis with otological involvement and reported on 38 believed to have no other causes for the hearing impairment identified. They found no common audiological pattern among the patients. Hearing loss appeared earlier in congenital cases. The commonest complaint was a gradual progressive sensorineural hearing loss over months, with occasional sudden hearing loss in a minority. Forty-seven per cent had tinnitus, while 42% reported episodic vertigo and 37% noticed unsteadiness. Improvement in hearing threshold levels was observed on treatment with high doses of corticosteroids. They noted a smaller incidence of endolymphatic hydrops than suggested by Karmody and Schuknecht in 1966. The pathogenesis of endolymphatic hydrops has been thought to be related to fibrous obliteration of the endolymphatic duct and sac. A diagnosis of otosyphilis should be suspected in any patient with a unilateral or bilateral hearing loss of obscure origin, a position also advocated by Darmstadt and Harris (1989). No prospective controlled trials supporting the efficacy of any specific treatment plan exist. Both penicillin and ampicillin have been used, orally or parenterally, with more prolonged treatment for late syphilis. For luetic hearing losses a combination of penicillin with steroids is recommended. Zoller, Wilson and Nadol (1979) found improvement to be mainly short-lived, with 15% retaining improved levels with therapy. Chan, Adams and Kerr (1995) have reported good long-term preservation of hearing with amoxycillin (or ampicillin) and steroids.

In patients with concomitant HIV infection the use of steroids should be avoided because of the risk of potentially lethal opportunistic infections. It has been suggested that with such cases, up to 24 million units of intravenous penicillin G daily for a period of 3 weeks should be considered (Smith and Canalis, 1989).

Meningitis

Sensorineural hearing loss in children with bacterial meningitis is well-documented, having a prevalence between 5 and 30%. *Streptococcus pneumoniae* infections have the highest incidence (31%), and *Haemophilus influenzae* the lowest, of the three bacterial organisms most frequently encountered with this condition (Dodge *et al.*, 1984). A more recent study by Fortnum and Davis (1993) in a group of 15 hearing-impaired children after bacterial meningitis showed no evidence that any one of the common bacterial organisms in this condition was different from any other with respect to the effect on hearing impairment. Nadol, in 1978, reported on 547 meningitis patients from infancy to adults. In his study of subjects over the age of 2.5 years, 21% suffered partial or complete hearing loss, with 77% of partial losses showing some degree of improvement. He described the temporal bones of a 45-year-old man who had shown recovery from his hearing impairment before dying from unrelated causes. No degeneration of the auditory or vestibular sense organs was noted. Another adult who died from pneumococcal meningitis had bacterial invasion and necrosis of the membranous labyrinth. Pfister, Feiden and Einhaupl (1993) in their prospective study of 86 adults with bacterial meningitis found intracerebral complications in 50%, but failed to detect any with a significant hearing loss. Cryptococcal meningitis is increasingly associated with a sudden sensorineural hearing loss, with the incidence as high as 27% (Maslan, Graham and Flood, 1985). The site of damage appears to be retrocochlear. Nadol (1978) reported cryptococcal granulomas involving the inner ear and the internal auditory canal in a 60-year-old patient with fungal neurolabyrinthitis.

Lyme disease

Lyme disease is an infection with *Borrelia burgdorferi*, a spirochaete, transmitted by the bite of a tick. The characteristic skin lesion is erythema chronicum migrans, followed weeks later by cardiac, neurological and musculoskeletal manifestations. Otological symptoms are less common and may be part of a more severe disease (Lesser, Dort and Simmen, 1990). Hanner, Rosenhall and Kaijser (1988), in a study of 73 patients with unilateral loss of vestibular function or Menière-like symptoms, found 14% had elevated levels of IgG antibodies against the Borrelia antigen. Four of these patients had sensorineural hearing loss. In a subsequent study, Hanner *et al.* (1990) found elevated antibodies to Borrelia antigen in 17% of 98 subjects with unilateral sudden or variable sensorineural hearing loss. Treatment of these 17 subjects with intravenous penicillin resulted in improvement of high frequency hearing loss in five patients. Mokry *et al.* (1990) reported a case of a 63-year-old man with an expanding granulomatous lesion in the cerebellopontine angle arising from chronic *B. burgdorferi* infection.

Post-chronic suppurative otitis media

The possible relationship between sensorineural hearing loss and chronic suppurative otitis media has been mooted for more than half a century. Several authors (English, Northern and Fria, 1973; Paparella, 1983; Paparella *et al.*, 1984; Kirtane *et al.*, 1985;

Cusimano, Cocita and D'Amico, 1989) have published work on various aspects of the relationship between sensorineural deafness and middle ear disease. Morrison (1969) indicated one quarter of cases with middle ear inflammation had sensorineural hearing loss.

Kirtane *et al.* (1985), in a survey of 100 patients, found sensorineural hearing loss in ears with attico-antral disease as well as in tubotympanic disease. English, Northern and Fria (1973), in a review of 404 patients with chronic otitis media, found a correlation between the duration of the disease and the extent of the sensorineural hearing loss. Cusimano, Cocita and D'Amico (1989), in a statistical study using linear regression, confirmed that the duration of the disease exerted an influence on the sensorineural hearing loss. The age of onset was not significant. Paparella *et al.* (1984) found a significant sensorineural hearing loss in experimental studies on chinchillas inoculated with *S. pneumoniae* via the superior bulla, as measured by electrocochleography. Temporal bone studies showed serous labyrinthine changes in the perilymph of the basal turn with serofibrous precipitate. In the same paper, a multicentre study involving 607 screened ears with recurrent otorrhoea showed significant levels of sensorineural hearing losses in such patients. Experimental studies on chinchillas by Schachern *et al.* (1992) showed that permeability of the round window membrane to *S. pneumoniae* was responsible for labyrinthitis and meningitis.

Margolis and Nelson (1993) reported a case of a sudden sensorineural hearing loss from acute otitis media that improved. Psychoacoustical tuning curves gave results consistent with a transient cochlear lesion. This suggests that the loss is due to an inner ear abnormality and not a mechanical disturbance of the middle ear. Similarly, Sheehy (1984) reported a case of improvement in hearing in a dead ear with chronic suppurative otitis media that, after reconstructive surgery, attained thresholds of 25 dB HL.

Goycoolea *et al.* (1980) demonstrated the permeability of the round window membrane to macromolecules and possibly to smaller molecules from experimental studies in cats. Cusimano, Cocita and D'Amico (1980) believed, in addition to round window permeability, other possible factors including circulatory disturbances of the round window mucosal vessels, blockage of lymphatic vessels on the round window, alteration of the constituents of the cochlear fluids, and reduction of oxygen diffusion from the middle ear into the perilymph, could result in sensorineural hearing loss with chronic otitis media.

Paparella (1991), in his review of interactive inner ear and middle ear disease, noted that bacterial infections as well as other agents could cause changes in both the endolymph as well as the perilymph thus resulting in endolymphatic hydrops.

Browning and Gatehouse (1989), in their study of 100 subjects with middle ear disease, believed that the poorer levels on bone conduction measurements in such subjects were due to a combination of the prevalence of sensorineural hearing impairment in the population, together with the artificial elevation of the bone conduction levels from a conductive hearing loss. The retrospective study by Walby, Barrera and Schuknecht (1983) on 87 unilateral uncomplicated cases of chronic suppurative otitis media, showed elevation of bone conduction levels across frequencies from 500 Hz to 4000 Hz by a maximum of 9.5 dB HL at the latter frequency. In the same study, analysis of temporal bones with unilateral disease revealed, 'no greater loss of specialized sensorineural structures in infected ears than in normal control ears'. They postulated that the poorer levels obtained on bone conduction measurement in such a condition were the result of changes in the mechanics of sound transmission.

Fungal infections

These can cause otitis externa, as well as sensorineural hearing loss. In subjects with a compromised immune system, such infections occur more frequently, as well as in subjects with AIDS.

Ischaemia
Ischaemic heart disease

The possible connection between ischaemic heart disease extends back to 1965 when in a review of the Mabaan tribe, Rosen and Olin postulated that the better thresholds from 500 to 6000 Hz could be due to a lower incidence of hypertension and atherosclerosis in tribespeople. Podoshin *et al.* (1975), in a study of 59 subjects with myocardial infarct compared with age-matched controls, found a significantly higher threshold at 4 and 8 kHz. They also noted a higher incidence of hypertension in the patient group. More recently Susmano and Rosenbush (1988) compared hearing threshold levels between 103 subjects with ischaemic heart disease, 29 subjects with organic heart disease and normal coronary arteries, and 101 age and sex-matched control group subjects. They found a significantly higher incidence of hearing loss in subjects with ischaemic heart disease. Multiple logistic regression analysis suggested that a patient with a hearing loss of unknown aetiology had an eightfold probability of having ischaemic heart disease. They also noted no significant differences in sex, hypertension, obesity or smoking when hearing-impaired subjects in both the control group and the ischaemic heart disease group were compared.

Gates *et al.* (1993), in a comparison of presbyacusis with cardiovascular disease based on patients in the Framingham cohort, found a relationship between low frequency sensorineural hearing loss (0.25 to 1 kHz) and cardiovascular problems in both sexes but more in females. In men, the age-adjusted loss over the low frequency range showed a correlation with coronary heart disease and cerebrovascular disorders. Male hypertensive subjects also had a greater age-adjusted loss than normotensive subjects. No information was available regarding previous middle ear disease or noise exposure in the subjects. They concluded that the relationship was primarily between cardiovascular disease and hearing impairment.

George *et al.* (1988) reported two subjects with acute myocardial infarction noted to have mild sensorineural hearing loss which improved within 3 days. They suggested that transient hearing loss might be an early indicator of coronary insufficiency.

Macrovascular disorders

Macrovascular causes of sensorineural hearing loss relate to pathology affecting vessels proximal to the labyrinthine artery, and those visible to the naked eye. Such causes for hearing impairment include posterior fossa aneurysms, ectasia of the vertebrobasilar artery, arteriovenous malformations arising from the brain or dura, and vascular loops. These vascular disorders causing compression of the root entry into the brain stem may also cause trigeminal neuralgia, hemifacial spasm, glossopharyngeal neuralgia and essential hypertension (Jannetta, 1980). The exact pathogenesis for the neuro-otological symptoms from these vascular disorders is believed to be pressure-related (Murphy, 1991). Applebaum and Valvassori (1984) found 10 subjects with unilateral anterior inferior cerebellar artery vascular loops with ipsilateral hearing loss, tinnitus and spontaneous nystagmus. They postulated that inner ear symptoms might arise from impaired blood flow through the vascular loop or its branches from compression by the VIIIth cranial nerve. Katayama, Tsubokawa and Yoshida (1987) reported on a subject with an angioma arising from the acoustic nerve and mimicking an acoustic neuroma in its neurological and radiological presentation.

Cerebrovascular accidents

Karp, Belmont and Birch (1969), among others, noted a unilateral hearing loss associated with hemiplegia arising from a cerebrovascular accident in a study involving 17 subjects. Formby, Phillips and Thomas (1987) in their review of 243 single stroke subjects showed no greater degree of hearing impairment in stroke patients than an age and sex matched group, and that aphasic patients were able to test accurately and did not have a greater degree of hearing loss than non-aphasic stroke subjects. However, it should be noted that not all of the 243 subjects were tested in sound proof booths.

Dorsolateral infarct from compromised blood supply from the anterior inferior cerebellar artery or its branches affects the vestibular and cochlear nucleus at the level of the lower pons. The clinical pattern is of an ipsilateral Horner's syndrome with loss of pain and temperature sensation to the contralateral body and limbs, and ipsilateral face area. There may also be ipsilateral cerebellar involvement. The onset is sudden, with vertigo and hearing impairment (Patten, 1977).

Bales (1989) reported a case of a 59-year-old woman with a lateral pontine stroke causing a unilateral moderate to severe hearing loss at high frequencies from a central conduction defect in the auditory pathway that recovered completely within 2 months.

Hypertension and postural hypotension

Blood pressure varies considerably in any one individual, depending on the demands of the circulation but is also subject to physiological factors including exertion, the circadian rhythm, ambient temperature, and emotional and physical arousal. Systemic blood pressure increases with age in developed countries, with a smaller increase for diastolic pressure (Tunstall Pedoe and Walker, 1990). Definition of hypertension varies, but a diastolic pressure at 90 mmHg and above is considered hypertensive (Williams and Braunwald, 1987).

Benign or essential hypertension affects the vast majority of hypertensive patients, and is estimated to occur in up to 20% of the middle-aged population in the UK. This diagnosis is based on the exclusion of known causes for hypertension. Secondary hypertension occurs in 5% of all hypertensive subjects and may be due to renal disease, endocrine disorders (e.g. Cushing's syndrome, Conn's syndrome) or may be drug-related (Tunstall Pedoe and Walker, 1990). Liu (1988) assessed the audiometric function of 32 patients (mean age 65.5 years) with hypertension and coronary heart disease and compared it with 23 normotensive subjects (mean age 65.0 years). The incidence of tinnitus was higher in the hypertensive group (62.5% versus 26.1%). Audiometric data indicated hearing threshold levels, after correction for age from ISO 7089 values, to be significantly higher in the hypertensive group. Tone decay and stapedial reflex decay were absent.

Short-term noise exposure above 90 dBA has been found to increase diastolic pressure and mean blood pressure transiently by up to 12%. Tarter and Robins (1990) found an interesting correlation between duration of noise exposure and hearing loss with hypertension among black workers but not among white workers. Talbott *et al.* (1990) noted a marginally significant relationship between severe noise-related hearing impairment and the prevalence of hypertension in subjects above the age of 64 years in a study of 245 retired workers in heavy industry. In an earlier study on the same population, Talbott *et al.* (1985) noted no difference in blood pressure between workers in two plants with ambient noise levels of 81 and 89 dBA respectively. They noted however that subjects with a severe noise-related hearing loss (loss > 65 dBHL averaged over 3, 4 and 6 kHz) had a greater likelihood of hypertension, and suggested that this could be the result of long-term noise exposure; it was also suggested that the converse was possible, namely that arteriosclerosis was a potentiator for noise-related hearing impairment.

In a review of the subject, Pillsbury (1986) reported experimental work by Borg with normotensive and hypertensive rats with and without noise exposure and found that hypertensive animals had a greater high frequency hearing loss with age, and had greater noise related hearing impairment, when compared with normotensive animals.

Hansen (1988) in a review of 158 subjects with postural hypotension found a hearing loss greater than expected for the subjects' age and sex, after excluding other possible causes.

Vasculitis

Wegener's granulomatosis a distinct condition characterized by necrotizing granulomas in the upper respiratory tract, together with vasculitis and glomerulonephritis. The mean age of onset is around 40 years, with a male:female ratio of 1.3:1. It has been reported to be associated with an increased prevalence of HLA-B8 and HLA-DR2. The upper airway and lung involvement suggests an aberrant response to exogenous or endogenous antigen entering via, or residing in, the respiratory tract. Some patients may demonstrate circulating or deposited immune complexes (Fauci, 1987).

The ear is frequently involved in this condition with otalgia, deafness and discharge; 20–40% of such patients have otological manifestations. Hearing loss is mainly conductive with occasional sensorineural hearing loss, thought to be caused by a vasculitis affecting the vasa nervorum of the VIIIth nerve, or the internal auditory artery or its cochlear branch. Histological studies have shown focal granulomas on the tympanic membrane, or necrotic areas in the temporal bones and mastoid air cells (Friedmann and Bauer, 1973). Kempf (1989) found antibodies to sarcolemma in four of six patients tested and antinuclear antibodies in one. Improvement in the sensorineural hearing loss following early treatment with cyclophosphamide and steroid has been reported by Clements *et al.* (1989) and by Guyot, Baud and Montandon (1990). Other manifestations include a rare syndrome of encephalopathy, sensorineural hearing loss and blindness in three young women recently reported by Bogousslavsky *et al.* (1989) thought to

be the result of an arteriolopathy possibly from a viral causation.

Coagulopathies

Hereditary coagulation disorder

Thomas *et al.* (1992) reported 10 subjects with an average age of 18 years with haemophilia A, haemophilia B or von Willebrand's disease. Testing included pure tone audiometry, impedance audiometry, reflex decay, speech audiometry and masking level difference testing. Results showed a predominantly high frequency loss greater than 4 kHz with 45% having a hearing threshold level greater than 15 dB HL. Central pathway tests suggested possible problems at the cortical, mid-brain or upper brain-stem level.

Earlier work by Fabiani *et al.* (1985) gave a puretone average over 2, 4 and 8 kHz in excess of 15 dB HL in 87% of their subjects. Hearing loss was greater in the mild coagulation disorder patients. Fabiani *et al.* (1985) suggested the possible cause was intracranial micro-haemorrhagic episodes.

Sickle cell anaemia

Sickle cell disease arises in homozygous individuals with HbS. It occurs mainly in black races of North and South America, the West Indies and in central Africa particularly where malaria is endemic as heterozygotes have a slight protection against falciparum malaria (Bunn, 1987). Clinical manifestations of sickle cell anaemia may occur after HbF is replaced by HbS by the sixth month of life. Patients are often plagued by sickle cell crises which are a result of thrombosis in capillaries. Upon deoxygenation, polymerization of HbS molecules occurs, forming thousands of 14-stranded fibres which align into long bundles, leading to sickle deformity. This increases cell rigidity which obstructs capillary flow further. Deoxygenation also increases blood viscosity, which in turn leads to further deoxygenation and sickling. This leads to thrombosis within the capillaries and the crises. By the time the patient reaches adulthood almost all organs, including the cochlea are affected.

Ajulo, Osiname and Myatt (1993), in a survey of 52 patients with homozygous sickle cell disease, found a hearing loss when compared with an age- and sex-matched control group. The site of damage is thought to be in the cochlea by Serjeant, Norman and Todd (1975) while Friedmann *et al.* (1980) and Odetoyinbo and Adekile (1987) postulated a neural contribution. Damage is mainly cochlear but a retro-cochlear contribution cannot be excluded. Abnormal auditory brain-stem response findings in sickle cell crises reported by Elwany and Kamel (1988) were thought to be due to brain-stem anoxia. Urban (1973) reported hair cell loss as well as the presence of sickle cells in the stria vascularis on autopsy.

Tavin, Rubin and Camacho (1993) reported on a case of a 43-year-old woman with HbSC disease (a heterozygous state with HbS and HbC genes) presenting with a sudden sensorineural hearing loss that improved on partial exchange transfusions.

Blood hyperviscosity

Browning and Gatehouse (1986) reported a relationship between increased high-shear blood viscosity and a greater degree of sensorineural hearing loss while increased plasma viscosity was associated with better hearing threshold levels. This was further supported by the work of Gatehouse *et al.* in 1989. Hildesheimer *et al.* (1990) found an increase in blood viscosity in 33 male subjects with a predominantly high frequency hearing loss compared to a control group. It was suggested that high blood viscosity may be a factor in the early development of hearing loss.

Inflammation
Autoimmune hearing loss

The inner ear is as susceptible to on-going autoimmune disease as any other part of the human body. Immunoglobulins within the perilymph may arise from the CSF through the cochlear aqueduct, the blood vessels around the perilymph sac or from local production (Hariri, 1993). Immunological activity appears to be limited to the endolymphatic sac. Autoimmune inner ear disease may be an organ-specific disorder or be part of a generalized autoimmune process. Stephens, Luxon and Hinchcliffe (1982) found cochleovestibular symptoms in a large number of autoimmune disease patients, while 20% of subjects with idiopathic cochleovestibular disorders developed autoimmune diseases within 10 years. It has been suggested that subjects with idiopathic cochleovestibular disorders should have a course of immunosuppressive therapy, as improvement in hearing was noted in 52 out of 56 subjects by McCabe (1989).

Rheumatoid arthritis

This is a multisystemic disease of unknown aetiology, with a female:male ratio of 3:1. A genetic predisposition is suspected – 30% of monozygous twins are concordant for rheumatoid arthritis compared with 5% of dizygous twins. This condition is also associated with HLA-DR4. The reported prevalence is 1% in the population with a variety of systemic manifestations. Prevalence increases with age, appearing around the fourth and fifth decades, usually affecting peripheral joints, with spread to the wrists, ankles, knees, elbows and shoulders. Rheumatoid nodules appear in 20–30% of subjects, while vasculitis affects most systems (Lipsky, 1987). The incidence of sensorineural hearing loss varies from 26% to 48% (Elwany, El Garf and Kamel, 1986). The previous authors also found reduced middle ear compliance; however, clinically significant conductive hearing loss was uncommon.

Cogan's syndrome

This condition originally reported by Cogan in 1945 includes non-syphilitic interstitial keratitis, acute sensorineural hearing loss and vestibular symptoms. Cogan's syndrome is believed to be one manifestation of a systemic autoimmune disorder mediated through cellular pathways. The pathogenesis is thought to be related to vasculitis. Findings are of non-syphilitic interstitial keratitis with vertigo, hearing loss and occasionally tinnitus. The common age of presentation is in the 20–40-year-old age group with an equal male to female ratio, usually following on an upper respiratory tract infection. No single diagnostic test is available, with canal paresis, and a moderate sensorineural hearing loss across all frequencies usually found. The sensorineural hearing loss in this condition is one of the few with a good likelihood of improvement with prompt steroid therapy. Haynes *et al.* (1980) performed meta-analysis on 60 reports encompassing 116 patients with reported Cogan's syndrome and determined that 78 had typical Cogan's syndrome with 38 atypical. Approximately 50% of subjects developed initial symptoms from 7 to 10 days after an upper respiratory tract infection. More than 90% of patients had acute rotatory vertigo associated with an interstitial keratitis presentation, while a sudden onset of hearing loss was seen in 100 of the 111 patients. Fidler and Jones (1989) suggested that pure tone audiometry and ESR measurements were useful in assessing activity of the condition.

Examination of the inner ear has shown endolymphatic hydrops, atrophy of the spiral ganglion, calcification of scala vestibuli, and oedema of the spiral ligament (Wolff *et al.*, 1965; Zechner, 1980).

Haynes *et al.* (1980) observed improvement in hearing threshold levels with early administration of corticosteroids, but noted that spontaneous improvement in hearing levels may occur up to 3 months after the onset of symptoms.

Systemic lupus erythematosus

This is an archetypal immunologically-mediated multisystem disease. Viral infections, genetic factors and abnormal immune responses are thought to interact to produce the disease. Clinical presentation is classically with a 'butterfly rash', myalgias, fatigue, weight loss and pyrexia; 90% of cases occur in women of child-bearing age.

Bowman *et al.* (1986) found moderate to severe hearing loss in 8% of a small group of 30 patients. They postulated the loss to be due to vasculitis or from direct attack on nucleoproteins in inner ear tissue. It has been suggested that an improvement may be obtained with immunosuppression or plasma exchange. Vestibular disturbances may also occur. However, Narula, Powell and Davis (1989) in their study of 20 subjects did not find significantly worse hearing when compared to a control group of 11 adults.

Other autoimmune disorders

Takayasu's disease

Takayasu's disease, often called aortic arch syndrome or 'pulseless disease', is an inflammatory and stenotic disease of middle-sized arteries, more common in Asians, and primarily affecting young women. It is suspected to have an immunopathogenic basis.

Siglock and Brookler (1987) observed bilateral and symmetrical high frequency sensorineural hearing loss, and reported temporal bone findings by Nomura and Kitamura showed well-demarcated hair cell losses in the basal turn of the cochlea, with normal blood vessels in the cochlea and internal auditory meatus. In five women Kunihiro *et al*. (1990) observed high frequency sloping sensorineural hearing loss with a conductive overlay postulated to be related to eustachian tube inflammation. Hearing improved with steroid ingestion.

IgA nephropathy

IgA nephropathy is an immune complex glomerulo-nephritis observed with various disorders, more common in young men. Ataya (1989) reported a case of sudden unilateral severe sensorineural hearing loss treated with corticosteroids with subsequent threshold improvement.

Behçet's syndrome

Behçet's syndrome is a multisystemic disorder with recurrent oral and genital ulcers, and uveitis. Andreoli and Savastano (1989) found bilateral moderate sensorineural hearing loss in 28% of a group of 14 subjects with this condition. Gemignani *et al*. (1991) in their assessment of 20 subjects found sensorineural hearing loss in 12, and vestibular disturbances in five. The HLA-B51 antigen was observed in 10 of the 14 subjects with ear involvement in the group. In a small study, 80% of 35 patients had a hearing loss greater than 25 dB HL. One quarter of patients given cyclosporin A (10 mg/kg reducing to 5 mg/kg per day) showed improvement in hearing threshold levels (Elidan *et al*., 1991).

Polyarteritis nodosa

Polyarteritis nodosa is a multisystem necrotizing vasculitis of small and medium-sized muscular arteries

resulting in non-specific signs of fever, weight loss, and malaise. Local signs follow, abdominal pains, angina, with renal involvement being the most common finding of a specific organ disorder. Middle ear disorder with conductive hearing loss has been reported. Sensorineural hearing loss, although rare, has been reported (Pietersen and Carlsen, 1966; Bakaar, 1978; Wolf *et al*., 1987). Pathological findings have included necrosis of the cochlea and vestibular system with fibrosis and bone formation (Gussen, 1977a), loss of organ of Corti with strial atrophy and reduction of spiral ganglia cells (Jenkins, Pollak and Fisch, 1981).

Another autoimmune disease associated with sensorineural hearing loss is *birdshot retinochoroidopathy* (Heaton and Mills, 1993).

Demyelination

Multiple sclerosis presents usually as recurrent attacks of focal or multifocal neurological dysfunction reflecting lesions within the central nervous system. In most cases it begins in early adult life, with an intermittent presentation but, in one-third, the disease is slowly progressive. The cause is unclear; it is commoner in whites, and in temperate zones. An HLA-linked genetic factor exists which predisposes towards multiple sclerosis. Excessive IgG production within the CNS is also seen in all stages of this disease. It is slightly more common in women, with the majority of cases presenting between the ages of 20 and 50 years (Antel and Arnason, 1987). Hearing loss is an uncommon presentation. Auditory brain stem response testing of patients with hearing loss shows little activity after wave I. The site of lesion is thought to be in the VIIIth nerve root-entry zone. Furman, Durrant and Hirsch (1989) reported a case of a sudden unilateral profound sensorineural hearing loss from such a lesion in a young woman with recovery of hearing levels to within normal limits within 10 days. Franklin, Coker and Jenkins (1989) reported two cases with a similar presentation of a sudden sensorineural hearing loss in young females, with deafness being the sole feature in one of them.

Neoplastic
Primary and secondary lesions

Primary tumours arising from the inner ear have not been reported, although neoplasia from the retrocochlear pathway is well-documented. Eleven per cent of patients with a unilateral sensorineural hearing loss have a neoplastic lesion, either metastatic or primary in origin. Irwin (1987) reported on the occurrence of sensorineural hearing loss with polycythaemia rubra vera, and with myelomatosis, as well as with Waldenstrom's macroglobulinaemia. Retrocochlear hearing loss may also arise as a consequence of the development of benign lipomas, epidermoids or meningiomas affecting the auditory pathway. Intramedullary tumours are uncommon and may include astrocytoma, glioblastoma, and tumours of the third ventricle including pineal body tumours.

The most common CNS tumours are metastatic, occurring in one-quarter of patients with systemic cancer. The largest percentage comes from the lung in men, and the breast in women, while melanomas have the highest probability of spread to the CNS.

Vestibular schwannoma (acoustic neuroma)

The vestibular schwannoma is a benign tumour arising from neoplastic proliferation of Schwann cells around the neurilemmal-glial junction (the Obersteiner-Redlich zone) most commonly from the sheath of the superior vestibular nerve. Vestibular schwannomas account for 5% of all intracranial tumours (Hochberg and Pruit, 1987). They are responsible for over 75% of all tumours of the cerebellopontine angle. The peak incidence is in the fourth decade with the majority of cases present between the fourth and sixth decades. The prevalence rate is one per 100 000 based on clinical findings (Monsell and Rock, 1990), but asymptomatic lesions account for the prevalence rate of 1% on post-mortem studies (Morrison, 1975). Vestibular schwannomas may be unilateral or bilateral. The latter condition is encountered in 96% of cases with central neurofibromatosis (Kanter *et al.*, 1980). Although it was previously believed that the same gene is responsible for formation of either peripheral neurofibromatosis (NF1) unilateral sporadic or central neurofibromatosis (NF2), bilateral hereditary vestibular schwannomas (Lanser, Sussman and Frazer, 1992), it is now known that both types of neurofibromatosis are genetically different entities. Recent work has shown that the central neurofibromatosis gene is located on chromosome 22 (Arai *et al.*, 1993), and functions as a tumour suppressor. The gene responsible for peripheral neurofibromatosis is found on chromosome 17 (Viskochil, White and Cawthorn, 1993), while Legius *et al.* (1992) recently identified a peripheral neurofibromatosis pseudogene on chromosome 15.

Unilateral vestibular schwannomas usually arising from the vestibular nerve displace the facial and cochlear nerves anteriorly, while in bilateral disease the tumour is usually a multilobulated mass with the VIIth nerve and the cochlear nerve entering it directly, making preservation of these nerve trunks more difficult (Baldwin and LeMaster, 1989). The commonest clinical presentation of vestibular schwannomas is unilateral deafness, either of a sudden or progressive nature. Other symptoms include unsteadiness on walking, and unilateral tinni-

tus. With expansion, involvement of adjacent cranial nerves occurs with typical clinical patterns appearing.

The growth rate of acoustic neuromas is difficult to determine but thought to be broadly divided into slow (0.02 cm/year axial diameter growth rate), medium (0.2 cm/year) or fast (1 cm/year), with peripheral neurofibromatosis being in the first two categories, while central neurofibromatosis patients are more often in the fast group (Lanser, Sussman and Frazer, 1992). In a review of 35 cases followed up where surgery was not performed, Valvassori and Guzman (1989) found that 57% of tumours grew, but observed no correlation between the growth of tumour and length of follow up or with age of patient. They believed that any potential tumour growth was manifested within the first year of detection of the neoplasm. A battery of audiovestibular investigations is required with varying degrees of positive results from the different procedures. Moffat *et al.* (1989b) found Unterberger's stepping test to be clinically more sensitive than the Romberg test in detection of vestibular abnormalities with vestibular schwannoma. Abnormal stapedial reflexes were seen in 69% of subjects and auditory brain-stem response abnormalities in 100% (Kanzaki, 1986), with abnormalities on contralateral auditory brain-stem responses reported in 19% (Moffat *et al.*, 1989a). However, normal caloric tests were observed between 4% and 8.5% (Kumar, Maudelonde and Mafee, 1986; Kanzaki, 1986). The 'gold standard' diagnostic test for the detection of vestibular schwannomas is magnetic resonance imaging with gadolinium contrast, which can detect tumours as small as 2–3 mm.

Strauss *et al.* (1991) reported on a series of seven patients who had delayed hearing loss after surgery for vestibular schwannoma finding that the best predictor for such cases was gradual deterioration of intraoperative auditory brain-stem potentials, especially of wave V. They observed improvement of hearing in four other patients with severe postoperative hearing loss when treated with low molecular weight Dextran. The pathogenesis was attributable to manipulation of the cochlear nerve causing disturbances of the microcirculation of the endoneurial vasa nervorum.

Leukaemia

Yabe, Kaga and Kodama (1989) reported on the temporal bones of a patient with chronic myeloid leukaemia presenting with sudden bilateral profound sensorineural hearing loss, with absent caloric responses on ice-water testing. Extensive leukaemic infiltration was noted of the perilymph and endolymph of both the cochlea and the labyrinthine system, with destruction of the organ of Corti and dilatation of Reissner's membrane. Paparella *et al.* (1973) in their earlier review of 45 temporal bones of patients with leukaemia found infiltration of internal auditory canal structures, but only one bone had involvement of the labyrinth. Haemorrhage into the middle ear and mastoid was a frequent finding. Forty-eight per cent of their patients had otological complications.

Metabolic disorders associated with hearing loss

Disorders of metabolism as well as endocrine disorders are reported to result in hearing impairment in diabetes mellitus, hypothyroidism, hyperlipoproteinaemia, renal failure, hyperuricaemia, acromegaly, Addison's disease and phaeochromocytoma.

Diabetes mellitus

Diabetes mellitus is classified as non-insulin-dependent diabetes mellitus or insulin-dependent diabetes mellitus, which corresponds to the previous labels of adult onset diabetes mellitus (type II) and juvenile onset diabetes mellitus (type I). They are suspected to be two separate entities from the pathogenesis, with the non-insulin type probably the result of breakdown of interaction of regulatory mechanisms, while insulin-dependent diabetes mellitus may be related to partial destruction of B cells in the pancreas and may be modified by polygenic (suspected to be a specific HLA antigen) and environmental (thought to be a viral infection) factors. An autoimmune component is thought to be responsible for the destruction of the B cells (Pickup and Williams, 1991).

Complications from insulin-dependent diabetes are microvascular, resulting in small vessel disease of the kidneys, retina and the skin as well as neuropathy, and less commonly macrovascular. An increased incidence of the disease has been noticed in the autumn and the winter.

Non-insulin-dependent diabetes is more common in obese and older patients, with a strong genetic predisposition. Fewer microvascular complications are seen; there is a higher risk of large vessel atherosclerosis, coronary disease and peripheral vascular disease.

The relationship between diabetes mellitus and hearing loss has been debatable and extends back to 1857 (Cullen and Cinnamond, 1993). Triana *et al.* (1991) carried out experimental studies on the spontaneous hypertensive/NIH corpulent (SHR/N-cp) rat being fed a sugar-rich or a starch-rich diet. They found a significant loss of outer hair cells in the diabetic obese animal when compared with non-obese control animals. The different diets had no significant effect on the extent of hair cell loss. There

was a statistically significant loss of outer hair cells in all diabetic obese ageing rats when compared with the non-diabetic obese ageing rats used as controls (Rust *et al.*, 1992). They also noted that neither diet nor gene expression for obesity affected the hair cell damage. They postulated that damage to the hair cells was the result of microangiopathy to the small vessels of the inner ear, leading to hypoxia. Taylor and Irwin (1978) had suggested that the microangiopathy caused deafness due to either direct means or to interference of supply of nutrients from vessel wall thickening. Other mechanisms may be neuropathic or a combination of angiopathy and neuropathy (Cullen and Cinnamond, 1993). Wackym and Linthicum (1986) postulated that the loss was due to microangiopathic involvement of the basilar membrane vessels and/or the endolymphatic sac, after comparison of temporal bones of diabetics with those from controls. They found a higher incidence of loss of hair cells and stria vascularis in diabetic patients with microangiopathy when compared to those without vascular disease.

Taylor and Irwin (1978) studied a group of 38 diabetic patients and 39 controls and concluded that the diabetic patients were 'drawn from a different, deafer population'. Kurien, Thomas and Bhanu (1989) found that diabetic subjects had a poorer high frequency hearing threshold than the non-diabetic population, with poorly controlled subjects showing a greater loss than the uncomplicated well-controlled diabetic patient. They, like Cullen and Cinnamond (1993), found no relationship between duration of diabetes and extent of hearing loss, in contrast to Edgar's conclusion of a relationship between the two (Jorgensen and Buch, 1961).

Huang *et al.* (1990) in a study of 43 diabetic subjects compared with age and sex-matched controls found statistically significant differences between the two groups for the average over 500, 1000 and 2000 Hz in addition to an increased incidence of recruitment, reduced speech discrimination scores, and prolongation of the I–V interval on auditory brain-stem response testing. They concluded that the damage was mainly cochlear, and high frequencies were predominantly affected.

Heinemann *et al.* (1992) concluded that non-insulin-dependent diabetic patients were not deafer than a control group and suggested that differing conclusions by other authors could be related to the different methods and criteria used. They could not exclude the possibility of a subclinical hearing loss. Parving *et al.* (1990) in a study of 39 diabetic subjects found no significant difference in hearing levels between diabetic patients with microangiopathy and those with no microangiopathy; nor was there a significant difference between diabetic patients and an age- and sex-matched control group. They noted abnormal auditory brain-stem responses in 40% of the subjects with long-term insulin-dependent diabetes compared with abnormalities in only 5% of the short-term insulin-dependent diabetic subjects.

Carmen *et al.* (1989) have suggested that a low frequency sensorineural hearing loss may be found in patients with diabetes mellitus, having found abnormally elevated plasma glucose in 47% of 45 subjects with such an audiometric configuration on oral glucose tolerance test. They postulated that significant glucose-insulin imbalance was more likely to affect the apical end of the cochlea due to the nature of the vascular supply.

Dieroff, Schuhmann and Westermann (1988) studied 44 young (less than 41 years of age) insulin-dependent diabetic patients and found abnormalities in distorted speech tests but normal thresholds at conventional pure tone audiometry. They believed that the early reduction of speech discrimination ability reflected the effect of diabetes mellitus on the entire hearing function.

Irwin (1987) postulated six possible mechanisms for diabetic labyrinthopathy, namely, microangiopathy of the cochlea, neuropathy, brain stem involvement, metabolic effect of hyperglycaemia or hypertriglyceridaemia, hyperviscosity resulting vascular problems, or a combination of the above.

Thyroid disorders

Much has been written about myxoedema and hearing impairment while in contrast little has been said about any link between hyperthyroidism and hearing disorders. The relationship between hypothyroidism and hearing loss was first mooted in 1888 by the Clinical Society of London. Several reports since then have suggested an incidence of deafness in myxoedema to be between 30 and 66% (Van't Hoff and Stuart, 1979). Bhatia *et al.* (1977) found a correlation between the severity of thyroid disorder with the degree of cochlear dysfunction. Parving, Parving and Lyngsoe (1983) in a small study of 15 myxoedema subjects found no significant hearing loss when compared to a control group, nor any improvement of thresholds on treatment of the thyroid disorder. On the other hand, Van't Hoff and Stuart (1979), in their study of 41 myxoedematous subjects with a sensorineural hearing loss, found improvement in hearing in 73% of affected ears, with thresholds returning to normal in 23%. Similarly, Anand *et al.* (1989) found a hearing loss in 80% of myxoedematous subjects. They believed that the lesion was at the level of the cochlea. After treatment, improvement in thresholds by more than 10 dB HL at one or more frequency in either or both ears was seen in three-quarters of the hearing impairment subjects. However, auditory brain-stem response audiometry showed no improvement suggesting that improvement in thresholds could be related to an overall improvement of the patient's general condition. Ben–

Tovim *et al.* (1985) noted abnormalities in wave III of auditory brain-stem responses in adult myxoedematous rats, and suggested a lesion at the level of the superior olivary complex in myxoedema. In humans with myxoedema, Himelfarb *et al.* (1981) found an increase in brain stem conduction times, with diminished amplitudes and poor synchronization. In hyperthyroidism they found hearing thresholds were normal in a small study of six patients but brain stem conduction time was reduced. They noted some correlation between conduction times and level of serum T4 for all thyroid dysfunction, and suggested that changes in conduction times reflected activity of the thyroid hormone in the nervous system.

Meyerhoff (1979), in a review of experimental studies, found elevated thresholds in chicks exposed to thiourea in gestation and hearing loss in cats and squirrel monkeys with thyroidectomy correctable with thyroid replacement. He observed middle ear pathology (stapes distortion, incus fusion) as well as inner ear disturbances (tectorial membrane distortion, inner hair cell and outer hair cell degeneration and distortion, lipid deposits of Hensen's cells and enlarged intracellular spaces in the stria vascularis).

Renal failure

There are similarities between the cochlea and the kidney, with ototoxicity and nephrotoxicity for aminoglycosides being well documented. In addition, the ionic exchange activity of the stria vascularis with sodium–potassium exchange pumping potassium into the scala media compares with the active reabsorption of sodium in the tubular epithelium of the ascending limb of Henle. Blockage of the sodium reabsorption with frusemide or ethacrynic acid exerts a diuretic effect but in higher doses causes reversible sensorineural hearing loss. Furthermore, animal experiments have shown an immunological connection between the kidney and the inner ear (Arnold, 1984). Gatland *et al.* (1991) found a high and a low frequency hearing loss in approximately 50% of 66 subjects with chronic renal disease. Interestingly, they observed significant improvement in low frequency thresholds after dialysis in 38% of 62 ears while, in their study of 290 patients with renal failure, Oda *et al.* (1974) found that hearing and vestibular disorders occurred in patients continuing on dialysis. They observed deposits within the stria vascularis, loss of hair cells, and spiral ganglion cells, with the severity of the temporal bone findings directly proportional to the number of dialyses or transplants of the patient.

Antonelli *et al.* (1991) found lengthening of the I–III interpeak interval when comparing auditory brain-stem response audiometry parameters of patients with chronic renal failure with an age and sex-matched control group. They postulated a subclinical disorder of VIIIth nerve function from axonal uraemic neuropathy.

Hyperlipoproteinaemia

Rosen and Olin (1965) discussed the correlation between the mean cholesterol levels of the Mabaan tribe in the Sudan with the average American value, and suggested that the lower levels in the tribespeople were linked to the better hearing at high frequencies. Subsequent research by Rosen, Olin and Rosen (1970) was carried out in which the diets of two mental hospitals in Finland were controlled for fat content. Individuals in the hospital with a low fat diet had significantly better hearing threshold levels. The diets were changed after 5 years and on retest 4 years later, the residents with the previous high fat diet had recovered their hearing acuity while those currently on the high fat diet had diminished auditory acuity compared with their previous results. Spencer (1973), in an uncontrolled study of 300 subjects, reported hyperlipoproteinaemia in 42% of his subjects with idiopathic sensorineural hearing loss. In a study of normotensive (WKY) and hypertensive (SHR) rats, Pillsbury (1986) clearly showed that an atherogenic diet was important in increasing susceptibility towards noise-related hearing loss in genetically predisposed animals. He found that diet and hypertension showed a synergistic effect on susceptibility to noise. However, hypertension and an atherogenic diet alone did not produce significant hearing loss in his study.

Ray (1991), in a review, was of the opinion that socioacusis contributed towards the significantly poorer hearing threshold levels in the average American, notwithstanding the differences in serum cholesterol.

Axelsson and Lindgren (1985) noted a synergistic effect between high serum cholesterol levels and noise exposure in causing a high frequency sensorineural hearing loss. They suggested that an elevated serum cholesterol could cause high frequency hearing loss by affecting blood viscosity, increased sludging of blood, or by resultant arteriosclerotic changes. Pyykko *et al.* (1988) in their longitudinal study of 199 noise-exposed forest workers, found a correlation between sensorineural hearing loss and elevated diastolic blood pressure, total cholesterol as well as low density lipid-cholesterol level. They concluded that elevated cholesterol level together with moderate noise exposure was sufficient to cause sensorineural hearing loss. The hearing loss from lipid metabolic dysfunction was not noticeable in subjects with 'heavy' noise exposure due to the greater effect of noise-related hearing impairment. Unfortunately, the authors did not offer their definition of moderate and heavy noise exposure. In a subsequent study, Starck, Pyykko and Pekkarinen (1988) found that smoking, in combination with elevated diastolic blood pressure

and/or occupationally-induced Raynaud's phenomenon in noise exposed forestry and shipyard workers, resulted in a higher risk of acquiring sensorineural hearing loss.

Hyperuricaemia

Delucci (1988) reported sensorineural hearing loss in 38 subjects with hyperuricaemia (serum uric acid level 70 mg/l or more) below 55 years of age, after exclusion of other known factors related to hearing impairment. The hearing impairment had a high frequency tendency with a 6 kHz notch. In one temporal bone, staining for uric acid was noted in all parts of the labyrinth.

Other metabolic disorders

Acromegaly is due to excess secretion of growth hormone with characteristic physical features. In addition, increased metabolic activity is common. Hearing loss in this condition has been reported by Crosara *et al.* (1985) who found a predominantly high frequency sensorineural hearing loss in a group of 15 subjects, which they postulated was due to vasculopathy.

Trauma and toxicity
Head injury

Injury to the skull may damage the ear by fractures of the temporal bones, by labyrinthine concussion without fracture, or by a combination of both. Longitudinal as opposed to transverse fractures of the temporal bone occur from blows to the temporal and parietal areas. The fracture line in a longitudinal fracture extends through the roof of the external canal, middle ear cavity, around the carotid artery, and the tensor tympani muscle ending in the vicinity of the foramen lacerum. Transverse fractures arise from blows to the occipital area, with immediate facial nerve paralysis in about half the cases. It is associated with haemotympanum without rupture of the tympanic membrane. In addition to facial palsy, vertigo with nystagmus and sensorineural hearing loss is common. Labyrinthine concussion can produce inner ear symptoms without any labyrinthine lesion identified on examination. Animal studies have shown bleeding into the perilymphatic space, as well as inner and outer hair cell loss (Gros, 1967). Vertigo is usually positional in nature, and may be peripheral or central.

Clinical evidence of post-traumatic endolymphatic hydrops is based on observation and from electrocochleography as well as from a positive glycerol dehydration test (Clark and Thomas, 1977). Murakami *et al.*

(1990) observed the temporal bone findings in two cases of head injury and found a picture of endolymphatic hydrops in one, but the case reported was affected by the absence of pre-morbid audiometry and vestibular assessment.

In 119 subjects with minor head injuries, abnormalities in interpeak latencies on auditory brain-stem responses were seen in 10% within 48 hours of trauma; more than half returned to normal on repeat testing 1 month later (Schoenhuber *et al.*, 1987). Montgomery, Fenton and McClelland (1984) reported abnormal central conduction times with delayed I–V latencies on auditory brain-stem potentials in 50% of minor head injury subjects, with persistent abnormalities 6 weeks later seen in the majority. On the other hand, Al-Hady *et al.* (1990) found abnormalities on auditory brain-stem responses in all their subjects with minor head injuries for wave V at a fast repetition rate. Similarly, Podoshin *et al.* (1990) found delay of wave V on auditory brain-stem responses only on rapid (55/s) stimulation rate and not with a rate of 10. They suggested that pathological findings at this stimulus rate were consistent with axonal damage, while pathological findings at more rapid rates were likely to have an ischaemic basis.

Elwany (1988) found abnormal auditory brain-stem responses in 60% of subjects with severe closed head injuries. Abnormalities ranged from delayed latencies to absent waves. He found the results from auditory brain-stem responses correlated with the neurological outcome of such patients. This was supported by Al-Hady *et al.* (1990). Hall, Huang-Fu and Gennarelli (1982), in addition to finding delayed waves and absent wave V patterns with auditory brain-stem responses, also observed abnormalities on impedance measurements on three-quarters of 25 patients with acute severe head injuries.

Barotrauma

Please refer to Chapter 7 in Volumes 1 and 3.

Radiotherapy

Radiotherapy, either primary or adjuvant, used for the treatment of localized neoplastic lesions in the head and neck is widely accepted, albeit with occasional complications from irradiation to local structures. Potential damage to the corneal lens is well recognized, while it is generally thought that mature bone is relatively resistant to harmful effects of irradiation. Ramsden, Bulman and Lorigan (1975) have described two patterns of temporal bone involvement: localized disease affecting primarily the temporal bone plate, or diffuse necrosis with possible effects to vital adjacent neurovascular structures. This was present with megavoltage as well as with orthovoltage

therapy, possibly occurring up to 20 years after treatment.

Singh and Slevin (1991) found a significant degree of ipsilateral sensorineural hearing loss in 15 of 28 subjects treated more than 5 years earlier with radiotherapy in divided doses over 20 days for parotid pleomorphic adenoma. They noted that a similar group of 18 subjects with the same total dosage given over twice the period for the same condition did not have significant hearing loss, as reported by Evans *et al.* (1988).

Lau *et al.* (1992) in a review of 49 patients with nasopharyngeal carcinoma treated with radiotherapy found hearing impairment from damage to middle ear, cochlea and to brain stem. Abnormalities on auditory brain-stem responses were present immediately after radiotherapy and persisted after 1 year.

More recently, Birzgalis *et al.* (1993) reported on seven cases of osteoradionecrosis following radiotherapy to the head and neck. Common presenting features included persistent otorrhoea, severe otalgia, facial palsy and hearing impairment.

Ototoxicity

Drug-induced ototoxicity is becoming increasingly important, due to the medico-legal implications arising from such a therapeutic accident. Medication commonly associated with adverse reports of ototoxicity, either causing tinnitus, deafness or vertigo, have been broadly categorized into antidepressants, nonsteroidal anti-inflammatory drugs, salicylates, betablockers, diuretics and aminoglycosides. To this list is added quinine, and cis-platinum. The latter drug frequently causes tinnitus and dose-related permanent sensorineural hearing loss. In addition, antiseptics used for preoperative sterilization, and topical antibiotics have been shown to be ototoxic in animal studies. The reader is invited to refer to Chapter 20 in Volume 3.

Acoustic trauma

Noise-induced hearing loss may arise from short intense periods of impact noise or from long-term exposure to excessive levels of noise. The extent of this disorder is suggested by the fact that one in 30 of the population in the USA have noise-related hearing impairment (Alberti, 1992), while one in 13 of the population have exposure to 'hazardous sound level'. Busis (1991) noted that workers' compensation for acoustic trauma exceeded 25 billion dollars in 1986, with the amount increasing annually. In addition to occupational noise exposure, there is an awareness of the expanding role of socioacusis towards noise-induced hearing loss developing. This is likely to be related to the use of personal stereos, leisure activities including home improvement work, as well as recreational vehicles, e.g. snow-mobiles and motorcycles. There is an increasing role of socioacusis in noise-related hearing impairment. The reader is invited to refer to Chapter 11 in this volume for a comprehensive review of this subject.

Degenerative
Age-related hearing impairment

Hearing loss due to chronological ageing is defined as presbyacusis. This was first reported in 1849 by Toynbee. Schuknecht (1974) has defined four types of presbyacusis; sensory, neural, strial, and cochlear conductive. These categories are based on a study of audiometric data and on histological findings from temporal bones. The possibility of central presbyacusis has been also raised by others.

Sensory presbyacusis is associated with an abruptly sloping high frequency loss above the speech frequency range, with slow progression. Temporal bone studies show loss of sensory cells in the basal turn of the cochlea, leading eventually to distortion and flattening of the organ of Corti (Schuknecht and Gacek, 1993).

Neural presbyacusis results in a greater degree of speech discrimination loss than the pure tone loss due to loss of cochlear neurons with a functional end-organ. Nadol (1988) observed typical findings on light microscopy but no significant pathology on electron microscopy. Pure tone thresholds are affected with 90% primary neuronal degeneration; with 50% degeneration, speech discrimination is still normal. Other central changes are also encountered, including weakness and lack of coordination.

Strial presbyacusis may be familial, with onset in the third to sixth decades. The pure tone audiogram shows a flat or slightly descending pattern with good speech discrimination. There is patchy atrophy of the stria vascularis in the middle and apical turns of the cochlea. Schuknecht and Gacek (1993) postulated the effect is due to alterations in the endolymph causing a detrimental effect.

Cochlear conductive presbyacusis is suggested by linear descending pure tone audiograms. Ramadan and Schuknecht (1989) were unable to find pathological correlates on light microscopy for this audiometric pattern and suggested a subcellular basis for the loss. It is also speculated that the loss is due to alterations in the resonant characteristics of the cochlear duct. However, the existence of this entity has been questioned.

Schuknecht and Gacek (1993) noted that patients commonly had a combination of some of the above four types, while other subjects had audiometric patterns which did not fit the pathological correlates. This postulate is not unequivocally accepted.

Stach, Spretnjak and Jerger (1990) in a study of 700 subjects estimated the prevalence of central auditory disorder in the elderly (central presbyacusis) and found that it increased with age, increasing from 17% in the 50–54 year age group up to 95% in the over 80 year age group. This increase with age was present after controlling for the degree of loss. Central presbyacusis was difficult to diagnose from conventional pure tone and speech audiometry procedures, but Fire, Lesner and Newman (1991) found a good correlation between the phonetically balanced words and synthetic sentence identification. They also noted a good correlation between self-perceived hearing disability and central auditory nervous system function.

Hearing loss from presbyacusis is often affected by noise exposure, both occupationally and socially related. Noise-related hearing loss is presented in detail in Chapter 11 of this volume. Rosenhall, Pedersen and Svanborg (1990) in a longitudinal study found a significant difference in high frequency hearing between noise exposed and non-exposed men at 70 and 75 years of age. However, by 79 years hearing acuity between 4 and 8 kHz was no longer significantly different. They also noted that the hearing loss in noise-exposed subjects extended to lower frequencies and postulated a possible contribution from other factors, including smoking. Macrae (1991) recently analysed longitudinal audiometric records from 240 ex-servicemen and found that the assumption that hearing loss from presbyacusis and noise damage being additive as advocated in International Standard ISO 1999 to be correct.

Jerger *et al.* (1993) found elderly men to have poorer hearing threshold levels above 1000 Hz, but at frequencies below 1000 Hz women had greater average loss. The effect increased with age, and persisted after excluding subjects with noise exposure. They postulated that the low frequency loss in females was related to microvascular disease affecting the stria vascularis (strial presbyacusis) and may be more likely in elderly women because of greater cardiovascular disease events. Gates and Cooper (1991) found more rapid deterioration in women at low frequencies with ageing, but a similar rate for men and women at high frequencies. In addition, the rate of acceleration increased with increasing age for low frequencies, but decreased for high frequencies. They believed strial atrophy to be responsible for the deterioration in the low frequency range, while hair cell degeneration was responsible for high frequency progressive loss.

Bonfils, Bertrand and Uziel (1988) found evoked otoacoustic emissions in all subjects tested until the age of 60; subsequently the incidence of evoked otoacoustic emissions fell to 35% in subjects over the age of 60 years. Elevation of the emission thresholds with increasing age was directly related to the decrease in hearing acuity. Reduction in measurable emissions were thought to be related to sensory presbyacusis.

Morrell and Brant (1991) reported on the largest current longitudinal study of hearing loss in hearing impaired and non-hearing impaired elderly men. Using the Newton–Raphson method for estimating parameters in the linear mixed-effects model for the 17 000 observations, they found the difference to be significant at 1000 Hz but not at higher frequencies. The rate of decline was similar for both subject groups.

Miscellaneous

Menière's syndrome

This condition is well presented in Chapter 19 of Volume 3 in this edition to which the reader should refer. Konigsmark and Gorlin (1976) noted the possibility of hereditary Menière's syndrome where the mode of transmission varied between recessive and dominant.

Bell's palsy

Auditory disorders have been reported in 5–20% of cases with idiopathic facial palsy. A study of the sequelae of Bell's palsy in 330 subjects (Yamamoto, Nishimura and Hirono, 1988) suggested that tinnitus and/or hearing loss observed during facial movement was seen in 2% of cases. Further audiological details were not available. Yagi, Yamaguchi and Nonaka (1988), however, reported hearing impairment and abnormal vestibular results on electronystagmographic and caloric testing in one-third of patients with Bell's palsy, despite the absence of auditory or vestibular symptoms. Abnormal auditory brain-stem response results have been found in approximately 20% of Bell's palsy patients (Gussen, 1977b); Welkoborsky *et al.* (1991) stated that it was possible for this to be due to compression of the VIIIth cranial nerve from oedema of the facial nerve in the internal acoustic meatus.

Sarcoidosis

Audiovestibular symptoms are unusual in this condition, with 50 cases reported having such symptoms over the past four decades. Bilateral fluctuating hearing loss was reported in half, often associated with uveitis and facial palsy (Moine *et al.*, 1990).

Sarcoid lesions are identifiable from the cochlea to the brain stem. Autopsy findings in a patient with sarcoid for 5 years from Babin, Liu and Aschenbrener (1984) included perivascular lymphocytic infiltration of the acoustic, vestibular and facial nerves in the internal auditory meatus with degeneration of the stria vascularis and neuroepithelium of the cochlea. Souliere *et al.* (1991) described two cases of sudden sensorineural hearing loss from neurosarcoidosis with no other cranial neuropathies in young adults. Good responses were obtained on prompt steroid therapy.

Obscure auditory dysfunction

Also known as the King–Kopetsky syndrome and auditory disability with normal hearing, among other titles for this condition, subjects present with hearing difficulties with normal thresholds on pure tone audiometry. This is thought to be a multifactorial disorder affecting a non-homogeneous group, with psychological, physiological and psychoacoustical factors being contributory (Hinchcliffe, 1992).

Abel, Krever and Alberti (1990) found such subjects to have greater difficulty in detecting pure tones in background low frequency high intensity noise, possibly due to an abnormal cochlear excitation pattern. This could be an early precursor to hearing loss of a particular aetiology.

Non-organic hearing loss

Although this condition, by definition, is outside the remit of this chapter, it is a relatively common finding of recent years, and is therefore mentioned here. Causes for this range from lack of attention during testing, to exaggeration of an organic loss. Synonyms for this condition include psychogenic hearing loss, functional hearing loss and malingering, while in the USA, the term pseudohypacusis was commonly used (Alberti, 1981). The commonest reason for this condition is financial, and related to claims for damages from the state, the employer, or the other party in accidental injuries. Such losses may also be associated with claims of tinnitus either developing or worsening with the incident or activity in question. The incidence of non-organic hearing loss has been reported by Alberti, Morgan and LeBlanc (1974) to be between 20 and 25% but varies depending on the patient population and the clinical acumen of the tester.

Detection may be difficult and is usually dependent on an alert and experienced tester. This is helped by the nature of the complaint, the possibility of compensation, and the patient's attitude during the assessment. Free field speech assessment is useful to detect the existence of a non-organic defect. Formal audiometric procedures to confirm the presence and quantify the extent of this defect should be undertaken, and include conventional pure tone audiometry, impedance audiometry, speech audiometry, transient click-evoked otoacoustic emission measurements, and cortical evoked response audiometry. Numerous publications about this condition are available for further perusal and are discussed in Chapter 11.

Sudden sensorineural hearing loss
(see Volume 3, Chapter 17)

Identifiable modalities associated with sudden sensorineural hearing loss are classified as vascular, haematological, inflammatory, toxic, traumatic or neoplastic. In addition, Cogan's syndrome, multiple sclerosis, systemic lupus erythematosus and Paget's disease have been implicated (Meyerhoff and Paparella, 1980). They believed that the pathogenesis was vascular based, with blood vessel narrowing, hypercoagulability, and/or thrombosis with subsequent necrosis of the end organ. They noted that this was more likely in patients with diabetes mellitus, arteriosclerotic vascular disease, hypertensive heart disease, hyperlipoproteinaemia, anxiety or allergic diathesis. A study of eustachian tube function of 50 patients with sudden onset of sensorineural hearing loss assessed impedance with exercises, including the Valsalva manoeuvre. There was no evidence of a patulous tubal function unlike previous reports suggesting that a patulous tube is responsible for sensorineural hearing loss (Maier, Hauser and Munker, 1992).

One-third of cases of sudden sensorineural hearing loss were associated with a preceding viral infection. This is reportedly not an unusual event in otolaryngological surgery. Non-otolaryngological surgical procedures have also been associated with this developing, and Journeaux *et al.* (1990) noted 21 such cases of sensorineural hearing loss, the majority after heart-lung bypass surgery. An embolic phenomenon is thought to be responsible. They also reported on a previously stapedectomized subject who developed a unilateral profound loss after undergoing adrenalectomy. It was postulated that in non-bypass surgical subjects, such a loss could develop as a result of fat embolism or from increased platelet adhesiveness postoperatively. Michel and Brusis (1992) observed that sudden hearing loss after lumbar puncture occurs in two per 1000 procedures. In a study of nine subjects following lumbar puncture, myelography and spinal anaesthesia they reported a hearing loss with subsequent hearing improvement in six. The loss was mainly low frequency and sensorineural, due to patent cochlear aqueducts with reverse flow of perilymph during lumbar puncture. Belal (1980) reported sudden sensorineural hearing loss after sacrifice of the labyrinthine artery during acoustic neuroma surgery with subsequent gradual ossification of the basal turn of the cochlea. In addition, he commented on two other temporal bones showing ossification following sudden sensorineural hearing loss unrelated to surgery, and postulated a vascular aetiology, based on experimental obstruction of the labyrinthine artery causing degenerative changes with ossification of the cochlea. He proposed that ossification of the cochlea was suggestive of a vascular cause for sudden sensorineural hearing loss. Colclasure and Graham (1981) reported sudden

hearing loss, tinnitus and vertigo secondary to an aneurysm of the posterior communicating artery, reversible on clipping of the aneurysm. Schuknecht and Donovan (1986) in a review of the literature on 10 temporal bone findings in cases of sudden sensorineural hearing loss, together with 12 others reported by Schuknecht, discussed the postulated causes for sudden deafness, namely membrane breaks, viral basis and vascular disorders. They concluded that the pathological findings from these temporal bones were most similar to those in clinically proven cases of viral labyrinthitis. No evidence of membrane breaks was noted, while fibrous and osseous proliferation associated with vascular causes was insignificant. Based on their findings they suggested that therapeutic regimens based on a vascular causation for sudden deafness were unlikely to be beneficial.

Conclusion

When attempting to establish the aetiology of hearing impairment, the history is essential as is the pure tone audiogram and an assessment of the ability to discriminate speech. Other investigations should be used selectively. Taking the time to find the cause will at the very least aid patient management as acceptance of disability is made easier by understanding the aetiology and prognosis. It is anticipated that fewer cases of sensorineural hearing losses will be left with an unknown diagnosis, as knowledge of possible causes continues to improve.

References

ABEL, S. M., KREVER, E. M. and ALBERTI, P. W. (1990) Auditory detection, discrimination and speech processing in ageing, noise-sensitive and hearing-impaired listeners. *Scandinavian Audiology*, **19**, 43–54

ABRAMOVICH, S. and PRASHER, D. K. (1986) Electrocochleography and brainstem potentials in Ramsay Hunt syndrome. *Archives of Otolaryngology – Head and Neck Surgery*, **112**, 925–928

AJULO, S. O., OSINAME, A. I. and MYATT, H. M. (1993) Sensorineural hearing loss in sickle cell anaemia – a United Kingdom study. *Journal of Laryngology and Otology*, **107**, 790–794

AL-HADY, M. R., SHEHATA, O., EL-MOUSLY, M. and SALLAM, F. S. (1990) Audiological findings following head trauma. *Journal of Laryngology and Otology*, **104**, 927–936

ALBERTI, P. W. (1981) Non-organic hearing loss in adults. In: *Audiology and Audiological Medicine*, edited by H. A. Beagley. Oxford: Oxford University Press. pp. 910–931

ALBERTI, P. W. (1992) Noise induced hearing loss. *British Medical Journal*, **304**, 522

ALBERTI, P. W., MORGAN, B. B. and LEBLANC, J. C. (1974) Occupational hearing loss: an otologist's view of a long-term study. *Laryngoscope*, **84**, 1822–1834

ANAND, V. T., MANN, S. B. S., DASH, R. J. and MEHRA, Y. N. (1989) Auditory investigations in hypothyroidism. *Acta Otolaryngologica*, **108**, 83–87

ANDREOLI, C. and SAVASTANO, M. (1989) Audiologic pathology in Behcet's syndrome. *American Journal of Otology*, 10, 466–467

ANON (1888) *Report of a Committee of the Clinical Society of London to Investigate the Subject of Myxoedema.* London: Longmans, Green and Co.

ANTEL, J. P. and ARNASON, B. G. W. (1987) Demyelinating diseases. In: *Harrison's Principles of Internal Medicine*, 11th edn, edited by E. Braunwald, K. J. Isselbacher, R. G. Petersdorf, J. D. Wilson, J. B. Martin, and A. S. Fauci. New York: McGraw-Hill. pp. 1995–1999

ANTONELLI, A. R., BONFIOLI, F., GARRUBBA, V., GHISELLINI, M., LAMORETTI, M. P., NICOLAI, P. *et al.* (1991) *Acta Otolaryngologica*, Suppl. 476, 54–68

APPLEBAUM, E. L. and VALVASSORI, G. E. (1984) Auditory and vestibular system findings in patients with vascular loops in the internal auditory canal. *Annals of Otology, Rhinology and Laryngology*, 93, 63–70

ARAI, E., TOKINO, T., IMAI, T., INAZAWA, J., IKEUCHI, T., TONOMURA, A. *et al.* (1993) Mapping the breakpoint of a constitutional translocation on chromosome 22 in a patient with NF2. *Genes, Chromosomes and Cancer*, 6, 235–238

ARNOLD, W. (1984) Inner ear and renal diseases. *Annals of Otology, Rhinology and Laryngology*, Suppl. 112, 119–124

ASBURY, A. K. (1987) Diseases of the peripheral nervous system. In: *Harrison's Principles of Internal Medicine*, 11th edn, edited by E. Braunwald, K. J. Isselbacher, R. G. Petersdorf, J. D. Wilson, J. B. Martin, and A. S. Fauci. New York: McGraw-Hill. pp. 2058–2069

ATAYA, N. L. (1989) Sensorineural deafness associated with IgA nephropathy. *Journal of Laryngology and Otology*, 103, 412

AXELSSON, A. and LINDGREN, F. (1985) Is there a relationship between hypercholesterolaemia and noise-induced hearing loss? *Acta Otolaryngologica*, 100, 379–386

BABIN, R. W., LIU, C. and ASCHENBRENER, C. (1984) Histopathology of neurosensory deafness in sarcoidosis. *Annals of Otology, Rhinology and Laryngology*, 93, 389–393

BAKAAR, L. G. (1978) Polyarteritis nodosa presented with nerve deafness. *Journal of the Royal Society of Medicine*, 71, 144–147

BALDWIN, R. L. and LEMASTER, K. (1989) Neurofibromatosis-2 and bilateral acoustic neuromas: distinctions from neurofibromatosis-1 (von Recklinghausen's disease). *American Journal of Otology*, 10, 439–442

BALES, J. D. (1989) Reversible sensorineural hearing loss in a stroke patient. *Ear and Hearing*, 10, 109–111

BELAL, A. JR (1980) Pathology of vascular sensorineural hearing impairment. *Laryngoscope*, 90, 1831–1839

BEN-TOVIM, R., ZOHAR, Y., ZOHIAR, S., LAURIAN, N. and LAURIAN, L. (1985) Auditory brain stem response in experimentally induced hypothyroidism in albino rats. *Laryngoscope*, 95, 982–985

BHATIA, P. L., GUPTA, O. P., AGRAWAL, M. K. and MISHR, S. K. (1977) Audiological and vestibular function tests in hypothyroidism. *Laryngoscope*, 87, 2082–2089

BIRCHALL, M. A., WIGHT, R. G., FRENCH, P. D., COCKBAIN, Z. and SMITH, S. J. M. (1992) Auditory function in patients infected with the human immunodeficiency virus. *Clinical Otolaryngology*, 17, 117–121

BIRZGALIS, A. R., RAMSDEN, R. T., FARRINGTON, W. T. and SMALL, M. (1993) Severe radionecrosis of the temporal bone. *Journal of Laryngology and Otology*, 107, 183–187

BLACKLEY, B., FRIEDMANN, I. and WRIGHT, I. (1967) Herpes zoster auris associated with facial nerve palsy and auditory nerve symptoms. *Acta Otolaryngologica*, 63, 533–550

BOGOUSSLAVSKY, J., GAIO, J-M., CAPLAN, L. R., REGLI, F., HOMMEL, M., HEDGES, T. R. *et al.* (1989) Encephalopathy, deafness and blindness in young women: a distinct retino-cochleocerebral arteriolopathy? *Journal of Neurology, Neurosurgery and Psychiatry*, 52, 43–46

BONFILS, P., BERTRAND, Y. and UZIEL, A. (1988) Evoked otoacoustic emissions: normative data and presbycusis. *Audiology*, 27, 27–35

BOWMAN, C. A., LINTHICUM, F. H., NELSON, R. A., MIKAMI, K. and QUISMORIO, F. (1986) Sensorineural hearing loss associated with systemic lupus erythematosus. *Otolaryngology – Head and Neck Surgery*, 94, 197–204

BROUWER, O. F., PADBERG, G. W., RUYS, C. J. M., BRAND, R., DE LAAT, J. A. P. M. and GROTE, J. J. (1991) Hearing loss in facioscapulohumeral muscular dystrophy. *Neurology*, 41, 1878–1880

BROWNING, G. and GATEHOUSE, S. (1986) Blood viscosity as a factor in sensorineural hearing impairment. *Lancet*, i, 121–123

BROWNING, G. and GATEHOUSE, S. (1989) Hearing in chronic suppurative otitis media. *Annals of Otology, Rhinology and Laryngology*, 98, 245–250

BUNN, H. F. (1987) Disorders of hemoglobin. In: *Harrison's Principles of Internal Medicine*, 11th edn, edited by E. Braunwald, K. J. Isselbacher, R. G. Petersdorf, J. D. Wilson, J. B. Martin and A. S. Fauci. New York: McGraw–Hill. pp. 1518–1527

BUSIS, S. N. (1991) Noise-induced hearing loss: the sixth question. *American Journal of Otology*, 12, 81–82

BYERS, P. H., WALLIS, G. A. and WILKINS, M. C. (1991) Osteogenesis imperfecta: translation of mutation to phenotype. *Journal of Medical Genetics*, 28, 433–442

CARMEN, R. E., SVIHOVEC, D. A., GOCKA, E. F., GAY, G. C. and HOUSE, L. R. (1989) Audiometric configuration as a reflection of low plasma glucose and diabetes. *American Journal of Otology*, 10, 372–379

CAUSSE, J. R., CAUSSE, J. B., BRETLAU, P., URIEL, J., BERGES, J., CHEVANCE, L. G. *et al.* (1989) Etiology of otospongiotic sensorineural loss. *American Journal of Otology*, 10, 99–105

CHAN, Y. M., ADAMS, D. A. and KERR. A. G. (1995) Syphilitic labyrinthitis – an update. *Journal of Larynyology and Otology*, 109, 719–725

CLARK, S. K and THOMAS, S. R. (1977) Posttraumatic endolymphatic hydrops. *Archives of Otolaryngology*, 103, 725–726

CLEMENTS, M. R., MISTRY, C. D., KEITH, A. O. and RAMSDEN, R. T. (1989) Recovery from sensorineural deafness in Wegener's granulomatosis. *Journal of Laryngology and Otology*, 103, 515–518

COGAN, D. G. (1945) Syndrome of non-syphilitic interstitial keratitis and vestibuloauditory symptoms. *Archives of Ophthalmology*, 33, 144–149

COLCLASURE, J. B. and GRAHAM, S. S. (1981) Intracranial aneurysm occurring as sensorineural hearing loss. *Otolaryngology – Head and Neck Surgery*, 89, 283–287

CROSARA, C., COLLETTI, V., SITTONI, V., BONANNI, G. and MOTTA, R. G. (1985) Analysis of auditory and brain stem function in acromegalic patients. In: *Disorders with Defective Hearing*, edited by V. Colletti and S. D. G. Stephens. *Advances in Audiology*, 3, 152–160. Basel: Karger

CULLEN, J. R. and CINNAHOND, M. J. (1993) Hearing loss in diabetics. *Journal of Laryngology and Otology*, 107, 179–182

CUMMINS, D., MCCORMICK, J. B., BENNETT, D., SAMBA, J. A., FARRAR, B., MACHIN, S. J. *et al.* (1990) Acute sensorineural deafness in Lassa fever. *Journal of the American Medical Association*, **264**, 2093–2096

CUSIMANO, F., COCITA, V. C. and d'AMICO, A. (1989) Sensorineural hearing loss in chronic suppurative otitis media. *Journal of Laryngology and Otology*, **103**, 158–163

DARMSTADT, G. L. and HARRIS, J. P. (1989) Luetic hearing loss. *American Journal of Otolaryngology*, **10**, 410–421

DAVIES, M., KANE, R. and VALENTINE, J. (1984) Impaired hearing in X-linked hypophosphataemic (vitamin-D-resistant) osteomalacia. *Annals of Internal Medicine*, **100**, 230–232

DEBRUYNE, F. (1992) Clinical observations on the on-off effect of the stapedial reflex. *Clinical Otolaryngology*, **17**, 10–12

DEVRIESE, P. P. (1968) Facial paralysis in cephalic herpes zoster. *Annals of Otology, Rhinology and Laryngology*, **77**, 1101–1109

DIEROFF, H. G., SCHUHMANN, G. and WESTERMANN, E. (1988) Hearing disease in diabetes mellitus. In: *Vertigo, Nausea, Tinnitus and Hypoacusia in Metabolic Disorders*, edited by C.-F. Claussen, M. V. Kirtane and K. Schlitter. Amsterdam: Excerpta Medica. pp. 361–364

DJUPESLAND, G., FLOTTORP, G. and REFSUM, S. (1983) Phytanic acid storage disease: hearing maintained after fifteen years of dietary treatment. *Neurology*, **33**, 237–240

DODGE, P. R., DAVIS, H., FEIGIN, R. D., HOLMES, S. J., KAPLAN, S. L., JUBELIRER, D. P. *et al.* (1984) Prospective evaluation of hearing impairment as a sequela of acute bacterial meningitis. *New England Journal of Medicine*, **311**, 869–874

EDWARDS, B. D., PATTON, M. A., DILLY, S. A. and EASTWOOD, J. B. (1989) A new syndrome of autosomal recessive nephropathy, deafness and hyperparathyroidism. *Journal of Medical Genetics*, **26**, 289–293

ELIDAN, J., LEVI, H., COHEN, E. and BENEZRA, D. (1991) Effect of cyclosporin A on the hearing loss in Behçet's disease. *Annals of Otology, Rhinology and Laryngology*, **100**, 464–468

ELL, J., PRASHER, D. and RUDGE, P. (1984) Neuro-otological abnormalities in Friedreich's ataxia. *Journal of Neurology, Neurosurgery and Psychiatry*, **47**, 26–32

ELUCCI, E. (1988) Tinnitus, hypoacusia and vertigo in hyperuricemia. In: *Vertigo, Nausea, Tinnitus and Hypoacusia in Metabolic Disorders*, edited by C.-F. Claussen, M. V. Kirtane and K. Schlitter. Amsterdam: Excerpta Medica. pp. 241–248

ELWANY, S. (1988) Auditory brain stem responses (ABR) in patients with acute severe closed head injuries. *Journal of Laryngology and Otology*, **102**, 755–759

ELWANY, S. and KAMEL, T. (1988) Sensorineural hearing loss in sickle cell crisis. *Laryngoscope*, **98**, 386–389

ELWANY, S., EL GARF, A. and KAMEL, T. (1986) Hearing and middle ear function in rheumatoid arthritis. *Journal of Rheumatology*, **13**, 878–881

ENGLISH, G. M., NORTHERN, J. L. and FRIA, T. J. (1973) Chronic otitis media as a cause of sensorineural hearing loss. *Archives of Otorhinolaryngology*, **98**, 18–22

EVANS, R. A., LIU, K. C., AZHAR, T. and SYMONS, R. P. (1988) Assessment of permanent hearing impairment following radical megavoltage radiotherapy. *Journal of Laryngology and Otology*, **102**, 588–589

FABIANI, M., DI GIROLAMO, A., MARIANI, G., CASINI, A., GIACOMINI, P. and CHISTOLINI, A. (1985) Hearing disorders in

haemophilia and von Willebrand's disease. *Advances in Audiology*, **3**, 161–168

FAUCI, A.S. (1987) The vasculitis syndromes. In: *Harrison's Principles of Internal Medicine*, 11th edn, edited by E. Braunwald, K. J. Isselbacher, R. G. Pedersdorf, J. D. Wilson, J. B. Martin and A. S. Fauci. New York: McGraw-Hill. pp. 1438–1444

FIDLER, H. and JONES, N. S. (1989) Late onset Cogan's syndrome. *Journal of Laryngology and Otology*, **103**, 512–514

FIRE, K. M., LESNER, S. A. and NEWMAN, C. (1991) Hearing handicap as a function of central auditory abilities in the elderly. *American Journal of Otology*, **12**, 105–108

FORMBY, C., PHILLIPS, D. E. and THOMAS, R. G. (1987) Hearing loss among stroke patients. *Ear and Hearing*, **8**, 326–332

FORQUER, B. D. and SHEEHY, J. L. (1981) Cochlear otosclerosis: acoustic reflex findings. *American Journal of Otology*, **2**, 297–300

FORTNUM, H. and DAVIS, A. (1993) Hearing impairment in children after bacterial meningitis: incidence and resource implications. *British Journal of Audiology*, **27**, 43–52

FRANKLIN, D. J., COKER, N. J. and JENKINS, H. A. (1989) Sudden sensorineural hearing loss as a presentation of multiple sclerosis. *Archives of Otolaryngology – Head and Neck Surgery*, **115**, 41–45

FRIEDMANN, E. M., LUBAN, N. L. C., HERER, G. R. and WILLIAMS, I. (1980) Sickle cell anaemia and hearing. *Annals of Otology, Rhinology and Laryngology*, **89**, 342–347

FRIEDMANN, I., and BAUER, F. (1973) Wegener's granulomatosis causing deafness. *Journal of Laryngology and Otology*, **87**, 449–464

FURMAN, J. M. R., DURRANT, J. D. and HIRSCH, W. L. (1989) Eighth nerve signs in a case of multiple sclerosis. *American Journal of Otolaryngology*, **10**, 376–381

GATEHOUSE, S., GALLCHER, J. E. J., LOWE, G. D. O., YARNELL, J. W. G., HUTTON, R. D. and ISING, I. (1989) Blood viscosity and hearing levels in the Caerphilly collaborative heart disease study. *Archives of Otolaryngology – Head and Neck Surgery*, **115**, 1227–1230

GATES, G. A., COBB, J. L., D'AGOSTINO, R. B. and WOLF, P. A. (1993) The relation of hearing in the elderly to the presence of cardiovascular disease and cardiovascular risk factors. *Archives of Otolaryngology – Head and Neck Surgery*, **119**, 156–161

GATES, G. A. and COOPER, J. C. (1991) Incidence of hearing decline in the elderly. *Acta Otolaryngologica*, **111**, 240–248

GATLAND, D., TUCKER, B., CHALSTREY, S., KEENE, B. M. and BAKER, L. (1991) Hearing loss in chronic renal failure – hearing threshold changes following haemodialysis. *Journal of the Royal Society of Medicine*, **84**, 587–589

GEMIGNANI, G., BERRETTINI, S., BRUSCHINI, P., SELLARI–FRANCESCHINI, S., FUSARI, P., PIRAGINE, F. *et al.* (1991) Hearing and vestibular disturbances in Behçet's syndrome. *Annals of Otology, Rhinology and Laryngology*, **100**, 459–463

GEORGE, G., SERAFIM, K., JACOB, P. and PASCAL, A. (1988) Sudden transient sensorineural deafness: sign of coronary insufficiency. In: *Vertigo, Nausea, Tinnitus and Hypoacusia in Metabolic Disorders*, edited by C.-F. Claussen, M. V. Kirtane and K. Schlitter. Amsterdam: Excerpta Medica. pp. 265–268

GLASSOCK, R. J. and BRENNER, B. M. (1987) Glomerulopathies associated with multisystem disease. In: *Harrison's Principles of Internal Medicine*, 11th edn, edited by E. Braunwald, K. J. Isselbacher, R. G. Petersdorf, J. D. Wilson, J. B. Martin, and A. S. Fauci. New York: McGraw–Hill: pp. 1183–1189

GOYCOOLEA, M. V., PAPARELLA, M. M., GOLDBERG, B. and CARPENTER, A.-M. (1980) Permeability of the round window membrane in otitis media. *Archives of Otorhinolaryngology*, **106**, 430–433

GROS, J. C. (1967) The ear in skull trauma. *Southern Medical Journal*, **60**, 705–711

GUSSEN, P. (1977a) Polyarteritis nodosa and deafness. A human temporal bone study. *Archives of Otorhinolaryngology*, **217**, 263–271

GUSSEN, R. (1977b) Pathogenesis of Bell's palsy: retrograde epineural edema and postedematous fibrous compression neuropathy of the facial nerve. *Annals of Otology, Rhinology and Laryngology*, **86**, 549–558

GUYOT, J.-P., BAUD, C. and MONTANDON, P. (1990) Wegener's granulomatosis with otological disorders as primary symptoms. *ORL*, **52**, 327–334

HALL, J. W. III, HUANG–FU, M. and GENNARELLI, T. A. (1982) Auditory function in acute severe head injury. *Laryngoscope*, **92**, 883–889

HALLPIKE, C. S. (1967) Observations on the structural basis of two rare varieties of hereditary deafness in myotatic, kinesthetic and vestibular mechanisms. *Ciba Foundation 19th Symposium*, edited by A. V. S. de Reuck and J. Knight. London: Churchill. p. 285

HANNER, P., ROSENHALL, U. and KAIJSER, B. (1988) Borrelia infection in patients with vertigo and sensorineural hearing loss. *Scandinavian Audiology*, Suppl. 30, 201–203

HANNER, P., ROSENHALL, U., EDSTROM, S. and KAIJSER, B. (1990) Hearing impairment in patients with antibody production against *Borrelia burgdorferi* antigen. *Lancet*, i, 13–15

HANSEN, S. (1988) Postural hypotension – cochleo-vestibular hypoxia – deafness. *Acta Otolaryngologica*, **449**, 165–169

HARIRI, M. A. (1993) Autoimmune inner-ear disease. *Journal of Audiological Medicine*, **2**, 41–52

HAYNES, B. F., KAISER–KUPFER, M. I., MASON, P. and FAUCI, A. S. (1980) Cogan syndrome: studies in thirteen patients, long term follow-up, and a review of the literature. *Medicine*, **59**, 426–441

HEATON, J. M. and MILLS, R. P. (1993) Sensorineural hearing loss associated with birdshot retinochoroidopathy. *Archives of Otolaryngology – Head and Neck Surgery*, **119**, 680–681

HEINEMANN, L., MULLER, J., KUHN, A. and LAMPRECHT, A. (1992) Type I diabetes does not influence hearing abilities. *Journal of Audiological Medicine*, **1**, 20–29

HILDESHEIMER, M., MAAYAN, Z., MUCHNIK, C., RUBINSTEIN, M. and GOODMAN, R. M. (1989) Auditory and vestibular findings in Waardenburg's type II syndrome. *Journal of Laryngology and Otology*, **103**, 1130–1133

HILDESHEIMER, M., BLOCH, F., MUCHNIK, C. and RUBINSTEIN, M. (1990) Blood viscosity and sensorineural hearing loss. *Archives of Otolaryngology – Head and Neck Surgery*, **116**, 820–824

HIMELFARB, M. Z., LAKRETZ, T., GOLD, S. and SHANON, E. (1981) Auditory brain stem responses in thyroid dysfunction. *Journal of Laryngology and Otology*, **95**, 679–686

HINCHCLIFFE, R. (1992) King–Kopetzky syndrome: an auditory stress disorder? *Journal of Audiological Medicine*, **1**, 89–98

HOCHBERG, F. and PRUIT, A. (1987) Neoplastic diseases of the central nervous system. In: *Harrison's Principles of Internal Medicine*, 11th edn, edited by E. Braunwald, K. J. Isselbacher, R. G. Petersdorf, J. D. Wilson, J. B. Martin, and A. S. Fauci. New York: McGraw–Hill. pp. 1968–1980

HUANG, Y. M., PAN C. Y., RUI, G., CAI, X. H., YU, L. M. and CHOU, C. Y. (1990) Study on the hearing impairment in diabetic patients. *Chinese Journal of Otorhinolaryngology*, **25**, 354–356

HUIZING, E. H., VAN BOLHUIS, A. H. and ODENTHAL, D. W. (1966) Studies on progressive hereditary perceptive deafness in a family of 355 members. *Acta Otolaryngologica*, **61**, 35–41, 161–167

IRWIN, J. (1987) Causes of hearing loss in adults. In: *Scott–Brown's Otolaryngology*, 5th edn, edited by A. G. Kerr, vol 2 *Adult Audiology*, edited by D. Stephens. London: Butterworths pp. 127–156

JANNETTA, P. J. (1980) Neurovascular compression in cranial nerve and systemic disease. *Annals of Surgery*, **192**, 518–525

JENKINS, H. A., POLLAK, A. M. and FISCH, U. (1981) Polyarteritis nodosa as a cause of sudden deafness. A human temporal bone study. *American Journal of Otolaryngology*, **2**, 99–107

JERGER, J., SCHMIEL, R., STACH, B. and SPRETNJAK, M. (1993) Gender affects audiometric shape in presbyacusis. *Journal of the American Academy of Audiology*, **4**, 42–49

JOHNS, D. R., TIERNEY, M. and FELSENSTEIN, D. (1987) Alteration in the natural history of neurosyphilis by concurrent infection with the human immunodeficiency virus. *New England Journal of Medicine*, **316**, 1569–1572

JORGENSEN, M. B. and BUCH, N. H. (1961) Studies on inner-ear function and cranial nerves in diabetics. *Acta Otolaryngologica*, **53**, 350–364

JOURNEAUX, S. F., MASTER, B., GREENHALGH, R. M. and BULL, T. R. (1990) Sudden sensorineural hearing loss as a compliction of non-otologic surgery. *Journal of Laryngology and Otology*, **104**, 711–712

KANTER, W. R., ELDRIDGE, R., FABRICANT, R., ALLEN, J. C. and KOERBER, T. (1980) Central neurofibromatosis with bilateral acoustic neuroma: genetic, clinical and biochemical distinctions from peripheral neurofibromatosis. *Neurology*, **30**, 851–859

KANZAKI, J. (1986) Present state of early neurotological diagnosis of acoustic neuroma. *Oto-rhino-laryngology* **48**, 193–198

KARMODY, C. S. and SCHUKNECHT, H. F. (1966) Deafness in congenital syphilis. *Archives of Otolaryngology*, **83**, 18–27

KARP, E., BELMONT, I. and BIRCH, H. G. (1969) Unilateral hearing loss in hemiplegic patients. *Journal of Nervous and Mental Diseases*, **148**, 83–86

KATAYAMA, Y., TSUBOKAWA, T. and YOSHIDA, K. (1987) Angioma of the cerebellopontine cistern simulating acoustic neurinomas. *Surgical Neurology*, **18**, 184–186

KEMPF, H.-G. (1989) Ear involvement in Wegener's granulomatosis. *Clinical Otolaryngology*, **14**, 451–456

KHETARPAL, U. (1993) Autosomal dominant sensorineural hearing loss – further temporal bone findings. *Archives of Otolaryngology – Head and Neck Surgery*, **119**, 106–108

KHETARPAL, U., SCHUKNECHT, H. F., GACEK, R. R. and HOLMES, L. B. (1991) Autosomal dominant sensorineural hearing loss. *Archives of Otolaryngology – Head and Neck Surgery*, **117**, 1032–1042

KIRTANE, M. V., MERCHANT, S. N., RAJE, A. R., ZANTYE, S. B. and SHAH, K. L. (1985) Sensorineural hearing loss in chronic otitis media – a statistical evaluation. *Journal of Postgraduate Medicine*, **31**, 183–186

KONIGSMARK, B. W. and GORLIN, R. J. (1976) *Genetic and Metabolic Deafness*. Philadelphia: W. B. Saunders Co

KONIGSMARK, B. W., MENGEL, M. and BERLIN, C. I. (1971)

Familial low frequency hearing loss. *Laryngoscope*, **81**, 759–771

KUMAR, A., MAUDELONDE, C. and MAFEE, M. (1986) Unilateral sensorineural hearing loss: analysis of 200 consecutive cases. *Laryngoscope*, **96**, 14–18

KUNIHIRO, T., KANZAKI, J., O-UCHI, T. and YOSHIDA, A. (1990) Steroid responsive sensorineural hearing loss associated with aortitis syndrome. *ORL*, **52**, 86–95

KURIEN, M., THOMAS, K. and BHANU, T. S. (1989) Hearing thresholds in patients with diabetes mellitus. *Journal of Laryngology and Otology*, **103**, 164–168

LANSER, M. J., SUSSMAN, S. A. and FRAZER, K. (1992) Epidemiology, pathogenesis and genetics of acoustic tumours. *Otolaryngologic Clinics of North America* **25**, 499–520

LAU, S. K., WEI, W. S., SHAM, J. S. T., CHOY, D. T. K. and HUI, Y. (1992) Early changes of auditory brain stem evoked response after radiotherapy for nasopharyngeal carcinoma. A prospective study. *Journal of Laryngology and Otology*, **106**, 887–892

LEGIUS, E., MARCHUK, D. A., HALL, B. K., ANDERSEN, L. B., WALLACE, M. R., COLLINS, F. S. *et al.* (1992) NF1-related locus on chromosome 15. *Genomics*, **13**, 1316–1318

LESSER, T. H. J., DORT, J. C. and SIMMEN, D. P. B. (1990) Ear, nose and throat manifestations of Lyme disease. *Journal of Laryngology and Otology*, **104**, 301–304

LIAO, B. S., BYL, F. M. and ADOUR, K. K. (1992) Audiometric comparison of Lassa fever hearing loss and idiopathic sudden hearing loss: evidence for viral cause. *Otolaryngology – Head and Neck Surgery*, **106**, 226–229

LIPSKY, P. E. (1987). Rheumatoid arthritis. In: *Harrison's Principles of Internal Medicine*, 11th edn, edited by E. Braunwald, K. J. Isselbacher, R. G. Petersdorf, J. D. Wilson, J. B. Martin and A. S. Fauci. New York: McGraw-Hill, pp. 1423–1428

LIU, D. (1988) Influence of hypertension and coronary heart disease on the hearing of the aged. *Chinese Journal of Otorhinolaryngology*, **23**, 342–345

MCCABE, B. F. (1989) Autoimmune inner ear disease: therapy. *American Journal of Otology*, **10**, 196–197

MCDONALD, T. J., ZINCKE, H., ANDERSON, C. F. and OTT, N. T. (1978) Reversal of deafness after renal transplantation in Alport's syndrome. *Laryngoscope*, **88**, 38–42

MACRAE, J. H. (1991) Presbycusis and noise-induced permanent threshold shift. *Journal of the Acoustical Society of America*, **90**, 2513–2516

MAIER, W., HAUSER, R., and MUNKER, G (1992) Eustachian tube function in sudden hearing loss and in healthy subjects. *Journal of Laryngology and Otology*, **106**, 322–325

MARGOLIS, R. H. and NELSON, D. A. (1993) Acute otitis media with transient sensorineural hearing loss: a case study. *Archives of Otolaryngology – Head and Neck Surgery*, **119**, 682–686

MASLAN, M. J., GRAHAM, M. D. and FLOOD, L. M. (1985) Cryptococcal meningitis presentation as sudden deafness. *American Journal of Otology*, **6**, 435–437

MAY, D. L. and WHITE, H. H. (1968) Familial myoclonus, cerebellar ataxia and deafness. Specific genetically-determined disease. *Archives of Neurology*, **19**, 331–338

MENDELL, J. R. and GRIGGS, R. C. (1987) Muscular dystrophy and other chronic myopathies. In: *Harrison's Principles of Internal Medicine*, 11th edn, edited by E. Braunwald, K. J. Isselbacher, R. G. Petersdorf, J. D. Wilson, J. B. Martin and A. S. Fauch. New York: McGraw–Hill pp. 2072–2079

MEYERHOFF, W. L. (1979) Hypothyroidism and the ear: electrophysiological, morphological, and chemical considerations. *Laryngoscope*, **89** (Suppl. 19), 1–25

MEYERHOFF, W. L. and PAPARELLA, M. M. (1980) Medical therapy for sudden deafness. In: *Controversy in Otolaryngology*, edited by J. B. Snow Jr. Philadelphia: W. B. Saunders Co. pp. 3–11

MEYERSON, M. D., LEWIS, E. and ILL, K. (1984) Facioscapulohumeral muscular dystrophy and accompanying hearing loss. *Archives of Otolaryngology*, **110**, 201–206

MICHAELS, L., SOUCEK, S. and LIANG, J. (1994) The ear in the acquired immunodeficiency syndrome: temporal bone histopathologic study. *Journal of Otology*, **15**, 515–522

MICHEL, O. and BRUSIS, T. (1992) Hearing loss as a sequel of lumbar puncture. *Annals of Otology, Rhinology and Laryngology*, **101**, 390–394

MISHELL, J. H. and APPELBAUM, E. L. (1990) Ramsay Hunt syndrome in a patient with HIV infection. *Otolaryngology – Head and Neck Surgery*, **102**, 177–179

MOFFAT, D. A., BAGULEY, D. M., HARDY, D. G. and TSUI, Y. N. (1989a) Contralateral auditory brainstem response abnormalities in acoustic neuroma. *Journal of Laryngology and Otology*, **103**, 835–838

MOFFAT, D. A., HARRIS, L. L., BAGULEY, D. M. and HARDY, D. G. (1989b) Unterberger's stepping test in acoustic neuroma. *Journal of Laryngology and Otology*, **103**, 839–841

MOINE, A., FRACHET, B., VAN DEN ABBEELE, T., TISON, P. and BATTESTI, J. P. (1990) Deafness and sarcoidosis. *Annales D'Otolaryngologie et de Chirurgie Cervico-Faciale*, **107**, 469–473

MOKRY, M., FLASCHKA, G., KLEINERT, G., KLEINERT, R., FAZEKAS, F. and KOPP, W. (1990) Chronic Lyme disease with an expansive granulomatous lesion in the cerebellopontine angle. *Neurosurgery*, **27**, 446–451

MONSELL, E. M. and ROCK, J. P. (1990) Sensorineural loss and the diagnosis of acoustic neuroma. *Henry Ford Hospital Medical Journal*, **38**, 9–12

MONTGOMERY, A., FENTON, G. W. and MCCLELLAND, R. J. (1984) Delayed brainstem conduction time in post-concussional syndrome. *Lancet*, i, 1011

MORGAN, D. W., ALDREN, M. B. and HOARE, T. J. (1990) Hearing loss due to cranio-metaphysial dysplasia. *Journal of Laryngology and Otology*, **104**, 807–808

MORRELL, C. H. and BRANT, L. J. (1991) Modelling hearing thresholds in the elderly. *Statistics in Medicine*, **10**, 1453–1464

MORRISON, A. W. (1969) Management of severe deafness in adults. *Proceedings of the Royal Society of Medicine*, **62**, 959–965

MORRISON, A. W. (1975) *Manual of Sensorineural Deafness*. London: Butterworths

MOSEWICH, R. K., DONAT, J. R., DIMAURO, S., CIAFALONI, E., SHANSKE, S., ERASMUS, M. *et al.* (1993) The syndrome of mitochondrial encephalomyopathy, lactic acidosis, and strokelike episodes presenting without stroke. *Archives of Neurology*, **50**, 275–278

MURAKAMI, M., OHTANI, I., AIKAWA, T. and ANZAI, T. (1990) Temporal bone findings in two cases of head injury. *Journal of Laryngology and Otology*, **104**, 986–989

MURPHY, T. P. (1991) Macrovascular sensorineural hearing loss. *American Journal of Otology*, **12**, 88–92

MYERS, G. J. and TYLER, H. R. (1972) The etiology of deafness in Alport's syndrome. *Archives of Otorhinolaryngology*, **96**, 333–340

NADOL, J. B. JR (1978) Hearing loss as a sequela of meningitis. *Laryngoscope*, **88**, 739–755

NADOL, J. B. JR (1988) Application of electron microscopy to human otopathology. *Acta Otolaryngologica*, **105**, 411–419

NARULA, A. A., POWELL, R. J. and DAVIS, A. (1989) Frequency-resolving ability in systemic lupus erythematosus. *British Journal of Audiology*, **23**, 69–72

ODA, M., PRECIADO, M. C., QUICK, C. A. and PAPARELLA, M. M. (1976) Labyrinthine pathology of chronic renal failure patients treated with hemodialysis and kidney transplantation. *Laryngoscope*, **84**, 1489–1506

ODETOYINBO, O. and ADEKILE, A. (1987) Sensorineural hearing loss in children with sickle cell anaemia. *Annals of Otology, Rhinology and Laryngology*, **96**, 258–260

OERTER, K. E., FRIEDMAN, T. C., ANDERSON, H. C. and CASSORIA, F. G. (1992) Familial syndrome of endocrine and neuroectodermal abnormalities. *American Journal of Medical Genetics*, **44**, 487–491

OHKOSHI, K., ISHIDA, N., YAMAGUCHI, T. and KANKI, K. (1989) Corneal endothelium in a case of mitochondrial encephalomyopathy (Kearns–Sayre syndrome). *Cornea*, **8**, 210–214

O'MALLEY, S. P., ADAMS, J. E., DAVIES, M. and RAMSDEN, R. T. (1988) The petrous temporal bone and deafness in X-linked hypophosphataemic osteomalacia. *Clinical Radiology*, **39**, 528–530

PAPARELLA, M. M. (1983) Quiet labyrinthine complications from otitis media. *Journal of Laryngology and Otology*, Suppl. **8**, 53–58

PAPARELLA, M. M. (1991) Interactive inner-ear/middle-ear disease including perilymphatic fistula. *Acta Otolaryngologica*, Suppl. **485**, 36–45

PAPARELLA, M. M., BERLINGER, N. T., ODA, M. and EL-FIKY, F. (1973) Otological manifestations of leukaemia. *Laryngoscope*, **83**, 1510–1526

PAPARELLA, M. M., MORIZONO, T., LE, T. C., MANCINI, F., SIPILA, P., CHOO, Y. B. *et al.* (1984) Sensorineural hearing loss in otitis media. *Annals of Otology, Rhinology and Laryngology*, **93**, 623–629

PARVING, A., ELBERLING, C., BALLE, V., PARBO, J., DEJGAARD, A. and PARVING, H-H. (1990) Hearing disorders in patients with insulin-dependent diabetes mellitus. *Audiology*, **29**, 113–121

PARVING, A., PARVING, H-H. and LYNSGOE, J. (1983) Hearing sensitivity in patients with myxoedema before and after treatment with L-thyroxine. *Acta Otolaryngologica*, **95**, 315–321

PATTEN, J. (1977) *Neurological Differential Diagnosis*, London: Harold Stahl Ltd. pp. 108–118

PEDERSEN, U. (1985) Osteogenesis imperfecta clinical features, hearing loss and stapedectomy-biochemical, osteodensitometric, corneometric and histological aspects in comparison with otosclerosis. *Acta Otolaryngologica*, Suppl. **415**, 6–36

PELLETIER, L. P. and TANGUAY, R. B. (1975) X-linked recessive inheritance of sensorineural hearing loss expressed during adolescence. *American Journal of Human Genetics*, **27**, 609–613

PFISTER, H-W., FEIDEN, W. and EINHAUPL, K.-M. (1993) Spectrum of complications during bacterial meningitis in adults. *Archives of Neurology*, **50**, 575–581

PICKUP, J. and WILLIAMS, G. (1991) *Textbook of Diabetes*. Oxford: Blackwell Scientific Publishers

PIETERSEN, E. and CARLSEN, B. H. (1966) Hearing impairment

as the initial sign of polyarteritis nodosa. *Acta Otolaryngologica*, **61**, 189–195

PILLSBURY, H. C. (1986) Hypertension, hyperlipoproteinemia, chronic noise exposure: is there synergism in cochlear pathology? *Laryngoscope*, **96**, 1112–1138

PODOSHIN, L., BEN-DAVID, Y., FRADIS, M., PRATT, H., SHARF, B. and SCHWARTS, M. (1990) Brainstem auditory evoked potential with increased stimulation rate in minor head trauma. *Journal of Laryngology and Otology*, **104**, 191–194

PODOSHIN, L., FRADIS, M., PILLAR, T. and ZISMAN, D. (1975) Sensorineural hearing loss as an expression of atherosclerosis in young people. *Eye, Ear, Nose and Throat Monthly*, **54**, 18–23

PYYKKO, I., STARCK, J., PEKKARINEN, J. and FARKKILA, M. (1988) Serum cholesterol and triglyceride in the etiology on sensorineural hearing loss. In: *Vertigo, Nausea, Tinnitus and Hypoacusia in Metabolic Disorders*, edited by C.-F. Claussen, M. V. Kirtane and K. Schlitter. Amsterdam: Excerpta Medica. pp. 335–338

PYYKKO, I., VESANEN, M., ASIKAINEN, K., KOSKINIEMI, M., AIRAKSINEN L. and VAHERI, A. (1994) Human spumaretrovirus in the etiology of sudden hearing loss. *Acta Otolaryngologica*, **114**, 224

RAMADAN, H. H. and SCHUKNECHT, H. F. (1989) Is there a conductive type of presbyacusis? *Otorhinolaryngology – Head and Neck Surgery*, **100**, 30–34

RAMSDEN, R. T., BULMAN, C. H. and LORIGAN, B. P. (1975) Osteoradionecrosis of the temporal bone. *Journal of Laryngology and Otology*, **89**, 941–955

RAY, J. (1991) Is there a relationship between presbyacusis and hyperlipoproteinemia? A literature review. *Journal of Otolaryngology*, **20**, 336–341

REAL, R., THOMAS, M. and GERWIN, J. M. (1987) Sudden hearing loss and acquired immunodeficiency syndrome. *Otolaryngology – Head and Neck Surgery*, **97**, 409–412

REARDON, W., MIDDLETON-PRICE, H. R., MALCOLM, S., PHELPS, P., BELLMAN, S., LUXON, L. *et al.* (1992) Clinical and genetic heterogeneity in X-linked deafness. *British Journal of Audiology*, **26**, 109–114

ROSEN, S. and OLIN, P. (1965) Hearing loss and coronary heart disease. *Archives of Otolaryngology*, **82**, 236–243

ROSEN, S., OLIN, P. and ROSEN, H. V. (1970) Dietary prevention of hearing loss. *Acta Otolaryngologica*, **70**, 242–247

ROSENHALL, U., PEDERSON, K. and SVANBORG, A. (1990) Presbycusis and noise-induced hearing loss. *Ear and Hearing*, **11**, 257–263

RUST, K. R., PRAZMA, J., TRIANA, R. J., MICHAELIS, O. E. and PILLSBURY, H. C. (1992) Inner ear damage secondary to diabetes mellitus. II. Changes in aging SHR/N-*cp* rats. *Archives of Otolaryngology – Head and Neck Surgery*, **118**, 397–400

SANDLER, E. D., SANDLER, J. M., LEBOIT, P. E., WENIG, B. M. and MORTENSEN, N. (1990) *Pneumocystis carinii* otitis media in AIDS: a case report and review of the literature regarding extrapulmonary pneumocystosis. *Otolaryngology – Head and Neck Surgery*, **103**, 817–821

SCHACHERN, P. A., PAPARELLA, M. M., HYBERTSON, R., SANO, S. and DUVALL, A. J. III (1992) Bacterial tympanogenic labyrinthitis, meningitis and sensorineural damage. *Archives of Otolaryngology – Head and Neck Surgery*, **118**, 53–57

SCHINELLA, R. A., BREDA, S. D. and HAMMERSCHLAG, P. E. (1987) Otic infection due to *Pneumocystis carinii* in an apparently healthy man with antibody to the human immunodeficiency virus. *Annals of Internal Medicine*, **106**, 399–400

SCHOENHUBER, R., GENTILINI, M., SCARANO, M. and BORTOLOTTI, P. (1987) Longitudinal study of auditory brain-stem response in patients with minor head injuries. *Archives of Neurology*, **44**, 1181–1182

SCHUKNECHT, H. F. (1974) *Pathology of the Ear*. Cambridge: Harvard University Press

SCHUKNECHT, H. F. and DONOVAN, E. D. (1986) The pathology of idiopathic sudden sensorineural hearing loss. *Archives of Otorhinolaryngology*, **243**, 1–15

SCHUKNECHT, H. F. and GACEK, M. R. (1993) Cochlear pathology in presbyacusis. *Annals of Otology, Rhinology and Laryngology*, **102**, 1–16

SERJEANT, G. R., NORMAN, W. and TODD, G. B. (1975) The internal auditory canal and sensorineural hearing loss in homozygous sickle cell disease. *Journal of Laryngology and Otology*, **89**, 453–455

SHEEHY, J. L. (1984) Dead ear? Not necessarily. *American Journal of Otology*, **4**, 238–239

SIGLOCK, T. J. and BROOKLER, K. H. (1987) Sensorineural hearing loss associated with Takayasu's disease. *Laryngoscope*, **97**, 797–800

SILLENCE, D. O., SENN, A. and DANKS, D. M. (1979) Genetic heterogeneity in osteogenesis imperfecta. *Journal of Medical Genetics*, **16**, 101–116

SINGH, I. P. and SLEVIN, N. J. (1991) Late audiovestibular consequences of radical radiotherapy to the parotid. *Clinical Oncology*, **3**, 217–219

SMITH, M. E. and CANALIS, R. F. (1989) Otologic manifestations of AIDS: the otosyphilis connection. *Laryngoscope*, **99**, 365–372

SORVINO, D. and LUCENTE, F. E. (1992) Acquired immunodeficiency syndrome – the epidemic. In: *Otorhinolaryngologic Manifestations of the Acquired Immunodeficiency Syndrome*. *Otolaryngologic Clinics of North America*, edited by T. A. Tami. **25**, 1147–1156

SOULIERE, C. R., KAVA, C. R., BARRS, D. M. and BELL, A. F. (1991) Sudden hearing loss as the sole manifestation of neurosarcoidosis. *Otolaryngology – Head and Neck Surgery*, **105**, 376–381

SPENCER, J. T. JR (1973) Hyperlipoproteinemia in the etiology of inner ear disease. *Laryngoscope*, **83**, 639–678

STACH, B. A., SPRETNJAK, M. L. and JERGER, J. (1990) The prevalence of central presbyacusis in a clinical population. *Journal of the American Academy of Audiology*, **1**, 109–115

STARCK, J., PYYKKO, I. and PEKKARINEN, J. (1988) Effect of smoking on sensory neural hearing loss. In: *Vertigo, Nausea, Tinnitus and Hypoacusia in Metabolic Disorders*, edited by C.-F. Claussen, M. V. Kirtane and K. Schlitter. Amsterdam: Excerpta Medica. pp. 347–350

STECKELBERG, J. M. and MCDONALD, T. J. (1984) Otologic involvement in late syphilis. *Laryngoscope*, **94**, 753–757

STEEL, K. P. and BOCK, G. R. (1985) Genetic factors affecting hearing development. *Acta Otolaryngologica*, Suppl. 421, 48–56

STEPHENS, S. D. G., LUXON, L. and HINCHCLIFFE, R. (1982) Immunological disorders and auditory lesions. *Audiology*, **21**, 128–148

STEWART, E. J. and O'REILLY, B. F. (1989) A clinical and audiological investigation of osteogenesis imperfecta. *Clinical Otolaryngology*, **14**, 509–514

STRAUSS, C., FAHLBUSCH, R., ROMSTOCK, J., SCHRAMM, J., WATANABE, E., TANIGUCHI, M. *et al.* (1991) Delayed hearing loss after surgery for acoustic neurinomas: clinical and electrophysiological observations. *Neurosurgery*, **28**, 559–565

SUSMANO, A. and ROSENBUSH, S. W. (1988) Hearing loss and ischaemic heart disease. *American Journal of Otology*, **9**, 403–408

SYLVEN, L., HAGENFELDT, K., BRONDUM-NIELSEN, K. and VON SCHOULTZ, B. (1991) Middle-aged women with Turner's syndrome. Medical status, hormonal treatment and social life. *Acta Endocrinologica*, **125**, 359–365

TALBOTT, E., HELMKAMP, J., MATTHEWS, K., KULLER, L., COTTINGTON, E. and REDMOND, G. (1985) Occupational noise exposure, noise induced hearing loss, and the epidemiology of high blood pressure. *American Journal of Epidemiology*, **121**, 501–514

TALBOTT, E. O., FINDLAY, R. C., KULLER, L. H., LENKNER, L., A., MATTHEWS, K. A., DAY, R. D. *et al.* (1990) Noise-induced hearing loss: a possible marker for high blood pressure in older noise-exposed populations. *Journal of Occupational Medicine*, **32**, 690–697

TARTER, S. K. and ROBINS, T. G. (1990) Chronic noise exposure, high frequency hearing loss, and hypertension among automotive assembly workers. *Journal of Occupational Medicine*, **32**, 685–689

TAVIN, M. E., RUBIN, J. S. and CAMACHO, F. J. (1993) Sudden sensorineural hearing loss in haemoglobin SC. *Journal of Laryngology and Otology*, **107**, 831–833

TAYLOR, I. G. and IRWIN, J. (1978) Some audiological aspects of diabetes mellitus. *Journal of Laryngology and Otology*, **92**, 99–113

TEIG, E. (1968) Hereditary progressive perceptive deafness in a family of 72 patients. *Acta Otolaryngologica*, **65**, 365–372

THOMAS, K., MCPHERSON, B., MCWHIRTER, W., MCGILL, J. and ROWELL, J. (1992) Hearing loss in patients with congenital coagulation disorders. *Journal of Audiological Medicine*, **1**, 176–184

TIMON, C.I. and WALSH, M. A. (1989) Sudden sensorineural hearing loss as a presentation of HIV infection. *Journal of Laryngology and Otology*, **103**, 1071–1072

TOYNBEE, J. (1849) On the pathology and treatment of the deafness attendant upon old age. *Monthly Journal of Medical Science Edinburgh*, **9**, 521–525

TRIANA, R. J., SUITS, G. W., GARRISON, S., PRAZMA, J., BRECHTELSBAUER, P. B., MICHAELIS, O. E. *et al.* (1991) Inner ear damage secondary to diabetes mellitus. I. Changes in adolescent SHR/N-cp Rats. *Archives of Otolaryngology – Head and Neck Surgery*, **117**, 635–640

TUNSTALL PEDOE, D. S. and WALKER, J. M. (1990) Cardiovascular disease. In: *Textbook of Medicine*, edited by R. L. Souhami and J. Moxham. Edinburgh: Churchill Livingstone pp. 329–450

TRYGGVASON, K., ZHOU, J., HOSTIKKA, S. L. and SHOWS, T. B. (1993) Molecular genetics of Alport syndrome. *Kidney International*, **43**, 38–44

URBAN, G. E. (1973) Reversible sensorineural hearing loss associated with sickle cell crisis. *Laryngoscope*, **83**, 633–638

VALVASSORI, G. E. and GUZMAN, M. (1989) Growth rate of acoustic neuromas. *American Journal of Otology*, **10**, 174–176

VAN'T HOFF, W. and STUART, D. W. (1979) Deafness in myxoedema. *Quarterly Journal of Medicine*, **190**, 361–367

VELTRI, R. W., WILSON, W. R., SPRINKLE, P. M., RODMAN S. M. and KAVESH, D. A., (1981) The implication of viruses in idiopathic sudden hearing loss. Primary infection or reactivation of latent viruses? *Otolaryngology – Head Neck Surgery*, **89**, 137–141

VISKOCHIL, D., WHITE, R. and CAWTHORN, R. (1993) The neurofibromatosis type I gene. *Annual Review of Neurosciences*, **16**, 183–205

WACKYM, P. A. and LINTHICUM, F. H. (1986) Diabetes mellitus and hearing loss: clinical and histopathological relationship. *American Journal of Otolaryngology*, **7**, 176–182

WALBY, A. P., BARRERA, A. and SCHUKNECHT, H. F. (1983) Cochlear pathology in chronic suppurative otitis media. *Laryngoscope*, **92** (Suppl. 103), 633–638

WALTON, J. N. (1977) *Brain's Diseases of the Nervous System*, 8th edn. Oxford: Oxford University Press

WATKIN, P. M. (1989) Otological disease in Turner's syndrome. *Journal of Laryngology and Otology*, **103**, 731–738

WAYMAN, D. M., PHAM, H. N., BYL, F. M. and ADDUR, K. K. (1990) Audiological manifestations of Ramsay Hunt syndrome. *Journal of Laryngology and Otology*, **104**, 104–108

WELKOBORSKY, H.-J., AMEDEE, R. G., ELKHATIEB, A. and MANN, W. J. (1991) Auditory-evoked brain-stem responses and auditory disorders in patients with Bell's palsy. *European Archives of Oto-rhino-laryngology*, **248**, 417–419

WILLIAMS, G. H. and BRAUNWALD, E. (1987) Hypertensive vascular disease. In: *Harrison's Principles of Internal Medicine*, 11th edn, edited by E. Braunwald, K. J. Isselbacher, R. G. Petersdorf, J. D. Wilson, J. B. Martin, and A. S. Fauci. New York: McGraw-Hill pp. 1024–1037

WILSON, W. R., BYL, F. M. and LAIRD, N. (1980) The efficacy of steroids in the treatment of idiopathic sudden hearing loss: a double-blind clinical study. *Archives of Otolaryngology*, **106**, 772–776

WINSHIP, I., GERICKE, G. and BEIGHTON, P. (1984) X-linked inheritance ocular albinism with late onset sensorineural deafness. *American Journal of Medical Genetics*, **19**, 797–803

WOLF, M., KRONENBERG, J., ENGELBERG, S. and LEVENTON, G. (1987) Rapidly progressive hearing loss as a symptom of polyarteritis nodosa. *American Journal of Otolaryngology*, **8**, 105–108

WOLFF, D., BERNHARD, W. G., TSUTSUMI, S., ROSSI, S. and NUSSBAUM, H. E. (1965) The pathology of Cogan's syndrome causing profound deafness. *Annals of Otology, Rhinology and Laryngology*, **74**, 507–520

YABE, T., KAGA, K. and KODAMA, A. (1989) Temporal bone pathology of a patient without hearing and caloric reaction, and with counter-rolling after chronic myeloid leukaemia. *Acta Otolaryngologica*, Suppl. 468, 307–312

YAGI, T., YAMAGUCHI, J. and NONAKA, M. (1988) Neurotological findings in Bell's palsy and Hunt's syndrome. *Acta Otolaryngologica*, Suppl. 446, 97–100

YAMAMOTO, E., NISHIMURA, H. and HIRONO, Y. (1988) Occurrence of sequelae in Bell's palsy. *Acta Otolaryngologica*, Suppl. 445, 93–96

YIH, J. S., WANG, S. J., SU, M. S., TSAI, S. C., LIN, R. H., LIN, K. N. and LIU, H. C. (1993) Hereditary spastic paraplegia associated with epilepsy, mental retardation and hearing impairment. *Paraplegia*, **31**, 408–411

ZECHNER, G. (1980) Zum Cogan syndrome. *Acta Otolaryngologica*, **89**, 310–316

ZOLLER, M., WILSON, W. R. and NADOL, J. B. (1979) Treatment of syphilitic hearing loss. *Annals of Otorhinolaryngology*, **88**, 160–165

11

Noise and the ear

Peter W. Alberti

This chapter deals with the effect of sound, particularly excessive sound, on hearing and the auditory system. Its effect on the organism as a whole, good and bad is discussed. Excessive sound is one of the most common causes of hearing loss in the world – from military, industrial and recreational sources. Developed countries are gradually bringing noise under control; not so the newly industrialized and middle level of developing nations where industrial and urban noise is rapidly increasing due to emerging industry, the use of large numbers of motorcycles, and the introduction of highly amplified music for advertising in the streets and bazaars. From Alexandria to Bangkok, urban sound levels have rapidly risen. The machinery of war has also become more devastating and more deafening. We are currently reaping the rewards of this unwanted increase in noise in an epidemic of hearing loss, which is incurable, but surely preventable.

Noise has physical, physiological and psychological connotations, all of which differ. Physically it is complex sound having little or no periodicity which can be measured or its characteristics analysed. Physiologically noise is defined as a signal that bears no information and whose intensity varies randomly in time. Psychologically noise is any sound, irrespective of its waveform, which is unpleasant or unwanted.

Noise, like any sound, is defined in terms of its duration, frequency spectrum (measured in Hz), and intensity measured in sound pressure level (SPL) and expressed in decibels (dB). It may be continuous, intermittent, impulsive or explosive. It may be steady-state or fluctuant.

Historical considerations

From the first use of metals hearing has been at risk from noise exposure. Gunpowder, discovered about 1300 AD, added to the problem. Ramazzini (1713) reported that workers who hammered copper for a living had their ears so injured by the perpetual din that they became hard of hearing. He recommended the use of hearing protectors to prevent deafness occurring. Nils Skragge, over 200 years ago, wrote a thesis on occupational deafness in coppersmiths and blacksmiths (Kylin, 1960), and Fosbroke in 1831 gave an accurate description of noise-induced hearing loss (NIHL) in blacksmiths, coining the expression 'blacksmith's deafness'. A good example of percussive noise injury was Admiral Lord Rodney who apparently became deaf for 14 days following the firing of 80 broadsides from his ship HMS Formidable in the year 1782.

It was necessary to construct machinery before man-made noise reached large scale deafening proportions. By the 1880s Roosa and Holt in America, Bezold in Germany and Barr in Great Britain had all recognized the importance of industrial noise as a cause of hearing loss, citing military and civil causes. Holt published a study of boilermaker deafness in 1882, and in 1886 Thomas Barr of Glasgow, wrote: 'it is familiarly known that boilermakers and others who work in very noisy surroundings are extremely liable to dullness of hearing. In Glasgow, we would have little difficulty in finding hundreds whose sense of hearing has thus been damaged, by the noisy character of their work. We have therefore in our city ample materials at hand for investigation on this subject'.

Barr's work was far ahead of its time; he undertook comparative studies of the hearing of boilermakers, iron founders and lettermen (postmen), made sound recordings, and established the study of occupational hearing loss on a scientific basis. Boilermaker's deafness is particularly interesting in that it did not exist until the invention of riveting, but has virtually disappeared again with the introduction of welding as a preferred method of joining sheets of metal, plus the use of hearing protection.

The site and nature of the lesion in the ear produced by noise was first described by Haberman (1890), in a 75-year-old blacksmith. Partial disappearance of the organ of Corti was found with destruction of the hair cells, the most extensive damage being in the lower basal coil. Soon after the introduction of audiometry, Fowler (1929) observed dips at 4 kHz and Bunch (1939) published probably the first audiometric data demonstrating the typical high frequency loss acquired by those exposed to noise. An excellent historical review is given by Hawkins (1976).

After the Second World War the results of technological and scientific discoveries of the 1930s, 1940s and 1950s were put into effect. Economies in size were made at the price of quantum increases in sound levels. Only in the past decade has there been any widespread attempt to manufacture quieter machinery and silence the workplace.

Effects of sound stimulation

Adaptation

Adaptation, or per-stimulatory fatigue, is an immediate phenomenon which occurs when a sound is presented to the ear somewhat elevating the threshold. For fatiguing sounds of up to about 80 dB sound pressure levels (SPL) the greatest adaptation is produced for an identical test tone of identical frequency. The amount of residual masking that remains after the fatigue tone ceases is proportional to the sound pressure level of the fatiguer, but independent of its duration. The recovery is exponential in nature, and for fatiguing sounds of up to 70 dB SPL occurs fully within 0.5 second. The sound intensity at which the crossover occurs between physiological fatigue and true temporary threshold shift (TTS) is variable. It is higher at low frequencies and ranges from 65 dB SPL for an octave band centred at 4 kHz to 75 dB SPL for an octave band centred at 250 Hz. There are electrophysiological correlates of this adaptation which can be measured in animals as reductions in the action potential; there are significant individual variations (Karja, 1968; Kryter, 1985; Botte and Monikheim, 1992).

Temporary threshold shift

This is post-stimulatory fatigue. Like adaptation, it has in the past been referred to as auditory fatigue.

Fatigue

The degree of temporary threshold shift increases

progressively with stimulus duration and intensity, a balance not being achieved until abnormal sound intensities are applied. Recovery is slow and related to the degree of temporary threshold shift. If the stimulus is strong enough, irreversible changes may occur. Although it was originally stated that the maximum temporary threshold shift occurs half an octave above the centre frequency of the stimulating sound (Figure 11.1), the story is more complex (McFadden, 1986). In the lower frequencies, maximum temporary threshold shift may occur more than an octave above the centre frequency of the stimulating sound; as the stimulus increases in frequency, the maximum point of the temporary threshold shift comes closer to the stimulating tone. For tones of equal intensity, the higher the frequency of the stimulating tone, the greater the temporary threshold shift, irrespective of the exposure frequency.

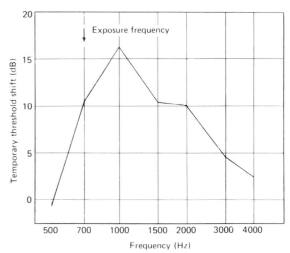

Figure 11.1 Temporary threshold shift at different frequencies 5 minutes after the end of exposure to a tone of 700 Hz for 5 minutes. Note the displacement upwards in frequency relative to the frequency of the exposure tone. (From Ward, 1962, reproduced by courtesy of the Editor of *Journal of the Acoustical Society of America*)

Most temporary threshold shift recovers within 16 hours; higher intensity sound produces temporary threshold shift which may take several days to recover. Temporary threshold shift greater than 40 dB is likely to be pathological and frequently associated with some degree of residual permanent threshold shift (PTS). Much work has been carried out to attempt to relate these longer periods of temporary threshold shift to long-term permanent threshold shift. Physiological fatigue should be limited to temporary threshold shift that lasts for more than 2 minutes, but that has completely recovered in less than 16 hours, for this covers the normal working experience.

The relationship between the auditory stimulus, temporary threshold shift and permanent threshold shift in humans has been extensively studied and well reviewed by Mills (1982), who, with his colleagues, exposed 300 young adults to noise for periods from minutes to 48 hours and studied the development of temporary threshold shift and its effect on certain psychophysical responses of the ear, such as temporal integration, simultaneous masking, forward masking and the psychophysical tuning curve. Exposure to a 4 kHz sound about a certain base level, 74 dB for this frequency, produced asymptotic threshold shift (ATS), that is that length of sound exposure at a given intensity above which no further temporary threshold shift occurred. The level of temporary threshold shift at asymptote rose by 1.7 dB for every 1 dB that the stimulus was raised above 74 dB. The lower the frequency of the sound stimulus the higher the base level above which temporary threshold shift occurs; thus temporary threshold shift was detected above 74 dB at 4 kHz, 78 dB at 2 kHz, and 82 dB at 1 and 0.5 kHz. Two assumptions are derived from this: that the risk to the inner ear from noise is extremely small beneath these levels, and that temporary threshold shift at asymptote produced by a given sound is the upper limit of permanent threshold shift that might be produced by that sound. As these levels vary from frequency to frequency, it makes it difficult to validate on scientific grounds risk levels for hearing based on decibels (A) for damage risk criteria. Figure 11.2 gives a graphic representation of the range of human audibility categorized according to risk. The cross-hatched area between the black area in which there is a high risk of damage to hearing, and the white where there is little or no damage to hearing is interesting. It represents a level of noise that will produce an asymptotic threshold shift between 0.1 and 5.0 dB but, more importantly, represents an area where exposure to these levels will delay the recovery of a temporary threshold shift produced by a high level sound (Ward, Cushing and Burns, 1976; Mills, 1976, 1982).

Recent animal studies have been summarized by Clark (1991a). He found that in the most commonly used laboratory animal, the chinchilla, continuous moderate noise exposure produces an asymptote in 18–24 hours. Permanent threshold shift depends on level, frequency and duration of exposure. Below 115 dB, permanent threshold shift and cell loss are related to the total energy of sound in continuous exposure but that periodic rest intervals are protective.

Melnick (1976, 1991) discussed human asymptotic threshold shift and concluded that it occurs in man for moderate levels of exposure to continuous noise, after 8–12 hours of noise exposure. He believed, however, that recovery from levels of asymptotic threshold shift of 30 dB or less is prolonged

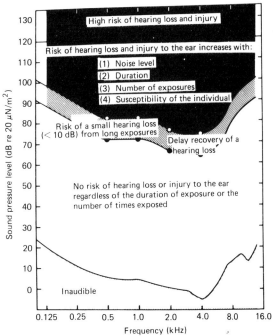

Figure 11.2 Most of the range of human audibility categorized with respect to the risk of injury and hearing loss. (From Mills, 1982, with permission)

when compared to the recovery from similar magnitudes of threshold shift produced by short-term high level exposure, and frequently is not complete within 24 hours of cessation. Clearly the matter is complex.

It is thus believed that recovery from temporary threshold shift may vary according to the conditions which produced it; even though different exposures produce the same temporary threshold shift, they may not be equally hazardous. Finally, asymptotic threshold shift produced by a given sound of this level and spectrum marks the upper bound of permanent threshold shift produced by that sound.

The relationship between the sound pressure levels of noise bands or pure tones and the amount of temporary threshold shift produced is also complex; criteria developed for pure tones do not necessarily cover noise bands or vice versa. Impulse noise also produces temporary threshold shift, which is similar to that for steady noise with the exception that temporary threshold shift for impulse noise grows linearly with time instead of exponentially, as found with steady noise.

Noise-induced permanent threshold shift

This is an irreversible elevation of the auditory threshold produced by noise exposure, associated with permanent pathological changes in the cochlea.

The anatomical correlates of acoustic injury

There have been many efforts to describe the anatomical consequences of acoustic trauma on the auditory system. These have concentrated largely on the cochlea and were initially light microscopic studies of the end result of severe damage. Bredberg and Hunter-Duvar (1975) provided a remarkably comprehensive survey of early work. Much recent work has concentrated on the ultrastructural changes in the cochlea and primary nerve fibres. It is now recognized that extensive study of high intensity exposures fails to reveal subtle early changes including the metabolic processes involved in the injury. Excellent, well referenced reviews have been published by Saunders *et al.* (Saunders, Dear and Schneider, 1985; Saunders, Cohen and Szymko, 1991). They pointed out that acoustic injury to the ear has a dynamic and a static phase. The former starts during acoustic stimulation, during which the cellular elements in the cochlea undergo structural and functional change which may be lethal or may initiate repair. After cessation of sound trauma the degenerative and reparative processes compete, leading to full recovery, partial recovery and scarring or destruction, and then the static phase, in which hearing is stable, is entered.

Knowledge of cochlear function had been dominated by the macromechanical model of Von Békésy. During the 1980s it was increasingly found wanting and, in the past few years, new models of cochlear function based on micromechanical models have emerged (Dallos, 1992).

From a macromechanical standpoint when a travelling wave passes, a radially directed shear stress develops in the cochlear partition, and the basilar membrane is flexed along each side of the spiral ligament, while the middle is not supported. This part is mobilized by the travelling wave with its maximal excursion somewhere near its centre. As the inner pillar cell is closely related to the fixed spiral lamina, with the outer pillar cell based on the more central part of the basilar membrane, the place of greatest movement, the whole triangle composed of both pillar cells and the structures attached to them will undergo a radially directed rocking movement, with the fulcrum near the base of the inner pillar cell. This may well explain why the supporting cells around the inner hair cells are so often damaged after extreme noise exposure and it is probably the reason why the outer hair cells in the first row, whose heads are attached to the phalangeal processes of both inner and outer pillar cells, are the ones most often injured (Beagley, 1965).

There is also a difference in the damage produced to inner and outer hair cells with the latter being much more susceptible to trauma, not only from noise but also from ototoxic drugs. This suggests strongly that their sensitivity is not purely mechanical but also metabolic. The inner row of outer hair cells is more susceptible to damage than the outer.

Progressively more severe damage with increases in the stimulating sound pressure level were found in the cochlea by Miller, Watson and Covell (1963). Their report is noteworthy for being one of the first also to describe late degeneration of spiral ganglion cells and peripheral nerve fibre as a result of excessive sound stimulation.

Scanning and transmission electron microscopy have added much new knowledge (Lim, 1986; Figure 11.3). These new observations have changed the thinking of auditory scientists from a macrodynamic to a microdynamic model in which subtle changes in movement between individual cells, and changes within individual cells themselves are studied closely.

Recently, there has been considerable emphasis on studying the functional integrity of hair cell and

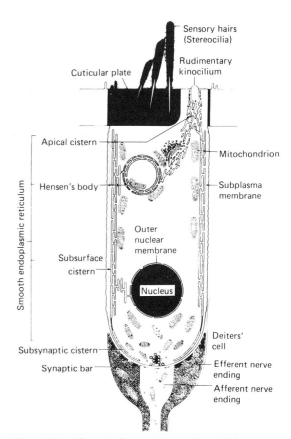

Figure 11.3 Schematic diagram of outer hair cell showing various organelles. Note interconnecting cisternal structures such as apical cistern, Hensen's body, subsurface cistern, subsynaptic cisternae. (Drawing by Nancy Sally, reproduced from Lim, 1986, by permission of the Editor, *Hearing Research*)

auditory nerve preparations following acoustic injury. Recordings are obtained from single hair cells and individual auditory nerve fibres whose characteristic frequency corresponds to the region of acoustic damage in the experimental animal. The use of horseradish peroxidase to label individual auditory nerve fibres enables correlations to be made between abnormal nerve physiology and specific injury to hair cells from which the fibre originates (Kiang *et al.*, 1986).

Hair cell injury

Recent interest in hair cell structure and function, and its disruption by excessive sound stimulation has centred around the contractility of outer hair cells (Zenner, Zimmerman and Glitter, 1988) in response to sound stimulation, about the micromechanics of individual cilia (Saunders, Dear and Schneider, 1985), their coupling to each other on the same cell by tip bands, and their role in gating the Na^+ and K^+ ions as initiators of cellular activity. Saunders, Cohen and Szymko (1991) presented a good recent review of structural and functional changes resulting from acoustic stimulation and over stimulation of the cochlea. How is mechanical energy transducted into an intracellular event that triggers the release of neurotransmitters? Between one and four transduction channels lie in the plasma membrane of each cilium, either at its tip or along the shaft, possibly controlled by the tip links, small bridges between the upper part of the cilia which link together the individual cilia of the cell. Mechanical motion of the bundle in the direction of the tallest row opens the channel, allowing an influx of K^+ and Ca^{++} and producing depolarization of the plasma membrane. Movement in the opposite direction closes channels and reduces the amount of membrane depolarization. When depolarization reaches a critical point intracellular events are triggered. The tips of the tallest cilia of the outer hair cells are embedded in the tectorial membrane.

It has long been known that the outer hair cells have little afferent but much efferent innervation. It is now believed that mechanical motion of the basilar membrane excites the outer hair cells which contract, thereby enhancing the motion at the point of stimulation and thus increasing the mechanical motion transmitted to the inner hair cell where neurotransmission occurs (Reuter *et al.*, 1992). Thus, damage to outer hair cells diminishes the sensitivity of the damaged area of the cochlea. How the efferent mechanism affects the fine tuning of the cochlea is not yet clear. The tuning curves of individual auditory nerve fibres in response to sound stimulation have been known for some time. A normal cochlear nerve fibre which is stimulated near the point of maximum sensitivity of the cells to which it is attached, has a very highly

tuned response which, as the stimulus intensity increases, spreads over a broader frequency band. It has now been shown that this sharp tuning also extends to individual hair cells (Cody and Russell, 1988).

Since cilia play such an important part in transduction they have been extensively studied. Stiffness of cilia appears related to the cilial bundle integrity, and particularly to the tip links which connect the cilia to each other and to the basal rootlets which extend through the cuticular plate of the hair cell into the basal part of the cilium. The importance of the latter was well shown by Liberman and Dodds, and Liberman in 1987, when they showed in acute and chronic preparations first shortening, and then with higher stimulation, fracture of the basal rootlet, and correlated this with loss of sensitivity of nerve response to sound. Fracture of the rootlet led to cell death (Figure 11.4).

Gao *et al.* (1992) produced temporary and permanent hearing loss in guinea pigs by stimulating them with 110 dB SPL white noise for 30 minutes, or 120 dB for 150 minutes. The auditory responses were monitored and the cochleae of the animals examined by scanning electron microscopy in the acute phase or after 80 days. The 110 dB group developed a reversible hearing loss, the 120 dB was generally irreversible (Figure 11.5, *a, b, c, d*). Lower levels of exposure produced minimal floppiness of the cilia, without fracture of the rootlet or extensive tip link damage; this recovered. Higher sound levels which broke the tip links produced severe floppiness, rootlet fracture and irreversible cellular changes.

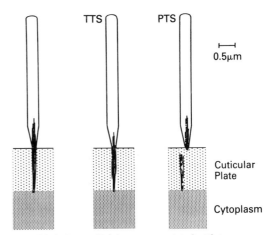

Figure 11.4 Stereocilial damage associated with temporary and permanent threshold shifts (TTS, PTS). In the former, a shortening of the supracuticular rootlet is the most obvious anatomical change. In PTS, rootlet fracture (or more severe damage) is usually evident. (Adapted from Liberman (1987) and Liberman and Dodds (1987) with permission)

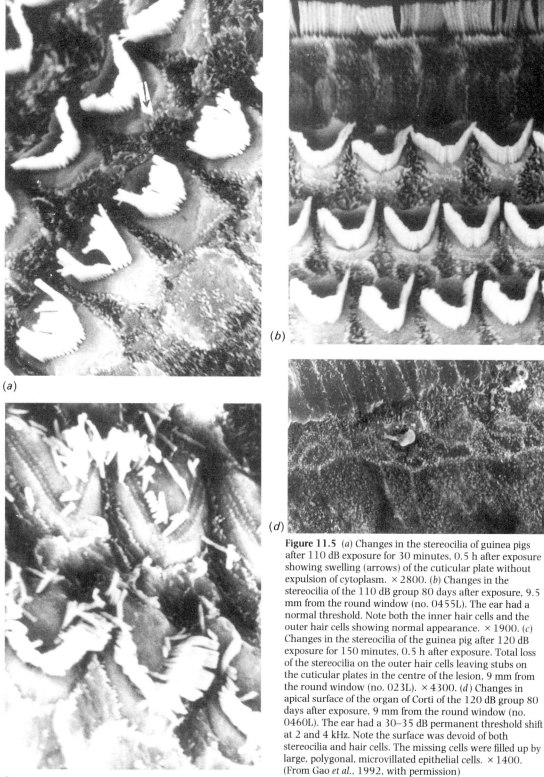

Figure 11.5 (*a*) Changes in the stereocilia of guinea pigs after 110 dB exposure for 30 minutes, 0.5 h after exposure showing swelling (arrows) of the cuticular plate without expulsion of cytoplasm. × 2800. (*b*) Changes in the stereocilia of the 110 dB group 80 days after exposure, 9.5 mm from the round window (no. 0455L). The ear had a normal threshold. Note both the inner hair cells and the outer hair cells showing normal appearance. × 1900. (*c*) Changes in the stereocilia of the guinea pig after 120 dB exposure for 150 minutes, 0.5 h after exposure. Total loss of the stereocilia on the outer hair cells leaving stubs on the cuticular plates in the centre of the lesion, 9 mm from the round window (no. 023L). × 4300. (*d*) Changes in apical surface of the organ of Corti of the 120 dB group 80 days after exposure, 9 mm from the round window (no. 0460L). The ear had a 30–35 dB permanent threshold shift at 2 and 4 kHz. Note the surface was devoid of both stereocilia and hair cells. The missing cells were filled up by large, polygonal, microvillated epithelial cells. × 1400. (From Gao *et al.*, 1992, with permission)

It was originally believed that the site of hair cell loss mirrored the threshold shift, i.e. high frequency hearing loss was measured by loss of hair cells in the basal parts of the cochlea. This is not totally correct; there appears to be a wide discrepancy between microscopic distribution of hair cell loss and the loss of sensitivity in the cochlea. The current view is that different patterns of over-stimulation leave unique footprints of hair cell injury and this may be related to peripheral features such as the middle ear muscle response to sound (see Saunders, Cohen and Szymko, 1991).

Biochemical changes

Wenthold *et al.* (1992) reviewed the putative biochemical processes in noise-induced hearing loss. They pointed out that not enough is known of the biochemical mechanism of normal hearing to detect changes with more exposure. True, if there is great cell damage from acoustic over-stimulation, then there are detectable chemical compounds associated with cell death. However, the goal in noise-induced permanent threshold shift studies is to identify chemical changes prior to microscopic changes being visible. These have not yet been found. They placed some hope in the study of heat shock proteins which are produced in response to cell shock, such as hyperthermia. They suggested a mild stress may lead to the production of heat shock proteins which prevents further damage with a later greater stress; i.e. a relatively benign loud sound may stimulate production of a protective untraceable protein to mitigate the effect of a following louder sound.

Auditory nerve and central changes

There has been significant experimentation analysing the effect of sound on single nerve units. Robertson and Johnstone (1979) and Cody and Johnstone (1980) showed that, after damage to the cochlea by ototoxic drugs or by noise, the most sensitive frequency of individual auditory neurons was lowered by half an octave and that the sensitive tip was lost (Figure 11.6).

A complementary approach is to study whole nerve action potentials; this has been undertaken extensively in animals and in humans. The findings effectively parallel those reported for single nerve fibres. In human subjects the tuning of the cochlear nerve became broader with increasing hearing loss. An excellent review by Patuzzi (1992) summarized knowledge in this area.

Central changes in noise-induced permanent threshold shift are similar to those that occur with any acquired sensorineural hearing loss. They are

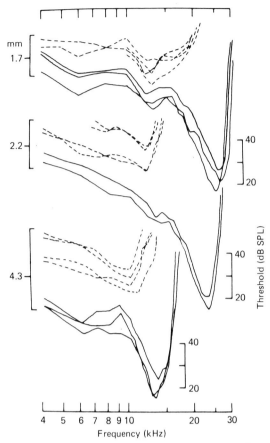

Figure 11.6 Frequency threshold curves (tuning curves) from single spiral ganglion cells in guinea pigs with and without cochlear pathology. The solid curves were obtained from normal cochleae, whereas the dashed curves are associated with cell bodies innervating regions of the basal turn devoid of outer hair cells. The three sets of curves correspond to three cochlear locations; from top to bottom the locations at 1.7, 2.2 and 4.3 mm from the basal end of the cochlear spiral. Note the pathology not only serves to desensitize the tip of the curve, but also lowers the best (most sensitive) frequency. These results are indirect evidence that the mechanical tuning of the organ of Corti can be changed with damage. (From Robertson and Johnstone, 1979, with permission)

outside the scope of this chapter. For recent reviews the reader should consult Dancer *et al.* (1992).

Noise-induced hearing loss

There are many causes of hearing loss produced by noise and occupation, and the following classification covers most:

1 Noise-induced temporary threshold shift
2 Noise-induced permanent threshold shift
3 Acute acoustic trauma.

The first two imply prior prolonged exposure to noise, which may be steady-state, impact or a mixture of the two; the latter is hearing loss caused by single intense sound sources as, for example, a rifle shot or, worse, blast trauma from an explosion. All produce variable hearing loss, some of which may recover. In acute acoustic trauma there may also be damage to the tympanic membrane and ossicles with a variable degree of injury to the cochlea.

Noise-induced temporary threshold shift

The usual initial change following hazardous noise exposure is a high frequency threshold shift. Classically this appears as a steep isolated audiometric dip, the 'acoustic notch', at 3, 4 (usually) or 6 kHz (Figure 11.7). In the early stages of exposure this occurs as a temporary threshold shift, also referred to as noise-induced temporary threshold shift. After a rest period away from the noise, the hearing usually returns to its former level.

Glorig (1958) noted that individuals with normal hearing whose ears have never previously undergone prolonged noise exposure (green ears) demonstrate greater temporary threshold shift than those whose ears have been exposed for long periods of time (ripe ears). More recently there has been a growing body of literature which describes acquired resistance to the ototraumatic affect of noise – a 'toughening up' of the ear, both in humans and animals. Such a resistance to noise-induced hearing loss is a consistent finding across species and techniques, which is found as a lessening of temporary threshold shift produced by a specific sound after repeated exposure. A low intensity sound, priming the ear prior to a subsequent high intensity sound reduces the temporary threshold shift produced. This occurs in the absence of the stapedius muscle (except in the rabbit)

and is not accompanied by reduction in hair cell damage. The mechanism may be related to efferent feedback, changes in the cilia, accumulation of protective protein (heat shock protein) and other mechanisms not yet known. The matter has been well reviewed by Henderson *et al.* (1992), Boettcher (1993) and Ryan *et al.* (1994).

The recovery of hearing from pathological temporary threshold shift was discussed in the previous section. Most recovery occurs in the first 2 days. It should be emphasized that this is not true of massive threshold shifts produced by explosions, for here significant recovery continues for some weeks (Figure 11.8).

Noise-induced permanent threshold shift

For practical purposes this is the most commonly encountered hearing loss caused by noise, one for which there are many synonyms: occupational hearing loss, industrial noise-induced deafness, chronic acoustic trauma, noise-induced hearing loss, permanent noise-induced hearing loss, stimulation deafness, occupational deafness, boilermaker's deafness, etc.

Although it is often stated that continuous employment in a potentially hazardous environment for 10–15 years is necessary for an initial temporary threshold shift to develop into noise-induced permanent threshold shift (Figure 11.9), the actual data vary. Two points of practical importance are the quite uneven noise levels in industry, both within a single work period of 8 hours and over a period of months or years, as the machinery and process vary, and the great individual variability in susceptibility to the effect of noise (Figure 11.10). Few studies have attempted to quantify the result

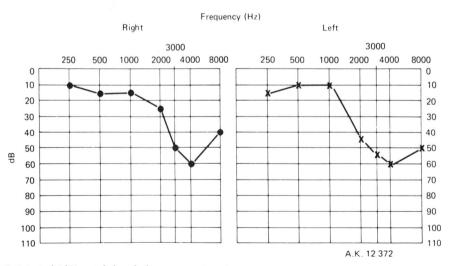

Figure 11.7 A typical 4-kHz notch found after exposure to noise

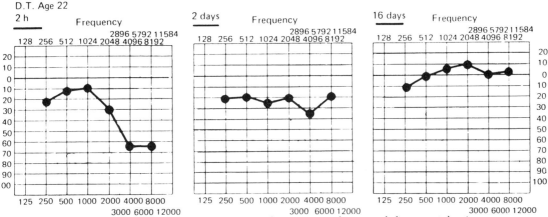

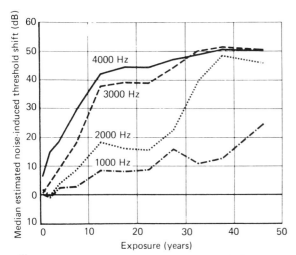

Figure 11.8 Serial audiograms of a 22-year-old laboratory technician exposed to an exploding report showing recovery over a 16-day period

Figure 11.9 Estimated noise-induced threshold shift as function of duration of exposure. (From Taylor *et al.*, 1965. In: *Noise and Man*, by W. Burns, 1968, London: John Murray, p. 174)

of prolonged constant industrial exposure, because there are singularly few industries where the noise level has remained constant over two or three decades. A notable exception is the extremely well studied group of jute workers in Dundee (Taylor *et al.*, 1965).

A major study by Burns and Robinson (1970) laid the scientific basis for the equal energy concept, which proposed that equal amounts of acoustic energy, between a level which is totally safe and one which is totally injurious, produce equal amounts of hearing loss. This hypothesis was adopted in Europe in the late 1970s. If one can compute the amount of noise exposure, one can predict the risk to hearing. As a doubling of energy represents an increase in noise levels of 3 dB, it follows that for equivalent risk,

the exposure time must be halved for each 3 dB increase in exposure. They coined the term 'noise immission level' as an index of the total noise energy incident on the ear over a period of time. This has also given rise to the expression 'equivalent continuous noise level' expressed as Leq. It is suggested that all noise exposure to steady-state noise, and indeed to much impulse noise (Martin, 1976) be related to a baseline 90 dB(A) weighting/40-hour working week, which allows for a good risk prediction. A comprehensive meta analysis by Passchier-Vermeer (1973), used data from 20 sets of subjects from 11 publications to study the effect of intermittent and varying noise exposure. She concluded that for equivalent continuous sound levels up to 100 dB(A) and noise immission levels up to 110 dB(A), the data agreed reasonably well with that for steady-state noise. These figures were incorporated into an international standard ISO 1999 designed to estimate risk to hearing from normal exposure, which has been frequently modified.

The equal energy concept is certainly valid if noise exposure is steady and consistent throughout the working day. However, regulations based on the equal energy concept do not take into account the effect of recovery periods on the ear in the presence of intermittent noise. Recognition that damage to the ear might be less for a given total amount of sound if presented intermittently (a common workplace occurrence) than if presented continuously, gave rise to the American Tables of Risk based on 5 dB halving and doubling known as L$_{OSHA}$. These were derived from a CHABA report in 1966, simplified by Botsford (1967) and codified in the Walsh-Healey Act of 1970. Here it is assumed that exposure to 95 dB(A) for 4 hours is equivalent to 90 dB(A) for 8 hours, whereas Leq assumed that 93 dB(A) for 4 hours is equivalent to 90 dB(A) for 8 hours. The controversy has been well reviewed by Ward (1991), who after more than a decade of animal experi-

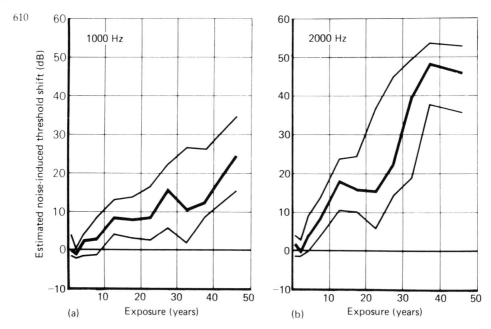

Figure 11.10 Estimated noise-induced threshold shift for particular frequencies, as median and quartile values, for different exposure durations (*a*) for 1000 Hz; (*b*) for 2000 Hz. (From Taylor *et al.*, 1965. In: *Noise and Man*, by W. Burns, 1968, London: John Murray, p. 174)

mentation suggested that neither view is correct; L_{OSHA} is too lax, equal energy too tough, and the truth lies somewhere between; 4 dB halving and doubling perhaps.

ISO 1999 is not applicable at noise levels above 100 dB, and in addition, the data that have been compressed to produce the standard have great interpersonal variation (Figure 11.11).

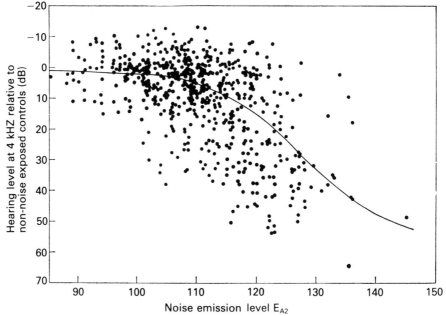

Figure 11.11 Individual age-corrected hearing levels, at 4 kHz, relative to controls unexposed to noise, plotted against noise emission level. Number of subjects 581. Noise emission level $E_{A2} = L_{A2} + 10 \log (T/1 \text{ month})$. (Attributed to Burns and Robinson)

Impact noise

So far most discussion has been concerned with steady-state noise. Impact noise is as dangerous and just as frequent in the military and industry; early examples were rifle shots and riveting. The characteristic of impact sounds varies enormously, rise and decay times range from abrupt to gently sloping and reverberation varies, all of which may alter the effect on the ear; contrast, for example, the crack of a high velocity rifle with the ring of a hammer hitting a metal tank.

The acoustic definition and measurement of impulse noise are the subject of a good recent review by Hamernik and Hsueh (1991) and as such will not be dealt with further.

There have been alarming reports of synergistic interactions between impact and steady-state noise (Hamernik and Henderson, 1976) at extremely high sound levels. More recent work suggests that within the limits of the regulation this does not happen. However, the concept of a critical level of impulse noise above which damage increases non-linearly and rapidly is probably valid. Hétu and Lazure (1982) provided some support for this in humans, although the response is not uniform.

This question of measurement of impulse noise, a difficult task, is crucial to establishing appropriate damage risk criteria. It is suggested that with impulsive, as with steady-state noise, there is biochemical damage produced by the lower levels and mechanical damage produced by the higher levels of damaging sound with a grey area in between. The belief that there is a break point above which there is permanent change has given rise to recommendations for damage risk criteria, based on dose and intensity. Within a limited range of industrial impulse noise an A weighted equal energy risk pattern has been suggested as a 'best fit', although Smoorenburg (1992) felt that for given exposures, impulse noise is more harmful than steady-state noise (see Sulkowski, Kowalska and Lipowcza, 1983). This certainly fits with clinical impressions.

Many studies have corroborated these results including a survey of 6835 workers exposed to industrial noise at General Motors (Baughn, 1966), a study of over 25000 Austrian industrial workers (Rop, Raber and Fischer, 1979), a study of British steelworkers (Burns *et al.*, 1979) and a study in three different Ontario industries (Abel and Haythornthwaite, 1984). It is unlikely that there will be any more because of the introduction of hearing conservation programmes.

A final word of caution is in order. The above studies of progression of hearing loss and regulations devised to control this are based on pure tone audiometric studies in humans. There is a good body of evidence which suggests that, during exposure to given damaging noise, hair cell damage continues even though the audiogram remains static, that is continuing damage to the cochlea may occur in the presence of an apparent asymptotic threshold shift. Indeed, the correlation between hair cell loss and permanent threshold shift is not good (Bohne and Clark, 1982; Ward, Turner and Fabry, 1983; Clark, 1991a). As more subtle cochlear damage resulting from acoustic over-stimulation is identified, some of these issues are being resolved (Erlandsson *et al.*, 1987; Saunders, Cohen and Szymko, 1991). Damage ceases when the noise exposure ceases.

Natural history of noise-induced permanent threshold shift

Within the broad range of noise levels described as hazardous, the average initial change is a temporary threshold shift which imperceptibly blends into noise-induced permanent threshold shift. There is no arbitrary period of exposure beneath which no noise-induced permanent threshold shift may occur, nor any maximum exposure beyond which no further shift will occur. However, the rate of progression varies according to frequency with maximum losses early in the high frequencies and late in the low frequencies.

Noise-induced permanent threshold shift usually commences between 3 and 6 kHz, often around 4 kHz, and gradually worsens at that frequency and spreads into neighbouring frequencies. At first it may be asymptomatic but if it spreads into the lower frequencies of 3 and 2 kHz, complaints begin. Initially, subjects experience difficulty in discriminating speech, particularly if there is any background noise. This may impact on the participation in meetings at work, and social gatherings. As the loss spreads into the lower frequencies they may have difficulty with sounds being too quiet. After a time, the high frequency recovery disappears so that the audiogram becomes flattened out in the uppermost ranges. While an audiometric notch is often present in noise-induced permanent threshold shift, it is not a prerequisite for the diagnosis, nor is noise the only cause of a notched audiogram. It is suggested that for predominantly impact noise the notch is centred at 6 kHz (Sulkowski, Kowalska and Lipowcza, 1983). Ylikoski (1987) has shown with impulse noise from weapons, the centre frequency of the notch varies with the acoustic characteristics of the weapon, lower with heavy weapons, higher with small ones. Also for steady-state tonal, or limited frequency range hazardous sounds, the audiogram may be quite atypical, and reflect maximum damage half an octave above the centre frequency of the sound.

'Typical' audiograms are frequently shown in texts, but they are typical only of the group to which they apply. The 'typical' audiogram shown in Figure 11.12 is quite different from the audiogram shown in

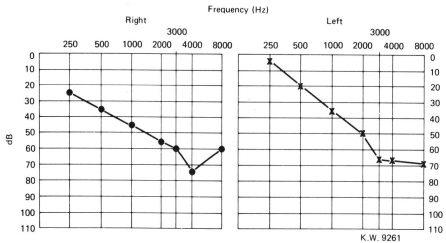

Figure 11.12 Audiogram of a 56-year-old nickel miner exposed to about 20 years of hard rock drilling. This audiogram is typical of rock miners after this exposure

Figure 11.7 and is typical of the hearing of male hard rock miners after 20 years of underground drilling with pneumatic tools. The loss in the miners is severe, but their noise exposure exceeds 100 dB(A) Leq8 for long periods, and is outside the prescribed range of ISO 1999e.

Hearing loss at 4 kHz progresses rapidly at first; with 100 dBA daily 8-hour exposure, it may reach 15–20 dB within 1–2 years. The loss continues to worsen fairly swiftly for about 10 years and then slows down, although it does not stop completely (Figure 11.13). The rate and total amount of loss are dose dependent. At lower frequencies the loss is less severe, and grows more slowly, although it is still greatest in the earlier years. As the years pass presby-

acusis begins to take its toll; indeed this was already pointed out by Baughn in 1973 who wrote, 'Intense noise produces such high losses so rapidly that the contribution of aging (which nevertheless is steadily producing its changes) is completely lost to view. In a number of years, however, the noise induced component decreases and then is lost to the age component – which has been steadily progressing at an accelerating rate – begins to catch up . . . Our figures indicate that if a whole population could be kept alive to age 86 it would make no difference what the exposure history of the members of that population has been . . .' (cited by Robinson, 1987).

It should be remembered that loss from noise is not the total hearing loss in an otherwise otologically

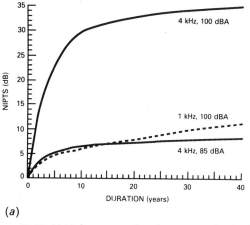

(*a*)

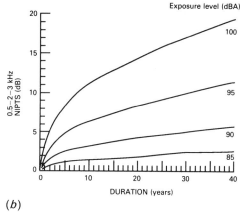

(*b*)

Figure 11.13 (*a*) Median noise-induced permanent threshold shift (NIPTS) as a function of exposure duration for 4 kHz (85 and 100 dBA) and 1 kHz (100 dBA). (*b*) Median NIPTS for the pure-tone average (0.5, 1, 2, 3 kHz) as a function of exposure duration, for different exposure levels (85–100 dBA). (From Dobie, 1993, with permission)

normal person, it is the difference between the normal hearing corrected for presbyacusis and the observed hearing loss.

Individual susceptibility varies enormously and unfortunately there is no good way of predicting this. Damage risk criteria predict the safety margins for a certain percentage of the population, but they do not help with protection of total populations. In unprotected ears the much-mentioned 90-dBA/40 hour exposure, which is described as 'safe', is so for about 85% of the population; conversely 15% of workers exposed to this level for a prolonged period will develop a demonstrable disabling hearing loss. In order to protect 95% of the population an 85-dB(A)/8 hour safe level must be adopted.

The rate of progression depends upon the type of noise and individual susceptibility. The type of progression for a particular noise is shown in Figure 11.9 and the range covered by these curves in Figures 11.10 and 11.14. Figure 11.9 shows quite clearly that, for that particular noise, the hearing loss at 3 and 4 kHz increases linearly at one rate for 12 years and then slowly tapers off while the hearing loss at 2 kHz behaves in an almost opposite way – slowly increasing for 25 years and then relatively more rapidly to reach the same level at the higher frequencies after 38 years of exposure. It is likely that the later deterioration is due to presbyacusis. At the end of a working lifetime the loss for 1 kHz is only just

making itself manifest. However, there is tremendous individual variation, e.g. at 2 kHz the loss after 30 years of exposure shows a 30-dB difference in permanent threshold shift between 25th and 75th percentiles. These graphs will vary with different noise exposures, and are confounded by presbyacusis. One of the difficulties of making predictions based on a given noise measurement is the changing nature of industrial noise – machinery may be changed or malfunction, a silencer may blow, a bearing break etc. There are numbers of well documented incidents of workers dating a sudden change in their hearing levels to such temporary changes in work noise.

There seems to be an intensity level above which noise produces dramatic changes which may not recover, usually associated with a single explosion or blast, but they may also be the result of exposure of an ear to an intense steady-state noise. Working long hours without sufficient recovery period between shifts may have the same effect. Some of the worst noise-induced hearing loss that the author has seen occurred in hard rock miners who worked back to back shifts drilling without hearing protectors during the Second World War with only 8 hour recovery periods. If workers are exposed to high exposure levels then administrative controls must be in place so that the temporary threshold shift has time to recover totally before the next acoustic assault on the ears.

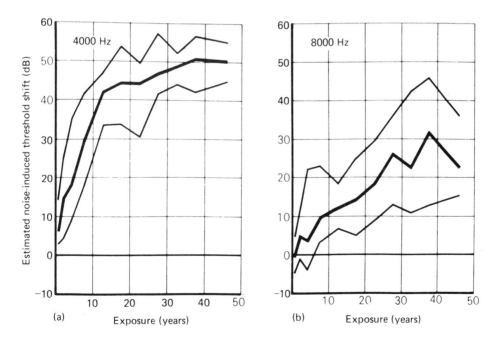

Figure 11.14 Estimated noise-induced threshold shift for particular frequencies, as median and quartile values, for different exposure durations (*a*) for 4000 Hz; (*b*) for 8000 Hz. (From Taylor *et al.*, 1965. In: *Noise and Man*, by W. Burns, 1968, London: John Murray, p. 174)

Individual susceptibility

There are some people with 'tough' ears who seem to be able to withstand higher levels of exposure better than the norm, and others with relatively 'tender' ears which are easily damaged. Audiograms of two such individuals are shown in Figure 11.15*a* and *b*. Both men had been hard rock drillers in a nickel mine for a similar number of years undertaking work which so far as could be ascertained was identical. Individual susceptibility to noise-induced hearing loss has recently been extensively reviewed by Henderson, Subramanian and Boettcher (1993). They concluded that the individual variations are real and have many causes such as interaction with other ototraumatic agents such as drugs. Non-auditory characteristics of a subject such as melanization and sex are unimportant. The relationship between temporary threshold shift and permanent threshold shift is not direct. The acoustic reflex may play a part and prior noise sensitization is also important as a protective agent. Early identification of those with tender ears has long been perceived as an important but elusive goal.

Otoacoustic emissions

Both transient and distortion product evoked otoacoustic emissions have been studied following acute

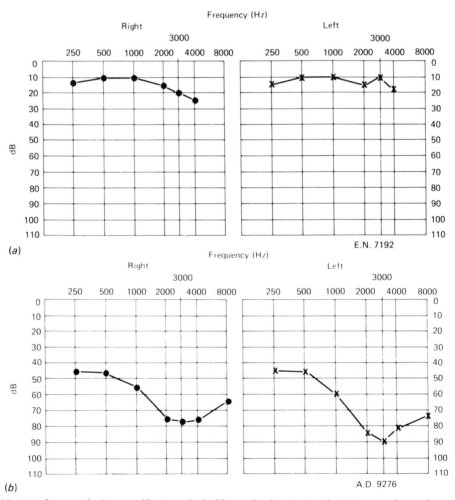

Figure 11.15 (*a*) Audiogram of a 50-year-old miner who had been a hard rock miner for 20 years and served as a tank driver during the Second World War; he shows little hearing loss and is an example of 'tough ears'; (*b*) audiogram of a 54-year-old miner with identical exposure to the man in (*a*). He has a profound loss and is an example of 'tender ears'. Both should be contrasted with Figure 11.12

acoustic over-stimulation and in chronic noise-induced hearing loss. With severe temporary threshold shift, transient otoacoustic emissions disappear (Wilson, 1992). They are a sensitive measure of presence or absence of hearing over 35–40 dB and have been used for this purpose including those with noise-induced permanent threshold shift (Kim *et al.*, 1992). Their practical use in noise-induced permanent threshold shift is as a screen for exaggerated hearing loss (their presence implies hearing better than 35 dB, whatever the admitted threshold), and as a sign of early noise changes. According to LePage and Murray (1993), the size of otoacoustic emissions diminishes even before there is a detectable pure tone threshold shift in overexposure to noise. If this is true (and it was not confirmed by Avan *et al.*, 1993), otoacoustic emissions might make a sensitive screen for susceptibility to noise damage.

Tinnitus

Tinnitus is a constant feature of an acute blast injury and is a fairly constant concomitant of industrial hearing loss; it is frequently present for some hours after noise exposure, but fortunately usually, but not always, disappears. However, after many years of exposure it may become permanent. This is a distressing symptom which is difficult to quantify and thus difficult to study. The prevalence of chronic tinnitus in workers exposed to noise is high, between 50 and 60%; both the series of Axelsson and McShane (McShane, Hyde and Alberti, 1988; Axelsson and Barrenäs, 1992) found it usually to be tonal, sometimes relieved by a hearing aid, and of greater prevalence in those exposed to impact noise. Tinnitus is such a ubiquitous symptom in the population at large that its relationship to noise exposure may only be incidental in some cases. Hinchcliffe and King (1992), in a recent study, suggested that it is frequently a symptom of compensation and pointed out that it used not to be a complaint. They also reviewed the history of the subject and its medico-legal implications. Their papers are a contrast to others related to tinnitus and noise-induced hearing loss, such as Axelsson and Barrenäs (1992) which are more accepting of tinnitus as a component of noise-induced permanent threshold shift. Both Alberti (1987) and Axelsson give good correlates of tinnitus in noise-induced permanent threshold shift with other aspects of the disorder.

Worsening of hearing after cessation of noise exposure?

It is generally accepted that when noise exposure ceases the hearing will not worsen, and indeed may even improve. In the long term hearing worsens as one gets older, and this is as true of the noise-exposed worker as the population at large. However, there is no evidence to suggest that the worsening is caused by prior noise exposure, so long as the exposure has ceased. In all people there is an additional central ageing effect making it more difficult to discriminate speech in a background of noise, which is not necessarily linked to a worsening of the pure tone threshold. So there may be general complaints about hearing becoming worse, even with no change in permanent threshold shift. Prior noise exposure plays no part. Tschopp and Probst (1989) undertook a longitudinal study of a large series of subjects with hearing loss from a single traumatic episode and found no evidence of progression from the accident.

Synergistic effect of ototraumatic agents

Various noxious agents may damage the ear. They include noise – steady-state, impact and explosive – a variety of drugs, head trauma, ageing, various ear diseases including the premature degeneration of the cochlea found in many familial hearing losses, and infectious degenerations of the ear. The question of how these various agents interact is complex and important. Is an ear which has already been damaged by noise more or less susceptible to further damage by an ototoxic antibiotic, or is the effect purely additive?

Drugs

There appears to be significant synergism between the toxic effects of certain aminoglycoside antibiotics, kanamycin and gentamicin and noise exposure, but only above a critical dosage of kanamycin and a specific level of noise – in the guinea pig this is 100 dB SPL. The damage from noise must be in the same area of the cochlea as that from kanamycin – the basal turn. The order in which the agents are given is important. If kanamycin is given after noise exposure the effects are synergistic, whereas if kanamycin is given first there is no synergism. Virtually all these experiments were undertaken in the guinea pig and it is difficult to know how far they can be generalized to humans. It is also suggested, but only demonstrated in one study, that neomycin is synergistic with noise. Aran *et al.* (1992) have undertaken a series of experiments to evaluate the relative roles of the diuretic ethacrynic acid and gentamicin in noise exposure. Ethacrynic acid facilitates the entry of gentamicin into the cell and makes it more susceptible to noise. Cisplatin is a fairly widely used cytotoxic drug which is also ototoxic, and acts synergistically with other ototoxic agents, including aminoglycoside antibiotics, diuretics and noise (Boettcher *et al.*, 1992).

Environmental hydrocarbons

There has been increasing concern about the ototoxic effects of organic solvents, and a variety of industrially-used chemicals. Odkvist, Møller and Thuomas (1992) reviewed the otoneurological disturbances caused by solvent pollution concentrating on hydrocarbon solvents, such as styrene and jet fuel which are implicated as the cause of the psycho-organic syndrome. Their main effect is on the vestibular system, especially centrally. Disturbances of central auditory processing were also found, more with jet fuel than styrene. Barregård and Axelsson (1984) had already suggested that there might be an interaction between the use of organic solvents and noise exposure. They found worse hearing than expected from noise exposure alone in some shipyard workers also exposed to organic solvent. Rybak (1992) also reviewed the subject exhaustively and is cautious in attributing a synergistic affect to the use of styrene with hazardous noise. He also reviewed the literature with regard to carbon disulphide used in the manufacture of rayon and suggested that the exposure to the compound may produce hearing loss, and that noise and CS_2 interact to produce worse hearing than exposure to noise alone (see also Morata, 1989).

Toluene is the most studied and so far the most ototoxic organic chemical in common use; 600 000 tons are used industrially in the manufacture of paints, in printing and leather tanning. It is also inhaled by glue and spray paint sniffers. On its own it produces hearing loss which is probably peripheral (Johnson and Canlon, 1994); it also acts synergistically with noise (Morata *et al.*, 1993).

Carbon monoxide poisoning may produce central hearing loss, and in the presence of noise may act as a facilitator of hair cell damage (see Rybak, 1992 and Boettcher *et al.*, 1992). The prevalence of hearing loss, and the mechanism of its production by organic compounds is neither well studied nor fully understood. Salicylates are of concern because of their widespread use. However, the effect appears to be slight (Boettcher *et al.*, 1992).

Vibration

There have been many attempts to relate vibration, and the combined affects of vibration and noise exposure to the development of hearing loss, dating back more than 60 years (Hamernik, Ahroon and Davis, 1989). Except when related to white hand, the findings are equivocal. Those subject to white hand (Raynaud's phenomenon), and exposed to excessive sound develop more hearing loss than those without white hand as in forestry workers who use chain saws in cold surroundings (Iki *et al.*, 1986; Pyykkö *et al.*, 1989) and ship builders, using noisy vibrating pneumatic tools in cold conditions (Stark, Pekkaimen and Pyykkö, 1988).

Noise and age

This subject has been much studied at two extremes: in the young and in the elderly. Is there a critical period in the development of the ear, or in its early life where it is particularly susceptible to noise damage? In a wide range of laboratory animals this appears to be so. The findings suggest that once the peripheral auditory system is fully developed, the younger the animal, the greater the damage from noise exposure. It has also been questioned whether interaction between noise and ototoxic drugs is greater in the young – a question of some practical importance in premature infants kept continuously for days in the relatively high sound levels of an incubator and frequently treated with gentamicin. Long-term studies of the hearing levels of children so treated are awaited with interest. However, if there is an effect, it is small.

At the other extreme of life, the question of interaction between industrial noise and ageing is frequently discussed. How does presbyacusis interact with noise: are they additive, synergistic or protective? The new noise standard ISO 1999 (1990) addresses the issue and suggests the two are additive, except in high levels of noise where there is slightly less additional affect from presbyacusis than predicted. McCrea (1991) has modelled the ISO formula based on a study of noise exposed Australian veterans and finds it to be correct. Dobie (1992) has used it to model a mechanism to apportion the affect of noise and ageing changes on a given hearing loss, which although based on group norms, is intuitively appealing and the best method currently available. Both Dobie (1992) and Robinson (1987) pointed out that ageing has a greater affect than hitherto appreciated. Robinson (1991a) pointed out that obvious fact that if all hearing is lost from noise then ageing cannot have an affect, and vice versa. Noise and ageing are only totally additive with moderate amounts of noise in young and middle-aged people (see also Bauer *et al.*, 1991). With higher noise levels the effects are less than additive, as they are also in the elderly. In later life ageing dominates. As Baughn suggested in 1973 and Rosenhall, Pedersen and Svanborg (1990) have shown, in the higher frequencies at any rate, by the age of 80 years, hearing is the same whether the ear is noise exposed or not (see also MaCrea, 1971; Novotny, 1975a,b; Welleschik and Raber, 1978; Corso, 1980). The matter has significant practical importance when attempting to evaluate hearing loss for pension purposes in elderly noise-exposed workers.

Previous noise-induced hearing loss

What is the interaction of further noise exposure on an ear which already shows damage from prior exposure? This is of importance in allotting the appropriate amount of hearing loss to the correct employer in compensation claims. Even if someone has worked continuously for one employer, there may be different insurers throughout the time and argument may ensue about apportionment of the loss. Both Dobie (1990) and Robinson (1991a) addressed this question and the reader is referred to their publications for details. In general terms it is possible to model group changes, using the latest ISO 1999 (1990) to predict the amount of hearing loss from noise in each segment of work.

Degree of melanization

It has been suggested that melanin is an important protective agent against noise and a degree of melanization is necessary for the appropriate functioning of the cochlea. The inference is therefore that albinos or blue-eyed people are more susceptible to noise damage than brown-eyed caucasians and black workers. The literature on eye colour is quite large and remains controversial; Henderson, Subramaniam and Boettcher (1993) believed it to be of little importance, while Barrenäs and Lindgren (1991) suggested that in previously normal subjects, there is more temporary threshold shift to a given noise in blue-eyed people than those with brown eyes. They carefully do not extrapolate their findings to permanent threshold shift.

The acoustic reflex

The acoustic reflex is a reflex contraction of the stapedius muscle in response to loud sound. Its dynamic characteristics have been admirably reviewed by Borg (1976). When contracted, the muscle can attenuate the passage of sound through the middle ear by up to 30 dB. However, the contracted muscle fatigues readily, particularly in response to high-frequency stimulation. The recovery is rapid and if the stimulus is repetitive then the muscle is believed to contract repetitively. It is therefore suggested that the middle ear muscle reflex may protect the ear against some of the harmful effects of noise, although the evidence is very contradictory. For impulse noise, the reflex is almost unfatiguable but with steady-state noise is quickly extinguished (Rossi, 1983a). This may account for some of the previously

reported incongruities. Coletti *et al.* (1992) reported experimental data and summarized their own work which seems to show some protective effect of the acoustic reflexes, which is less effective with severe physical exertion (see also Henderson, Subramaniam and Boettcher, 1993). One function of the acoustic reflex appears to be to compensate against hearing damage from one's own voice; it may have an as yet not fully defined role in protecting against noise exposure.

Complex interactions

Much of the above has described specific effects of noise and at most how this may be modified by a single other factor, such as vibration. It is becoming more obvious that complex interactions are the rule rather than the exception. The interaction between environment – heat, humidity and the like – atmospheric toxins, smoking, psychological factors (is a pleasurable sound less damaging than an annoying one?) and noise is slowly being unravelled (see for example Boettcher *et al.*, 1989).

Acoustic trauma

That explosions can produce hearing loss is well known. However, single loud sounds unassociated with explosion can also cause cochlear damage which may be temporary or permanent. Early examples were 'telephone-ear' produced by atmospheric static and thus limiters were placed on telephones (Bunch, 1929; Fowler, 1939). The modern variant is caused by occasional inadvertent ringing of a portable telephone while the hand piece is held close to the ear (Gerling and Jerger, 1985; Guyot, 1988). The writer is unaware of any recorded cases of hearing loss due to the use of cellular telephones.

Industrial examples include workers inside tanks which are inadvertently struck by a sledge hammer on the outside which can produce devastating hearing loss.

Otitic blast injury

In this form of trauma, external, middle and inner ear structures can all be damaged. Blast is the sudden explosive force generated by bursting shells, bombs or other explosives. There is a qualitative similarity between a bomb explosion and a gun report. However, the shock waves from an explosion are three times longer than those from the report of a 2 cm gun.

Kerr and Byrne (1975) gave a graphic and remarkably well documented account of the effect of a lethal bomb blast in a restaurant in Belfast in which there were multiple injuries. Eighty people were identified, present in the restaurant at the time, who were examined later. In general, the closer the person was to the bomb, the more likelihood of ear perforation, and in people with unilateral perforations the membrane perforated was usually the one facing the bomb. At least 60 tympanic membrane perforations were identified, which had protean characteristics; they were linear, cleanly punched or ragged, large or small and occasionally double, and the edges were both inverted and everted. Most victims complained of severe temporary deafness which verged on total for those most badly affected. Virtually all complained of severe tinnitus following the blast. These findings agree with those from the Vietnam war. Kerr and Byrne advocated conservative management, with surgical repair reserved for those which did not heal spontaneously – 80% healed spontaneously and the remaining ears were successfully closed by surgery.

The inner ear damage was also variable. Initially, most had some degree of sensorineural loss which usually cleared quickly and completely. Many of the subjects who had a residual high frequency hearing loss were unaware of its presence. Tympanic membrane rupture did not protect the inner ear from sensorineural hearing loss. The present author has similar experience with an unfortunately large number of miners exposed to accidental dynamite blasts underground who, almost uniformly, complained of an immediate profound hearing loss accompanied by tinnitus, which usually, but not always, recovers. Several patients have now been seen in whom one ear became permanently deaf after a blast, while the other recovered significantly.

Specific non-industrial noise hazards
Guns

Coles (1963) found an intensity of 174 dB at the firer's head with an automatic gun; Glorig and Wheeler (1955) found that noise from firearms might attain 180 dB; Yarington (1968) recorded impulse noise attaining 190 dB from 105 mm howitzers and Salmivalli (1967) 188 dB from field cannons and 185.6 dB from antitank guns.

The maximum permissible level which the ear can tolerate without sustaining permanent damage is dependent on the exposure time. Pfander (1975) considered 165 dB permissible for 0.003 second/day, but for 0.3 second only 145 dB can be tolerated. The matter is complex. For example, Patterson and Johnson (1993), in a series of recently reported experiments, showed that under certain circumstances 180 dB SPL can be safe. Permanent damage may be caused on initial exposure. The same is true for small arms fire (Ylikoski, 1987). Sudden deafness after short exposure to gunfire, even if causing a 60 dB

loss, usually recovered in 48 hours, although it might take 60 hours, and occasionally 20 days. An asymmetrical hearing loss is characteristic of rifle and shotgun fire where the ear nearest the muzzle has up to 25 dB worse hearing at the depth of the notch. Acoustic trauma has become much more prevalent in the modern army as weapons have become noisier, and to this is added the high background noise of armoured personnel carriers and troop transporting helicopters.

The amount of recreational shooting undertaken in the western world, including the UK and Europe is great; in the USA, Lankford, Mikiut and Jackson (1991) found about 20% of a group of male and 10% of female high school students used firearms regularly and in the UK, Fearn and Hanson (1989) found that 9% of 13–17-year old pop concert goers had been exposed to firearms. Those exposed to acceptable levels of workplace noise may have an unacceptable 24 hour total noise exposure because of transportation and leisure pursuits.

Socioacusis

Hearing loss from the cumulative effect of social noise exposure has been termed 'socioacusis', and should be taken into account in evaluating the cause of hearing loss, along with industrial and military exposure to noise, and presbyacusis (see Davis, 1983).

Recreational noise exposure

Hazardous sound levels are an accompaniment of many enjoyable playthings of young and old alike; model aeroplane engines (Bess and Powell, 1972), motor cycles (Van Moorhen *et al.*, 1981), snowmobiles, sports cars, all share high levels of noise. A recent review has been published by Clark (1991b), which emphasizes common North American social and leisure noise hazards, including gardening equipment and power tools.

Fireworks and cap pistols

Gjaevenes, Moseng and Nordahl (1974) examined the hearing of 791 Norwegian schoolchildren aged 12–14 years before and after the Constitutional Day holiday, at which time firecrackers are exploded with abandon. Follow-up examination showed that 0.7% of the boys had considerable permanent hearing loss. They extrapolated that 75 boys living in Oslo aged 12–15 years acquired a permanent hearing loss that day. Similar findings were made by Gupta and Vishwarama (1989) related to the Indian Festival of Deepavali; of 600 volunteer subjects aged 3 to 31 years, 3.8% developed temporary threshold shift, and 2% a permanent loss. Cap pistols may be just as harmful as fireworks (Axelsson *et al.*, 1991).

Snowmobiles

Baxter and Ling (1974) found that up to 85% of the adult male Inuit population had a sensorineural hearing loss caused by repeated 12-hour snowmobile safaris at full throttle on unsilenced machines, accompanied by rapid firing of powerful rifles from the shoulder. Sami (Laplanders) suffer similarly (Sorri *et al.*, 1983).

Sports

Motorcycle riding, drag racing, sport shooting and boxing may produce hearing loss (Fletcher and Gross, 1977; McCombe, Binnington and McCombe, 1993).

Aircraft

Sound levels within most commercial airliners are safe; this is not so in many small private propeller-driven airplanes (Jha and Catherines, 1978a, b). Cockpit sound levels may be in the low 90s dB(A) at cruising speeds and higher in take-off and climb. The high levels of background noise both have a deleterious effect on communication and require even higher radio levels. The present author has seen several flyers, particularly instructors, with significant sensorineural hearing losses attributed to the planes themselves.

Hobbies

Home hobbies may be harmful: gardening equipment – lawnmowers, edgers, leaf blowers (112 dBA) – chain saws and workshop power tools may produce sound levels well in excess of safe levels. Hearing protection should be used (Davis, 1983; Clark, 1991b). Noise-induced hearing loss occurs too often in teenage boys, due to firearms, farm and horticultural machinery (Kramer and Wood, 1982).

'Pop' music and its effect

Whether music gives pleasure or not is a subjective question. That it may be a source of high intensity sound, is however, beyond debate. The purpose of high intensity sound is to produce vegetative effects of a general kind quite apart from imposing the sound on the listener. In order to have a musical 'trip' it seems necessary to listen to sounds at a sufficiently high intensity which may be above safe levels for hearing.

There has been considerable discussion in the literature about the potentially harmful effect of amplified music both on the ears of the musician and the audience. In the case of the musician and disc jockeys the question is no different from any other form of occupational noise exposure. Here the introduction of level attenuating ear plugs has been a boon (see below). Audience sound levels at rock concerts are well summarized by Clark (1991b) – levels in excess of 100 dB are common. Many rock concerts produce temporary threshold shift and tinnitus in some of the audience, which usually clears by the next day. Rice, Rossi and Aina (1987) put the risk of permanent hearing loss from regular rock concerts attendance at less than 1/4000. There are however those with hypersensitive ears who can be permanently damaged (Ulrich and Pinheiro, 1974; Tomioka, 1982; but see also Carter *et al.*, 1982).

Personal cassette players and radios

There is concern that personal cassette players are a hearing hazard. These ubiquitous devices can produce intense sound levels but it is questionable whether they are listened to for periods of time long enough for damage to occur. Turunen-Rise, Flottorp and Trete (1991) gave a balanced review of the issues. It is accepted that listening to personal cassette players may produce temporary threshold shift but it is very rarely long lived. Acoustical measures made of different recordings and different headphones show the weighted sound fields produced by personal cassette players only rarely exceed Leq8 of 85 dB(A). School children listen at relatively low settings which the authors attributed to equipment distortion at higher intensities. Bradley, Fortnum and Coles (1987) found that a large sample (1443) of British school children were conservative listeners. This corroborates the exhaustive review of the British MRC centre (Davis *et al.*, 1985) and is substantiated by the work of Rice, Rossi and Aina (1987), who concluded that the risk of a hearing loss following regular listening with personal cassette players (if continued over a 10-year period), is one in 1500 users. Royster (1985) has come to similar conclusions in North America. However, there are sensitive individuals. Anyone suffering from regular postexposure tinnitus and/or fullness of hearing should be cautioned that these are warning signs of early hearing loss.

Classical music

Sound levels in symphony orchestras are high, particularly in the percussion section and for those musicians seated in front of the brass instruments where there are transient peaks of well over 100 dB (see review by Royster, Royster and Killion, 1991). Solo violinists may expose the left ear (in right-handed musicians) to levels as high as

105 dB and many have asymmetrical hearing losses. The risks to hearing from orchestra playing alone are not high, although instrumentalists who play in several ensembles, teach and practise much, may exceed damage risk criteria. Flat response protectors (Killion, DeVilbiss and Stewart, 1988) are recommended.

Community noise exposure

The levels of noise experienced in the community are orders of magnitude less than those in industry, but they affect many more people, and add to the daily quota of sound exposure.

Noise levels within aircraft, buses, and underground trains are harsh. Many commuters spend considerable periods daily on underground trains where the sound levels may be 90 dB(A) or even higher. On highways heavy vehicles represent only 10% of the traffic stream but produce almost 70% of sound. Thus, efforts aimed at their noise control should be cost effective. In warm climates, where it is the norm to have windows open the noise of music in the bazaars, motorcycles and unsilenced engines can be a tyranny. For example the motor rickshaws and 'long tailed' boats in Bangkok may expose the driver to over 100 dB of sound.

The emerging technology of active noise reduction has great promise in reducing low frequency sounds by electronic phase cancelling and is likely to be applied widely in areas such as air conditioning units, refrigerators, and automobile exhausts during the late 1990s. The principles are well reviewed by Alper (1991).

Full discussion of community noise levels, their effect, their measurement and their control, is beyond the scope of this chapter. The books by Burns (1973) and by Kryter (1985), which deal with noise as a nuisance, together with the successive conference proceedings, *Noise as a Public Health Problem*, give good background summaries (Rossi, 1983b; Berglund *et al.*, 1988; Vallet, 1993).

Compression chambers and diving

The sound from air entry valves in compression chambers may be hazardous (Hughes, 1976). Deep sea commercial diving can be extremely noisy. The ear is less sensitive under water and most sound conduction is by the bone route, but noise levels from tools are extremely high – up to 200 dB SPL. The maximum point of hearing loss is in the mid frequencies rather than at 4 kHz (Al-Masri, Martin and Nedwell, 1993). Molvaer (1991) described sound levels of over 145 dB inside hard helmets of divers operating high pressure water jet lances as deafening and possibly affecting balance.

Medical noise

Hazards from hearing aids

Hearing aids may rarely damage hearing (Studebaker, Bess and Beck, 1991). Temporary threshold shift is undesirable because it increases the amplification need and permanent threshold shift is unacceptable (Macrae, 1994).

Hospital noise

Hospitals themselves can be extremely noisy and the source both of inconvenience and of hearing loss. In open plan intensive care units (ICUs), the sounds from monitoring equipment, respirators, suction pumps, and a variety of life support systems are certainly sufficient to disturb patients and staff. In addition, in the background noise of an ICU, the many audible warning signals can be easily confused, and difficult to localize. Thus silencing an ICU and paying attention to the ergonomics of warning signals may save lives.

Service areas in hospitals may have unacceptable sound levels, especially laboratory and kitchen dishwashers and heating plants (see Ducel, Suter and Dupont, 1976; Bentley, Murphy and Dudley, 1977; Borenzi and Collareta, 1984).

Magnetic resonance imaging units may produce sound levels at the patient's head exceeding 90 dBA (Brummett, Talbot and Charuhas, 1988). Cases of temporary threshold shift have been reported, and hearing protectors recommended for patients. Some newer devices have active noise reduction built in.

Drills and suction units

There is a lengthy literature about affects of high speed drills used in ear surgery, which produce high levels of air and bone conducted sound to both ears of the patient. Large cutting burrs produce more sound than small ones, diamond burrs produce least. It is unlikely that drill noise damages the hearing of patients. Suction units, too, may produce high sound levels in the ear (see Paulsen and Vietor, 1975a, b; Kylen and Arlinger, 1976; 1977; Parkin *et al.*, 1980; Man and Winerman, 1985; Spencer and Reid, 1985).

Dental drills have been implicated as a potential noise hazard; current devices do not appear to be damaging (Coles and Hoare, 1985).

Effects of infrasound, vibration and ultrasound

There are still wide gaps in our knowledge of the effects of acoustical stimuli above and below the normal range of human auditory perception. Normally noise is heard and vibration is felt, but physically they are similar (Westin, 1975) and it is sometimes quite difficult to differentiate between the two.

Sources of infrasound

Most infrasound is from geophysical phenomena, such as thunder, high winds, ocean waves, and earthquakes (see Westin, 1975; Von Gierke and Nixon, 1976). Man-made infrasound is common but infrequently detected, for most sound measuring surveys do not extend the range of investigation into frequencies below 60 Hz. The automobile is one of the most common sources, it is responsible for some of the unpleasant sensations experienced when driving at speed with windows open. Much heavy industrial machinery produces infrasound, including air conditioning plants, fans, and many forms of transportation. Crew of spaceships are subjected to intense infrasound at the time of launching.

Non-auditory effects of infrasound have been hotly debated but are nebulous (Nussbaum and Reinis, 1985). Infrasound with higher harmonics may be associated with headache and fatigue, whereas pure infrasounds may be associated with dizziness and nausea.

Ultrasound

Sources of ultrasound are fairly widespread, both in jet aircraft and, among other industrial sources, sonic cleaners and dental drills. There is no hard evidence that any of these are harmful.

Non-auditory effects of noise

Sound has extra-auditory effects. It has an alerting value which produces reflex responses, unconditioned and conditioned. The startle response in the infant to a loud sound is an example of the former; the downing of tools as the lunchtime buzzer goes in a plant is an example of the latter.

There have been many suggestions that community and industrial noise have an adverse effect on health, although it is extremely difficult to differentiate the effect of the sound itself from other stressful stimuli. Kryter (1985) has written extensively on the subject. Sound may directly stimulate or cause activation of the autonomic nervous system to such an extent that it endangers health. Cohen (1973) studied the injury and illness rates in a noisy and a relatively quiet plant, and found that both were higher in the noisy plant. However, whether these were the direct result of noise or other factors in the plant remains open.

The effect of noise on sleep has been extensively studied, both in the laboratory and, in more recent years, in the home. The results are well summarized by Thiessen (1976), Kryter (1985) and by Stevenson and McKellar (1989). They suggested that for moderate intermittent levels of noise repeated through several nights, the probability of awakening as a result of the noise diminishes, i.e. there is a subconscious adaptation to the noise which becomes less disturbing although, even if the subject does not wake, the alpha rhythm is disturbed by noise. Certainly the higher the background noise, the more the likelihood of a shift in sleep level.

Noise and health

The report of an increased incidence of mental hospital admission among those subjected to high levels of aircraft noise has been widely quoted (Abey-Wickram *et al.*, 1969). This study has spawned much controversy and other derivative studies in the USA and the UK, which have been extensively analysed by Kryter (1985). The original conclusions are probably not valid. An excellent review by Stansfeld *et al.* (1993) of the effect of noise on a carefully chosen population in Caerphilly, part of a larger European study, concluded that there is no association between noise exposure and psychiatric disorder. There is, however, an association between noise sensitivity and future psychiatric disorder. Noise sensitivity is also a secondary symptom of depression. A larger study of the risks of heart disease related to noise exposure (Babisch, Elwood and Ising, 1994) in Berlin and Caerphilly concluded that there is possible evidence of a 1.2:1 increased risk in the highest noise areas, especially if the noise is annoying. More work is needed.

Other non-auditory effects of noise

Evans (1990) described the direct and indirect non-auditory effects of chronic noise exposure on children's health and behavioural development, including delayed cognitive development because of interference with speech perception and strategies to tune out unwanted auditory stimuli; learning helplessness is an important final outcome. The behaviour of teachers may also be affected by noise, thus leading to less competent instruction (Mills, 1975; see also Hétu, Truchon-Gagnon and Biloda, 1990). Studies in Sweden (Hygge, 1993) showed that recall of items presented earlier was impaired in teenagers who were exposed to aircraft and road noise during the learning period but not by train and other verbal noise. In New York, Bronzaft (1991) showed that children taught in classrooms facing the tracks of elevated trains had worse reading abilities than children of the same socioeconomic background in the same school taught away from the trains. There are similar aircraft related reports.

Clinical features of noise-induced permanent threshold shift

The diagnosis of noise-induced permanent threshold shift is based on a full evaluation of history, physical examination and laboratory tests, including the audiogram. The diagnosis is usually circumstantial. It should be remembered that noise-induced permanent threshold shift and other ear disease may coexist. In the author's own series (Alberti and Blair, 1982), of 1222 consecutive workers evaluated for noise-induced permanent threshold shift, 5% had other ear disease as the major cause of hearing loss – otosclerosis, chronic otitis media, Menière's disease, etc. Conversely, the presence of other pathology does not preclude a diagnosis of noise-induced permanent threshold shift – the two may coexist. The patient with a mid frequency familial hearing loss may have an additional noise loss.

A careful history is necessary, both personal and familial, of past and present occupational, recreational and accidental noise exposure. Enquiry must be made of illnesses associated with or known to cause deafness; head injuries and ototoxic drug exposure; haematological, serological, radiological, and other investigative procedures may be indicated, and a complete examination of the ears, nose and throat must be made. As social and military noise exposure has increased, so has its importance in the history. It becomes a matter of exquisite judgment to attribute various percentages of loss to current employment, past employment, military service and social events! If there are asymmetrical hearing thresholds the worker should be asked about asymmetrical noise exposure.

Any history or physical signs, including audiometric findings, suggestive of other cochlear or retrocochlear lesions such as Menières' disease, acoustic neuroma, meningioma etc. should be investigated as indicated on clinical grounds. When the results of the history and physical findings, together with laboratory tests and audiograms are evaluated, it is usually possible to decide whether an individual is suffering from hearing loss attributable to noise.

Audiometric configuration

Much is made of the shape of the audiogram in noise-induced hearing loss, with the suggestion that a notch centred at about 4 kHz with some recovery above this frequency is a prerequisite for the diagnosis. This is not invariably true. First, notched audiograms may occur in the absence of noise, e.g. as a response to ototoxic drug exposure, or sudden hearing loss. Second, the notch of noise-induced hearing loss may range between 3 and 6 kHz and, after a period of time, the high frequency recovery above the notch disappears, leaving a non-descript high frequency loss. The slope may be abrupt, the ski-slope type of loss, with normal hearing to 1000 or 1500 Hz followed by a drop of as much as 30 dB/octave, or it may be shallower. By contrast, the loss may show a gentle slope, a relatively common finding after many years in drop forging or high noise exposure. Thus, audiometric shape is only a guide to diagnosis. With so many different types of noise exposure added to ears of different susceptibilities, this should not be surprising. However, flat audiograms, or those which are upsloping are quite unlikely to be caused by noise.

Exceptions may occur. In the presence of a pure tone, or narrow band noise, without other background sounds, the greatest loss is half an octave above the centre frequency of the noise. This is a rare industrial situation. A major American text (Sataloff and Sataloff, 1993) illustrated such an audiogram with a notch at 1 kHz. The author has seen others. Full sound measurements must be available if such a rare diagnosis is to be sustained. It has already been noted that underwater sound produces a notch based at 1–2 kHz as does high speed motorcycle driving, with and without a helmet.

Guidance as to whether a given audiogram fits the parameters of the claimed sound exposure is given by the International Standard 1999 (ISO, 1990) but this covers only sound levels up to Leq8 100 dB. There are many industries, particularly resource industries such as hard rock mining and heavy equipment operating where this sound level is exceeded, and even if hearing protection has been worn (not common until recently), the daily exposure may be above this level. In these circumstances the evaluation becomes one of exquisite judgement.

Asymmetrical hearing loss

Epidemiologically, normal males have hearing at 4 kHz which is 5 dB worse in the left ear (Pirila, Jounio-Ervasti and Sorri, 1991; Pirila 1991). It is usually stated that in noise-induced permanent threshold shift the audiogram must be symmetrical. This is based on the assumption that the binaural noise exposure is equal. However, unequal hearing thresholds in claimants for noise-induced permanent threshold shift, far from being a curiosity, are fairly common, about 15% in the author's experience (Alberti, Symons and Hyde, 1979). Many are due to other ear disease, middle and inner ear, sometimes to asymmetrical noise exposure and sometimes they are unexplained.

Most sound surveys are static measures of environmental sound levels. They do not indicate the total sound exposure of a worker who may move in and out of the sound. Even less do they indicate the exposure of the ears individually. It is possible to perform dosimetry studies with a microphone at each ear of the worker; remarkable differences may be shown. A recent study by Sinclair (1992), found a 9 dB SPL difference between the sound falling on the right and left ears of a worker using a heavy electric drill, to perforate a concrete wall. Many other similar, but smaller differences were noted in other trades. Chung *et al.* (1983) in a study of shinglers found asymmetrical exposure of each ear. Other causes include rifle and shotgun shooting where the ear nearest the muzzle is most affected, rock drills in mines, various types of mobile metal forming machines, and even such seemingly innocuous devices as older farm tractors and combine harvesters, where one ear is chronically exposed to more sound than the other from the exhaust pipe, and where hearing loss develops at different rates in the two ears. Similar findings have been documented in truck drivers who drive with one window open (Dufresne, Alleyne and Reesal, 1988). Pilots of older twin-engined piston planes often flew with one ear covered by the headset and the other ear uncovered to listen to the motor through an open window, developing a loss in that ear.

If there is a history of acoustic trauma or blast, such as the use of explosives in mining or construction, a tank or tyre exploding, the one ear may be more affected than the other because of the protection afforded by the head shadow, or even if both are equally affected initially, one may recover more fully than the other.

If the audiometric configuration is similar in both ears, although worse in one than the other and the history suggests an asymmetrical exposure, the author tends to attribute the loss to the noise exposure. If not these are diagnosed as hearing loss of unknown cause. Full investigation is warranted whenever it is indicated on clinical grounds. The author's current practice is to screen, using brain stem audiometry, all unequal sensorineural hearing loss in pension assessments and initiate further investigation as required. One vestibular schwannoma has been found for approximately each 700 claims seen (Figure 11.16). Asymmetrical thresholds from noise make up less than 5% of the total.

Concomitant conductive loss

There is considerable controversy as to whether a concomitant conductive hearing loss provides protection from noise injury. Intuitively it is widely accepted that otosclerosis or other long standing middle ear lesions should act like a hearing protector. The present author has undertaken two studies on the interaction between otosclerosis and noise in separate cohorts of compensation claimants for presumed noise damage to the ear. One group had bilateral otosclerosis, unilateral surgery, and continued to work in noise after the operation for lengthy periods; the bone conduction curves of both ears remained similar, suggesting that the otosclerosis did not provide protection in the unoperated ear (Alberti *et al.*, 1980). In the second series noise exposed workers with unilateral unoperated conductive hearing loss presumed to be due to otosclerosis were evalu-

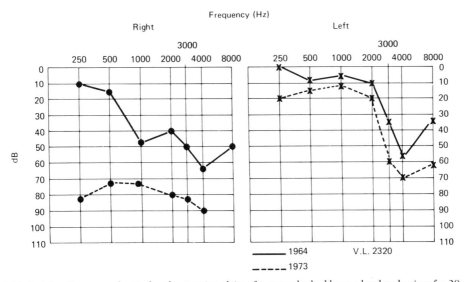

Figure 11.16 Serial audiograms submitted with a pension claim of a man who had been a hard rock miner for 20 years. The asymmetry was investigated, and found to be due to a vestibular schwannoma which was successfully removed

ated. The only protective affect that was observed was about 4 dB at 4 kHz (McShane *et al.*, 1991). Similar results were found in a study of workers with chronic middle ear disease by Simpson and O'Reilly (1991). Only Nilsson and Borg (1983) have found a protective effect. There is no explanation for these findings (Figure 11.17).

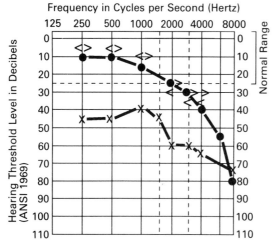

Figure 11.17 Audiogram of a 61-year-old car worker with 34 years of high level occupational noise exposure; 20 years earlier he had a right stapedectomy. Note bone conduction curves are the same in both ears

Audiometry

Authorities vary enormously in the period of time for which a worker must be away from noise (because of temporary threshold shift) in order to quantify hearing for medico-legal purposes. The present author recommends 48 hours minimum for noise exposure and 3 months for a major blasting accident or head injury.

The basis of most compensation assessments for noise-induced permanent threshold shift is the pure tone audiogram, and thus it must be extremely reliable. The degree of accuracy required, if financial compensation is at stake, is much greater than that required for pure diagnostic audiometry. There are many techniques for obtaining a pure tone audiogram which include conventional behaviourial threshold audiometry, automatic recording audiometry of discrete and continuous frequency type (Békésy), various forms of electrical response audiometry (ERA) including slow vertex response (SVR) audiometry and more recently brain stem audiometry (ABR) and electrocochleography (ECoG). Of these, only slow vertex response audiometry is currently in widespread use in threshold determinations in adults. Conventional pure tone audiometry is quite a complicated psychoacoustical

task which, for extreme accuracy, requires skills often beyond the experience of the patient, who may well be ill educated, not fluent in the language of the tester, and tired from travelling for the test. It is hardly surprising that inaccurate results frequently occur. The addition of the frank dissembler to these ranks makes this type of hearing testing a considerable challenge. It is the present author's practice never to rely upon results of one test for pension purposes, and the author only feels happy if the results of several conventional tests match.

If the 500 Hz threshold is 40 dB or worse, it is unlikely to be caused by noise (Klockoff, Drettner and Svedberg, 1974; Alberti, Morgan and Czuba, 1978). Considerable reliance is placed on this finding and a fairly extensive battery of tests including electric response audiometry is routinely undertaken in people whose hearing at 500 Hz is poor. Likewise a discrepancy between the speech reception threshold (SRT) and the pure tone threshold is looked for. The yield of dissemblers and other ear disease is extremely high in these circumstances. If there is a discrepancy between findings, the patient should be carefully reinstructed and re-tested; confrontation should be avoided. The techniques of forensic audiology have been extensively reviewed by Alberti (1981), and of the relative merits of various electric response audiometric tests by Hyde *et al.* (1986).

Therapy for noise-induced hearing loss

In acute acoustic trauma it has been suggested that the use of hyperbaric oxygen (Demaertelaere and Van Opstal, 1981) or carbogen, a 10% carbon dioxide −90% oxygen mixture (Witter *et al.*, 1980), has a vasodilating effect in the cochlea and is of help in preventing noise-induced permanent threshold shift, either if taken before exposure, or if used as first aid for an accidental high noise exposure. The animal evidence is convincing (Dengerink *et al.*, 1984), its application in humans less so.

Rehabilitation

Noise-induced permanent threshold shift can be helped by various rehabilitative manoeuvres. As the early symptoms are largely caused by the loss of ability to inhibit unwanted sound, the remedial efforts are directed towards increasing the signal-to-noise ratio (S/N) of various signals such as a personal television amplifier, a telephone handset amplifier and louder telephone and doorbells. Such devices, known as assistive listening devices, are described further in Chapter 13.

As the loss becomes more severe a hearing aid will be indicated and is frequently fitted with success, in spite of possibly difficult audiometric configurations. Even in those with a 'ski-slope' type of loss, a modern high frequency emphasis aid, with an open or vented ear mould (which further filters out low frequencies) is often of considerable help.

The psychological aspects and impact on family life of noise-induced permanent threshold shift is significant (Hétu, Lalonde and Getty, 1987; Hétu *et al.*, 1988; Hallberg and Barrenås, 1993). Withdrawal from oral interaction and the denial of any problem is common and makes rehabilitation difficult. Family relationships may be disrupted. These psychological aspects have been inadequately studied.

Hearing conservation programmes

The current emphasis on prevention and compensation of noise-induced hearing loss has led to more and more plants and industries establishing hearing conservation programmes. The typical hearing conservation programme is a multidisciplinary project requiring engineering, managerial, audiological, and medical skills. Ideally it has eight phases:

1 Noise hazard identification
2 Engineering controls
3 Personal hearing protection
4 Monitoring audiometry
5 Record keeping
6 Health education
7 Enforcement
8 Programme evaluation.

Good short guides have been produced by Royster and Royster (1990) and by NIOSH (Suter and Franks, 1990).

Sound measurement

It is necessary to know both whether workplace sound levels are potentially hazardous and the workers' sound exposure. The former is undertaken by means of sound surveys, the latter by personal sound dosimetry. Sound surveys should trigger engineering changes, administrative controls and the use of personal protective devices. Sound levels frequently fluctuate through a work cycle so that it is important to sample a total cycle. Noise measurements require skill and special equipment and are outside the scope of this chapter. It is customary after a sound survey is taken to draw a sound contour of the plant and indicate areas where levels are above the local trigger for hearing conservation, usually 85 dB. These vary from jurisdiction to jurisdiction; in some places are 85 dB and in others 90 dB.

Individual exposure is measured by personal noise dosimeters which are quite sophisticated (and expensive) devices worn by the worker during a shift. They store sound levels which, at the end of the period of observation, can be printed out from a master unit, providing records of sound levels sampled every minute or so throughout the work shift. They can also integrate the information to provide a direct reading of Leq8 or L$_{OSHA8}$.

Sound control

If it is established that sound levels are hazardous, then steps are taken to control the amount of sound to which workers are exposed, both by engineering and by personal protection. The engineering controls range from quite simple modifications to redesigning machinery or encasing it. It is usually impractical to make major modifications to an existing machine, although noise specifications should be written with new or replacement orders. Operators may be separated from the machines by placing controls in an observation booth similar to an audiometric sound-proof booth; this has been used in many industries. Noisy machinery should be isolated: too often a workman is harmed by vicarious noise from a neighbouring machine. For further details a noise control manual should be consulted.

Hétu (1992) has emphasized the importance of the acoustic environment in the workplace which he described as potentially hostile. 'Safe' sound levels from a hearing standpoint may still be high enough to interfere with communication, and inhibit sound localization, a critical issue in identifying the source of warning signals, which by themselves may be confusing because a work site may contain many.

Hearing screening

Industrial hearing testing involves screening and identification audiometry – it is not diagnostic. Testers, frequently industrial nurses whose hearing testing training consists of a 3- or 4-day course, usually have limited skills. The function of the hearing test is:

1 To identify those with a hearing loss
2 To identify those whose hearing alters
3 To determine whether the hearing conservation programme is effective.

New employees should be screened and those with a hearing loss identified, referred for accurate quantification of the loss and diagnosis of its cause. This will limit an employer's liability only to further hearing loss, excluding pre-existing problems. There is controversy about annual hearing tests. Arguments range from an extreme that annual screening interferes with the freedom of the individual to a belief that it should be mandatory. More critical issues surround the validity of annual testing. What constitutes a significant threshold shift (STS)? How can this be distinguished from the test/retest error of audiometry?

(see Draft American National Standard 5.12.13 – 1991; Hétu, Quoz and Duguay, 1990). In spite of these doubts, the present author believes that annual audiometry is a valid tool; it demonstrates management interest; it provides an opportunity to discuss problems related to hearing protective devices; it may identify other ear disease and it may identify areas of a plant where the programme is ineffective because a cohort of workers shows change. Who has access to the results should be negotiated before the programme starts.

Timing of tests is not critical. In the presence of an adequate hearing conservation programme, using hearing protective devices if noise levels are high, there should be no threshold shift in the workplace, and therefore testing can be done at anytime of the day. If workers' hearing has changed significantly then they should be retested with rested ears.

The question of record storage, particularly in middle-sized plants, has bedevilled hearing conservation programmes. In small plants manual record keeping is adequate so long as the serial audiograms are stored in digital form, preferably on one piece of paper, so that changes can be readily appreciated. There are now several relatively cheap industrial computerized audiometry programmes available which automatically store the record, compare it with previous tests, flag changes, and produce batch data for a total plant or an individual section. They are so cost effective that they should be the norm.

Do hearing conservation programmes work? The few reports that exist show that hearing loss can be prevented (Pell, 1973; Nilsson and Lindgren, 1980; Royster, Royster and Cecich, 1984; Savell and Tootham, 1987; Franks, Davis and Kreig, 1989; Bertrand and Zeidan, 1993). Full details of an industrial hearing conservation programme are outside the scope of this chapter. The reader should consult appropriate industrial hygiene manuals such as Gasaway (1985) and Royster and Royster (1990).

Personal hearing protection

Where noise levels remain hazardous and the worker cannot be isolated, a programme of personal hearing protection should be initiated. To be accepted these require considerable education, although where both labour and management give their full backing, it is surprising how well they are received.

The basic hearing protective device prevents sound from reaching the ear either by blocking the ear canal (ear plugs), or by putting a sound barrier around the ear (ear muff). These devices are usually passive protectors, which attenuate sound more in the high than the low frequencies. There have been several recent advances in the practical design and application of hearing protective devices. Passive protectors have been modified by the addition of acoustic filters

to be level dependent or to produce a flat response. The former attenuates more in extremely high levels of sound, the latter attenuates equally across frequencies. Active protectors are widely marketed which incorporate electronic circuitry akin to a hearing aid with a good automatic gain control; they are fitted to a muff, which has a microphone and amplifier which allow low intensity sound to pass, but which cut out at a predetermined intensity, usually about 85 dB, to act as a passive muff. Speech and environmental sounds can be heard – indeed are slightly amplified – until the external sound level is high, then the device acts as a good muff. They are particularly useful in the military and wherever there is intermittent high level sound. Finally active noise reduction headsets combine a good headset for high frequency attenuation with a noise cancelling circuit which minimizes low frequency sound, producing virtually flat attenuation. These are now much used in small aircraft and military jets (Alberti, 1990; Nixon, McKinley and Steuver, 1992). Many factors enter into the choice of the appropriate type of protector including individual preference, the need to wear other protective devices, durability, hygiene, price etc.

The cheapest and most commonly used type of protector is a prefabricated earplug. These are usually made of soft plastic. The so-called 'fircone' or 'Comfit' which, in its various forms, has two or three soft flanges which effectively seal the ear canal. The disposable foam polyurethane plug is in common use. These cylindrical plugs can be compressed so that they fit easily into the ear canal and, over a period 2 minutes, expand to fit the shape of the canal, sealing it comfortably but tightly. Care must be taken that they are inserted far enough so that jaw movements do not work them out, and that they are held in place while expansion occurs. Although effective, they may be difficult to remove.

Many workers find earplugs uncomfortable, at least initially, and care must be taken to ensure that they use plugs of adequate size, which may be relatively uncomfortable at first fitting; fortunately users quickly adapt to them.

Semi-insert hearing protectors which consist of earplugs on a spring, are used where muffs or plugs are unacceptable. They are used in the food handling industry where a muff would be inappropriate because of the need to wear a net over the hair, but where the fear of dropping plugs into food is real.

Theoretically the most effective type of hearing protector is the ear muff. This consists of a cup filled with a sound absorbing material worn around the ear, sealed to the side of the head by a malleable gasket which accommodates the uneven shape of the head. The muffs must be pressed to the side of the head, and are therefore worn with spring bands. There are many types of muffs available including ones that fit under hard hats, either by having a separate spring band behind the neck or by being fixed directly to the hard hat. Anything that breaks the seal between an earmuff and side of the head such as long hair, or thick plastic temple bars of safety glasses, reduces the attenuation provided. The most sophisticated, effective, and expensive muffs are those built directly into the flying helmets of modern jet fighter pilots.

The theoretical limitations of personal hearing protection is the level at which bone conduction becomes the dominant factor. In sufficiently high sound levels both the ear plug and ear muff vibrate and conduct sound to the ear both by bone and air. In theory no more than 25 dB in the lower frequencies and 40 dB in the higher frequencies is possible with a plug, or 30 dB in the lower frequencies and 50 dB in the higher frequencies with a muff. In practice these levels are virtually never attained.

The attenuation results published with the devices, expressed in the USA and other parts of the world as a noise reduction rating (NRR) and given in dB, are the best that can be obtained under controlled laboratory conditions. It is accepted practice to halve the figure to arrive at the protection available within the workplace. Thus a protector with an noise reduction rating of 30, can be assumed to provide on average, 15 dB of effective protection. Even this figure may be optimistic because there is considerable variation in the amount of protection provided among individuals. Thus the lowest quartile of the workforce may have protection of only 7 or 8 dB even though using protectors with an noise reduction rating of 30! If plugs and muffs are worn together, as is the practice in some very heavy industry, the additional protection provided is between 5 and 7 dB. Thus in practical terms using one protector it is possible to provide 10–15 dB of attenuation, using two, 15–20 dB (Figure 11.18).

The reasons for this are manifold. Plugs may be of the wrong size, or more commonly are incorrectly inserted. The custom-moulded plugs shrink with age,

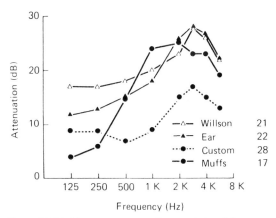

Figure 11.18 Mean attenuation characteristics of three types of ear plugs and a group of ear muffs, as issued to industrial workers and fitted by them. (From Riko, K., Abel, S. M. and Alberti, P. W., 1978, *Journal of Otolaryngology*, with permission)

foam rubber plugs are not inserted far enough or come out with jaw movement. Muffs may have broken seals or large dents where safety glasses had been applied or springs bent back to relieve pressure on the head (Riko and Alberti, 1981).

Any programme of hearing conservation requires constant maintenance and monitoring of the use of the protective devices. The plant nurse must be skilled in fitting, training, and encouraging workers to use the devices appropriately. Muffs require change of seal and liner, plugs require cleaning.

Education is essential in hearing conservation as in all other health and safety practices. A work force that appreciates the need for these measures and understands how they are applied will show much greater compliance with a hearing conservation programme.

The question of communication in noise is frequently raised. There are two issues: workers fear that they will be unable to hear warning signals and believe they cannot hear conversation, or machinery when wearing protective devices. As Laroche *et al.* (1991) stated, 'Every year fatal injuries occur in noisy workplace because a warning signal is not heard'. This results from the interaction of warning signal design and the worker hearing. Wilkins and Martin (1987) concluded that the effectiveness of some warning signals is reduced for hearing impaired listeners using hearing protectors. They summarized their findings:

1 Hearing protectors do not remove all sound, they may be likened to sunglasses which remove some of the brightness from vision
2 If a signal is loud enough to be heard above background noise, then it will be heard by those wearing hearing protectors
3 A signal of sound spectrum totally different from the background noise may be discernible to the unprotected ear at a low intensity and be masked by hearing protectors
4 Workers with a hearing loss may be at a considerable disadvantage.

In those with a pre-existing high frequency hearing loss, who use a hearing protective device, the additional predominantly high frequency attenuation of the protector, produces a precipitous high frequency drop. Abel *et al.* (1982) showed that speech discrimination in a background of noise by the hearing impaired is markedly worse when compared with normally hearing subjects both with and without hearing protection, but is probably worsened by the hearing protector. Thus the person with a pre-existing hearing loss introduced into a hearing protection programme may suffer real deterioration in communication. Flat response devices, in which the attenuation is the same across the frequencies are better because they eliminate the high frequency distortion introduced by the protectors.

Medicolegal and social implications

Here there are many complicated and interrelated questions. What is a safe level of noise at which no hearing loss occurs? What is the probability for any given noise that any particular amount of hearing loss occurs? How should one define social handicap in terms of hearing loss? If compensation laws are introduced, what should be compensated? Hearing loss? Disability? Social handicap? Loss of earning power? Von Gierke and Johnson (1976) summarized many of these points and Noble (1978) made a strong argument for using handicap/disability scales for assessment.

It should be remembered that the pure tone audiogram is only a surrogate measure of disability and a quite inadequate surrogate for handicap. It is used because it is easy to apply, not because it is an accurate measure of human function. The reader will recognize that people with identical audiometric configurations may cope very differently with auditory tasks (disability), and in every day life (handicap).

Unfortunately even the terms impairment, disability and handicap are used differently in various parts of the world. A trenchant plea for the adoption of the WHO definitions (Table 11.1) was made by Stephens and Hétu (1991). (The USA currently uses different definitions.) With its use it is easier to understand the real life difficulty of the hearing impaired and the effect on their families (Hétu, Lalonde, and Getty, 1987; Hétu *et al.*, 1988).

Table 11.1 Definitions of impairment, disability and handicap (WHO, 1980)

Impairment is: 'any loss or abnormality of psychological, physiological, or anatomical structure or function', i.e. which is measured by audiometry.
Disability is: 'any restriction or lack of ability to perform an activity in the manner or within the range considered normal for a human being', i.e. a description of everyday sounds that cannot be heard.
Handicap is: 'the disadvantage for a given individual, resulting from impairment or disability that limits or prevents the fulfilment of a role that is normal for that individual', i.e. the impact of the disability on everyday function.

Compensation

Traumatic hearing loss – that caused by head injury or a single traumatic episode – has been pensionable in many parts of the world since the early parts of the twentieth century. Hearing loss from prolonged noise exposure became pensionable in many developed countries in the last two decades. Legislators have faced several problems. How should hearing loss be measured for compensation purposes? How was handicap to be defined, and was hearing loss or handicap to be compensated? Most jurisdictions have opted to compensate hearing disability (handicap in US terminology), so the concept of a low fence was introduced, a level of hearing beneath which no 'disability' existed, even though the hearing level itself was not normal.

Over the years many schemes for measuring percentage hearing loss and percentage disability for compensation purposes have been applied (see Noble, 1978). Currently, in the USA, the American Medical Association and the American Academy of Otolaryngology – Head and Neck Surgery recommend beginning hearing handicap at 25 dB average at 500, 1000, 2000 and 3000 Hz, although certain states and certain federal agencies use hearing loss averages at 1, 2 and 3 kHz as does the UK. Whether and where a low fence for compensation is placed is a matter of philosophy and economics which appears to bear little relationship to the science of hearing disability/handicap measurement. The recent British study (King *et al.*, 1992) addressed these issues head on. It rejected a low fence, used a sigmoid function for increasing disability related to worsening hearing and addressed binaural hearing loss in a less simplistic way than many schemes. This is an important document, both because of its philosophy and its practical application.

The effect of ageing is well discussed and modelled by Robinson (1991a, b). This remains a contentious issue, but agreement seems gradually to be emerging that the effects of noise and age should be pro rated in compensation schemes, rather than subtracted (see also Dobie, 1992).

The whole issue of how to compensate, for what, and for how long is such an individual issue, varying between and within countries, that no attempt will be made to review it.

Conclusions

Excessive noise is obnoxious: it destroys hearing and interferes with normal human intercourse. It must not be concluded, however, that all sound is bad – indeed the aim of the otologist working with excessive noise is to preserve hearing so that wanted sounds can be heard.

References

ABEL, S. M. and HAYTHORNTHWAITE, C. A. (1984) The progression of noise induced hearing loss – survey of workers in selected Canadian industries. *Journal of Otolaryngology*, **13**, (suppl. 13), 1–36

ABEL, S. M., ALBERTI, P. W., HAYTHORNTHWAITE, C. and RIKO, K. (1982) Speech intelligibility in noise: effects of fluency and hearing protector type. *Journal of the Acoustical Society of America*, **71**, 708–715

ABEY-WICKRAM, I., A'BROOK, M. F., GATTONI, F. E. G. and HERRIDGE, C. F. (1969) Mental hospital admissions and aircraft noise. *Lancet*, ii, 1275–1277

ALBERTI, P. W. (1981) Non organic hearing loss in adults. In: *Audiology and Audiological Medicine*, edited by H. Beagley. London: Oxford University Press. pp. 910–930

ALBERTI, P. W. (1987) Tinnitus in occupational hearing loss: nosological aspects. *Journal of Otolaryngology*, **16**, 34–35

ALBERTI, P. W. (1990) Active hearing protectors. In: *Noise as a Public Health Problem*, part I, edited by V. Berglund, J. Karlsson and T. Lindvall. Stockholm: Swedish Council for Building Research. pp. 79–87

ALBERTI, P. W. and BLAIR, R. L. (1982) Occupational hearing loss: an Ontario perspective. *Laryngoscope*, **92**, 535–539

ALBERTI, P. W., MORGAN, P. P. and CZUBA, I. (1978) Speech and pure tone audiometry as a screen for exaggerated hearing loss. *Acta Otolaryngologica*, **88**, 328–321

ALBERTI, P. W., MORGAN, P. P. and LEBLANC, J. C. (1974) Occupational hearing loss – an otologist's view of a long term study. *Laryngoscope*, **84**, 1822–1834

ALBERTI. P. W., SYMONS, F. and HYDE, M. L. (1979) The significances of asymmetrical hearing thresholds. *Archives of Otolaryngology*, **87**, 255–263

ALBERTI, P. W., HYDE, M. L., SYMONS, F. M. and MILLER, R. B. (1980) The effect of prolonged exposure to industrial noise on otosclerosis. *Laryngoscope*, **90**, 407–413

AL-MASRI, M., MARTIN, A. and NEDWELL, J. (1993) Underwater hearing and occupational noise exposure limits. In: *Noise as a Public Health Problem*, vol. 2, edited by M. Vallet. Bron: INRETS pp. 5–8

ALPER, J. (1991) Antinoise creates the sounds of silence. *Science*, **252**, 508–509

ARAN, J. M., HIEL, H., HAYASHIDA, T., ERIE, P., AUROUSSEAN, C., GUILHAUME, A. *et al.* (1992) Noise, aminoglycosides and diuretics. In: *Noise Induced Hearing Loss*, edited by A. L. Dancer, D. Henderson, R. J. Salvi and R. P. Hamernick. St Louis: Mosby Year Book. pp. 188–195

AVAN, P., LOTH, D., BONFILS, P., MENGUY, C. and TEYSSON, M. (1993) Otoacoustic emissions, physiopathology and early diagnosis of noise induced hearing loss. *Proceedings of the 6th International Congress of Noise as a Public Health Problem*, edited by M. Vallet. Bron: INRETS. pp. 13–16

AXELSSON, A. and BARRENÄS, M. L. (1992) Tinnitus in noise induced hearing loss. In: *Noise Induced Hearing Loss*, edited by A. L. Dancer, D. Henderson, R. J. Salvi and R. P. Hamernick. St Louis: Mosby Year Book. pp. 269–276

AXELSSON, A., HELLSTROM, P. A., ALTSCHULLER, R. and MILLER, J. M. (1991) Inner ear damage from toy cap pistols and firecrackers. *International Journal of Paediatric Otolaryngology*, **21**, 143–148

BABISCH, W., ELWOOD, P. C. and ISING, H. (1994) Road traffic noise and heart disease risk: results of the epidemiological studies in Caerphilly, Speedwell and Berlin. In: *Noise as a Public Health Hazard*, vol. 3 edited by M. Vallet. Bron: INRETS. pp. 260–267

BARR, T. (1886) Enquiry into the effects of loud sound upon the hearing of boiler makers and others who work amid noisy surroundings. *Transactions of the Philosophical Society of Glasgow*, **17**, 223–239

BARREGÅRD, L. and AXELSSON, A. (1984) Is there an ototraumatic interaction between noise and solvents? *Scandinavian Audiology*, **13**, 151–155

BARRENÅS, M. L. and LINDGREN, F. (1991) The influence of eye colour on susceptibility to TTS in humans. *British Journal of Audiology*, **25**, 303–307

BAUER, P., KORPERT, K., NEUBERGER, M., RABER, A. and SCHWETZ, F. (1991) Risk factors for hearing loss at different frequencies in a population of 47 388 noise exposed workers. *Journal of the Acoustical Society of America*, **90**, 3086–3098

BAUGHN, W. L. (1966) Noise control. Percent of population protected. *International Audiology*, **5**, 331–338

BAUGHN, W. L. (1973) Relation between daily noise exposure and hearing loss based on the evaluation of 6835 industrial noise exposure cases. *AMRL-TR-73-53*. Wright-Patterson Air Force Base, Aerospace Medical Research Laboratory. Cited by Robinson, D. W. (1987)

BAXTER, J. D. and LING, D. (1974) Ear disease and hearing loss among the Eskimo population of the Baffin zone. *Canadian Journal of Otolaryngology*, **3**, 110–122

BEAGLEY, H. A. (1965) Acoustic trauma in the guinea pig. II Electron microscopy including the morphology of cell functions in the organ of Corti. *Acta Otolaryngologica*, **60**, 479–495

BENTLEY, S., MURPHY, F. and DUDLEY, H. (1977) Perceived noise in surgical wards and an intensive care area: an objective analysis. *British Medical Journal*, **2**, 1503–1506

BERGLUND, B., BERGLUND, V., KARLSSON, J. and LINDVALL. T. (1988) *Noise as a Public Health Problem*. 5 volumes. Stockholm: Swedish Council for Building Research

BERTRAND, R. A. and ZEIDAN, J. (1993) Retrospective field evaluation of HPD based on evaluation of hearing. In: *Noise as a Public Health Hazard*, vol 2, edited by M. Vallet. Bron: INRETS. pp. 21–24

BESS, F. H. and POWELL, R. L. (1972) Hearing hazard from model airplanes. *Clinical Paediatrics*, **11**, 61–64

BOETTCHER, F. A. (1993) Auditory brainstem response correlates of resistance to noise induced hearing loss in Mongolian gerbils. *Journal of the Acoustical Society of America*, **94**, 3207–3214

BOETTCHER, F. A., HENDERSON, D., GRATTON, M. A., BYRNE, C. and BANCROFT, B. (1989) Recent understandings of noise interactions. *ACES*, **1**, 15–21

BOETTCHER, F. A., GRATTON, M. A., BANCROFT, B. R. and SPONGR, V. (1992) Interaction of noise and other agents: recent advances. In: *Noise Induced Hearing Loss*, edited by A. L. Dancer, D. Henderson, R. J. Salvi and R. P. Hamernick. St Louis: Mosby Year Book. pp. 175–187

BOHNE, D. A. and CLARK, W. W. (1982) Growth of hearing loss and cochlear lesion increases of noise exposure. In: *New Perspectives on Noise Induced Hearing Loss*, edited by R. P. Hamernik, D. Henderson and R. Salvi. New York: Raven Press. pp. 283–302

BORENZI, M. and COLLARETA, J. (1984) Noise levels in a hospital. *Industrial Health*, **22**, 75–82

BORG, E. (1976) Dynamic characteristics of the intra-aural muscle reflex. In: *Acoustic Impedance and Admittance*, edited by A. S. Feldman and L. A. Wilber. Baltimore: Williams and Wilkins. pp. 236–299

BOTSFORD, J. H. (1967) A simple method for identifying acceptable noise exposures. *Journal of the Acoustical Society of America*, **42**, 810–819

BOTTE, M. C. and MONIKHEIM, S. (1992) Psychoacoustic characterization of two types of auditory fatigue. In: *Noise Induced Hearing Loss*, edited by A. L. Dancer, D. Henderson, R. J. Salvi and R. P. Hamerick. St Louis: Mosby Year Book. pp. 259–268

BRADLEY, R., FORTNUM, H. and COLES, R. (1987) Research

note: patterns exposure of schoolchildren to amplified music. *British Journal of Audiology*, 21, 119–125

BREDBERG, G. and HUNTER-DUVAR, I. M. (1975) Behaviourial tests of inner ear damage. In: *Handbook of Sensory Physiology*, vol. 5, part II edited by W. D. Keidl and W. D. Neff. New York: Springer-Verlag. pp. 261–306

BRONZAFT, A. L. (1991) The effects of noise on learning, cognitive development and social behaviour. In: *Noise and Health*, edited by T. H. Fay. New York: New York Academy of Medicine. pp. 87–92

BRUMMETT, R. E., TALBOT, J. M. and CHARUHAS, P. (1988) Potential hearing loss resulting from MR imaging. *Radiology*, 169, 539–540

BUNCH, C. C. (1929) Age variations in auditory acuity. *Archives of Otolaryngology*, 9, 625–636

BUNCH, C. C. (1939) Traumatic deafness. In: *Nelson Loose Leaf Medicine of the Ear*, edited by E. P. Fowler Jr. New York: Thos. Nelson. pp. 349–367

BURNS, W. (1973) *Noise and Man*, 2nd edn. London: John Murray

BURNS, W. and ROBINSON, D. W. (1970) *Hearing and Noise in Industry*. London: HMSO

BURNS, W., ROBINSON, D. W., SHIPTON, M. S. and SINCLAIR, A. (1979) Hearing hazards from occupational noise: observations on a population from heavy industry. *Acoustic Report AC 18*, National Physics Laboratory

CARTER, N. L., WAUGH, R. L., KEEN, K., MURRAY, N. and BULTEAU, V. G. (1982) Amplified music and young people's hearing: review and report of Australian findings. *Medical Journal of Australia*, 2, 125–128

CHABA (1966) Hazardous exposure to intermittent and steady state noise. *Report of Working Group 46*. Washington, DC

CHADWICK, D. L. (1971) Noise and the ear. In: *Scott-Brown's Diseases of the Ear, Nose and Throat*, 3rd edn, vol. 2, edited by J. Groves and J. Ballantyne. London: Butterworths. pp. 475–539

CHUNG, D. Y., MASON, K., WILLSON, G. N. and GANNON, R. P. (1983) Asymmetrical noise exposure and hearing loss among shingle sawyers. *Journal of Occupational Medicine*, 25, 541–543

CLARK, W. W. (1991a) Recent studies of temporary threshold shift (TTS) and permanent threshold shift (PTS) in animals. *Journal of the Acoustical Society of America*, 90, 155–163

CLARK, W. W. (1991b) Noise exposure from leisure activities: A review. *Journal of the Acoustical Society of America*, 91, 175–181

CODY, A. R. and JOHNSTONE, B. M. (1980) Single auditory neuron response during acute acoustic trauma. *Hearing Research*, 3, 3–16

CODY, A. R. and RUSSELL, I. J. (1988) Acoustically induced hearing loss: intracellular studies in the guinea pig cochlea. *Hearing Research*, 35, 59–70

COHEN, A. (1973) Industrial noise and medical accident record data on exposed workers. *Proceedings of the International Congress on Noise as a Public Health Problem*. Washington, DC: US Environmental Protection Agency. pp. 441–453

COLES, R. R. A. (1963) *Journal of the Royal Navy Medical Service*, 49, 1; cited by Chadwick (1971)

COLES, R. R. and HOARE, N. W. (1985) Noise induced hearing loss and the dentist. *British Dental Journal*, 159, 209–218

COLLETTI, V., FIORINO, F. G., VERLATO, G. and MONTRESOR, G. Z. (1992) Physical exercise and active protection from temporary threshold shift. In: *Noise Induced Hearing Loss*, edited

by A. L. Dancer, D. Henderson, R. J. Salvi and R. P. Hamerick. St Louis: Mosby Year Book. pp. 500–510

CORSO, J. F. (1980) Age correction factor in noise induced hearing loss: a quantitative model. *Audiology*, 19, 221–232

DALLOS, P. (1992) Neurobiology of cochlear hair cells. In: *Auditory Physiology and Perception*, edited by by Y. Cazals, K. Horner and L. Demany. Oxford: Pergamon Press. pp. 3–17

DANCER, A. L., HENDERSON, D., SALVI, R. J. and HAMERNIK, R. P. (eds) (1992) *Noise Induced Hearing Loss*. St Louis: Mosby Year Book

DAVIS, A. C. (1983) Effects of noise and socioeconomic factors of hearing impairment. *Proceedings of the Fourth International Congress on Noise as a Public Health Hazard*, edited by G. Rossi. Milan: Centro Richerche e Studi Amplifon. pp. 201–211

DAVIS, A. C., FORTNUM, H. M., COLES, R. R. A., HAGGARD, M. P. and LITMAN, M. E. (1985) *Damaged Hearing from Leisure Noise: a Review of the Literature*. University of Nottingham, Nottingham: MRC Institute of Hearing Research

DEMAERTELAERE, L. and VAN OPSTAL, M. (1981) Treatment of acoustic trauma with hyperbaric oxygen. *Acta Oto-Rhinologica Belgica*, 35, 303–314

DENGERINK, H. A., AXELSSON, A., MILLER, J. M. and WRIGHT, J. W. (1984) The effect of noise and carbogen on cochlear vasculature. *Acta Otolaryngologica*, 98, 81–88

DOBIE, R. A. (1990) A method for allocation of hearing handicap. *Otolaryngology – Head and Neck Surgery*, 103, 733–739

DOBIE, R. A. (1992) The relative contributions of occupational noise and aging in individual loss of hearing loss. *Ear and Hearing*, 13, 19–27

DOBIE, R. A. (1993) Noise induced hearing loss. In: *Head and Neck Surgery – Otolaryngology*, edited by B. J. Bailey. Philadelphia: J. B. Lippincott. pp. 1782–1792

DRAFT AMERICAN NATIONAL STANDARD – Evaluating the effectiveness of hearing conservation programmes 1991. *ANSI*, 512. 13–1991

DUCEL, G., SUTER, T. and DUPONT, B. (1976) The noise in an intensive care unit. *Sozial Praventiv Medizin*, 21, 135

DUFRESNE, R. M., ALLEYNE, B. C. and REESAL, M. R. (1988) Asymmetric hearing loss in truck drivers. *Ear and Hearing*, 9, 41–42

ERLANDSSON, B., HAKANSON, H., IVANSSON, A., NILSSON, I. and WERSALL, J. (1987) Hair cell damage in the inner ear of the guinea pig due to noise in a workshop. *Acta Otolaryngologica*, 103, 204–211

EVANS, G. W. (1990) The non auditory effects of noise on child development. In: *Noise as a Public Health Problem*, 4, edited by B. Berglund, V. Berglund, J. Karlsson, and T. Lindvall. Stockholm: Swedish Council for Building Research. pp. 425–453

FEARN, R. W and HANSON, D. R. (1989) Hearing level of young subjects exposed to gunfire noise. *Journal of Sound and Vibration*, 131, 157–159

FLETCHER, J. L. and GROSS, C. W. (1977) Effects on hearing in sports related noise or trauma. *Sound and Vibration*, 11, 26–27

FOSBROKE, J. (1831) Practical observations on the pathology and treatment of deafness II. *Lancet*, 654–648

FOWLER, E. P. (1929) Limited lesions of basilar membrane. *Transactions of the American Otolaryngological Society*, 19, 182

FOWLER, E. P. (1939) (ed.) Diseases of the neural mechanism of hearing: cochlea, auditory nerve, and its center in the medulla and cortex. In: *Nelson's Loose Leaf Medicine of the Ear*. Nelson, New York

FRANKS, J. R., DAVIS, R. R. and KREIG, E. R. (1989) Analysis of a hearing conservation programme data base. Factors other than workplace noise. *Ear and Hearing*, **10**, 273–280

GAO, W-Y., DING, D-L., ZHENG, X-Y., RUAN, F-M. and LIU, Y-J. (1992) A comparison of changes in the streocilia between temporary and permanent hearing losses in acoustic trauma. *Hearing Research*, **62**, 27–41

GASAWAY, D. C. (1985) *Hearing Conservation – A Practical Manual and Guide*. Englewood Cliffs: Prentice Hall

GERLING, I. J. and JERGER, A. F. (1985) Cordless telephones and acoustic trauma: case study. *The Ear*, **6**, 203–205

GJAEVENES, K., MOSENG, J. and NORDAHL, T. (1974) Hearing loss in children caused by the impulse noise of Chinese crackers. *Scandinavian Audiology*, **3**, 153–156

GLORIG, A. (1958) *Noise and Your Ear*. New York: Grune and Stratton

GLORIG, A. and WHEELER, E. (1955) An introduction to the industrial noise problem. *Illinois Medical Journal*, **107**, 10–16

GUPTA, D. and VISHWARAMA, S. K. (1989) Toy weapons and firecrackers: A source of hearing loss. *Laryngoscope*, **99**, 330–334

GUYOT, J. P. (1988) Acoustic trauma caused by the telephone: a report of two cases. *Otorhinolaryngology*, **50**, 313–318

HABERMAN, J. (1890) Uber die Schwerhorigkeit des kesselschmiede. *Archiv für Ohrenheilkunde*, **30**, 1–25

HALLBERG, L. R-M. and BARRENÅS, M. L. (1993), Living with a male with noise induced hearing loss: experiences from the perspective of spouses. *British Journal of Audiology*, **27**, 255–261

HAMERNIK, R. P. and HENDERSON, D. (1976) The potentiation of noise by other ototraumatic agents. In: *Effects of Noise on Hearing*, edited by D. Henderson, R. P. Hamernik, D. S. Dosanj and J. H. Mills. New York: Raven Press. pp. 291–307

HAMERNICK, R. P. and HSUEH, K. D. (1991) Impulse noise: some definitions, physical acoustics and other considerations. *Journal of the Acoustical Society of America*, **90**, 189–196

HAMERNICK, R. P., AHROON W. A. and DAVIS, R. I. (1989) Noise and vibration interactions: effects on hearing. *Journal of the Acoustical Society of America*, **86**, 2129–2137

HAWKINS, J. E. JR (1976) Experimental noise deafness: recollections and ruminations. In: *Hearing and Davis*, edited by S. K. Hirsch, D. H. Eldridge, J. J. Hirsch and S. R. Silverman. Washington DC: Washington University Press. pp. 73–84

HENDERSON, D., SUBRAMANIAM, M. and BOETTCHER, F. A. (1993) Individual susceptibility to noise induced hearing loss: an old topic revisited. *Ear and Hearing*, **14**, 153–168

HENDERSON, D., CAMPO, P., SUBRAMANIAM, M. and FIORINO, F. (1992) Development of resistance to noise. In: *Noise Induced Hearing Loss*, edited by A. L. Dancer, D. Henderson, R. J. Salvi and R. P. Hamernick. St Louis: Mosby Year Book. pp. 476–488

HÉTU, R. (1992) Hearing in the industrial work environment. *21st International Congress on Audiology*

HÉTU, R. and LAZURE, R. (1982) La dosimetrie et bruits: effet de l'interaction dose d'impacts dose de bruit continu. *Doc IRSST N/D–25–80–25*

HÉTU, R., LALONDE, M. and GETTY, L. (1987) Psychosocial disadvantages associated with occupational hearing loss as experienced in the family. *Audiology*, **26**, 141–152

HÉTU, R., QUOZ, H. T. and DUGUAY, P. (1990) The likelihood of detecting significant hearing threshold shift amongst noise exposed workers subject to annual audiometric testing. *Annals of Occupational Hygiene*, **34**, 361–370

HÉTU, R., TRUCHON-GAGNON, C. and BILODAU, S. A. (1990) Problems of noise in school settings. *Journal of Speech, Language Pathology and Audiology*, **14**, 31–39

HÉTU, R., RIVERIN, L., LALONDE, N., GETTY, L. and ST CYR, C. (1988) Qualitative analysis of the handicap associated with occupational hearing loss. *British Journal of Audiology*, **22**, 251–264

HINCHLIFFE, R. and KING, P. F. (1992) Medicolegal aspects of tinnitus. I, II, III. *Journal of Audiological Medicine*, **1**, 38–58, 59–79, 127–147

HOLT, E. E. (1882) Boilermaker's deafness and hearing in noise. *Transactions of the American Otological Society*, **3**, 34–44

HUGHES, K. B. (1976) Sensorineural deafness due to compression chamber noise. *Journal Laryngology and Otology*, **90**, 803–807

HYDE, M. L., ALBERTI, P. W., MATSUMOTO, N. and LI, Y. (1986) Auditory evoked potentials in audiometric assessment of compensation and medical-legal patients. *Annals of Otology, Rhinology and Laryngology*, **95**, 514–519

HYGGE, S. (1993) Classroom experiments on the effects of aircraft, traffic, train and verbal noise on long term recall and recognition in children aged twelve to fourteen years. In: *Noise as a Public Health Problem, Proceedings of the 6th International Congress*, edited by M. Vallet, vol. 2. Bron: INRETS. pp. 531–534

IKI, M., KURUMATAMI, N., HIRATA, K., MORIYAMA, T., ITOH, J. and ARAI, T. (1986). An association between vibration induced white finger and hearing loss in forestry workers. *Scandinavia Journal of Work and Environmental Health*, **12**, 365–370

ISO 1999 (1990) International Organisation for Standardisation. *Acoustic determination of occupational noise exposure and estimation of noise-induced hearing loss*. Geneva, ISO

JHA, S. K. and CATHERINES, J. J. (1978a) Interior noise studies for general aviation types of aircraft. Part 1: Field studies. *Journal of Sound and Vibration*, **58**, 375–390

JHA, S. K. and CATHERINES, J. J. (1978b) Interior noise studies for general aviation type of aircraft. Part 2: Laboratory studies. *Journal of Sound and Vibration*, **58**, 391–406

JOHNSON, A. C. and CANLON, B. (1994) Toluene exposure affects the functional activity of the outer hair cells. *Hearing Research*, **72**, 189–196

KARJA, J. (1968) Perstimulatory suprathreshold adaptation for pure tones. I Basic studies on normal hearing persons. *Acta Oto-Laryngologica*, (Suppl. 241), 1–68

KERR, A. G. and BYRNE, J. E. T. (1975) Concussive effects of bomb blast on the ear. *Journal of Laryngology and Otology*, **89**, 131–143

KIANG, N. Y. S., LIBERMAN, M. C., SEWELL, W. F. and GUINAN, J. J. (1986) Single unit clues to cochlear mechanisms. *Hearing Research*, **22**, 171–182

KILLION, M. C., DEVILBISS, E. and STEWART, J. (1988) An ear plug with a 15 dB attenuation. *Hearing Journal*, **41**, 14–17

KIM, D. O., LEONARD, G., SMURZYNSKI, J. and JUNG, M. D. (1992) Otoacoustic emissions and noise induced hearing loss: human studies. In: *Noise Induced Hearing Loss*, edited by A. L. Dancer, D. Henderson, R. J. Salvi and R. P. Hamernick. St Louis: Mosby Year Book. pp. 98–105

KING, P. F., COLES, R. R. A., LUTMAN, M. E. and ROBINSON, D. W. (1992) *Assessment of Hearing Disability*. London: Whurr Publishers

KLOCKHOFF, I., DRETTNER, B. and SVEDBERG, A. (1974) Computerized classification of the results of screening audiometry in groups of persons exposed to noise. *Audiology*, **13**, 323–334

KRAMER, M. B. and WOOD, D. (1982). Noise induced hearing loss in rural school children. *Scandinavian Audiology*, **11**, 279–280

KRYTER, K. D. (1985) *The Effects of Noise on Man*, 2nd edn. New York: Academic Press

KYLEN, P. and ARLINGER, S. (1976). Drill generated noise levels in ear surgery. *Acta Otolaryngologica*, **82**, 252–259

KYLEN, P., STERNVALL, J. E. and ARLINGER, S. (1977) Variables affecting the drill generated noise in ear surgery. *Acta Otolaryngologica*, **84**, 252–259

KYLIN, B. (1960) Temporary threshold shift and auditory trauma following exposure to steady-state noise. An experimental and field study. *Acta Otolaryngologica* (Suppl.) 152, 1–93

LANKFORD, J. E., MIKIUT, T. A. and JACKSON, P. L. (1991) Noise exposure of high school students. *Hearing Instruments*, **42**, 19–24

LAROCHE, C., QUOC, H. T., HETU, R. and MCDUFF, S. (1991) 'Detectsound': a computerised model for predicting the detectability of warning signals in noisy workplaces. *Applied Acoustics*, **32**, 193–214

LEPAGE, E. and MURRAY, N. (1993) Otoacoustic emissions and hearing conservation screening. Poster, *Proceedings of the NHCA conference*, Albuquerque

LIBERMAN, M. C. (1987) Chronic ultrastructural changes in acoustic trauma: serial section reconstruction of stereocilia and cuticular plates. *Hearing Research*, **26**, 25–88

LIBERMAN, M. C. and DODDS, L. W. (1987) Acute ultrastructural changes in acoustic trauma: serial section of stereocilia and cuticular plates. *Hearing Research*, **26**, 45–64

LIM, D. J. (1986) Functional structure of the organ of Corti: a review. *Hearing Research*, **22**, 117–146

MCCOMBE, A. W., BINNINGTON, J. and MCCOMBE, T. S. (1993) Hearing protection of motorcyclists. *Clinical Otolaryngology*, **18**, 465–469

MCFADDEN, D. (1986). The curious half octave shift: evidence for a basalward migration of the traveling wave envelope with increasing intensity. In: *Basic and Applied Aspects of Noise Induced Hearing Loss*, edited by R. J. Salvi, D. Henderson, R. P. Hamernik and V. Colletti. New York: Plenum Publishing Co. pp. 295–312

MACREA, J. H. (1971) Noise induced hearing loss and presbycusis. *Audiology*, **10**, 323–333

MACREA, J. H. (1991) Presbyacusis and noise induced permanent threshold shift. *Journal of the Acoustical Society of America*, **90**, 2513–2516

MACREA, J. H. (1994) An investigation of temporary threshold shift caused by hearing and use. *Journal of Speech and Hearing Research*, **37**, 227–237

MCSHANE, D. P., HYDE, M. L. and ALBERTI, P. W. (1988) Tinnitus prevalence in industrial hearing loss compensation claimants. *Clinical Otolaryngology*, **13**, 323–330

MCSHANE, D. P., HYDE, M. L., FINKELSTEIN, D. M. and ALBERTI, P. W. (1991) Unilateral otosclerosis in noise induced hearing loss. *Clinical Otolaryngology*, **16**, 70–75

MAN, A. and WINERMAN, I. (1985) Does drill noise during mastoid surgery affect the contralateral ear? *American Journal of Otology*, **6**, 334–335

MARTIN, A. M. (1976) The equal energy concept applies to impulse noise. In: *Effects of Noise on Hearing*, edited by D. Henderson, R. P. Hamernik, D. S. Dosanj and J. Mills. New York: Raven Press. pp. 421–449

MELNICK, W. (1976) Human asymptotic threshold shift. In: *Effects of Noise on Hearing*, edited by D. Henderson, R. P. Hamernik, D. S. Dosanj and J. H. Mills. New York: Raven Press. pp. 277–289

MELNICK, W. (1991) Human temporary threshold shift (TTS) and damage risk. *Journal of the Acoustical Society of America*, **90**, 147–164

MILLER, J. D., WATSON, C. S. and COVELL, W. P. (1963) Deafening effects of noise on the cat. *Acta Otolaryngologica* (Suppl.), **176**, 1–91

MILLS, J. H. (1975) Noise and children. *Journal of the Acoustical Society of America*, **58**, 767–779

MILLS, J. H. (1976), Threshold shifts as produced by a 90 day exposure to noise. In: *Effects of Noise on Hearing*, edited by D. Henderson, R. P. Hamernik, D. S. Dosanj and J. H. Mills. New York: Raven Press. pp. 265–275

MILLS, J. H. (1982) Effects of noise on auditory sensitivity, psychophysical tuning curves and suppression. In: *New Perspectives on Noise Induced Hearing Loss*, edited by R. P. Hamernik, D. Henderson and R. Salvi. New York: Raven Press. pp. 249–263

MORATA, T. C. (1989) Study of the effects of the simultaneous exposure to noise and carbon disulphide on workers' hearing. *Scandinavian Audiology*, **18**, 53–58

MORATA, T. C., DUNN, D. E., KRETSCHMER, L. W., LEMASTER G. K. and KEITH, R. W. (1993) Effects of occupational exposure to organic solvents and noise on hearing. *Scandinavian Journal of Environmental Health*, **19**, 245–254

MOLVAER, O. I. (1991) Vestibular problems in diving and in space. *Scandinavian Audiology (suppl.)*, **34**, 163–170

NILSSON, R. and LINDGREN, F. (1980). The effects of long term use of hearing protectors in industrial noise. In: *Proceedings of International Symposium on Effects of impulse noise on hearing*, edited by P. Nillson and S. Arlinger. *Scandinavian Audiology* (suppl. 12), 204–211

NILSSON, R. and BORG, E. (1983) Noise induced hearing loss in shipyard workers with unilateral hearing loss. *Scandinavian Audiology*, **12**, 125–140

NIXON, C. W., MCKINLEY, R. L. and STEUVER, J. W. (1992) Performance of active noise reduction headsets. In: *Noise Induced Hearing Loss*, edited by A. L. Dancer, D. Henderson, R. J. Salvi and R. P. Hamernick. St Louis: Mosby Year Book. pp. 389–400

NOBLE, W. G. (1978) *Assessment of Impaired Hearing*. New York: Academic Press

NOVOTNY, Z. (1975a) Age factor in auditory fatigue in occupational hearing disorders due to noise. *Csekoslovenska Otolaryngologie*, **24**, 5–9

NOVOTNY, Z. (1975b) Development of occupational deafness after entering into noisy job at an advance age. *Ceskoslovenska Otolaryngologie*, **24**, 151–154

NUSSBAUM, D. S. and REINIS, S. (1985) University of Toronto Institute of Aerospace. Report 282 CNISSN 0082–5255

ODKVIST, L. M., MØLLER, C. and THUOMAS, K. A. (1992) Otoneurologic disturbances caused by solvent pollution. *Otolaryngology, Head and Neck Surgery*, **106**, 687–692

PARKIN, J. L., WOOD, G. S., WOOD, R. D. and MCCANDLESS, G. A. (1980) Drill and suction generated noise in mastoid surgery. *Archives of Otolaryngology*, **106**, 92–96

PASSCHIER-VERMIER, W. (1973) Noise induced hearing loss from intermittent and varying noise. In: *Proceedings of Noise as a Public Health Problem*, edited by W. D. Ward. Washington, DC. EPA

PATTERSON, J. H. and JOHNSON, D. L. (1993) Actual effectiveness of hearing protection in high level impulse noise. In: *Noise as a Public Health Problem*, vol. 3, edited by M. Vallet. Bron: INRETS. pp. 122–127

PATUZZI, R. (1992) Effect of noise on cranial nerve VIII responses. In: *Noise Induced Hearing Loss*, edited by A. L. Dancer, D. Henderson, R. J. Salvi and R. P. Hamernick. St Louis: Mosby Year Book. pp. 45–59

PAULSEN, K. and VIETOR, K. (1975a) Measurement of sound transmitted through the body while drilling and grinding in fresh isolated temporal bones. *Archives of Otorhinolaryngology*, 209, 159–168

PAULSEN, K. and VIETOR, K. (1975b) Noise level measurements of the air noise during drilling and grinding in fresh isolated temporal bones. *Laryngologie, Rhinologie und Otology*, 54, 824–834

PELL, S. (1973) An evaluation of a hearing conservation programme – a five year longitudinal study. *American Industrial Hygiene Association Journal*, 34, 82–91

PFANDER, F. (1975) Discussion of the progressive nature of acoustic trauma. In: *Das Knalltrauma*. Berlin: Springer-Verlag. pp. 97–101

PIRILA, T. (1991) Left-right asymmetry in the human response to noise exposure I. Intraaural correlation of the temporary threshold shift at 4 kHz frequency. *Acta Otolaryngologica*, 111, 677–683

PIRILA, T., JOUNIO-ERVASTI, J. and SORRI, M. (1991) Hearing asymmetry in left and right handed persons in a random population. *Scandinavian Audiology*, 20, 223–226

PYYKKO, I., KOSKIMIES, K., STARK, J., PEKKARMEN, J., FARKILLA, M. and DRABA, R. (1989) Risk factors in the genesis of sensorineural hearing loss in Finnish factory workers. *British Journal of Industrial Medicine*, 40, 439–440

RAMAZZINI, B. (1713). *Diseases of Workers*. Translated from the Latin *De Morbis Artificum* by W. C. Wright (1964). New York: Hafner. pp. 438–439

REUTER, G., GITTER, A. H., THURM, U. and ZENNER, H. P. (1992) High frequency radial movements of the reticular lamina induced by outer hair cell mobility. *Hearing Research*, 60, 236–246

RICE, C. G., ROSSI, G. and AINA, M. (1987) Damage risk from personal cassette players. *British Journal of Audiology*, 21, 279–288

RIKO, K. and ALBERTI, P. W. (1981) How ear protectors fail: a practical guide. In: *Personal Hearing Protection in Industry*, edited by P. W. Alberti. New York: Raven Press. pp. 323–338

ROBERTSON, D. and JOHNSTONE, B. M. (1979) Aberrant tonotopic organization in the inner ear damaged by kanamycin. *Journal of the Acoustical Society of America*, 66, 466–469

ROBINSON, D. W. (1987) Noise exposure and hearing. A new look at the experimental data. *HSE Contract Research Report* 1/1987

ROBINSON, D. W. (1991a) Relation between hearing threshold level and its component parts. *British Journal of Audiology*, 25, 93–103

ROBINSON, D. W. (1991b) Impairment and disability in noise induced hearing loss. *Advances in Audiology*, 5, 71–81

ROP, I., RABER, A. and FISCHER, G. H. (1979) Study of hearing losses of industrial workers with occupational noise exposure using statistical methods for the analysis of qualitative data. *Audiology*, 18, 181–196

ROSENHALL, U., PEDERSEN, K. and SVANBORG, A. (1990) Presbycusis and noise induced hearing loss. *Ear and Hearing*, 11, 257–263

ROSSI, G. (1983a) (ed.) Acoustic reflex amplitude and response to continuous noise and impulse noise with the same energy content. In: *Proceedings of the 4th International Congress on Noise as a Public Health Hazard*. Milan: Amplifon. pp. 183–192

ROSSI, G. (1983b) (ed). *Noise as a Public Health Problem*, vol. 2. Milan: Amplifon

ROYSTER, J. D. and ROYSTER, L. H. (1990) *Hearing Conservation Programs*. Chelsea, Michigan: Lewis Publishers

ROYSTER, J. D., ROYSTER, L. H. and KILLION, M. D. (1991) Sound exposures and hearing thresholds of symphony orchestra musicians. *Journal of the Acoustical Society of America*, 89, 2793–2803

ROYSTER, L. H. (1985) Should the Walkman take a walk? (editorial). *Sound and Vibration*, 19, 5

ROYSTER, L. H., ROYSTER, J. D. and CECICH, T. F. (1984) An evaluation of the effectiveness of the hearing protection devices at an industrial facility with a TWA of 107 dB. *Journal of the Acoustical Society of America*, 76, 485–497

RYAN, A. F., BENNETT, T. M., WOOLF, N. K. and AXELSSON, A. (1994) Protection from noise induced hearing loss by prior exposure to a non traumatic stimulus: role of the middle ear muscles. *Hearing Research*, 72, 23–28

RYBAK, L. P. (1992) Hearing: The effects of chemicals. *Otolaryngology, Head and Neck Surgery*, 106, 677–686

SALMIVALLI, A. (1967) Acoustic trauma in regular army personnel. *Acta Otolaryngologica*, Suppl. 222

SATALOFF, R. T. and SATALOFF, J. (1993) *Occupational Hearing Loss*. New York: Dekker. p. 251

SAUNDERS, J. C., COHEN, Y. E. and SZYMKO, Y. M. (1991) The structural and functional consequences of acoustic injury in the cochlea and peripheral auditory system: a five year update. *Journal of the Acoustical Society of America*, 90, 136–146

SAUNDERS, J. C., DEAR, S. P. and SCHNEIDER, M. E. (1985) The anatomical consequences of acoustic injury: a review and tutorial. *Journal of the Acoustical Society of America*, 78, 833–860

SAVELL, J. F. and TOOTHAM, E. H. (1987) Group mean hearing threshold changes in a noise exposed industrial population using personal hearing protectors. *American Industrial Hygiene Association Journal*, 48, 23–27

SIMPSON, D. C. and O'REILLY, B. F. (1991) The protective effect of a conductive hearing loss in workers exposed to industrial noise. *Clinical Otolaryngology*, 16, 274–277

SINCLAIR, J. (1992) *Unpublished thesis*. Masters in Occupational Hygiene. Toronto: University of Toronto

SMOORENBURG, G. F. (1992) Damage risk for low frequency impulse noise: the spectral factor in noise induced hearing loss. In: *Noise Induced Hearing Loss*, edited by A. L. Dancer, D. Henderson, R. J. Salvi and R. P. Hamernik. St Louis: Mosby Year Book. pp. 313–324

SORRI, M., SIPILA, R., PIRILA, T. and KARJALAINEN, H. (1983) Use of snowmobiles and hearing loss among reindeer herders. In: *Proceedings of the 4th International Congress on Noise as a Public Health Problem*, edited by G. Rossi. Milan: Centre Richerche e Studi Amplifon. pp. 395–398

SPENCER, M. G. and REID, A. (1985) Drill generated noise levels in mastoid surgery. *Journal of Laryngology and Otology*, 99, 967–972

STANSFELD, S., GULLACHER, J., BABISCH, W. and ELWOOD, P. C. (1993) Road traffic noise, noise sensitivity and psychiatric disorder: preliminary prospective findings from the Caerphilly study. In: *Noise as a Public Health Problem*, vol. 3, edited by M. Vallet. Bron: INRETS. pp. 268–273

STARK, J., PEKKAIMEN, J. and PYYKKO, I. (1988) Impulse noise and hand arm vibration in relation to sensorineural hearing loss. *Scandinavia Journal of Work and Environmental Health*, **14**, 265–271

STEPHENS, S. D. G. and HÉTU, R. (1991) Impairment, disability and handicap in audiology: towards a consensus. *Audiology*, **30**, 185–200

STEVENSON, D. C. and MCKELLAR, N. R. (1989) The effect of traffic noise on sleep of young adults in their homes. *Journal of the Acoustical Society of America*, **85**, 768–771

STUDEBAKER, G. A., BESS, F. H. and BECK, L. B. (1991) *The Vanderbilt Hearing Air Report, II.* Timonium, MD: York Press

SULKOWSKI, W. J., KOWALSKA, S. and LIPOWCZA, A. (1983) Hearing loss in weavers and drop forge hammermen: comparative study on the effects of steady state impulse noise. In: *Proceedings of the 4th International Congress: Noise as a Public Health Problem*, edited by G. Rossi, vol. 1. Milan: Centre Recherche e Studi Amplifon. pp. 171–184

SUTER, A. H. and FRANKS, J. R. (1990) *A Practical Guide to Effective Hearing Conservation in the Workplace.* US Dept of Health & Human Services. NIOSH publ. 90–120

TAYLOR, C. F. (1976) Hearing loss in new apprentices due to exposure to non industrial noise. *Journal of Social and Occupational Medicine*, **26**, 57–58

TAYLOR, W., PEARSON, J., MAIR, A. and BURNS, W. (1965) Study of noise and hearing in the jute weaving industry. *Journal of the Acoustical Society of America*, **33**, 113–120

THIESSEN, G. J. (1976) *Effects of Noise on Man.* National Research Council of Canada, publication no. 15383, Ottawa: Canada

TOMIOKA, S. (1982) Two cases of acute bilateral hearing loss from exposure to rock and roll music. *Otolaryngology*, **54**, 1005–1011

TSCHOPP, K. and PROBST, R. (1989) Acute acoustic trauma. A retrospective study of influencing factors in different therapies in 268 patients. *Acta Otolaryngologica*, **108**, 378–384

TURUNEN-RISE, I., FLOTTORP, G. and TRETE, O. (1991) A study of the possibility of acquiring noise induced hearing loss by the 'use of' personal cassette players (Walkman). *Scandinavian Audiology* (suppl. 34), 144

ULRICH, R. F. and PINHEIRO, M. L. (1974) Temporary hearing losses in teenagers attending repeated rock and roll sessions. *Acta Otolaryngologica*, **77**, 51–55

VALLET, M. (1993) (ed.) *Noise as a Public Health Problem*, 3 vol. Bron: INRETS

VAN MOORHEN, W. K., SHEPHERD, K. P., MAGLEBY, T. D. and TORIAN, G. E. (1981) The effects of motorcycle helmets on hearing and the detection of warning signals. *Journal of Sound and Vibration*, **77**, 39–49

VON GIERKE, H. E. and JOHNSON, L. (1976) Summary of present damage criteria. In: *Effects of Noise on Hearing*, edited by D. Henderson, R. P. Hamernik, D. S. Dosanj and J. H. Mills. New York: Raven Press. pp. 457–560

VON GIERKE, H. E. and NIXON, W. C. (1976) The effects of intense infrasound on man. In: *Infrasound on Low Frequency Vibrations*, edited by W. Tempest. London: Academic Press. pp. 129–153

WARD, W. D. (1962) *Journal of the Acoustical Society of America*, **34**, 1230

WARD, W. D. (1991) The role of intermittence in PTS. *Journal of the Acoustical Society of America*, **90**, 164–169

WARD, W. D., CUSHING, E. M. and BURNS, E. M. (1976) Effective quiet and moderate TTS: implications for noise exposure standards. *Journal of the Acoustical Society of America*, **59**, 160–165

WARD, W. D., TURNER, C. W. and FABRY, D. A. (1983) The total energy and equal energy principles in the chinchilla. *Proceedings of 4th International Congress on Noise as a Public Health Problem*, edited by G. Rossi, vol. 1. Milan: Centre Richerche e Studi Amplifon. pp. 399-405

WELLESCHIK, B. and RABER, A. (1978) Einfluss von Expositionszeit und Alter Auf Den Irmbedingten Horverlust. *Laryngology, Rhinology and Otology*, **57**, 1037–1048

WENTHOLD, R. J., SCHNEIDER, M. E., KIM. H. N. and DECHESNE, C. J. (1992) Putative biochemical processes in noise induced hearing loss. In: *Noise Induced Hearing Loss*, edited by A. L. Dancer, D. Henderson, R. J. Salvi and R. P. Hamernick. St Louis: Mosby Year Book. pp. 28–37

WESTIN, J. B. (1975) Infrasound. A short review of effects on man. *Aviation Space and Environmental Medicine*, **46**, 1135–1143

WHO (1980) *International Classification of Impairments, Disabilities and Handicaps.* Geneva: World Health Organisation

WILKINS, P. and MARTIN, A. M. (1987) Healing protection and warning sounds in industry – a review. *Applied Acoustics*, **21**, 267–293

WILSON, J. P. (1992) Otoacoustic emissions and noise induced hearing loss. In: *Noise Induced Hearing Loss*, edited by A. L. Dancer, D. Henderson, R. J. Salvi and R. P. Hamernick. St Louis: Mosby Year Book. pp. 89–97

WITTER, H. L., DEKO, R. C., LIPSCOMB, D. M. and SHAMBAUGH, G. E. (1980) Effects of pre-stimulatory carbogen inhalation on noise induced temporary threshold shifts in humans and chinchilla. *American Journal of Otology*, **1**, 227–232

YARINGTON, C. T. JR (1968) Military noise induced hearing loss: problems in conservation programs. *Laryngoscope*, **78**, 685–692

YLIKOSKI, J. (1987) Audiometric configurations in acute acoustic trauma carried by firearms. *Scandinavian Audiology*, **16**, 115–120

ZENNER, H. P., ZIMMERMAN, R. and GLITTER, A. H. (1988) Active movements of the cuticular plate induce sensory hair motion in mammalian outer hair cells. *Hearing Research*, **34**, 233–240

12

Diagnostic audiometry

M. E. Lutman

This chapter outlines the major tests of hearing function used in the routine audiology clinic, the term *audiometry* being taken to mean measurement of hearing in its most general sense. Most of the tests are based on voluntary responses, the patient being required to respond to sound stimuli according to instruction but, increasingly, diagnostic audiology is becoming dependent on investigations using involuntary responses, including electrophysiological tests. The increasing availability of imaging techniques, especially magnetic resonance imaging (see Volumes 1 and 3), has further shifted emphasis away from diagnostic procedures based on voluntary responses. This chapter attempts to reflect this picture of changing priorities relating to the differential diagnosis of peripheral hearing disorders.

The involuntary tests of auditory function included in the present chapter are those using the otoadmittance (impedance) technique, electrophysiological tests and otoacoustic emissions. They are included here because they can now be conducted in the routine audiology clinic and because their interpretation in practice has become so interwoven with that of the others. Although many of the tests may be used with children, in some cases with an appropriately modified procedure, specialized tests for children are outside the scope of this chapter (see Volume 6).

It is useful at the outset to distinguish between the domains of pathology, impairment and disability. The majority of the clinical tests described measure impairment of hearing function, e.g. the pure-tone audiogram measures loss of sensitivity. Some tests give a specific indication of pathology, e.g. the tympanogram gives a measure of middle-ear pressure which is directly related to nasopharyngeal (eustachian) tube function. Lastly, speech tests, while being dependent on sensitivity, discrimination and resolution, may be considered to reflect an aspect of disability – the inability to perform certain basic and useful skills. For diagnostic purposes, pathology and impairment are paramount, whereas disability is more relevant to rehabilitation, dealt with in Chapter 13. The aim of this chapter is to concentrate on diagnostic aspects of audiometry, with particular emphasis on the basic tests of pure-tone audiometry, tympanometry and acoustic reflex measurement.

Diagnostic categories

Attempts to identify the cause of a hearing impairment are often unsuccessful, especially in cases of sensorineural hearing loss, even after extensive supplementary investigations (e.g. vestibular, electrophysiological, biochemical, haematological, radiological). The causative factor may well have disappeared by the time of testing, leaving the hearing loss as its only evidence. *Post hoc* diagnosis is frequently extremely presumptive and depends on possibly coincidental factors such as age, noise exposure, drug administration or viral infection. Furthermore, with one or two exceptions, there are no accepted medical or surgical treatments when the hearing loss is sensorineural. Therefore, there will often be no useful diagnosis in the aetiological sense, although pragmatic considerations also apply. By attaching a label, patient expectations may be fulfilled, which may in turn promote confidence in the medical profession, reassurance of the patient and acceptance of any advice given. Also, this may avoid fruitless requests for further medical opinions. The lack of definitive diagnosis in most cases has led to the implicit classification of hearing impairment into clinical *types* rather than specific diseases or conditions. Although these types are not always defined formally, they are based upon combinations of assumed sites of lesion and clusters or ranges of values on impairment measures; types are therefore hybrid functional-anatomical categories. The most commonly used types are *conductive, sensory, neural* (divided into *peripheral neural* and *central neural*), *non-organic* and *mixed*. Mixed is simply a mixture of conductive and sensory or neural.

The term *conductive* relates to external-ear and middle-ear disorders where the transmission of sound to the cochlea is impaired. Our knowledge and ability to diagnose conductive disorders is fairly comprehensive and robust as a consequence of their mechanical and relatively peripheral nature and the possibility of visual observation or surgical confirmation.

Sensorineural implies an organic disorder of the cochlea and/or subsequent parts of the auditory system. *Sensory* is intended to relate to the cochlea and *neural* to the subsequent sections (peripheral and central) of the auditory pathways, but it must be remembered that these terms refer to the audiological types rather than individually confirmed sites of lesion. Until recent decades, it was not customary to distinguish sensory from neural and the superordinate category *sensorineural* is still used to distinguish these two jointly from conductive, for the good reason that their pathologies and audiological manifestation generally occur together. The type is defined by a combination of impairment measures; the relation to anatomical site in an individual case may be by inference only. As knowledge of the respective functions of the inner and outer hair cells of the cochlea increases, there may become a need further to subdivide sensory into two categories reflecting dysfunction of the two types of hair cell; loss of outer hair cell function would entail loss of the enhanced sensitivity conferred by their electromotile properties, whereas loss of inner hair cell function would entail a general loss of sensitivity of the cochlea as a transducer converting mechanical input into afferent neural activity. At the present time it is not known to what extent these two types of cochlear dysfunction are mutually interdependent and hence a formal subdivision of the *cochlear* type at the present time would be premature.

The term *central neural* is used to describe hearing disorders where there is a defect in auditory pattern processing, usually without appreciable hearing loss. The disorder is often most evident when speech stimuli are used. The site of lesion may, in some cases, be inferred as the auditory cortex or brain stem, in that tests involving specifically binaural phenomena show abnormalities.

Non-organic hearing loss is used to describe conditions where audiological tests give rise to doubt regarding the presence of an organic disorder. By implication these include, but are not synonymous with, psychogenic hearing loss and deliberate feigning. The dividing line between central neural and non-organic can be difficult to define in individual cases.

Much clinical research in audiology has revolved around the relationships between individual test results and the above types, and to a lesser extent between types and *confirmed diagnoses*. Investigation of such relationships forms the basis of the diagnostic principles described later in this chapter, but has been constrained by the general lack of confirmed diagnoses except in certain conditions, such as acoustic neuromas (vestibulocochlear schwannomas). The availability of confirmation in such cases has given rise to some overemphasis of the peripheral neural type in relation to its prevalence. Furthermore, the peripheral neural type has been characterized predominantly on the basis of acoustic neuroma cases for the same reason.

Characterization of ears into one or more of the above types is based on measurement of hearing functions, which can conveniently be grouped and defined as follows.

Sensitivity is defined by the least intense sound that can be heard (auditory threshold), most commonly for pure tones as a function of frequency.

Discrimination is the ability to distinguish between similar acoustic waveforms and is often measured using speech stimuli. Speech tests often require subjects to repeat words from an open set and, in such circumstances, the term *identification* is more appropriate to describe the task used. Alternatively, the term *recognition* is being preferred by international standards on speech audiometry.

Intensity resolution involves the ability of the ear to resolve sounds of different intensities. Most people can also assign subjective magnitude (loudness) to a sound of a given intensity or at least make comparative loudness judgements. The term *loudness recruitment* is widely used to describe the steep loudness function that is entailed by an elevated threshold and relatively normal loudness of sounds in the upper intensity range. Corresponding indices of recruitment are available from electroacoustic and electrophysiological measures of the magnitude of activity in the auditory system.

Frequency resolution is the ability of the ear to detect a sound of one frequency in the presence of competing sounds at other frequencies.

Temporal resolution is the ability to detect rapid changes in the waveform envelope of a sound signal.

Adaptation is a reduction with time in sensitivity to a prolonged stimulus. With pure tones, the term *decay* is often used, as in tone decay or acoustic reflex decay. Adaptation can be distinguished from fatigue of the auditory system (e.g. temporary threshold shift) by momentary cessation of stimulation which abolishes adaptation but only has a minor effect on fatigue.

In the following sections, tests which assess the above functions are described, together with the variations to be expected with the different hearing loss types. Considerable space is devoted to pure-tone audiometry, speech audiometry and otoadmittance testing, which are fundamental to basic clinical evaluations. Only limited space is devoted to less common or newer procedures for which fewer data are available or for which the diagnostic potential is not established. In particular, thorough coverage is given to bone-conduction audiometry and to masking of the non-test ear in pure-tone audiometry because these techniques are so often poorly executed and understood, leading to erroneous conclusions. For similar reasons, the description of otoadmittance measurement is relatively detailed. Speech audiometry is emphasized because of its multiple use as a differential diagnostic test, as an indicator of non-organic hearing loss and as a reflection of disability. Measurement of otoacoustic emissions is included in view of its developing potential as a tool in the diagnostic armamentarium, particularly its potential roles in distinguishing cochlear and retrocochlear disorders and distinguishing outer hair cell and inner hair cell dysfunction. There is insufficient space in a chapter of this general nature to do justice to every measurement technique; the reader is referred to one of the excellent textbooks available on clinical audiology (e.g. Katz, 1994).

Instrumentation and calibration

The human ear responds to sound over a remarkably wide range of intensities, from a sound pressure level of approximately 0 dB at normal threshold in the mid-frequencies to at least 120 dB at the upper end of the dynamic range. This corresponds to a pressure amplitude ratio of one to one million. Instrumentation to generate stimuli over such a wide range requires specialized construction, with emphasis being placed on achieving a high signal-to-noise ratio. Amplifier noise that would be acceptable in a domestic environment, where the level of ambient noise is much higher than in an audiometry suite, is unacceptable in an audiometer and would lead to masking of the absolute threshold in some subjects. Furthermore, harmonic distortion must be kept as low as possible when using pure-tone stimuli to avoid the spread of acoustical excitation to frequencies other than those it is intended to test. Fortunately, there are specific international standards governing the specification of the more common types of instrumentation used in audiology (e.g. audiometers, otoadmittance meters) and it is a relatively simple matter to choose instruments that satisfy the standards. Pure-tone audiometers for use in the diagnostic audiology clinic should conform with the specification for type 1 audiometers given in IEC 645-1 (1992). Speech audiometers are covered by IEC 645-2 (1993) whereas impedance meters are the subject of IEC 1027 (1991).

Type testing of instrument models does not remove the need for calibration of the actual instruments used. This must be carried out at regular intervals according to a rigorous procedure. The principle of calibration is to check that the instrument produces the correct output, within tolerances, and to make adjustments as necessary. For pure-tone audiometers, the most important characteristics to check are the frequencies and intensities of pure tones, the amount of harmonic distortion, the linearity of output with alteration of the hearing level control, and output levels of masking noise. Both acoustic output via earphones and vibratory output via the bone vibrator must be checked. A three-tier system of checks and calibrations has been adopted by ISO 389 (1991), consisting of daily routine checks and subjective testing (stage A), periodic objective checks (stage B), and baseline calibration (stage C). Stage B entails detailed objective measurements and should only be carried out by a competent technician with the necessary measuring equipment having verified performance with reference to a national standardizing laboratory. Typically, stage B would be carried out every 6 months, and certainly the interval between stage B checks should not exceed 1 year. Stage C checks are required when instrumentation is newly acquired or modified, when stage A or B checks indicate a fault that cannot be rectified by simple adjustment, or after an extended period of use (e.g. 5 years).

The acoustical environment in which audiometric tests are conducted should be treated as an extension of the instrumentation, i.e. subject to the same system of checks and calibrations. In particular, the level of ambient noise must be sufficiently low to avoid interference with test results. Minimal acceptable levels of background noise are tabulated in ISO 8253-1 (1989) for audiometry by air conduction or by bone conduction. Adherence to those specifications ensures that hearing threshold levels can be obtained down to 0 dB with an error due to background noise masking not exceeding 2 dB. This requirement is a compromise between the ideal of being able to measure down to −10 dB with negligible error and the high cost of reaching the ideal.

Pure-tone audiometry
Measurement of sensitivity: the audiogram

The extent of hearing impairment is usually measured primarily in terms of loss of sensitivity. Because of the fundamental differences in the causes, characteristics and management of conductive and sensorineural types of hearing loss, it is desirable to enumerate separately the loss of sensitivity caused by conductive or sensorineural components. Essentially, this reduces to measurement of both the sensitivity at the cochlea and the overall sensitivity of the ear, the conductive loss being the difference between the two (in decibels).

Measurement of the overall sensitivity of the ear is relatively straightforward; the only major difficulty arises out of the need to distinguish between responses of the left and right ears (see below: cross-hearing). However, measurement of sensitivity at the cochlea is much more problematic, requiring a stimulus which bypasses the outer and middle ear and stimulates the cochlea directly. The method almost universally adopted is to present a vibration stimulus to the skull (usually over the mastoid process) with the underlying but incorrect assumption that vibration will travel directly through the bones of the skull to the cochlear fluids independent of the outer and middle ear. This mechanism is referred to as *bone conduction.*

Before discussing the actual methods of measurement, it is worth examining the validity of this assumption in some detail. Tonndorf (1972) made exhaustive measurements of the routes taken by bone-conducted sounds in the cat, using several surgical alterations of the anatomy of the ear in order to quantify the components travelling by no less than eight routes! His conclusions may be simplified as delimiting three routes (each of which in fact has one or more component). These three routes are:

1 The direct osseous route
2 The route passing from the skull to the middle ear and thence to the cochlea via the ossicles and the air of the middle-ear cavity, part of which is termed

the *inertial* component and arises from the inertia of the mass of the ossicles
3 The route passing from the skull to the ear canal and middle ear.

Figure 12.1 illustrates the relative magnitudes of transmission via these three routes in the cat and also the vector sum of the three components, which takes into account differences in phase between components. Notice that the assumption that vibration travels predominantly via the osseous route is not upheld.

Unfortunately, the extrapolation of these relative contributions to humans is difficult to validate and, given differences in anatomy, humans should not be assumed to be the same. Furthermore, the use of different types of vibrator, different vibrator location and a different direction of vibrating force can be presumed to contaminate the transfer of results from cat to human. However, sensitivity to vibration applied to the skull is not necessarily equivalent to the sensitivity of the cochlea and the use of bone-conduction thresholds in the interpretation of audiometric results is subject to significant errors (Coles, Lutman and Robinson, 1991). Such considerations apply equally to the interpretation of tuning fork tests, such as the Rinne test.

For clinical purposes, the contaminating effect of outer- and middle-ear bone-conduction routes might be tractable if the direction of their interaction with

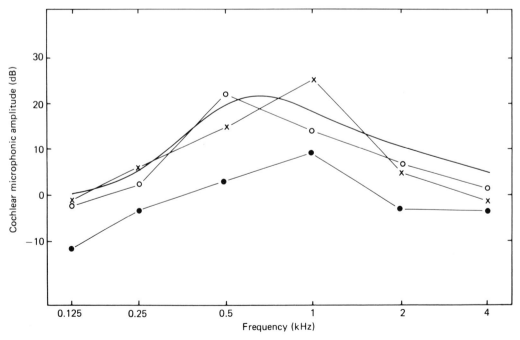

Figure 12.1 Comparison of the principal routes of bone conduction in the cat (X, outer ear; ○, middle-ear; ●, osseous; —, composite, see text). (Modified from Tonndorf, 1972, by courtesy of the publisher)

middle-ear pathology were predictable; e.g. if middle-ear pathologies always reduced the middle- and outer-ear components. However, abnormalities may have either an enhancing or depressing effect. Increased mass of the ossicular chain theoretically causes a reduction in resonance frequency resulting in an increase in sensitivity at some frequencies and a decrease at others, as demonstrated by Tonndorf (1966). Added stiffness caused by otosclerosis for example, is likely to increase the resonance fre- quency, and physiological experiments seem to indi- cate that added stiffness generally reduces sensitivity (Smith, 1943; Tonndorf and Tabor, 1962). In addi- tion, because of the different phases seen at the basilar membrane for the signals conducted by the different routes, the reduction of bone conduction by one particular route does not necessarily lead to an overall reduction in sensitivity, because of the com- plex interaction between the various components. In fact, it is possible that a particular form of pathology may remove the phase cancellation between two components leading to an increase in sensitivity, at least at certain frequencies.

Despite the important qualifications outlined above, the use of bone-conduction measurements in clinical audiology is unavoidable at present, mainly because no acceptable alternative exists. The magnitude of error thereby introduced can only be ascertained directly in certain circumstances, but it is instructive to examine such a case. Figure 12.2 illustrates typical audiograms which were obtained pre- and postopera- tively with successful stapedectomy for otosclerosis (see below for details of audiometric technique and the audiogram). The overall sensitivity of the ear given by the air-conduction thresholds improves by an average of approximately 40 dB as a result of provision of a more effective sound conduction path to the cochlea. The bone-conduction thresholds im- prove by an average of approximately 10 dB, depend- ing considerably on frequency. Obviously, there is unlikely to be an actual improvement in cochlear sensitivity; rather the outer- and middle-ear bone- conduction routes have been enhanced leading to improved bone-conduction thresholds. The improve- ment is an artefact of the method of measurement. Such effects are unlikely to be restricted to cases of otosclerosis; their association with otosclerosis (the Carhart effect, named after Carhart, 1950, and often less aptly termed a *notch*) is probably connected more with the fact that stapedectomy provides an elegant circumstance in which to demonstrate the effect, rather than with otosclerosis as a specific aetiology. Gatehouse and Browning (1982) suggested that such pre- and postoperative demonstrations actually under- estimate the magnitude of the effect. Evidence that other middle-ear abnormalities have similar effects has been provided, e.g. with radical mastoidectomy (Békésy, 1939; Tonndorf, 1966), mallear fixation (Goodhill, 1965; Dirks and Malmquist, 1969), secre- tory otitis media (Naunton and Fernandez, 1961) and ossicular discontinuity (Priede, 1970).

Methodology of pure-tone audiometry

Pure-tone audiometry involves estimating the thresh- old of hearing for certain standardized stimuli, usually via the air-conduction (a-c) and bone-conduction (b-c) routes. Threshold of hearing is variously defined but it is often taken to be 'the lowest sound pressure or alternating force level at which, under specified conditions, a person gives a predetermined percent- age of correct detection responses on repeated trials' (International Organization for Standardization, 1991). Threshold definitions are usually based on 50% correct detection. The stimuli used are calibrated on the hearing level (HL) scale which has been obtained from normalization studies involving large numbers of subjects, and is deemed to have the 0 dB hearing level point at the modal value of hearing threshold levels measured in otologically normal sub- jects aged between 18 and 30 years.[1] Because it is impractical to obtain a biological calibration for every audiometer, the biological baseline is defined objec- tively in national and international standards for certain combinations of earphone or bone vibrator

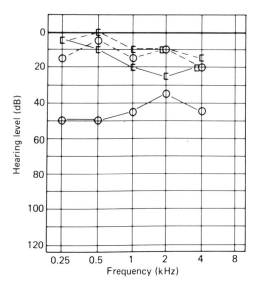

Figure 12.2 Changes in air-conduction and bone - conduction threshold due to successful stapedectomy for otosclerosis (——, preoperative; - - -, postoperative)

---

[1] Normative investigations on which the hearing level scale are based were mainly conducted in the 1950s and have only a tenuous connection with the earphones and couplers used nowadays. Recent evidence suggests that the standard is too strict for general populations of otologically normal young subjects (Lutman and Davis, 1994).

and acoustic or mechanical coupler. The standards are also specific to particular audiometric test frequencies. For air-conduction, frequencies of 0.125, 0.25, 0.5, 1, 1.5, 2, 3, 4, 6 and 8 kHz are included;[2] for bone-conduction, at least the following are included: 0.25, 0.5, 1, 2, 3 and 4 kHz, although there is some variation between national standards. This effectively restricts the frequencies which are useful in audiometry. It should be noted that bone-vibrator output is generally limited to about 80 dB hearing level at most frequencies – much less at low frequencies where there is also more harmonic distortion. Figure 12.3 illustrates the standard audiogram format used for plotting results. Note the use of particular symbols for air conduction and bone conduction for the (R) and (L) ears. Those shown in the figure are the accepted symbols for use in the UK and several other countries. They are also used in the international standard ISO 8253–1 (International Organization for Standardization, 1989).

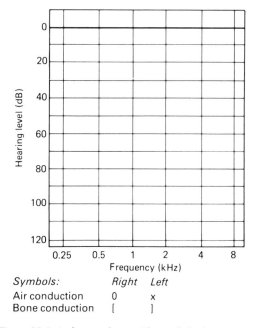

Figure 12.3 Audiogram format. The symbols shown are consistent with draft international standard ISO 8253–1 (International Organization for Standardization, 1989)

Apart from the use of properly calibrated stimuli, the test conditions for pure-tone audiometry are important. As described above, the audiometer itself must conform to appropriate standards and the acous-

tic environment must be sufficiently quiet not to mask the stimuli. In effect this usually means the subject must be seated in an acoustically treated room or enclosure. In common with all psychoacoustical tests, the psychophysical procedure used to determine thresholds is important. Most recommended procedures utilize an adaptive form of bracketing whereby the stimulus is presented at levels above and below threshold to 'home in' on the threshold region. Examples of recommended procedures are British Society of Audiology/British Association of Otolaryngologists (1981) and ISO 8253–1 (International Organization for Standardization, 1989). All procedures must ensure that non-auditory cues such as sight of the tester and rhythmic stimulus presentation do not yield thresholds that are too sensitive; likewise vibration from the earphone must not elicit artefactual responses. As an alternative to manually operated procedures, self-recording audiometers automate the bracketing of stimulus levels and plot out the pattern of presentation levels for each frequency, as illustrated in Figure 12.4.

This method had limited applicability in diagnostic audiometry because the instruments are seldom able to counteract the effects of cross-hearing (see below) and, consequently, self-recording bone-conduction audiometry is inappropriate. It is used mainly for screening by air conduction only. However, the procedure does have a clinically useful variant for diagnostic purposes (see below: Békésy audiometry). Computer-controlled audiometers are currently becoming available which overcome some of the limitations of current self-recording instruments (Chapter 18). However, the complexity of reasoning involved in conducting audiometry with masking makes the task of programming a fully automatic clinical audiometer suitable for all patients exceedingly difficult and it is unlikely that manually-operated instruments will be replaced in the foreseeable future.

A variant of the Békésy procedure has been developed for use on the Audioscan instrument. Instead of following an adaptive procedure while frequency is slowly swept, the Audioscan presents stimuli at fixed hearing levels and scans the frequency range in a large number of small discrete steps. The procedure starts at a low stimulus intensity. According to the responses of the subject, the instrument determines those frequency ranges in which the subject can hear the stimulus at the current level. These frequency ranges are excluded from subsequent sweeps. The intensity is raised for further sweeps which are evaluated the same way until all frequencies have been heard. The aim is to eliminate redundancy by only testing at frequencies where the threshold has not yet been determined, and also to obtain measurements of sensitivity that are highly resolved in the frequency domain. At the present time there has been only limited validation of the psychophysical properties of the technique (Laroche and Hétu, 1991);

---

[2] Work by the International Organization for Standardization is under way to define the hearing level scale for air conduction up to a frequency of 16 kHz.

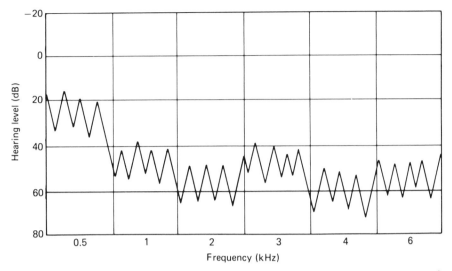

Figure 12.4 A self-recording audiogram. The stimulus frequency is held constant within each of the six intervals on the horizontal scale

the influence of spurious or slow responses by the subject could potentially play havoc with the results. Further validation in clinical populations is required before it can be recommended.

The problem of cross-hearing

Nature of the problem

It is natural to assume that, when sound is presented to the earphone on the left ear, it is the sensitivity of the left ear which is being measured; likewise for the right ear. Unfortunately, this assumption does not hold true under all circumstances because the earphone also transmits a certain amount of energy into the skull as vibration, albeit at a much lower level than the acoustic signal. The vibration energy travels through the skull almost equally to both cochleae. Considering as an example a patient with no hearing in the left ear and normal hearing in the right ear, when the sound presented to his left ear reaches a certain intensity, he will perceive the sound via the right cochlea. The level of sound necessary to overcome the transmission loss from the left earphone to the right cochlea varies considerably between individuals, in the range 40–85 dB (Lidén, Nilsson and Anderson, 1959; Chaiklin, 1967; Coles and Priede, 1970; Smith and Markides, 1981). It also varies with frequency. Thus, if − 10 dB hearing level is accepted to be the lower end of the range of practicably measurable thresholds in the non-test ear, whenever the stimulus in the test ear is raised to 30 dB hearing level in an individual, there is theoretically a possibility of cross-hearing, depending on the sensitivity of the non-test cochlea. In general, when there is no

conductive component to the hearing loss on either ear, it can be assumed that cross-hearing will not interfere with threshold measurement if there is less than a 40 dB asymmetry between the ears at each frequency. However, because it is the sensitivity of the non-test *cochlea* which determines the level at which cross-hearing occurs, the presence of a conductive component on the non-test ear reduces the allowable asymmetry by a corresponding amount. Audiometric procedures must recognize such circumstances and indicate the need to use appropriate masking to combat cross-hearing as described below.

Incidentally, regardless of the effect of the non-test ear, the transmission of stimulus energy from the earphone to the ipsilateral cochlea via bone conduction sets an upper limit to the conductive hearing loss that can be measured. For supra-aural earphone stimuli this is between 40 and 85 dB, depending on the individual and the stimulus frequency.

So far only air-conduction stimuli have been considered. For bone conduction the situation is more extreme. The transmission loss from ipsilateral mastoid process to contralateral cochlea varies between − 5 and + 15 dB (Studebaker, 1964), but for most practical purposes should be treated as zero. Therefore, bone-conduction stimuli are always potentially cross-heard and masking is always necessary to determine the separate thresholds of the right and left cochleae. Despite this, in many cases it is possible to determine a range of possible cochlear sensitivity for each frequency and ear without the use of masking, which may be adequate for clinical diagnostic purposes. The opportunity occurs because neither cochlea can be appreciably more sensitive than the bone-conduction threshold measured without masking and the cochlea on each side cannot be less sensitive than the overall sensitivity of that ear measured by air conduction.

The use of masking to combat cross-hearing

By presenting a suitable continuous masking noise to the non-test ear, the signal-to-noise ratio of the cross-heard sound can be reduced sufficiently to prevent the patient from hearing it. For cross-conducted pure-tone stimuli and narrow-band noise on the non-test ear, the signal-to-noise ratio on *that ear* must be kept below about −5 dB (International Organization for Standardization, 1987), to prevent cross-hearing, and preferably below −15 dB, thus allowing a further safety margin of about 10 dB. The art of successful masking is to use only sufficient masking to prevent cross-hearing, because the use of excessive masking has two major undesirable consequences. First, for the same reasons that the pure-tone stimulus may be cross-heard, the masking noise may travel across the skull and mask the test tone directly on the test ear. This is termed *cross-masking* (or sometimes *over-masking*); it occurs mainly when there is a conductive component to the hearing loss on the non-test ear. It can also occur in purely sensorineural cases if grossly excessive masking is used. The second undesirable consequence is termed *central masking* and is an elevation of threshold due to the presentation of the masking to the non-test ear independent of the effect of cross-masking. It is presumed to be a result of competition for neural channels within the central auditory system.

As a consequence of the complexity of cross-hearing, cross-masking and central masking effects, it is usually not possible to predict the necessary level of masking noise without some prior knowledge of the quantities to be established, namely the sensitivities of the cochleae on both sides. A two-pass approach is therefore required which, in essence, involves determining the correct threshold after first determining the correct masking level. A commonly used procedure is the plateau-seeking method, whereby the masking noise is presented at successively higher levels and responses to pure tones obtained at each level. The idealized pattern of change of pure-tone threshold with masking level is illustrated in Figure 12.5. Initially there is a *pro rata* increase in the threshold as a result of peripheral masking of the cross-heard signal in the non-test ear. Subsequently, the threshold remains constant with increases in masking as the signal is heard in the test ear independent of the masking presented to the non-test ear. This is the *plateau*. Finally, there is a further *pro rata* increase caused by the peripheral masking of the signal in the test ear by the cross-masking noise. The threshold measured on the plateau is the true threshold. In addition, there may be a portion of the curve with a slope less than that for the peripheral masking as a result of central masking, as illustrated in Figure 12.5. In some patients with conductive components to their hearing loss(es), the plateau may become so short that it is not identifiable. This is the so-called *masking dilemma*; in such cases it is impossible to evaluate hearing sensitivity fully using conventional masking methods.

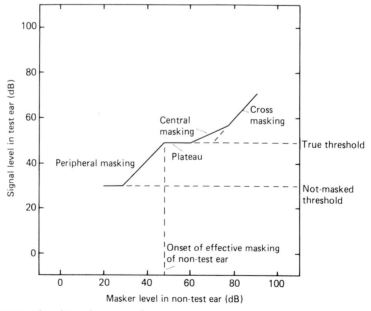

Figure 12.5 Idealized pattern of masking when a stimulus tone is presented to the test ear and a narrow-band masker is presented to the non-test ear. The signal level at the plateau represents the true threshold of the test ear

The possibility of a masking dilemma is reduced if the amount of cross-masking can be reduced. The main practicable method of achieving this is to use an insert earphone to deliver the masking noise. By virtue of the fact that a smaller area of the head is exposed to the masking noise, less energy is transmitted into the skull allowing a greater range of masking levels to be used (Studebaker, 1962). Killion (1985) has developed the ER-3A insert earphone system which gives approximately 40 dB more interaural attenuation at 0.25 and 0.5 kHz than a TDH-39 earphone, reducing to approximately 10 dB more at frequencies above 2 kHz. The main disadvantage of insert earphones in general is that their sensitivity is difficult to calibrate meaningfully as their output level depends on the individual ear canal characteristics, including the depth of insertion and the amount of acoustic leakage. Therefore, the masking procedure cannot rely on calibrated masking levels, but requires an individual biological calibration for each ear. In practice, the advantages of an insert receiver and the convenience of its use in conjunction with a bone-vibrator headband probably justify the small change in masking procedure necessary to accommodate its lack of calibration when measuring bone-conduction thresholds; given the problems with masking in bone-conduction audiometry, an increasing use of insert earphones may be expected. The use of ER-3A insert earphones will probably become more common following the inclusion of suitable calibration data in ISO 389 (International Organization for Standardization, 1991). For air conduction, the convenience of using a standard pair of earphones for signal and masker and the lesser incidence of air-conduction masking dilemmas probably militate against insert earphones for routine purposes.

Typical audiograms

Figure 12.6 illustrates several audiograms (all for right ears) which might be obtained in a typical clinic. Audiogram (*a*) depicts air-conduction and bone-conduction thresholds varying with frequencies between − 5 and + 10 dB hearing level which might be obtained in a normally hearing subject. Notice that the bone-conduction thresholds in this ear are systematically less sensitive than the air-conduction thresholds, giving negative values to the air-bone gap. This simply illustrates normal variation in the air-bone gap which is only an inexact measurement of the transmission loss through the middle ear, the true loss itself cannot be negative for purely physical reasons. Audiogram (*b*) shows a conductive hearing loss, which might have been caused by otitis media with effusion. Audiogram (*c*) illustrates a sensorineural hearing loss which increases steadily as a function of frequency, as sometimes found in age-related hearing loss. Audiogram (*d*) also shows a sensorineural loss at high frequencies, but sensitivity

is greater at 8 kHz than at 3, 4 or 6 kHz (that is the audiogram pattern shows a dip). This finding is common with sensorineural losses resulting from excessive noise exposure, but may occur for many other presumed aetiologies. Audiogram (*e*) indicates a profound hearing loss where hearing is only measurable at frequencies below 1 kHz. Even these threshold estimates must be treated with caution because of the possibility of vibration artefacts producing a tactile sensation (Boothroyd and Cawkwell, 1970), especially in the bone-conduction thresholds at lower test frequencies. Bone-conduction output was insufficient to give any response above 0.5 kHz as indicated by the arrows attached to the bone-conduction symbols. Such an audiogram might be obtained from an ear with a congenital impairment (e.g. caused by rubella) or accidental injury to the cochlea (e.g. the result of a skull fracture or failed ear surgery).

In addition to artefacts caused by tactile sensation, commercially available bone-vibrators cause significant air-borne radiation, particularly at 3 and 4 kHz. Data regarding air-borne radiation from the most common models of vibrator are given by Lightfoot (1979), Bell, Goodsell and Thornton (1980) and Shipton, John and Robinson (1980) together with suggestions for overcoming this problem in clinical practice, i.e. insertion of an earplug in the external auditory meatus of the test ear during bone-conduction measurements at 3 and 4 kHz (only).

Stenger check for non-organic hearing loss

Audiometric procedures assume that the patient responds genuinely to presented stimuli, as instructed. Clearly, if this assumption is not met, the audiometric results are of little value. Many social and psychological conditions can lead to a non-organic hearing loss, so the clinician must always be aware of the possibility. Often suspicion is justified if patients' communication abilities are inconsistent with the audiogram or if their responses are erratic. (Methods of checking the validity of audiometric thresholds are described in a later section.)

However, the existence of a unilateral non-organic hearing loss is more difficult to detect informally and can lead to a great deal of confusion and wasted time in attempts to obtain masked thresholds. Therefore, it is wise to use a simple check whenever asymmetry in air-conduction threshold of 20 dB or more occurs. This is the Stenger check (Coles and Priede, 1971) based on the more lengthy Stenger test described by Chaiklin and Ventry (1965), and involves presenting in-phase tones at the same frequency simultaneously to both ears (see also Chapter 17). In the ear with the better threshold, the tone is presented 5 dB above its apparent threshold and in the ear with the worse threshold it is presented 5 dB below its apparent

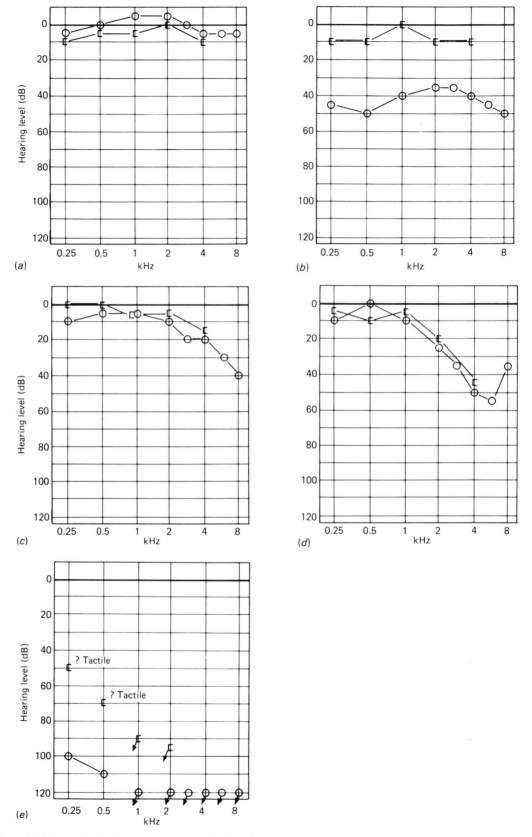

Figure 12.6 Examples of audiogram patterns, all for the right ear only (see text)

threshold. If the thresholds are genuine, the patient will respond because the tone in the better ear is above threshold. If the threshold in the worse ear is above his true threshold by more than 15 dB, the tone in the worse ear will dominate his perception and it will appear to him that the only stimulus is the one in his worse ear at a level below that at which he has chosen to respond. He will therefore not respond. Progressive reductions in the worse ear stimulus level and subsequent re-checks can be made until the patient eventually acknowledges hearing the signal (when the level in the worse ear is low enough for the tone to be heard in the better ear). This gives a rough estimate of the true difference in thresholds between ears. The method is by no means foolproof but is well worth the expenditure of about one minute for the check to reduce the possibility of confusion when carrying out the more difficult bone-conduction testing entailed by air-conduction asymmetries. It is important, however, that the test be carried out as an immediate extension of the audiometric procedure without indicating to the patient that a new test is commencing.

High-frequency audiometry

Conventional audiometric procedures and equipment are usually constrained to frequencies up to 8 kHz, although the normal young human ear can detect tones at frequencies up to approximately 20 kHz. Several studies have highlighted the importance of monitoring at frequencies in the 8–20 kHz range in patients receiving various ototoxic drugs (e.g. Jacobson, Downs and Fletcher, 1969; Osterhammel, 1980). It appears that the first signs of ototoxicity are usually evident at frequencies above 8 kHz and such changes have been recorded prospectively by Rappaport *et al.* (1986). It has also been suggested that high-frequency audiometry may be used as an indicator of hyperlipidaemia (Cunningham and Goetzinger, 1974).

The major constraint imposed by conventional audiometers involves the earphones. Typical supra-aural earphones have their major resonance frequency in the region of 6 kHz and they become much less sensitive as frequency increases beyond resonance. Despite the fact that they are only designed to operate at frequencies up to 8 kHz, by using a separate oscillator to generate the signal, conventional audiometers can be used to record thresholds reliably at frequencies up to 12 kHz (Rendell and Miller, 1983), despite some limitations on maximum output. At higher frequencies, a different type of earphone is essential. An audiometer is now commercially available which allows audiometry to be performed between 8 and 18 kHz. International Technical Commission (1994) specifies equipment for high-frequency audiometry, but no international

standards yet exist for calibration of output levels at these frequencies, although work is in progress on this matter. In the meantime, assessment of individuals must depend on biological baseline data obtained with the type of equipment in use.

Otoadmittance measurements (impedance)

After pure-tone audiometry, admittance measurements of the ear form the most commonly used set of tests in clinical audiology. They provide a simple and rapid method of obtaining objective information in a normal clinical environment using relatively simple equipment, as briefly reviewed by Lutman (1986).

Concepts of admittance and impedance

It is important for the clinician to have a basic understanding of the physical concepts which make possible the measurement of the mobility of middle-ear structures using the admittance technique in order that interpretation of the results can cater for all cases rather than just the few particular cases described in the textbooks. The term *acoustic admittance* as applied to the ear describes the mobility of the vibrating structures. Strictly, it is the ratio of the velocity of the middle-ear displacements to the applied sound pressure. It is measured at a low frequency, typically 220 Hz. A highly mobile ear will present a high admittance to an incoming sound wave (the probe tone) and an immobile ear will present a low admittance. The physical parameters governing the mobility (mass, stiffness, damping) influence the phase of the measured admittance as well as its amplitude; examination of admittance amplitude and phase together makes it possible to determine whether the motion of the ear structure is controlled mainly by mass, stiffness or damping (Lutman, 1985b; Lutman, McKenzie and Swan, 1985). The measured admittance contains contributions from the ear canal air volume, the tympanic membrane itself, the ossicular chain and ligaments and the loading of the ossicular chain by the cochlear fluids and the oval window membrane, although a more sophisticated type of analysis is necessary to estimate the contributions of the latter items separately. In most clinical instruments, phase information is discarded and admittance amplitude (modulus) is displayed. At low frequencies, the measured admittance is dominated by the stiffness-controlled component (positive susceptance). This is often referred to as *compliance* which is really a misnomer. However, the terminological error is unimportant here and it can be accepted that, *for low-frequency probe tones*, compliance and admittance modulus are practically synonymous. In fact, virtually all instruments which display readings on a compliance scale actually measure the admittance modulus.

The relevant unit of admittance is the c.g.s. millimho (mmho), but since hard-walled cavities are used to calibrate admittance meters and because 1 ml of air has an admittance very close to 1 mmho at 220 Hz, it is common practice to use only that frequency and to mark admittance meter scales in millilitres 'equivalent air volume'. This is acceptable for low-frequency probe tones for which the measured admittance is stiffness controlled, but causes difficulties for higher probe tone frequencies. The general class of otoadmittance meters is often referred to as impedance meters, impedance being the reciprocal of admittance. However, since most modern instruments give a reading of admittance modulus, the term *admittance* is more appropriate and is used throughout this chapter.

Measurement of admittance

A typical otoadmittance meter has a small probe unit which is sealed hermetically to the ear canal by means of a soft plastic cuff. The unit contains a miniature earphone, a microphone and an air line (Figure 12.7). The earphone generates the 220 Hz probe tone and the microphone measures the sound pressure level (SPL) in the ear canal. Circuitry in the instrument automatically adjusts the driving signal to the earphone in order to maintain a set level of approximately 85 dB. Because the sound pressure is kept constant, the admittance modulus at the tip of the probe is simply proportional to the earphone

driving signal required to maintain the set sound pressure level; for an ear with a high admittance, a large driving signal is required, and vice versa. Its amplitude is displayed by a meter against a calibrated scale.

Tympanometry

The admittance at the probe tip is the sum of the admittance of the ear-canal air volume and the admittance at the tympanic membrane. Strictly speaking, this is the complex (or vector) summation, but at 220 Hz it is sufficiently accurate to ignore phase and consider admittance modulus only. To obtain the admittance at the tympanic membrane it is first necessary to measure the ear canal admittance alone. This may be achieved by forcing the tympanic membrane admittance to decrease to near zero. This latter condition can be obtained practically by introducing a static pressure differential between the ear canal and the middle-ear cavity. This stresses the tympanic membrane and greatly reduces its mobility.

Once the ear canal admittance has been measured in this way, it can be subtracted from subsequent measurements to give the admittance in the plane of the tympanic membrane. The actual procedure to obtain these values is termed *tympanometry*. Usually the ear canal pressure is swept from approximately + 200 daPa (1 daPa = 1.02 mm H$_2$O) to − 200 daPa to plot out admittance as a function of ear canal pressure. This curve is the tympanogram (Figure 12.8). The peak of the curve corresponds to the condition where the tympanic membrane is most

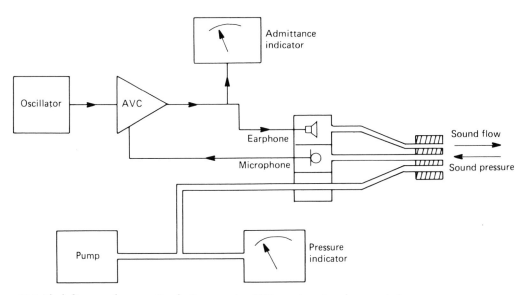

Figure 12.7 Block diagram of an acoustic admittance meter. AVC = automatic volume control

mobile, that is when the pressure differential across it is zero. By reading the ear canal pressure at which the peak occurs, an accurate estimate of the middle-ear pressure is obtained. The admittance at each end of the tympanogram curve approximates that of the ear canal air volume. The difference between the admittance at the peak and that at either end is a measure of middle-ear admittance. Obviously, if the eardrum is perforated, no dependence upon the pressure differential is obtained and a flat curve at a level representing the admittance of the combined volume of the ear canal and middle-ear cavity is obtained. Similarly a blocked probe gives a flat curve close to zero (see Figure 12.8).

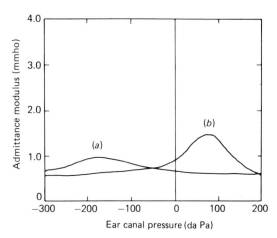

Figure 12.9 Typical tympanograms showing (*a*) negative and (*b*) positive middle-ear pressure

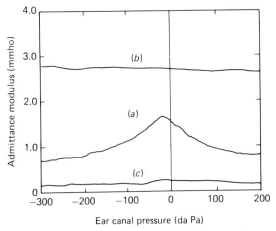

Figure 12.8 Typical tympanograms for (*a*) a normal ear, (*b*) an open tympanic membrane perforation and (*c*) a blocked admittance meter probe

The main abnormalities of the ear which affect the tympanogram involve dysfunction of the eustachian tube. Negative middle-ear pressure is observable directly from the tympanogram, as is the positive middle-ear pressure that occurs after autoinflation in the presence of a 'sticky' eustachian tube. Figure 12.9 illustrates these two conditions. The presence of fluid in the middle ear is also evident from the tympanogram as it reduces mobility leading to a rounded and flattened curve (Figure 12.9). The stapedial fixation occurring in otosclerosis causes a slight reduction in middle-ear admittance. However, because of the wide range obtained from normal ears (0.25–1.6 mmho; 90% range), otosclerotic ears are indistinguishable from normal, individually. Figure 12.10 is included to make this cautionary point; it shows tympanograms from a patient with subsequently confirmed bilateral otosclerosis where the middle-ear admittance is abnormally *high*, contrary to the expectation of reduced middle-ear admittance; in such a case, it is coincident hypermobility of the tympanic membrane (not observable otoscopically) which dominates the admittance measurement. It is possible that

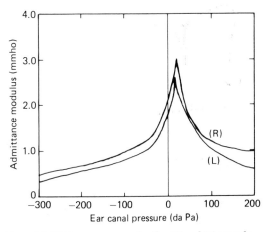

Figure 12.10 Tympanograms for the (R) and (L) ears of a 37-year-old woman with tympanic membranes of normal appearance and a bilateral conductive hearing loss. The clinical diagnosis was otosclerosis, which was later confirmed surgically

the hypermobility resulted from generalized thinning of tissues, including the tympanic membrane as part of the disease which is thought to be of mesenchymal origin (Bentzen, 1967).

A parallel situation occurs in osteogenesis imperfecta which Carruth, Lutman and Stephens (1978) have shown to be associated with hypermobility of the tympanic membrane. Patients with osteogenesis imperfecta have abnormally blue sclerae caused by their thinness allowing the pigmented choroid to show through, while blue sclerae have also been observed in patients with otosclerosis (Beales, 1981). It is evident that otosclerosis cannot be diagnosed on the basis of a shallow tympanogram, at least when a low-frequency probe tone is used. The situation may be more favourable when tympanograms recorded at both 220 and 660 Hz are available (Van Camp and Vogeleer, 1986).

Ossicular discontinuity reduces the loading on the tympanic membrane leading to increased middle-ear admittance, although the exact location of the disruption governs the magnitude of the effect. Discontinuities involving the malleus, incus, incudostapedial joint or both stapedial crura have a marked effect on the tympanic membrane, displaying abnormally high peaks. When only one crus is fractured, results within the normal range may be recorded. Table 12.1 gives a summary of the great diversity of diagnostic indications available from the tympanogram. Notice that a healed tympanic membrane perforation can have a profound effect on the middle-ear admittance as a consequence of the presence of a 'two-layer drum'. This is an example that can limit the diagnostic interpretation of middle-ear admittance measurements, and of which the clinician has to be aware, particularly as it is the more laterally located abnormality which dominates the tympanometric results from ears with multiple abnormalities. Nevertheless, the potential relevance of many features of the tympanogram to diagnosis has contributed to its routine use. The admittance meter is truly remarkable in being able to furnish this diversity while also, in appropriately simplified field versions, meeting the requirements of speed and simplicity necessary for screening tests.

In some clinics it has become common practice to categorize tympanograms with respect to shape, location of the peak and middle-ear admittance, using a classification scheme initially described by Jerger (1970). Their patterns are only applicable to low-frequency probe tones and are designated types A, B and C with some subclassifications of the A type. In the opinion of the present author, the use of such classification is unhelpful as it tends to camouflage

the underlying dimensions which the tympanogram describes. For a detailed description the reader is referred to the original article, or to the lucid explanation given by Hannley (1986). Further investigations of eustachian tube function are available using the impedance meter but are beyond the scope of this chapter. They have been reviewed by Holmquist (1976).

The acoustic reflex

A further powerful set of tests using the otoadmittance meter is a result of the fact that reflex middle-ear muscle contractions can be detected as a concomitant reduction in admittance. Most important is the reflex contraction of the stapedius muscle in response to sound stimulation – the acoustic reflex (for a review see Silman, 1984). The tendon of the stapedius muscle, which is situated in a bony cavity close to the oval window, passes out of the cavity and attaches to the neck of the stapes (Volume 1, Chapter 1). When the muscle contracts, it pulls in a direction perpendicular to the main axis of the ossicular chain so as to stiffen the chain, thus decreasing the admittance measured at the tympanic membrane. It is innervated by the stapedial branch of the facial nerve. Figure 12.11 illustrates, in an idealized form, the main components in the acoustic reflex arc as described by Borg (1973). The reflex is consensual in that sound stimulation of one side stimulates almost equal stapedius muscle contractions on both sides. Its purpose is not entirely clear, although at its present stage of evolution it probably has had more than one. Many theories have been presented and these are reviewed by Borg, Counter and Rosler (1984). There is little doubt that, when high intensity sounds are presented, the reflex acts to attenuate the transmission of low frequencies (Møller, 1964; Rabinowitz, 1977), so

Table 12.1 Summary of diagnostic information available from the tympanogram

Pathology	Tympanometric characteristics (220 Hz probe tone)
Otitis media with effusion	Negative middle-ear pressure. Flattened, rounded shape
Eustachian tube deficiency	Negative middle-ear pressure, occasionally positive after autoinflation
Patent eustachian tube	Pulsatile variation synchronous with respiration
Open perforation	Flat curve at high admittance value
Thinly healed perforation	Sharp high peak
Ossicular discontinuity	High peak, generally not so sharp as thinly healed perforation
Otosclerosis	Usually indistinguishable from normal
Sensorineural hearing impairment	Normal curve
Glomus tumour	Markedly pulsatile variations synchronous with heartbeat
Totally obstructed ear canal	Flat curve at low admittance value, or zero if the probe tube impinges on obstruction (or is blocked)
Tympanic membrane damped by wax, foreign body or debris	Flattened rounded shape, at normal middle-ear pressure (if normal eustachian tube function)
Palatal myoclonus	Irregular marked twitching in the admittance recordings
Osteogenesis imperfecta	Normal or high-peaked curve

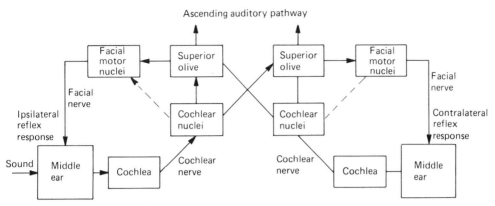

Figure 12.11 Block diagram showing the major direct pathways of the contralateral and ipsilateral acoustic reflexes. The arrows show the effect of stimulating the ear to the left of the figure which produces reflex contractions of the stapedius muscles on both sides. The dashed lines show a minor direct pathway on each side contributing only to ipsilateral reflexes

as to restrict the upward spread of masking from those frequencies; thus one function appears to be to maintain resolution in the presence of intense sound.

Acoustic reflex contractions of the stapedius muscle occur in normal ears for tones above approximately 85 dB hearing level, the strength of contraction increasing with stimulus intensity. The resultant admittance changes can be recorded on the ipsilateral or contralateral side with almost equal sensitivity (Green and Margolis, 1984).

For ipsilateral recording, the reflex-eliciting signal must be presented by way of the admittance meter probe and the instrument must therefore incorporate circuitry to prevent unwanted interactions between the signal and probe tone (artefacts). In practice, such artefacts are quite common for ipsilateral stimuli and can usually be identified because the instrument indicator 'goes the wrong way', apparently showing an admittance increase (Lutman and Leis, 1980). Contralateral artefacts due to interaural sound conduction (see above: cross-hearing) occur occasionally for stimulus frequencies of 0.5 and 1 kHz at intensities above about 105 dB hearing level using supra-aural earphones (Niswander and Ruth, 1976) and are more difficult to detect because the indicator 'goes the right way'. Lutman (1985a) has described a method of isolating contralateral artefacts with certain instrumentation capable of pulsing the stimulus. Essentially, since such instruments are able to measure admittance during the interpulse intervals, the artefact is avoided. Changing from the steady to the pulsed mode causes an artefactual indication to disappear, whereas a true response remains.

The diagnostic importance of acoustic reflex measurements should be considered in two separate ways. First, there is the ability to record reflex contractions of the stapedius muscle in the 'probe ear' which is a function of the efferent branch of the reflex arc governed mainly by the status of the middle ear on the

probe side, but also by the efferent innervation. Second, there is the effect of an impairment of the afferent portion of the reflex arc, that is the conductive apparatus, cochlea and auditory nerve on the 'stimulus ear'. Rarely, there may also be an identifiable central effect due to brain stem abnormality.

Effects on the acoustic reflex of pathology of the probe ear

Reduced mobility of the middle-ear structures, as caused by many types of conductive hearing loss, prevents the stapedius muscle contraction registering any further admittance decrease. As the magnitude of the conductive impairment increases, the likelihood of recording an acoustic reflex contraction decreases (Jerger *et al.*, 1974a; Lutman, 1984). Table 12.2 shows that an air-bone gap of 20 dB is associated with 50% incidence of abnormal reflexes, whereas for air-bone gaps over 35 dB the incidence increases to over 90%. Interestingly, a material incidence of

Table 12.2 Cross-tabulation of numbers of ears in each reflex presence category against air-bone gap

Air-bone gap (dB)	Acoustic reflex presence (ears)		
	Normal	*Elevated*	*Absent*
$\leqslant 0$	1312 (92%)	47 (3%)	72 (5%)
1–5	70 (89%)	2 (3%)	7 (9%)
6–10	43 (70%)	4 (7%)	14 (23%)
11–15	33 (65%)	3 (6%)	15 (29%)
16–20	24 (52%)	2 (4%)	20 (43%)
21–25	15 (43%)	1 (3%)	19 (54%)
26–30	5 (20%)	3 (12%)	17 (68%)
> 30	3 (6%)	0	45 (94%)

From Lutman (1984)

acoustic reflex abnormalities occurs with air-bone gaps that are clinically indistinguishable from normal, even when the afferent portion of the reflex arc is shown to be functional. This suggests that testing the efferent section of the acoustic reflex provides a more sensitive indicator of middle-ear abnormality than the air-bone gap. In this context, early otosclerosis has been coupled with a particular 'biphasic' pattern of acoustic reflex response (Flottorp and Djupesland, 1970). Table 12.2 also shows that reflexes are sometimes recorded in the presence of a large air-bone gap. In a few instances this has been shown to occur with ossicular discontinuity medial to the insertion of the stapedius tendon on the neck of the stapes, although such cases are too rare to explain the incidence in Table 12.2. Although the most common type of disorder in the probe ear affecting the measurement of acoustic reflexes is a conductive hearing loss, it should be remembered that neuromuscular disease affecting the stapedial branch of the facial nerve or the neuromuscular transmission at the stapedial muscle itself can also abolish the reflex. Examples are Bell's palsy and myasthenia gravis respectively.

Effect on the acoustic reflex of pathology of the stimulated ear

The main indicator of the functioning of the stimulated ear is the acoustic reflex threshold. Normal ranges are given in Table 12.3. Conductive impairment of the stimulated side can be considered as simple attenuation of the stimulus with consequent elevation of the acoustic reflex threshold, although 'conductive recruitment' has been demonstrated (Anderson and Barr, 1966), in which the elevation of the acoustic reflex threshold is less than the magnitude of the air-bone gap. With a sensory impairment of the stimulated side, the acoustic reflex threshold elevation is far less than the auditory threshold elevation, as shown in Table 12.4, in a manner analogous

to loudness recruitment (see below). However, with a peripheral neural type of loss, acoustic reflex thresholds are relatively more elevated as indicated in Table 12.4 and reflexes may well be unobtainable. Diagnostic criteria involving the acoustic reflex threshold have been proposed by Hirsch and Anderson (1980).

Further diagnostic information can be obtained by recording the reflex response to a prolonged stimulus. Neural types of disorder tend to display rapid adaption (reflex decay), possibly as a result of a mechanism similar to that involved in threshold tone decay (see below). Anderson, Barr and Wedenberg (1970) have suggested that 50% adaptation in less than 5 s for tones at 0.5 or 1 kHz presented at acoustic reflex threshold + 10 dB is indicative of a peripheral neural lesion (Figure 12.12), while some authors suggest a time of 10 s instead (Jerger *et al.*, 1974c; Olsen, Stach and Kurdziel, 1981). The former criterion has been coupled with acoustic reflex threshold criteria by Hirsch and Anderson (1980), and Cleaver and Stephens (1977) have extended the decay criterion to encompass wide-band noise stimulation. Reflex decay amounting to 50% in 5 s at frequencies of 2 kHz and above occasionally occurs in normal ears or ears with sensory types of hearing loss and hence has no significance as an indicator of neural involvement (Fowler and Wilson, 1984).

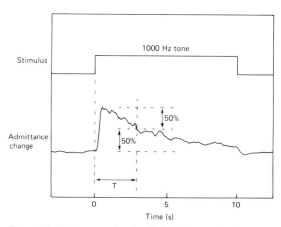

Figure 12.12 An example of pathological acoustic reflex decay. If the time *T* is less than 5 s, reflex decay is considered to be indicative of a peripheral neural lesion

Finally, an estimate of auditory threshold may be obtained by comparing acoustic reflex thresholds for different types of stimulus, provided the possibility of a conductive element has been excluded. (It is tacitly assumed that neural types of loss are sufficiently rare to be ignored in this context.) Most predictive methods utilize the principle of Niemeyer and Sesterhenn (1974) and Jerger *et al.* (1974b) of comparing acoustic reflex thresholds for pure tones and for noise stimuli – the larger the tonal-noise acoustic reflex threshold difference, the better the predicted thresh-

Table 12.3 Normal range of contralateral acoustic reflex threshold measured under laboratory conditions

	Frequency (kHz) (dB HL)				Wide-band noise (dB SPL)
	0.5	1	2	4	
Mean	83	84	83	85	76
Standard deviation (dB)	5	5	5	6	8

Under typical clinical conditions, using 5-dB steps, acoustic reflex threshold is approximately 4–5 dB less sensitive than above for pure tones and 8–9 dB less sensitive for noise (Gelfand, 1984)

Table 12.4 Effect of cochlear hearing losses on the acoustic reflex threshold level

	Pure tone hearing threshold (dB)							
	20/25	*30/35*	*40/45*	*50/55*	*60/65*	*70/75*	*80/85*	*90/95*
Acoustic reflex threshold (dB HL)								
Lower quartile	80	80	80	85	90	95	100	105
Median	85	90	95	100	105	110	115	120

Neural lesions: Acoustic reflex threshold virtually always above C_{25}. Acoustic reflex threshold above C_{60} in over 80% of neural lesions.
Modified from Priede and Coles (1974)

old. A wide variety of formulae has been developed and these are extensively reviewed by Popelka (1981) and by Silman *et al.* (1984). It should be noted that while these formulae may be accurate in discriminating between normal and impaired ears when the subject pool has bimodal distribution of normal and moderately/severely impaired ears, a high proportion of errors is to be expected if they are used in an unselected population, where there is likely to be a preponderance of normal and mildly impaired ears.

Effects on the acoustic reflex of central nervous system pathology

The central section of the acoustic reflex involves the cochlear nuclei and superior olive (see Figure 12.11). There are also probably other polysynaptic pathways involving other regions of the central nervous system. One particular pattern of acoustic reflex results is strongly indicative of a central abnormality: when ipsilateral reflex responses are recorded normally on both sides, abnormalities of a contralaterally stimulated reflex must arise in the central crossing pathways. Several such case studies are presented by Hall (1985) based on studies by Jerger and Jerger (1977). Similarly, contralateral acoustic reflex decay has been shown to be excessive with brain stem lesions in the absence of cochlear nerve involvement. A useful future development would be to compare ipsilateral and contralateral reflex decay in the same individual for this purpose.

Brain stem pathology has also been associated with alterations to the dynamics of the acoustic reflex response (Borg, 1973; Bosatra, Russolo and Poli, 1975; Colletti, 1975; Jerger and Jerger, 1977). However, most of these studies have been contaminated by instrumentation limitations whereby reduced response amplitude may have been the cause of the reported latency increases. Until apparatus with more rapid response characteristics is developed, this promising area of research will be difficult to interpret. More detailed consideration of central nervous system pathology is given in Chapter 11.

Speech audiometry
Speech audiometry in quiet

While hearing impairment in general may be adequately characterized in most cases by the pure-tone audiogram, there are certain types of disorder in which speech discrimination and the audiogram are discrepant. Excessive loss of discrimination, for example, is a feature of neural types of hearing loss; this makes comparison of pure-tone and speech test results a potentially useful tool in differential diagnosis. Also, since the patient will usually judge his own hearing acuity, at least in part, by his ability to understand speech, it is appropriate to measure this ability directly.

Clinical speech audiometry in most countries involves obtaining word-identification scores for pre-recorded lists of phonetically balanced monosyllables (usually consonant-vowel-consonant), or spondees, at various intensity levels. Examples of frequently used English word lists are the Boothroyd (1968) and CID W-22 (Newby, 1979) lists. Figure 12.13 illustrates the type of chart used to plot the results. Scoring may be in terms of phonemes or words correctly repeated. A performance-intensity curve for a normally hearing ear rises steeply from low to high scores as speech intensity increases (Figure 12.13, curve *a*). Notice that the abscissa is graduated in relative decibels, the actual values being a function of the method of scoring, as well as the characteristics of the equipment, tape recording and method of connecting the tape recorder output to the audiometer. It is convenient to include the stereotype normal curve on the chart to aid interpretation for persons not familiar with the procedure and equipment used. Curve (*b*) is typical of a sensory hearing loss. The shift to the right compared with normal reflects the loss of sensitivity, while the fact that the curve does not reach 100% indicates a lack of discrimination. Curve (*c*) indicates a loss of sensitivity coupled with a very low maximum discrimination score, typical of a peripheral-neural type of loss. The sensitivity feature of the speech audiogram is usually measured at the 50% point on the performance-

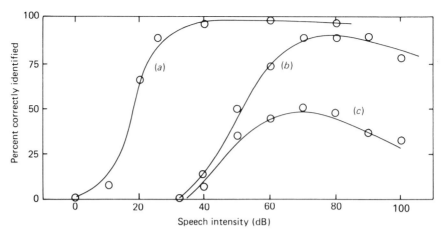

Figure 12.13 Typical speech audiograms for (*a*) a normal ear, (*b*) an ear with a sensory type of impairment, and (*c*) an ear with a peripheral-neural type of impairment. Adequate masking of the non-test ear is assumed

intensity curve, the speech reception threshold. Alternatively, it may be measured at a point corresponding to a score which is half of the maximum obtained for that ear, the half-peak level. This allows the neural type curves, as shown in Figure 12.13, to be categorized more conveniently.

The loss of discrimination may be characterized by the maximum score obtained, the optimal discrimination score, sometimes referred to as PB-max, when phonetically balanced word lists are used, usually tested at 35 dB above the speech reception threshold. The assessment of PB-max is often used as a quick test of speech discrimination ability. The decrement of this point from 100%, the discrimination loss, is also used to describe the maximum score.

Conductive hearing losses cause an elevation of the speech reception threshold or half-peak level without a concomitant reduction in optimal discrimination score. Most types of sensorineural loss cause speech reception or half-peak level elevations together with reductions in optimal discrimination score, the principal exception being sensory hearing losses restricted to frequencies above 1 kHz for which the speech reception threshold is often normal. The distinction between sensory and neural types is merely probabilistic and is most clearly illustrated by plotting individual data against bivariate coordinates such as shown in Figure 12.14. The curve in Figure 12.14 divides the bivariate space into sensory and peripheral-neural regions and allows individual results to be interpreted accordingly. A further indication of peripheral-neural involvement is given by the shape of the performance-intensity curve at high intensities. A marked reduction in score with increasing intensity ('rollover') is suggestive of a peripheral-neural type of loss (Jerger and Jerger, 1971).

The possibility of cross-hearing applies equally to speech audiometry and pure-tone audiometry; this is often overlooked. For speech stimuli and supra-aural audiometric earphones, it can be assumed that the effective interaural attenuation will not fall below 50 dB. Given that pure-tone sensitivity of each ear has been fully established, the level of masking noise can be calculated for each speech level, using this assumption, by means of a formula which takes into account the calibration of the speech and noise materials and the characteristics of the broad-band masking noise (usually 'speech-shaped' in its frequency spectrum). Cross-hearing can have particularly adverse consequences when the worse ear has poor discrimination; the leakage of even a severely attenuated signal to the better cochlea can boost the identification score markedly. Thus, masking must be used in *all* patients according to the formula.

Comparison of the pure-tone audiogram and the sensitivity loss evident on the speech audiogram provides a check for non-organic hearing loss (see also Chapters 8 and 17), and often indicates the true threshold of hearing in cases where the pure-tone thresholds are spurious, especially in children (Coles, 1982). The elevation of the half-peak level is generally within ± 10 dB of the average of the best two pure-tone thresholds in the range 0.25–4 kHz in organic disorders (Coles, Markides and Priede, 1973; Markides, 1980; Coles, 1982).

Speech-in-noise tests

Speech-in-noise tests are thought to give a better indication of potential disability than speech-in-quiet because they represent more faithfully the circumstances in which difficulties are encountered. They

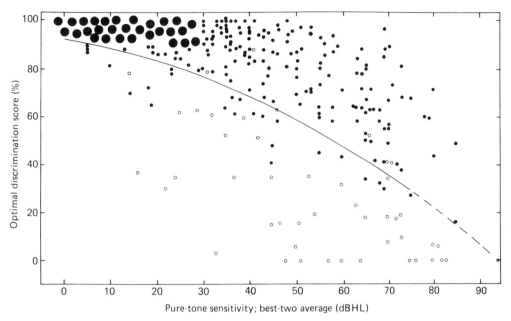

Figure 12.14 Optimal discrimination scores as a function of pure-tone sensitivity for ears with primarily sensory (● = 1 case, ⬤ = 10 cases) and primarily neural (○ = 1 case) cases. Pure-tone sensitivity is measured as the average of the best two pure-tone thresholds (500–2000 Hz). The solid curve represents the criterion which divides the two groups of data. (Modified from Coles, Markides and Priede, 1973, by courtesy of the authors and publisher)

also tap hearing functions such as frequency and temporal resolution to a much greater extent than does speech-in-quiet. However, self-reported disability does not seem to relate particularly well to scores on speech-in-noise tests when compared with the pure-tone audiogram (Tyler and Smith, 1983; Lutman, Brown and Coles, 1987), nor to frequency resolution ability (Lutman, 1983). Furthermore, little standardization of speech-in-noise tests has yet been achieved. Speech-in-noise tests are therefore of somewhat limited clinical utility at present, particularly in the context of diagnostic audiometry, although they have been used in the identification of central-neural types of disorder and obscure auditory dysfunction/auditory disability with normal hearing (see Chapter 11). The use of speech testing for the assessment of disability has been reviewed by Lutman (1987).

Further voluntary test techniques for differential diagnosis

Pure-tone audiometry, otoadmittance tests and speech audiometry form the main armoury of tests for basic audiological investigations. They are capable of distinguishing between conductive and sensorineural types of impairment. They also provide an opportunity to identify peripheral-neural and non-organic types of dysfunction. In addition, a wider array

of voluntary test techniques is available which may add information that can be used to differentiate further between sensory, peripheral-neural and central-neural types. However, they are of limited diagnostic accuracy and have been largely supplanted by objective test techniques, mainly involving auditory brain stem responses (ABR), and are outlined only briefly below. Nonetheless, in so far as such tests describe the functional performance of the auditory system, they may also be used to assist rehabilitation, especially definition of the required characteristics of hearing aids. They are grouped below under headings of intensity resolution, frequency and temporal resolution, adaptation and tests of central auditory processing, although there are inevitable overlaps since many tests measure more than one function.

Intensity resolution

Intensity resolution involves the ability of the ear to resolve sounds at different intensities. Also in the intensity domain is the assignment of loudness to sounds of different intensities. *Loudness recruitment* is the term applied to the abnormally steep growth of loudness with increasing intensity, usually associated with sensorineural hearing loss. In cochlear disorders, it has been claimed to result from the loss of tuning within the cochlea resulting from malfunction of the hair cells (Evans, 1975; Salvi *et al.*, 1983), but more recent evidence indicates that recruitment is independent of tuning (Moore *et al.*, 1985) and is probably present in the non-linear micromechanical behaviour of the cochlear partition (see below: otoacoustic emissions). As a result of recruitment, a tone at (say) 50 dB in a sensorineurally impaired ear may be close to threshold and have minimal loudness, whereas a tone at 90 dB may be just as loud as in a normal ear. Thus, the dynamic range of the ear is compressed. A practical consequence of this is that simple amplification of sound, for example by a basic hearing aid, cannot restore normal loudness to all sounds; if enough amplification is provided to compensate for the threshold loss, more intense sounds will be too loud.

Several types of test may be used to give a measure of the amount of loudness recruitment, either directly or indirectly. It is the *amount* of recruitment which is the critical diagnostic factor, not merely the presence or absence of recruitment. These tests include the alternate binaural loudness balance test (Fowler, 1936), which identifies intensities of sound presented to each ear that are equally loud, and measuring the lower and upper limits of the dynamic range (i.e. absolute threshold and threshold of uncomfortable loudness). A more direct indicator of intensity resolution is the short-increment sensitivity index which measures the ability of the subject to detect 1-dB intensity modulations in a suprathreshold tone (Jerger, Shedd and Harford, 1959).

As in the interpretation of speech audiograms, the distinction between sensory and neural types is a probabilistic one. In general, the greater the amount of recruitment, the less is the probability of a peripheral-neural disorder. However, because the tests themselves are not very specific, and also because sensory and peripheral-neural pathology commonly occur together, tests of recruitment have severely limited diagnostic accuracy. The reason for their development and use arises primarily from the lack of practical alternatives in previous decades.

Frequency and temporal resolution

In recent years, attention has been focused on the measurement of several aspects of auditory processing and the manner in which they vary with hearing impairment. A great deal of research has concentrated on their measurement in normally hearing subjects and on methodological developments. Of particular interest are the properties of frequency resolution and temporal resolution (see above for definitions), in so far as they appear to be related to speech discrimination. Methods of measurement have also been adapted to suit clinical circumstances (Zwicker and Schorn, 1978; Lutman and Wood, 1985). Many studies have demonstrated that both frequency resolution and temporal resolution are impaired in cases of

sensorineural hearing loss (e.g. de Boer and Bouwmeester, 1974; Pick, Evans and Wilson, 1977; Wightman, McGee and Kramer, 1977) and that in such cases speech discrimination is also impaired (e.g. Leshowitz, 1977; Tyler *et al.*, 1982; Festen and Plomp, 1983). Whether the loss of speech discrimination ability is a result of the loss of sensitivity, the loss of resolution, or both is extremely difficult to determine unequivocally (Lutman and Clark, 1986; Lutman, 1991), given that all of these effects tend to covary. However, at present it appears that most of the speech discrimination loss can be accounted for by correlation with the loss of sensitivity in cases of moderate sensorineural hearing loss with possibly a lesser independent resolution factor also having some influence.

Very few studies have compared these resolution measures in patients with different types of hearing loss and therefore their diagnostic utility at present is limited. Temporal resolution deteriorates with sensorineural hearing loss, and Efron *et al.* (1985) have shown a monaural degradation of gap detection in the ear contralateral to temporal lobe insult. If there is an association between frequency resolution and recruitment, as has been proposed on theoretical grounds (Evans, 1975; Salvi *et al.*, 1983), it is to be expected that abnormal frequency resolution should occur in sensory types of hearing loss, but not in conductive nor in peripheral-neural types. The limited data available to date confirm the expectation for conductive impairments. However, critical band measures of frequency resolution in 11 cases of acoustic neuroma tested by Bonding (1979) were indistinguishable from those in Menières disorder, although there was some correlation between critical bandwidth and recruitment. However, the fact that the critical bandwidth procedure used by Bonding was also unable to distinguish between ears with moderate-severe hearing loss due to Menière's disorder and normal ears cast some doubt on the sensitivity of the method, and consequently on the validity of this null result. The association between measures of recruitment and frequency resolution in patients undergoing neuro-otological investigation has been addressed directly by Smith and Ferguson (1994), who were unable to show any correlation once the effects of covariation with hearing threshold level had been accounted for. Hence, the diagnostic utility of frequency resolution tests, although theoretically promising, is unsupported by experimental evidence to date. There are stronger grounds for believing that such measures are useful in assessment prior to rehabilitation. For example, Haggard, Lindbald and Foster (1986) indicated that frequency resolution is at least as powerful a predictor as pure-tone threshold of the hearing-aid frequency response giving the higher speech discrimination score, when a 'flat' and a 'rising' response are compared.

Auditory adaptation (tone decay)

Adaptation is the decrease with time in sensitivity or responsiveness of a system during prolonged stimulation and is traditionally measured for clinical audiological purposes by threshold tone decay tests. It has been known for more than a century that patients with tumours affecting the auditory nerve demonstrate abnormally rapid adaptation to a crude audiometric stimulus (Gradenigo, 1893). Modern tests employ the pure-tone output of an audiometer. The tone is presented continuously at a level at, or slightly above, threshold while the patient indicates whether it is heard. In the procedure described by Carhart (1957), each time the tone becomes inaudible, its level is immediately increased in level by 5 dB without switching off the tone. The test continues until one level is heard for 60 seconds. An alternative procedure has been described by Hood (1956). The result of the test has been expressed as the total of the 5 dB increments. In normal ears, some adaptation is measurable at high frequencies (e.g. 4 kHz). However, at lower frequencies the test gives more useful diagnostic results, with neural types of loss being characterized by tone decay in excess of 25 dB (Rosenberg, 1969). In some neural cases adaptation may be extremely rapid as well as excessive. For the same reason as for speech audiometry, masking of the non-test ear is essential. An objective analogue of the threshold tone decay test is the acoustic reflex decay test (see above).

As an alternative to tone decay tests, adaptation may be assessed by means of Békésy audiometry (Jerger, 1960). This is a form of self-recording (tracking) audiometry in which the tone frequency is swept continuously from low to high over a period of several minutes. Two modes of signal presentation are used on separate sweeps. Using a continuous tone, adaptation takes place and the apparent threshold at any point is the sum of the actual threshold at the tone frequency and the cumulative adaptation within the relevant frequency band. When the tone is pulsed, in the intermittent mode, adaptation is effectively obliterated by the silent intervals between the tone pulses. A measure of adaptation is, therefore, the elevation of threshold in the continuous mode compared with the intermittent mode, although it is difficult to determine quantitatively for a particular frequency because of indeterminate factors such as the spread of adaptation from low frequencies to high and the variations in actual stimulus level during the procedure. The former difficulty is removed if a fixed frequency test is performed, as described by Jerger (1960). The width of the Békésy tracing is claimed to give an indirect measure of recruitment (see above). Better thresholds for the continuous than for the intermittent presentation are taken as an indication of non-organic hearing loss (Jerger and Herer, 1961). As with other behavioural tests, differential diagnostic accuracy is limited, and tests of adaptation have been largely superseded by objective tests, especially ABR measurement.

Auditory evoked potential tests

Advances in knowledge of auditory evoked potentials (AEP) and of technology for their measurement have made it possible to conduct various types of AEP tests in the audiology clinic. Increasingly AEP tests are being used as an adjunct to routine diagnostic testing, in addition to their use as a further diagnostic test performed by specialist departments. This section focuses on the two most commonly used types of AEP, the auditory brain stem response (ABR) and the auditory cortical response (ACR) measured during cortical electrical response audiometry (CERA). The former is used for objective threshold estimation and differential diagnostic purposes, whereas the latter is restricted primarily to threshold estimation. Detailed description of the origins of the various AEPs and methodology for their measurement is outside the scope of this short section, which concentrates on the practical use of CERA and ABR measurement and broad interpretation of their results. A fuller description of AEP testing generally is given by Hyde (1987) and an excellent account of ABR measurement has recently been published by Mason (1993).

As employed for routine audiological assessment, AEP measurements involve recording from surface electrodes placed on the scalp or other parts of the head. Hence, the recorded potentials are in the far field, well displaced from the generator sites in the brain stem and cortex. As a consequence, the potentials are small compared with other ongoing electrical activity, and specialized apparatus is required to record satisfactory waveforms. Three parallel approaches are used to improve signal-to-noise ratio. First, filtering is employed to restrict the recording bandwidth to that containing the important components of the signal. Second, repeated stimulation with synchronous time-domain averaging is used to increase the amplitude of components that are time-locked to the stimulus (signal) relative to other random components (noise). In practice these two processes are achieved by connecting the electrodes to a special pre-amplifier with appropriate filter settings and passing the output to a time-domain averager. Many proprietary systems are available to achieve this, some being based on general-purpose microcomputers. Third, stimulus polarity is alternated. This leads to polarity alternation of any recorded components that are directly related to the stimulus waveform, but not of neurological response components. The former include electrical artefacts generated by the stimulus earphone. The effect of averaging is to eliminate such components without diminishing the neurological responses. The standard electrode configuration for both ABR and CERA testing involves a non-inverting electrode placed on the vertex of the head and an inverting electrode placed on the earlobe or mastoid prominence of the test ear. For two-channel recording of bilateral responses, inverting electrodes are placed on both sides of the head, while a common non-inverting electrode is used for both channels. A further electrode referred to as the 'earth' or 'guard' is generally required for the proper functioning of the pre-amplifier, and is usually placed on the forehead.

As suggested by its name, the ABR is considered to originate from the auditory brain stem. It has several components, as seen by the standard electrode configuration, consisting of a series of peaks and troughs, as illustrated in Figure 12.15. The positive peaks (vertex positive) are commonly referred to by the roman numerals I–VII, and are considered to originate from the following anatomical sites in man (Møller and Jannetta, 1985): cochlear nerve (waves I and II), cochlear nucleus (III), superior olivary complex (IV), nuclei of lateral lemniscus (V), inferior colliculus (VI and VII). These peaks occur most readily in response to click stimulation over a period from approximately 1 to 10 ms after the stimulus in ears of adults with normal hearing. By contrast, the ACR is a more generalized response originating from the cortex with components occurring between 50 and 300 ms after the onset of stimulation. The ACR is generally elicited with a tone burst lasting approximately 200 ms. Hence, CERA gives responses that are frequency specific. By contrast, ABR measurement has limited frequency specificity, although the response is considered to arise primarily from activity generated by the high-frequency components of the broadband stimulus.

Threshold estimation

Objective threshold estimation is required in cases where results from behavioural (subjective) tests may be in doubt. CERA is the procedure of choice because of its frequency specificity and the close correlation between behavioural threshold and the minimum stimulus level that gives a recordable response. However, CERA has certain limitations that are important in practice. It can only be carried out satisfactorily in unsedated awake subjects who are prepared to cooperate by keeping still. This effectively precludes its use in children below the age of about 8 years and occasionally in some adults. The ABR technique is the most appropriate for use in such subjects.

Interpretation of CERA is relatively straightforward. Threshold is defined as the minimum stimulus level that gives a consistently identifiable response component in the recorded waveform on repeated averaging runs. One strategy is to conduct three averaging runs and also form a grand average by combining the three sub-averages. For the response

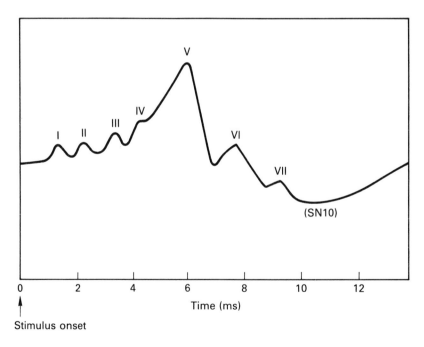

Figure 12.15 Typical auditory brain stem response (ABR) waveform showing the various identifiable peaks, indicated by roman numerals I–VII. Vertex positive potential shown upwards

to be counted as present, a waveform component in the grand average must be present in at least two of the sub-averages. Provided the stimuli are presented via appropriately calibrated earphones, CERA thresholds can be compared directly with thresholds determined by (behavioural) pure tone audiometry. Agreement within ± 10 dB is to be expected in more than 90% of cases when averaged across a number of frequencies.

Requirements for masking of the non-test ear are identical to those for pure-tone audiometry. However, it is inappropriate to use a plateau-seeking method to determine the amount of masking used, in view of the extended time necessary to measure each CERA threshold. Instead, a procedure similar to that used for speech audiometry (see above) based on a formula is used, although narrow-band noise masking is required. Particular care is required when there may be a conductive component to the hearing loss on the non-test ear, but behavioural pure tone thresholds are in doubt. In such cases it is useful to use tympanometry and acoustic reflex testing (see above) to gain further information about the possibility of a conductive hearing loss before conducting CERA. When the results of pure-tone audiometry are unknown or of doubtful validity, it is acceptable to use a level of masking noise that is between 30 and 40 dB below the level of the stimulus.

When CERA cannot be used, ABR measurement can be used to estimate threshold by measuring the lowest stimulus level at which it is possible to identify a response. The largest and most robust component of the ABR is the wave V and SN10 complex. Recording bandwidth can be set to emphasize this component at the expense of the fine detail of other waves. Because the ABR is resistant to the effects of sleep, sedation and anaesthesia, it is suitable for children and for adults who are not able to cooperate for CERA. The subject can be tested while lying quietly awake, in sleep entered naturally or under sedation, or anaesthetized, as appropriate. Under good recording conditions, click ABR threshold should be within 10 dB of behavioural threshold for the click. A degree of frequency specificity can be obtained by using tone-pip stimuli, which is useful to add some information about hearing in the mid-frequencies, say at 1 kHz. However, correspondence with behavioural threshold is poorer for such stimuli.

For all types of AEP measurement, it is important to obtain the best possible recording conditions. In particular, the electrodes should be applied in such a way as to give a low contact impedance and the subject should be positioned, either sitting or lying, to be comfortable and to minimize muscular activity that may interfere with the signal. Contact impedance should be measured for every pair of electrodes and must be below 5 kΩ (preferably 2 kΩ). In all instances, the results should be accompanied by a report of the recording conditions that were achieved.

Electrophysiological tests for differential diagnosis

The use of objective testing for differential diagnostic purposes encompasses a range of complexity from simple to highly specialized. This section is restricted to consideration of simple electrophysiological testing by measurement of the ABR that can be accomplished in the routine audiology clinic. As such, it may be considered to be primarily a screening test. Patients found to be unequivocally 'normal' will be considered to have passed the screen, whereas patients who have marginal or abnormal results will be referred for further testing by more specialized electrophysiological or other tests. As with all such tests, accuracy of screening depends on an adequate degree of skill to administer the test properly, to make appropriate contingent decisions during testing and to interpret the results. Frequent performance of the test is necessary to maintain an adequate level of skill.

One of the most important dimensions of diagnostic distinction facing the audiologist is between cochlear and retrocochlear disease. The former is far more prevalent, but the latter has such potentially severe consequences for the patient that it deserves special attention. In particular, retrocochlear disease includes cerebellopontine angle tumours of which the acoustic neuroma (vestibulocochlear schwannoma) is the most common. The clinical presentation of cerebellopontine angle tumours typically involves progressive unilateral hearing loss or tinnitus without obvious cause, although presentation is variable and may alternatively involve neurological signs such as facial weakness or dysequilibrium, or combinations of the above. Any of these signs are an indication for appropriate differential diagnostic screening. A suitable criterion for asymmetry of hearing would be a difference between the ears of 15 dB averaged over the frequencies 0.5–4 kHz, or 20 dB averaged over any two adjacent audiometric frequencies. The relative efficiency of electrophysiological and other tests in screening for cerebellopontine angle tumours is addressed later in this chapter.

Screening entails measurement of the ABR elicited by clicks at a typical rate of 10 per second and at a relatively high intensity, typically 80–90 dB normal hearing level (nHL).[3] The objective is to obtain a clear waveform allowing peaks I to V to be identified on both sides and measured in terms of amplitude and latency. In practice, it is often not possible to identify all peaks. As a minimum, wave V must be identifiable

---

[3] Normal hearing level is the intensity relative to behavioural threshold obtained in an adequately large sample of young adults with normal hearing threshold levels for the particular equipment and stimulus characteristics in use (i.e. a biological baseline).

and preferably wave I should also be evident. The principle of the test is based on knowledge that retrocochlear lesions lead to a reduction in amplitude and an attendant increase in latency of responses originating from sections of the auditory pathway central to the lesion. Reference to the sites of origin of the various waves constituting the ABR (see above) indicates that cerebellopontine angle tumours will affect waves III–VII. In practice, increased latency of wave V provides the most robust indicator. The performance of the screening test can be improved in either of two ways by using the subject as his own control. First, assuming that lesions will be unilateral in most cases, comparison of wave V latencies of the two ears is more sensitive than comparing one ear with appropriate control subjects. Second, examination of the difference in latency between waves I and V removes the effect of intersubject variation of processes peripheral to the lesion.

It is not possible to state universal criteria for any of the above test outcomes. Both latency and amplitude measures depend critically on characteristics of the stimulus and, more importantly, the recording apparatus. In particular, the phase response of filters affects measured latencies in a way that is difficult to correct for *post hoc*. Hence, interpretation of results inevitably involves reference to a sample of control subjects tested on the same equipment under similar conditions and with identical stimuli. Ideally, separate control groups of males and females should be gathered, and their results applied separately according to the sex of the test subject.

However, as a general guide, normal interaural latency differences (ILD) have been reported to have a mean of zero and a standard deviation of 0.2 ms (Selters and Brackman, 1979). Values in the range ±0.3 ms might be regarded as normal. Latency differences between waves I and V are typically reported to be of the order of 4 ms. Deviations from the control population mean in excess of approximately 0.3 ms could be considered to constitute a fail of the screening test. A similar criterion could be applied to deviations of absolute wave V latency from the control population mean.

Interpretation of ABR results is complicated by coexistence of either conductive or sensory (cochlear) impairment. Conductive hearing loss leads to a reduction in effective stimulus intensity. Either this or sensory impairment leads to reduced response amplitude and increased latency. Various methods have been proposed to allow for such coexistence, but in the screening context they are best avoided. The effects of conductive or sensory hearing loss on the performance of the screen will be a loss of specificity: more patients will be referred for further testing than otherwise. This is preferable to the loss of sensitivity that might occur if inappropriate corrections were applied.

Otoacoustic emissions

The term otoacoustic emission describes releases of acoustic energy from the cochlea recorded in the external ear. They have been reviewed by Probst, Lonsbury-Martin and Martin (1991) and Cope and Lutman (1993). The release of energy may be spontaneous or evoked by sound stimulation. Otoacoustic emissions are considered to originate from active processes involving motile properties of the outer hair cells of the cochlea that are part of their normal function. Spontaneous otoacoustic emissions are generally continuous low-intensity tones that are not heard by the subject and are recordable in approximately half the population of ears with normal hearing. Evoked otoacoustic emissions are recordable in three categories: transient otoacoustic emissions or 'cochlear echoes' follow stimulation by a click or brief tone burst; distortion-product otoacoustic emissions occur at intermodulation frequencies when two or more tones are presented to the ear simultaneously; stimulus-frequency otoacoustic emissions occur at the same frequency as a stimulus and are most readily demonstrated by sweeping a low-intensity tone across a range of frequencies to reveal a pattern of peaks and troughs as stimulus and stimulus-frequency otoacostic emissions reinforce and cancel. Evoked otoacostic emissions are present in virtually all ears with normal hearing, given adequate recording conditions. Of these three types, the transient otoacoustic emissions have been studied most widely in clinical populations and are the principal contender as a diagnostic tool at the present time. The following paragraphs are restricted to the clinical application of transient otoacoustic emissions.

The diagnostic possibilities of transient otoacoustic emissions lie in their association with normal outer hair cell function and the fact that they are abolished by cochlear impairments exceeding approximately 25 dB HL (e.g. Probst *et al.*, 1987; Lutman, 1989). At the simplest level, recording of evoked acoustic emissions may be used as a screening test, or cross-check, of normal hearing. The most widely used clinical application has involved recording transient otoacoustic emissions in neonates as a hearing screening test (Stevens *et al.*, 1991). The presence of a transient otoacoustic emission in response to click stimulation indicates normal cochlear function at least at some frequencies, most likely in the 1–3 kHz range. Hence, neonates demonstrating transient otoacostic emissions can be considered to have functionally adequate hearing and are therefore not candidates for early hearing aid fitting. A similar logic can be applied to the use of transient otoacoustic emissions as a cross-check of pure tone thresholds to screen for non-organic hearing loss.

Transient otoacoustic emissions may also be used for differential diagnosis of cochlear and retrocochlear disorder. In cases of substantial retrocochlear disorder without cochlear involvement transient otoacoustic emissions should be recordable because outer hair cell function is unaffected. This may occur despite the presence of sensorineural hearing loss that would abolish the transient otoacoustic emissions if the disorder were cochlear. The fact that such cases exist was demonstrated by Lutman, Mason and Sheppard (1989) who recorded strong transient otoacoustic emissions in an ear with a profound (retrocochlear) hearing loss. The possibility of using transient otoacoustic emissions to assist in the diagnosis of cerebellopontine angle tumours has been explored by Bonfils and Uziel (1988). This application is complicated by the fact that the tumour often leads to collateral cochlear damage by reducing its blood supply via the internal auditory artery. Cane, Lutman and O'Donoghue (1994) examined 45 cases of confirmed cerebellopontine angle tumours. Twenty-four had no recordable transient otoacoustic emissions, while nine had recordable transient otoacoustic emissions and best-hearing thresholds consistent with either a cochlear or a retrocochlear disorder. However, 12 cases had recordable transient otoacoustic emissions despite best-hearing thresholds in excess of 25 dB HL. This latter combination provides definitive evidence of retrocochlear disorder. In several of the cases that had been studied prospectively, this had been the strongest indication of a cerebellopontine angle tumour, prior to electrophysiological and imaging studies.

Transient otoacoustic emissions can be recorded easily and rapidly in the routine audiology clinic, without active participation by the subject. It is recommended that all patients with a sensorineural hearing impairment of unknown origin should undergo testing for transient otoacoustic emissions. In the vast majority with hearing threshold levels exceeding 25 dB at all frequencies transient otoacoustic emissions will be absent. However, in the small number that demonstrate transient otoacoustic emissions, despite hearing threshold levels exceeding 25 dB, there is a strong indication of retrocochlear disease.

A further potential diagnostic application of transient otoacoustic emissions relies upon the fact that their amplitude is influenced by contralateral sound stimulation (Collet *et al.*, 1990), presumably due to efferent activity via the crossed olivocochlear pathway. Thus, demonstration of such a reduction constitutes a test of the integrity of the crossing pathway. Ryan, Kemp and Hinchcliffe (1991) have demonstrated how this can be abolished in a case study of one patient with a congenital cholesteatoma within the posterior fossa.

Further research into the properties of the various types of evoked otoacoustic emissions will contribute to the understanding of cochlear function, and in particular the relative roles of the inner and outer hair cells. Evoked otoacoustic emissions are directly related to outer hair cell function and may be somewhat independent of the inner hair cells. Hence, improved understanding may lead to differentiation of disorders affecting primarily either the inner hair cells or the outer hair cells, based on evoked otoacoustic emission properties. This would entail an enhanced taxonomy of hearing impairment, with subdivision of the current cochlear or sensory type. At the present time there is insufficient evidence to indicate whether inner and outer hair cell disorders can exist separately, and if they can, whether they are so strongly correlated statistically that the distinction is meaningless. Application of evoked otoacoustic emission testing in clinical populations is an important route to furthering this understanding.

Integration of findings and interpretation

This section briefly outlines the typical characteristics (or stereotypes) associated with the main types of hearing impairment. It will be immediately apparent that they are not all mutually exclusive and therefore integration of test battery findings in individual clinical cases cannot be straightforward.

Interpretation in diagnostic audiology is inevitably holistic, contingent, probabilistic and heuristic: *holistic* in that all of the information available must be considered together to establish an overall pattern; *contingent* in that the relationship between the findings and the likely aetiology or site-of-lesion type depends on the characteristics of the patient (e.g. age) and of the clinical population being tested (e.g. referral patterns); *probabilistic* in that, as in most areas of medicine, diagnostic classification is subject to a degree of error; and *heuristic* in that the clinician must search for relationships between variables to establish useful rules of thumb for future reference. It goes without saying that a comprehensive history is a most important aspect of the information. Results from the other examinations and tests outside the scope of this chapter (e.g. vestibular function tests, radiology) should also be taken into account.

For the present purposes, interpretation will be confined to attributing a hearing loss to one (or more) of the major types outlined, either conductive, sensory, peripheral-neural or non-organic. Central-neural disorders are dealt with in Chapter 11.

Conductive hearing loss is principally identified by an air-bone gap or absence of acoustic reflexes. Otoscopic and tympanometric results give information about the details of the pathology.

Sensory hearing loss is distinguished from peripheral-neural hearing loss in terms of three dimensions of discrimination, recruitment and adaptation. There are also important distinctions based on electrophysiological characteristics. The sensory hearing loss is typified by good discrimination, marked recruitment and little adaptation, with ABR waves close to normal in latency for high-intensity clicks.

Peripheral-neural hearing loss is typified by poor discrimination, little recruitment and excessive (and rapid) adaptation, although often only one or two of these characteristics may be present. ABR waves central to the lesion are delayed and reduced in amplitude. Concomitant sensory damage is common, giving a mixture of sensory and peripheral-neural characteristics (Priede and Coles, 1974; Tonndorf, 1980, 1981).

Non-organic hearing loss does not have a single definitive characteristic, but can be identified from inconsistency between tests (e.g. repeated threshold determinations, the Stenger test, sensitivity loss on speech audiogram less than pure-tone loss, acoustic reflexes inconsistent with pure-tone audiometry). The principal means of establishing the definite presence of an non-organic hearing loss is to compare pure-tone audiometric thresholds with those obtained by cortical electric response audiometry (Coles and Mason, 1984). Methods of evaluating non-organic hearing loss have been reviewed by Coles (1982).

As with many other disciplines, individuals do not necessarily fall neatly into one or another of the above categories. The diagnostic process is fundamentally statistical and the value of undertaking further steps to reach a more firm diagnostic conclusion depends greatly upon the possible outcome in terms of management. At a very simplistic level, the priority is to identify patients for whom a remedial form of management is necessary or feasible; the remainder, who in many clinics comprise the vast majority, are candidates for rehabilitation. The main remedial treatments are surgical at present, most commonly for middle-ear disorders. However, the major life-threatening condition presenting with audiological symptoms is the acoustic neuroma (vestibular schwannoma), and it is the low but significant incidence of acoustic neuromas and other neoplasms in the brain stem region which has justified the attention paid to distinguishing between sensory and peripheral-neural types of loss that might result from an acoustic neuroma. The ready availability of high-resolution radiological and magnetic resonance imaging techniques has radically changed clinical practice in this area of diagnostics over the past decade, to the extent that they have largely displaced other approaches to the identification of cerebellopontine angle tumours. This is especially so in the case of MRI. Nonetheless, it is instructive to examine briefly the evidence leading to the above changed practice.

Many studies published during the last three decades have examined the accuracy of various tests in correctly identifying peripheral-neural lesions. More recently, attempts have been made to develop statistical models which help in this comparison of tests. In a series of three articles, Turner, Frazer and Shepard (1984), Turner and Neilsen, (1984), Turner, Shepard and Frazer (1984) have applied the techniques of clinical decision analysis to data regarding the performance of 26 tests from 107 studies published since 1968. Those articles form a convenient synthesis of the knowledge available in the mid-1980s. Any implementation of a screening test involves a compromise between sensitivity and specificity; the sensitivity can be increased at the expense of specificity by shifting the referral criterion, and vice versa. Usually, the performance of the test is measured in terms of the percentage of correct detections (hits) and the percentage of false referrals (false alarms). However, because these percentages depend on the criterion used, there is a need for a measure which is independent of the criterion and is therefore fundamental to the test itself. Turner and his co-authors utilized the theory of signal detection to derive the measure of d' for each of the 26 tests after pooling data across relevant studies. The higher the value of d', the higher is the sensitivity of a test for a given specificity. Table 12.5 lists values for d' for various audiological/vestibular, electrophysiological (auditory brain stem response) and radiological tests obtained by Turner, Shepard and Frazer (1984). Their results indicated three main clusters whereby the more sophisticated radiological tests yield relatively high values of d', auditory brain stem response and intravenous enhancement computerized tomography yield intermediate values and the audiological/vestibular tests, plain X-ray and tomography yield low values. Speech discrimination gave an exceptionally low value. From this it is apparent that none of the audiological/vestibular tests is of much value.

Table 12.5 Values of d' for various diagnostic tests

	d'
Posterior fossa cisternography	> 5
Computerized tomography, gas cisternography	> 4
Computerized tomography, metrizanide cisternography	> 4
Auditory brain stem response	2.9
Computerized tomography, intravenous enhancement	2.6
Combined acoustic reflex threshold/decay	2.0
Tomography	1.8
Threshold tone decay	1.6
Alternate binaural loudness balance	1.5
Bithermic caloric	1.5
Békésy audiometry (sweep frequency)	1.4
Short increment sensitivity index	1.4
Plain X-ray	1.3
Speech discrimination	0.6

Modified from Turner, Shepard and Frazer (1984)

The analysis presented by Turner and his colleagues is extremely useful in that it provides a formal basis for discussing matters which are more commonly dealt with intuitively. However, their analysis represents an early stage in such modelling and is subject to some limitations. First, the outcome of each test is dichotomized, whereas in clinical practice most tests give a graduated result with more confidence being placed in more extreme results. Second, for several of the audiological/vestibular tests their criterion chosen to dichotomize the outcome does not represent the optimum and in some instances is quite inappropriate (e.g. the caloric test is treated as positive for peripheral-neural pathology when there is a canal paresis of 25% or more; this could equally well occur for a sensory type of lesion). Third, the population assessed by audiological/vestibular testing is considered to be equivalent to that assessed radiologically, whereas it is likely the prevalence of peripheral-neural lesions is far higher in the latter group, particularly those referred for the more invasive procedures. Fourth, the cost of each test and of each possible outcome is not included in the analysis. In response to these articles, Dobie (1985) has suggested a method by which costs can be attached to the outcomes (e.g. he puts the cost of a missed peripheral-neural lesion at five times that of a false alarm). By using this approach, the interpretation of the original data of Turner, Shepard and Frazer (1984) is altered considerably. Fifth, the analysis does not acknowledge the significance of *changes* in the measured variables with time which are characteristic of a progressive disorder, as caused by a growing space-occupying lesion.

In order to examine the criteria used by Turner and his co-authors, two studies which they had not included and which have led to differential diagnostic criteria widely used in the UK were selected here for similar analysis. The alternate binaural loudness balance criteria developed by Priede and Coles (1974) and the speech audiometric criterion of Coles, Markides and Priede (1973) (see Figure 12.14), both alter with the sensitivity of the ear in a fashion which describes extreme results obtained from control subjects with a sensory type of impairment. Values of d' obtained from these two studies were 3.6 and 3.3 respectively, which are superior to the performances of all but the most sophisticated radiological tests shown in Table 12.5. While independent evaluation of these two criteria on a second test population might reduce the values of d', it does appear as though the studies contributing to Table 12.5 may not have been fully optimized. Furthermore, these findings strongly suggest that referral criteria should be contingent, as described above, and aim to identify extreme cases *in the light of other known measures* (e.g. the pure-tone audiogram). In the alternate binaural loudness balance example, to refer on the basis of the presence or absence of recruitment according to a fixed criterion would have been far less effective.

The weakness of the two values of d' given above is that the criteria used to calculate d' were selected *a*

posteriori, and hence they have only limited predictive value. Furthermore, there is a tendency for patient groups used in such studies to be distributed bimodally; comprising mainly unambiguous sensory or unambiguous peripheral-neural cases, with few intermediate examples. Evaluation of predictive accuracy requires prospective study of unselected new cases from a representative clinical population using diagnostic criteria stated *a priori*. As yet unpublished data from the Nottingham neuro-otology clinic provide such a prospective evaluation of many of the tests included in the Turner *et al.* study, plus transient otoacoustic emissions. The study group of 237 patients with symptoms suggestive of a cerebellopontine angle tumour included 18 who were ultimately found to have a tumour. Of the tests examined, only ABR produced a moderately respectable value of d' (1.9). Even this test, conducted by a specialist department with extensive relevant experience, missed two cases: a small (1 cm) vestibular schwannoma and a large congenital petrous apex cholesteatoma. The promise of transient otoacoustic emissions described above did not turn out to have a practical benefit for screening in this context. Hence, it can be concluded that the preferred diagnostic route for patients suspected of a cerellopontine angle tumour involves imaging, using high-resolution CT, or preferably MRI, methods. When this route is not readily available, resort may have to be made to ABR testing to identify those patients with normal results who might forego imaging studies. However, when this route is followed, there is a small but not insignificant risk that target cases may be missed. None of the other audiological tests has sufficient diagnostic accuracy to be used in this way.

The above statements should not be taken to imply that diagnostic audiological tests have no value at all. Not all peripheral-neural hearing losses arise from cerebellopontine angle tumours, and clear-cut peripheral-neural findings can occur when there is no radiological evidence of any space-occupying lesion. In such cases, the audiological results, *in combination with imaging studies*, provide the relevant diagnostic information and suggest appropriate forms of treatment. For example, a patient with a peripheral-neural hearing loss and very poor speech discrimination would not be an ideal candidate for a hearing aid.

The vast majority of adult patients needing any form of management do not require any medical or surgical treatment, but fall into the rehabilitation category, many of them being elderly (Chapter 4). Although rehabilitation is outside the scope of this chapter, information regarding the necessity for, or form of, hearing aid provision is available from the diagnostic tests which can be utilized alongside other assessments of the patient's needs and aspirations. Principally, the pure-tone audiogram indicates the severity of the hearing loss and the extent to which it is a conductive attenuation of sound; recruitment measures illustrate the dynamic range available for aided hearing; speech tests verify the actual hearing ability and show the residual discrimination ability. All of these measures can suggest the likely success to be obtained by means of an amplifying hearing aid, the ear or ears which may provide greater success and the type of hearing aid which may be tried initially.

Concluding remarks

Diagnostic audiometry is not a precise science and requires consideration of a diverse array of test results to arrive at a satisfactory conclusion. Several individuals may be involved in the testing, each able to apply expertise in specific areas. Attaching appropriate weight to possibly conflicting data is the main challenge to the clinician. A major difficulty is the fact that, even in skilled hands, many of the tests used can provide potentially misleading or artefactual results and most are subject to considerable variability. In particular, errors arising out of the incorrect use of masking of the non-test ear are difficult to detect *post hoc*. As more new tests are developed, the possibility of errors is bound to increase. It is therefore incumbent on the clinician to keep abreast of developments and to understand fully the principles and characteristics of the tests being employed, together with their pitfalls. This requires continual study and devotion of significant amounts of time to learn the techniques; however, for the sake of accurate diagnosis the effort is well spent.

References

ANDERSON, H. and BARR, B. (1966) Conductive recruitment. *Acta Oto-Laryngologica*, **62**, 171–184

ANDERSON, H., BARR, B. and WEDENBERG, E. (1970) The early detection of acoustic tumours by the stapedial reflex test. In: *Sensorineural Hearing Loss*, edited by G. Wolstenholme and J. Knight, London: Churchill. pp. 278–289

BEALES, P. H. (1981) *Otosclerosis*. Bristol: John Wright. p. 2

BÉKÉSY, G. V. (1939) Uber die piezoelectrische messung der absoluten horschwelle bei knockenleitung. *Akustische Zeitung*, **4**, 113–125

BELL, I., GOODSELL, S. and THORNTON, A. R. D. (1980) A brief communication on bone conduction artefacts. *British Journal of Audiology*, **14**, 73–75

BENTZEN, O. (1967) The otosclerotic syndrome. *Acta Oto-Laryngologica*, Suppl. **224**, 124–132

BONDING, P. (1979) Critical bandwidth in patients with acoustic neuroma. *Scandinavian Audiology*, **8**, 15–22

BONFILS, A. and UZIEL, A. (1988) Evoked otoacoustic emissions in patients with acoustic neuromas. *American Journal of Otology*, **9**, 412–417

BOOTHROYD, A. (1968) Developments in speech audiometry. *Sound*, **2**, 3–10

BOOTHROYD, A. and CAWKWELL, S. (1970) Vibrotactile thresholds in pure tone audiometry. *Acta Oto-Laryngologica*, **69**, 381–387

BORG, E. (1973) On the neuronal organisation of the acoustic middle ear reflex. A physiological and anatomic study. *Brain Research*, **49**, 101–123

BORG, E., COUNTER, S. E. and ROSLER, G. (1984) Theories of middle-ear muscle function. In: *The Acoustic Reflex. Basic Principles and Clinical Applications*, edited by S. Silman. Orlando: Academic Press. pp. 63–99

BOSATRA, A., RUSSOLO, M. and POLI, P. (1975) Modifications of the stapedius muscle reflex under spontaneous and experimental brain-stem impairment. *Acta Oto-Laryngologica*, **80**, 61–66

BRITISH SOCIETY OF AUDIOLOGY/BRITISH ASSOCIATION OF OTOLARYNGOLOGISTS (1981) Recommended procedures for pure-tone audiometry using a manually operated instrument. *British Journal of Audiology*, **15**, 213–216

CANE, M. A., LUTMAN, M. E. and O'DONOGHUE, G. M. (1994) Transient evoked otoacoustic emissions in patients with cerebello-pontine angle tumours. *American Journal of Otology*, **15**, 207–216

CARHART, R. (1950) Clinical application of bone conduction. *Archives of Otolaryngology*, **51**, 798–807

CARHART, R. (1957) Clinical determination of abnormal auditory adaptation. *Archives of Otolaryngology*, **65**, 32–39

CARRUTH, J. A. S., LUTMAN, M. E. and STEPHENS, S. D. G. (1978) An audiological investigation of osteogenesis imperfecta. *Journal of Laryngology and Otology*, **92**, 853–860

CHAIKLIN, J. B. (1967) Interaural attenuation and cross-hearing in air conduction audiometry. *Journal of Auditory Research*, **7**, 413–424

CHAIKLIN, J. B. and VENTRY, I. M. (1965) The efficiency of audiometric measures used to identify functional hearing loss. *Journal of Auditory Research*, **5**, 196–211

CLEAVER, V. G. C. and STEPHENS, S. D. G. (1977) Observations on the clinical use of broad-band noise as an acoustic reflex stimulus. *British Journal of Audiology*, **11**, 22–24

COLES, R. R. A. (1982) Non-organic hearing loss. In: *Otology*, edited by A. G. Gibb and M. F. W. Smith. London: Butterworths. pp. 150–176

COLES, R. R. A. and MASON, S. M. (1984) The results of cortical electric responses audiometry in medico-legal investigation. *British Journal of Audiology*, **18**, 71–78

COLES, R. R. A. and PRIEDE, V. M. (1970) On the mis-diagnoses resulting from incorrect use of masking. *Journal of Laryngology and Otology*, **84**, 41–63

COLES, R. R. A. and PRIEDE, V. M. (1971) Non-organic overlay in noise-induced hearing loss. *Proceedings of the Royal Society of Medicine*, **64**, 194–199

COLES R. R. A., LUTMAN M. E. and ROBINSON D. W. (1991) The limited accuracy of bone-conduction audiometry: its significance in medicolegal assessments. *Journal of Laryngology and Otology*, **105**, 518–521

COLES, R. R. A., MARKIDES, A. and PRIEDE, V. M. (1973) Uses and abuses of speech audiometry. In: *Disorders of Auditory Function*, edited by W. Taylor. London: Academic Press. pp. 181–202

COLLET, L., KEMP, D. T., VEUILLET, E., DUCLAUX, R., MOULIN, A. and MORGON, A. (1990) Effects of contralateral auditory stimuli on active cochlear micromechanical properties in human subjects. *Hearing Research*, **43**, 251–262

COLLETTI, V. (1975) Stapedius abnormalities in multiple sclerosis. *Audiology*, **14**, 63–71

COPE, Y. and LUTMAN, M. E. (1993) Otoacoustic emissions.

In: *Paediatric Audiology 0–5 years*, edited by B. McCormick. London: Whurr Publishers. pp. 250–290

CUNNINGHAM, D. R. and GOETZINGER, C. P. (1974) Extra-high-frequency hearing loss and hyperlipidaemia. *Audiology*, 13, 470–484

DE BOER, E. and BOUWMEESTER, J. (1974) Critical bands and sensorineural hearing loss. *Audiology*, 13, 236–259

DIRKS, D. and MALMQUIST, C. (1969) Comparison of frontal and mastoid bone conduction threshold in various conduction lesions. *Journal of Speech and Hearing Research*, 12, 725–746

DOBIE, R. A. (1985) The use of relative cost ratios in choosing a diagnostic test. *Ear and Hearing*, 6, 113–116

EFRON, R., YUND, E. W., NICHOLS, D. and CRANDALL, P. H. (1985) An ear asymmetry for gap detection following anterior temporal lobectomy. *Neurophysiologica*, 23, 43–50

EVANS. E. F. (1975) Normal and abnormal functions of the cochlear nerve. In: *Sound Reception in Mammals*, edited by R. J. Bench., A. Pye and J. D. Pye. London: Academic Press. pp. 133–165

FESTEN, J. M. and PLOMP, R. (1983) Relations between auditory functions in impaired hearing. *Journal of the Acoustical Society of America*, 73, 652–662

FLOTTORP, G. and DJUPESLAND, G. (1970) Diphasic impedance change and its applicability in clinical work. *Acta Oto-Laryngologica*, Suppl. 263, 200–204

FOWLER, C. G. and WILSON. R. H. (1984) Adaptation of the acoustic reflex. *Ear and Hearing*, 5, 281–288

FOWLER, E. P. (1936) A method for the early detection of otosclerosis. *Archives of Otolaryngology*, 24, 731–741

GATEHOUSE, S. and BROWNING, G. G. (1982) A re-examination of the Carhart effect. *British Journal of Audiology*, 16, 215–220

GELFAND, S. A. (1984) The contralateral acoustic-reflex threshold. In: *The Acoustic Reflex. Basic Principles and Clinical Applications*, edited by S. Silman. Orlando: Academic Press. pp. 137–186

GOODHILL, V. (1965) The fixed malleus syndrome: surgical and audiological considerations. *Transactions of the American Academy of Ophthalmology and Otolaryngology*, 79, 797 (abstract)

GRADENIGO, G. (1893) On the clinical signs of the affections of the auditory nerve. *Archives of Otolaryngology*, 22, 213–215

GREEN, K. W. and MARGOLIS, R. H. (1984) The ipsilateral acoustic reflex. In: *The Acoustic Reflex. Basic Principles and Clinical Applications*, edited by S. Silman, Orlando: Academic Press. pp. 275–299

HAGGARD, M. P., LINBALD, A. C. and FOSTER, J. R. (1986) Psychoacoustical and audiometric prediction of auditory disability at listener-adjusted presentation levels. *Audiology*, 25, 277–298

HALL, J. W. (1985) The acoustic reflex in central auditory dysfunction. In: *Assessment of Central Auditory Dysfunction. Foundations and Clinical Correlates*, edited by M. L. Pinheiro and F. G. Musiek. Baltimore: Williams and Wilkins. pp. 103–130

HANNLEY, M. (1986) *Basic Principles of Auditory Assessment*. London: Taylor and Francis

HIRSCH, A. and ANDERSON, H. (1980) Audiologic test results in 96 patients with tumours effecting the eighth nerve. *Acta Oto-laryngologica*, Suppl. 369, 1–26

HOLMQUIST, J. (1976) Eustachian tube evaluation. In: *Acoustic Impedance and Admittance – the Measurement of Middle Ear Function*, edited by A. S. Feldman and L. A. Wilber. Baltimore: Williams and Wilkins. pp. 156–174

HOOD, J. D. (1956) Fatigue and adaptation of hearing. *British Medical Bulletin*, 12, 125–130

HYDE, M. L. (1987) Objective tests of hearing. In: *Scott-Brown's Otolaryngology*, Vol. 2. *Adult Audiology*, edited by D. Stephens. London: Butterworths. pp. 272–303

INTERNATIONAL ELECTROTECHNICAL COMMISSION (1991) *Instruments for the Measurement of Aural Acoustic Impedance/Admittance*. (IEC 1027). Geneva: IEC

INTERNATIONAL ELECTROTECHNICAL COMMISSION (1992) *Audiometers. Part 1. Pure Tone Audiometers*. (IEC 645–1). Geneva: IEC

INTERNATIONAL ELECTROTECHNICAL COMMISSION (1993) *Audiometers. Part 2. Equipment for Speech Audiometry*. (IEC 645–2). Geneva: IEC

INTERNATIONAL ELECTROTECHNICAL COMMISSION (1994) *Audiometers. Part 4. Equipment for Extended High Frequency Audiometry*. (IEC 645–4). Geneva: IEC

INTERNATIONAL ORGANIZATION FOR STANDARDIZATION (1987) *Acoustics – Reference Level for Narrow Band Masking*. (ISO 8798). Geneva: ISO

INTERNATIONAL ORGANIZATION FOR STANDARDIZATION (1989) *Acoustics – Pure-tone Audiometric Test Methods – Part 1: Basic Pure Tone Air and Bone Conduction Threshold Audiometry (ISO 8253–1)*. Geneva: *ISO*

INTERNATIONAL ORGANIZATION FOR STANDARDIZATION (1991) *Acoustics – Standard Reference Zero for the Calibration of Pure-tone Audiometers (ISO 389)*. Geneva: ISO

JACOBSON, E. J., DOWNS, M. P. and FLETCHER, J. L. (1969) Clinical findings in high-frequency threshold during known ototoxic drug usage. *Journal of Auditory Research*, 9, 379–385

JERGER, J. (1960) Békésy audiometry in analysis of auditory disorders. *Journal of Speech and Hearing Research*, 3, 257–287

JERGER, J. (1970) Clinical experience with impedance audiometry. *Archives of Otolaryngology*, 92, 311–334

JERGER, J. and HERER, G. (1961) An unexpected dividend in Békésy audiometry. *Journal of Speech and Hearing Disorders*, 26, 390–391

JERGER, J. and JERGER, S. (1971) Diagnostic significance of PB word functions. *Archives of Otolaryngology*, 93, 573–580

JERGER, J., SHEDD, J. and HARFORD, E. (1959) On the detection of extremely small changes in sound intensity. *Archives of Otolaryngology*, 69, 200–211

JERGER, J., ANTHONY, L., JERGER, S. and MAULDIN, L. (1974a) Studies in impedance audiometry. III. Middle ear disorders. *Archives of Otolaryngology*, 99, 165–171

JERGER, J., BURNEY, P., MAUDLIN, L. and CRUMP, B. (1974b) Predicting hearing loss from the acoustic reflex. *Journal of Hearing and Speech Disorders*, 39, 11–22

JERGER, J., HARFORD, J., CLEMIS, J. and ALFORD, B. (1974c) The acoustic reflex in eighth nerve disorders. *Archives of Otolaryngology*, 96, 513–523

JERGER, S. and JERGER, J. (1977) Diagnostic value of crossed versus uncrossed acoustic reflexes. Eighth nerve and brain-stem disorders. *Archives of Otolaryngology*, 103, 445–453

KATZ, J. (1994) Editor. *Handbook of Clinical Audiology*, 4th edn. Baltimore: Williams and Wilkins

KILLION, M. C. (1985) Insert earphones for more interaural attenuation. *Hearing Instruments*, 36, 34–36

LAROCHE, C. and HÉTU, R. (1991) Etude de Fidélité de l'audiométrie automatique pour balayage fréquentiel asservi

(Audioscan). *Research Report*. Quebec: Institut de Recherche en Santé et en Sécurité du Travail

LESHOWITZ, B. (1977) Speech intelligibility in noise for listeners with sensorineural hearing damage. *Instituut voor Perceptie Onderzoek Annual Progress Report*, **12**, 11–23

LIDÉN, G., NILSSON, F. and ANDERSON, H. (1959) Narrow band masking with white noise. *Acta Oto-Laryngologica*, **50**, 125–136

LIGHTFOOT, G. R. (1979) Air-borne radiation from bone conduction transducers. *British Journal of Audiology*, **13**, 53–56

LUTMAN, M. E. (1983) Frequency resolution, auditory disability, and handicap. *Journal of the Acoustical Society of America*, **73**, 51 (abstract)

LUTMAN, M. E. (1984) The relationship between acoustic reflex threshold and air-bone gap. *British Journal of Audiology*, **18**, 223–229

LUTMAN, M. E. (1985a) Cross-talk in stapedial reflex measurement. *Audiology in Practice*, **2**(1), 7

LUTMAN, M. E. (1985b) Phasor admittance measurement of the middle ear. I. Theoretical approach. *Scandinavian Audiology*, **13**, 253–264

LUTMAN, M. E. (1986) Acoustic impedance audiometry. In: *Physics in Medicine and Biology Encyclopedia*, edited by T. F. McAinsh. Oxford: Pergamon Press. pp. 1–4

LUTMAN, M. E. (1987) Speech tests in quiet and in noise as measures of auditory processing. In: *Speech Audiometry*, edited by M. C. Martin. London: Taylor and Francis. pp. 63–73

LUTMAN, M. E. (1989) Evoked otoacoustic emissions in adults: implications for screening. *Audiology in Practice*, **6**(3), 6–8

LUTMAN, M. E., (1991) Degradations in frequency and temporal resolution with age and their impact on speech identification. *Acta Oto-Laryngologica*, Suppl. **476**, 120–126

LUTMAN, M. E. and CLARK, J. (1986) Speech identification under simulated hearing aid frequency response characteristics in relation to sensitivity, frequency resolution and temporal resolution. *Journal of the Acoustical Society of America*, **80**, 1030–1040

LUTMAN, M. E. and DAVIS, A. C. (1994) The distribution of hearing threshold levels in the general population aged 18–30 years. *Audiology*, **33**, 327–350

LUTMAN, M. E. and LEIS, B. R. (1980) Ipsilateral acoustic reflex artefacts measured in cadavers. *Scandinavian Audiology*, **9**, 33–39

LUTMAN, M. E. and WOOD, E. J. (1985) A simple clinical measure of frequency resolution. *British Journal of Audiology*, **19**, 1–8

LUTMAN, M. E., BROWN, E. J. and COLES, R. R. A. (1987) Self-reported disability and handicap in the population in relation to pure-tone threshold, age, sex and type of hearing loss. *British Journal of Audiology*, **21**, 45–58

LUTMAN, M. E., MCKENZIE, H. and SWAN, I. R. C. (1985) Phasor admittance measurements of the middle ear. II Normal phasor tympanograms and acoustic reflexes. *Scandinavian Audiology*, **13**, 265–274

LUTMAN, M. E., MASON, S. M. and SHEPPARD, S. (1989) Differential diagnostic potential of otoacoustic emissions: a case study. *Audiology*, **28**, 205–210

MARKIDES, A. (1980) The relation between hearing loss for pure tones and hearing loss for speech among hearing-impaired children. *British Journal of Audiology*, **14**, 115–121

MASON, S. M. (1993) Electric response audiometry. In: *Paediatric Audiology 0–5 Years*, edited by B. McCormick. London: Whurr. pp. 187–249

MØLLER, A. R. (1964) Effect of tympanic muscle activity on movement of the eardrum, acoustic impedance and cochlear microphonics. *Acta Oto-Laryngologica*, **57**, 525–534

MØLLER, A. R. and JANNETTA, P. J. (1985) Neural generators of the auditory brainstem response. In: *The Auditory Brainstem Response*, edited by J. T. Jacobson. San Diego: College-Hill Press. pp. 13–32

MOORE, B. C. J., GLASBERG, B. R., HESS, R. F. and BIRCHALL, J. P. (1985) Effects of flanking noise bands on the rate of growth of loudness of tones in normal and recruiting ears. *Journal of the Acoustical Society of America*, **77**, 1501–1513

NAUNTON, R. F. and FERNANDEZ, C. (1961) Prolonged bone conduction; observations on man and animals. *Laryngoscope*, **71**, 306–318

NEWBY, H. A. (1979) *Audiology*, 4th edn. New York: Appleton-Century-Crofts

NIEMEYER, W. and SESTERHENN, G. (1974) Calculating the hearing threshold from the stapedius reflex threshold for different sound stimuli. *Audiology*, **13**, 421–427

NISWANDER, P. S. and RUTH, R. A. (1976) An artifact in acoustic reflex measurement: some further observations. *Journal of the American Audiological Society*, **1**, 209–214

OLSEN, W., STACH, B. and KURDZEIL, S. (1981) Acoustic reflex decay in 10 seconds and in 5 seconds for Menière's disease patients and for VIIIth nerve tumour patients. *Ear and Hearing*, **2**, 180–181

OSTERHAMMEL, D. (1980) High-frequency audiometry: clinical aspects. *Scandinavian Audiology*, **9**, 249–256

PICK, G. F., EVANS, E. F. and WILSON, J. P. (1977) Frequency resolution in patients with hearing loss of cochlear origin. In: *Psychophysics and Physiology of Hearing*, edited by E. F. Evans and J. P. Wilson. London: Academic Press. pp. 273–281

POPELKA, G. (1981) Editor. *Hearing Assessment with the Acoustic Reflex*. New York: Grune and Stratton

PRIEDE, V. M. (1970) Acoustic impedance in two cases of ossicular discontinuity. *International Audiology*, **9**, 127–136

PRIEDE, V. M. and COLES, R. R. A. (1974) Interpretation of loudness recruitment tests – some new concepts and criteria. *Journal of Laryngology and Otology*, **88**, 641–661

PROBST, R., LONSBURY-MARTIN, B. L. and MARTIN, G. K. (1991) A review of otoacoustic emissions. *Journal of the Acoustical Society of America*, **89**, 2027–2067

PROBST, R., LONSBURY-MARTIN, B. L., MARTIN, G. K. and COATS, A. C. (1987) Otoacoustic emissions in ears with hearing loss. *American Journal of Otolaryngology*, **8**, 73–81

RABINOWITZ, W. M. (1977) Acoustic-reflex effects on the input admittance and transfer characteristics of the human middle ear. *PhD Thesis*. Cambridge: Massachusetts Institute of Technology

RAPPAPORT, B. Z., FAUSTI, S. A., SCHECHTER, M. A. and FREY, R. H. (1986) A prospective study of high-frequency auditory function in patients receiving oral neomycin. *Scandinavian Audiology*, **15**, 67–71

RENDELL, R. J. and MILLER, J. J. (1983) An evaluation of high-frequency audiometry suitable for routine clinical use. *British Journal of Audiology*, **17**, 81–85

ROSENBERG, P. E. (1969) Tone decay. *Maico Audiologic Library Series*, **7**, report 6

RYAN, S., KEMP, D. T. and HINCHCLIFFE, R. (1991) The influence of contralateral stimulation on click-evoked otoacoustic emissions in humans. *British Journal of Audiology*, **25**, 391–397

SALVI, R. J., HENDERSON, D., HAMERNIK, R. and AHROON, W. A. (1983) Survey paper: neurological correlates of sensorineural hearing loss. *Ear and Hearing*, **4**, 115–129

SELTERS, W. A. and BRACKMAN, D. E. (1979) Brainstem electric response audiometry in acoustic tumour detection. In: *Acoustic Tumours*, volume I: *Diagnosis*, edited by W. F. House and C. M. Luetje. Baltimore: University Park Press pp. 225–236

SHIPTON, M. S., JOHN, A. J. and ROBINSON, D. W. (1980) Air-radiated sound from bone vibration transducers and its implications for bone conduction audiometry. *British Journal of Audiology*, **13**, 53–56

SILMAN, S. (1984) Editor. *The Acoustic Reflex. Basic Principles and Clinical Applications*. Orlando: Academic Press

SILMAN, S., GELFAND, S. A., PIPER, N., SILVERMAN. C. A. and VAN FRANK, L. (1984) Prediction of hearing loss from the acoustic-reflex threshold. In: *The Acoustic Reflex. Basic Principles and Clinical Applications*, edited by S. Silman. Orlando: Academic Press. pp. 187–223

SMITH, B. L. and MARKIDES, A. (1981) Interaural attenuation for pure tones and speech. *British Journal of Audiology*, **15**, 49–54

SMITH, K. R. (1943) Bone conduction during experimental fixation of the stapes. *Journal of Experimental Psychology*, **33**, 96–107

SMITH, P. A. and FERGUSON, M. A. (1994) Comparison of measures of frequency resolution and recruitment in patients undergoing neuro-otological investigation. *British Journal of Audiology*, **28**, 155–163

STEVENS, J. C., WEBB, H. D., HUTCHINSON, J., CONNELL, J., SMITH, M. F. and BUFFIN, J. T. (1991) Evaluation of click-evoked oto-acoustic emissions in the newborn. *British Journal of Audiology*, **25**, 11–14

STUDEBAKER, G. (1962) Clinical placement of vibrator in bone conduction testing. *Journal of Speech and Hearing Disorders*, **29**, 23–25

STUDEBAKER, G. (1964) Clinical masking of air and bone-conducted stimuli. *Journal of Speech and Hearing Disorders*, **29**, 23–25

TONNDORF, J. (1966) Bone conduction; studies in experimental animals. *Acta Oto-Laryngologica*, Suppl. 213, 1–132

TONNDORF, J. (1972) Bone conduction. In: *Foundations of Modern Auditory Theory*; vol. II, edited by J. V. Tobias. New York: Academic Press. pp. 195–237

TONNDORF, J. (1980) Acute cochlear disorders: the combination of hearing loss, recruitment, poor speech discrimination and tinnitus. *Annals of Oto-Rhino-Laryngology*, **89**, 353–358

TONNDORF, J. (1981) Stereociliary dysfunction, a cause of sensorineural hearing loss, recruitment, poor speech discrimination and tinnitus. *Acta Oto-Laryngologica*, **91**, 469–480

TONNDORF, J. and TABOR, J. R. (1962) Closure of the cochlear windows; its effect upon air and bone conduction. *Annals of Otolaryngology*, **71**, 5–29

TURNER, R. G. and NEILSEN, D. W. (1984) Application of clinical decision analysis to audiological tests. *Ear and Hearing*, **5**, 125–133

TURNER, R. G., FRAZER, G. L. and SHEPARD, N. T. (1984) Formulating and evaluating audiological test protocols. *Ear and Hearing*, **5**, 321–330

TURNER, R. G., SHEPARD, N. T. and FRAZER, G. L. (1984) Clinical performance of audiological and related diagnostic tests. *Ear and Hearing*, **5**, 187–194

TYLER, R. S. and SMITH, P. A. (1983) Sentence identification in noise and hearing-handicap questionnaires. *Scandinavian Audiology*, **12**, 285–292

TYLER, R. S., SUMMERFIELD, Q., WOOD, E. J. and FERNANDES, M. A. (1982) Psychoacoustical and phonetic temporal processing in normal and hearing-impaired listeners. *Journal of the Acoustical Society of America*, **73**, 740–752

VAN CAMP, K. J. and VOGELEER, M. (1986) A tympanometric approach to otosclerosis. *Scandinavian Audiology*, **15**, 109–114

WIGHTMAN, F. L., MCGEE, T. and KRAMER, M. (1977) Factors influencing frequency selectivity in normal and hearing-impaired listeners. In: *Psychophysics and Physiology of Hearing*, edited by E. F. Evans and J. P. Wilson. London: Academic Press. pp. 295–306

ZWICKER, E. and SCHORN, K. (1978) Psychoacoustical tuning curves in audiology. *Audiology*, **17**, 120–140

13

Audiological rehabilitation

Dafydd Stephens

In its broadest sense, audiological rehabilitation involves all aspects apart from surgery and pharmacological treatment, of the management of the patient with hearing difficulties. In the first edition of this textbook (1952) it was defined by Edith Whetnall in her chapter on hearing aids in the following way: 'Rehabilitation consists in teaching the patient to adopt the right attitude towards his handicap. At the same time the patient is given instruction in auditory training and lip reading. The training is of the greatest importance; under no circumstances should a patient receive an aid and then be left to his own devices in learning to use it'. She continued to discuss the importance of the attitude and adjustment of the patient and wrote, 'To overcome the handicap the deaf patient must first admit to himself that he is deaf, and secondly agree to learn everything he can about deafness and how to overcome it. He must realize that not only is he deaf, but that it is quite apparent to other people that he is so and that his handicap will, in fact, be noticed less if he uses a hearing aid. He must be helped to realize the effects of his deafness. It is explained that he is anxious and irritable because he is continually afraid of making mistakes through not hearing correctly'.

I shall return repeatedly to these aspects of adjustment and attitude throughout this chapter.

Altogether, while some of Whetnall's terminology is dated, given the advances of the past 44 years, most is as applicable today as it was then. She, together with other pioneers such as Carhart (1946), Bergman (1950), and others in the USA were writing at the time when it was first reasonably feasible to incorporate the unique contribution of wearable hearing aids with other aspects of rehabilitation to provide a meaningful and effective package for people with hearing disabilities. Many of the insights of these early authors were profound and we can all still learn much from reading their pioneering works.

I shall discuss the concepts of disability and handi-

cap below; I shall indicate that hearing disability comprises the hearing difficulties experienced by the patient and that the handicap is the effects of his impairments and disabilities on his general life. I shall follow throughout this chapter the general definition of audiological rehabilitation as a 'problem solving process aimed at minimizing disability and avoiding or reducing handicap'. This statement encompasses the concept that the process be orientated towards the individual concerned and aimed at meeting his specific needs within his particular environment. In that context a most important part of the environment is that created by significant others (spouse, parents, children, workmates, carers, etc.) and Hétu et al. (1988) have widely discussed the role of the significant others in the development of or amelioration of handicap.

These concepts may be applied to the rehabilitation of all types of disabilities and Chamberlain (1989) has equally broadly defined rehabilitation, in its general respect, as: 'The process designed to maximize a patient's physical, mental, social and vocational potential'. Earlier the World Health Organization (WHO, 1980) defined the process of rehabilitation as: 'An *active* process by which those disabled by injury/disease achieve a full recovery or if full recovery is not possible, realize their optimal physical, mental and social potential and are integrated into their most appropriate environment'.

In all domains of disability and handicap, psychosocial factors have a most important role. Both psychological and social factors interact with factors such as the age of onset, type, severity, mode of onset and progression of the disability. They will depend on social class, family type and network, and the reaction of others. Stigma may be experienced or imagined by the patient and family, and the individual's personality with his coping style, self-image and self-esteem will have important roles which must be addressed (Coughlan, 1988; Davies, 1988).

Impairment, disability and handicap

These terms, collectively known as disablements, have been very loosely used by different authors in the past. Now, however, a growing consensus is focusing on the application of the World Health Organization ICIDH (International Classification of Impairments, Disabilities and Handicaps) definitions, formulated initially by Philip Wood (WHO, 1980; Wood, 1980). The ICIDH definitions in general terms are specified as follows:

Impairment: any disturbance of the normal structure and functioning of the body, including the systems of mental function.
Disability: the loss or reduction of functional ability and activity consequent upon impairment.
Handicap: the disadvantage experienced as a result of impairment or disability.

Broadly these reflect a sequence of effects (Figure 13.1) but when examined in detail, there may be some complex interactions between them, in their production and also as a result of successful rehabilitation.

These definitions have been applied in the audiological domain for a number of years (Thomas and Gilhome Herbst, 1980; Davis, 1983) and have been discussed at some length by Stephens and Hétu (1991).

Impairment

Stephens and Hétu (1991) developed the definition of impairment within the audiological field to defective function which may be measured using psychoacoustical or physiological techniques.

These measures are essentially independent of psychosocial factors although certain aspects of personality (Stephens, 1973) and cognitive function may influence their measurement. They are an indication of the potentialities of the individual rather than his actual behaviour in a real life environment.

While auditory impairments form a continuum from the inability to hear the most simple to the most complex sound, they may be broadly divided into simple and complex impairments. These are shown in Table 13.1. A characteristic of all the impairments covered in Table 13.1 is that they can be measured in a reliable and repeatable form in any laboratory or clinic with a well defined test–retest variability. Although the results may be influenced by individual differences (Stephens, 1973; Gatehouse and Davis, 1992), in general, such effects are small.

Table 13.1 Types of hearing impairment

Simple	*Complex*
Tonal threshold sensitivity	Speech recognition in the quiet
Frequency resolution	Speech recognition in noise
Temporal resolution	Music recognition
Spatial resolution	Discrimination of specific environmental sounds
Speech component resolution	

The tests range from the use of acoustically very simple stimuli such as clicks or tone bursts to very complex recognition tasks, such as the discrimination of speech in noise, and are designed to tap different levels and types of impairment in different parts of the auditory system. Even speech tests have a range of complexity ranging from synthetic measures of speech components (Fourcin, 1980) through consonant or vowel confusion tests, to single words in quiet and sentences in noise with different degrees of complexity and redundancy (e.g. the Spin test – Kalikow, Stevens and Elliott, 1977). Most measures are behavioural measuring the recognition or discrimination of particular stimuli, whereas others are electrophysiological, requiring no conscious participation on the part of the listener. Yet others may use measures such as response or reaction times to assess the processing ability of the auditory system (Gatehouse and Gordon, 1990).

Hearing disability

Hearing disability implies the problems which the individual experiences with his hearing in a real life environment. This will depend on the activities indulged in by the hearing impaired person and his previous experience. Thus three people may have a high frequency hearing loss. One may not be conscious of any abnormality or difficulty, a second may notice problems in group situations and in a noisy environment, whereas a third person, for whom hearing is particularly important, such as a musician, will find the loss incapacitating.

A prelingually deaf person, even with a severe hearing loss, who has never experienced the ability

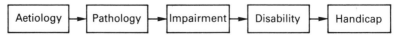

Figure 13.1 Factors in the establishment of handicap

to hear under a variety of circumstances will often report no disability. However, if such a person finds himself in a situation which he has not previously experienced, and is in that environment with hearing friends, he may become aware of a certain disability such as the difficulty in hearing a singer in a bar.

Other people with apparently normal hearing (auditory disability with normal hearing, ADN; obscure auditory dysfunction, OAD; King-Kopetzky syndrome, see Stephens, 1992) may report hearing difficulties, particularly hearing speech in noisy places. While on extensive audiometric evaluation of the impairment, some of these individuals may be found to have subtle cochlear or central auditory dysfunction, many will be found to have no impairment, yet for them the disability will be very real. For this reason Hinchcliffe (1992) has argued that this condition is primarily a stress-related disorder.

The disabilities experienced are generally related to difficulties in hearing specific sounds but also include a hypersensitivity to or intolerance of sounds (phonophobia). This is dealt with further in Chapter 18.

The difficulties range from hearing speech to environmental sounds and specific difficulties related to the particular occupation of the individual concerned. These are shown in Table 13.2 based on Stephens and Hétu (1991) which was in turn derived from a compilation of the WHO (1980) proposals and other suggestions (Davis, 1983).

The disability experienced by a person may alter according to a change in the environment of the individual. Thus he may be unaware of any problems while his wife is alive, she taking all action in response to the telephone, knocks at door and tolerating the loudness of the television. However, if she dies or is taken into hospital, he may be made aware of his disabilities by his friends who cannot make him hear when they come to the door, by relatives who complain that he does not hear the telephone bell, and by his children and grandchildren who cannot tolerate the loudness of his television.

Table 13.2 Classification of auditory disabilities

1   Disability listening to speech and discriminating in quiet or in noise

   a Live voice
       one to one
       in groups/meetings
       theatre/opera
       from one side in the car
       strangers/dialects
       religious services

   b Non-live voice
       telephone
       TV/video
       radio
       public address systems
       cinema

2   Disability receiving other audible signals in quiet or in noise

     Telephone bell
     Door bell
     Other warning
     Music
     Water boiling

3   Disability relating to auditory localization in space
     Warning signals
     Footsteps
     Birds, etc.

4   Identification disability
     Music
     Birdsong
     Stethoscope
     Acoustical signals for crossroads

5   Environmental awareness
     Clock/watch
     Birdsong
     Wind
     Traffic, etc.

6   Intolerance of noise

After Stephens and Hétu (1991)

Handicap

Handicap is not 'hearing handicap'. Rather, it is the effects of the impairment and disability on the individual's life. This entails the non-auditory effects of the hearing loss on employment, psychological state and social relationships. Hearing handicap does not exist.

The handicap experienced by the individual is very much a function of his environment, both animate and inanimate. It is particularly influenced by significant others, people who play an important role in the life of the hearing impaired person. Thus Hétu and his colleagues (1990) have argued the case for the secondary handicap experienced by hearing impaired people stemming from the efforts made by the individual to

overcome the experienced disability and primary handicap. There is then a strong interaction with the effect of their hearing disability on their significant others (their primary handicap), which then leads to an alteration of their behaviour and attitude towards the hearing impaired individuals and further alteration in the handicap. Jones, Kyle and Wood (1987) have shown that the whole family structure may be affected by the hearing impairment and have highlighted the handicap experienced by the partner of the hearing impaired person which needs to be addressed if any rehabilitation programme is to be effective. In addition, the handicap will be very much influenced by factors such as the personality, occupation and interests of the individual, together with the cultural environment within which he lives.

Recently Hétu *et al.* (1990) have proposed a model for the development of handicap as a result of the interaction between the hearing impaired person and his partner. While the work was based essentially on noise-exposed workers and their wives, the model is equally applicable to other groups. Kerr and Cowie (1992) extended it to include positive experiences arising from the hearing disability which were highlighted in their studies on individuals with profound acquired hearing loss. These experiences included the experience of people being caring and helpful to them because of their disability, giving them a better understanding of human nature, religious feelings, and the finding that 'some people behave better when they know you are deaf'.

These concepts have been incorporated into a revised version of their models shown in Figure 13.2. In this figure continuing the line from aetiology, pathology and impairment through disability we encounter the primary handicaps of the impaired individual which includes direct effects of the disabilities experienced, such as reduced quality of social interactions, anxiety and negative self-image. The individual then tries to compensate/adjust for this by speech-reading (lip reading), by positioning himself better, changing the pattern of telephone use, etc. While these may have a direct effect on reducing some of the handicap in social interaction, e.g. the effort needed may result in greater fatigue and the behavioural changes in greater stigma. These will then contribute to increasing the individual's overall handicap.

On the other hand, the positive experiences will result in a sense of well-being and reduce the overall handicap.

The interaction with the significant other is even more complex. Such individuals will be affected primarily by the disabilities experienced by the patient and develop primary handicaps themselves. These will include stress, reduced quality of social interactions and reduced satisfaction which then contribute to and reinforce the patient's primary handicap. The patient's disabilities do, however, trigger adjustments in the behaviour of the significant other, such as acting as an interpreter, tolerating television at a higher level, and raising their voice which, again, while reducing the patient's primary handicap will produce a secondary handicap for the significant other. These will stem from the fatiguing effect of the effort involved, and their embarrassment, and this results in a secondary handicap reflected in an alteration in their attitude towards the patient. This will again increase the patient's overall handicap.

Figure 13.2 also shows a line going from the patient's *impairment* towards causing a primary handicap for the significant other, together with various adjustments. This occurs in the case of patients who may be unaware of their hearing impairment and not conscious of any disability. This will be because a caring partner has compensated for their difficulties, either consciously or subconsciously, by adjusting the television loudness, answering on their behalf, and so on. This can result in a global handicap of a deterioration of the social relationship between the

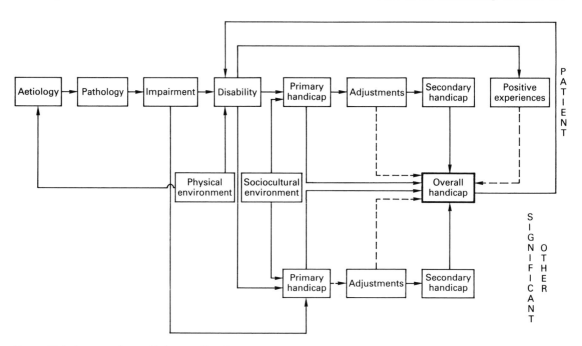

Figure 13.2 Factors in the establishment of handicap. - - - - Reduction of handicap

two without the hearing impaired person being aware that it results from that hearing impairment.

The final points shown in Figure 13.2 comprise the other effects of the environment in which the individual lives, the physical environment and the sociocultural environment. Noble (1983) has highlighted these effects in his concepts of 'ecological audiology' and this work has been extended in terms of disablements by Noble and Hétu (1994).

The physical environment in which the individual lives, such as the noise levels, lighting, reverberance, etc., has its main effects on disablements by affecting the level of disabilities experienced. Thus a patient with a cochlear hearing loss living in a quiet environment will experience far fewer disabilities than his counterpart with a noisy family living in drab dingy tenement block and working in a noisy factory. The noise of the environment will also have a more indirect effect on disablement by causing the hearing loss in the first instance or by aggravating an underlying hearing loss.

The sociocultural environment, on the other hand, influences the primary handicap, both of the individual and of any significant others which will consequently contribute to the individual's overall handicap. Factors which come into play here are prejudices, intolerances and lack of understanding of the problems of the hearing impaired person, the stigma within the society of using a hearing aid, etc. These will have bearings on both the patient and any significant others, and influence the type and degree of adjustments they may make to compensate for or hide the patient's disabilities.

A final line links back from handicap to disability. This is necessary if we are to consider the process as a dynamic model with potential changes taking place in the sociocultural environment and the patient's significant others. Thus, as illustrated in the next section, such changes may result in psychological disorders which in turn can influence the disability experienced by the patient.

The different primary and secondary handicaps experienced by the patient and the significant other are illustrated by Hétu *et al.* (1990) and by Stephens and Hétu (1991). The overall range of handicaps experienced, based on the WHO (1980) classification is shown in Table 13.3. It is particularly important to emphasize here that we should be referring to an individual suffering from specific disabilities and handicaps rather than using the label of a disabled or handicapped person.

Changes in disablements

Disablements are not static and may be altered by life event changes and alterations in the work, domestic or social environment of the individual. This has been discussed elsewhere in the context of prelingually deaf individuals who may be so well adjusted

Table 13.3 Domains of handicap

1 Orientation handicap: the individual's abiity to orientate themselves in relation to their surroundings
2 Physical independence handicap: the individual's ability to sustain a customarily effective independent existence
3 Occupation handicap: the individual's ability to occupy their time in the manner customary to their age, sex and culture
4 Economic self-sufficiency handicap: the individual's ability to sustain customary socio-economic activity and independence
5 Social integration handicap: the individual's ability to participate in and maintain customary social relationships
6 Emotional handicap: the psychological disturbances experienced by the individual consequential to his impairment and disability

that they are unaware or certainly unwilling to articulate and define any disability or handicap. However, even a relatively minor change may create havoc with this adjustment.

This may be illustrated by the case of a 53-year-old man who became deaf from meningitis at the age of 7 years and was subsequently educated in and identified with the deaf community. He has a deaf wife, but his sister, who was close to him and has normal hearing, signs fluently and acts as an interpreter. He had worked as a painter and decorator all his professional life and was well adjusted until the introduction of metrication by his employers. Unlike his workmates he was not able to adjust following a retraining course, and this difficulty was enhanced as his wife was thoroughly confused by metrication herself and unable to support him. This led to him losing his job resulting in an economic self-sufficiency handicap and reactive depression. This depression was increased by the difficulty he had communicating with colleagues in a new job, and in turn increased his speech communication disability.

These last problems were alleviated by appropriate hearing aid fitting and counselling coupled with liaison with the Disability Employment Advisor to organize more specific retraining matching his needs.

These alterations are illustrated in Figure 13.3.

Evaluation of disablements

Various measures of *impairment* of auditory function are described elsewhere in this volume (Chapter 12) and in the psychoacoustical chapter of Volume 1. Here I shall deal specifically with the evaluation of disability and handicap.

Both are inherently subjective matters experienced by the individual and can normally be tapped only by questionning or questionnaires. It is possible, however, in a limited way to assess them within the

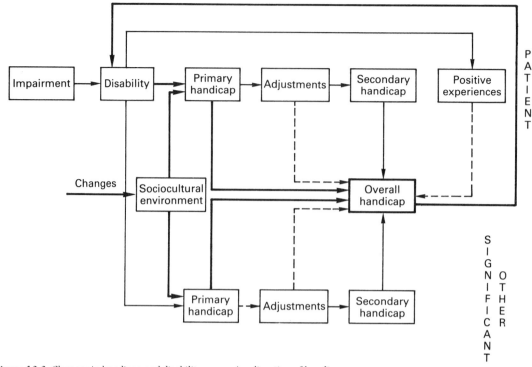

Figure 13.3 Changes in handicap and disability. ----- Amelioration of handicap

individual's own environment, but to the present time such approaches have been extremely limited. More commonly, disability and handicap are assessed by the use of questionnaires. Such questionnaires may be open-ended, asking the patient to list the disabilities and handicaps experienced, or by closed-set questionnaires in which the patient is required to respond to a predefined set of questions. The best of these are themselves derived from piloting with interviews and open-set questionnaires. There are difficulties with these stemming from the fact that they restrict the individual's responses. In addition there is a number of terminological confusions.

One of the main areas of confusion arises from the terminology used. Although in Australia, Quebec and most of western Europe this now follows the WHO model (1980), many authors in the USA still persist with the American Academy of Otolaryngology (AAO) (1979) terminology derived from medicolegal applications, which is not relevant to a rehabilitative context. The questionnaires as a whole will be discussed in a later section concerned with the evaluation of the effectiveness of the rehabilitative process.

Open-set evaluation

The open-set approach was pioneered by Barcham and Stephens (1980) with the problem questionnaire

which simply states: 'Please make a list of the problems which you have as a result of your hearing loss. List them in order of importance starting with the biggest problem. Write down as many as you can think of'. This gives rise to a range of responses which, while specific for the particular individual may be grouped into a number of categories. These have been replicated by various authors (Tyler, Baker and Armstrong Bednall, 1983; Golabek *et al.*, 1989). The technique has also been applied to tinnitus (Tyler and Baker, 1983) and to vertigo and dysacuses (Stephens, 1990). Tyler, Baker and Armstrong Bednall (1983) have also compared such results for those awaiting hearing aids with those already fitted. Plummer (1985) has compared the results of such a questionnaire with those of interviews, and Hickin (1986) and Lormore and Stephens (1994) have considered the different responses given by patients and their significant others. More recently, in order to define the contribution handicap derives from the significant other we have asked both the patient and significant other to specify what they consider the effects of the patient's hearing loss to be on the significant other. This will be considered further below.

While the overall pattern of patient disability/handicap categories has been described in detail (Barcham and Stephens, 1980; Stephens, 1980; Tyler, Baker and Armstrong Bednall, 1983), they were later considered in terms of disability and handicap (Stephens, 1987a). These results are summarized in Tables 13.4 and 13.5 which list the main groups of responses for disabilities (Table 13.4) and for handicaps (Table 13.5). The tables also show the mean importance

Table 13.4 Disabilities reported in the problem questionnaire

Disability group	Specific complaints	Main weighting for group
Live speech	General conversation Group conversation Speech in noise Meetings Speech from one side Quiet voices Speech with no lip reading Conversation with strangers Discrimination Children's voices Speech from a distance One to one conversation Accents/dialects	3.4
Electronic speech	TV/radio Telephone conversation Cinema PA systems	2.6
Alerting/warning sounds	Doorbell Telephone bell Alarms/sirens/horns Kettle, etc.	2.7
Environmental noises	Clock/watch General	1.7
Music		2.9
Localization		3.1
Hearing when called		2.7

After Stephens (1987a)

Table 13.5 Handicaps complained of in the problem questionnaire

Handicap group	Specific complaints	Mean weighting
Employment problems		4.3
Psychological problems	Embarrassment Depression/strain Loneliness Family strain Lack of confidence	2.9

After Stephens (1987a)

weightings given to the different groups on the basis of the order in which the responses were given. While the psychological aspects of handicap were given a relatively low rating, this may stem in part from the difficulty which many patients experience in identifying a direct relationship between the hearing loss and its consequences, or perhaps from an unwillingness on the part of the patient to express it. Within this group of responses it is also interesting to note that in the author's experience of several thousands of such problem questionnaires, no patient has directly expressed any paranoid feelings in their responses.

The patient's problem questionnaire was also administered to significant others accompanying patients to the clinic to evaluate how they saw the patient's disability and handicap (Hickin, 1986; Lormore and Stephens, 1994). In these studies we rephrased the questionnaire to read, 'Please make a list of the problems which your spouse/friend/relative has as a result of his/her hearing loss . . .'.

In the primary study Hickin (1986) found that the significant others were more likely to report psychological problems and less likely to report problems with the doorbell or telephone bell, etc. than the patient, but that otherwise the broad perceptions of the significant other closely reflected those of the patient. More extensive studies (Lormore and Stephens, 1994; Siwiek *et al.*, 1996), however, indicated more subtle differences in attitude between the patient and significant other. Thus the patient noted the problems in a remediative manner, whereas the significant others refer to their burdensome implications. So, while the patients report general difficulties in hearing the television the significant others report that the patient frequently turns it up loud.

This indicates, however, that useful insights can be obtained into the strategy to be adopted in the rehabilitation, particularly of patients with complex problems. It also emphasizes the importance of incorporating significant others in the rehabilitation process.

More recently we have extended this questionnaire to ask the significant other to list the problems which he experiences as a result of the patient's hearing loss and also to ask the patient to list those problems that the significant other experiences (Stephens, France and Lormore, 1995). This gives insights into the production of handicap in the patient (see Figure 13.2) and also provides an important entrée to counselling and in depth rehabilitation of the more complex patients.

The effects of the patient's disability on the significant other as viewed by both the significant other (wife) and her hearing impaired husband are illustrated by the responses shown in Table 13.6 from a 66-year-old patient and his wife. This couple showed a fair insight into each other's problems but others show much less.

Table 13.6 Effects of patient's hearing loss on wife

Wife's account	*Patient's account*
A Conversation together quite difficult – my husband tries to guess sometimes what I'm saying rather than admit he can't hear, then when questioned says that I'm speaking too quietly – this sometimes after I've repeated what I'm saying a few times and looking at him face to face	A Wife gets very frustrated if I cannot hear her
	B Also gets annoyed as I tend to shout
B I get very frustrated at times. His lack of hearing causes arguments between us. His not being able to hear the TV and having to have the sound turned up and down continuously some evenings makes for frustration and nerves on edge	C If I'm listening to a friend talking and can't hear properly I generally tend to nod as if I can which annoys my wife as she knows I have not heard properly
C When he's driving the car I sometimes forget he cannot hear and end up carrying on a conversation that I suddenly realize he hasn't heard	
D When out in company he has now started to look to me to 'see' how I answer rather than keep saying he cannot hear	
E I sometimes say – I'm sorry he hasn't heard you – and then am firmly told by my husband that he has heard. Frustrating!	

Who enters the rehabilitation process?

Many studies both in the UK (Davis, 1983, 1993) and the USA (Garsteki, 1993) indicated that only between one-tenth and one-quarter of the patients who could benefit from hearing aids actually possess and use them.

Furthermore, related to this, the average person attending a hearing aid clinic for the first time is aged about 70 and has had a hearing loss for 10–20 years (Brooks, 1976; Thomas and Gilhome Herbst, 1980; Stephens *et al.*, 1980). While Brooks (1981) did report a small reduction in the average age of those being fitted for the first time following the introduction of postaural hearing aids by the UK National Health Service, the change was small. In the USA, Garstecki (1993) reported a static hearing aid market despite the initial increase of popular interest in hearing aids when ex-President Reagan was fitted with in-the-ear hearing aids.

The delay between the patient experiencing hearing disability and seeking hearing aid help to overcome it has consequential effects both for the patient, his family, and the professionals concerned with his eventual rehabilitation.

The delay has resulted in the fact that the mean better ear hearing level at time of fitting is some 50 dB (Stephens *et al.*, 1980) so that most individuals affected will be experiencing quite significant disability. This will have effects on significant others in terms of television loudness, the individual not hearing the telephone bell or doorbell, withdrawal from social activities and the like. The long period of partial sensory deprivation will lead the individual to take considerably longer to adjust to amplification in the form of hearing aids aimed at reducing the disability. The increased age of the patient will also lead to increased sensory and fine motor difficulties and hence problems in learning new tasks involved such as fitting the earmould/hearing aid to the ear and manipulating the controls. On the other hand, if those skills are acquired earlier they are usually well retained even if the ability to learn new skills subsequently becomes impaired.

Why then is there such a delay? This stems in part from the individual concerned and in part from the professionals encountered on the way towards obtaining help. The stigmata perceived by the patient associated with hearing loss and, perhaps even more, with the use of hearing aids remain very strong. Other factors such as his physical and psychological status, social and experiential factors and the accessibility of rehabilitative facilities have been discussed elsewhere (Stephens, 1983).

Humphrey, Gilhome Herbst and Faruqi (1981) and Gilhome Herbst, Meredith and Stephens (1991) have found that less than one-half (44%) of patients aged 70 or over with a better ear hearing loss of 35 dB or worse who consult their general practitioner or primary physician are subsequently referred on for rehabilitative help (Table 13.7). This was despite the fact that both practices studied were very well run with a positive attitude towards helping their patients, so that it can be surmised that the situation may be

Table 13.7 Percentages of patients aged 70 years and ≥ 35 dB HL in better ear seeking help

	Inner London	*Wales*
Admit no hearing loss	26	25
Admit loss but not consulted GP	25	19
Consulted GP but not referred for hearing aid	27	32
Have hearing aid	21	25

After Gilhome Herbst, Meredith and Stephens (1991)

worse in other places. We have subsequently questioned a number of the patients who were not referred on to the audiology clinics, and in the majority of cases it appeared that they had little motivation themselves for seeking help, often consulting their doctor because of family pressures. Hence, the doctor may well have felt that they were unlikely to wear a hearing aid even were they to accept referral to an appropriate hospital department.

This indicates a need for health education directed both at the health professionals whom they will encounter, together with a case finding approach oriented via general practitioners.

The first approach to this was initiated by Adrian Davis (Davis *et al.*, 1992). Within that study all patients in the 50–65 year age group in a general practice in Cardiff were studied and either sent a questionnaire or offered a home visit to screen for hearing loss. Those with over 30 dB HL in their worse ear (averaged over 500, 1000, 2000 and 4000 Hz) were offered a hearing aid fitting. Ultimately the pick-up rate in terms of fittings was the same with the two approaches to case finding, so further studies have concentrated on the questionnaire-based approach which is more cost-effective.

The reason for targetting this age group is that it is within this group that the prevalence of hearing impairment begins to increase dramatically. In older people, Herbst's studies (1983) have indicated that intervention might be less effective. Furthermore, the National Study of Hearing (Davis, 1987) has indicated that some 35% of the over 50s in the UK have a significant impairment, and that about 90% of the hearing impaired adult population are aged 50 or over. Stephens, Lewis and Charny (1991) found in the Cardiff Health Survey, that 22% of this age group responded affirmatively to the question, 'Do you have any problems with your hearing?'.

Subsequent case-finding studies have concentrated on examining and refining the techniques of the earlier study, based on the initial finding that hearing aid use on the initial study population increased

threefold (3% to 9%) following intervention, together with improved speech in noise discrimination performance by those patients aided. The later studies have been summarized by Stephens and Meredith (1991a) who found that, even in a socially deprived area, the hearing aid use, following intervention increased dramatically from 8% to 23% in this same age group. They also found that a very much simplified questionnaire involving two questions: 'Do you have any difficulty with your hearing?' and 'Do you have problems with noise(s) in your ear(s) or head?' are as good, in terms of sensitivity at detecting those ultimately being successfully fitted with hearing aids, as the complex multiquestion approach used in the initial study (Stephens *et al.*, 1990). Among those patients responding that they had hearing disability/tinnitus, the inability to hear a forced whisper at 70 cm was a good predictor of subsequent acceptance of a hearing aid (Davies, John and Stephens, 1991). Among those who had a hearing loss greater than 30 dB in their better hearing ear, the level of emotional handicap was a better predictor of whether they would accept and use a hearing aid than either impairment or disability (Stephens *et al.*, 1991). Subsequent long-term follow up of those individuals shows good on going hearing aid use with greater reduction in disability and handicap in those individuals using their hearing aids regularly.

The one disappointing result in these studies is the small overall reduction in disability and handicap following intervention. This highlights the need for further consideration of non-instrumental aspects of the rehabilitative process, and this is being further explored.

The overall message, however, is that such early intervention on a case finding basis is broadly effective, markedly increasing hearing aid use and resulting in some reduction in disability and handicap. Furthermore, in a non-life-threatening condition such as hearing loss, acceptance of intervention is a very individual matter and is determined by the individual's handicap and disability, rather than impairment.

The process of audiological rehabilitation

Once the hearing impaired patient arrives at an audiological department in a hospital, the first stage is obviously one of defining the aetiology of the hearing loss and, where possible, treating it. For most patients, however, such as those with noise-induced hearing loss, genetic loss or age-related hearing loss, there is no medical or surgical management to improve the hearing. Even in those cases which are treatable there is generally some residual hearing impairment and consequent disability. In all such circumstances in which treatment is appropriate or unlikely to relieve completely the condition, the rehabilitative process must be started as early as possible. It is essential to avoid building up any false hopes of a cure in the patient, as anticipation of such a cure will impede the patient's acceptance of rehabilitation.

The rehabilitative process itself must involve a consideration of all relevant factors in the evaluation of the patient and all possible interventions to ensure nothing appropriate is missed. Some such factors may be immediately dismissed as not pertinent to the particular individual concerned, but that is better than omitting something relevant for particular individuals. In this I shall follow the approach of the rehabilitative model developed by Goldstein and Stephens (1981) with some changes of detail and presentation.

Within that model we endeavoured to break away from the divorce of hearing aids and other components of the rehabilitative process, as was common before that time, instead integrating the different components into a coordinated whole. As mentioned earlier, such an approach was pioneered by Whetnall (1952), Bergman (1950) and the other pioneers of the immediate post-World War Two era, but largely ignored by many subsequent practitioners.

The widespread introduction of cochlear implants and the rehabilitative 'packages' associated with them (see Chapter 15) has helped to emphasize and publicize the need for such a comprehensive approach.

Within such an approach the personal instrument(s), be they hearing aids or cochlear implants, usually have a unique and pivotal role in the process, like the axle of a wheel, but cannot function appropriately without the other components of the rehabilitative process. For some patients (e.g. auditory disability with normal hearing, prelingually totally deaf adults), such instruments may be unacceptable or irrelevant and in others may comprise almost the entirety of the remedial process, but in isolation of other elements optimal benefit will not be derived by the patient.

Where we differ from the pioneers is in the concept that not all patients will require the same approach. Some will take the fast lane, others a more prolonged systematic approach, others a somewhat devious approach, and in others, direct intervention will be considered inappropriate, any efforts being concentrated on their significant others.

In all cases, however, the philosophy behind the approach is that it should be orientated towards the specific needs of the particular patient concerned. We also need to consider the situation of the patient in the context of particular significant others.

The model is applicable to any and every sociomedical system with the components differing in degree of emphasis, but not in need, according to the characteristics of the particular system. All it assumes is a patient-orientated, holistic approach.

A management model of audiological rehabilitation

Within this amended model there are four components: evaluation, integration and decision making, short-term remedial processes, and on-going rehabilitation (Figure 13.4). What was previously the remedial process has been split into three components in order to highlight the importance and difference of

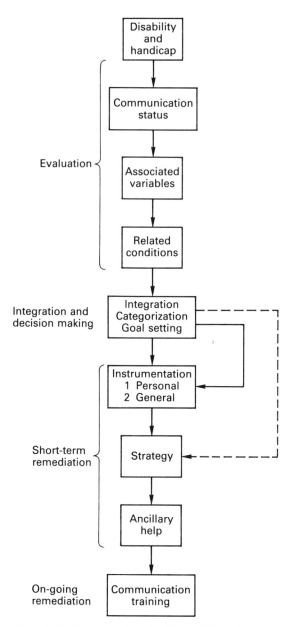

Figure 13.4 Management model of the audiological rehabilitation process

these three components. Thus the integration/decision making section emphasizes the need for the professional(s) to reflect on the information obtained about the patient, collect any necessary further information, decide on the categorization of the patient and define the specific goals which are important for the patients and considered to be realistically achievable by the professional. They must together discuss openly how these goals can be best achieved.

The short-term remediation deals with the remedial steps which can be implemented immediately, or at least within one or two sessions. Obviously in the particular cases of the bone anchored hearing aids or cochlear implants, this step will extend to cover the period of surgery and recovery, but otherwise there is no fundamental difference from the vast majority of more straightforward cases.

The on-going remediation is something which may potentially last the rest of the individual's life. It may be a quick check that the patient is coping well with his hearing aid(s) and has no further problems, following which he will be discharged from regular follow up, to return should he experience new problems. On the other hand, for example in patients with severe central processing disorders, such as after brain stem injury, and for those with cochlear implants or vibrotactile aids, this rehabilitation may well continue for months and even years until the professional and patient between them decide that as much as can be done for the individual has been done. This would then be followed by regular if infrequent follow up. In audiological rehabilitation our patients are with us for life.

Evaluation

Before considering the components of this essential stage of the rehabilitative process, it is important to consider how an evaluation may be performed and what it comprises. This will, obviously, vary from one circumstance to another and within different parts of the evaluation for audiological rehabilitation. Furthermore each component may be evaluated differently in different centres according to the facilities available. What is important, however, is that a question should be asked about each component in each patient, the depth and format of such an evaluation varying.

The possible approaches to evaluation are shown in Table 13.8. There are three general methods of evaluation: by observation, by questioning and by testing (Table 13.8A). Each of these may be performed in different ways. Thus *observation* may be performed directly by the clinician, by the use of video recordings, or on the basis of observations provided to the clinician by others. *Questioning* may be likewise a face-to-face exercise, may be performed using questionnaires, or on the basis of computer interrogation.

Finally, *testing* may be on the basis of subjective responses provided voluntarily by the subject or objective responses measured electrophysiologically.

Table 13.8 Evaluation

A Modes of evaluation

Observation	Direct
	Video recording
	Reports
Questioning	Direct
	Questionnaires
	Computer administered
Testing	Subjective
	Objective

B Characteristics of evaluations

Formal	Informal
Systematic	Non-systematic
Qualitative	Quantitative
Binary	Multiply variable
Standardized	Non-standardized

A set of characteristics of each of these modes is outlined in Table 13.8B, which can apply to any of the modes of evaluation. Thus a pure tone audiogram is a form of subjective testing. It is standardized, multiply variable, quantitative, systematic and formal. A direct observation that a patient who arrives in the clinic has no auricles (pinnae) is informal, non-systematic and qualitative. Each approach has its relevance in the assessment of the patient, and some approaches may lead on to others.

Thus, a simple direct question to the patient, 'Do you know any sign language?', may be presented systematically as a formal part of the qualitative assessment of the patient expecting a binary response – yes or no. If yes, then multiply variable quantitative information may be obtained by systematic questioning or even by standardized testing.

Again, different approaches may be used where relevant to different parts of the evaluation process and also for different individuals being evaluated. Thus the question about sign language might be quite perfunctory in the case of an elderly person with a mild age-related hearing loss, but would be more detailed from the start in an adolescent with a profound congenital hearing loss. However, it is important to tap it even in the most unlikely case as this can give insight into the individual and open up possible lines of approach to the global management of the particular individual.

The evaluation process

This process may be divided into four distinct components which must be assessed to manage the patient appropriately. The first, *disability and handicap* is critical, tapping the reasons why the individual has come to the clinic in the first instance and what he feels in need of help to overcome.

Communication status is concerned with the raw materials with which the therapist will have to work; the hearing, visual and speech abilities of the patient, signing skills and the like.

Associated variables on the other hand, predominantly the psychosocial variables, will determine the overall approach which the therapist will have to adopt to the remedial process, given the attitudes and feelings of the patient and those around him. Finally, on the other hand, the *related conditions*, including particularly other aural conditions and upper limb function, will determine the important details of what is done, particularly with regard to instrumentation, within the overall approach determined by the associated variables.

Disability and handicap

These are normally assessed by simply asking the patient what difficulties or problems they have because of their hearing loss. That question is one of the most important questions which the patient will be asked.

Unfortunately, however, for many patients a visit to the clinic is a stressful experience, no matter how hard the staff may try to put them at ease, and they may omit to mention crucial problems, or even the most important. In that context we find it useful to send the problem questionnaire (see above) to the patient with the appointment letter, so giving them a chance to think about their problems, discuss them with significant others, where relevant, and to bring the form with them to their clinic appointment. In practice now we discount the order of listing of problems as we find that the patient may specify the problems in different orders according to their more recent experiences. Completing the questionnaire at home helps in this way, but also has its shortcomings as dominant significant others may prevail on the patient to list what they see as the problems rather than what the patient themselves see as problems.

It is, however, important to tap the reaction and responses of the significant other(s) because, as was indicated earlier, this will be an important determinant of the patient's ultimate handicap. Again this may be achieved simply by asking the individual directly, or by giving them a questionnaire: 'Please make a list of the problems you have because of your spouse/friend/relative/carer's hearing loss. Write down as many as you can think of'. This can easily be administered to the significant other while the patient is being tested, but such administration should always have the permission of the patient.

In this way the patient's disabilities and handicaps may be tapped both separately and in conjunction with the significant other, and an idea of the handi-

caps experienced by the significant other also defined. This information can then be invaluable in the subsequent structuring of the rehabilitation programme.

It is possible at this stage to administer disability and handicap questionnaires (e.g. Hearing Measurement Scale, Noble and Atherley, 1970) to obtain quantitative measures of various components of the individual's different disabilities and handicaps. While these may have a useful role as broad outcome measures, being administered before and after the rehabilitative process, they are generally too insensitive to the specific problems of the individual patient under consideration to be particularly useful here. Alternatively they are so complicated that they would take an inordinately long time to administer, although approaches using adaptive computer presentation may have a role here in the future.

What we have found useful in certain patients who are likely to have an extensive rehabilitative programme is to ask them to rate the severity of the individual disabilities or handicaps listed on a scale of 1 to 100, as used by Habib and Hinchcliffe (1978) or on a visual analogue scale (Sim, Stephens and Meredith, 1996). These can then be used subsequent to the rehabilitative process as personalized outcome measures as well as giving valuable information as to which aspects of the patient's disabilities/handicaps should be the focus of the initial attention.

Communication status

The components of communication status are shown in Table 13.9. It may be seen that they comprise the different elements and potentials for communication which the individual has at the time of assessment. The *audition* component reflects the measures of hearing relevant to rehabilitation. *Visual skills* covers not only visual acuity and the use of spectacles but also speech reading (lip reading) abilities. *Speech production* is self-explanatory as is *manual communication*. *Non-verbal skills* covers those other aspects of non-verbal communication not covered by sign language systems. *Previous rehabilitation* is important to allow for what has been done previously to help the individual's communication, and *overall* integrates these various components together with cognitive factors into the total communication skills of the patient which may often be very different from the sum of its component parts.

Table 13.9 Communication status

Audition
Visual skills
Speech production
Manual communication
Non-verbal skills
Previous rehabilitation
Overall

Audition

It must be emphasized that the concerns are those aspects of auditory function relevant to the individual's function in the real world, rather than diagnostic audiometric tests. There is, however, inevitably some overlap between the two. These will be important for determining the level and type of amplification required, and the optimal performance which it might be expected that the patient could achieve in different listening situations. The range of types of measures being considered is shown in Table 13.10.

Table 13.10 Relevant elements of audition

Auditory acuity
Dynamic range
Speech discrimination
Binaural interaction

Other signal processing abilities

Dynamic range for electroauditory stimulation

? Vibrotactile

The auditory acuity will normally be assessed by pure tone audiometry giving measures of hearing levels across a wide range of frequencies. There is much to be said for measures sweeping in detail across the frequencies such as Békésy audiometry or Audioscan testing (Meyer-Bisch, 1990) as major abnormalities (e.g. dips or peaks) in the audiogram may be easily missed with octave frequency testing. Peakiness of audiograms together with hearing aid resonances can cause problems with tolerance of the aid and hence its rejection.

For most patients, seen in a rehabilitative context, bone conduction thresholds are of little direct relevance. However, for the small groups with congenital defects of the outer and/or middle ears or unmanageable chronic suppurative otitis media or otitis externa, in whom either bone conduction or bone-anchored hearing aids are to be considered, they are critical. In these individuals speech discrimination measures using bone conduction presentation will also be indicated.

Two dynamic range measures are commonly used and may be used in certain hearing aid prescription procedures (Berger, 1976; see also Chapter 14). These are the most comfortable loudness level (MCLL) and the uncomfortable loudness level (ULL), two concepts introduced by Bangs and Mullins (1953). The most comfortable loudness level shows very large intra-subject and inter-subject variability (Stephens, Blegvad and Krogh, 1979) and may be calculated approximately as being one-half to two-thirds of the distance

(in dB) between the threshold and the uncomfortable loudness level. Because of this variability, much recent work in this field has concentrated on the most comfortable range of loudness rather than focusing on a somewhat arbitrary single level. The most comfortable loudness level measures are important in defining the gain necessary for amplification.

The uncomfortable loudness level (threshold of uncomfortable loudness (TUL) or loudness discomfort level (LDL)) is the lowest intensity of sound which the individual finds uncomfortably loud. It often has to be emphasized to the patient that it is not a test of their ability to tolerate loud sounds, and should be regarded as the softest level they could tolerate for a significant period of time, and hence gives an indication of the maximum output levels of any amplification which should not be exceeded.

While most measures of most comfortable loudness level or uncomfortable loudness level are based on tonal measures, speech material is sometimes used on the premise that it more closely represents what the patient will be having to tolerate via the amplification. However, on the other hand, it gives little frequency-specific information, and in certain circumstances, it may be necessary to define detailed frequency characteristics of the uncomfortable loudness level using Békésy tracking.

Speech discrimination measures are widely used in audiological rehabilitation, although it is debatable how much they influence any decision making in the process. Certainly, in patients with very asymmetrical hearing losses or severe losses, they may influence the decision as to which ear to aid or whether or not an ear should be aided, but in routine testing of individuals with symmetrical hearing losses the procedure contributes little to any rehabilitative decisions.

Where speech discrimination is less than optimal, discrimination scores may give an indication as to how much emphasis should be put on audiovisual rehabilitation. If there is little or no correct speech discrimination by both ears, even at high intensity levels, this may be an indication for further consideration of a cochlear implant.

A plethora of speech in noise tests also exists. While these may be useful in hearing aid selection processes (see Chapter 14), the results are generally predictable from pure tone testing and contribute little to management decisions.

Binaural integration measures may give some indication as to which patients will benefit from binaural hearing aid fitting. Indeed, although some early studies suggested that a poor binaural masking level difference indicated limited benefit to be derived from binaural aiding in terms of speech in noise discrimination, more recent studies have suggested that patients should not be denied binaural aiding just on this basis (e.g. Chung and Stephens, 1986). Improved speech in noise discrimination is only one of the potential benefits of binaural aiding, and more work is needed in this domain.

Gradually more sophisticated signal processing hearing aids are being developed and relevant assessment of different aspects of psychophysical performance are being incorporated in patient assessment batteries prior to fitting with such aids. Certainly discrimination of fundamental frequencies may be relevant to aids such as the Sivo aid (Rosen *et al.*, 1987) and duration discrimination measures may define which patients with profound hearing losses will and will not derive benefit from acoustical hearing aids.

This leads on to a use of the same approaches by electroacoustical stimulation as an assessment of potential candidates for cochlear implants. Certainly those with poor temporal resolution are often poor candidates for implantation.

Within the field of cochlear implantation general measures of frequency dependent thresholds and dynamic range measures will also give an indication as to which ear should be implanted and, perhaps, which implant system (single or multichannel) should be used.

Visual skills

Within this section there are three factors relevant to rehabilitation: the individual's visual acuity, whether or not spectacles are worn and if so how often, and their speechreading (lipreading) skills.

Visual acuity is relevant to the patient's ability to speech read. The simplest and most effective way to help a patient to be able to communicate better is to improve his visual acuity by the use of more appropriate spectacles. Many patients will spontaneously report that they 'hear' better when they are wearing their spectacles if they do not wear them all the time. Thus it is important to ensure that the individuals have their vision optimally corrected as far as possible for their middle distance vision when they are involved in communication. Usually their 'television' spectacles will be optimal under those circumstances.

Many patients, particularly the elderly, will have such severe visual impairments that they cannot be adequately corrected, and may indeed be totally blind. It is important to be aware of this as such severe visual impairment will be an additional indication for binaural fitting of hearing aids to provide auditory localization ability to compensate for the lack of visual localization ability.

Finally, appropriate vision for close work, corrected or otherwise, will be necessary for reading and adjusting controls on the hearing aids and other devices.

Furthermore, it is important to know whether the individual uses spectacles, and if so how much of the time with how many different pairs, to be aware of the interaction between such spectacles and any postaural hearing aids which may be used. This may influence the decision to fit in-the-ear hearing aids, spectacle aids, spectacle adapters or postaural aids according to the type(s) of spectacles used and the frequency of use. Within a sociomedical system in which most hearing aids fitted are in-the-ear aids, this will be a less important consideration.

Speechreading or lipreading is an important skill which entails the recognition of speech by the observation of the mouth patterns and expressions of the speaker. Most speechreading skills are acquired subconsciously, particularly among those working in noisy environments and the evidence that it can be effectively taught is somewhat limited (Binnie, 1977). However, when scheduling a rehabilitative programme, particularly for a severely hearing impaired patient it is important to have a basic assessment of his speechreading skills. The problem arises as to how this assessment can best be made. Should we be assessing the most basic components of speech, the visemes (the visual equivalent of phonemes), or should we be assessing running speech as in connected discourse tracking (CDT) (de Filippo and Scott, 1978)? Furthermore, there is the argument as to whether the testing should use visual stimulation alone, or whether an audiovisual presentation should be used.

The answer generally is that it will depend very much on the needs of the patient. It is often better to start with simple tasks like speech reading high redundancy material such as groups of numbers on which most individuals will score well, before progressing to more complex tasks such as sentences with or without redundancy. Connected discourse tracking is generally presented in a non-standardized form, although more recently efforts have been made to use more sophisticated programmed learning methodology, using a computer linked to a video disc, to administer such testing in a controlled standardized way. The basic principle of such testing is that the therapist (or the videotape) presents material from a text, a phrase at a time, and the patient has to repeat what is being said. If the text is correctly repeated the presenter continues with the next phrase. If not, it is repeated with increasing degrees of simplification until the testee is able correctly to repeat it. The patient is scored on the basis of the number of words correctly repeated per minute. This technique is useful for monitoring changes in the individual's performance with time and with and without different instrumentation. With live presentations it is also possible to select test material within the language skills and interest of the patient being tested.

At the present time the test materials most commonly used for patient evaluation, to provide a general overview, are usually either consonant or vowel confusion tests or sentence lists. The consonant confusion lists, e.g. aba/ata/aka/ama/, can be presented either in the quiet or with sound present from video recordings, and can be used to generate a confusion matrix with scores for place, manner and voicing errors together with total correct scales. The groups of consonants to be used will depend on the groups of consonants present in the particular language of the test, with the balance of consonants differing from language to language. Thus for example, even within the British Isles, Welsh has three consonants not found in English and a number of English consonants are not found in Welsh (Meredith, Stephens and Jones, 1990).

Vowel confusion tests are more difficult to generate but may be useful under certain circumstances. An example of such a list is BID – BAD – BAWD – BED – BEED – BUD – BIDE – BARD – BODE – BAYED – BUDE.

Consonant or vowel discrimination may also be assessed using a four alternative choice procedure with video recording such as the FADAST test (Summerfield and Foster, 1983) in which, for example the patient has to choose between CAT – CUT – BAT – BUT. Following a number of different presentations, particular error scores can be generated.

Among sentence lists the most widely used in English are the BKB (Bamford-Kowal-Bench) lists (Bench and Bamford, 1979), while the CID (Central Institute for the Deaf) sentence lists are still widely used in the USA. The BKB lists have been standardized (Rosen and Corcoran, 1982; McLeod and Summerfield, 1987) and may be used both auditorily and audiovisually in the presence of different levels of background noise.

Signal noise ratios have been extensively manipulated by MacLeod and Summerfield (1990) and others to give reliable and repeatable tests which may be adjusted to provide a standard baseline for measuring standardized improvements. They have also used techniques of manipulating the clarity of the visual image within this (MacLeod and Summerfield, 1987).

Lyxell (1989) has extensively studied the cognitive and conceptual factors involved in speechreading. He has also repeated the earlier studies relating speechreading skills to the latency of visual evoked responses, with less encouraging results than those suggested in previous studies (Shepherd *et al.*, 1977).

Speech production skills

This section is not concerned with all aspects of speech and language disorders, rather, it deals with linguistic problems relevant to the audiological rehabilitation of the patient concerned. Thus while an individual who stammers may have a hearing loss associated with an intermittent tinnitus which can aggravate his stammering, this is only of borderline relevance to the question which we are considering here.

The factors which are particularly relevant to the

rehabilitative process are shown in Table 13.11. They comprise those which are largely independent of the hearing loss, those which are abnormal usually only in cases of prelingual hearing loss and those which may be influenced by both prelingual and postlingual hearing loss.

Table 13.11 Speech production skills

1　Largely independent of hearing loss
　　a　First language
　　b　Dialect
　　c　Lexicon

2　Normally affected by prelingual hearing loss
　　a　Morphology
　　b　Syntax

3　Affected by both prelingual and postlingual hearing loss
　　a　Phonology
　　b　Pragmatics

Initially it is important to be aware of the first language of the patient and to be aware whether or not the rehabilitation can be provided within that language. Thus for example in a bilingual country like Wales, a young person who lost her hearing due to meningitis at an age when all her communication and education was via the medium of Welsh, her rehabilitation with a cochlear implant should largely be conducted in Welsh rather than in English, which she had acquired in the interim.

If the department does not have a speaker of the individual's first language, it is important to assess broadly the level of the individual's communication in any of the languages used in the department. If this is very limited, as with a profoundly deafened Somali speaker, it is essential that a good interpreter is present during the rehabilitation sessions.

Dialect differences are less important, but need to be borne in mind by any therapist working with the individual. Lexical differences, the range of vocabulary and specific aspects of the vocabulary of the individual, need to be borne in mind in the detailed planning of the rehabilitative process.

Thus, examples and training in communication skills will have a different orientation and context for a farm labourer than for a computer programmer.

Morphology, word structure, is unlikely to be altered in patients with a postlingual hearing loss. Those with a prelingual hearing loss may have difficulty, for example, in differentiating between the pronounciation of licked/lɪkt/ and wicked/wɪkɪd/, and also with verb endings.

Syntax, the grammatical structure of language, will be normal in most individuals with acquired hearing loss except in certain patients with brain lesions after cerebrovascular accidents or injuries. In prelingually deaf individuals, the sentence structure may be different from the normal syntax, and in some cases may be influenced by the syntax of the sign language to which they are exposed.

Phonology, the sound pattern of the language, may be grossly abnormal in prelingually deaf individuals. It may also be affected particularly in people with severe acquired hearing losses which can have a marked effect especially on intonation patterns. However, even moderate high frequency hearing losses can affect the pronunciation of voiceless consonants (e.g. s, sh, f, th) due to the lack of auditory feedback to the individual concerned. There may be particular problems when the individual is learning a new language to which they have not previously been exposed.

Pragmatics is the social use of language. The same word phrase or sentence may convey different messages according to the intention of the speaker, depending on factors such as context and intonation patterns. Thus the word 'really' may convey approval, disapproval, sarcasm etc., according to the intonation pattern. Hearing loss may interfere with the recognition of these, and lack appropriate auditory feedback in particular individual's ability to differentiate appropriately between them in productive speech.

Manual communication

In most patients seen with mild to severe acquired hearing loss this is of little relevance, but it is important to enquire as to whether or not the patient knows or is learning some form of sign language. In the prelingually deaf this is much more important, and it may well have a role in the postlingually profoundly deaf.

If the individual does have some knowledge or skills in signing, it is important to know which system they know, whether it is an autonomous system, or one which supplements speechreading, and if autonomous whether it has syntax close to the dominant language of the hearing society.

Thus American (ASL), British (BSL) and French sign languages have their own syntax independent of English or French. Signed English, however, and the Paget-Gorman system are based on the syntax of English.

The mouth hand system (MHS) (Forchammer, 1903) was developed in Denmark mainly for individuals with severe acquired hearing loss and is essentially a supplement to speechreading, providing information not easily accessible from lip patterns. Cued speech (Cornett, Beadles and Wilson, 1982) is an American system which, again, is designed to supplement speechreading but has been used with deaf children. The different types of sign languages are shown in Table 13.12.

Finally, finger spelling is used in conjunction with BSL to sign proper names or word(s) for which the individual may not know the sign. It may also be

Table 13.12 Types of manual communication

Sign languages	e.g.	British Sign Language American Sign Language
Sign languages based on language of hearing society	e.g.	Signed English Paget Gorman
Supports speech reading	e.g.	Cued speech Mouth-hand system (finger spelling)

used to supplement speechreading, and as such is probably more applicable in societies in which MHS is not widely known, to help deafened people differentiate between words difficult to speechread, e.g. MAT – PAT – BAT, by the communicator finger-spelling the first letter to the listener.

If the individual does know one or more manual communication systems it is important to ascertain his level of competence in both receptive and productive communication with the system, either by questioning or by testing the skills. Formal tests have been developed for ASL and there is a need for a more systematic approach to BSL in this respect.

Non-verbal communication

This comprises the use of eye and facial movements, body posture and gesture, paralinguistic variables, personal appearance and environmental factors (Rustin and Kuhr, 1989). The ability to use these varies considerably from person to person even in those people with normal hearing, and training in the good use of non-verbal communication may be important for someone with poor skills who develops a hearing impairment.

In most people with acquired hearing loss the non-verbal skills will be comparable with others within their community, apart from the paralinguistic variables which may degrade following the abolition, reduction or alteration in feedback which the individual receives. Paralinguistic variables include emotional tone, timing of speech, use of silence, pitch, volume, speed, fluency and personal accent. Retraining in some of these may be important in the rehabilitative process.

Many individuals with prelingual hearing loss have never acquired or been taught the importance of non-verbal communication and such training may be important in helping them adapt to a hearing environment after they leave school.

Non-verbal communication behaviour is not normally formally assessed, but may be evaluated in the course of clinical interview and other evaluative and remedial sessions.

Previous rehabilitation

Before starting any rehabilitative programme, it is essential to know what habilitation/rehabilitation the individual has received or been exposed to previously. In this respect it is important to define the strengths and weaknesses of what has been done before, to build on the strengths and to overcome any negative attitudes the patient may have because of the weaknesses of what has been done before.

Within this context it is important to probe for previous instrumental help, hearing aids and environmental aids, any particular communication training, manual communication, and educational orientation.

If one aspect of the individual's rehabilitation has already been dealt with optimally with an appropriate hearing aid fitting, for example, there is no point in altering that and efforts should be concentrated on other aspects of the remedial process.

Overall

While each of the components of the communication status is important in itself, it is essential not to overlook the patient's total communication skills which may be more or less than the sum of the components.

It is important to assess the patients using their optimum mode of communication in order to assess how well they can communicate at the present time so that there are no misconceptions about the outcome of the rehabilitative process.

It is particularly important to take account of the individual's audiovisual skills and compare them with his auditory and speechreading skills alone. There may be very poor integration of the two especially among some patients with prelingual hearing loss.

Finally, it is important to be aware that hearing impaired people have to work hard to hear. They are always listening, not hearing passively, and the degree of this extra effort should be assessed.

Associated variables

These concern the overall approach of the individual towards his hearing loss and the pressures upon him. They cover primarily *psychological* and *sociological* factors, but *work* and *educational* factors may have an important role. These sets of variables will determine the individual's acceptance of or attitude towards his hearing loss and possible remedial intervention, and have a major influence in determining the broad rehabilitative approach to be adopted.

Playing a key role within these factors will be the individual's significant others, individuals such as spouse, parents or children who may play an important, and often dominant role within the patient's domestic and social life, together with close work-

mates, schoolmates or friends who may strongly influence other aspects of his life.

Psychological factors

The individual's attitude towards the rehabilitative process is one of the primary determinants of its outcome. The motivation behind attendance at the clinic and help-seeking is a critical factor. Indeed the second major question which is essential to ask any patient seeking rehabilitative help after determining their disability and handicap, is, 'what made you decide to do something about your hearing problems?'. The astute clinician must always be aware of the misleading answers which some individuals may give to this question and be prepared to probe further to determine the reality of the situation.

McKenna (1991) has highlighted the importance of the individual's motivation in determining the outcome of cochlear implantation, and we have all seen patients in whom much waste of time and expense could have been avoided by more careful probing in this respect.

Related to this as a factor in the individual's attitude are his expectations in terms of the outcome of the rehabilitation process and his acceptance of his hearing loss. These factors will be discussed further in a later section.

The individual's personality has been considered by a number of authors, and will determine the approach and interaction of the professional *vis-à-vis* the patient. Depressive illnesses or anxiety states may lead to the process being introduced in a different way or at a different pace but will not necessarily have major effects on the overall approach. Indeed many authors have highlighted the fact that some hearing impaired patients are more depressed and/or neurotic than hearing controls (Thomas and Gilhome Herbst, 1980) but such deviations will tend to normalize following therapy (Gildston and Gildston, 1972; McKenna, 1991).

On the other hand, serious psychological illness such as manic depressive or paranoid psychoses may need care and attention in the orientation of the rehabilitative approach which should usually be organized in close liaison with psychiatric services.

The conformity and assertiveness of the individual will have to be taken into consideration in developing rehabilitative strategies and may have a strong influence on the individual's attitude towards instrumentation or manual communication.

Finally, the patient's intelligence will have a bearing on the way in which aspects of the rehabilitation are discussed and presented but should not have a major influence on the rehabilitative decisions, which must be made according to the individual's needs.

Sociological factors

These are highlighted by the role of any significant others in the patient's life. In certain cases they have a predominant role in the patient's attitude towards the rehabilitative process. Other factors which come into play are stigma, life-style and, to a lesser extent, social class.

The role of the significant others has been highlighted by a number of authors (Jones, Kyle and Wood, 1987; Hétu *et al.*, 1990; Hallberg and Barrenäs, 1993). While their work has been based on interviews conducted either together with or separate from the hearing impaired patient, they have all highlighted the elements of co-acting, minimizing, mediating or distancing strategies as elaborated by Hallberg and Barrenäs (1993).

The interaction between the significant others and the patient in relation to the ultimate handicap experienced is illustrated in Figure 13.2, but many details of this interaction require more detailed investigation, and most studies have been confined to the interaction between the patient and his spouse who will be the dominant significant other for many of our hearing impaired patients. However, for others the person may be another partner, a child, a parent, a sibling or a carer. Until we understand better the nature of some of these interactions it will be difficult to structure an optimal rehabilitative process.

Without in depth interviews some leads can be obtained by the use of a problem questionnaire targetted at the significant others as mentioned earlier with wording along the lines, 'Please make a list of the problems which you have because of your spouse/friend/parent's hearing difficulties'.

Responses from this may vary from statements such as 'Repeat conversations', 'TV too loud', 'People call and get no answer' to more extensive responses as in Table 13.6. However, in all cases they can provide useful leads to probe for problems in greater depth.

Stigma associated with hearing loss dates back to classical times and to early Jewish and Christian texts in which hearing impaired people were considered incapable of playing a full role in society. They were often regarded as less intelligent, and even in modern day African tribes hearing impairment is regarded as something which provokes scorn, whereas blindness attracts sympathy.

There have been various hypotheses as to the origins of this stigmatization of hearing impaired people, mainly based on the difficulties which they create for hearing people trying to communicate with them. It may also be related to the fact that the prevalence of hearing loss increases with advancing age. The extent of the stigma varies from country to country and also within different societies within any one country. Thus for example, in an area in which there has long been a noisy industry, such as the jute workers of Dundee, hearing impairment was regarded as a normal occurrence, a fact of life and the associated stigma minimal. Similarly in Martha's Vineyard, in the USA where in the last century the prevalence

of profound congenital recessive hearing loss was very common, it was so accepted within the society that many of the normally hearing people learned sign language (Groce, 1985).

In other societies there is a less tolerant attitude and people with acquired hearing loss may have been intolerant themselves before acquiring such a loss. Often many hearing impaired people may have a disproportionate view of the stigmatizing aspects of hearing loss within their society.

The individual's life-style will have obvious effects on their disability and handicap stemming from any impairment. Thus the gregarious individual who takes part in many meetings and social events will be affected differently from the quiet individual who spends his retirement gardening and watching the television. It is, however, important to probe for any changes in life-style, such as social withdrawal, which are consequent upon the hearing loss. It is also important to take into account the general life-style of the patient when planning an appropriate rehabilitation programme.

Social class affects this less and will usually be mediated by influences of stigma and life-style. Prejudices may be found in all social classes even though they may be more openly articulated among manual workers. Furthermore, as hearing impairment and disability are more commonly found among manual classes (Davis, 1983; Stephens, Lewis and Charny, 1991) this can reduce its personal impact on the individual concerned.

Employment/vocational factors

Employment factors may also intervene with hearing loss in a complex way. For some individuals such as musicians, gamekeepers, psychiatrists, their livelihood depends very largely on their ability to hear clearly and an acquired hearing loss may be disastrous leading to a complete change in direction of their working life. This will depend very much on their training and background and the nature and severity of the hearing loss. The lesion may only need to cause a mild distortion for the musician's career to be destroyed, whereas with appropriate rehabilitation a physician may be able to continue his work, having perhaps to switch his orientation to pathology or radiology if his loss is sufficient to preclude normal one-to-one communication with his patients.

Generally, the individual's occupation will influence the orientation of the rehabilitation and many of the major problems will be highlighted during the assessment of disability and handicap. It is always well to be aware, however, that the individual may be unhappy with his chosen career or changes which have taken place within it, and use his disabilities as means of changing career or taking early retirement, actions which he might have hesitated to take without this additional stimulus. The feelings of the patient in these changes must be respected.

It is also important to be aware of the impact of changes in the individual's work on the disability and handicap arising from this impairment. Thus an individual with a moderate hearing loss who is able to perform well as an accountant may be promoted to a management post which entails business meetings and more telephoning, and consequently finds it difficult to cope and loses self-confidence.

The attitude of others in the workplace may have a considerable influence on the individual. Some may have supportive colleagues, and employers who will install environmental aids (assistive listening devices) to help their hearing impaired colleagues. Others may find themselves victimized by the prejudices of their supervisors who find it difficult to cope with the new communicative situation. Yet others may fear the reaction of their superiors who might in fact be very sympathetic and supportive should the individual be prepared to articulate his problems.

Educational factors

While these apply particularly to individuals whose hearing loss arose in childhood, this is not always true. Thus attitudes towards hearing loss inculcated in the individual from being educated alongside and becoming friendly with hearing impaired children may foster a positive attitude towards hearing loss in later life. Many hearing children may even learn different types of sign language from such schools in order to enter more into the world of the deaf child and have a language not understandable by others.

Furthermore, many individuals continue with education throughout their adult lives and it is important to remember that even people in their 70s and 80s may wish to learn a new language to use on their holidays or with their grandchildren. This again merits consideration when planning rehabilitative programmes. Frequently, language classes are conducted with poor quality sound recordings in highly resonant classrooms.

The educational upbringing of the deaf child can have a very important bearing on his subsequent communication skills. All too often the education of hearing impaired children has rigidly followed a particular oral or signing dogma rather than being keyed into a pragmatic determination of the educational approach necessary for the particular child. Such an oral system may lead to an inappropriately educated individual barely able to communicate even with his family in any communicative mode. On the other hand, a manual obsession by the system may leave an individual with good residual hearing totally unable to use his voice. Even the drive towards full integration into normal schools with good support can lead to social difficulties for the individual concerned, particularly the less able of the deaf children. These, because of their difficulties in the classroom, may mix socially with children less able and more disruptive than themselves, which can then have a further deleterious effect on their development.

Related conditions

This section is concerned with factors which have an important influence on the detail of the remedial process. Here the concern is with the characteristics of the individual which influence ability to cope with different types of instrumentation used to help them, and consequently the selection of the appropriate instrumentation. It will also influence the use of supplementary means of communication in cases in which that might be appropriate.

The factors coming in here are somewhat disparate, but all act on this level. They cover *mobility*, how well the individual is able to get around, *upper limb function*, particularly tactile sensitivity and fine motor skills, and finally *related aural pathology*. This last includes tinnitus, otorrhoea, pressure feelings in the ear, otalgia and associated problems.

Mobility

This is concerned with gross limitations of the mobility of the patient. For example the approach to a fully mobile active patient will differ from that for one who is able to leave the house only with aid, to one who is largely chair or bed-bound.

Particularly for those who rarely leave the room, such a fact will influence the rehabilitative process in terms of a greater orientation towards environmental aids and less towards wearable hearing aids, unless the former will not meet the needs of the patient.

Upper limb function

This will influence the ability of the patient to manipulate fine controls on hearing aids and other devices and influence the type of aid/ear mould which may be used in their particular circumstances.

At one extreme we have to consider the amputee who will be unable to control normal hearing aids at all. While the aid(s) may be fitted to his ear(s) by a significant other or carer, it is essential that sophisticated compression and other processing systems be incorporated into the aid to avoid tolerance problems when the individual moves from quiet to more noisy surroundings. With the introduction of programmable aids or those controllable by infrared signals, this problem is more amenable to maintaining the individual's independence than it was a few years ago.

A far more common problem is that of reduced fine manipulative skills and tactile sensitivity found particularly in elderly people. This may be extreme in individuals after cerebrovascular accidents, severe osteoarthritis or rheumatoid arthritis, and in neuro-degenerative conditions. However, to a lesser extent it is common in many elderly people, particularly women (Upfold, May and Battaglia, 1990; Meredith and Stephens, 1993). This leads to difficulties in manipulating controls on hearing aids, particularly the volume control (Roberts, 1992), and in fitting ear moulds in the ears (Meredith and Stephens, 1993). While gross abnormalities may be detected by most audiologists, we have found that two simple tasks, recognizing shapes by touch alone, and undoing and redoing a screw and washer (Figure 13.5), are good predictors of manipulative performance in elderly first-time hearing aid users (Meredith and Stephens, 1993).

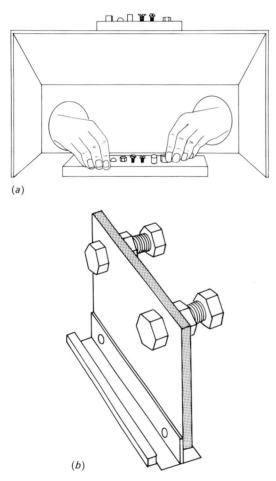

(a)

(b)

Figure 13.5 Devices for testing (a) tactile sensitivity and (b) manipulative skills (from Sperling *et al.*, 1980; Meredith and Stephens, 1993)

Related aural pathology

Here we are concerned about other aural symptoms which can affect the ability of an individual to tolerate a hearing aid/ear mould system within the ear. These include the presence of tinnitus, a pressure sensation, pain, discharge, perforation and the Tullio phenomenon. External ear problems include deformed pinnae and ear canals and the presence of bony osteomas.

Tinnitus is a very common phenomenon (see Chapters 3 and 18) and Coles, Davis and Smith (1991) have reported that about one-third of all individuals with hearing loss have significant tinnitus. Most commonly, well fitted hearing aids can reduce such tinnitus, although occluding moulds may increase it in many cases (Hazell *et al.*, 1985). It is therefore important in patients with significant tinnitus in addition to the hearing loss, to be aware of this and, wherever possible use non-occluding ear moulds. This will generally improve both the hearing and the tinnitus, although in some cases, even with a good fit, the tinnitus may be exacerbated (Stephens and Meredith, 1991b).

Pressure sensation in the ears may be due to either eustachian tube dysfunction or endolymphatic hydrops. When fitting hearing aids, if medical treatment has not successfully abolished the sensation, it is important again that, wherever possible, any ear moulds should be non-occluding with a pressure vent if necessary. A tightly fitting ear mould will often accentuate or exacerbate any underlying discomfort in this respect.

Reports of pain in the ears must be carefully probed and investigated. It may stem from the external or middle ears or the trigeminal nerve (e.g. herpes zoster, vestibular schwannoma). In addition, some individuals may report the pressure sensation of endolymphatic hydrops as pain.

The underlying cause of the pain should be treated and such a report should always be taken seriously. Anything in the way of a hearing aid fitting which aggravates the pain will make the individual turn against such a fitting. In individuals with chronic idiopathic otalgia an open ear mould or non-occluding fitting will generally be more acceptable than a standard fitting.

Otorrhoea from otitis externa or chronic suppurative otitis media is normally a contraindication to an air-conduction hearing aid fitting to that ear until it is brought under control. When that is achieved, and also in the case of persistent perforations of the tympanic membrane, open or vented ear moulds will have to be used, with a filter (French St George and Barr Hamilton, 1975) where feedback is a problem. The presence of a persistent perforation may also be a good indication for a myringoplasty, where feasible, to facilitate a hearing aid fitting.

In some individuals recurrent infections (both otitis externa and chronic suppurative otitis media) cannot be effectively controlled, and bone anchored hearing aids may be indicated, provided that the bone conduction thresholds are not markedly elevated. These will also be indicated in gross deformities of the external meatus such as may be found in Treacher Collins syndrome.

In less severe deformities, with a normal external meatus and abnormal pinna, a good fitting may well be achieved with in-the-ear or in-the-canal aids in patients where any postural hearing aid fitting will be impossible.

Finally, in some individuals loud acoustical stimulation may give rise to vertigo, as in Tullio's phenomenon. This is found in patients who had fenestrations, some 20% of patients with Menière's disorder, and in certain other patients. In such individuals, it is essential to determine the sound pressure levels and the different frequencies which will trigger such vertigo, and then to ensure that the maximum output level of any hearing aid to be fitted does not exceed these levels.

Integration and decision making

This is the stage at which the first and most important decisions are made as to the most appropriate line of management of the patient. Within this section the audiologist must pull together the relevant attitudinal aspects of the patient, modify them in the course of discussion when that is possible, and decide on the broad categorization of the patient and hence the most relevant approach to management. Finally, bearing that in mind, some initial goals must be negotiated between the patient and professional to determine the particular orientation within the decided approach.

Integration

This entails determining the attitude of the patient and attempting to nudge it in an appropriate direction, when it is likely to be counterproductive to the outcome of the rehabilitative process. The attitude may be regarded as comprising three components of *acceptance*, *understanding* and *expectation*. It is important that the individual *accepts* that his hearing loss is likely to be permanent and is not going to recover to normality, and that without appropriate rehabilitative help (and perhaps even with it) there are certain activities which he will find difficult or impossible. Without such an acceptance, the rehabilitative programme is going to be a failure.

Hallberg, Johnsson and Axelsson (1993) have recently applied a modified version of the 'Acceptance of Illness Scale' (Felton, Revenson and Hinrichsen, 1984) to individuals with noise-induced hearing loss and found that acceptance of hearing problems was negatively correlated with handicap but not related to audiometric thresholds (Hallberg, 1994).

The scale is an eight question instrument and merits examination in the outcome of the rehabilitative programme.

Understanding entails some comprehension of what has caused the hearing loss, the mechanism involved, and the changes in the aural function and its consequences in terms of disability and handicap. These can be clarified with the patient and the time taken to do this by the professional often pays big dividends in terms of the patient's overall motivation.

The *expectations* of the patient must be appropriate. It is as bad for the patient to expect too much from the rehabilitative process as to have too low an expectation. The individual who thinks that he will be able to function completely normally as a result of the rehabilitation may become disillusioned and reject the process altogether when it fails to meet these expectations. Persistence would, however, have given tangible benefits.

Equally, a patient with low expectations may not persist with the process. For example, coming in with limited expectations of any benefit he is going to obtain from a hearing aid, he is likely to reject the aid altogether as soon as he encounters the slightest problem.

Thus again time taken by the professional in helping the patient to have realistic expectations can be invaluable in improving the outcome of any rehabilitative process.

Categorization

Here decisions must be made. Will the patient be for the fast track and have rapid straight-forward and successful rehabilitation (category 1); does he have complicating factors so that, despite his positive motivation he requires a more extensive rehabilitative programme (category 2); does he want help but reject an important part of the rehabilitative process (category 3); or does he deny disability and reject all help (category 4)?

Fortunately most patients come within categories 1 and 2 (Stephens, 1987b; Stephens and Meredith, 1991c). The differentiation between the two has important resource implications in terms of professional time taken to achieve optimum rehabilitation, and planning must be made taking this into account.

The details of the rehabilitative types have been discussed at length elsewhere (Goldstein and Stephens, 1981). The *category 1* patients will require few clinic visits, usually one visit following the fitting will be adequate to check that all is well, making any necessary adjustments and giving advice about environmental aids and hearing tactics. The patient can then usually be discharged on the understanding that he will return should he encounter any problems with hearing or the aid(s).

The reasons for *type 2* categorization are outlined in Table 13.13. The balance of these will depend on the type of clinic population being seen. The proportion of category 2 patients increases with age, Stephens and Meredith (1991c) finding a proportion

Table 13.13 Reasons for type 2 categorization

Tactile and manipulative problems
Cognitive difficulties
Chronic middle ear disease
Annoying tinnitus
Otitis externa
Psychological problems
Relatively low motivation
Mild or very severe impairment
Prelingual hearing loss

of 37% in patients of less than 65 years of age, increasing to 77% in those aged 85 and over. The understanding of this balance of patients within the particular population being seen can have important implications in costing any service.

Category 3 patients may want help but reject an important part of the process. For example they may reject a hearing aid, even though it may be essential in order to achieve optimum rehabilitation. Others may expect a cochlear implant to resolve all their psychosocial problems and be unprepared to accept the counselling which they really need in that context before cochlear implantation can be appropriately considered.

In such cases, following an orthodox approach will be doomed to failure. What has to be done, in the case of those refusing a hearing aid, is to pursue a reasonable approach adopting appropriate aspects of the rehabilitative process acceptable to the patient, and introducing the hearing aid as 'something worth trying' in a non-threatening way when the individual's disability has been put in better perspective at a later stage.

For those with inappropriate expectations of instrumentation – cochlear implants or hearing aids – these should not be pursued directly until, using various approaches, the individual has been brought round to having more realistic expectations. Without this, the patient will undoubtedly reject the instrumentation on finding that it does not resolve all his problems.

Category 4 patients are those who refuse to admit disability, coming to the clinic as a result of pressure from family and friends. Attempting to intervene is both ethically and practically inappropriate. What must be done with the individual is to accept in discussion with him that if he experiences no disability there should be no intervention, but leaving the door open should he experience (or admit to) a disability at a later stage. The significant others, for whom this may be a considerable problem, should however, be offered advice on communication tactics and environmental aids.

One of the problems with category 4 patients is that sometimes they do not overtly express their feelings, and it is important to be alert for such individuals, particularly in the course of discussing with the patient his reasons for attending the clinic.

Goal setting

At this stage it is important to define the principal goals which the rehabilitation process is to aim at achieving. These emerge from a frank discussion with the patient, taking as a starting point the main elements of disability and handicap already defined and the individual's current communication status. The therapist must tease out from these the most important goals which the patient wishes to achieve, at the same time counselling him with regard to goals which are not achievable, given his auditory status. Thus an individual with a total unilateral hearing loss who wants to be able to localize birds is always going to be disappointed.

Once the goals have been defined, most category 1 and 2 patients will proceed with a hearing aid/instrumental fitting. Some category 2 patients with minimal hearing loss and specific needs may go straight to consideration of environmental aids. The same path may be followed by some physically infirm patients with a moderate hearing loss whose goals can be most effectively met by appropriate environmental aids. For some people, such as many of those with auditory disability and normal audiograms (see Chapter 17), it may be appropriate to pass straight to defining better communication strategies, bypassing instrumentation altogether.

Category 3 patients will also generally follow the same route, bypassing personal instrumentation, until that is felt to be appropriate, and starting with environmental aids and strategy, according to the goals defined in discussion. Likewise, the significant others of category 4 patients may be given some advice along the same route.

Short-term remediation

Instrumentation

The devices discussed in this section have a unique role in the rehabilitative process. It is, however, essential to remember that they remain only tools to help the patient and professional achieve the goals which they have set themselves. The instruments are not ends in themselves.

Secondly, it is essential to remember that any provision of instrumentation must be accompanied by appropriate instruction to ensure that the patient obtains optimum benefit from the device(s). While this is particularly true for the personal instruments (hearing aids, cochlear implants, vibrotactile aids), it is also true to a lesser extent of the simplest environmental aids. For this reason, instruction is specified as a key section of this component of the rehabilitative process.

The section is summarized in Table 13.14.

Personal instrumentation

This section, while arguably the most important single component of the rehabilitation process will be

Table 13.14 Instrumentation

1   Personal instrumentation
    a Hearing aid systems
       i hearing aid(s)
      ii ear moulds
    b Bone anchored hearing aids
    c Vibrotactile aids
    d Cochlear implants
    e Brain-stem implants

2   General instrumentation/environmental aids (assistive listening devices)
    a Communication systems
       i telephone
      ii radio/hifi/TV/video
     iii FM radio systems
     iv PA systems/ticket office systems
    b Alerting and warning systems
       i doorbells
      ii telephone bells
     iii alarm clocks
     iv baby alarms
      v fire/smoke/burglar alarms

3   Instruction

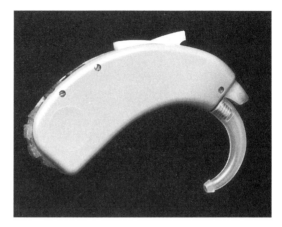

Figure 13.6 A prototype ergonomic postaural hearing aid. Note the large push-on/push-off switch and the volume control built around the battery compartment (after Roberts, 1992)

Table 13.15 Factors determining choice of ear mould

Factor		Consequences
1	Hearing loss	
	a Severity	Severe hearing losses lead to a need for tight fitting soft moulds to reduce feedback
	b Configuration	High frequency losses indicate a need for vented/horned moulds
2	Self-consciousness	A need for inconspicuous, skeleton type, colourless moulds
3	Tactile/manipulative problems	Avoid moulds with 'top prongs'. Use moulds with a firm connecting tube facilitating handling
4	Tinnitus	Use as open a mould as possible, given the hearing loss
5	Perforation	Ensure that the mould is open or vented with a sintered filter where necessary
6	Pressure sensations	As 5
7	Allergy	Once it has been determined that the problem is truly allergic, use non-allergenic materials, progressing to a silver or gold mould if necessary

discussed only very briefly here, being covered in detail in Chapters 15 and 16.

Hearing aid systems

These are generally considered in terms of the electroacoustical characteristics of the devices concerned, together with cosmetic elements. It is, however, essential to consider them also in terms of the individual's ability to use them, to fit them in their ear(s) and to manipulate their controls. These factors are rarely taken into account by manufacturers but, particularly with demographic changes resulting in a larger proportion of elderly people within the population, will assume a greater profile in the future. Various studies have indicated that, after the problems of fitting the ear mould (or in-the-ear aid) into the ear, the greatest difficulty experienced by most elderly patients is with the volume control (Roberts, 1992). This may be overcome using sophisticated, hence expensive, technology such as infrared or ultrasonic hand-held control boxes, but can also be facilitated by the application of simple engineering technology (Figure 13.6). This low cost approach is particularly important given the financial status of most elderly patients and the unwillingness of health care systems to support an expensive option.

Ear moulds are particularly important both in terms of difficulties experienced by patients in fitting the hearing aid system to their ears and also in terms of comfort, in addition to the acoustical effects they can have on the hearing aid system.

The factors from the evaluation part of the process which can influence the particular choice of ear-mould fitting have been discussed elsewhere (Stephens, 1985), and an amended version of this is shown in Table 13.15. Here it is very important to bear in mind that a very simple modification to the ear mould (Meredith and Stephens, 1993) can have a dramatic effect on whether or not the patient is able to fit the hearing aid system to his ear and can become a major determinant in whether or not he continues to use the hearing aid.

A variety of non-auditory factors will also influence the choice of hearing aid fittings and these have been discussed elsewhere (Stephens, 1984).

Other types of personal instrumentation

While hearing aids constitute the vast majority of personal instruments fitted, some 600 000 per year in the UK (Davis, 1993), vibrotactile aids, bone anchored hearing aids, and cochlear implants are being increasingly successful, used with small selected client groups. Thus several hundred vibrotactile aids, 100–200 bone anchored hearing aids and some 200 cochlear implants are fitted per year to adults within the UK. There are unlikely to be more than single figures of brain-stem implants (Shannon *et al.*, 1993) per year, the first in the UK being performed in 1994.

The choice of different systems is often very difficult and should always be based on the needs and capacities of the individual patient, bearing in mind the different components of the evaluative process, and it is easy to implant an inappropriate patient who has a suitable hearing loss but a completely unsuitable set of psychosocial problems (McKenna, 1991).

General instrumentation

Within this section, I shall consider the use of *environmental aids* or *assistive listening devices*. The interest in these devices as a part of the rehabilitative process has increased markedly in the last decade, although many have been available since the time of Edith Whetnall.

The range and application of devices available in the USA has been extensively discussed by Compton (1993) and the various technologies which may be used summarized elsewhere (Stephens, 1987b).

The main fact which differentiates these devices from personal aids is that while they may be used by one individual alone, they may equally be used by a group of individuals within a house, a school or a public place.

The collective name for these devices has in the UK usually been 'environmental aids' which will be used here. With the recent interest in them in USA, the term 'assistive listening devices' has become widely accepted and is sometimes also used in other English speaking countries.

The devices may be broadly separated into those which facilitate communication, enabling the listener to receive speech or other meaningful signals, and those which facilitate alerting/warning signals.

Communication systems

These have a common factor in being aimed at making the signal (usually speech) recognizable by the hearing impaired person. Usually they will entail some form of additional amplification or coupling of the source of speech to the patient, or a means of improving the signal-noise ratio and reducing the inverse square law effect. An alternative approach is to transmit the message, either in its entirety or as a supplement to other forms of communication, using the printed word. These are summarized in Table 13.16.

Table 13.16 Communication aid systems

Using sound
1   Additional speaker/receiver
2   Additional amplifier
3   Direct hardwire link to patient
    a   additional headset
    b   link to hearing aids
4   Induction coil systems
5   Infrared or FM transmission

Using visual information
1   Text telephones
2   Subtitled TV/videos
3   Video telephones
4   Text TV announcements in airports/stations, etc.

Enhancement of Loudness and Clarity

This is a simple process using either an amplifier system coupling the television/radio to the patient, or an additional amplifier on the telephone handset (usually around 15 dB). An alternative approach with the television is to use an extension speaker with good sound quality situated by the hearing impaired person's chair, to supplement or replace the small poor-quality speaker in the TV itself. This is analogous in some ways to the additional earpiece available on some telephones, which can also be used by a significant other.

Coupling systems may be direct links to the patient via an additional amplifier and headset, as with many television listening devices. These may be either directly plugged into the television, or have a microphone which may be stuck on to the front of the TV loudspeaker. The sound quality is obviously superior with the first of these.

The second system is to link the sound source directly to the 'audio input' of the hearing aid. This requires considerable supervision and care because of potential dangers of linking the aid to a high voltage system.

An induction coil coupling system may be used with the hearing aid switched to the telecoil input. This may be achieved by a loop within a telephone handset or an induction coil system which can be clipped onto it. For television, radio and a variety of public address, church or theatre systems, a range of electromagnetic loop systems may be used. These can range from a personalized loop silhouette which can be placed on the ear alongside the hearing aid, a neck loop around the patient's neck to a pillow or chair loop, to having a loop system covering a section or all of a public place. With such large systems involving an electromagnetic field within a room, care has to be taken because of lack of uniformity of the field strength in different parts of the room.

Finally, infrared or FM radio transmission can be used from the sound source, e.g. television or public speaker to the individual. These necessitate a purpose-built receiver which is then linked to the individual's hearing aid via a direct audio-input or neck-loop system. The sound quality is better with these than with electromagnetic systems, but apart from the considerably greater cost, there are problems if the receiver is trained away from the light source or if there is bright light in the room with the infrared systems. With the FM radio system problems may arise from a 'spill over' of the signal to and from adjacent rooms.

Use of Visual Information

Messages may be transmitted in written form through a telephone either directly with text telephones (Minicom in the UK) or via computer terminals linked with modems. These systems need either both parties to the communication having such a system, or being linked via an interpreter on a switchboard as was developed in the UK by the Royal National Institute for the Deaf. Text telephone and interpreter systems have the problems of expense and that such a system is much slower than acoustical communication. Computer based systems reduce that problem but preclude the immediate interactive spontaneity of a normal two-way conversation.

Work is rapidly developing on the use of the video telephone which will complement many of the existing systems.

Subtitling is being increasingly used with television programmes and video throughout the world, and certainly is invaluable for many hearing impaired viewers. However, recent studies in the UK (Sancho-Aldridge and Davis, 1993) have indicated that relatively few people with acquired hearing loss use such a system, and Kyle (1992) has highlighted problems with it for prelingually deaf people, related in part to limited reading skills. This can be overcome by the use of a simultaneous signer shown on the screen, although at present such an approach is generally limited to a small number of news programmes.

Whichever system is to be adopted, particularly for severely impaired people using the telephone, considerable instruction and training may be needed. While this has been highlighted in the case of patients with cochlear implants, it is equally true for many hearing aid users, and a valuable approach to this problem has been developed by Burdo and Poggia (1991) who have produced specific training programmes as well as highlighting the choices between different systems.

Finally, technology in the field of electronic speech recognition systems is advancing rapidly and is likely to be increasingly available in the next few years, with obvious applications for hearing impaired people.

Alerting and warning systems

A common approach is also applicable through these systems. This entails either making the sound louder, bringing it closer to the patient, changing the nature of the sound to one more likely to be heard, or by using a sensory substitution system.

The sound of bells and alarms can easily be increased by changing the system. This may still cause problems for the patient with a high frequency hearing loss who has an alarm system which is predominantly high frequency. Substituting a low frequency buzzer, generally very cheap, can be invaluable in such a case.

The other major problem is that of individuals who spend much of their life listening to television and are unable to hear the bell(s) because of their poor signal-in-noise discrimination. Installation of an extension bell in their living room is a cheap and effective way of resolving these problems.

Patients with more severe hearing loss may need the use of sensory substitution devices. These normally use visual stimuli either with specially installed lights, as in a telephone handset or smoke alarm, or linkage to a system which flashes on and off all the lights in the house. There may even be different flashing systems here according to whether it is the doorbell or the telephone bell which is ringing.

Vibratory stimuli are commonly used for alarm clocks with the vibrator installed under the individual's pillow. This is a particularly important situation as the vast majority of hearing aid users remove them at night. An alternative used in these situations is a fan alongside the patient's bed which blows cold air on the sleeper's face when triggered by the alarm.

Finally an alarm system may be alive! Many patients have long reported that their dog warns them when there is someone at the door, a burglar or the telephone is ringing. Over the past 10–20 years specially trained dogs, 'Hearing dogs for the deaf', have been made available for needy individuals by charities, the dogs being trained to respond in different ways according to the signal ringing.

Strategy

Within this section we return to the goals which were considered in the integration/categorization section and reconsider how they can be best achieved by modification of the patient's behaviour.

In order to achieve this it is first important to define or review the patient's personality and the attitudes of his significant others and then discuss tactics to achieve the goals bearing these factors in mind.

Hearing tactics, developed in Denmark (Von der Lieth, 1972; Vognsen, 1976) and applied in many other parts of the world, are most useful in themselves, but need to take into account the individual's personality and life situation, in particular his interaction with significant others. It would be useless to discuss a particular set of tactics to achieve an aim, e.g. functioning adequately in a business meeting by the individual assertively announcing his hearing disability and how the others at the meeting can help him overcome it, if the patient is a shy withdrawn person. Likewise the development of tactics for hearing better within the home must bear in mind the personality and attitudes of the individual's spouse and children.

The overall strategy to be negotiated with the patient thus is to define the goals and to clarify the best tactics to use bearing in mind his personality and those of his significant others.

Personality

Within this section it is mainly important to decide whether the individual is an assertive, outward going individual or a timid introverted person both of which may lead to the use of a particular set of tactics. Thus, at a meeting, the assertive extrovert may publicly announce to the meeting how the others can facilitate his communication and do it in such a way that they feel good in themselves about helping. The shy introvert, on the other hand, may arrange the papers which he will have carefully pre-read, arrange the seating so that he is facing the principal participants whose faces should be well illuminated, and record the whole meeting, getting the agreement of the chairman privately to do that before hand.

Unfortunately the situation is not always so clear cut as an individual may be reasonably assertive in one set of circumstances and feel threatened in others, so that tactics will have to be discussed bearing this apparent dichotomy in mind.

Significant others

This section is concerned with the most important significant others in the patient's life. Their attitude and approach to the patient's hearing loss is critical in defining appropriate tactics and they should be involved in discussions between the patient and therapist from an early stage. However, it is essential that the initial discussions are with the patient alone. Without this, dominating assertive significant others can completely overwhelm the patient in the course of discussions.

While the spouse or other family member is the most important significant other for the vast majority of patients, a significant other from the workplace or from the patient's leisure pursuits may also be of some relevance, and more than one significant other

can be involved in discussions for different goals which are important to the patient.

The different responses for the significant others have been discussed by Jones (1987), Hétu *et al.* (1988) and Hallberg and Barrenäs (1993). These last authors, who specifically investigated 10 wives of men with noise-induced hearing loss, identified four strategies which the significant others may adopt. They defined these as:

1 Co-acting: pretending with the patient that there is no real problem
2 Minimizing: playing down the problems arising from the patient's hearing loss
3 Mediating:
   a controlling – taking over control of the situation
   b navigating – keeping the patient away from auditorily stressful circumstances
   c Advising – getting the patient to tell others about his hearing loss, etc
4 Distancing: separating themselves from the patient as far as possible.

It is essential that a feeling for such approaches adopted by the significant other are borne in mind when defining appropriate tactics. Any attempt to modify an approach which seems inappropriate can be considered in counselling sessions during the communication training process.

Hearing tactics

These involve manipulating the individual's environment (animate and inanimate) to improve the listening conditions. They may involve basic matters like positioning themselves so that the light is in the speaker's face and not the patient's, reducing background noise (e.g. turning off the radio) when speaking with the family, to aspects of observing nonverbal communication.

They have been investigated by Field and Haggard (1989) who listed them in three categories involving manipulating social interaction, manipulating the physical environment and observation. These are summarized in Table 13.17, and may be complemented by other approaches specific to particular situations.

Ancillary help

In the course of their habilitative process, needs of the patient will often emerge which come outside the expertise of the rehabilitative team. Under these circumstances it is important to involve the relevant professionals who can provide help in other domains to complement that provided 'in-house'.

Within this context particular domains include *social work* and *educational support, aid with employment, medical* and *psychological help*. The last may, in part, be encompassed by physicians and psychologists

Table 13.17 Types of hearing tactics

Manipulating social interaction

1 Asking talker to speak slowly, clearly and loudly but without shouting
2 Asking talker to catch your attention before speaking
3 Asking talker to face you
4 Asking significant other to specify topic
5 Asking significant other to repeat/rephrase difficult phrases/sentences
6 Repeat back phrase/sentence to confirm details
7 Give feedback with non-verbal gestures
8 Point out that you are hard of hearing

Manipulating physical environment

1 Ensure speaker's face is well illuminated and not obscured
2 Move closer to the talker
3 Reduce/avoid background noise, e.g. radio, TV, traffic
4 Have soft furnishings to reduce resonance
5 Position yourself close to loudspeaker, with your better ear facing it
6 Adjust tuning/tone control of radio/TV to optimum listening condition

Observation

1 Watch the lips/face of speaker
2 Take note of non-verbal communication
3 Fill in gaps in conversation from background knowledge
4 Keep calm and patient

After Field and Haggard, 1989

within the rehabilitative team, but they will encounter problems requiring other medical and psychological expertise for management of related neurological conditions or offering family therapy, etc.

Social work support can help in the context of rehousing and the provision of environmental aids, and in many cases, social workers for the deaf have a unique role in support services for the prelingually deaf community. In this context, as well as general support, they can provide interpreting services and often organize centres/clubs for the deaf.

Educational and employment services, the latter via the disability employment advisors, can provide appropriate advice and support in the form of environmental aids in the workplace, radio aids in education, and can organize appropriate retraining courses for the deafened. The educational services are increasingly extending their cover to further and higher education, and university facilities for the deaf are gradually increasing.

Communication training

While the preceding sections have usually entailed a relatively short duration component of management, lasting one or two sessions, communication training involves the on-going rehabilitative management which may continue over months or years. In other cases (category 1 patients) it may last only a part of one session.

In every case there are four main components of communication which need to be considered: *information provision*; *skill building*; *instrumental modification* and *counselling*. Each one of these is a broad area which will be very different for each patient and group of patients. In every case what is done must be relevant and planned within the context of the individual's goals which have been discussed earlier. A major defect of many rehabilitative programmes in the past has been that patients have often been slotted into a standardized programme regardless of their specific needs. For some it has been excessive and unnecessary, for others insufficient and often inappropriate.

Information provision

Information is provided to the patient with regard to the cause and prognosis of the hearing loss, so far as is possible, together with what can and is to be done to alleviate its effects. This last section may include a broad discussion of what hearing tactics comprises, a presentation of what may be offered to the individual with poor manual dexterity, or an outline of the benefits and limitations of different types of cochlear implants. In every case the aim of this section is to provide information to the patients which increases their confidence and their ability to benefit optimally from the on going rehabilitative process.

The provision of information will progress with the patient in long duration rehabilitation sessions. Thus with a patient having a cochlear implant, for example, while the first session may be, as mentioned above, a presentation of different types of implants, successive sessions may outline the particular characteristics of the chosen implant, ways in which it can be used to complement speechreading, a discussion of its use in hearing without visual cues, and a presentation of its use in telephone communication.

Provision of information with regard to other facilities within the community to help the hearing impaired person, together with self-help groups comes within this domain.

Skill building

The provision of information leads into the skill building section which entails training the patient in the skills which are necessary to acquire in order to have optimum rehabilitation. Again the areas of skill building will depend upon what is important to the individual to meet the agreed goals.

These will vary from developing and practising handling skills in terms of fitting a hearing aid to the ear and adjusting the controls, to extracting various aspects of speech information from a vibrotactile stimulator. Each procedure needs to be performed in a carefully staged way with the stages organized according to the individual's capabilities. The progress should be carefully monitored with progression to successive stages being contingent on success at the preceding stage. This question of staged skill building is common to all educational/rehabilitative processes and has been discussed in the audiological context by McKenna (1987) and by Dillon *et al.* (1991).

The skill building has often been carried out in groups bringing together patients with broadly similar sets of problems for speechreading classes or auditory training. While group sessions are beneficial in terms of economic considerations and peer group motivation, they have to be very carefully structured with supplementary sessions on a one-to-one basis to meet the individual patient's needs. Merely putting a group of individuals together whose only common feature is a moderate acquired hearing loss, and trying to teach them speechreading is doomed to failure. Indeed many studies have indicated that acquisition of speechreading skills on such a basis is minimal. What must be done is to structure the training to the vocabulary and individuals to be encountered by the patient, possibly on an interactive video basis (e.g. Tye-Murray *et al.*, 1988) in order to enable them to meet their specific needs.

It is beyond the scope of this chapter to discuss in detail the techniques of speechreading, auditory or audiovisual training and the reader is referred to such general texts as Jeffers and Barley (1978), Berger (1972) and for a brief and succinct overview to Montgomery (1993). Useful further information may be found in the training manual for cochlear implant users (Cochlear, 1991) and for use with telephone systems to Burdo and Poggia (1991).

Skill building applies to the achievement of specific goals defined together by the patient and therapist. When such goals have been achieved, they must be discussed together to determine whether they should define and proceed to further goals or whether patient and therapist are satisfied with the progress which has been made and agree to terminate the on-going programme.

Instrumental modification

In this stage the instrumentation with which the patient has been provided is reviewed to determine whether or not he is obtaining optimum benefit from it. Adjustments may need to be made to hearing aid frequency responses with Barfod (1979) and Gatehouse (1992) having highlighted the fact that adjustment to appropriate amplification is a long-term process. Initially patients prefer to listen to a frequency response which matches their habitual listening situation, whereas, ideally, they may need more high

frequency or more low frequency input to obtain optimum speech discrimination. Such frequency characteristics may be unacceptable at first and they must gradually be weaned over to such a configuration over a period of months.

Other necessary adjustments to hearing aids or cochlear implants will depend on the experiences of the patient as described to the therapist, and will include adjustment of output levels, physical comfort and general acceptability of the sound quality. The basis of adjustment to the use of the device will generally have been covered in the context of the fitting and skill-building sessions and should also be reviewed at this stage.

The provision of appropriate environmental aids should also be reviewed at this stage. Some devices such as alarm clock, baby alarm or smoke alarm systems will be independent of any wearable aid system and need only be briefly reviewed. Others, such as television and telephone aids, and even doorbell or telephone bell systems will be contingent on the efficacy of the hearing aid system in meeting the patient's needs. Thus one individual may find that he is able to hear the television adequately without any disturbance to his significant others when using his hearing aid, and require no further help. Others may find persistent problems and alternative approaches with loop systems, additional amplifiers or speakers, or subtitling should be considered and tested.

Should the overall hearing aid/implant system with which the patient has been fitted prove to be unsatisfactory at this stage, it may be necessary to return to the instrumentation section of the rehabilitative process to select an alternative system with careful comparisons between the existing and new systems.

Counselling

This is an on-going interactive process between the patient (with or without significant other) and therapist aimed at discussing any problems, highlighting solutions together with the patient describing appropriate positive aspects of the rehabilitation which has so far occurred.

The overall approach together with different frameworks which may be used have been extensively discussed by Erdman (1993). Table 13.18 summarizes her classification of the different approaches to counselling and the reader is referred to her chapter for detailed references.

The exact approach to be adopted depends very much on the therapist concerned and must be attuned to their own feelings and skills. Overall the cognitive approaches are most generally favoured at the present time, there having been a general reaction among the more mechanistic approaches based on behavioural therapy.

Table 13.18 Approaches to counselling

Cognitive approaches
 Individual psychology
 Cognitive therapy
 Rational emotive therapy
 Transactional analysis

Behavioural approaches
 Behaviour therapy
 Social learning models
 Multimodel therapy
 Cognitive behaviour modification

Humanistic approaches
 Person-centred therapy
 Gestalt therapy
 Existential psychotherapy

After Erdman, 1993

It is important that any audiological therapist who will be working with on-going rehabilitative procedures has training in an appropriate counselling system. This is essential to provide a framework ranging from the development of empathy with the patient through the various interactive stages as appropriate, always with the aim of reducing the individual's disabilities and handicaps.

Evaluation of the rehabilitative process

In common with all interventions, it is essential to evaluate the effectiveness of the rehabilitation which is being conducted. This is necessary not only in order to increase the relevance of what is being done and to improve any rehabilitative approaches, but also to justify the programme to those paying for it. This last point is equally relevant whether the purchasers of the service are the state, insurance companies, or the individual concerned.

How then can this be evaluated? Given the aims of rehabilitation being to minimize disability and handicap, the obvious solution is to assess how well such aims have been achieved. However, for a variety of reasons this is often difficult to achieve and other approaches used have included satisfaction measures, problem-benefit measures, a variety of measures related to hearing aid or implant use and benefits (see Chapters 14 and 15) and changes in psychological variables.

Perhaps the simplest way to evaluate changes in disability and handicap at different stages of the rehabilitative process is to ask the subject simply to rate his levels of disablements at different stages of the rehabilitative process following either the technique of Habib and Hinchcliffe (1978) discussed earlier, or using visual analogue scales. Unfortunately, however, some patients have difficulties with such concepts and the results may depend upon how the task is presented to them, but useful results may be obtained both on an individual and on a group basis (Figure 13.7).

These are gross overall responses and may be insensitive to small changes or the degree of change, particularly in disability in patients with profound hearing loss all of whom will normally rate their preintervention disability as 100 or maximum. It therefore makes sense to look at components of disability and handicap. This may be achieved either by the use of established disability and handicap scales or by creating individual measures for the patient concerned using his self-reports from the problem questionnaire or from non-directive questioning. The disability and handicap scales will be considered further below.

We may take the problems listed by a patient together with any others mentioned in response to a question along the lines of, 'Are there any other problems which you have as a result of your hearing loss?'. These are then listed for the patient who is asked to rate each on a 1 to 100 scale, or a visual analogue scale, running from no problem = 0 to a very severe problem = 100. The same list can then be readministered after intervention and the ratings compared. Table 13.19 shows such results for two patients before and after cochlear implantation, and is derived from the study of Sim, Stephens and Meredith (1996).

Table 13.19 Rating of spontaneously listed problems by two patients before and after cochlear implants

	Pre	*Post*
Patient 8		
Overall		
Disability	100	50
Handicap	100	24
Life quality effect	75	25
Specific problems		
Can't go shopping alone	100	50
Can't hear the children	100	25
Can't hear the television	100	50
Can't hear on the telephone	100	25
Need to rely on others	100	75
Patient 10		
Overall		
Disability	80	15
Handicap	75	10
Life quality effect	65	10
Specific problems		
Understanding people at work	95	30
Loss of job satisfaction	75	10
Understanding strangers	55	10
Frustration at missing out		
on fishing trips	40	30
Not hearing on the telephone	60	50

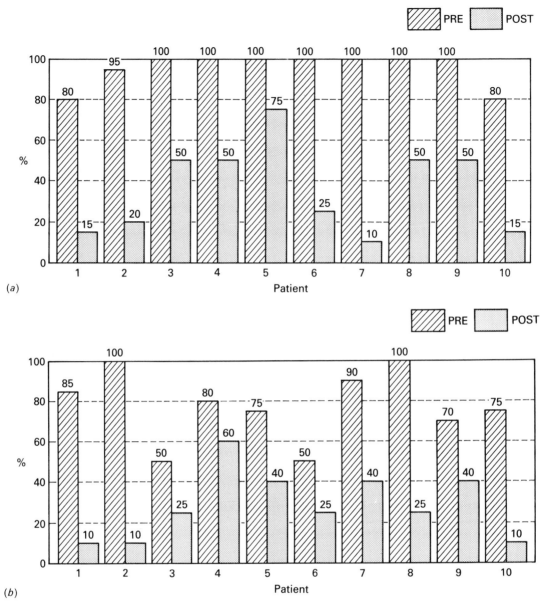

Figure 13.7 Ratings of (*a*) disability and (*b*) handicap by patients before and after cochlear implants (from Sim, Stephens and Meredith, 1996)

If repeated assessments are made, the individual may be probed for additional disabilities/handicaps of which he becomes aware as the more severe disablements are reduced, and these in their turn may be incorporated into the on going assessments.

The further area which has been neglected in the past is assessing the handicap experienced by significant others of the patients. Again it is possible to ask them to rate the severity of their various problems

before and after intervention as this will have important ramifications on the outcome of the rehabilitation of the patient.

General measures of disability and handicap

A variety of standardized questionnaire measures of aspects of disability and handicap have been available since the hearing handicap scale was developed by High, Fairbanks and Glorig (1964). There are two major problems in the use of such scales before and after rehabilitation, even if they have been well standardized, which has not always been the case. The first and fundamental problem is that they can measure only general aspects of disability and handicap which may not be particularly relevant to the individual concerned. Thus the situation may arise when only one or two items in a questionnaire may be applicable to his set of problems and hence any changes in score as a result of rehabilitation will be minimal.

The second difficulty stems from a terminological problem in that most studies in the USA use definitions related to medicolegal work in the 1950s rather than following the WHO definitions (1980) which have been widely adopted elsewhere. This has consequently led to considerable confusion.

A final major weakness arises in the question of a 'universal' scale which can be administered to all patients. With existing scales, individuals with a profound hearing loss will score very high on disability before and even after rehabilitation. Others with a mild loss but very specific disabilities will score minimally before intervention giving little scope for improvement. This leads to an argument for different scales for different patient groups, which in turn leads to a negation of the value of standardized scales.

Table 13.20 represents an update of an approach used in an earlier review (Stephens, 1987b) which looks at different scales in terms of how many questions tap into various dimensions of disability and handicap.

In the selection of a particular scale a decision has to be made on an *a priori* basis as to those dimensions which are most important in the auditing of the outcome of a particular rehabilitative programme, and how universally applied such measures should be. Here there is always a balance between having a short measure which will ensure high compliance by the patients and a longer measure which may potentially give more information, but which, because of its length, leads to poor compliance by many, so that the results may not be representative of the population of patients being rehabilitated.

Recently, Hétu *et al.* (1994), in cross-cultural studies, have endeavoured to develop a short (20 question) scale tapping two dimensions of disability (disability for speech and non-speech sounds) and of handicap (emotional response and social isolation). However, while the two dimensions of disability have proved to be robust, the handicap scales are not sufficiently distinct to be separated. This has been validated in English language populations, in two countries and in French speakers in Quebec and is now being tested in various other languages, so could potentially provide a reliable basic scale for wide application.

Table 13.20 Number of questions on different components of disability and handicap in various published scales

	Disability				Handicap		
	Live speech	Electronic speech	Localization	Non-speech	Emotional response	Social withdrawal	Reaction of others
HHS	15	3	0	2	0	0	0
SHHI	18	3	0	0	0	0	0
HMS	6	5	7	8	4	2	2
DS	0	0	0	1	9	5	5
SAC	4	2	0	3	1	1	1
HPI	44	7	0	0	3	4	1
HDHS	3	2	0	5	5	3	2
CPHI	24	2	0	0	45	12	21
HHIA	5	1	0	0	10	9	0
McCASH	0	0	0	0	11	8	9

HHS = Hearing handicap scale, High, Fairbanks and Glorig (1964)
SHHI = Social hearing handicap index, Ewertsen and Birk-Nielsen (1973)
HMS = Hearing measurement scale, Noble and Atherley (1970)
DS = Denver scale, Alpiner and McCarthy (1993)
SAC = Self-assessment of communication, Alpiner and McCarthy (1993)
HPI = Hearing performance inventory, Giolas (1982)
HDHS = Hearing disability and handicap scale, Hétu *et al.* (1994)
CPHI = Communication profile for the hearing impaired, Demorest and Erdman (1987)
HHIA = Hearing handicap inventory for adults, Alpiner and McCarthy (1993)
McCASH = McCarthy-Alpiner scale of hearing handicap, Alpiner and McCarthy (1993)

Satisfaction measures

Much care has to be taken in the development of such questionnaires, as the average patient who has been treated well has a strong tendency to want to please. Such an individual will tend to answer in the affirmative all questions seeking his opinion as to the benefit of the rehabilitative programme. Other approaches have adopted specific questions on change in disability/handicap, hearing aid use etc., and as such are not really satisfaction measures.

Recently, arising from some work in Poland (Golabek *et al.*, 1988), we have been using a benefit/problem questionnaire to examine different aspects of outcome. This comprises two simple questions based on the problem questionnaire: 'Please make a list of any benefits which you have had as a result of your hearing aid. List them in order of importance starting with the greatest benefit. Write down as many as you can think of' and 'Please make a list of any shortcomings of your hearing aid and list them . . .'. While this was originally applied to specific hearing aid benefits (Stephens and Meredith, 1991b), it has subsequently been extended to broader aspects of the rehabilitative benefit experienced by individuals suffering from hearing loss and tinnitus. Examples of the results of a study on reported benefits and shortcomings of bone anchored hearing aids (Stephens *et al.*, 1996) are shown in Table 13.21.

Behavioural measures

This is an area largely neglected at the present time. Here the hypothesis is that appropriate rehabilitative intervention will reduce the number of days of sick leave taken by the specific individual and this can be measured easily before and after intervention (Ringdahl *et al.*, 1993).

A second approach is in recording social interactions between the target patient and other individuals before and after rehabilitation, again on the premise that good rehabilitation will increase the number of interactions. This is a procedure that has been successfully used in studies on the effects of intervention in patients with intellectual disabilities (Repp and Felce, 1990) but has not been systematically applied in the hearing loss domain.

Specific benefits

There is an extensive literature on the patient benefits in terms of improved speech discrimination, speech in noise and audiovisual discrimination in patients fitted with hearing aids or cochlear implants and these are discussed in Chapters 14 and 15.

The problem remains how these improvements relate to perceived benefits, and to reductions in disability and handicap. Table 13.22 illustrates that there is not a simple relationship between the two, in

Table 13.21 Most common benefits and shortcomings listed with bone anchored hearing aids

Benefits	n	% Reporting	Shortcomings	n	% Reporting
Better hearing	18	46	Telephone	9	23
Ease of use	15	38	Wind noise	8	21
Better clarity	13	33	Speech in noise	8	21
Less noticeable	12	31	Easily dislodged	8	21
More confident	11	28	Size	6	15
More comfortable	8	21			
Fewer infections	7	18			

Table 13.22 Correlation matrix between change in various measures following cochlear implants

	DIS	HAND	QUAL	PROBS	AB[S]	BKB	CDT
DIS	1.00	0.35	0.36	0.33	0.36	− 0.14	0.31
HAND		1.00	0.75**	0.58*	0.78**	0.33	0.92**
QUAL			1.00	0.20	0.78**	0.31	0.72*
PROBS				1.00	0.07	− 0.35	0.40
AB[S]					1.00	0.64*	0.80**
BKB						1.00	0.56
CDT							1.00

DIS = Rated disability; HAND = Rated handicap; QUAL = Rated quality of life; PROBS = Mean rated value of problems; AB[S] = Boothroyd word lists; BKB = Bamford-Kowal-Bench audiovisual sentence lists; CDT = Connected discourse tracking. (** = $P < 0.01$; * = $P < 0.05$)

that individuals showing little benefit from their implants in terms of their performance based measures, may report good benefit in terms of well-being and social activities (Sim, Stephens and Meredith, 1996).

It is therefore apparent that there is no simple answer to the assessment of rehabilitative outcome. As in the whole process of rehabilitation it must be primarily focused on the individual patient and the extent that as a result of our intervention he is able to function more as he would wish to do than before. This has been addressed on a multidimensional basis by McKenna (1991) in cochlear implant patients. His results do however leave us with the caveat that individuals's ideas of his ideal function may bear little relationship to how they were realistically functioning before.

An in depth approach to the way forward in this field has recently been outlined by Hyde and Riko (1994), highlighting the relevance of different measures and how they relate to the individual's real needs.

References

ALPINER, J. G. and MCCARTHY, P. A. (eds) (1993) *Rehabilitative Audiology: Children and Adults*, 2nd edn. Baltimore: Williams and Wilkins

AMERICAN ACADEMY OF OTOLARYNGOLOGY (1979) Guide for the evaluation of hearing handicap. *Journal of the American Medical Association*, **241**, 2055–2059

BANGS, J. L. and MULLINS, C. J. (1953) Recruitment testing and its applications. *Archives of Otolaryngology*, **58**, 582–592

BARFOD, J. (1979) Speech perception processes and fitting of hearing aids. *Audiology*, **18**, 430–441

BARCHAM, L. J. and STEPHENS, S. D. G. (1980) The use of an open-ended problems questionnaire in auditory rehabilitation. *British Journal of Audiology*, **14**, 49–54

BENCH, J. and BAMFORD, J. (eds) (1979) *Speech-Hearing Tests and the Spoken Language of Hearing-Impaired Children*. London: Academic Press

BERGER, K. W. (1972) *Speechreading: Principles and Methods*. Kent, Ohio: Herald

BERGER, K. W. (1976) Prescription of hearing aids: a rationale. *Journal of the American Audiological Society*, **2**, 71–78

BERGMAN, M. (1950) The audiology clinic. *Acta Otolaryngologica*, Suppl. 89, 1–107

BINNIE, C. A. (1977) Attitude changes following speechreading training. *Scandinavian Audiology*, **6**, 13–19

BROOKS, D. N. (1976) The use of hearing aids by the hearing impaired: In: *Disorders of Auditory Function* II, edited by S. D. G. Stephens. London: Academic Press. pp. 255–263

BROOKS, D. N. (1981) Use of postaural aids by National Health Service. *British Journal of Audiology*, **15**, 79–86

BURDO, S. and POGGIA, C. (1991) *Sordità e Telefono*. Daverio: Arte Stampa

CARHART, R. (1946) Selection of hearing aids. *Archives of Otolaryngology*, **44**, 1

CHAMBERLAIN, M. A. (1989) What is rehabilitation? *British Journal of Hospital Medicine*, **41**, 311

CHUNG, S.M. and STEPHENS, S. D. G. (1986) Factors influencing binaural hearing aid use. *British Journal of Audiology*, **20**, 129–140

COCHLEAR (1991) *Mini System 22 Rehabilitation Manual*. Melbourne: Cochlear Ltd

COLES, R., DAVIS, A. and SMITH, P. (1991) Tinnitus: its epidemiology and management. In: *Presbyacusis*, edited by J. Hartvig-Jensen. Copenhagen: Danavox. pp. 377–402

COMPTON, C. L. (1993) Assistive technology for deaf and hard of hearing people. In: *Rehabilitative Audiology: Children and Adults*, 2nd edn, edited by J. G. Alpiner and P. A. McCarthy. Baltimore: Williams & Wilkins. pp. 441–469

CORNETT, R. D., BEADLES, R. and WILSON, B. (1982) Automatic cued speech. In: *Papers from the Research Conference on Speech-Processing Aids for the Deaf*, edited by J. M. Pickette. Washington, DC: Gallaudet College. pp. 224–239

COUGHLAN, A. (1988) Psychological aspects of disability. In: *Rehabilitation of the Physically Disabled Adult*, edited by G. J. Goodwill and M. A. Chamberlain. London: Croom Helm. pp. 35–48

DAVIES, B. M. (1988) Social factors in disability. In: *Rehabilitation of the Physically Disabled Adult*, edited by C. J. Goodwill and M. A. Chamberlain. London: Croom Helm. pp. 35–48

DAVIES, J. E., JOHN, D. G. and STEPHENS, S. D. G. (1991) Intermediate hearing tests as predictors of hearing aid acceptance. *Clinical Otolaryngology*, **16**, 76–83

DAVIS, A. C. (1983) Hearing disorders in the population: first phase findings of the MRC National Study of Hearing. In: *Hearing Science and Hearing Disorders*, edited by H. E. Lutman and M. P. Haggard. London: Academic Press. pp. 35–60

DAVIS, A. C. (1987) Epidemiology of hearing disorders. In: *Scott Brown's Otolaryngology*, 5th edn, vol 2, edited by D. Stephens. London: Butterworths. pp. 90–126

DAVIS, A. C. (1993) Public health issues and hearing aids. *British Society of Audiology Annual Conference*, Bath

DAVIS, A., STEPHENS, D., RAYMENT A. and THOMAS, K. (1992) Hearing impairments in middle age: the acceptability, benefit and cost of detection (ABCD). *British Journal of Audiology*, **26**, 1–14

DE FILIPPO, C. L. and SCOTT, B. L. (1978) A method for training and evaluating the reception of ongoing speech. *Journal of the Acoustical Society of America*, **63**, 1186–1192

DEMOREST, M. E. and ERDMAN, S. A. (1987) Development of the communication profile for the hearing impaired. *Journal of Speech and Hearing Disorders*, **52**, 129–143

DILLON, H., KORITSHONE, R., BATTAGLIA, J., LOVEGROVE, L., DINIS, J., MAVRIAS, G. *et al.* (1991) Rehabilitation effectiveness 1: assessing the needs of clients entering a national rehabilitation program. *Australian Journal of Audiology*, **13**, 55–65

ERDMAN, S. A. (1993) Counselling hearing-impaired adults. In: *Rehabilitative Audiology: Children and Adults*, 2nd edn, edited by J. G. Alpine and P. A. McCarthy. Baltimore: Williams & Wilkins. pp. 374–413

EWERTSON, H. W. and BIRK-NIELSEN, H. (1973) Social hearing handicap index. *Audiology*, **12**, 180–187

FELTON, B. J., REVENSON, T. A. and HINRICHSEN, G. A. (1984) Stress and coping in the explanation of psychological adjustment among chronically ill adults. *Social Science Medicine*, **18**, 889–898

FIELD, D. L. and HAGGARD, M. P. (1989) Knowledge of hearing tactics 1: assessment by questionnaire and inventory. *British Journal of Audiology*, **23**, 349–354

FORCHAMMER, G. (1903) *Orm nodvendigheden af sikre meddelelsesmidler i Dovestummeundervisningen.* Kobenhavn: J. Frimodt

FOURCIN, A. J. (1980) Speech pattern audiometry. In: *Auditory Investigation: the Scientific and Technological Basis,* edited by H. A. Beagley. Oxford: Oxford University Press. pp. 170–208

FRENCH ST GEORGE, M. and BARR-HAMILTON, R. (1975) Relief of the occluded ear sensation to improve earmould comfort. *Journal of the American Auditory Society,* **4,** 30–35

GARSTECKI, D. C. (1993) Rehabilitative audiologists and the hearing impaired population: continuing and new relationships. In: *Rehabilitative Audiology: Children and Adults,* 2nd edn, edited by J. G. Alpiner and P. A. McCarthy. Baltimore: Williams & Wilkins. pp. 17–34

GATEHOUSE, S. (1992) The time course and magnitude of perceptual acclimatization to frequency responses: evidence from monaural fitting of hearing aids. *Journal of the Acoustical Society of America,* **92,** 1258

GATEHOUSE, S. and DAVIS, A. C. (1992) Clinical pure tone versus three interval forced choice thresholds: effects of hearing level and age. *Audiology,* **31,** 30–44

GATEHOUSE, S. and GORDON, J. (1990) Response times to speech stimuli as measures of benefit from amplification. *British Journal of Audiology,* **24,** 63–68

GILDSTON, H. and GILDSTON, P. (1972) Personality changes associated with surgically corrected hypoacusis. *Audiology,* **11,** 354–367

GILHOME HERBST, K. R., MEREDITH, R. and STEPHENS, S. D. G. (1991) Implications of hearing impairment for elderly people in London and in Wales. *Acta Otolaryngologica,* Suppl. 476, 209–214

GIOLAS, T. G. (1982) *Hearing Handicapped Adults.* Englewood Cliffs: Prentice Hall

GOLABEK, W., NOWAKOWSKA, M., SIWIEK, H. and STEPHENS, S. D. G. (1988) Self-reported benefits of-hearing aids by the hearing impaired. *British Journal of Audiology,* **22,** 183–186

GOLABEK, W., NOWAKOWSKA, M., SIWIEK, H. and STEPHENS, S. D. G. (1989) Problems of the hearing impaired in Poland. *British Journal of Audiology,* **23,** 73–75

GOLDSTEIN, D. P. and STEPHENS, S. D. G. (1981) Audiological rehabilitation: management model I. *Audiology,* **20,** 432–452

GROCE, M. E. (1985) *Everyone Here Spoke Sign Language.* Cambridge, Massachusetts: Harvard University Press

HABIB, R. G. and HINCHCLIFFE, R. (1978) Subjective magnitude of auditory impairment. *Audiology,* **17,** 68–76

HALLBERG, L.R.-M. (1994) Psychometric evaluation of a Swedish version of the Acceptance Scale, an instrument intended to measure acceptance of illness scale. *Journal of Audiological Medicine,* **3,** 23–34

HALLBERG, L. R.-M. and BARRENÄS, M. L. (1993) Living with a male with noise-induced hearing loss: experiences from the perspective of spouses. *British Journal of Audiology,* **27,** 253–261

HALLBERG, L. R.-M., JOHNSSON, T. and AXELSSON, A. (1993) Structure of perceived handicap in middle-aged males with noise-induced hearing loss, with and without tinnitus. *Audiology,* **32,** 137–152

HAZELL, J. W. P., WOOD, S. M., COOPER, H. R., STEPHENS, S. D. G., CORCORAN, A. L., COLES, R. R. A. *et al.* (1985) A clinical study of tinnitus maskers. *British Journal of Audiology,* **19,** 65–146

HERBST, K. G. (1983) Psycho-social consequences of disorders of hearing in the elderly. In: *Hearing and Balance in the Elderly,* edited by R. Hinchcliffe. Edinburgh: Churchill Livingstone. pp. 174–200

HÉTU, R., RIVERIN, L., LALANDE, N., GETTY, L. and ST CYR, C. (1988) Qualitative analysis of the handicap associated with occupational hearing loss. *British Journal of Audiology,* **22,** 251–164

HÉTU, R., RIVERIN, L., GETTY, L., LALANDE, N. and ST CYR, C. (1990) The reluctance to acknowledge hearing difficulties among hearing impaired workers. *British Journal of Audiology,* **24,** 265–276

HÉTU, R., GETTY, L., PHILBERT, L., DESILETS, F., NOBLE, W. and STEPHENS, D. (1994) Mise au point d'un outil clinique pour la mesure d'in capacités auditives et de handicaps. *Journal of Speech-language Pathology and Audiology,* **18,** 83–95

HICKIN, J. (1986) An investigation of the perception of hearing disability by the hearing impaired and their significant others. *Undergraduate dissertation.* London: University of London

HIGH, W. S., FAIRBANKS, G. and GLORIG, A. (1964) Scale for the self assessment of hearing handicap. *Journal of Speech and Hearing Disorders,* **19,** 215–230

HINCHCLIFFE, R. (1992) King-Kopetzky syndrome: an auditory stress disorder? *Journal of Audiological Medicine,* **1,** 89–98

HUMPHREY, C., GILHOME HERBST, K. and FARUQI, S. (1981) Some chacteristics of the hearing impaired elderly who do not present themselves for rehabilitation. *British Journal of Audiology,* **15,** 23–30

HYDE, M. L. and RIKO, K. (1994) A decision-analytic approach to audiological rehabilitation. *Journal of the Academy of Rehabilitative Audiology,* **27,** Monograph, pp. 337–374

JEFFERS, J. and BARLEY, M. (1978) *Speechreading (Lipreading),* 6th printing. Springfield: Charles Thomas

JONES, L. (1987) Living with hearing loss. In: *Adjustment to Acquired Hearing Loss,* edited by J. Kyle. Bristol: Centre for Deaf Studies. pp. 126–139

JONES, L., KYLE, J. and WOOD, P. L. (1987) *Words Apart. Losing your Hearing as an Adult.* London: Tavistock

KALIKOW, D., STEVENS, K. and ELLIOTT, L. (1977) Development of a test of speech intelligibility in noise using sentence material with controlled word predictability. *Journal of the Acoustical Society of America,* **61,** 1337–1351

KERR, P. and COWIE, R. (1992) A quantitative analysis of the experience of acquired deafness. In: *Proceedings of the 2nd International Conference on Tactile Aids, Hearing Aids and Cochlear Implants,* edited by A. Risberg, S. Felicetti, G. Plant and K. A. Spens. Stockholm: KTH. pp. 11–17

KYLE, J. (1992) *Switched on: Deaf People's Views on Television Subtitling.* Bristol: Deaf Studies Trust

LORMORE, K. A. and STEPHENS, S. D. G. (1994) Use of openended questionnaire with patients and their significant others. *British Journal of Audiology,* **28,** 81–89

LYXELL, B. (1989) *Beyond Lips: Components of Speechreading Skills.* Umeå: University of Umeå

MCKENNA, L. (1987) Goal planning in audiological rehabilitation. *British Journal of Audiology,* **21,** 5–11

MCKENNA, L. (1991) The assessment of psychological variables in cochlear implant patients. In: *Cochlear Implants: a Practical Guide,* edited by H. Cooper. London: Whurr. pp. 125–145

MCLEOD, A. and SUMMERFIELD, Q. (1987) Quantifying the contribution of vision to speech perception in noise. *British Journal of Audiology,* **21,** 131–141

MACLEOD, A. and SUMMERFIELD, Q. (1990) A procedure for measuring auditory and audio-visual speech-reception thresholds for sentences in noise: rationale, evaluation and recommendations for use. *British Journal of Audiology*, **24**, 29–44

MEREDITH, R. and STEPHENS, D. (1993) In the ear and behind the ear hearing aids in the elderly. *Scandinavian Audiology*, **22**, 211–216

MEREDITH, R., STEPHENS, S. D. G. and JONES, G. E. (1990) Investigations on viseme groups in Welsh. *Clinical Linguistics and Phonetics*, **4**, 253–265

MEYER-BISCH, C. (1990) Audiometrie automatique de depistage preventif: le balayage frequentiel asservi (audioscan). *Notes de Cahiers Documentaires*, pp. 139, 335–345

MONTGOMERY, A. A. (1993) Management of the hearing impaired adult. In: *Rehabiliative Audiology: Children and Adults*, edited by J. G. Alpiner and P. A. McCarthy. Baltimore: Williams & Wilkins. pp. 311–330

NOBLE, W. (1983) Hearing, hearing impairment and the audible world: a theoretical essay. *Audiology*, **22**, 325–338

NOBLE, W. G. and ATHERLEY, G. R. C. (1970) The hearing measurement scale: a questionnaire for the assessment of auditory disability. *Journal of Auditory Research*, **10**, 229–250

NOBLE, W. and HÉTU, R. (1994) An ecological approach to disability and handicap in relation to impaired hearing. *Audiology*, **33**, 117–126

PLUMMER, D. (1985) The use of self report questionnaires in the assessment of hearing handicap – a comparison of two questionnaires with home vists and interviews. *Undergraduate dissertation*. London: University of London

REPP, A. C. and FELCE, D. (1990) A microcomputer system used for evaluative and experimental behavioural research in mental handicap. *Mental Handicap Research*, **3**, 21–32

RINGDAHL, A., ERIKSSON-MANGOLD, M., BERENSTAAF, E., CAPRIN, S., LYCHE, S., SIMONSSON, S. *et al.* (1993) Evaluation of a 4 week audiological rehabilitation program. *Paper presented at 7th International Symposium on Audiological Medicine*, Cardiff

ROBERTS, P. (1992) An ergonomic investigation into the design of a behind the ear (BTE) hearing aid to overcome handling difficulties experienced by elderly users. *Undergraduate dissertation*. Pontypridd: University of Glamorgan

ROSEN, S. and CORCORAN, T. (1982) A video-recorded test of lipreading for British English. *British Journal of Audiology*, **16**, 245–254

ROSEN, S., WALLIKER, J. R., FOURCIN, A. and BALL, V. (1987) A microprocessor-based acoustic hearing aid for the profoundly impaired listener. *Journal of Rehabilitation Research and Development*, **24**, 239–260

RUSTIN, L. and KUHR, A. (1989) *Social Skills and the Speech Impaired*. London: Taylor & Francis

SANCHO-ALDRIDGE, J. and DAVIS, A. (1993) The impact of hearing impairment on television viewing in the UK. *British Journal of Audiology*, **27**, 163–173

SHANNON, R. V., FAYAD, G., MOORE, J., LO, W. W., OTTO, S., NELSON, R. A. *et al.* (1993) Auditory brainstem implants: 2. postsurgical issues and performances. *Otolaryngology, Head and Neck Surgery*, **108**, 634–642

SHEPHERD, D. C., DELAVERGNE, R. W., FRUEH, F. X., and CLOBRIDGE, C. (1977) Visual-neural correlate of speechread-ing ability in normal hearing adults. *Journal of Speech and Hearing Research*, **20**, 752–765

SIM, S. W., STEPHENS, S. D. G. and MEREDITH, R. (1996) A comparative study of self rating and performance measures in cochlear implant patients (in preparation)

SIWIEK, H., LORMORE, K., STEPHENS, D. and HICKIN, J. (1996) Uses of open-ended interview and questionnaires in patients and significant others. (in preparation)

SPERLING, L., JONSSON, B., HOLMER, I. and LEWIN, T. (1980) Test program for work gloves. *Report for the Department of Occupational Safety, Labor Physiology Unit, Umeå, Sweden*, no. 18

STEPHENS, D. (1983) Rehabilitation and service needs. In: *Hearing Science and Hearing Disorders*, edited by M. E. Lutman and M. P. Haggard. London: Academic Press. pp. 283–324

STEPHENS, D. (1992) The King-Kopetzky syndrome. *Journal of Audiological Medicine*, **1**, ii–iii

STEPHENS, D. and HÉTU, R. (1991) Impairment, disability and handicaip in audiology: towards a consensus. *Audiology*, **30**, 185–200

STEPHENS, D. and MEREDITH R. (1991a) The Afan Valley audiological rehabilitation studies. In: *Presbyacusis and Other Age Related Aspects*, edited by J. H. Jensen. Copenhagen: Danavol. pp. 323–335

STEPHENS, D., FRANCE, L. and LORMORE, K. (1995) The effect of hearing impairment on the patient's family and friends. *Acta Otolaryngologica*, **115**, 165–167

STEPHENS, D., BOARD, T., HOBSON, J. and COOPER, H. (1996) Reported benefits and problems experienced with bone-anchored hearing aids (in preparation)

STEPHENS, S. D. G. (1973) Hearing and personality: a review. *Journal of Sound and Vibration*, **20**, 287–298

STEPHENS, S. D. G. (1980) Evaluating the problems of the hearing impaired. *Audiology*, **19**, 205–220

STEPHENS, S. D. G. (1984) Hearing aid selection: an integrated approach. *British Journal of Audiology*, **18**, 199–210

STEPHENS, S. D. G. (1985) Non-acoustical aspects of earmould selection. *Audiology in Practice*, **2**, 7–8

STEPHENS, S. D. G. (1987a) People's complaints of hearing difficulties. In: *Adjustment to Acquired Hearing Loss*, edited by J. G. Kyle. Bristol: Centre for Deaf Studies. pp. 37–47

STEPHENS, S. D. G. (1987b) Auditory rehabilitation. *British Medical Bulletin*, **43**, 999–1026

STEPHENS, S. D. G. (1990) Auditory and vestibular rehabilitation of the adult. In: *Horizons in Medicine 2*, edited by K. K. Borysiewicz. Tunbridge Wells: Transmedica. pp. 220–228

STEPHENS, S. D. G. and MEREDITH R. (1991b) Qualitative reports of hearing aid benefit. *Clinical Rehabilitation*, **5**, 225–229

STEPHENS, S. D. G. and MEREDITH R. (1991c) Physical handling of hearing aids by the elderly. *Acta Otolaryngologica*, Suppl. 476, 281–285

STEPHENS, S. D. G., BARCHAM, L. J., CORCORAN, A. L. and PARSONS, N. (1980) Evaluation of an auditory rehabilitation scheme. In: *Disorders of Auditory Function III*, edited by I. G. Taylor and A. Markides. London: Academic Press. pp. 265–273

STEPHENS, S. D. G., BLEGVAD, B. and KROGH, H. J. (1979) The value of some suprathreshold auditory measures. *Scandinavian Audiology*, **6**, 213–221

STEPHENS, S. D. G., CALLAGHAN, D. E., HOGAN, S., MEREDITH, R., RAYMENT, A. and DAVIS, A. (1990) Hearing disability in people aged 50–65: effectiveness and acceptability of rehabilitative intervention. *British Medical Journal,* **300,** 508–511

STEPHENS, S. D. G., LEWIS, P. A. and CHARNY, M. (1991) Assessing hearing problems within a community survey. *British Journal of Audiology,* **25,** 337–343

STEPHENS, S. D. G., MEREDITH, R., CALLAGHAN, D. E., HOGAN, S. and RAYMENT, A. (1991) Early intervention and rehabilitation: factors influencing outcome. *Acta Otolaryngologica,* Suppl. 476, 221–225

SUMMERFIELD, A. Q. and FOSTER, J. R. (1983) Assessing audio-visual speech reception disability. In: *High-technology Aids for Disabled People,* edited by W. J. Perkins. London: Butterworth. pp. 33–41

THOMAS, A. and GILHOME HERBST, K. (1980) Social and psychological implications of acquired deafness for adults of employment age. *British Journal of Audiology,* **14,** 76–85

TYE-MURRAY, N., TYLER, R. S., BONG, B. and NARES, T. (1988) Computerised laser videodisc programs for training speechreading and assertive communication behaviours. *Journal of the Academy of Rehabilitative Audiology,* **21,** 143–152

TYLER, R. S., and BAKER, L. J. (1983) Difficulties experienced by tinnitus sufferers. *Journal of Speech and Hearing Disorders,* **48,** 150–154

TYLER, R. S., BAKER, L. J. and ARMSTRONG BEDNALL, G. (1983) Difficulties experienced by hearing-aid candidates and hearing aid users. *British Journal of Audiology,* **17,** 191–201

UPFOLD, L. J., MAY, A. E. and BATTAGLIA, J. A. (1990) Hearing aid manipulation skills in an elderly population: a comparison of ITE, BTE and ITC aids. *British Journal of Audiology,* **24,** 311–318

VOGNSEN, S. (ed.) (1976) *Hearing Tactics.* Copenhaven, Oticon

VON DER LIETH, L. (1972) Hearing tactics I & II. *Scandinavian Audiology,* **1,** 155–160

WHETNALL, E. (1952) Hearing aids. In: *Diseases of the Ear, Nose and Throat,* vol 2, edited by W. G. Scott-Brown. London: Butterworth. pp. 361–377

WORLD HEALTH ORGANIZATION (1980) *International Classification of Impairments Disabilities and Handicaps.* Geneva: WHO

WOOD, P. H. N. (1980) The language of disablement – a glossary relating to disease and its consequences. *International Rehabilitation Medicine,* **2,** 86–92

14

Hearing aids

S. Gatehouse

Hearing loss in the population is predominantly sensorineural in origin and is not usually amenable to either medical or surgical management. Thus the disabling and handicapping effects of a hearing impairment can often only be alleviated by some structured programme of rehabilitation. Usually a major component of this rehabilitation process is the provision of personal amplification, via a hearing aid or aids. Although substantial advances in our understanding of the impaired auditory system are being made, for the foreseeable future the hearing aid will remain one of the cornerstones of the alleviation of auditory disability and therefore an important component of the practice of otolaryngology. It was perhaps the case some 15–20 years ago that the technological limitations of hearing aids resulted in the situation that virtually all devices had the same characteristics and degree of functionality. This, however, is no longer the case, and while there are still limitations imposed by technological capabilities, the situation has now arrived where, if the practitioner were able to converge upon a set of characteristics for a hearing aid, then their practical realization and delivery to the hearing impaired ear should be possible.

This technological flexibility has led to a substantial literature on the functioning and fitting of hearing aids, whose detailed understanding requires expertise not only in practical audiology but electronics, electroacoustics, physiology and psychoacoustics. Therefore, in formulating a contribution for practising otolaryngologists and audiological physicians, some way of dealing with this technological complexity is required. This chapter aims to satisfy this need by concentrating on and emphasizing the rational concepts and overall functions that different types of modern hearing aids aim to embody, without addressing the technological detail of how those functions are achieved via an engineering solution. Rather, it

attempts to point to the more detailed scientific literature for the reader whose requirements are not satisfied by this level of detail.

Consequences of sensorineural hearing impairment

While hearing aids are usually thought of as appropriate management for sensorineural hearing loss they can, of course, serve the same purpose for conductive conditions where surgical intervention is either not desired nor appropriate. However, because of the additional complexity of sensorineural conditions, the limitations of and demand on hearing aids are greater and, in general, hearing aids are more successful in conductive conditions (Carlin and Browning, 1990). Given that a conductive hearing loss can be represented almost entirely by a simple attenuation (i.e. everyday sounds are decreased in intensity without any accompanying distortions) the hearing aid there has a relatively simple job to do and it is merely required to overcome the attenuation due to the conductive condition by providing amplification which mirrors to an extent the usually flat or low frequency hearing loss.

Sensorineural conditions, however, cannot be represented so simply. The great majority of sensorineural conditions result from damage to hair cells in the cochlea, and these structures are essential components in the auditory system's abilities to process different frequencies as well as sounds of different intensity. In the normally functioning auditory system it is possible for the ear to be presented with frequencies (e.g. in a broad band signal such as speech or music) which are very close together, but both of which carry important and useful information. The hearing mechanism can detect and process these frequencies simultaneously. Numerous physiological and behavioural studies have shown that this ability is degraded, or perhaps entirely absent, in sensorineural hearing loss due to hair cell damage in the cochlea. This can have the effect that the adjacent frequencies may be indistinguishable and the information contained in them therefore confused, or even that one relatively intense frequency may physically mask the perception of another frequency close by. Given that almost all hearing aids make no attempt to overcome the various physiological deficits that accompany sensorineural hearing loss, it is clear that they are unlikely to return all auditory abilities to the levels of performance enjoyed by individuals with normal hearing. However, for advantageous listening conditions, such as understanding a conversation on a one-to-one basis at a favourable signal-to-noise ratio, the fact that a speech signal contains a high degree of redundancy (i.e. there is a lot more information available than is needed to understand the message), then with suitable amplification, most hearing impaired listeners can function quite well. The same argument however, cannot be made in the case of listening in adverse conditions such as when background noise or other competing speakers are present.

Even individuals with normally functioning auditory systems can have severe difficulties in understanding speech in a background of noise, but if hearing impaired listeners and hearing aid users are interviewed about the situations which cause them most difficulty, then they almost uniformly report the situation where interfering noise is present. This is because, although the desired signal may be brought above the listener's hearing threshold, the presence of competing noise interacts with the non-linear distortions due to a sensorineural hearing loss, to produce performance that falls well below that enjoyed by normally hearing listeners. Thus one of the most important circumstances for consideration with hearing aids is the noisy background, even when the hearing aid itself makes no attempt to separate the speech from the noise.

Aspects of the auditory world

Any sound signal may be characterized by its overall level (i.e the intensity of the stimulus), how the sound is constructed out of different frequency components, and how the sound varies as a function of time. For a meaningful stimulus, examples of which could be alerting sounds, music or speech, each of these parameters carries with it potentially important information. Thus in a passage of music a change of intensity carries with it some implication about the interpretation of the music. Similarly in an alerting sound (such as a car alarm) a change in frequency implies to the listener that some external event has

occurred. Again using music as an example, the temporal or melodic aspects of a passage of music themselves carry implications for the listener. Thus in considering what we would like to present to the impaired auditory system, all three aspects of intensity, frequency and temporal changes in the acoustical signal have to be considered.

These three aspects manifest themselves most clearly when speech is considered as the particular signal of interest. Certainly, for human beings the prime function of their auditory system is to allow the transmission of information between two individuals via the medium of the speech signal. This, does not imply that other signals are not important, but rather that a very heavy emphasis should be placed upon speech processing and understanding. Thus, in the rehabilitation of hearing impaired listeners and the provision of hearing aids, there has been an overwhelming concentration of making speech available to the impaired listener, perhaps to the exclusion of other signals in some circumstances. For example, it could well be an important component of a hearing impaired listener's auditory disability and consequent handicap that they were unable to hear the ringing of the doorbell or the ringing of the telephone, and making that acoustical information available may well have different demands upon an amplifying device and consequences for the management of the individual. Similarly, an important component of auditory disability is to localize in space the origin of a particular sound source (Noble and Byrne, 1991; Byrne, Noble and Lepage, 1992) and, to make available to the impaired auditory system the cues that enable localization, could place different demands upon an amplifying system.

However, in considering the primary role of a hearing aid, it is likely that, for the great majority of listeners, understanding speech will be the overwhelmingly important component of their hearing problems and, while provision of the hearing aid may have to consider other matters on a secondary basis, making the speech signal available is likely to be the prime requirement.

Characteristics of speech

Speech is a signal which changes rapidly in both intensity, frequency and time. For any given speaker in a particular listening environment, the speech may be characterized by its average level in dB sound pressure level (SPL). This is the average root mean square level at which the speech is produced at any given distance from the speaker. It is generally accepted that normal conversational speech in a quiet background achieves a level of some 60 to 65 dB SPL at a distance of 1 m from the speaker and that this may range in intensity from 50 to 80 dB SPL over a range of quiet to loud speech for different communication circumstances. Thus the average level over which a hearing aid could be reasonably expected to perform could range on average from 50 dB SPL to approximately 80 dB SPL, though this of course will depend upon individual speakers and listening circumstances.

It is also important to realize that while average conversational speech may achieve an overall level of some 62 dB SPL for example, that for any given speaker this is only an average level, and that an utterance such as a sentence will contain some elements which are louder and some elements which are quieter than this overall average. It is usually accepted that across a range of speakers, the peaks in speech can be some 12 dB greater than the average and the quieter components of speech some 18 dB less than the average. Thus, for any given range of speech, the individual elements can vary by some 30 dB. This is illustrated by the data in Table 14.1 which is drawn from Pavlovic (1990) and shows the contributions of the different frequency bands to speech of a variety of overall levels (vocal efforts). It can be seen that speech has greater intensity at low rather than high frequencies, and that some of the speech information, as illustrated by the lower 1% of the distribution, can take values for which the SPL is, in fact, below 0. The Table also shows the effect whereby, as an individual raises vocal effort (remembering that one reason for raising vocal effort will be

increases in background competing noise), the increases in the low frequency energy can be relatively modest, while increases in high frequencies can be observed in an attempt to make sure that the relatively less intense high frequencies are not physically masked by the more intense low frequencies.

The above discussion concentrates purely on the physical distribution of the elements of speech without any consideration of their contribution to intelligibility. Speech is made up of different phonetic and phonemic structures, some of which can be thought of as relatively low frequency, relatively intense elements (e.g. vowel sounds), and others of which can be characterized as relatively more intense, relatively high frequency components (such as consonants). Unfortunately the information content of speech does not equate directly to the energy content of speech, and, in particular, the high frequency less intense consonant sounds can be of greater importance for understanding speech than the relatively less intense lower frequencies. This is illustrated in Table 14.2 (from Studebaker, Pavlovic and Sherbecoe, 1987) which shows the band importance to the understanding of speech of the different frequency components for an average conversational speech over a number of speakers and number of different languages. The Table illustrates quite clearly that speech contains important information for intelligibility at frequencies, say, above 4000 Hz which are not usually

Table 14.1 The distribution of energy as a function of frequency for a number of vocal efforts

Frequency band (Hz)	Overall level = 62 dB SPL (normal effort)			Overall level = 68 dB SPL (raised effort)			Overall level = 75 dB SPL (loud effort)			Overall level = 82 dB SPL (shout effort)		
	Mean dB SPL	Lower 1%	Upper 1%	Mean dB SPL	Lower 1%	Upper 1%	Mean dB SPL	Lower 1%	Upper 1%	Mean dB SPL	Lower 1%	Upper 1%
100– 200	31	43	13	34	46	16	34	46	16	28	40	10
200– 300	34	46	16	38	50	20	41	53	23	42	54	24
300– 400	34	46	16	38	50	20	43	55	25	47	59	29
400– 510	34	46	16	39	51	21	44	56	26	48	60	30
510– 630	33	45	15	39	51	21	45	57	27	50	62	32
630– 770	30	42	12	37	49	19	45	57	27	51	63	33
770– 920	27	39	09	35	47	17	43	55	25	51	63	33
920–1080	25	37	07	33	45	15	42	54	24	51	63	33
1080–1270	23	35	05	32	44	14	41	53	23	49	61	31
1270–1480	22	34	04	30	42	12	39	51	21	49	61	31
1480–1720	20	32	02	28	40	10	37	49	19	47	59	29
1720–2000	18	30	00	26	38	08	35	47	17	45	57	27
2000–2320	16	28	– 2	24	36	06	33	45	15	43	55	25
2320–2700	13	25	– 5	22	34	04	30	42	12	40	52	22
2700–3150	12	24	– 6	21	33	03	29	41	11	39	51	21
3150–3700	11	23	– 7	19	31	01	27	39	07	37	39	19
3700–4400	09	21	– 9	16	28	– 2	25	37	07	34	46	16
4400–5300	05	17	– 13	12	24	– 6	19	31	01	29	41	11
5300–6400	03	15	– 15	09	21	– 9	15	27	– 3	25	37	07
6400–7700	01	13	– 17	6	18	– 12	12	24	– 6	22	34	04
7700–9500	0	12	– 18	3	15	– 15	9	27	– 9	18	30	0

Table 14.2 The relative importance of frequency bands to the intelligibility of conversational speech

Frequency band (Hz)	Band importance for average speech
100– 200	0.01
200– 300	0.02
300– 400	0.03
400– 510	0.04
510– 630	0.04
630– 770	0.04
770– 920	0.04
920–1080	0.04
1080–1270	0.05
1270–1480	0.05
1480–1720	0.05
1720–2000	0.06
2000–2320	0.07
2320–2700	0.07
2700–3150	0.06
3150–3700	0.06
3700–4400	0.06
4400–5300	0.06
5300–6400	0.05
6400–7700	0.02
7700–9500	0.00

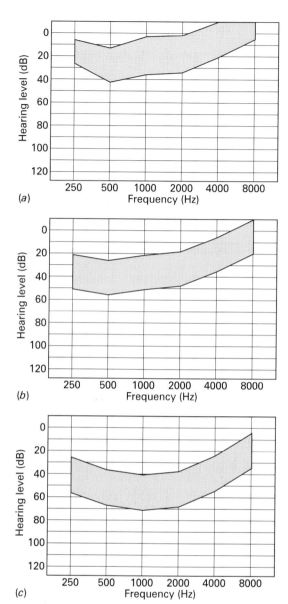

(a)

(b)

(c)

Figure 14.1 The spectrum of speech plotted on a clinical audiogram format corresponding to mean levels of (a) 50 dB SPL, (b) 65 dB SPL and (c) 80 dB SPL

considered important for hearing aid fitting. Certainly, when frequencies in the 2000–4000 Hz region are taken into account, the band importance functions show how much of the speech signal is likely to be degraded by inattention to the high frequency components.

This consideration of the physical properties of speech in terms of its distribution as a function of level and frequency and the importance to speech intelligibility of different frequencies has important consequences for the effects of a sensorineural hearing loss, first on the audibility of speech and second on its intelligibility.

Audibility of speech

These considerations concerning the range and spread of intensities and frequencies contained in a speech signal lead directly to an understanding of how different configurations and degrees of hearing loss can affect the understanding of speech. Figure 14.1 shows the distribution of speech now plotted on a conventional audiogram format for speech at levels of 50, 65 and 80 dB SPL. It is not possible to incorporate the band importance functions into these diagrams but it should be remembered that the relatively less intense high frequencies do contain important contributions. It can be seen that relatively small deficits at the high frequencies can lead to parts of the speech spectrum not being available to the impaired auditory system. As the overall level of

the hearing loss increases (e.g. a hearing loss of 45 dB HL), for conversational speech substantial elements of all of the speech spectrum including the more intense low frequencies becoming unavailable.

At this point it becomes possible to construct a rule for the major role of a hearing aid and that is to 'make the speech spectrum to the largest possible extent available to the impaired auditory system without being uncomfortably loud'. There are a number of aspects to this rule which deserve consideration.

The first of these is, what is 'the speech spectrum'? Different individuals will experience different auditory environments and hence will place different demands upon the auditory abilities. It is normal in considering hearing aid fittings to take the speech spectrum at normal conversational speech, usually around 65 dB SPL. However, it is certainly the case that the auditory range of acoustical stimuli will be outside this, and this has implications for more detailed fitting of hearing aids both in groups and across individuals which will be considered later in the chapter. The second point of consideration is the amplification that is required to make the speech audible, but not uncomfortably loud (British Society of Audiology, 1987). It would be relatively easy to prescribe (and using modern technology to deliver) amplification which made all of the speech spectrum above threshold. However, it is an almost inevitable consequence of sensorineural hearing loss that, while thresholds are elevated, the ear suffers from what is commonly termed 'clinical recruitment'. This is an abnormally rapid growth of loudness such that, while substantial deficits at threshold may be present, the upper end of the dynamic range (often characterized by the threshold of uncomfortable loudness) is elevated only marginally, if at all. Thus there is a limited dynamic range available for the speech spectrum to be mapped into. It then becomes the task of the hearing aid, having identified the speech spectrum of interest, to provide sufficient amplification to convert the speech spectrum from below threshold to the range of audibility without reaching uncomfortable listening levels.

It is not possible to overemphasize at this stage this important concept of audibility, as it becomes the driving force and standard by which hearing aid fitting and evaluation procedure may be assessed and also the criterion for which different types of processing can be rationally analysed.

Dimensions of choice in a hearing aid

There are a number of dimensions along which a hearing aid can be characterized and therefore the choice for an individual or a group of individuals can be made. These can either be physical parameters, such as the layout of the components, or can be more associated with the type of transducers or processing that is involved. At the simplest level they consist of decisions of how and where the sound is going to be picked up by the hearing aid, how the sound is processed or amplified before delivery to the impaired ear, and how and where the processed acoustical signal is delivered to the impaired auditory system. In making these considerations it is helpful to draw up some form of 'standard' hearing aid and then discuss differences from that standard. Given the organization of hearing services in the UK National Health Service, this chapter has chosen as its

standard hearing aid a postaural (behind-the-ear, BTE) device with an omnidirectional microphone fed to the impaired ear via a customized earmould, the device having simple linear circuitry with output limiting achieved by peak clipping. Such a device has a single microphone which is sensitive to sounds arriving at the transducer from all spatial locations (i.e. it is not directionally sensitive in terms of its orientation either towards or away from the sound source). It is important to realize that the eventual frequency response of the hearing aid device can be no better and is often determined by the frequency response of the microphone itself. This can have an important effect both on the overall bandwidth of the hearing aid (i.e. the lowest and highest frequencies that the hearing aid can transmit), but also the shape of the frequency response (particularly in terms of peaks or resonances in the response). The electrical signal from the microphone is fed to an amplifier (similar in concept to those found in hi-fi systems) which often has control over three functions: the low frequency or base response; the high frequency or treble response; and the gain or volume setting of the device. Although the extent to which low and high frequency controls are available will vary from device to device they do provide, to a limited extent, the ability to alter and therefore tailor the overall frequency characteristics of the hearing aid. Hearing aids usually come in a range of power or strength suitable for different degrees of hearing loss. The gain or volume control on the hearing aid provides a degree of fine control over the sound level delivered by the device, so that the user can compensate for changes in the acoustical environment. The maximum output that can be achieved by a hearing aid is often determined by the hearing aid amplifier and its associated power supply (commonly called a battery but more properly a single cell) and further control is usually available at this stage. Earlier it was suggested that the hearing aid should not have the capacity to make signals louder than the threshold of uncomfortable listening for the impaired ear. The device therefore usually has a way of limiting the maximum output via a process of simple peak clipping. This is a process whereby when the output attempts to go beyond a certain predetermined level, the circuitry simply clips or flattens the output of the waveform so that this situation does not arise. Finally, the now amplified electrical signal is converted back into sound by the hearing aid earphone (sometimes called the receiver) and coupled by one means or another to the listener's auditory system.

There is then a number of variations available on this basic configuration.

Directional microphones

It is possible to construct microphones suitable for hearing aid use which are more sensitive to sound arriving from one direction (usually the direction in which the microphone is pointing) than from others. Although these microphones can be difficult to miniaturize, and their performance is usually superior for postaural or body worn devices, it is possible to apply them in smaller units such as is found in in-the-ear hearing aids. The directionality is often achieved by a second port or inlet into the microphone which faces in a direction away from the sound source of interest. Thereafter, careful mechanical construction and tuning leads to the situation whereby a degree of enhanced sensitivity is achieved for the forward direction because sounds coming from other directions are in effect cancelled out across the two mechanical ports or inputs to the device (Hawkins and Yacullo, 1984). The degree of directionality that can be achieved is usually limited to the lower frequencies (up to 1.5–2 kHz) so does not apply equally across the range of sounds of interest. This can either be regarded as a positive advantage in terms of shaping the frequency response towards greater high frequency emphasis, or as a disadvantage in that the degree of directionality achieved can be reduced for a hearing aid with a sloping frequency response.

It has not been routine practice to fit directional microphones to hearing aids by default, but rather to regard them as a special case for difficult-to-fit listeners. Part of the reason for this could be the increased potential cost, but is more likely to arise from the realization that, while a directional microphone may be advantageous for some listening situations, this is not always the case. Where the acoustical stimulus of interest consists of a single source, a directional microphone can be used to advantage to focus in on that source at the expense of other competing noise sources. As such, a directional microphone can achieve an improved signal-to-noise ratio of 3–6 dB – a benefit of material advantage to the understanding of speech. However, there are other listening circumstances where directionality could be a positive disadvantage, such as listening to music from an orchestra or for certain occupational circumstances such as trying to understand speech in a car, or other situations where the speaker's interest cannot be necessarily located directly in front of the listener.

Thus to date the theoretical advantages of directional microphones have not often been realized in everyday hearing aid fitting. However, it is now possible to achieve a directional microphone using a pair of omnidirectional microphones and cancelling the signals between the forward facing and noise detecting microphone by electronic means. This has the advantage of being able to switch easily between directional and non-directional modes, achieving the benefits of directionality without the penalties.

In addition, some of the signal processing techniques using multi-microphone arrays can be thought of as an advanced form of directional microphone where the electronic processing that takes place upon the input achieves a form of 'electronic focusing' which can exceed the properties of a more traditional device. Some of the potential benefits of this approach are discussed later in the chapter.

Body-worn devices

Historically, body-worn hearing aids preceded the development of ear level devices because of the extra space available for power supplies and the associated electronics. In current technology, there is little in terms of simple linear amplification that can be achieved in a body worn device that cannot be achieved in an ear level device, and the role of body worn aids has declined steadily over the years. There are two minor exceptions to this progression which arise from the very high gains that some users may require to overcome a deficit or the very limited manipulative skills due to other conditions (such as arthritis in the elderly) which may limit the listener's ability to manipulate the physically smaller ear level device. The limitations imposed by feedback can usually be overcome in ear level devices using appropriate earmould techniques but, particularly in individuals with large conductive components to their hearing loss (often accompanied by anatomical deficits in the ear canal making appropriately fitting earmoulds difficult) and the high gains required, such conditions can lead to feedback being an insuperable problem in ear level devices. In this case, a body-worn device may be a viable alternative. Similarly, there will be a small number of individuals who, with appropriate training and counselling, cannot cope with the small controls on a postaural device and may have to be fitted with a body-worn device. However, these situations are rare and body-worn devices are usually only fitted following an unsuccessful trial with ear level devices.

Spectacle aids

At one stage of the development of hearing aids, it was common practice to build the hearing aid electronics into one arm of a pair of spectacles and to deliver the acoustical signal via a conventional ear piece. The miniaturization of electronics has made this situation no longer necessary, and in current practice spectacle aids are rarely employed except as bone conduction devices (see below).

In-the-ear hearing aids

Throughout the development of hearing aids there has been continued pressure from consumers and efforts from designers to make the devices smaller and, hence, theoretically less conspicuous. It is generally accepted that one of the contributory reasons to the relatively low take-up of hearing aids among candidates is the perception that a degree of stigma is associated with the wearing of the physical prosthesis. It is, therefore, assumed that the less obvious the prosthesis, the more likely is the hearing impaired individual prepared to make use of them. During the 1970s and 1980s it became possible to embed the hearing aid electronics and associated transducers, first of all into full shell concha aids, then into in-the-ear devices and, more latterly, into completely in-the-canal devices. The pressures for this development arose largely out of the cosmetic considerations, and actually had rather little to do with any electroacoustic advantages, though advertising claims for in-the-ear devices did, of course, attempt to dwell on this aspect.

In the push for in-the-ear devices, hearing impaired listeners did, until very recently, pay a significant penalty in terms of the electroacoustic performance, sound quality, battery life and adjustments/facilities available on the device for the hearing aids which were in-the-ear rather than postaural. It is instructive to note that in countries where the free market reigns supreme (such as in North America) the proportion of sales met by in-the-ear devices rapidly rose to over 80% (Kirkwood, 1990), because of the pressure from consumers who perceived the advantages of in-the-ear devices.

However, as technology and manufacturing capabilities have increased, a simple linear hearing aid which contains appropriate degrees of frequency shaping via high and low frequency controls and output limiting via peak clipping, can be manufactured as an in-the-ear device, which carries the same electroacoustic performance and sound quality as current postaural devices (Cole, 1993). Thus the situation now arises in which hearing impaired listeners could be fitted with either postaural or in-the-ear devices without regard to the differences in hearing aid performance and specification. The use of in-the-ear devices by a number of patient groups is steadily increasing throughout the world (Clasen, Vesterager and Parving, 1987; Henrichsen *et al.*, 1988, 1991; May, Upfold and Battaglia, 1990; Upfold, May and Battaglia, 1990; Tonning, Warland and Tonning, 1991).

One of the problems with the widespread application of in-the-ear devices, particularly in large scale enterprises such as the National Health Service, has been that they have to be customized for each individual ear because the electronics and transducers are inherently embedded in the shell which is configured to the individual anatomical characteristics of each ear canal. Modular in-the-ear devices are now available which contain the hardware inside a standard housing (in fact, there are two standard housings in most implementations, one for left ears and one for right ears) which is then coupled to a minimal shell mould and fitted to the individual listener's ear canal. Such devices potentially carry the advantages of standard-ized hardware and the ability to supply off-the-shelf replacements with the perceived cosmetic advantages of in-the-ear devices, though their application, for example to National Health Service clinics, is only just beginning to receive detailed scrutiny.

In any in-the-ear device, the microphone and the earphone are closer together than in either the post-aural device or a body-worn device. As such, they are always going to be more susceptible to feedback problems than the alternatives and, therefore, the gain that can be delivered via an in-the-ear device will continue to be more limited than that from a postaural device. The actual degree of gain that can be delivered before the onset of oscillatory feedback will depend upon the quality of the fit but, in general terms, in-the-ear devices are suitable for mild and moderate hearing impairments, and prescribing them for severe hearing losses becomes much more problematical.

Bone conduction hearing aids

A bone conduction hearing aid can be regarded as similar in concept to a conventional linear air conduction device where the hearing aid earphone is replaced with a mechanical vibrator similar to that employed for bone conduction tests in clinical audiometry. Here, the intention is to bypass the middle ear and to stimulate directly the cochlea via the temporal bone (though, of course, in actual practice there are middle ear components to bone conduction transmission). Bone conduction hearing aids are usually only regarded as an appropriate management when the wearing of a conventional air conduction device becomes problematical or impracticable. If an individual has a congenital abnormality of the middle or external ear it may not be possible, even after repeated surgical intervention, for that individual successfully to wear a conventional earmould. Alternatively any attempted earmould may either produce constant feedback because of the anatomical abnormalities or may lead to the exacerbation of any middle or external ear pathology that might be present. For example, it is not usually regarded as good practice to wear a conventional earmould in an ear with active chronic otitis media (Alvard, Doxey and Smith, 1989). In these circumstances, bone conduction hearing aids may be the only available form of management. Early bone conduction hearing aids were body-worn devices, but have since developed into spectacle devices or devices with postaural amplifiers. The transducer (bone conductor) has to be held in firm contact with the temporal bone via the mastoid process if reasonably efficient transduction of the stimulus is to be achieved. The problems associated with bone conduction hearing aids are those that are familiar from bone conduction testing in clinical audiometry. The pressure of contact has to be high and, therefore, leads to irritation and discomfort from prolonged use, the maximum output of a bone conduction device is around 40 dB HL at low frequencies and 75–80 dB HL at higher frequencies, and the distortion characteristics of bone conduction transducers, particularly for wide band signals such as speech, are extremely poor. It is, therefore, not surprising that success using conventional bone conduction devices has been extremely limited, and this has led to efforts to improve the quality of the signal delivered.

The configuration of a conventional bone conduction hearing aid is shown in Figure 14.2*a* where the electrical signal from the hearing aid is coupled to a mechanical vibrator which is placed in contact with the skin surface, thereby transmitting mechanical energy to the temporal bone. Historically, the next development consisted of a pair of magnets. The first of these was a permanent rare earth magnet which was attached to a screw and implanted in the temporal bone below the skin surface on the mastoid process (Figure 14.2*b*). The skin surface was then closed. Energy is transmitted to the implanted magnet by an external electromagnet which is held in position by the attraction between the internal and external components. An oscillatory magnetic field produced by the external magnet induces a force in the internal implanted magnet and, hence, bone conduction vibrations in the temporal bone. The development of this device took place primarily in North America where, for some years, it was a popular alternative to conventional bone conduction transducers. Its applications, however, have been limited by a number of factors. Perhaps the most important of these has been the inefficiency of the energy transfer which leads to the device having a very limited maximum output

(Browning, 1990), so that even with a body-worn processor and power supply, the device is really suitable only for candidates who have essentially normal bone conduction thresholds. Given that, with age, an individual is likely to acquire sensorineural components to the hearing loss, the number of candidates for this device has been limited. It is also the case that the degree of force to keep the external and internal magnets in close contact leads to potential problems of discomfort on the skin and even erosion of the skin surface. Recent years has seen a decline in the use of this device and the relative increase of an alternative which relies on more direct coupling.

The direct coupling bone conduction device (known as the bone anchored hearing aid) was developed in Sweden and is illustrated in Figure 14.2*c*. It consists of a titanium peg which passes through the skin surface and is embedded in the temporal bone. This is coupled to a mechanical vibrator which is directly attached to the implanted screw (Håkansson *et al.*, 1985; Håkansson, Tjellström and Carlsson, 1990). This form of coupling has some direct implications. First, the transfer of energy is relatively efficient, even compared with the conventional bone conduction coupling situation because the energy no longer passes through the soft tissue interface (the skin surface) but directly to the temporal bone. The devices currently commercially available can be coupled either to an ear level processor and transducer array or to a body-worn processor with a more conventional ear level bone conduction type transducer. For the ear level implementation, the maximum output available from the device makes it a

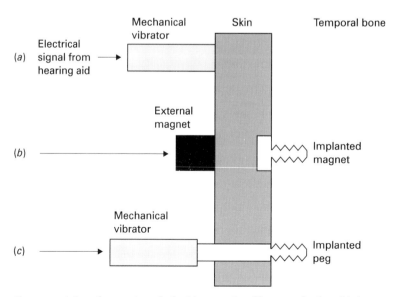

Figure 14.2 Schematic representation of energy transfer for (*a*) conventional bone conduction, (*b*) electromagnetic couplers and (*c*) direct coupling to the bone anchored hearing aid

suitable treatment for individuals with bone conduction thresholds on average better than 50 dB HL, whereas in the body-worn implementation candidates up to 65 dB HL can be accommodated. Although application of this device throughout the world is still developing, it does appear to be a much more successful method of transferring electroacoustical energy to the temporal bone in subjects for whom bone conduction aids are required (Albrektsson *et al.*, 1987; Bonding, 1990; Bonding, Holm Jonsson and Salomon, 1990; Candela-Cano, Aguado-Blass and Sada-Garcia-Lomas, 1990; Cremers, Snik and Benyon, 1991, 1992; Bonding *et al.*, 1992; Mylanus *et al.*, 1994a, b; Tjellstrom and Granstrom, 1994). It must be recognized, however, that there are medical problems associated with such a transcutaneous device because of potential infection around the site of the implanted coupling. The candidature criteria for such devices are still under investigation, but where an individual could only previously be managed by a conventional bone conduction amplification system, it is likely that the benefits of the bone anchored hearing aid are likely to be marked and certainly more beneficial than the implanted magnet configuration (Wade, Halik and Chasin, 1992).

Specifying the characteristics of a hearing aid

When a hearing aid is received at the clinic from the manufacturer, it will be accompanied by an array of specifications, in both graphical and tabular form, which attempt to summarize its performance under a variety of electroacoustic conditions which conform to one or more of the national or international standards currently in use (e.g. ANSI S3.22 – 1982). For those who are not technically inclined, the array of graphs and figures provided can be somewhat daunting and difficult to interpret. Table 14.3 shows a summary of the tests recommended by the appropriate American National Standard. In attempting to understand the data in Table 14.3 it is useful to isolate and concentrate on three of the most important components in specifying the characteristics of any particular device.

Gain

The gain of a hearing aid attempts to describe what the device does to typical sound arriving at the hear-

Table 14.3 A summary of the specifications of hearing aid performance

Characteristic	Input SPL (dBO re 20 μPa)	Frequency (Hz)	Gain control setting	Presentation
SSPL90 (Saturation)	90	200–5000	Full on	Curve
Maximum SSPL90	90	Any frequency between 200 and 5000	Full on	Number (dB)
Average SSPL90	90	1000, 1600, 2500	Full on	Number (dB)
Average full on gain	60 or 50 (State which) 50 for AGC	1000, 1600, 2500	Full on	Number (dB)
Reference test gain	60	1000, 1600, 2500	Set gain control to give output SPL 17 dB less than average SSPL90, or full on for low gain aids	
Frequency response	60 (linear) 50 (AGC)	200—500 or to 20 dB below 3 frequency average	Reference test position	Curve
Total harmonic distortion	70 65	500, 800, 1600	Reference test position	Number (%)
Equivalent input noise level, L	50 (AGC)	1000, 1600, 2500 Avg. To get L_{av}	Reference test position	Number (dB)
Telephone pickup (induction coil)	10 mA/m rms magnetic field	1000	Full on	Number (dB)
Battery current	65	1000	Reference test	Number (mA)
Input-output curves (AGC only)	50 to 90	2000	Full on	Curve Input-abscissa Output-ordinate
Attack and release times (AGC only)	Abrupt 55 to 80 80 to 55	2000	Full on	Numbers (ms)

ing aid microphone. In particular it attempts to describe by how much, as a function of frequency, the sound is amplified at the output of the hearing aid compared with the sound level arising at the hearing aid microphone. It is usually presented graphically (e.g. Figure 14.3) in the form of a frequency response curve, though various summary indices which are the gain averaged over a number of particular frequencies (dependent on the standard) may be provided in tabular form. Important parameters to be specified when considering and interpreting the gain of a particular device are the level of the signal presented to the hearing aid microphone and the gain setting on the device itself.

much sound energy, and how it is distributed, that the hearing aid could conceivably deliver. The most common term for the maximum output is the SSPL90 which is a shortform description for the measure which is usually conducted using an input signal of 90 dB SPL and the gain control set at maximum. It is presented in graphical form (Figure 14.4) with summary indices extracted at particular point frequencies. It is usually important to specify the adjustment of any control for limiting the maximum output of the hearing aid, though often this is assumed to be also set at the maximum value.

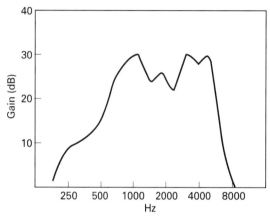

Figure 14.3 Example of the gain of a hearing aid as a function of frequency

Maximum output

In assessing the maximum output of the hearing aid, the specifications attempt to summarize how

Distortion

The distortion parameters attempt to summarize how well the hearing aid does the job of taking the input signal, amplifying it, and delivering it to the output without adding any unwanted components to the signal. If a single frequency (a pure tone or sinusoid) is presented to the hearing aid, an ideal device would amplify that single frequency without introducing energy at any other frequencies. However, any real device can introduce a degree of harmonic distortion. That is, for an input signal of 1000 Hz, the output signal would say contain elements at its harmonic frequencies of 2000, 3000, 4000 Hz, etc. The harmonic distortion is expressed either in per cent or dB. For total harmonic distortion expressed in per cent a low value indicates that the energy at frequencies other than the primary is small compared to the primary, where for total harmonic distortion expressed in dB, a high value represents good performance, being a measure of how much reduced from the level of the primary 1000 Hz tone the other components are.

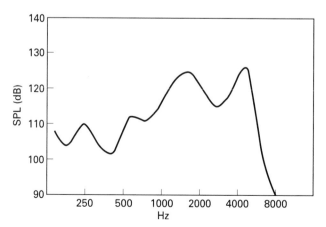

Figure 14.4 Example of the output of the hearing aid as a function of frequency

Hearing aid specifications in relation to performance

It is now relevant to consider the uses to which the manufacturer's specification of hearing aid characteristics should be put. The first of these in any clinical or commercial setting is to act as part of a quality control system. Thus, if an individual device differs significantly from the manufacturer's specifications for a particular parameter, this implies that the device is likely to be faulty and therefore should be replaced or withdrawn from circulation for repair. Thus, many of the standard specifications contain a tolerance limit for the parameters of summary performance.

A second use to which hearing aid specifications may be put is to provide a preliminary comparison of likely performance between devices which apparently differ materially in one or other respect. Thus a hearing aid might specify its frequency range at 200–5000 Hz while an alternative be specified as 200–8500 Hz. The reader can then reasonably expect the latter device potentially to provide more amplification to the high frequency components of speech than the former (although of course whether this could be achieved in practice could depend upon the earmould delivery system). Likewise the SSPL90 or maximum power output can give an indication of the suitability of a particular device for an individual with given audiological characteristics. As will be seen later, the gain required by a particular hearing loss can be estimated in the first instance from the pure tone thresholds, while the maximum output required from a hearing aid can be estimated from the uncomfortable loudness levels.

Perhaps one of the most difficult parameters to interpret in hearing aid specifications are the measures of distortion characteristics. Given that distortion measures attempt to describe the quality of amplification provided by the device, it would be expected that a close relationship to assessments of sound quality would be apparent. While it is the case that very poor harmonic distortion can lead to poor sound quality and speech intelligibility, the parameter is insensitive as many hearing aids with apparently similar characteristics in terms of harmonic distortion are reported as having a wide range of sound quality by both normal and hearing impaired listeners (Bode and Kasten, 1971; Agnew, 1988). Although not necessarily yet part of standard specifications, more complex and perhaps appropriate measures of distortion characteristics based on intermodulation distortion and the hearing aid's ability to deal with time varying wide band signals are under development (American National Standard, 1992), but again the link to receptual attributes such as speech identification and sound quality judgements remains to be established (Dyrlund, 1989a; Preves, 1990; Kates, 1992).

Equipment for measuring hearing aid characteristics

The hearing aid test box is a familiar sight in audiology departments, although its complexity can range from simple portable devices the size of a small briefcase to sound chambers and associated equipment which, in themselves, constitute a small laboratory. The objective in measuring hearing aid characteristics is an attempt to specify the output of the hearing aid compared to the input of the the hearing aid (American National Standards Institute/Acoustical Society of America, 1982) and, as described previously, the original motivation for this was part of the quality control of the physical devices. In order to achieve this, a number of decisions have to be taken at the outset and historically the signals that have been traditionally used for this specification have been simple pure tones or sinusoids. A schematic layout of a test situation is shown in Figure 14.5, although commercial realizations may well differ in their components, orientation and organization. The sound that is delivered to the hearing aid is usually a pure tone whose frequency can be controlled by the external equipment. This is delivered to a loudspeaker enclosed in a measuring chamber which attempts to isolate the measurement from the ambient noise outside. The level of the pure tone delivered to the hearing aid has to be measured and controlled in some way, and this is often achieved by having a calibrated reference microphone placed close to the hearing aid in the test chamber. The reference microphone can measure the level of the tone being presented to the hearing aid microphone and can be used to adjust the level of the pure tone delivered to the external loudspeaker so that the desired test level is obtained. This configuration is often adopted as equipment is used to sweep the pure tones from low to high frequencies, either in steps or in a continuous manner to generate the frequency response curves, and can therefore compensate for changes in the sensitivity of the loudspeaker. Thus a calibrated signal is delivered to the hearing aid microphone.

The next consideration is how to couple the output of the hearing aid to the test equipment so that the output characteristics of the hearing aid can be measured. There is a variety of couplers in use in audiological practice often based on the simple 2cc coupler which is a simple test chamber and makes little or no attempt to reproduce the complex acoustical characteristics of the human ear. Alternatives that may be used include an occluded ear simulator (often the Zwislocki coupler) which better attempts to represent the acoustics of the ear but, unless the subject's individual earmould is used in some way in the assessment, cannot take its own acoustical properties into account. The important factor from an interpretation point of view is that when a measurement characteristic is given, the conditions under which it

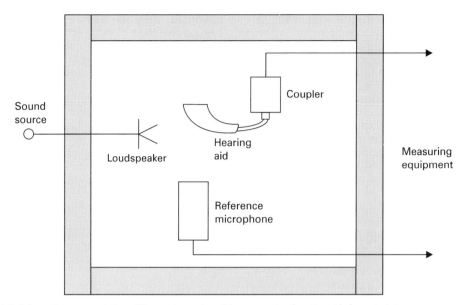

Figure 14.5 Schematic representation of the equipment used for measuring hearing aid characteristics

was derived are clearly stated so that the coupler in use and method of attaching the hearing aid to the coupler is readily available. Once the sound has been fed in to the standard coupler, it may be processed by the measuring equipment and represented on a display screen, chart recorder, printer, etc.

For many years pure tones were the only signals that were used to specify the characteristics of a hearing aid. However, the advent of more complex circuitry and processing has prompted more detailed examination of some of the assumptions which underlie the use of sinusoids and it has become apparent that hearing aids do not necessarily perform in the same way for a broad band signal as they do for simple pure tones. This is true even for simple linear hearing aids where, for example, if one part of the wide band signal is driving the hearing aid into saturation, then the performance of the device at other remote frequencies may not be what one had expected from the characteristics derived from pure tones. Where more complex devices are used, it is totally unrealistic to extrapolate from characteristics derived from pure tones to those for broad band signals. Therefore, more modern equipment and measuring techniques use signals which are closer in content to those that the hearing aid will be dealing with in real life, i.e. speech. These signals usually contain the same overall spectrum of speech and consist either of noise shaped to have the same spectrum as speech or a harmonic complex with that same spectrum (American National Standard, 1992). Using these signals with modern instrumentation it is possible to derive hearing aid characteristics which

more closely resemble the real world performance of devices under a variety of conditions of signal level and settings on the hearing aid. Use of these speech-like signals has also enabled more appropriate measures of hearing aid distortion to be implemented, based on coherence analysis which attempt to give a measure of how faithfully the speech signal would be reproduced, and therefore more closely related to the perceptual attributes of speech itself.

Coupler versus real ear measures

Over the years the emphasis on hearing aid characteristics and specifications has moved from that of quality control to the desire to relate how the hearing aid might perform when fitted to an individual hearing impaired listener. As technology has advanced it has become possible to measure the characteristics of the hearing aid as worn by the hearing impaired listener (Barlow *et al.*, 1988). Previously, the only way that the hearing aid characteristics could be measured *in situ* were by measures of so-called functional gain. Here the free-field (or sound field) thresholds were measured without the hearing aid in place, then repeated with the hearing aid, the difference then being the gain delivered by the hearing aid – the functional gain. In some circumstances these could also be measured by changes in acoustic reflex thresholds. To anyone familiar with the accuracy and repeatability of audiological test methods, it will be apparent that the difference in the two threshold measures will have a relatively high degree of variance and therefore limited potential clinical utility. The motivation for performing these sorts of measurements has been the growing realization of the dissociation of measurements taken in standard couplers (even where they attempt to mimic the average acoustical performance of real ears) and those that apply when hearing aids are worn in real ears with appropriate earmoulds, although before the improvements in technological capability many attempts have been made to predict from coupler measurements (perhaps using the subject's own earmoulds) the performance in the real ear environment (Dillon and Murray, 1987; Bentler and Pavlovic, 1989).

The stage has now been reached where instrumentation and the associated test procedures are available that are sufficiently robust for application in clinical settings, of comparable cost to other audiological equipment, and for whom the accuracy of the measures approaches clinical requirements. For a review of the development and application of real ear measures, see Mueller, Hawkins and Northern (1992).

Although by no means in routine clinical use throughout the world, it is predicted that, when the role of the measurements is associated with the selection, verification or evaluation of hearing aids, the procedures are likely to rely increasingly on real ear measures rather than predictions from those ascertained from standard couplers. There is one deviation from this general trend which is interesting and bears examination and is concerned with the fitting of hearing aids to young children. It is well recognized that the differences between what a hearing aid delivers in a standard coupler and in a real ear are greatest when the acoustical characteristics of the real ear differ significantly from those of the average human adult – the acoustical properties of children's, and particularly young children's ears change materially as they mature. Clinical practice also suggests that the time available during which the child will cooperate in real ear measures is extremely limited, and therefore repeated testing during which time the audiologist makes changes and adjustments to the hearing aids is likely to lead to an alienation between the child and the fitting process. It has therefore been suggested that a process be adopted whereby a single measure of the real ear coupler difference (i.e. the difference between what a hearing aid delivers to a coupler and to a real ear for that individual) be taken using transducers and earmould similar to those which would be employed eventually, and that this individually measured correction factor be applied thereafter to all coupler measures (Zelisko, Seewald and Gagne, 1992). This approach has been shown to be successful. Based upon the individually tailored real ear to coupler differences, the predicted response in the real ear closely matches that actually delivered. However, it is only likely to find application in children where the subject tolerance is low.

Thus for purposes of hearing aid fitting rather than quality control, the measure of clinical interest has now become the real ear insertion gain, which may be thought of as the difference between the characteristics of sound arriving at the tympanic membrane when the hearing aid is not in place from those characteristics when the hearing aid is worn by the hearing impaired listener. This has obvious advantages in including the effects of any earmould/tubing system and takes into account the loss of natural resonance from the listener's external ear canal, both of which can materially affect the sound delivered to the tympanic membrane. In terms of hearing aid fitting and evaluation, similar sets of measures to those shown in Table 14.3 from couplers can, of course, be derived for real ear measures.

Alternative hearing aid architecture

To date consideration has been focused on the conventional personal amplifier which is commonly thought of as the hearing aid, though there are of course many other aids to hearing and variations upon the conventional device.

Vibrotactile aids

In individuals with profound hearing impairment, it is often not possible to deliver acoustical signals above threshold. Sometimes even when this is feasible, the auditory system may be sufficiently damaged that reasonable speech perception abilities cannot be maintained. Under these circumstances, the listener's requirement can sometimes be at least in part satisfied by a device which delivers the energy via a vibration transducer, often worn on the forearm. There are some devices clinically available and the area remains the focus of some research activity (Weisenberger, Broadstone and Saunders, 1989) but, because of the limited capacity of the vibrotactile sense to convey information which is complex and changes rapidly in terms of intensity, frequency and time (the important parameters of speech and other complex acoustic signals), the application of such vibrotactile stimuli is restricted mainly to providing the hearing impaired wearer with notification of warning or alerting signals. It is possible via a vibrotactile sense for the hearing impaired listener to receive the information, e.g. that the doorbell is ringing. However, as a communication channel it is unlikely that they are going to find widespread use in the near future. For further information see Chapter 16.

Implants

Cochlear implants are dealt with in detail in Chapter 15, but briefly consist of a delivery system whereby the mechanisms of the ear are bypassed entirely and electrical stimulation of the auditory nerve or brain stem is achieved. The application of cochlear implants has expanded greatly in recent years and will probably continue to do so with considerable benefit to individuals with severe and profound hearing losses. Other forms of implants for the auditory system have been attempted, in particular middle ear devices. Here some form of transducer is attached to a component of the ossicular chain and stimulated from an external source. The transducer is a small magnet or a piezoelectric crystal. The potential advantage (compared to the problems with any transfer in bone conduction stimuli) is that the force required to stimulate reasonably movement on the ossicular chain is very much smaller and therefore the energy requirements that much less severe. These implants are still undergoing experimental development (Gyo and Yanagihara, 1985; Gyo, Goode and Miller, 1987; Saiki, Gyo and Yanagihara, 1990; Goode, 1991). The patient population to whom they would be applicable is restricted but coming years will probably see their continued development and application in clinical practice.

Assistive listening devices (environmental aids)

Earlier in this chapter, it was suggested that while the primary aim of a hearing aid is to facilitate understanding of speech, there might be other components of a hearing impaired individual's auditory disability that deserve attention. It is usually to these other aspects or specialized situations that assistive listening devices are directed. In the UK, because of the separation between the hospital services (responsible for hearing aids and associated rehabilitation) and the local authority social services departments (responsible for advice and provision of assistive listening devices), an integration of approach has been difficult to achieve, and hearing impaired individuals often have to rely on the voluntary sector for information, such as the Royal National Institute for Deaf People. It is outside the scope of this chapter to provide a comprehensive description of the types, performance, availability and cost of the various assistive listening devices which are also considered in Chapter 13. However, devices do exist which can, for example, alert the hearing impaired listener to the telephone ringing, or doorbell via a flashing light, provide information about alarm clocks via visual stimuli or vibrating pillow pads, or provide specialized *in situ* amplification from fixed devices such as televisions or telephones.

Educational or radio aids

These devices were developed primarily in an attempt to meet the needs of educating hearing impaired children and facilitating communication in the classroom situation. The speaker (usually the teacher or lecturer) wears a microphone which is remote from the hearing impaired listener, and coupled via radio frequency transmission to the listener or listeners using a specialized coding scheme. This has the advantage that the signal-to-noise ratio at the microphone will be good compared to the signal-to-noise ratio arriving at the listener's hearing aid, because of all of the extraneous acoustical stimuli present in a typical classroom. Arrangements can be made so that the child also receives input from the conventional microphone and is not restricted to input from the single teacher or lecturer. Such devices have found widespread application in specialized schools for the deaf and also for hearing impaired individuals who are integrated into conventional educational programmes. They do achieve advantageous signal-to-noise ratio and therefore greatly improve the communication of information from the teacher to the student.

Remote microphones

Many modern hearing aids contain a facility for a so-called direct input. This is a socket on the hearing aid into which a separate microphone may be plugged which can then be placed further away from the listener and closer to the sound source. One example of an application of this arrangement is in a meeting room whereby the microphone can be made available to the speaker and hence improve communication with the hearing impaired listener. Their application has been largely restricted to individuals with specialized demanding acoustical needs but, where those needs do occur, it can be very effective in meeting them.

Telecoil

At present all standard hearing aids provided by the National Health Service in the UK have a facility for a telecoil switch. This bypasses or supplements the acoustical input by picking up electromagnetic signals from the telecoil. It is useful in buildings where a loop system has been fitted, such as cinemas, theatres, churches, etc. and also where it is incorporated into a telephone handset. Here the sound stimuli are fed to the telecoil and therefore available as electromagnetic information to the hearing aid. Hearing impaired listeners report telecoil facilities as extremely advantageous where they are available and, although their application is spreading, the effectiveness of this facility depends both on the availability of loop systems and the awareness of hearing impaired listeners of their existence.

Binaural hearing aids

The issue of whether and when to fit one or two hearing aids to a hearing impaired listener has been a source of contention in audiological circles for many years and there are perhaps three components that require consideration: what are the audiological benefits of binaural fitting?; will hearing impaired listeners accept binaural hearing aids? and is the extra cost worthwhile?

The huge literature of binaural abilities in normally hearing subjects and hearing impaired subjects can lead to a variety of interpretations about the applicability of binaural amplification. This author has a simple philosophy – if a hearing impaired listener has two ears, each of which has a hearing impairment that could benefit from the provision of amplification (taking no account at all of the state of the other ear), then there will be acoustical environments under which the listener will benefit from two hearing aids as opposed to a single one. Thus the issue now becomes not so much centred around whether the hearing impaired individual could conceivably benefit from two devices, but whether the demands placed upon the hearing impaired listener's hearing by their acoustical environment are such as to justify two devices.

Not all hearing impaired listeners will accept binaural amplification, reacting rather in the manner of 'Surely I'm not that deaf doctor?'. The acceptability in the clinical population of binaural amplification will vary (Chung and Stephens, 1986; Balfour and Hawkins, 1992) and may well depend upon the way in which binaural amplification is offered. For example, an initial attempt to fit two hearing aids when a subject first presents may result in failure, but suggestion to an established user after say 6–12 months of use of a single hearing aid, that a second device would confer additional benefits may meet with approval. Differing health care systems have evolved different traditions of monaural versus binaural amplification, some of which arise out of advertising pressure and some out of the economics of state schemes of hearing aid provision. It is undoubtedly the case that, for many hearing impaired listeners, the benefits of wearing two relatively simple hearing aids far outweigh the benefits of a single such device and may provide superior performance to a single more sophisticated and hence more expensive hearing aid. However, it is likely to continue that the issue of binaural versus monaural provision is dictated by factors other than the subject's ability to benefit – factors more associated with the market economics and politics rather than audiological benefit.

A subsidiary issue which has arisen in recent years has been the demonstration that, in long-term users of a single hearing aid, the speech identification abilities of the normally not aided ear decline relative to those of the normally aided ear (Gelfand, Silman and Ross, 1987; Silman *et al.*, 1992), and that these deficits may or may not be reversible on provision of a second aid (Silman, Gelfand and Silverman, 1984). These findings are being used in the USA to advance the argument that fitting only a single hearing aid to an individual with bilateral hearing impairment could be regarded as unethical and thereby open to claims of professional negligence. Fortunately, this argument has not spread outside North America and, in fact, consists only of one of a number of reasons as to why binaural amplification is likely to be superior to a single device.

Hearing aid selection

In selecting a particular device for a hearing impaired individual, some reference must be made to the technological options that are likely to be available. These can vary enormously from the situation in a state health care system with limited access to different devices to the case in private practice where there may be consumer pressure to consider more advanced options. It is often the case in the National Health Service in the UK that a limited range of devices is available with relatively restricted control over the overall bandwidth and the adjustments to the frequency response. However, the underlying concepts of selecting a device are common to all linear instrumentation and in configuring this section it has been assumed that the choice has been made to fit a linear hearing aid with some method of limiting the maximum output, while no reference is made to the frequency range over which the hearing aid will operate as this is independent of the various rationales adopted.

The choice of physical configuration of the device (i.e. a postaural device, in-the-ear device or a body-worn device) will depend upon the particular setting but does not necessarily interact with the choice of electroacoustic parameters. It is also assumed here that a range of devices with suitable power handling capabilities are available to fit the range of hearing losses that are likely to be met in practice, i.e. lower powered aids suited to mild to moderate hearing losses ranging to higher powered aids to moderate to severe impairments. So the question then arises, given the audiometric characteristics of a hearing loss, what are the underlying concepts that guide the selection and adjustment of a particular device?

Although in the early days of hearing aid development the pragmatic assumption was made that a single type of frequency characteristic would be broadly appropriate for the majority of hearing impaired subjects, it has now become more accepted audiological practice to attempt to compensate for the different audiological parameters of the hearing loss by appropriate selection of the characteristics of the instrument. There is, theoretically, available a large number of approaches to this particular problem which can perhaps be usefully classified into four overall areas:

1 Methods by which measures can be taken of the hearing function of impaired listeners so that targets for the amplification characteristics of the hearing aid may be derived.
2 Methodologies whereby hearing impaired listeners may be presented with different hearing aid characteristics and be able reliably to choose between them and converge on an optimum.
3 Tests of speech identification ability which are sufficiently rapid to perform and reliable in distinguishing between hearing aids so that an optimum characteristic can be derived.
4 Methods of assessing hearing disability and consequent handicap that can be used to distinguish between alternatives.

Although these approaches are not necessarily mutually exclusive, throughout the world, audiological practice has concentrated on the first due to some of the inherent weaknesses in the tools available for the other approaches (for a discussion see Gatehouse, 1993b).

Therefore, it is reasonable to examine in some detail the various alternatives for deriving a set of target characteristics from audiological data which can then serve as the initial adjustment parameters for the fitted device. The audiological literature concerning hearing aid selection has multiplied in recent years (Byrne, 1983; Byrne and Dillon, 1986; Skinner, 1988; Byrne, Parkinson and Newall, 1990). Each of the competing methodologies has its committed supporters and, unfortunately, few comparative studies have been conducted to validate the different approaches and compare their relative effectiveness. This issue might be considered academic if the competing regimens all produced targets that were similar or were within the range of measurement errors. However, this is not the case. Skinner (1988) has shown that, among six of the most commonly advocated prescription strategies for listeners with not atypical threshold values, the differences with frequency of prescribed gain (e.g. the slope of the frequency response) for the six procedures can cover a range of 20–25 dB. Thus there are clearly important differences between the available prescriptive regimens. For a description of the detailed application of different regimens, reference should be made to Skinner (1988) and here we consider, in summary form, the underlying rationale of the approaches.

Procedures based on pure tone thresholds alone

It is intuitively obvious that, in some way and to some degree, the ideal amplification for a particular configuration of hearing loss is likely to be greater at those frequencies where the hearing loss is greatest.

The earlier assumptions taken in hearing aid fitting were that the degree of amplification should be a direct image of the degree of hearing loss. Therefore a hearing loss of 70 dB HL should need amplification of 70 dB. However, even a very early understanding of the consequences of sensorineural hearing impairment had identified the phenomenon of abnormally rapid growth of loudness (clinically referred to as recruitment) whereby individuals with sensorineural hearing impairment have a loss of threshold sensitivity but little or no loss of loudness sensation at high levels. This leads to the natural consequence that the amplification required is somewhat less than the degree of the hearing loss. An early formulation was the 'half gain' rule, whereby subjects were deemed to require amplification consisting of half the degree of the hearing loss. Most of the later modifications of threshold based procedures have been based upon the gains that users actually select when presented with bands of noise or speech at different frequencies. Perhaps the most systematically derived and validated of these prescriptive regimens is that originating from the National Acoustic Laboratories (NAL, Byrne and Dillon, 1986) which leads to an arithmetic formula, whereby the hearing loss at a particular frequency combined with that at adjacent frequencies leads to a prediction of the gain required. Modern hearing aid test equipment designed to perform real ear measures now contains several of the prescriptive regimens as part of the associated software, so that when the equipment has access to the hearing thresholds of the impaired ear, it can produce the target gain (in the real ear or perhaps alternatively in a coupler) for that particular hearing loss according to one of a number of prescriptive regimens. Thus, for example, if one is attempting to fit a hearing aid according to the NAL prescription (which is probably the most widely used prescriptive regimen worldwide) then it is possible either by applying the algebraic formula on a pocket calculator or laboratory computer, or using the facilities of the audiological hearing aid test equipment, to provide a target in terms of the real ear measures which one can then attempt to match. Hence with the hearing aid in place in the subject's ear and the probe to measurement system active, it is possible to ascertain the extent to which the target has been reached and to make the appropriate adjustments to the hearing aid in an attempt to overcome any deficiencies.

Procedures based on measures of the auditory dynamic range

If the goal of a hearing aid is to make the desired signals audible but not uncomfortably loud, then some consideration has to be given to audiological parameters other than threshold, and these are usually referred to as suprathreshold measures of the hearing function. A clinically available measure of the upper limits of the dynamic range is the threshold of uncomfortable loudness, sometimes referred to as loudness discomfort level. An example of the clinical procedure given to ascertain these measures in a clinical setting is given in BSA (British Society of Audiology, 1987). These measures are usually taken using pure tones as stimuli and represent the lowest sound levels which the subject finds uncomfortably loud for long-term listening. The assumption is then made that the hearing aid should be adjusted so that it cannot deliver sound levels which exceed the threshold of uncomfortable loudness, and the SSPL90 (i.e. the sound delivered by the hearing aid with full on gain for an input level of 90 dB SPL) is adjusted to be below the threshold of uncomfortable loudness (though of course account has to be taken of the differences between stimulation using sinusoids and wide band signals such as speech). This is an example of using suprathreshold measures to set one of the characteristics of a hearing aid, the maximum power output.

However, suprathreshold measures can also be used as a way of deriving the likely frequency response that is going to be required. Figure 14.6 shows the unaided speech spectrum for normal conversational speech plotted on an audiogram format along with the hearing threshold levels of the ear to be aided and its uncomfortable loudness level. It is now clear that the aim of the hearing aid should be to amplify the speech spectrum by a certain amount at each frequency so that each portion of the speech spectrum now falls above threshold but does not exceed the threshold of uncomfortable loudness. This can then give a frequency response characteristic which one can attempt to verify. A more rigorous representation of Figure 14.6 is to plot all the data in sound pressure level rather than hearing level and to derive the threshold measures and threshold of un-

comfortable loudness through the same sort of transducer and coupling system as is used for delivering the hearing aid signals (Zelisko, Seewald and Gagne, 1992). This is in use in a small number of clinics throughout the world and has many advantages from a technical point of view. However, the representation is unfamiliar to clinicians and therefore the more usual units of hearing level have been retained here. The representation of speech spectrum threshold and uncomfortable loudness levels can of course also be used for setting the maximum power output of the instrument.

A further refinement is an attempt to decide where in the available dynamic range the speech spectrum should be located via a measurement of the most comfortable listening levels. Audiological procedures attempt to identify for each frequency band the level at which the subject would find long-term listening to acoustic stimuli most comfortable. The example is repeated (Figure 14.7) with a representation of the most comfortable listening levels as a function of frequency which now gives an explicit target for the frequency gain characteristic of the device, while the thresholds of uncomfortable loudness produce targets for the maximum power output.

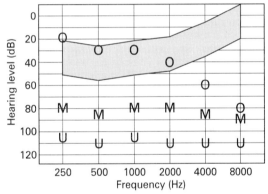

Figure 14.7 Example of a clinical audiogram containing hearing threshold levels, uncomfortable listening levels and most comfortable listening levels for the same speech. O, Hearing threshold; U, uncomfortable loudness level; M, most comfortable listening level

It is argued here that these forms of representation are much more intuitive than targets based on abstract algebraic formulae which have been derived as an average across a large number of hearing impaired subjects who may differ in their characteristics. For example, the NAL formula contains an element whereby the degree of air-bone gap can alter the predicted amplification required, and indeed there is a separate target formula for individuals with severe to profound losses as opposed to mild to moderate losses (Byrne, Parkinson and Newall, 1990).

It is confidently predicted (irrespective of whether the data are presented in sound pressure level units

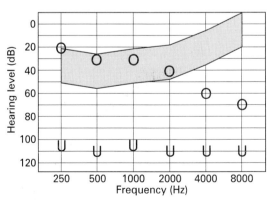

Figure 14.6 Example of a clinical audiogram containing hearing thresholds, uncomfortable listening levels and the spectrum of speech for a mean level of 65 dB SPL. O, Hearing threshold; U, uncomfortable loudness level

or hearing level units) that as the use of real ear measurement systems increases in clinical practice, the audiologist attempting to select and adjust a hearing aid will have available to him an indication of the lower limits of the auditory dynamic range (the hearing thresholds), an indication of the upper limits of the dynamic range (thresholds of loudness discomfort) which, when coupled with a representation of the average speech spectrum (or perhaps even in the future an individually tailored speech spectrum), will lead to a direct indication of the simple amplification characteristics required, the extent to which a given device is meeting them and will point the way for remedial action.

Earmoulds

In this discussion the earmould has been largely regarded as a device whose sole function is to conduct the sound from the output of the hearing aid to the subject's ear. While it is certainly the case that the prime requirements of a earmould are that it be comfortable to the wearer and that it not leak acoustic energy and lead to oscillatory feedback, it must be remembered that the earmould does, in fact, have acoustical properties. A tube conducts sound from the output of a postaural device to the earmould through the internal bore of the earmould and then via the remaining portion of the external auditory canal to the eardrum. As such the earmould can be regarded as an acoustical filter which will modify the sound produced by the hearing aid. This is one of the primary reasons why the characteristics of a hearing aid in a standard coupler do not necessarily represent how the hearing aid processes sound to an individual ear.

Earmould acoustics are complex, but a small number of general statements may be made. First, if tubing is used this is likely to reduce the high frequencies that are delivered to the ear, and the narrower the bore of the tube the more will be the reduction in the high frequency energy (Burgess and Brooks, 1991). The absence of the tube coupling with in-the-ear hearing aids is one of the main contributors to their improved high frequency characteristics. A second general principle is that each element of the earmould system is likely to cause resonances or peaks in the frequency response and that the more of these elements that exist the greater is the degree of disturbance to the frequency response with a consequent effect upon sound quality (Cox and Gilmore, 1986).

Unfortunately, in most clinical practice relatively little attention is paid to the acoustical characteristics of the earmould, first because they are complex, and second, because they are somewhat unpredictable, with the result that many clinics fit earmoulds which have the effect of reducing the effectiveness of the

high frequencies which may or may not be delivered by the hearing aid.

A rough guide to good practice is to ensure that all tubing is of the maximum diameter possible, that the internal bore of the earmould itself be of as large a diameter as possible, and that the length of tubing involved be kept to a minimum (usually of course dictated by anatomy).

It is only when real ear measures of hearing aid performance are made that it is possible to identify the unwanted and perhaps unexpected effects of a particular earmould configuration (e.g. if the high frequency response of the hearing aid-earmould combination is less than one would have expected from coupler measures, or if there are undue peaks and troughs in the frequency response). Unfortunately, given the complexity of earmould acoustics, modification tends to be on a trial and error basis using different types of tube and horns in the mould with acoustical filters or dampers in attempts to smooth out the frequency response.

It is, however, important to return to the prime function of an earmould. There is little point in paying attention to the acoustical properties of the earmould if the result is that problems with earmould comfort or acoustical feedback occur (Dyrlund, 1989b). Such problems will almost certainly lead to underuse or even rejection of the aid by the hearing impaired listener and have to be regarded as more important and relevant than the detailed acoustics. If an aid is not comfortable to wear or it whistles, the subject will not wear it. Fortunately, true allergic reactions to earmould materials are rare (Burgess and Brooks, 1991; Oliwiecki, Beck and Chalmers, 1991; Meding and Ringdahl, 1992).

One of the prime complaints of hearing aid users is of the feeling of occlusion from the earmould itself (Dillon and Murray, 1987). There are two components to this feeling of occlusion, one of which is actual blockage of the external auditory canal. It is often common practice to provide a vent in the earmould to allow pressure equalization between the eardrum and the external environment. The degree of venting that can be achieved is closely related to the amount of gain that the hearing aid is attempting to deliver, as of course sound can exit through the vent, be picked up by the hearing aid microphone and lead to acoustical feedback. Thus the greater the amplification, the smaller the vent that can be achieved (and indeed above certain gains no venting is possible) (Gatehouse, 1989). For very mild hearing losses it is possible to achieve an 'open mould' where there is little, if any, occlusion with the hearing aid tubing being merely located in the ear canal.

A second effect of venting is to reduce the low frequency content of the signal delivered, thereby achieving a relative emphasis in the high frequency response. This effect is, however (like all earmould acoustics), variable and, if sufficient controls are available in the electronics of the hearing aid, might be more conveniently achieved via that route. A second component to the occlusion effect is itself acoustic whereby the earmould, which lies against the cartilaginous section of the external canal, can generate noise via movements of the listener's jaw. This can easily be reproduced in normal hearing listeners by placing one's finger in one's ear canal and chewing. A further component of the acoustic occlusion problem arises from the subject's perception of his own voice via bone conduction stimuli. This component of occlusion can also be replicated by placing one's finger in one's ear and speaking. It will be observed than one's own voice changes in pitch and in amplitude as the external ear is occluded. It is therefore not surprising that hearing aid wearers complain of occlusion problems resulting from the earmould.

There are anecdotal reports that some of the very small in-the-canal hearing aids (so-called completely in-the-canal devices or deep-fitting devices) which pass beyond the cartilaginous portion of the ear canal towards the bony portion, suffer from reduced occlusion problems but these are as yet unsubstantiated by large scale field trials.

In summary, the earmould is an important component of the hearing aid delivery system both from the acoustical and patient comfort/acceptance point of view. The acoustics are somewhat complex and unpredictable and can only really be managed on a trial and error basis, and are only amenable to solution when real ear measures are available. However, acoustical modifications should not be made which compromise the integrity of the earmould as a comfortable coupling device which does not lead to feedback.

Outcome measures for hearing aids

Much of the audiological literature concentrates on hearing aid selection while calling it evaluation, with little regard to overall outcome (i.e. the extent to which the hearing impaired individual's problems have been solved by the provision of a hearing aid as part of a process of rehabilitation). A preliminary stage prior to ultimate evaluation can be regarded as the process during which it is verified that the hearing aid is doing what was intended.

Verification of hearing aid characteristics

If a purely prescriptive approach is adopted (e.g. based solely on pure tone thresholds), then an entirely separate verification stage is likely to be required whereby the degree to which the hearing aid characteristics are performing correctly are assessed (Cox and Alexander, 1990). If the sort of system outlined earlier is available, whereby real ear measures are used adaptively with the particular target (which may be based on thresholds, or on measures of dynamic range, etc.), then the verification process becomes part of the cycle whereby the target and the degree to which the hearing aid meets the target are available to the audiologist as part of a continuing process of adjustment and selection.

It is, however, reasonable to suggest that in both of these instances a further process of verification is desirable, although in practice it is often ignored or perhaps conducted only informally. A reasonable approach to verification is to configure a system whereby a variety of relevant acoustical stimuli could be presented to the hearing impaired listener wearing the hearing aid. These could include, for example, levels of normal conversational speech, music, and perhaps environmental sounds relevant to the listener. They should also include some representation of speech which is intended to drive the hearing aid into saturation so that checks to ensure that uncomfortable loudness levels are not exceeded can be made. Such materials are currently available, e.g. on compact discs and are relatively easy and inexpensive to set up in clinic. Thus a process, whereby the verification of a reasonable electroacoustical set of characteristics can be achieved relatively rapidly in the clinic, is possible. Many audiologists conduct the verification stage informally via their own conversation with the hearing impaired client, but as aids become more complex and attempt to deal with different acoustical circumstances, a move to a more formalized structure is both desirable and likely.

Hearing aid evaluation

Hearing aid evaluation is the process by which one attempts to determine whether the provision of a hearing aid (and all that goes with it) has been successful in overcoming the auditory disabilities and handicaps suffered by the listener. It is possible to conceive of hearing aid evaluation as either technical (i.e. device centred) or related to disability and handicap (i.e. client centred). Both approaches have their adherents but it is argued here that a reasonable evaluation process should contain elements of each.

The characteristic that differentiates the evaluation from the selection and verification processes is that it is not comparative (i.e. it is not comparing two different devices or alternatives) but attempts to assess the performance of the device and the hearing impaired individual's abilities on direct scales. In the technical domain the most attractive outcome measure to employ would be a measure of the extent to which the hearing aid has returned the speech identification abilities of hearing impaired subjects to those enjoyed by normal hearing listeners under appropriate presentation conditions. Unfortunately, speech intelligibility measures have a checkered history in both hearing aid evaluation and hearing aid selection (Gatehouse, 1993b; Walden, Schwartz and Williams, 1983) and because of the time that is required to gather sufficiently stable and sensitive measures, speech identification tests are unlikely to find application in a routine clinical environment as opposed to research studies. It is suggested here that an appropriate outcome measure in the technical domain could be derived from the real ear measures of the hearing aid performance.

Earlier in this chapter we considered the degree to which a speech spectrum might be above threshold and the relative importance of the different frequency bands in speech. It is possible to combine these considerations into a single number called the Articulation Index which varies between 0 and 1. An articulation index of 0 indicates that none of the speech spectrum is available to the auditory system, while an articulation index of 1 indicates that all of the speech information is available for processing by the auditory system – i.e. this is a measure of *audibility* of speech. Note that the articulation index is not a measure of the *intelligibility* of speech. Audibility is concerned with how much information is available for processing by the auditory system, intelligibility is the degree to which the auditory system can make use of the information. The articulation index has a history of application to both hearing aid selection and evaluation (Studebaker, Pavlovic and Sherbecoe, 1987; Pavlovic, 1988, 1990; Berger, 1990; Fabry and Van Tasell, 1990; Rankovic, 1991) and in its later manifestations contains many elements appropriate to sensorineural hearing loss, such as masking of one speech band by another and distortions due to excess amplification. Although still in its infancy as a detailed evaluation tool, it is suggested here that if a technical measure of the outcome of fitting a hearing aid is required (and it is suggested that such a measure is likely to be both required and useful in future), then the aided articulation index as a single simple outcome measure in the performance domain could find application in clinical practice.

In the disability and handicap domains the evaluation process is perhaps more developed (e.g. Oja and Schow, 1984; Newman and Weinstein, 1988; Cox and Gilmore, 1990; Weinstein, 1990; Dillon *et al.*, 1991). Prior to deciding to fit a hearing aid, some assessment will be made of the disabilities and handicaps suffered by the individual hearing impaired listener. Based upon these it will have been decided that a hearing aid as part of a course of rehabilitation is an appropriate way to try to overcome these disabilities and handicaps. It is therefore incumbent upon the person responsible for managing the hearing impaired listener that, following the management, he should attempt to assess the extent to which the intervention has been successful in alleviating those disabilities and handicaps. This is not merely a useful performance indicator for the service and intervention, but acts as a guidance tool for further intervention. If primary problems of the hearing impaired listener have not been overcome or substantially alleviated by the management, then further action may be required, either by provision of more complex technology or by further rehabilitation strategies to attempt to reduce the residual disability. Only if such information is available can realistic decisions be taken about the degree to which current services are successful in alleviating disability and handicap and considerations for changes in the content and organization of services be made.

In the organization of evaluation procedures, there arises the question of when the evaluation should take place. In many countries throughout the world, the eventual evaluation takes place some 4–6 weeks after hearing aid fitting. Recent research has produced data which undermine this timescale because it shows that systematic changes in the benefits delivered by hearing aids can be demonstrated over a period of 8–16 weeks. This is not the acknowledged process of individuals adjusting to a hearing aid, but an apparently underlying perceptual process whereby the individual's impaired auditory system can take time to realize the benefits of a particular hearing aid characteristic. Thus it is not necessarily possible to determine whether an optimal selection has been made if the timescales involved have been sufficiently short that the perceptual changes have not stabilized (Gatehouse, 1993a). Such findings perhaps have more implications for research and field trials of new devices rather than for current clinical practice, but they can be used to encourage individuals that material improvements are possible with time.

Advanced processing in hearing aids

The current hearing aid market and research literature contains many descriptions of devices which purport to implement novel processing schemes whose claims and rationale can be difficult for the non-specialist to follow. Part of this difficulty is due to confusion and sometimes misrepresentation of the aims of the processing, and no attempt is made here to cover each and every processing scheme. Rather it is intended to cover the major classes of processing in use.

Compression aids

Hearing aids which contain some form of compression have been available for many years, and among technical audiologists there is much discussion of the relative merits and effects of input compression, output compression, compression kneepoint settings, compression ratio, attack and release times, etc. Such language is impenetrable to the non-specialist and does disguise the fact that compression aids can contain one or more of three functions (Moore and Glasberg, 1988):

1 Output limiting achieved by compression
2 Automatic volume control
3 Syllabic compression.

For a detailed description of the relationship between these functional aspects and the technical parameters see Hickson (1994).

Output limiting is built into hearing aids in an attempt to ensure that sounds do not become uncomfortably loud, and is usually achieved by a process of peak clipping. Any system which clips the acoustic signal will introduce distortions which can then have an adverse effect on speech perception. A compression limiting hearing aid attempts to curtail the output of the device without introducing significant degrees of distortion. In considering compression limiting we encounter the first of the parameters associated with such systems, that of the compression ratio. For a simple linear device, for every 10 dB increase in the input, the output also increases by 10 dB, which corresponds to a compression ratio of one as shown in Figure 14.8a. Figure 14.8b shows the same linear aid with output limiting achieved by peak clipping. Here, no matter by how much we increase the input, the output remains constant. Therefore, for a device which achieves output limiting by compression, the compression ratio should be high. That is, for a given increase in the input level, the output only increases by a small amount (Figure 14.8c).

A second consideration of the requirements for output limiting, is that the threshold of compression (i.e. the input level at which the compression starts to take effect), sometimes referred to as the compression kneepoint, should be high and close to the threshold of uncomfortable listening. At this point it is necessary to introduce a second parameter of the compression limiter and that is the time it takes to come into effect. If we wish to protect the hearing impaired listener against sharp transients (such as a door slamming or cup breaking) then the compressor has to act rapidly to changes in the level of the sound arriving at the hearing aid, if the sound is not to exceed an uncomfortable listening level for a significant period of time. This is illustrated in Figure 14.9 which shows the envelope of the sound stimulus arriving at the hearing aid microphone and the envelope of the sound stimulus delivered by the hearing aid. Times of the order of 1–2 ms are required if the ear is to be adequately protected. A variant is called adaptive time constants where, for example, the release time (i.e. the time taken for the output to restabilize following the cessation of the transient) might be dependent on how long the intense stimulus was applied. For a hearing aid to act as a compression limiter it should not affect quiet sounds, but attenuate loud sounds, should have

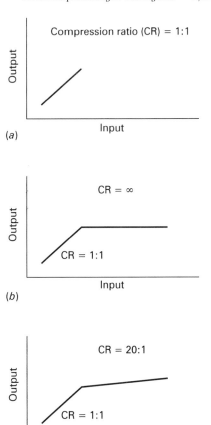

Figure 14.8 Input/output functions to illustrate the concept of the compression ratio

a high compression ratio and should act rapidly. Well configured compression limiting systems have been shown to confer advantages for the majority of hearing impaired listeners (e.g. Preves, 1991). A possible exception to this is for individuals with severe and profound hearing losses. One of the consequences of implementing compression limiting is that the gain and output available can be reduced (note that this is not the result of the concept of compression, but rather its engineering implementation) and it is suggested that some individuals with severe and profound impairments prefer output limiting because of the trade-off between distortion from the peak clipping and reduction in available gain from the compression circuit. However, in general, output limiting via compression is advantageous.

The second use of a compression aid is to act as an automatic volume control (Moore and Glasberg, 1988). As discussed earlier, the input signal to a hearing aid can vary in overall level from 50 dB SPL to 80 dB SPL as speech varies from quiet to loud.

Transient

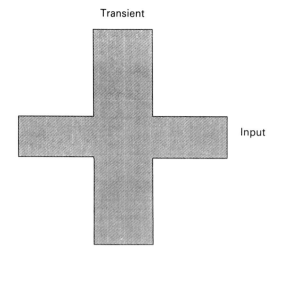

Input

Output

Attack time

Release time

Figure 14.9 The time course of compression limiting

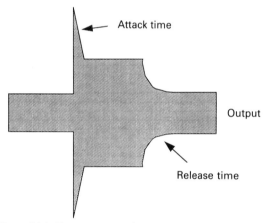

Syllabic compression is a more complex concept. It is sometimes represented as an attempt to overcome problems of limited dynamic range. This is illustrated in Figure 14.10 where it is evident that no simple linear amplification can map the conversational speech spectrum (even without allowing the overall level to vary) into the available dynamic range between threshold and uncomfortable listening. Therefore, in some way the speech has to be squashed or compressed into the available range. This form of processing has to act relatively rapidly as the different elements of speech change from moment to moment (usually over 10–20 ms) which determines the eventual time constant. Given that the range of speech for a given mean level is 30 dB, if the available dynamic range is 15–20 dB, then the compression ratio will be low (often around 2:1). Syllabic compression has been the subject of much attention, although the results have often been contradictory. Much of the conflicting evidence can be attributed to different engineering implementations and test conditions, but recent results suggest that well engineered implementations can be advantageous to individuals with limited dynamic range (Moore *et al.*, 1992).

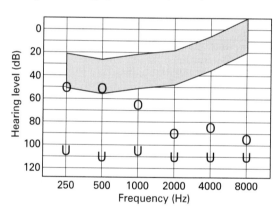

Figure 14.10 Example of a hearing loss with very limited dynamic range. O, Hearing threshold; U, uncomfortable loudness level

Hearing impaired listeners usually compensate for these changes by adjusting the volume control on the aid, though this option may not always be available to individuals with limited manipulative skills. The aim of automatic volume control is to adjust the overall level of speech delivered to the ear so that it is above threshold but not uncomfortably loud. An automatic volume control system should act relatively slowly (over a period of several hundred milliseconds) to take account of the changes in input as different speakers are encountered and as the overall ambient noise level changes. Although such devices are unlikely to confer significant advantages to listeners when the hearing aid characteristics can be individually adjusted to a given acoustical stimulus (e.g. a given speech level), when a range of speech levels is encountered, the advantages can be demonstrated.

Another way of viewing syllabic compression systems is as a method of overcoming some of the non-linear distortions that are inherent in a sensorineural hearing loss, e.g. temporal masking. It is possible for an intense stimulus (such as a vowel sound) physically to mask out a relative weak sound which follows it (e.g. a consonant in vowel-consonant utterance). Here the intention is to reduce the level of the preceding vowel, so that the subsequent consonant can be perceived.

The results of experimental studies are equivocal (Moore and Glasberg, 1986; Bustamante and Braida, 1987; Moore, 1987, 1990; Plomp, 1988; Dreschler, 1989; Benson, Clark and Johnson, 1992; Moore *et al.*, 1992; Festen, Van Dijkhuizen and Plomp, 1993;

Kollmeier, Peissig and Hohmann, 1993; Verschuure *et al.*, 1993) but a reasonable interpretation would be that syllabic compression systems can confer advantages for some hearing impaired listeners but, as yet, candidature is unclear.

In this consideration of compression systems, we have ignored the number of bands or channels within which the compression is required to act. Some devices act in the same way for all frequencies, while others act in two or three separate frequency bands. There are good reasons to suppose that for each of the functions that compression systems attempt to fulfil, there are advantages to be gained from having more than one channel, but that if too many bands are employed (usually more than two or three), then there are perceptual disadvantages.

When considering candidature for compression systems, it should be possible to adopt various informal rules in considering the different options. If an individual is unduly disturbed by the distortions resulting from loud transients, then output compression limiting could be beneficial. If the listener is routinely exposed to a wide range of input levels (e.g. quiet speakers are inaudible, but loud speech distorted) then an automatic volume control might be appropriate. In individuals for whom there is a very narrow dynamic range between hearing thresholds and thresholds of loudness discomfort, then some form of syllabic compression may be appropriate.

Noise reduction systems

It was stated earlier in this chapter that individuals with sensorineural hearing loss are unduly susceptible to the interfering effects of ambient noise. Many processing schemes have been tried which attempt physically to improve the signal-to-noise ratio presented to the impaired listener's ear. Many of these have been based upon multimicrophone techniques which can be reasonably thought of as electronic directional microphones which attempt to 'focus in' on a particular point in space from which the hearing-impaired listener wishes to receive sound and to exclude sound from other directions (Kollmeier, 1990; Peterson *et al.*, 1990; Greenberg and Zurek, 1991; Bilsen, Soede and Berkhout, 1993; Soede, Bilsen and Berkhout, 1993). An overall summary of these implementations would suggest that such processing can work in a limited number of acoustical environments (e.g. they tend to break down in reverberant environments) but that, as yet, they require more processing capability than is likely to be found in wearable hearing aids.

Other attempts have been made to overcome some of the deficit in sensorineural hearing impairment (e.g. due to impaired frequency resolution) by algorithms which attempt to 'sharpen up' the elements of the acoustical signal which correspond to the speech sound so that problems of masking of one frequency by an adjacent frequency do not occur. Examples of this process have been reported by Baer, Moore and Gatehouse (1993), but the results, while they can be shown to be beneficial over a range of listening conditions using rather specialized test methods, do not suggest that these are likely to find wide application to hearing aids for large numbers of people in the foreseeable future.

Level dependent or adaptive frequency responses

In the commercial advertising literature there are several references to automatic signal processing (ASP), a label which is almost entirely meaningless, and certainly does not describe what the hearing aid attempts to do. Two types of level dependent frequency response have been implemented:

1 The BILL (base increases at low levels) device which has a frequency characteristic relatively flatter for low input levels and more sloping towards the high frequencies for high input levels. This is an attempt to overcome the consequence of sensorineural hearing impairment whereby relatively intense low frequency sounds can mask out relatively weak high frequency sounds. In the evaluation studies that have been conducted, there do appear to be some subjects who can benefit from such processing schemes.

2 A directly contradictory processing scheme, that of the TILL (treble increases at low levels) response, is a hearing aid which has a sloping frequency response for low input levels and is flat or essentially transparent at high input levels. In many implementations this can actually be thought of as a compression device with the compression acting primarily in the high frequencies (Killion, 1990). Such devices are likely to be of benefit to individuals with steeply sloping hearing losses as a function of frequency but for whom the uncomfortable listening levels are relatively flat. However, the evaluation studies to date are extremely patchy and suggest that, on paired comparison trials, only around half of individuals who might reasonably be thought to be candidates for such devices say they prefer them over conventional linear processing.

A slightly different form of processing is where the hearing aid attempts to detect what form of frequency response is appropriate for a particular acoustical environment and, in particular, the hearing aid attempts to detect the presence of low frequency noise and to institute a low frequency attenuation on the hearing impairment. It is argued that such devices are particularly suitable for individuals who suffer from the upward spread of masking from low frequencies to high frequencies.

Multi-memory devices

Although not strictly advanced signal processing, these are hearing aids for which it is possible to select a number of frequency responses usually via a remote control device. The rationale for this approach is that for differing listening environments individuals will require a different frequency response. For example, when an individual listener encounters an environment where there is much low frequency noise, then it would be sensible to attenuate the low frequencies relative to a quiet background. Such approaches do appear to be successful (Ringdahl *et al.*, 1990; Mangold *et al.*, 1991; Kuk, 1992), although research has yet to show how many different programmes are appropriate for different environments and types of hearing impaired listeners. It is certainly possible to regard the multi-memory devices as a form of level dependent or adaptive frequency response where the frequency response is under the control of the user rather than the processing occurring automatically.

Feedback suppression

With careful earmould techniques, for the great majority of hearing impaired listeners, feedback is not a particular problem. However, for individuals for whom high gains are required, the presence of feedback may limit the gain that the user is able to employ to lower levels that are required for speech understanding. Using digital technology, it is now becoming possible to use processing techniques to cancel out the feedback in such a way that leads to circumstances where the hearing impaired listener can use 10–15 dB more gain with the feedback suppression active than without the processing available (Engebretson, French-St. George and O'Connel, 1993; French-St. George, Wood and Engebretson, 1993; Henningsen *et al.*, 1994). The application of such devices is in its infancy, but should not be regarded as a substitute for good earmould technique.

Applications to severe and profound hearing losses

Individuals with severe and profound hearing losses may have damage to the auditory system which can make it impossible for them to understand speech even if the information may be brought above threshold. Such individuals often have measurable hearing capability only at low frequencies. One of the potential processing options for such individuals is, first of all, to ensure that the hearing aids one fits have very good low frequencies characteristics (this is often the opposite of what one is trying to achieve in sloping sensorineural hearing losses) and then to simplify the speech signal by extracting only the elements which match the residual capacity of the impaired auditory system to process them (Faulkner, 1989; Faulkner *et al.*, 1992). This approach is successful in some listeners with profound sensorineural hearing impairment who might not necessarily be suitable candidates for cochlear implants, although it is an expectation that cochlear implants will become more widely available in the future.

An additional form of processing for individuals who have residual capabilities at low frequencies, but no hearing capability at high frequencies, is to transpose the high frequency information and present it to the residual low frequencies. Thus, the impaired auditory system is now presented with what can be regarded as a 'scrambled' signal which it has to learn to decode. Although experimental implementations of frequency transposition devices have been in research environments for some time, they have not reached wide clinical application.

The future of hearing aid provision

The future of hearing aids and their provision, particularly in the context of the National Health Service in the UK, is likely to change in a number of ways. The technological possibilities and, indeed, current availability, is such that the audiologist will have at his disposal a range of adjustments and processing options which far exceed those available today, independent of the physical configuration on fitting of the devices, in terms of postaural or in-the-ear units. This technology is likely to impose severe demands upon the procedures that are used, first of all, to select and then to evaluate the efficacy of hearing aids. It is the role of research to provide indications whereby different types of processing can be matched to different types of deficits in the auditory system in attempts to overcome them. However, in all of these considerations, the primary role of audibility cannot be overemphasized. It is the job of the hearing aid to make audible to the auditory system that which the hearing impaired listener wants to be able to hear. It is unlikely that sufficiently robust candidature criteria for different processing regimens that will allow simple mapping of technology on to individual listeners will be available. Rather, it is suggested that the current divorce between technological expertise and concerns with disability and handicap will have to be bridged if an individual listener's needs are going to be matched appropriately to the technological options.

References

AGNEW, J. (1988) Hearing instrument distortion: what does it mean for the listener. *Hearing Instruments*, **39**(10), 10–20

ALBREKTSSON, T., BRANEMARK, P. I., JACOBSSON, M. and TJELL-STROM, A. (1987) Present clinical applications of osseointegrated percutaneous implants. *Plastic and Reconstructive Surgery*, **79**, 721–731

ALVARD, L. S., DOXEY, G. P. and SMITH, D. M. (1989) Hearing aids worn with tympanic membrane perforation: complications and solutions. *American Journal of Otology*, **10**, 277–280

AMERICAN NATIONAL STANDARDS INSTITUTE/ACOUSTICAL SOCIETY OF AMERICA (1982) Specifications for hearing aid characteristics. *ANSI, S3.22 – 1982*. New York: ANSI

AMERICAN NATIONAL STANDARD (1992) Testing hearing aids with a broad-band noise signal. *ANSI, S3.42*

BAER, T., MOORE, B. C. J. and GATEHOUSE, S. (1993) Spectral contrast enhancement of speech in noise for listeners with sensorineural hearing impairment: effects on intelligibility, quality, and response times. *Journal of Rehabilitation Research and Development*, **30**, 49–72

BALFOUR, P. B. and HAWKINS, D. B. (1992) A comparison of sound quality judgements for monaural and binaural hearing aid processed stimuli. *Ear and Hearing*, **13**, 331–339

BARLOW, N. L. N., AUSLANDER, M. C., RINES, D. and STELMACHO-WICZ, P. G. (1988) Probe-tube microphone measures in hearing-impaired children and adults. *Ear and Hearing*, **9**, 243–247

BENSON, D., CLARK, T. M. and JOHNSON, J. S. (1992) Patient experiences with multiband full dynamic range compression. *Ear and Hearing*, **13**, 320–330

BENTLER, R. A. and PAVLOVIC, C. V. (1989) Transfer functions and correction factors used in hearing aid evaluation and research. *Ear and Hearing*, **10**, 58–63

BERGER, K. W. (1990) The use of an articulation index to compare three hearing aid prescriptive methods. *Audecibel*, **39**, 16–19

BILSEN, F. A., SOEDE, W. and BERKHOUT, A. J. (1993) Development and assessment of two fixed-array microphones for use with hearing aids. *Journal of Rehabilitation Research and Development*, **30**, 73–81

BODE, D. L. and KASTEN, R. N. (1971) Hearing aid distortion and consonant identification. *Journal of Speech and Hearing Research*, **14**, 323–331

BONDING, P. (1990) Permanent, percutaneous osseointegrated titanium implants. A review and preliminary results. *Ugeskr-Laeger*, **152**, 664–667

BONDING, P., HOLM JONSSON, M. and SALOMON, G. (1990) Bone-anchored hearing aids. Preliminary results. *Ugeskr-Laeger*, **152**, 667–670

BONDING, P., HOLM JONSSON, M., SALOMON, G. and AHLGREN, P. (1992) The bone-anchored hearing aid. Osseointegration and audiological effect. *Acta Otolaryngologica*, Suppl. 492, 42–45

BRITISH SOCIETY OF AUDIOLOGY (1987) Technical note. Recommended procedure for uncomfortable loudness level (ULL). *British Journal of Audiology*, **21**, 231

BROWNING, G. G. (1990) The British experience of an implantable, subcutaneous bone conduction hearing aid (Xomed Audiant). *Journal of Laryngology and Otology*, **104**, 534–538

BURGESS, N. and BROOKS, D. N. (1991) Earmoulds: some benefits from horn fitting. *British Journal of Audiology*, **25**, 309–315

BUSTAMANTE, D. K. and BRAIDA, L. D. (1987) Principal component amplitude compression for the hearing impaired. *Journal of the Acoustical Society of America*, **82**, 1227–1242

BYRNE, D. (1983) Theoretical prescriptive approaches to select the gain and frequency repairs of a hearing aid. *Contemporary Audiology*, **4**, 1–40

BYRNE, D. and DILLON, H. (1986) The National Acoustic Laboratories (NAL) new procedure for selecting the gain and frequency response of a hearing aid. *Ear and Hearing*, **7**, 257–265

BYRNE, D., PARKINSON, A. and NEWALL, P. (1990) Hearing aid gain and frequency response requirements for the severely/profoundly hearing impaired. *Ear and Hearing*, **11**, 40–49

BYRNE, D., NOBLE, W. and LEPAGE, B. (1992) Effects of long-term bilateral and unilateral fitting of different hearing aid types on the ability to locate sounds. *Journal of the American Academy of Audiology*, **3**, 369–382

CANDELA-CANO, F. A., AGUADO-BLASS, F. and SADA-GARCIA-LOMAS, J. (1990) Branemark-type osteo-integrated implants for the adaption of endosseous hearing aids. *Acta Otolaryngologica*, **41**, 61–64

CARLIN, W. V. and BROWNING, G. G. (1990) Hearing disability and hearing aid benefit related to type of hearing impairment. *Clinical Otolaryngology*, **15**, 63–67

CHUNG, S. M. and STEPHENS, S. D. G. (1986) Factors influencing binaural hearing aid use. *British Journal of Audiology*, **20**, 129–140

CLASEN, T., VESTERAGER, V. and PARVING, A. (1987) In-the-ear hearing aids. A comparative investigation of the use of custom-made versus modular type aids. *Scandinavian Audiology*, **16**, 195–200

COLE, W. A. (1993) Current design options and criteria for hearing aids. *Journal of the Speech and Language Pathology Association*, **1**, 7–14

COX, R. M. and ALEXANDER, G. C. (1990) Evaluation of an in-situ output probe-microphone method for hearing aid fitting verification. *Ear and Hearing*, **11**, 31–39

COX, R. M. and GILMORE, C. (1986) Damping the hearing aid frequency response: effects on speech clarity and preferred listening level. *Journal of Speech and Hearing Research*, **29**, 357–365

COX, R. M. and GILMORE, C. (1990) Development of the profile of hearing aid performance (PHAP). *Journal of Speech and Hearing Research*, **33**, 343–357

CREMERS, C. W., SNIK, F. M. and BENYON, A. J. (1991) A hearing aid anchored in the cranial bone for amplification of bone conduction. *Ned-Tijdschr-Geneeskd.*, **135**, 468–471

CREMERS, C. W., SNIK, F. M. and BENYON, A. J. (1992) Hearing with the bone-anchored hearing aid (BAHA, HC 200) compared to a conventional bone-conduction hearing aid. *Clinical Otolaryngology*, **17**, 275–279

DILLON, H. and MURRAY, N. (1987) Accuracy of twelve methods for estimating the real ear gain of hearing aids. *Ear and Hearing*, **8**, 2–11

DILLON, H., KORITSCHONER, E., BATTAGLIA, J., LOVEGROVE, R., GINIS, J., MAVRIAS, G. *et al.* (1991) Rehabilitation effectiveness. 1: assessing the needs of clients entering a national hearing rehabilitation program. *Australian Journal of Audiology*, **13**, 55–65

DRESCHLER, W. A. (1989) Phoneme perception via hearing

aids with and without compression and the role of temporal resolution. *Audiology*, **28**, 49–60

DYRLUND, O. (1989a) Characterization of non-linear distortion in hearing aids using coherence analysis. A pilot study. *Scandinavian Audiology*, **18**, 143–148

DYRLUND, O. (1989b) Acoustical feedback associated with the use of post aural hearing aids for profoundly deaf children. *Scandinavian Audiology*, **18**, 237–241

ENGEBRETSON, A. M., FRENCH-ST. GEORGE, M. and O'CONNEL, M. P. (1993) Adaptive feedback stabilization of hearing aids. *Scandinavian Audiology*, Suppl. 38, 56–64

FABRY, D. A. and VAN TASELL, D. J. (1990) Evaluation of an articulation-index based model for predicting the effects of adaptive frequency response hearing aids. *Journal of Speech and Hearing Research*, **33**, 676–689

FAULKNER, A. (1989) Psychoacoustic aspects of speech pattern coding for the deaf. Hearing impairment and signal processing hearing aids. *Acta Otolaryngologica*, **469**, 172

FAULKNER, A., BALL, V., ROSEN, S., MOORE, B. C. J. and FOURCIN, A. (1992) Speech pattern hearing aids for the profoundly hearing-impaired: speech perception and auditory abilities. *Journal of the Acoustical Society of America*, **91**, 2136–2155

FEDERAL DRUG ADMINISTRATION (1994) *Guidance to Hearing Aid Manufacturers for Substantiation of Claims*. Washington, DC: Federal Drug Administration

FESTEN, J. M., VAN DIJKHUIZEN, J. N. and PLOMP, R. (1993) The efficacy of a multichannel hearing aid in which the gain is controlled by the minima in the temporal signal envelope. *Scandinavian Audiology*, Suppl. 38, 101–110

FRENCH-ST GEORGE, M., WOOD, D. J. and ENGEBRETSON, A. M. (1993) Behavioural assessment of adaptive feedback equalization in a digital hearing aid. *Journal of Rehabilitation Research and Development*, **30**, 17–25

GATEHOUSE, S. (1989) Limitations on insertion gains with vented earmoulds imposed by oscillatory feedback. *British Journal of Audiology*, **23**, 133–136

GATEHOUSE, S. (1993a) Role of perceptual acclimatization in the selection of frequency responses for hearing aids. *Journal of the American Academy of Audiology*, **4**, 296–306

GATEHOUSE, S. (1993b) Hearing aid evaluation: limitations of present procedures and future requirements. *Journal of Speech Language Pathology and Audiology*, Suppl. 1, 50–57

GELFAND, A., SILMAN, S. and ROSS, L. (1987) Long-term effects of monaural, binaural and no amplification in subjects with bilateral hearing loss. *Scandinavian Audiology*, **16**, 201–207

GOODE, R. (1991) Implantable hearing devices. *Medical Clinics of North America*, **75**, 1261–1266

GREENBERG, J. B. and ZUREK, P. M. (1991) Evaluation of an adaptive beamforming method for hearing aids. *Journal of the Acoustical Society of America*, **91**, 1662–1676

GYO, K. and YANAGIHARA, N. (1985) Clinical application of an implantable, miniaturized hearing aid (artificial middle ear). *Kango Gijutsu*, **31**, 662–664

GYO, K., GOODE, R. L. and MILLER, C. (1987) Stapes vibration produced by the output transducer of an implantable hearing aid. *Archives of Otolaryngology – Head and Neck Surgery*, **113**, 1078–1081

HÅKANSSON, B., TJELLSTRÖM, A., ROSENHALL, U. and CARLSSON, P. (1985) The bone-anchored hearing aid. Principal design and a psychoacoustical evaluation. *Acta Otolaryngologica*, **100**, 229–239

HÅKANSSON, B., TJELLSTRÖM, A. and CARLSSON, P. (1990) Percutaneous vs transcutaneous transducers for hearing

by direct bone conduction. *Otolaryngology – Head and Neck Surgery*, **102**, 339–344

HAWKINS, D. B. and YACULLO, W. S. (1984) Signal-to-noise ratio advantage of binaural hearing aids and directional microphones under different levels of reverbation. *Journal of Speech and Hearing Disorders*, **49**, 278–285

HENNINGSEN, L. B., DYRLUND, O., BISGAARD, N. and BRING, B. (1994) Digital feedback suppression (DFS). Clinical experiences when fitting a DFS hearing instrument on children. *Scandinavian Audiology*, **23**, 117–122

HENRICHSEN, J., NORING, E., CHRISTENSEN, B., PEDERSEN, F. and PARVING, A. (1988) In-the-ear hearing aids. The use and benefit in the elderly hearing impaired. *Scandinavian Audiology*, **17**, 200–212

HENRICHSEN, J., NORING, E., LINDEMANN, L., CHRISTENSEN, B. and PARVING, A. (1991) The use and benefit of in-the-ear hearing aids. A four-year follow-up examination. *Scandinavian Audiology*, **20**, 55–59

HICKSON, L. M. H. (1994) Compression amplification in hearing aids. *American Journal of Audiology*, **3**, 51–65

KATES, J. M. (1992) On using coherence to measure distortion in hearing aids. *Journal of the Acoustical Society of America*, **91**, 2236–2244

KILLION, M. C. (1990) A high fidelity hearing aid. *Hearing Instruments*, **41**(8), 38–39

KIRKWOOD, D. H. (1990) 1990 US hearing aid sales summary. *Hearing Journal*, **43**(12), 7–9, 12–13

KOLLMEIER, B. (1990) Speech enhancement by filtering in the loudness domain. *Acta Otolaryngologica*, Suppl. 469, 207–214

KOLLMEIER, B., PEISSIG, J. and HOHMANN, V. (1993) Real-time multiband dynamic compression and noise reduction for binaural hearing aids. *Journal of Rehabilitation Research and Development*, **30**, 82–94

KUK, F. K. (1992) Evaluation of the efficacy of a multimemory hearing aid. *Journal of the American Academy of Audiology*, **3**, 338–348

MANGOLD, S., ERIKSSON–MANGOLD, M., ISRAELSSON, B., LEIJON, A. and RINGDAHL, A. (1991) Multi-programmable hearing aid. *Acta Otolaryngologica*, Suppl. 469, 70–75

MAY, A. E., UPFOLD, L. J. and BATTAGLIA, J. A. (1990) The advantages and disadvantages of ITC, ITE and BTE hearing aids: diary and interview reports from elderly users. *British Journal of Audiology*, **24**, 301–309

MEDING, B. and RINGDAHL, A. (1992) Allergic contact dermatitis from the earmolds of hearing aids. *Ear and Hearing*, **13**, 122–124

MOORE, B. C. (1987) Design and evaluation of a two-channel compression hearing aid. *Journal of Rehabilitation Research and Development*, **24**, 181–192

MOORE, B. C. J. (1990) How much do we gain by gain control in hearing aids? *Acta Otolaryngologica*, Suppl. 469, 250–256

MOORE, B. C. J. and GLASBERG, B. R. (1986) A comparison of two-channel and single-channel compression hearing aids. *Audiology*, **25**, 210–226

MOORE, B. C. J. and GLASBERG, B. R. (1988) A comparison of four methods of implementing automatic gain control (AGC) in hearing aids. *British Journal of Audiology*, **22**, 93–104

MOORE, B. C. J., JOHNSON, J. S., CLARK, T. M. and PLUVINAGE, V. (1992) Evaluation of a dual-channel full dynamic range compression system for people with sensorineural hearing loss. *Ear and Hearing*, **13**, 349–370

MUELLER, H. G., HAWKINS, D. B. and NORTHERN, J. L. (1992)

Probe Microphone Measurements: Hearing Aid Selection and Assessment. San Diego: Singular Publishing Group

MYLANUS, E. A. M., SNIK, A. F. M., JORRITSMA, F. F. and CREMERS, C. W. R. J. (1994a) Audiological results for the bone anchored hearing aid. *Ear and Hearing*, **15**, 87–92

MYLANUS, E. A. M., SNIK, A. F. M., JORRITSMA, F. F., CREMERS, C. W. R. J. and VERSCHUURE, H. (1994b) Audiological results for the bone anchored hearing aid: multi-centre results. *Annals of Otology, Rhinology and Laryngology*, **103**, 368–374

NEWMAN, C. W. and WEINSTEIN, B. E. (1988) The hearing handicap inventory for the elderly as a measure of hearing aid benefit. *Ear and Hearing*, **9**, 81–85

NOBLE, W. and BYRNE, D. (1991) Auditory localization under conditions of unilateral fitting of different hearing aid systems. *British Journal of Audiology*, **24**, 237–250

OJA, G. L. and SCHOW, R. L. (1984) Hearing aid evaluation based on measures of benefit, use and satisfaction. *Ear and Hearing*, **5**, 77–86

OLIWIECKI, S., BECK, M. H. and CHALMERS, R. J. (1991) Contact dermatitis from spectacle frames and hearing aid containing diethyl phthalate. *Contact Dermatitis*, **25**, 264–265

PAVLOVIC, C. V. (1988) Articulation index predictions of speech intelligibility in hearing aid selection. *American Speech and Hearing Association*, 30(6–7), 63–65

PAVLOVIC, C. V. (1990) Statistical distribution of speech for various languages. 120th Meeting of the Acoustical Society of America, Sandiago, California. *Journal of the Acoustical Society of America*, **88**, 8SP10, abstract

PETERSON, P. M., WEI, S-M., RABINOWITZ, W. M. and ZUREK, P. M. (1990) Robustness of an adaptive beamforming method for hearing aids. *Acta Otolaryngologica*, Suppl. 469, 85–90

PLOMP, R. (1988) The negative effect of amplitude compression in multichannel hearing aids in the light of the modulation-transfer function. *Journal of the Acoustical Society of America*, **83**, 2322–2327

PREVES, D. A. (1990) Expressing hearing aid noise and distortion with coherence measurements. *American Speech and Hearing Association*, 32(6–7), 56–59

PREVES, D. A. (1991) Output limiting and speech enhancement. In: *The Vanderbilt Hearing Aid Report II*, edited by G. A. Studebaker, F. H. Bess and L. B. Beck. Parkton, MD: York Press. pp. 35–51

RANKOVIC, C. M. (1991) An application of the articulation index to hearing aid fitting. *Journal of Speech and Hearing Research*, **34**, 391–402

RINGDAHL, A., ERIKSSON–MANGOLD, M., ISRAELSSON, B., LINDKVIST, A. and MANGOLD, S. (1990) Clinical trials with a programmable hearing aid set for various listening environments. *British Journal of Audiology*, **24**, 235–242

SAIKI, T., GYO, K. and YANAGIHARA, N. (1990) Audiological evaluation of the middle ear implant – speech discrimination under noise circumstances. *Nippon–Jibiinkoka–Gakkai–Kaiho*, **93**, 566–571

SILMAN, S., GELFAND, S. A. and SILVERMAN, C. A. (1984) Late onset auditory deprivation: effects of monaural versus binaural hearing aids. *Journal of the Acoustical Society of America*, **76**, 1357–1362

SILMAN, S., SILVERMAN, C. A., EMMER, M. B. and GELFAND, S. A. (1992) Adult-onset auditory deprivation. *Journal of the American Academy of Audiology*, **3**, 390–396

SKINNER, M. W. (1988) *Hearing Aid Evaluation*. Englewood Cliffs, New Jersey: Prentice Hall

SOEDE, W., BILSEN, F. A. and BERKHOUT, A. J. (1993) Assessment of a directional microphone array for hearing-impaired listeners. *Journal of the Acoustical Society of America*, **92**, 799–808

STUDEBAKER, G. A., PAVLOVIC, C. V. and SHERBECOE, R. L. (1987) A frequency importance function for continuous discourse. *Journal of the Acoustical Society of America*, **81**, 1130–1138

TJELLSTROM, A. and GRANSTROM, G. (1994) Long-term follow-up with the bone-anchored hearing aid: a review of the first 100 patients between 1977 and 1985. *Ear, Nose and Throat Journal*, **73**, 112–114

TONNING, F., WARLAND, H. and TONNING, K. (1991) Hearing instruments for the elderly hearing-impaired – a comparison of in-the-canal and behind-the-ear hearing instruments in 1st time users. *Scandinavian Audiology*, **20**, 69–74

UPFOLD, L. J., MAY, A. E. and BATTAGLIA, J. A. (1990) Hearing aid manipulation skills in an elderly population: a comparison of ITE, BTE, and ITC aids. *British Journal of Audiology*, **24**, 311–318

VERSCHUURE, J., DRESCHLER, W. A., DE HAAN, E. H., VAN CAPPELLEN, N., HAMMERSCHLAG, R., MARE, M. J. *et al.* (1993) Syllabic compression and speech intelligibility in hearing impaired listeners. *Scandinavian Audiology*, Suppl. 38, 92–100

WADE, P. S., HALIK, J. J. and CHASIN, M. (1992) Bone conduction implants: transcutaneous vs. percutaneous. *Otolaryngology – Head and Neck Surgery*, **106**, 68–74

WALDEN, B. E., SCHWARTZ, D. M. and WILLIAMS, D. L. (1983) Test of the assumptions underlying comparative hearing aid evaluations. *Journal of Speech and Hearing Disorders*, **48**, 264–273

WEINSTEIN, B. E. (1990) The quantification of hearing aid benefit in the elderly: the role of self-assessment measures. *Acta Otolaryngologica*, Suppl. 476, 257–261

WEISENBERGER, J. M., BROADSTONE, S. M. and SAUNDERS, F. A. (1989) Evaluation of 2 multichannel tactile aids for the hearing-impaired. *Journal of the Acoustical Society of America*, **86**, 1764–1775

ZELISKO, D. L. C., SEEWALD, R. C. and GAGNE, J. P. (1992) Signal delivery/real ear measurement system for hearing aid selection and fitting. *Ear and Hearing*, **13**, 460–463

15

Cochlear implants

Stuart Rosen

Most hearing impaired people can be provided with acoustical hearing aids that provide reasonable degrees of benefit in everyday life. There are some, however, with so little hearing that even the most powerful of hearing aids is of little practical use. In such cases, two main approaches have been developed. *Cochlear implants*, the subject of this chapter, bypass the transduction mechanisms of the cochlea by electrically stimulating the auditory nerve directly. Perhaps a more radical approach, insofar as it avoids the use of the auditory system altogether, is taken by *tactile aids* (see Chapter 16). Tactile aids attempt to recode acoustic information into vibratory patterns on the skin – a true sensory substitution.

Each method has relative advantages and disadvantages, and both have seen increasing use over the last decade. In such circumstances, review chapters like this one can quickly become outdated. In an attempt to avoid this, greater emphasis has been placed on underlying principles than on current experimental results, although the latter are discussed as well. It is also important to note that although these topics are of clear clinical importance, there are many fundamental theoretical issues at stake. For example: is the ability to adapt to a radically different kind of 'hearing' strongly dependent on the age at which it is introduced? To what extent does speech perception depend upon the frequency analysis exacted in the cochlea? I begin with a brief history, while noting that the discussion will focus solely on results with adults, as opposed to children.

Historical background

Reviews of cochlear implant research commonly begin with the discomforting observations of Volta who, at the end of the 18th century, placed metal rods in his ear canals and connected them to the terminals of a group of electrolytic cells. He reported a sensation of a blow to the head, followed by the sound of boiling liquid, but evidently did not wish to continue his researches into electrically-induced auditory sensations (Volta, 1800). In fact, the first publication of any relevance for the use of electrical stimulation as a way to restore some sense of hearing to a deafened person appeared less than 40 years ago. Djourno and Eyries (1957) found that direct electrical stimulation of the auditory nerve could induce auditory sensations. This paper served as the initial impetus to three groups, all working in California in the 1960s, to attempt the development of a practical method of electrical stimulation for routine use in the treatment of total and near-total deafness (for personal reminiscences by three of the first experimenters involved, see House, 1985; Michelson, 1985; Simmons, 1985; also, for an extensive review of the literature prior to the early 1960s, see Simmons, 1966).

During the 1970s, work on implants spread to a number of other countries and centres, and implant research ceased to be a uniquely Californian phenomenon. Very quickly thereafter, a number of commercial companies became involved in the field (most notably 3M of the USA) and began to produce and market devices for sale to otologists. A landmark at this time was the first approval by the United States Food and Drug Administration (FDA) in 1984 of an implant (known as the House/3M device) for sale as part of a recognized clinical procedure whose safety and efficacy was considered acceptable enough for routine use. Other devices have since been approved.

Although there was important research being done in the UK, the clinical application of implants was rather slow in getting off the ground, not only in comparison to the USA, but also with regard to

France, Germany, Austria and Australia. In 1990, however, the Department of Health announced the funding of six regional centres in England as part of the National Health Service Cochlear Implant Programme (other centres have been set up in Wales, Scotland and Northern Ireland). Cochlear implants have now been recognized the world over as fairly standard clinical procedures (at least for postlingually deafened adults). In May 1988, it was estimated that there were nearly 4000 users of cochlear implants throughout the world (National Institutes of Health, 1988), with the rate of implantation still increasing significantly. Current estimates (as of June, 1994) put the total closer to 10 000 worldwide.

What makes up a cochlear implant?

Cochlear implant systems are made up of three main components:

1 A *processor* to convert acoustical waveforms (primarily speech) into appropriate electrical currents
2 *Electrodes* through which current is delivered to or near the stimulable neural elements
3 A *connection* between the speech processor and electrodes.

I shall now describe the ways in which each of these components can vary, before going on to describe a number of complete systems. Because the characteristics of the electrode play such an important role in determining the other two components of any implant system, I begin by discussing those.

Electrodes

There are four major ways in which electrode systems vary: in the number of individual electrodes, in their implanted position, in the mechanical properties of the electrode array, and in the shape and placement of electrodes in the carrier.

Multichannel versus single channel

Multichannel systems typically use at least four active electrodes in an attempt to mimic (at least roughly) the frequency analysing capabilities of the normal ear. As is well known, the basilar membrane responds differentially to different frequencies, such that the high-frequency energy in a sound causes vibration at more basal locations than the low-frequency energy. Because the vast majority of auditory nerve afferents appear to synapse with a single hair cell along the basilar membrane, the pattern of activity across the afferent fibres is related directly to the frequency content of the stimulating sound (Ruggero, 1992). Analogously, multichannel cochlear implants deliver

current corresponding to higher frequency energy in a sound to cochlear locations more basal than it delivers current corresponding to lower frequency sounds.

Note, though, that it is not typically possible to map frequencies onto their appropriate place in the nerve fibre array. Current electrode designs allow currents to be delivered no more than about 25 mm from the base of the cochlea, corresponding to a place most sensitive to frequencies of about 1 kHz. The fact that patients can do quite well with such stimulation indicates that it is the *pattern* of the distribution of energies in frequency that is crucial, not a particular correspondence between the frequency content of a signal and and its delivery to a particular place in the auditory nerve fibre array. This principle, that the perception of speech depends upon the appropriate *patterning* of acoustic information, is perhaps the single most important factor in the success of implant systems as a whole. If usable electroauditory percepts only resulted from an accurate emulation of normal auditory nerve firing patterns, cochlear implant systems would be of little use.

Single channel systems, on the other hand, use a single pair of electrodes (signal and ground) through which current is passed. It is not then possible to emulate to any degree the frequency analysing capabilities of the normal ear, because it appears that the so-called 'place principle' is based almost totally on the vibratory patterns of the basilar membrane/organ of Corti system. Therefore, how could electrical stimulation, which is understood to bypass the normal transduction mechanism of the cochlea and stimulate the afferent fibres directly, lead to selective stimulation of populations of those fibres? More directly, Kiang and Moxon (1972) have measured frequency tuning curves to electrical stimulation in auditory nerve fibres of the cat, and found the shape of the curve to be independent of where in the cochlea the fibres synapse with the hair cells. To acoustical stimulation sharply-pointed 'V'-shaped curves are found, with the tip of the 'V' being predictable from the position along the basilar membrane of hair cell synapse (being lower in frequency for more apical positions along the membrane). Behaviourally, too, no place principle operates (Shannon, 1983). In short, whatever patients receive from single-channel devices must be based purely on the the *temporal* properties of the waveform. What is surprising is the extent to which patients can be aided in speech perception through a single channel, even if performance does not generally reach the standards achievable with a multichannel implant.

Intra- versus extracochlear

Although there are a number of possible placements, the vast majority of electrodes are placed either in the scala tympani through the round window, or at the round window itself. An intrascalar approach has the advantages that the auditory nerve is arrayed in a clear tonotopic fashion, for ready exploitation by electrodes spaced along a carrier. Although there has been some work with extracochlear placements of multiple electrodes, such an approach appears to have few or no advantages over intrascalar placements. In particular, there appears to be considerably more overlap in the neural elements stimulated by different electrodes than is typically the case with intrascalar electrodes. It thus becomes more difficult to emulate the frequency-analysing properties of the normal ear, the main aim of using multiple electrodes.

Extracochlear approaches may have an important advantage in allowing access to apical regions of the cochlea not accessible from the round window. Not only is important speech information coded near the apex in the normal ear, it is also the region in which nerve survival tends to be best (Johnsson, 1985). Due to the spiralling of the cochlea, it appears to be nearly impossible to thread an electrode via the round window any further than the 25 mm or so currently used in multichannel electrodes. The apex is much more readily accessible by drilling through the medial wall of the middle ear cavity (Douek, personal communication) or from the external ear canal (Hochmair-Desoyer *et al.*, 1989). Such approaches may also be

preferable for implanting severely ossified cochleae. There have been a number of promising reports concerning the use of titanium to anchor electrodes in the cochlear wall, both in animals and humans (Pfingst *et al.*, 1985, 1989; Miller *et al.*, 1987; Niparko *et al.*, 1993).

For a more detailed review of the entire issue of electrode placements see Rosen (1990).

Electrode construction

The fabrication of single-channel electrodes presents little difficulty nowadays, as there is a relatively good understanding of the kinds of materials that should be used, and few other constraints on their design. Multichannel electrodes, on the other hand, present a variety of difficult design problems because they are almost exclusively inserted some 25 mm or so through the round window and around the first turn of the cochlea. Thus the electrode carrier must be flexible and smooth enough to negotiate the first turn of the cochlea without causing extensive damage (Clark *et al.*, 1983). Alternatively, some other means of 'getting round the bend' must be provided. One group has taken the route of making a spiral electrode carrier (currently used in the Clarion system; Figure 15.1), which when straightened for

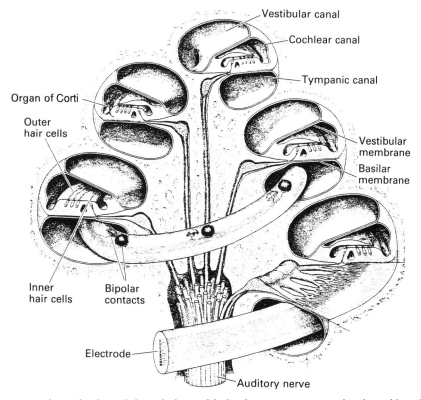

Figure 15.1 Illustration of an eight-channel electrode designed for bipolar use, in position within the cochlea. This design is similar to that used in the Clarion device. (Redrawn with permission from Loeb, 1985)

insertion, resumes its original form (Rebscher, 1985). At least one electrode design (used with the Ineraid) has been found, both in post-mortem studies of three patients, and in a further 12 living patients using computerized tomography, to pass from scala tympani into scala media for some part of its length (Ketten, personal communication; Ketten and Nadol, 1990; Ketten, Nadol and Burgess, 1990). Although such damage clearly does not preclude good performance, it seems likely that minimizing it can only be beneficial. Further studies will make it clear whether the insertion of other multichannel electrodes is as innocuous as has sometimes been claimed (e.g. by Shepherd *et al.* (1984) in connection with the Nucleus device).

There are also important differences among systems in the shape and placement of the electrode contacts themselves. The Nucleus device, for example, uses a set of 22 bands wrapped entirely around the electrode carrier, whereas other designs use mushroom-shaped contacts placed radially on the surface of the carrier (Rebscher, 1985).

Summary and current practice

There is little doubt now that multichannel systems generally lead to better performance. Therefore, the primary interest in single channel systems arises from:

1 Their use in patients with severely ossified cochleae which can prevent a significant insertion depth for the electrode carrier
2 The possibility of using an ear-level device in place of a body-worn 'box' (Hochmair-Desoyer, Zierhofer and Hochmair, 1993)
3 Situations where simplicity of construction and low cost are paramount.

For multichannel stimulation, however, there is still much controversy regarding the best electrode design. Although systems differ considerably, often for specific theoretical reasons, there are few empirical data suggesting the advantages of one design over another, except perhaps in ease of insertion and in limiting the degree of mechanical damage. Developing improved access to the apical regions of the cochlea is likely to lead to improved patient performance.

Connecting the electrodes and processor

There are two main possibilities for the route by which electrical signals from the processor are delivered to the electrodes: via a *percutaneous* connector or *transcutaneous* transmission.

Percutaneous connectors

A percutaneous connector is constructed out of some biocompatible material, and passes directly through the skin. In so doing, it allows direct access to the electrodes, and therefore imposes no constraints on the kinds of waveforms that may be presented. Major changes in processing schemes require, therefore, no surgical intervention. It is also readily possible to *measure* what happens at the electrodes, which may have some diagnostic value. Finally, there are no implanted electronics to fail. On the other hand, even the best currently available percutaneous connectors appear to require regular cleaning and monitoring, with minor infections and crusting occurring relatively frequently (Parkin, 1990; Gray *et al.*, 1993). There is also, unfortunately, a history of serious failures with percutaneous connectors, but avoiding such failures appears to be simply (or perhaps not so simply) a matter of appropriate design. Current percutaneous devices rarely lead to major problems.

Only one implant system with a percutaneous connector has been used to any great extent – the Ineraid system which uses a pyrolysed carbon connector (Parkin, 1990). A number of groups have shown interest in developing connectors based on titanium, as these have been successfully used in bone-anchored hearing aids. However, a review of the relevant literature shows titanium to have similar drawbacks to pyrolysed carbon, minor as they are (Rosen, 1994). It may be that coatings of a more bioactive material on to titanium would encourage more stable soft tissue adhesion (Faulkner *et al.*, 1992b).

Transcutaneous connectors

Transcutaneous transmission, in contrast, employs a receiver that is completely implanted under the skin. A transmitter is then placed on the surface of the skin, directly over the buried receiver. Magnets in both the receiver and transmitter are typically used in order to ensure accurate alignment. Signals can be transferred either in analogue form (when waveforms are coded directly in varying electromagnetic fields) or digitally (when waveforms are coded as numbers in such fields). Transcutaneous systems differ greatly in their degree of *transparency*, i.e. the extent to which signals of arbitrary form can be transmitted to the electrodes. All transcutaneous systems must place some restrictions on the waveforms they can deliver, but the degree of constraint varies widely. Transcutaneous systems also can make allowance for the relaying of information *from* the electrodes to the outside world, but typically do not. Note that percutaneous connectors represent the ideal as regards transparency and access to events at the electrode.

The advantages of transcutaneous systems lie primarily in their being more resistant to infection (insofar as the skin is sealed over the implant) and in their cosmetic appeal (insofar as nothing sticks out through the skin). They are not without medical risk, however. A recent survey of complications associated with the Nucleus device reported a 4.8% incidence of flap breakdown or infection in 459 cases (Cohen, Hoffman and Stroschein, 1988). However, much of this appears to arise from surgical inexperience – 80% of the complications arose within the first three operations by a particular surgeon. Also, most complications can be resolved by various means.

Summary and current practice

The vast majority of systems implanted today use transcutaneous transmission, with relatively few problems. Older devices can, however, impose serious limitations on the ability to upgrade processors as they develop. Newer transcutaneous systems are avoiding such difficulties by becoming more transparent (e.g. the Clarion device described below). On the other hand, percutaneous systems appear to have a much worse reputation than is deserved. There are over 2000 patients using percutaneous connectors, either for bone-conduction hearing aids, or cochlear implants, with low rates of moderate or serious complications. It appears likely that percutaneous connectors will be used in at least small numbers, as they still provide the best basis for exploring different speech processing schemes. They are also, of course, more efficient of battery power, as no energy is lost in transmission. Thus it may be possible to utilize ear-level devices (whose size is usually constrained by the batteries needed) more readily with percutaneous connectors.

Sound processor

The sound processor performs three distinct functions, which can be at least partially separated. First, it *transduces* the acoustic pressure variations via a microphone into electrical currents. This stage is common to all implant systems, although there may be differences in the location of the microphone, and whether auxiliary equipment can be plugged directly in to the processor. Second, the relevant acoustic information must be *processed* or *transformed* in some way. Implant systems differ greatly in this stage, particularly in the complexity of the transformations involved. Finally, the selected information must be *coded* in an appropriate form for presentation to the the electrode(s). Although it is not always easy to separate the processing and coding stages (and such a distinction is not typical in the implant literature), it will prove useful in our discussion below.

Sound processing

Sound processing schemes differ along a number of dimensions. All implant systems face the problem of mapping the enormous range of acoustic intensities present in the environment onto the restricted range possible with electrical stimulation (see below). Therefore, it is necessary to *compress* the range of stimulation in some way. This can be done either by some kind of automatic gain control (AGC) or by instantaneous compression.

Of course, there is also the obvious distinction between schemes for multichannel, and schemes for single-channel stimulation. By definition, single-channel schemes output a single electrical waveform, upon which all information must be coded in a purely temporal fashion. Multichannel schemes, on the other hand, always try to code some frequency-varying feature of the acoustic input onto different electrode places, preserving at least the relative ordering of frequency information. Hence, as noted above, higher frequency information in the acoustic input is delivered to more basally placed electrodes (for the most typical case of scala tympani electrodes).

The final major way in which speech processing schemes differ concerns their general philosophy as regards the advisability of 'tampering' with the signal. Two main strands of thought exist on this issue. The 'whole signal' approach is by far the most commonly used. Its underlying rationale seems to be of an agnostic type: given that so little is known about the properties of electrical hearing, and of what patients are able to make use, transmit *all* the information available. The signal processing employed in such systems tends to be confined to some degree of frequency shaping, compression or automatic gain control, and, particularly in the case of multichannel implants, band-pass filtering.

For single-channel implants, the 'whole signal' approach is exemplified by the device designed by a team in Austria (Hochmair and Hochmair-Desoyer, 1983, 1985; Hochmair-Desoyer *et al.*, 1989; Hochmair-Desoyer, Zierhofer and Hochmair, 1993). Here, a moderate degree of automatic gain control and frequency shaping is applied to the microphone-sensed acoustic signal, which would not affect to a great degree the intelligibility to normal listeners of signals so processed. A good example of the 'whole-signal' approach in a multichannel implant is the Ineraid device (based on the work of Eddington *et al.* (1978); Eddington (1983)). In addition to automatic gain control and frequency shaping, four band-pass filters are used to direct the energy in different frequency bands of the signal to different electrodes. In order to mimic the frequency-analysing properties of the normal ear, the signal from the highest frequency filter band is sent to the most basal electrode, while the waveform from the lowest frequency band is sent to the most apical electrode.

A radically different approach to signal processing in cochlear implants has been advocated by the External Pattern Input (EPI) Group in London (Fourcin *et al.*, 1979). They argued that patients would be better served by an explicit extraction of acoustic features that are matched both to the patients' needs and to their new sensory abilities. This is known as the 'feature extraction' approach or, since discussion centres mostly around the coding of speech sounds, the 'speech pattern' approach.

The EPI Group has developed a single-channel system based on this idea. Arguing that the range of auditory sensations elicited by single-channel electro-cochlear stimulation is so limited, EPI have set as their goal, *not* the understanding of speech through auditory means alone (as most groups have), but optimal speech reception *with* lip-reading. They thus focused attention on those speech patterns that are relatively invisible, and have been shown to be important aids to lip-reading. Most of the work of the EPI Group has concerned devices that transmit only the fundamental frequency of the voice. Hence, patients primarily receive information about the segmental aspects of voicing, through the presence or absence of stimulation, as well as the prosodic cues signalled through changes in voice fundamental frequency. This approach is not limited to the use of fundamental frequency, however, and more recent work has explored cues to overall amplitude and voiceless sounds like /s/ and /f/. Straightforward extensions to the signalling of vowel colour and place of articulation (both through contrasts in spectral shape) have also been discussed.

Insofar as it is now clear that multichannel systems are likely to lead to better performance in most patients, this single-channel work has lost some of its impetus. The same ideas have been extensively applied, however, in acoustic speech-pattern hearing aids for use in profound hearing impairment (Rosen *et al.*, 1987; Faulkner *et al.*, 1992a), in tactile aids, and in a multichannel system.

Only one commercial implant system has used a speech pattern approach in a multichannel device. This is known as the Nucleus system, which has been based at least partly on the principles and advice of the EPI Group (Tong *et al.*, 1980; Dowell *et al.*, 1985, 1987; Clark *et al.*, 1987). In the initial version of the speech processor, the frequency of a spectral peak in the second formant (F_2) frequency region was used to control which electrode was stimulated. Only one stimulating pulse per voicing period occurred, based on the fundamental frequency of the incoming speech. Thus the rate of stimulation was always at the speech fundamental. A low pulse rate was used for voiceless sounds, while a measure of the overall amplitude of the original speech wave controlled the overall charge of the pulses delivered (by varying pulse width and amplitude).

Although this scheme has undergone a number of revisions, its principles have remained in place (until recently, see below). In a later version of the device, information was given about the first and second formant (F_1 and F_2) frequencies. Here, two peaks of

spectral energy in the regions of the first and second formants of speech were determined. The estimated frequency peak in the lower frequency region was used to select an electrode within a more apical set of electrodes, while the estimated frequency peak in the second formant range was used to select an electrode within a more basal set of electrodes. Two closely spaced pulses were presented per voicing period. For voiceless sounds, a random pulse rate was used. An important feature of the Nucleus device, and one first proposed in connection with it, is the use of non-simultaneous pulses as a way to minimize the physical interaction of electrical currents across electrodes, thus preserving control over the loudness generated at individual electrodes (Clark *et al.*, 1987). Thus, in a yet later version of the speech processing scheme, four electrodes were stimulated sequentially, to represent various combinations of F_1, F_2 and higher frequency spectral information (Skinner *et al.*, 1991).

As will be described below, there have been recent developments in this device which have led to the introduction of a distinctly different speech processing scheme which has clearly been motivated by the success of what has become known as *continuous interleaved sampling* (CIS). Continuous interleaved sampling integrates a number of features of previously implemented schemes, including band-pass filtering, logarithmic compression of waveform amplitudes, and the presentation of interleaved pulses, with one essential difference – the use of high stimulation rates (Wilson *et al.*, 1991, 1993, 1994). The details of this scheme follow.

The incoming speech is first passed through a bank of band-pass filters, each filter output being rectified and smoothed by a low-pass filter (typically with a cut-off of 400 Hz). The resulting envelopes are then mapped appropriately into the dynamic range of the patient (using a logarithmic or power law transformation), and used to modulate pulse trains at fairly high rates (typically > 500 pulses per second in each channel). Crucially, as indicated above, pulses on different channels are interleaved (Figure 15.2),

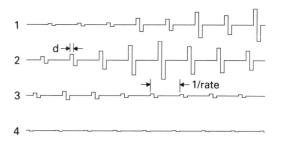

Figure 15.2 An example of interleaving of pulses in a continuous interleaved sampling scheme using four channels. Note that the biphasic pulses are only present on one electrode at any given time. (Courtesy of Blake Wilson)

in order to minimize channel interactions. (The name *continuous interleaved sampling* arises because the interleaved pulse trains can be considered to be sampling the transformed envelopes.) Figure 15.3 compares continuous interleaved sampling outputs to those obtained from a so-called *compressed analogue* (CA) scheme, as used in the Ineraid device. In the compressed analogue scheme, the speech is compressed before being filtered and presented to the electrodes.

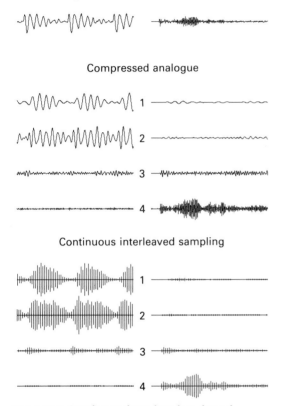

Figure 15.3 Sample waveforms from four-channel compressed analogue (CA) and continuous interleaved sampling (CIS) speech processing schemes for two speech segments. The speech pressure waveforms are shown at top. In the left column are a few cycles of the vowel 'aw', while at the right is the release burst and aspiration of a 't'. The numbers indicate the waveforms output to each electrode, with increasing numbers indicating channels with higher centre frequencies (corresponding to more basal cochlear positions). (Courtesy of Blake Wilson)

Extremely impressive results have been reported for continuous interleaved sampling in comparison to the compressed analogue scheme, even though the patients had little experience of the former (Wilson *et al.*, 1991, 1993, 1994). More recent work reports performance in noise backgrounds, and with the use of 'virtual channels', created by simultaneous stimulation of two or more electrodes (Wilson *et al.*, 1994).

Wilson and his colleagues have worked primarily with the Ineraid device, because its percutaneous connector presents no constraints on the waveforms presented. Dillier *et al.* (Dillier, Bögli and Spillman, 1993b; Dillier *et al.*, 1993), however, have been working on modifications of continuous interleaved sampling schemes that are appropriate for the Nucleus device. They too report improved performance with continuous interleaved sampling-like processing in comparison to the commercially-available schemes (see also McKay *et al.*, 1992; McKay and McDermott, 1993). Although it is clear that improvements to the Nucleus speech processing are possible, and are in progress, it remains to be seen how much of an an impediment to further developments in speech processing the current hardware will be.

Coding

Once the acoustical information has been processed, it must be *coded* into a form appropriate for presenting to the electrode array. There are two main dimensions along which implant systems differ: the exact form the electrical waveforms take, and (for multichannel systems) the way in which the stimulating and ground electrodes are arranged.

All systems can choose to present the information in either a continuously-varying form, or as pulses (separated in time by periods, however short, where stimulation is at zero). This distinction should not be confused with the difference between analogue and digital signals. All waveforms presented to an electrode are analogue by nature, even if they have been processed by digital electronics.

With one crucial exception, the choice of continuously-varying versus pulsatile stimulation appears to have relatively little influence on the overall performance of an implant. The single (and important) exception concerns multichannel implants which can, as mentioned above, avoid the problem of physical interaction of currents across electrodes by using pulsatile stimulation in which only a single electrode is stimulated at any given time (Favre and Pelizzone, 1993).

Electrode configuration

Once the exact form of stimulation is chosen, there is a final decision, concerning only multichannel implants, as to the exact electrode configuration to use. Generally speaking, there are three distinct modes. In *bipolar* stimulation, current is passed between electrodes relatively close to one another in the electrode array. For example, the stimulating and ground electrode may be adjacent to one another, or separated by one, two or more electrodes. Thus each stimulating electrode typically has a unique ground. In *monopolar* stimulation, the ground electrode remains the same for all stimulating electrodes, and is usually remote from all the intracochlear electrodes (typically somewhere in the middle ear). In *common ground* stimulation, all the electrodes except the stimulating electrode are connected together to serve as a ground – hence the name.

Insofar as these different electrode configurations lead to different current distributions through the cochlea, we might expect important differences among them. Early interest in different configurations was sparked by physiological findings that bipolar stimulation appeared to lead to much more discrete stimulation than monopolar stimulation (van den Honert and Stypulkowski, 1987).

In fact, electrode configuration has not turned out to be a very important factor in determining the performance of patients in speech tasks. For one thing, there is the evident success of users of the monopolar Ineraid device, and the yet greater success of users of the monopolar implementation of continuous interleaved sampling. Lehnhardt *et al.* (1992) have reported no differences in speech perceptual performance between monopolar and bipolar stimulation even for the Nucleus device.

Interestingly, different electrode configurations do lead to clear differences in detection thresholds and comfortable listening levels, and sometimes to changes in perceived pitch (Busby *et al.*, 1994). What is not yet at all clear is the relationship of these findings to the perception of speech.

Details of specific systems

Many different implant systems have been developed, some of which have only seen use in a few patients. Here we focus on those systems that have been used in significant numbers of patients.

House/3M

The House/3M device, no longer manufactured, was a single-channel device manufactured by 3M, based on a device first developed at what is now known as the House Ear Institute (House *et al.*, 1976). It consisted of an active electrode implanted in the scala tympani of the cochlea and a ground electrode placed in the eustachian tube or temporalis muscle. Both electrodes were attached to an induction coil (acting as the receiver) implanted subcutaneously behind the auricle. A second induction coil (acting as the transmitter) was worn externally and aligned directly over the internal coil. A miniature, omnidirectional electret microphone sensed the sound-pressure, and routed it to a signal processor where it was amplified, band-pass filtered (340–2700 Hz, with filter slopes of about 12 dB/octave) and used to amplitude modulate a 16-kHz sinusoidal carrier. The operation of this modulator was highly non-linear, one of its most important characteristics being a hard-clipping of its

output level for sound-pressure inputs greater than 65–75 dB SPL, depending upon the setting of the user-operated 'sensitivity' control. (For more details on the effects this processing has on acoustic signals, see Edgerton *et al.* (1983); Edgerton and Brimacombe (1984); Fretz and Fravel (1985); Rosen *et al.* (1989).) The modulator output was then amplified and transferred via electromagnetic induction across the skin to the internal coil and the active cochlear electrode. Further technical details may be found in Fretz and Fravel (1985) and Danley and Fretz (1982). Although no longer implanted, this device was the first to be used in any significant numbers in both adults and children.

Vienna/Innsbruck

Now based at Innsbruck and working with the manufacturer Med-El, the group in Vienna had their initial successes with a family of single-channel implants that shared many features. In the most commonly used device, the acoustical signal picked up by a microphone was amplitude-compressed, frequency-equalized and then modulated onto a radio-frequency (rf) carrier for transmission across the skin. A coil in the implanted receiver picked up the radio-frequency signal, demodulated it with a simple diode detector, and passed the result to a single electrode. This electrode could be placed intracochlearly, or (equipped with a ball-end) placed in the round window niche (further details may be found in Hochmair–Desoyer *et al.*, 1980; Hochmair and Hochmair–Desoyer, 1983, 1985). Such a system was highly transparent, albeit limited to single-channel stimulation. The 3M company in the USA manufactured a version of this device at one time (but no longer), and it also served as a model for the most commonly used single-channel implant in the UK (Fraser *et al.*, 1989). The Innsbruck group is still quite active, having moved on to multichannel work, while continuously developing their single-channel device (Hochmair–Desoyer, Zierhofer and Hochmair, 1993).

Currently, there is a single-channel device (with speech processing and transcutaneous transmission similar to that described above) with a speech processor contained in the shell of a behind-the-ear hearing aid. Thus there need no longer be a cable running from the transmitter to a body-worn 'box'. The batteries last 7–12 days before needing replacement.

Symbion/Ineraid

Based on work begun at the University of Utah (Eddington *et al.*, 1978), the Ineraid is a multichannel device with a percutaneous connector (Parkin, Randolph and Parkin, 1993). Although the electrode has six platinum intracochlear electrodes (plus two separate extracochlear ones used as electrical grounds), only four are used in the current speech processors (monopolar four-channel compressed analogue). The transparency of this system, though, has been crucial in the development of continuous interleaved sampling (see above).

Nucleus/Cochlear

The Nucleus multichannel device has resulted from a fruitful collaboration between the Department of Otolaryngology at the University of Melbourne, and a manufacturer with expertise in pacemakers (Clark *et al.*, 1987). The electrode consists of 22 platinum bands wrapped around a flexible silicon rubber electrode carrier. Signal transmission is transcutaneous, again with alignment assured by magnets. The system is anything but transparent, with strong constraints on the waveforms that can be delivered. Stimulation is always pulsatile, and to a single electrode at any one time. The pulses can be controlled in amplitude, duration and in which electrode will be stimulated. Both monopolar and bipolar stimulation are supported, with the ability to control the number of electrodes separating bipolar pairs. The maximum stimulation rate is rather low, on the order of a maximum of 300–600 pulses per channel when six electrodes are being stimulated (Dillier, Bögli and Spillmann, 1993a).

As mentioned above, speech processing schemes have been based primarily on a speech-pattern approach (Brimacombe and Beiter, 1994). Very recently, processors that can also implement a scheme related to continuous interleaved sampling (but with important differences) have been introduced. Here, each electrode is associated with a bandpass filter, more apical electrode positions corresponding to lower centre frequencies for the filter. The filter bank is scanned continuously, with an average of six maxima selected at any given time (but limited to 10). Then the six or so associated electrodes (representing the six or so spectral maxima) are stimulated sequentially, before beginning the next round of scanning the filter bank. Stimulation rates depend on a host of factors, but are generally within the range 180–300 (average 250) stimulation cycles per second (Cochlear Corporation, 1994; Skinner *et al.*, 1994).

Clarion

The Clarion device (Schindler and Kessler, 1993; Kessler and Schindler, 1994) draws heavily on the many years of work done at the University of California at San Francisco, particularly in its electrode design. This consists of 16 near-radial contacts held in a 25 mm silicone rubber carrier (Rebscher, 1985).

Communication between the electrodes and the outside world is by transcutaneous means (aligned by magnets), and designed to be reasonably transparent. The waveforms output by the device consist of pulses controllable in amplitude and width, thus enabling the close approximation of continuously variable signals by signals with discrete steps. With all eight channels driven simultaneously, the channels can be updated 13 500 times per second. Stimulation can be either in bipolar or monopolar mode. Information about electrode impedances can also be relayed from the electrodes to the external device. In these ways, the Clarion tries to avoid some of the more serious constraints of transcutaneous systems.

An important design goal of the Clarion system is to allow the use of a variety of speech processing schemes. To that end, two popular schemes have so far been implemented: compressed analogue (similar to that used in the Ineraid) and a version of continuous interleaved sampling.

What can be 'heard' through an implant?

Although we are a long way from understanding fully the relationship between electrical stimulation and evoked auditory percepts, much *is* known about the relationship between stimulation parameters and people's experiences.

Detection of sounds

First, there is no doubt that, when stimulated, people who have had some experience of normal hearing before being deafened report that they hear *sounds*. Of course, it is also possible to induce other sensations (tactile, pain, or facial twitching), but these are the exception in well-placed intracochlear electrodes. Such sounds may have a very different quality to the sounds remembered from periods of acoustical hearing, but they are sounds nevertheless. This follows, of course, from what has been known as *The Law of Specific Nerve Energies*. When the optic nerve fires, we report seeing something. When the auditory nerve fires, we report hearing something.

Loudness

When the current level of stimulation is increased, people report increases in *loudness*. So, it is usually possible, for any particular stimulation waveform, in the absence of extra-auditory effects, to find a range of currents over which the stimulation is undetectable, quiet, comfortable and too loud. It is not uncommon to engender extra-auditory sensations before reaching the level of 'too loud'. The ability to detect changes in intensity is roughly normal, with about a 1-dB just noticeable difference. Most importantly, the dynamic range of stimulation (i.e. the range between detection and discomfort) is very narrow, varying from only a few, to a maximum of about 20 dB. This contrasts with the normal-hearing dynamic range of over 100 dB (depending upon frequency). Thus normal listeners have many more discriminable steps of loudness available within their dynamic range.

Rate pitch

Stimulation with relatively low frequency periodic waveforms typically leads to a 'buzzy' percept with a distinct pitch. By varying the fundamental frequency of such waveforms in the appropriate range, melodies can be recognized, and intonation contours perceived. Strikingly unlike normal hearing is the limited frequency range over which changes in fundamental frequency can evoke changes in pitch – up to about 300–500 Hz. In normal hearing, there is a clear sense of pitch that continues to change over at least a few thousands of hertz. Insofar as this type of pitch can only relate to changes in temporal cues for implant users (by definition), it is interesting to note that normal listeners appear to be limited to the same rates for auditory stimulation that lacks spectral variation. For example, normal listeners presented with sinusoidally amplitude-modulated white noises, which contain temporal, but no spectral variations, can only discriminate (in a musical sense) rates up to about 500 Hz (Burns and Viemeister, 1976).

Timbre or quality

There are, unfortunately, many misunderstandings concerning the perception of timbre by implant users, not the least of which are terminological. Let us first be perfectly clear what it is we mean by 'timbre' – essentially any attribute of an auditory stimulus which lets us distinguish between two stimuli of identical duration, loudness and melodic pitch. Schouten (1968) lists five acoustic correlates of timbre: spectral envelope variations; the range between tonal and noiselike character; the time envelope in terms of rise, duration and decay; the gradual changes both in spectral envelope and fundamental frequency; and, the prefix, an onset of a sound quite dissimilar to the ensuing lasting vibration. However, because of its importance in speech, and its clear relevance to multichannel stimulation, we will only discuss here spectral envelope variations.

There is also another semantic difficulty, which has to do with the variety of percepts we label with the word 'pitch'. On the one hand is the melodic pitch as discussed above, which seems clearly related

to the fundamental frequency of complex sounds; on the other is the kind of 'timbral pitch' we might associate with a sound with a single spectral peak (like the single formant of a vowel). There is no doubt that we can use the same words to describe variations in frequency for these two kinds of attributes (running from 'low pitch' to 'high pitch'), but that does not mean they refer to the same thing, a confusion which is perhaps all too common. The fact is that although we use the word 'pitch' in at least these two ways, there is clear evidence from normal listeners (Plomp and Steeneken, 1971), and at least anecdotal evidence from users of multichannel implants (Tong *et al.*, 1982), that the two types of perceptual attributes are essentially independent of one another.

Whatever terminology we use, it is clear that many users of multichannel implants are able to hear changes in place of stimulation as changes in timbre, and use them in everyday situations (see Shannon (1993) for a review). Tong *et al.* (1983) have also shown that stimulation of two electrodes leads clearly to perceptual attributes that vary in two dimensions. These findings are a clear confirmation of the initial idea behind multichannel implants – that restoring anything like normal-hearing sensations requires the independent stimulation of neural elements across the basilar membrane (the place principle). But further, the findings confirm that it is indeed possible to simulate through electrical stimulation, at least roughly, the frequency-analysing properties of the normal auditory system.

For single-channel implants, the range of timbral contrasts that can be signalled is much more limited. Given the total lack of a 'place' mechanism, and thus the complete reliance on temporal features of stimulation, what is perhaps more surprising is the fact that *some* variation in timbre is found. Generally speaking, such variations appear not to be typically used by the majority of single-channel patients, and are limited to frequencies below 1 kHz or so in those that do (Rosen *et al.*, 1989; Rosen, 1992).

Temporal features

Generally speaking, the temporal features of acoustical stimulation are those that are most 'normal' for users of cochlear implants (Shannon, 1993). So, for example, implant users can detect 2–5 ms gaps in otherwise continuous stimulation, so long as the stimulation is sufficiently intense. This value is close to that found for normal listeners operating with acoustic stimuli. Implant users are also about 'normal' at detecting amplitude modulations imposed on an auditory signal. It would thus appear that good use could be made of the envelope and periodicity features of speech and other acoustic stimuli (see below).

The perception of environmental sounds

Although most investigations of implant use focus on the perception of speech (a reasonable focus given the unique role of language for humans), there has been some degree of interest in the perception of environmental sounds. Implant users often note the importance of such sounds to them, and it is easy to appreciate their utility. For these reasons, overall studies of implant patient performance have often included a test of environmental sounds. Here, patients are played a set of sounds which they are asked to identify, usually without knowing the possibilities.

Given only the wide variation in temporal features among environmental sounds (features we know to be processed well by most implant users), it is perhaps not surprising that patients can do quite well on such tests. Generally speaking, performance is better with multichannel implants than with a single-channel (from which it can be inferred that temporal features are not the only crucial cues), and better with the Ineraid device than with the Nucleus (Gantz et al., 1988; Tyler, Moore and Kuk, 1989). Presumably this arises not only from the fact that the Nucleus device was designed explicitly for speech signals, but also that the feature-extracting capabilities of the Nucleus device are not as good as they could be.

How well can speech be perceived through an implant?

Although the perception of environmental sounds is clearly an important benefit of cochlear implants (and often under-rated), much more attention is focused on the reception of speech. This arises from the realization that the primary difficulty of acquired deafness (which has been the case with the majority of implant patients) concerns everyday communication in a mostly hearing world. A wide variety of tests has been applied to implant patients, not always with a firm theoretical basis (see Rosen et al. (1985) for a fuller discussion). Rather than describing in detail the tests used, I shall again try to focus on the main trends in the results, restricting my discussion primarily to results obtained with adults who have been deafened after linguistic maturity.

Single-channel implants

As discussed above, all information passing through a single channel must be based on the temporal properties of the stimulation. Because the study of speech perception developed primarily in the context of normal hearing, with its fine-grained frequency analysis, there has been a gap in appropriate terminology for discussions of purely temporal speech percep-

tion. In an attempt to fill this terminological vacuum, Rosen (1989, 1992) has introduced a three way classification of the temporal structure of speech, based on dominant fluctuation rates:

1 *Envelope* – Fluctuations in overall amplitude, existing primarily in the region of a few hertz to some tens of hertz, which can convey prosodic cues about stress, syllabicity and timing, and segmental cues as to manner of articulation and voicing.
2 *Periodicity* – The presence of periodic or aperiodic stimulation, and if periodic, the rate of stimulation. Existing in the region of 50–500 Hz for periodic (voiced) sounds, and to considerably higher rates for voiceless ones, this cue directly conveys segmental aspects of manner and voicing, and the prosodic feature of intonation.
3 *Fine-structure* – Temporal detail within single periods of voiced sounds and short stretches of voiceless ones (with dominant fluctuations from about 600–800 Hz and upwards). Fine-structure conveys information about the spectral content of a sound, and hence can signal place of articulation and vowel quality.

Note that while envelope and periodicity can act as important aids to lip-reading (Summerfield, 1983), the understanding of speech without visual cues requires access to the information in fine structure.

Before applying this framework to the results of single-channel users, there is an added consideration – the extent to which temporal features are modified by the patient's speech processor. This can range from the relatively innocuous automatic gain control of the Vienna device (which has little effect on any of the features) to the hard-clipping of the House/3M device (which has drastic effects on envelope and fine-structure, leaving perhaps only periodicity unaffected). These modifications of temporal features may be advantageous or disadvantageous, of course. There is evidence, for instance, that the House/3M device may make certain envelope features (e.g. plosive release bursts) more salient, while severely distorting the fine structure (Rosen et al., 1989).

Without worrying too much about differences between devices for the moment, it appears that most users of analogue single-channel implants are sensitive to envelope and periodicity, but the relative importance of each cue is not yet clear (Rosen and Ball, 1986; Tyler et al., 1987; Agelfors and Risberg, 1989; Cooper et al., 1989; Rosen et al., 1989). Also, some patients may only be sensitive to the low-frequency periodicity of voiced sounds, missing out voiceless sounds completely (Rosen and Ball, 1986). In many, if not most, patients there is also sensitivity to temporal fine-structure (in the sense that stimuli with different fine structure can be discriminated from one another), but this is relatively rarely used in the perception of natural speech.

However, there do appear to be at least some

patients who can understand unknown sentences by auditory means alone, a feat which requires some linguistic use of the temporal fine-structure of speech (Hochmair-Desoyer *et al.*, 1980; White, 1983; Hochmair and Hochmair-Desoyer, 1985; Rosen and Ball, 1986; Agelfors and Risberg, 1987, 1989; Cooper *et al.*, 1989; Rosen *et al.*, 1989; Tartter, Hellman and Chute, 1992; Hochmair-Desoyer, Zierhofer and Hochmair, 1993; Cohen *et al.*, 1993). Interestingly, no person implanted as an adult with the House/3M device has ever shown this level of performance, although a small number of implanted children have (Luxford *et al.*, 1987; Tartter, Hellman and Chute, 1992).

The difference in results between the Vienna and House/3M device are not, perhaps, all that surprising given the vast differences in the waveforms they present to the patient. What is perhaps more surprising is the extent to which results from the two devices have been so similar, at least for patients implanted outside Austria.

The unexplained fact remains that most groups using the single-channel Vienna device (or one like it) find that approximately 10% of the implanted patients are able to understand some speech without lip-reading (Agelfors and Risberg, 1989; Cooper *et al.*, 1989; Cohen *et al.*, 1993), whereas the group at Innsbruck report speech perception without lip-reading in at least half of their patients. This level of performance is roughly equivalent to that obtained with multichannel implants, a result that has been corroborated by outside investigators testing the Vienna/Innsbruck patients (Tyler, Moore and Kuk, 1989; Tyler and Moore, 1992).

There have been speculations that the Vienna/Innsbruck patients typically have more preoperative residual hearing than patients implanted elsewhere; but there has been little hard evidence that this explains the result. There is, for example, no indication of more extensive residual hearing in the Vienna/Innsbruck group (compared to other devices) among the better performing patients studied by Tyler, Moore and Kuk (1989).

Multichannel implants

Although originally developed for single-channel implants, the three-way division of the temporal structure of speech outlined above can still serve well for organizing the discussion of results, even with multichannel implants. Insofar as the frequency analysis possible with even the most advanced multichannel implant is likely to remain far inferior to the frequency analysis exacted by the normal peripheral auditory system, we should expect the temporal features of stimulation to be more important for implant users than for normally hearing listeners.

In the first instance, envelope and periodicity will almost certainly be coded by temporal means for implant patients. Envelope is coded in such a way even for normal listeners. Although there remains an important controversy about the respective role of time- and place-based analyses for periodicity perception in normal listeners, no cochlear implant now, or in the foreseeable future, is likely to be able to resolve in frequency the harmonic structure of speech. Therefore, periodicity too, will be cued by temporal aspects. (For speech extraction schemes like the earlier Nucleus schemes described above, there is an explicit coding of speech fundamental frequency into a temporal form.)

It is only the consideration of fine-structure that warrants a major change of outlook from that appropriate for single-channel implants. For multichannel implants, changes in fine-structure will now be represented as changes in the frequency spectra of sounds, and hence in changes in the distribution of excitation across the electrode array. As was indicated above, most users of multichannel implant systems can distinguish stimulation that differs only in which electrode it is delivered to, and these percepts change in quality that is usually related sensibly to the relative position of the electrode along the cochlea.

Again speaking in a general way, users of multichannel implants (at least for the most commonly used devices, the Nucleus and the Symbion) typically show some degree of sensitivity to all three kinds of speech information: envelope, periodicity and spectral shape. Thus about one-half of patients are able to understand some speech without lip-reading, with a significant proportion even able to use the telephone (Dorman, 1993). A much greater proportion, of course, find the implant useful in aiding lip-reading.

Although few surprises arose in its outcome, a particularly convincing study of the relative advantages of multichannel implants was that funded by the Department of Veterans' Affairs in the USA (Waltzman, 1992; Cohen *et al.*, 1993). Three different implant systems (the Nucleus, the Ineraid, and the single-channel Vienna/3M) were randomly implanted in a total of 82 patients. About 60% (37/60) of patients who received a multichannel system were able to understand some words and sentences without lip-reading 2 years after implantation. In contrast, only 5% (1/20) of the single-channel users could do this. Interestingly, it was not possible to find a statistically significant difference between implant systems for two of the three tasks concerning lip-reading plus electrical stimulation, although this was a common result for tests *not* involving lip-reading (Waltzman, Cohen and Fisher, 1992).

Of course, current clinical practice does not necessarily represent the best that can be done. As mentioned above, there have been very promising results from a variety of schemes based upon continuous interleaved sampling, and results from these are just beginning to be available in quantity.

Effects on speech production

Although the primary effect of deafness in the deafened adult is an impairment to receptive processes, it has long been recognized that articulatory control can also be degraded. This issue has received relatively little attention (in comparison to the assessment of receptive potential), but its importance should not be underestimated, especially to the patient. Generally speaking, it has not been hard to find beneficial effects of implant use on speech production, although the effects vary greatly from one individual to another. An excellent review of available results may be found in Tobey (1993).

Patient selection

For the adult candidate, a number of selection criteria have become fairly standard (Tye-Murray, 1993). Patients should have profound bilateral sensorineural hearing losses, with minimal ability to benefit from an acoustical hearing aid (but see below). Best results are obtained from those patients who had good hearing at least until the age of 6 years, and preferably later. There are also, of course, a number of medical criteria, one of which is crucial to the success of a multichannel implant – an unobstructed cochlea.

Although implants have traditionally been reserved for patients with essentially no residual hearing, in the light of generally good results there have recently been attempts to broaden the criteria for implantation. With some exceptions, this work has proceeded in a relatively conservative way, primarily because it became clear early on that the implantation of long intrascalar electrodes (as is necessary for intracochlear multichannel stimulation) leads to a severe loss of whatever residual hearing is present (Rizer *et al.*, 1988; Boggess, Baker and Balkany, 1989).

Perhaps the most complete study of this sort is one currently underway using the Nucleus 22-channel device (Arndt, Brimacombe and Staller, 1993). Here a group of 61 postlingually deafened adults with aided open-set sentence recognition ≤ 30% were implanted. Mean preoperative aided thresholds in the implanted ear were about: 75 dB HL at 125 Hz, 85 dB HL at 250 Hz, 100 dB HL at 500 Hz, and greater than 110 dB HL for 1 kHz and above. As was expected from earlier work, audiometric thresholds in the implanted ear worsened considerably postoperatively, with average thresholds greater than 115 dB HL at all frequencies.

Balanced against this loss of residual hearing were clear improvements in speech perception found for most of the patients. For example, on a test of open-set sentence recognition, preoperative mean scores were 11% for the non-implanted ear, 6% for the implanted ear and 17% for a binaural presentation. Postoperatively, they jumped to 48% for the implanted ear and 59% binaurally, with little change in the non-implanted ear (to 16%). The majority of users (82%) improved significantly in the implanted ear, and binaural conditions. Qualitatively similar results were found with an open-set test of word recognition.

There is another crucial question that can be addressed by this study: do users with greater degrees of residual hearing perform better, on average, than those with less residual hearing? Brimacombe *et al.* (1994) looked at the same group of patients, but subdivided them into two groups varying in preoperative performance on the open-set sentence test. These two groups also differed, unsurprisingly, in audiometric thresholds. And indeed, the users with better residual hearing did appear to perform better with implants.

This finding is also confirmed in some work by Boothroyd and his colleagues (reviewed in Boothroyd, 1993). Here, the claim is made that the average implant user does about as well as a hearing aid user with a hearing loss of 100 dB (averaged at 0.5, 1 and 2 kHz). Given that the severe-to-profound users discussed above have losses of about 100 dB and 110 dB in the non-implanted and implanted ear respectively, and do considerably better with implants than they do with hearing aids in either ear, it would appear again that a greater degree of residual hearing does indeed lead to better implant performance. Of course, it is not yet clear to what extent these limits on audiometric criteria can be pushed. What is clear is that the actuarial approach favoured by Boothroyd and his colleagues will lead to quite conservative limits insofar as there is any positive correlation between the extent of residual acoustic hearing and implant performance (as demonstrated in Brimacombe *et al.*, 1994).

These studies clearly have important implications for implant patient selection criteria, and by inference, for other interventions aimed at the profoundly hearing-impaired adult. For example, there have been a number of promising studies of speech processing hearing aids for severe-to-profound hearing-impaired listeners (Rosen *et al.*, 1987; Faulkner *et al.*, 1992a), and there is also much interest in tactile aids (see Chapter 16). It seems fairly clear that the average results now being obtained by implant patients are better than those that would be obtained through such acoustical or tactile means, at least for this group of patients. Balancing this consideration is the fact that acoustic and tactile aids are at least an order of magnitude cheaper, and require no surgery. Furthermore, both kinds of prostheses are still very much in their infancy and could develop significantly. It is also difficult to know from average results which particular approach will be more successful for any particular patient, especially when other factors are present (e.g. bone growth in the cochlea preventing insertion of a multichannel electrode). Availability is also an issue – acoustic speech-processing hearing aids are not yet commercially available, whereas implants and tactile aids are. In short, it seems likely that a variety of approaches will remain useful, even if implants come to be applied in a wider range of situations.

Individual differences and prediction of clinical outcome

Closely allied to the issue of patient selection (but not synonymous with it), is the extent to which we can predict, from preoperative results, the eventual performance any particular patient is likely to achieve. Although we have tended to generalize enormously in our discussion of results, it is a cliché in the implant area that patients vary widely in outcome, in a way which is not readily predictable (even for patients using the same implant). So, for example, one implant user may be able to engage in conversation on the telephone, while another would even have difficulty when visual cues were available in face-to-face conversation. This should not be surprising. If we take a sample of normally-hearing listeners, with normal vision, and give them a lip-reading test, we find scores (on the basis of lists of 16 sentences containing 50 key words each) that can vary from an average of two words to 28 words correctly identified (Rosen and Corcoran, 1982). Clearly then, any test involving lip-reading would have a great deal of variability even if an implant worked equally well for all patients. But there are probably related factors even for tests of sound alone. Presumably, tests of lip-reading are also tests of the linguistic ability of a person to make sense of incomplete information. Insofar as a cochlear implant is far from providing perfectly normal auditory sensations, the ability of patients to use incomplete and imperfect information will be an important factor in their overall performance.

For clinical practice, however, it would be a great advantage if it were possible to predict preoperatively how well an implant patient would do. For one thing, it could help clarify patient selection criteria, and also aid in the choice of prosthesis – tactile, acoustic or electrical.

A number of groups has tackled this issue, and with some success. One of the early studies (Fritze and Eisenwort, 1989) led to few surprises in its conclusions, even though its methods for assessing outcome were fairly vague. Based on 28 patients using a single-channel device (with the prediction procedure then applied to 19 further patients), language competence was found to be the most important predictor of patient performance. This factor clearly separated pre-, peri- and postlingually deafened patients, along with another important predictor – the duration of deafness before implantation. Also

of predictive value was preoperative performance on an aided speech task (identification of numbers), even though this did not correlate with pure tone thresholds.

More recent adult studies have restricted their investigations to postlingually deafened adults, in recognition of the overwhelming importance of linguistic competence to performance. Blamey *et al.* (1992) studied 64 users of the Nucleus implant, in order to decide which variables predicted performance in an open-set test of sentence perception. Two preoperative predictors were found:

1 Combined performance in frequency discrimination and gap detection during promontory single-channel stimulation (a confirmation of a similar finding by Hochmair–Desoyer, Hochmair and Stiglbrunner, 1985)
2 Duration of profound deafness prior to implantation.

Along with two other predictors that could only be determined postoperatively (the dynamic range on the middle electrode, and the number of intracochlear electrodes used for coding speech), 43% of the variance in performance could be accounted for. Unfortunately, predictive accuracy for purely preoperative measures was not reported.

Taking quite a different tack, Knutson *et al.* (1991) have focused attention on a number of psychological predictors of patient performance. They reported that a combination of a cognitive (non-auditory) visual monitoring task and a measure of patient compliance can account for 25% of the variance in multichannel implant performance with sentence material (sound alone). At the same time, IQ scores appear to have no predictive power in this situation.

To summarize, although much headway has been made in this area, we are still far from predicting accurately eventual patient performance. It appears likely that the combination of patient histories, psychological and audiological measures, possibly with the addition of electrophysiological tests that require no response from the patients (Abbas, 1993), could improve predictive accuracy further.

The role of rehabilitation

In the entire field of audiology, there has been an increasing emphasis on the role of rehabilitation in assuring optimal use of an auditory prosthesis. Because cochlear implants seem to be so different from traditional hearing aids, and the adaptation to them has appeared to be more difficult, patients receiving cochlear implants typically receive much more in the way of auditory rehabilitation than do users of acoustical hearing aids. Although there appears to be general agreement that a significant degree of counselling and rehabilitation is beneficial, there are important disagreements about the extent to which the various components of the rehabilitation process are indeed necessary. Unfortunately, there are few controlled studies of these components.

There have been some assessments, however, of the role of explicit speech-perceptual training in improving implant patient performance (reviewed in Tye-Murray, 1993). Generally speaking, the effects seem to be present, but not necessarily large. Such training appears to have the greatest benefit early on in implant use. Also clear are the large individual differences in acclimatizing to an implant. Some users do well almost immediately, while others take many months for their performance to level off. Sorely needed are guidelines to deal with the wide range of patient behaviour, and in matching rehabilitation to the patients' needs.

Tinnitus

For many years, there has been considerable interest in the possibility of tinnitus suppression by electrical stimulation, both as an added benefit of cochlear implants (Tyler and Kelsay, 1990; Souliere *et al.*, 1992) and as a primary clinical treatment (Hazell *et al.*, 1993; Okusa *et al.*, 1993). It appears that electrical tinnitus suppression is somehow intimately connected with evoked auditory sensations, as indicated by findings that it is not possible to suppress tinnitus with a subthreshold stimulus (Dauman, Tyler and Aran, 1993; Hazell *et al.*, 1993). In fact, there appears to be a strong correlation (across patients and frequencies) between the level of stimulation needed for tinnitus suppression, and the detection threshold (Hazell *et al.*, 1993).

Perhaps the most confusing aspect of this area concerns *residual inhibition*, i.e. suppression of tinnitus after the electrical stimulation is turned off. Although there are statements in the literature that residual inhibition is rare (Dauman, Tyler and Aran, 1993), it appears to occur frequently both in implant users implanted primarily for their deafness (Souliere *et al.*, 1992) and in patients with varying degrees of hearing loss treated acutely (Okusa *et al.*, 1993). Jastreboff and Hazell (1993) have recently provided a more general approach to the understanding of tinnitus, stressing the importance of central processing, which may lend insight into this problem.

Making strong generalizations in this area is not helped by the wide variation in hearing loss, place, type and duration of stimulation used. Perhaps surprisingly, there does appear to be one constant among this variation – tinnitus appears to be suppressed best by the lowest frequencies used (Dauman, Tyler and Aran, 1993; Hazell *et al.*, 1993; Okusa *et al.*, 1993).

Auditory brain stem implants

Although cochlear implants can play an important role in the treatment of many types of profound and total deafness, there are situations that demand other, albeit related, approaches. In particular, patients who have no remaining auditory nerve (arising typically from surgical removal of an acoustic neuroma (Kveton, 1993)) must be stimulated elsewhere in the auditory pathway. A reasonable assumption is that stimulation as far out into the periphery as is possible should be advantageous, in order to make use of the remaining higher neural processing. As the cochlear nucleus is the normal termination site for all auditory nerve fibres, and as such the most 'peripheral' of the 'central' structures, it is an obvious choice for stimulation.

A group based at the House Ear Institute has been investigating the use of auditory brain stem stimulation in adult patients with neurofibromatosis type 2 undergoing resection of acoustic neuromas (Brackmann *et al.*, 1993; Shannon *et al.*, 1993). The electrode carrier is placed within the lateral recess of the fourth ventricle adjacent to the dorsal cochlear nucleus and the inferior portion of the ventral cochlear nucleus. Although it might be thought that stimulation of the anteroventral cochlear nucleus would be most desirable (insofar as units in that area respond most like the reasonably well-understood and homogeneous auditory nerve fibres), stimulation directly over the ventral cochlear nucleus appears to lead to more non-auditory effects (e.g. facial movement, a tickling or constriction in the throat, tingling in the shoulder or arm, or a feeling of vibration in the eye).

The initial series of patients were implanted with electrodes meant to be used in a single-channel mode (Brackmann *et al.*, 1993), and most patients were able to be fitted with the House/3M speech processor designed for single-channel cochlear stimulation (Shannon *et al.*, 1993). Generally speaking, the use of such a processor leads to rudimentary (but vital) auditory percepts that can significantly improve lip-reading ability, but will not allow the understanding of speech without lip-reading. Performance, in fact, is similar to that obtained with the same processor in conjunction with a single-channel cochlear implant. It must be stressed that, although the auditory information is limited, the patients in these studies would typically have been totally deaf after such surgery. Even a modicum of appropriate auditory information can have surprisingly large benefits, as has long been known from work with single-channel cochlear implants.

The most recent work in this area has been in two complementary directions. First, there has been some effort in optimizing single-channel processing schemes, in particular with single-channel variants of the continuous interleaved sampling scheme described above (Shannon, Zeng and Wygonski, 1992).

Here, the wide-band speech signal is rectified and smoothed, with the resulting envelope mapped in amplitude and used to modulate a single pulse train (hereinafter referred to as continuous interleaved sampling (1-channel)). The one patient tested with this scheme did markedly better than any patient with the House/3M processing scheme (to the extent of understanding unknown sentences and words without lip-reading), but few implications can be drawn from such a small study. For one thing, as noted above, it is well known that a small proportion of single-channel users, perhaps 5–10% (Cooper *et al.*, 1989; Cohen *et al.*, 1993) can understand speech without lip-reading on the basis of a relatively unprocessed speech signal quite unlike the one delivered by the House/3M device (although much better performances have been claimed by one group (Hochmair-Desoyer, Zierhofer and Hochmair, 1993)). It is therefore not at all clear if continuous interleaved sampling (1-channel) led to any advantages over a simple frequency-equalized speech signal. My own pilot studies of single-channel variants of continuous interleaved sampling suggest it has no advantages over presenting the unprocessed speech signal. In fact, it appeared that the smoothing associated with continuous interleaved sampling (1-channel) makes fricatives much more difficult to identify (as the amplitude variation so typical of the fricatives is eliminated).

Second, there has been a considerable investment in constructing multichannel electrodes for brain stem stimulation, and in testing patients for the extent to which multichannel stimulation is genuinely feasible (Shannon *et al.*, 1994). The current design uses eight electrodes on a carrier designed, as was the earlier implant, to be placed in the lateral recess of the fourth ventricle. Three patients have so far received this device. Initial psychophysical studies suggested that stimulation of at least some electrodes can lead to distinct pitches. Initial speech-perceptual results with the Nucleus type of multichannel processors (based on extraction of speech fundamental frequency and one or two of the lowest formant frequencies) were quite encouraging, although it is not yet clear to what extent the patients were actually making use of multichannel stimulation.

Certainly, this is an area that is ripe for development, with a number of promising research leads. Perhaps the most obvious and simple approach, of using the relatively raw speech signal (which, as mentioned above, is available in an ear-level device (Hochmair-Desoyer, Zierhofer and Hochmair, 1993)), would also be worth a serious look.

Dedication

This chapter is dedicated to Graham Fraser (1936–1994) for his work in bringing the clinical use of cochlear implants to the UK.

Suggestions for further reading

For the prospective patient or interested layperson, the National Association of Deafened People (in the UK) has produced an informative booklet, *An Introduction to Cochlear Implants*, edited by Alison Heath, herself a user of a cochlear implant.

The excellent volume edited by Tyler (1993) provides a number of contributions from leading researchers in the field, covering aspects of speech production and perception, patient selection and rehabilitation. An extremely useful book aimed at a more clinical audience is that edited by Cooper (1991).

The most up-to-date research findings may be found in a volume consisting of the proceedings of a recent conference (Hochmair–Desoyer and Hochmair, 1994).

References

ABBAS, P. J. (1993) Electrophysiology. In: *Cochlear Implants: Audiological Foundations*, edited by R. S. Tyler. London: Whurr. pp. 317–355

AGELFORS, E. and RISBERG, A. (1987) The identification of synthetic vowels by patients using a single-channel cochlear implant. In: *Proceedings of the XIth International Congress of Phonetic Sciences*. Tallinn: Academy of Sciences of the Estonian SSR. **4**, 181–184

AGELFORS, E. and RISBERG, A. (1989) Speech feature perception by patients using a single-channel Vienna 3M extracochlear implant. In: *Proceedings of the Speech Research '89 International Conference* (Budapest). Budapest: Linguistics Institute of the Hungarian Academy of Sciences, pp. 149–152. Also in (1989) *Speech Transmission Laboratory – Quarterly Progress and Status Report*. Stockholm. Royal Institute of Technology. **1**, pp. 145–149

ARNDT, P. L., BRIMACOMBE, J. A. and STALLER, S. J. (1993) Multichannel cochlear implantation in adults with residual hearing. Paper presented at the *American Speech-Language-Hearing Association* (Anaheim, California)

BLAMEY, P. J., PYMAN, B. C., CLARK, G. M., DOWELL, R. C., GORDON, M., BROWN, A. M. *et al* (1992) Factors predicting postoperative sentence scores in postlinguistically deaf adult cochlear implant patients. *Annals of Otology, Rhinology and Laryngology*, **101**, 342–348

BOGGESS, W. J., BAKER, J. E. and BALKANY, T. J. (1989) Loss of residual hearing after cochlear implantation. *Laryngoscope*, **99**, 1002–1005

BOOTHROYD, A. (1993) Profound deafness. In: *Cochlear Implants: Audiological Foundations*, edited by R. S. Tyler. London: Whurr, pp. 1–33

BRACKMANN, D., HITSELBERGER, W., NELSON, R., MOORE, J., WARING, M., PORTILLO, F. *et al.* (1993) Auditory brainstem implant: I. Issues in surgical implantation. *Otolaryngology – Head Neck Surgery*, **108**, 624–633

BRIMACOMBE, J. A., ARNDT, P. L., STALLER, S. J. and BEITER, A. L. (1994) Multichannel cochlear implantation in adults with severe-to-profound sensorineural hearing loss. In: *Advances in Cochlear Implants*, edited by I. J. Hochmair-Desoyer and E. S. Hochmair. Vienna: Manz. pp. 387–392

BRIMACOMBE, J. A. and BEITER, A. L. (1994) The application of digital technology to cochlear implants. In: *Understand-*

ing Digitally Programmable Hearing Aids, edited by R. E. Sandlin. Boston: Allyn and Bacon. pp. 151–170

BURNS, E. M. and VIEMEISTER, N. F. (1976) Nonspectral pitch. *Journal of the Acoustical Society of America*, **60**, 863–869

BUSBY, P. A., WHITFORD, L. A., BLAMEY, P. J., RICHARDSON, L. M. and CLARK, G. M. (1994) Pitch perception for different modes of stimulation using the Cochlear multiple-electrode prosthesis. *Journal of the Acoustical Society of America*, **95**, 2658–2669

CLARK, G. M., SHEPHERD, R. K., PATRICK, J. F., BLACK, R. C. and TONG, Y. C. (1983) Design and fabrication of the banded electrode array. *Annals of the New York Academy of Science*, **405**, 191–201

CLARK, G. M., BLAMEY, P. J., BROWN, A. M., BUSBY, P. A., DOWELL, R. C., FRANZ, B. K.-H. *et al.* (1987) *The University of Melbourne – Nucleus Multi-Electrode Cochlear Implant* Basel: Karger.

COCHLEAR CORPORATION (1994) FDA releases new SPEAK Coding Strategy and Spectra 22 processor. *Clinical Bulletin*

COHEN, N., WALTZMAN, S., FISHER, S., TYLER, R., DOBIE, R., JENKINS, H. *et al.* (1993) A prospective, randomized study of cochlear implants. *New England Journal of Medicine*, **328**, 233–237

COHEN, N. L., HOFFMAN, R. A. and STROSCHEIN, M. (1988) Medical or surgical complications related to the Nucleus multichannel cochlear implant. *Annals of Otology, Rhinology and Laryngology*, **97** (suppl. 135), 8–13

COOPER, H. (ed.) (1991) *Cochlear Implants: A Practical Guide.* London: Whurr

COOPER, H., CARPENTER, L., ALEKSY, W., BOOTH, C., READ, T., GRAHAM, J. *et al.* (1989) UCH/RNID single channel extracochlear implant: results in thirty profoundly deafened adults. *Journal of Laryngology and Otology*, Suppl. 18, 22–38

DANLEY, M. J. and FRETZ, R. J. (1982) Design and functioning of the single-electrode cochlear implant. *Annals of Otology, Rhinology and Laryngology*, **91** (Suppl. 91), 21–26

DAUMAN, R., TYLER, R. and ARAN, J. (1993) Intracochlear electrical tinnitus reduction. *Acta Otolaryngologica*, **113**, 291–295

DILLIER, N., BÖGLI, H. and SPILLMAN, T. (1993a) Speech discrimination via cochlear implants with two different digital speech processing strategies: preliminary results for 7 patients. *Scandinavian Audiology*, Suppl. 38, 145–153

DILLIER, N., BÖGLI, H. and SPILLMAN, T. (1993b) Speech encoding strategies for multielectrode cochlear implants: a digital signal processor approach. *Progress in Brain Research*, **97**, 301–311

DILLIER, N., FRÖLICH, T., KOMPIS, M., BÖGLI, H. and WAIKONG, K. L. (1993) Digital signal processing (DSP) applications for multiband loudness correction digital hearing aids and cochlear implants. *Journal of Rehabilitation Research and Development*, **30**, 95–109

DJOURNO, A. and EYRIES, C. (1957) Prothèse auditive par excitation électrique à distance du nerf sensoriel à l'aide d'un bobinage inclus à demeure. *La Presse Médicale*, **63**, 14–17

DORMAN, M. F. (1993) Speech perception by adults. In: *Cochlear Implants: Audiological Foundations*, edited R. S. Tyler. London Whurr. pp. 145–190

DOWELL, R. C., SELIGMAN, P. M., BLAMEY, P. J. and CLARK, G. M. (1987) Evaluation of a two-formant speech-processing strategy for a multichannel cochlear prosthesis. *Annals of*

Otology, Rhinology and Laryngology, **96** (suppl. 128), 132–134

DOWELL, R. C., TONG, Y. C., BLAMEY, P. J. and CLARK, G. M. (1985) Psychophysics of multiple-channel stimulation. In: *Cochlear Implants*, edited by R. A. Schindler and M. M. Merzenich. New York: Raven Press. pp. 283–290

EDDINGTON, D. K. (1983) Speech recognition in deaf subjects with multichannel intracochlear electrodes. *Annals of the New York Academy of Science*, **405**, 241–258

EDDINGTON, D. K., DOBELLE, W. H., BRACKMANN, D. E., MLADEJOVSKY, M. G. and PARKIN, J. L. (1978) Auditory prostheses research with multiple channel intracochlear stimulation in man. *Annals of Otology, Rhinology and Laryngology*, **87** (suppl. 53), 1–39

EDGERTON, B. J. and BRIMACOMBE, J. A. (1984) Effects of signal processing by the House-3M Cochlear Implant on consonant perception. *Acta Otolaryngologica*, Suppl. 411, 115–123

EDGERTON, B. J., DOYLE, K. J., BRIMACOMBE, J. A., DANLEY, M. J. and FRETZ, R. J. (1983) The effects of signal processing by the House–Urban single-channel stimulator on auditory perception of patients with cochlear implants. *Annals of the New York Academy of Science*, **405**, 311–322

FAULKNER, A., BALL, V., ROSEN, S., MOORE, B. C. J. and FOURCIN, A. (1992a) Speech pattern hearing aids for the profoundly hearing-impaired: speech perception and auditory abilities. *Journal of the Acoustical Society of America*, **91**, 2136–2155

FAULKNER, A., WALLIKER, J., ROSEN, S., DOUEK, E. and FOURCIN, A. (1992b) Psychoacoustic performance with a Bioglass-based multi-channel extra-cochlear implant. *Speech, Hearing and Language: Work in Progress*, **6**, 35–44

FAVRE, E. and PELIZZONE, M. (1993) Channel interactions in patients using the Ineraid multichannel cochlear implant. *Hearing Research*, **66**, 150–156

FOURCIN, A. J., ROSEN, S., MOORE, B. C. J., DOUEK, E. E., CLARKE, G. P., DODSON, H. *et al.* (1979) External electrical stimulation of the cochlea: clinical, psychophysical, speech-perceptual and histological findings. *British Journal of Audiology*, **13**, 85–107

FRASER, J. G., CONWAY, M. J., BOYLE, P., RYAN, R. M., GRAHAM, J. M., EAST, C. A. *et al.* (1989) The University College Hospital/RNID Cochlear Implant Program. *Journal of Laryngology and Otology*, Suppl. 18, 1–57

FRETZ, R. J. and FRAVEL, R. P. (1985) Design and function: a physical and electrical description of the 3M House Cochlear Implant System. *Ear and Hearing*, **6**, 14S–19s

FRITZE, W. and EISENWORT, B. (1989) Statistical procedure for the preoperative prediction of cochlear implantation. *British Journal of Audiology*, **23**, 293–297

GANTZ, B., TYLER, R., KNUTSON, J., WOODWORTH, G., ABBAS, P., MCCABE, B. *et al.* (1988) Evaluation of five different cochlear implant designs: audiologic assessment and predictors of performance. *Laryngoscope*, **98**, 1100–1106

GRAY, R., BAGULEY, D., HARRIES, M., COURT, I. and LYNCH, C. (1993) Profound deafness treated by the Ineraid multichannel intracochlear implant. *Jounal of Laryngology and Otology*, **107**, 673–680

HAZELL, J., JASTREBOFF, P., MEERTON, L. and CONWAY, M. (1993) Electrical tinnitus suppression: frequency dependence of effects. *Audiology*, **32**, 68–77

HOCHMAIR, E. S. and HOCHMAIR–DESOYER, I. J. (1983) Percepts elicited by different speech-coding strategies. *Annals of the New York Academy of Sciences*, **405**, 268–279

HOCHMAIR, E. S. and HOCHMAIR–DESOYER, I. J. (1985) Aspects

of sound signal processing using the Vienna intra- and extracochlear implants. In: *Cochlear Implants*, edited by R. A. Schindler and M. M. Merzenich. New York: Raven Press. pp. 101–110

HOCHMAIR–DESOYER, I. J. and HOCHMAIR, E. S. (eds) (1994) *Advances in Cochlear Implants*. Vienna: Manz

HOCHMAIR–DESOYER, I., ZIERHOFER, C. and HOCHMAIR, E. (1993) New hardware for analog and combined analog and pulsatile sound-encoding strategies. *Progress in Brain Research*, **97**, 291–300

HOCHMAIR–DESOYER, I. J., HOCHMAIR, E. S., FISCHER, R. E. and BURIAN, K. (1980) Cochlear prostheses in use: recent speech comprehension results. *Archives of Oto–Rhino–Laryngology*, **229**, 81–98

HOCHMAIR–DESOYER, I. J., HOCHMAIR, E. S. and STIGLBRUNNER, H. K. (1985) Psychoacoustic temporal processing and speech understanding in cochlear implant patients. In: *Cochlear Implants*, edited by R. A. Schindler and M. M. Merzenich. New York: Raven Press. pp. 291–304

HOCHMAIR–DESOYER, I. J., HOCHMAIR, E. S., ZIERHOFER, C. and STIGLBRUNNER, H. (1989) A family of extra- and intracochlear implant systems. In: *Cochlear Implant: Acquisitions and Controversies*, edited by B. Fraysse and N. Cochard. Basel: Cochlear AG. pp. 361–372

HOUSE, W. F. (1985) A personal perspective on cochlear implants. In: *Cochlear Implants*, edited by R. A. Schindler and M. M. Merzenich. New York: Raven Press. pp. 13–16

HOUSE, W. F., BERLINER, K., CRARY, W., GRAHAM, M., LUCKEY, R., NORTON, N. *et al.* (1976) Cochlear implants. *Annals of Otology, Rhinology and Laryngology*, **85** (suppl. 27), 1–93

JASTREBOFF, P. and HAZELL, J. (1993) A neurophysiological approach to tinnitus: clinical implications. *British Journal of Audiology*, **27**, 7–17

JOHNSSON, L.-G. (1985) Cochlear anatomy and histopathology. In: *Cochlear Implants*, edited by R. F. Gray. London: Croom Helm. pp. 50–73

KESSLER, D. K. and SCHINDLER, R. A. (1994) Progress with the multi-strategy cochlear implant system: The Clarion™. In: *Advances in Cochlear Implants*, edited by I. J. Hochmair–Desoyer and E. S. Hochmair. Vienna: Manz. pp. 354–362

KETTEN, D. R. and NADOL, J. B. (1990) Imaging and temporal bone diagnostics in cochlear implantation. Paper presented at *The Second International Cochlear Implant Symposium* (Iowa City, Iowa)

KETTEN, D. R., NADOL, J. B. and BURGESS, B. J. (1990) In situ sectioning of multiple electrode implants: techniques for histology, morphometry and reconstruction. Paper presented at *The Second International Cochlear Implant Symposium* (Iowa City, Iowa)

KIANG, N. Y. S. and MOXON, E. C. (1972) Physiological considerations in artificial stimulation of the inner ear. *Annals of Otology, Rhinology and Laryngology*, **81**, 714–730

KNUTSON, J. F., HINRICHS, J. V., TYLER, R. S., GANTZ, B. J., SCHARTZ, H. A. and WOODWORTH, G. (1991) Psychological predictors of audiological outcomes of multichannel cochlear implants: preliminary findings. *Annals of Otology, Rhinology and Laryngology*, **100**, 817–822

KVETON, J. (1993) Evaluation and management of acoustic neuroma. *Current Opinion in Otolaryngology and Head and Neck Surgery*, **1**, 53–63

LEHNHARDT, E., GNADEBERG, D., BATTMER, R. and VON WALLENBERG, E. (1992) Experience with the Cochlear miniature speech processor in adults and children together with a comparison of unipolar and bipolar modes. *ORL*, **54**, 308–313

LOEB, G. E. (1985) The functional replacement of the ear. *Scientific American*, **252**, 86–92

LUXFORD, W. M., BERLINER, K. I., EISENBERG, L. S. and HOUSE, W. F. (1987) Cochlear implants in children. *Annals of Otology, Rhinology and Laryngology*, **96** (suppl. 128), 136–138

MCKAY, C. M. and MCDERMOTT, H. J. (1993) Perceptual performance of subjects with cochlear implants using the Spectral Maxima Sound Processor (SMSP) and the Mini Speech Processor (MSP). *Ear and Hearing*, **14**, 350–367

MCKAY, C., MCDERMOTT, H., VANDALI, A. and CLARK, G. (1992) A comparison of speech perception of cochlear implantees using the Spectral Maxima Sound Processor (SMSP) and the MSP (MULTIPEAK) processor. *Acta Otolaryngologica*, **112**, 752–761

MICHELSON, R. P. (1985) Cochlear implants: personal perspectives. In: *Cochlear Implants*, edited by R. A. Schindler and M. M. Merzenich. New York: Raven Press. pp. 9–11

MILLER, J. M., PFINGST, B. E., TJELLSTRÖM, A., ALBREKTSSON, T., THOMPSON, P. and KEMINK, J. L. (1987) Titanium implants in the otic capsule: development of a new multichannel extracochlear implant. *American Journal of Otology*, **8**, 230–233

NATIONAL INSTITUTES OF HEALTH (1988) Cochlear Implants. *Consensus Development Conference Statement*, 7

NIPARKO, J., PFINGST, B., JOHANSSON, C., KILENY, P., KEMINK, J. and TJELLSTROM, A. (1993) Cochlear wall titanium implants for auditory nerve stimulation. *Annals of Otology, Rhinology and Laryngology*, **102**, 447–454

OKUSA, M., SHIRAISHI, T., KUBO, T. and MATSUNAGA, T. (1993) Tinnitus suppression by electrical promontory stimulation in sensorineural deaf patients. *Acta Otolaryngologica*, Suppl. 501, 54–58

PARKIN, J., RANDOLPH, L. and PARKIN, B. (1993) Multichannel (Ineraid(R)) cochlear implant update. *Laryngoscope*, **103**, 835–840

PARKIN, J. L. (1990) Perutaneous pedestal in cochlear implantation. *Annals of Otology, Rhinology and Laryngology*, **99**, 796–800

PFINGST, B. E., GLASS, I., SPELMAN, F. A. and SUTTON, D. (1985) Psychophysical studies of cochlear implants in monkeys: clinical implications. In: *Cochlear Implants*, edited by R. A. Schindler and M. M. Merzenich. New York: Raven Press. pp. 305–321

PFINGST, B. E., MILLER, J. M., TJELLSTRÖM, A., ALBREKTSSON, T. and CARLISLE, L. (1989) Development of cochlear wall implants for electrical stimulation of the auditory nerve. *Acta Otolaryngologica*, **107**, 210–218

PLOMP, R. and STEENEKEN, H. J. M. (1971) Pitch versus timbre. In: *Proceedings of the 7th International Congress on Acoustics*, (Budapest), pp. 377–380

REBSCHER, S. J. (1985) Cochlear implant design and construction. In: *Cochlear Implants*, edited by R. F. Gray. London: Croom Helm. pp. 74–123

RIZER, F. M., ARKIS, P. N., LIPPY, W. H. and SCHURING, A. G. (1988) A postoperative audiometric evaluation of cochlear implant patients. *Otolaryngology – Head and Neck Surgery*, **98**, 203–206

ROSEN, S. (1989) Temporal information in speech and its relevance for cochlear implants. In: *Cochlear Implant: Acquisitions and Controversies*, edited by B. Fraysse and N. Cochard. Basel: Cochlear AG. pp. 3–26

ROSEN, S. (1990) Electrode placements for cochlear implants: a review. *British Journal of Audiology*, **24**, 411–418

ROSEN, S. (1992) Temporal information in speech: acoustic, auditory and linguistic aspects. *Philosophical Transactions of the Royal Society London B*, **336**, 367–373

ROSEN, S. (1994) Implantable electroacoustic prostheses. *Current Opinion in Otolaryngology and Head and Neck Surgery*, **2**, 209–216

ROSEN, S. and BALL, V. (1986) Speech perception with the Vienna extra-cochlear single-channel implant: a comparison of two approaches to speech coding. *British Journal of Audiology*, **20**, 61–83

ROSEN, S. and CORCORAN, T. (1982) A video-recorded test of lipreading for British English. *British Journal of Audiology*, **16**, 245–254

ROSEN, S., FOURCIN, A. J., ABBERTON, E., WALLIKER, J. R., HOWARD, D. M., MOORE, B. C. J. *et al.* (1985) Assessing assesment. In: *Cochlear Implants*, edited by R. A. Schindler and M. M. Merzenich. New York: Raven Press. pp. 479–498

ROSEN, S., WALLIKER, J. R., FOURCIN, A. J. and BALL, V. (1987) A microprocessor-based acoustic hearing aid for the profoundly impaired listener. *Journal of Rehabilitation Research and Development*, **24**, 239–260

ROSEN, S., WALLIKER, J. R., BRIMACOMBE, J. A. and EDGERTON, B. J. (1989) Prosodic and segmental aspects of speech perception with the House/3m single-channel implant. *Journal of Speech and Hearing Research*, **32**, 93–111

RUGGERO, M. A. (1992) Physiology and coding of sound in the auditory nerve. In: *The Mammalian Auditory Pathway: Neurophysiology*, edited by A. N. Popper and R. R. Fay. New York: Springer-Verlag. pp. 34–93

SCHINDLER, R. and KESSLER, D. (1993) Clarion cochlear implant: Phase I investigational results. *American Journal of Otology*, **14**, 263–272

SCHOUTEN, J. F. (1968) The perception of timbre. *IPO Annual Progress Report (Institute for Perception Research, Eindhoven)*, **3**, 32–34

SHANNON, R., FAYAD, J., MOORE, J., LO, W., OTTO, S., NELSON, R. *et al.* (1993) Auditory brainstem implant: II. Postsurgical issues and performance. *Otolaryngology – Head and Neck Surgery*, **108**, 634–642

SHANNON, R., ZENG, F.-G. and WYGONSKI, J. (1992) Speech recognition using only temporal cues. In: *The Auditory Processing of Speech: From Sounds to Words*, edited by M. E. H. Schouten. New York: Mouton-Gruyer. pp. 263–274

SHANNON, R. V. (1983) Multichannel electrical stimulation of the auditory nerve in man. I. Basic psychophysics. *Human Research*, **11**, 157–189

SHANNON, R. V. (1993) Psychophysics. In: *Cochlear Implants: Audiological Foundations*, edited by R. S. Tyler. London: Whurr. pp. 357–388

SHANNON, R. V., OTTO, S., KUZMA, J. and HELLER, J. (1994) Multi-channel electrical stimulation of the human cochlear nucleus: A preliminary report. In: *Advances in Cochlear Implants*, edited by I. L. Hochmair-Desoyer and E. S. Hochmair. Vienna: Manz. pp. 175–177

SHEPHERD, R. K., WEBB, R. L., CLARK, G. M., PYMAN, B. C., HIRSHORN, M. S., MURRAY, M. T. *et al.* (1984) Implanted material tolerance studies for a multiple-channel cochlear prosthesis. *Acta Otolaryngologica*, Suppl. **411**, 71–81

SIMMONS, F. B. (1966) Electrical stimulation of the auditory nerve in man. *Archives of Otolaryngology*, **84**, 2–54

SIMMONS, F. B. (1985) History of cochlear implants in the United States: a personal perspective. In: *Cochlear Implants*, edited by R. A. Schindler and M. M. Merzenich. New York: Raven Press. pp. 1–7

SKINNER, M. W., HOLDEN, L. K., HOLDEN, T. A., DOWELL, R. C., SELIGMAN, P. M., BRIMACOMBE, J. *et al.* (1991) Performance of postlinguistically deaf adults with the Wearable Speech Processor (WSP III) and Mini Speech Processor (MSP) of the Nucleus Multi-Electrode Cochlear Implant. *Ear and Hearing*, **12**, 3–22

SKINNER, M. W., CLARK, G. M., WHITFORD, L. A., SELIGMAN, P. M., STALLER, S. J., SHIPP, D. B. *et al.* (1994) Evaluation of a new spectral peak (SPEAK) coding strategy for the Nucleus 22 channel cochlear implant system. *American Journal of Otology*, **15** (suppl. 2), 15–27

SOULIERE, C. R., KILENY, P. R., ZWOLAN, T. A. and KEMINK, J. L. (1992) Tinnitus suppression following cochlear implantation. A multifactorial investigation. *Archives of Otolaryngology – Head and Neck Surgery*, **118**, 1291–1297

SUMMERFIELD, Q. (1983) Audio-visual speech perception, lipreading and artificial stimulation. In: *Hearing Science and Hearing Disorders*, edited by M. P. Haggard and M. E. Lutman. London: Academic Press. pp. 131–182

TARTTER, V. C., HELLMAN, S. A. and CHUTE, P. M. (1992) Vowel perception strategies of normal-hearing subjects and patients using Nucleus multichannel and 3M/House cochlear implants. *Journal of the Acoustical Society of America*, **92**, 1269–1283

TOBEY, E. A. (1993) Speech production. In: *Cochlear Implants: Audiological Foundations*, edited by R. S. Tyler. London: Whurr. pp. 257–316

TONG, Y. C., MILLAR, J. B., CLARK, G. M., MARTIN, L. F., BUSBY, P. A. and PATRICK, J. F. (1980) Psychophysical and speech perception studies on two multiple channel cochlear implant patients. *Journal of Laryngology and Otology*, **94**, 1241–1256

TONG, Y. C., CLARK, G. M., BLAMEY, P. J., BUSBY, P. A. and DOWELL, R. C. (1982) Psychophysical studies on two multiple channel cochlear implant patients. *Journal of the Acoustical Society of America*, **71**, 153–160

TONG, Y. C., DOWELL, R. C., BLAMEY, P. J. and CLARK, G. M. (1983) Two component hearing sensations produced by two-electrode stimulation in the cochlea of a totally deaf patient. *Science*, **219**, 993–994

TYE–MURRAY, N. (1993) Aural rehabilitation and patient management. In: *Cochlear Implants: Audiological Foundations*, edited by R. S. Tyler. London: Whurr. pp. 87–143

TYLER, R. S. (ed.) (1993) *Cochlear Implants: Audiological Foundations*. London: Whurr.

TYLER, R. S. and KELSAY, D. (1990) Advantages and disadvantages reported by some of the better cochlear-implant patients. *American Journal of Otology*, **11**, 282–289

TYLER, R. S. and MOORE, B. C. J. (1992) Consonant recognition by some of the better cochlear-implant patients. *Journal of the Acoustical Society of America*, **92**, 3068–3077

TYLER, R. S., MOORE, B. C. J. and KUK, F. K. (1989) Performance of some of the better cochlear-implant patients. *Journal of Speech and Hearing Research*, **32**, 887–911

TYLER, R. S., TYE–MURRAY, N., PREECE, J. P., GANTZ, B. J. and MCCABE, B. F. (1987) Vowel and consonant confusions among cochlear implant patients: do different implants make a difference? *Annals of Otology, Rhinology and Laryngology*, **96** (Suppl. 128), 141–144

VAN DEN HONERT, C. and STYPULKOWSKI, P. H. (1987) Single fiber mapping of spatial excitation patterns in the electrically stimulated auditory nerve. *Hearing Research*, **29**, 195–206

VOLTA, A. (1800) On the electricity excited by mere contact of conducting substances of different kinds. *Transactions of the Royal Society of Philosophy*, **90**, 403–431

WALTZMAN, S. B. (ed.) (1992) A comprehensive evaluation of cochlear implants in adults. *Seminars in Hearing*, **13**, 191–270

WALTZMAN, S. B., COHEN, N. L. and FISHER, S. G. (1992) An experimental comparison of cochlear implant systems. *Seminars in Hearing*, **13**, 195–207

WHITE, M. W. (1983) Formant frequency discrimination and recognition in subjects implanted with intracochlear stimulating electrodes. *Annals of the New York Academy of Science*, **405**, 348–359

WILSON, B., FINLEY, C., LAWSON, D., WOLFORD, R., EDDINGTON, D. and RABINOWITZ, W. (1991) Better speech recognition with cochlear implants. *Nature*, **352**, 236–238

WILSON, B., LAWSON, D., FINLEY, C. and WOLFORD, R. (1993) Importance of patient and processor variables in determining outcomes with cochlear implants. *Journal of Speech and Hearing Research*, **36**, 373–379

WILSON, B., LAWSON, D., ZERBI, M. and FINLEY, C. (1994) Recent developments with the CIS strategies. In: *Advances in Cochlear Implants*, edited by I. J. Hochmair–Desoyer and E. S. Hochmair. Vienna: Manz. pp. 103–112

16

Tactile aids

John C. Stevens

The idea of using the sense of touch as a substitute for hearing in the profoundly or totally hearing impaired is not a new one. Indeed, the profoundly hearing impaired have long made use of vibrotactile sensations to help their awareness of the acoustic environment. One group who has pioneered the use of the tactile sense for communication has been the deaf-blind, together with those involved in their education and rehabilitation. The result has been the development of several methods, of which perhaps the Tadoma technique is best known. Its origins can be traced to the nineteenth century being introduced to the USA in the 1920s by Alcorn (1932). Communication takes place by the listener monitoring with his hand the movements of the faces of the speaker and airflow around the mouth. Although this method of communication applies only to the deaf-blind, the interest for those developing tactile aids for the profoundly hearing impaired is that a significant level of communication is possible. For example, Reed, Durlach and Delhorne (1992) reported that users of Tadoma can achieve good intelligibility at about 60–75% of normal speaking rates for conversational sentence materials.

Many psychophysical studies have been carried out in order to measure the capacity of the sense of touch to convey information. In particular, the ability of the tactile sense to discriminate between different amplitudes, frequency and the timing of vibratory stimuli has been studied. This work was reviewed by Verrillo and Gescheider (1992). In summary, the range of frequencies that can be usefully used in a tactile aid is between 20 and 500 Hz. Sensitivity rapidly reduces above 500 Hz and it is unlikely that valid thresholds are obtainable above 1000 Hz. For sinusoidal stimulation, values of around 25% are reported (Figure 16.1) for the frequency difference limen, which compares very poorly with the ear

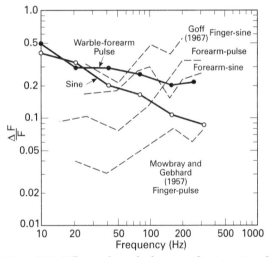

Figure 16.1 Difference limen for frequency discrimination of pulses and sinusoids measured on the volar forearm and finger (----). The results are plotted as the Weber fraction (ΔF/F). In general, the ability to discriminate between frequencies diminishes as frequency increases. However the opposite is true for detection of whether stimuli are frequency modulated (warble tones on the forearm: ——). (From Rothenberg *et al.*, 1977, courtesy of Whurr Publishers Ltd)

which has a frequency difference limen of about 0.3%.

The dynamic range of intensity for vibrotactile stimulation is about 55 dB, which is much smaller than the range for the auditory system. Reports on the smallest detectable intensity difference have varied from 0.4 to 2.3 dB (Verrillo and Gescheider, 1992) which is comparable to that for hearing.

Temporal resolution is often measured by the ability to detect a gap in a continuous stimulus. Verrillo and Gescheider (1992) reported values of around 10 ms in the literature, although there is a lack of experimental data in this area. They reported that these are substantially higher than for the auditory system and suggested that much of the temporally modulated information in speech may fail to be transmitted by a tactile aid.

From this evidence it is clear that the tactile sense can be used for communication, although it has a much smaller information transfer capacity than the auditory system. It is interesting to compare this capacity with cochlear implants as, clearly, the tactile aid offers an alternative to an implant for patients who obtain little or no input through their auditory system, even with maximum amplification. A full discussion of this is given by Blamey and Cowan (1992). They described results of a comparison between the tickle talker (an electrotactile device) and the Nucleus implant. The dynamic range for amplitude and the ability to describe the location of stimuli were comparable. However, pulse rate discrimination was better with the implant except for the best users of the tickle talker. They concluded that a tactile device may offer real advantages over a cochlear implant for certain categories of patients, in particular, those who are prelingually deafened, resulting in poor auditory skills, who are thus less likely to benefit from a cochlear implant.

Electrotactile and vibrotactile devices

Much laboratory experimentation with electrotactile and vibrotactile devices has been carried out over recent decades, although the number of devices that have become commercially available has remained small. Given the options of electrotactile or vibrotactile, single or multi-channel, choice of stimulus location and all the possible options in coding the acoustic signal into a tactile stimulation, it is not surprising that a large number of different devices has been developed.

Electrotactile devices

Lindner (1937) developed a 'teletactor' for deaf mutes. This used audio filters to present high and low frequency stimulation to two fingers. Saunders, in 1973, described a device which presented frequency patterns of sounds to the abdomen via an array of electrodes. He used bursts of pulses where the number of pulses in each burst determined the perceived intensity of the stimulus. A similar device was produced by Spark *et al.* (1979) who used an array of 288 electrodes with the frequency of the sound presented in one dimension and amplitude in the other.

Dodgson *et al.* (1983) produced a wrist-worn device which presented electrical stimulation between two wrist bands. This had the advantage of being entirely self-contained. Tillman and Prioth (1986) produced a 16-channel device to be worn on the forearm with stimulus patterns corresponding to articulatory movements in speech. Lastly, the 'tickle talker', as noted above, of Blamey *et al.* (1988) was developed as an alternative to the Nucleus cochlear implant. This device is shown in Figure 16.2 and has eight electrodes placed over the digital nerve bundles of one hand.

Vibrotactile devices

Gault (1924) pioneered the use of vibrotactile stimulation in deafened subjects. His initial experiments involved subjects placing their palm at the end of a tube, down which words were spoken. He then moved on to develop the teletactor, which was the first multichannel system and used the principle of frequency to place by presenting the output from bandpass filters to vibrators applied to the fingers of one hand. This principle has been used in many subsequent devices such as the 'Felix' developed by Wiener and Wiesner (1949). One important development was the attempt to match the output to the tactile frequency range of the skin.

Guelke and Huyssen (1959) developed a 160-channel device using tuned reed oscillators to stimulate the fingers. Again the principle of frequency to place of stimulation was used.

One device which has received a considerable amount of evaluation is the device produced by Mason, Scilley and Frost (1981). This system consisted of a 16-channel vocoder where the acoustic signal was divided into one-third octave bands across the frequency range 200–8000 Hz. The amplitude was logarithmically compressed before being used to drive one of the 16 vibrators located on the forearm. Brooks *et al.* (1986) described some of the results obtained with this device. One subject was able to acquire a 250-word vocabulary using the tactile aid alone and showed considerable benefits to lipreading.

The vibrotactile devices described so far have not attempted to extract 'speech features' from the acoustic signal and then use these signals to drive the tactile transducers. Several vibrotactile devices of this type have been developed. Kirman (1974) described a device whereby the fundamental voice frequency (F_0) and first formant (F_1) were extracted every 10 ms and presented to one column of a 15 by 15 array on the fingers. The complete array contained the F_0 and F_1 output for the previous 150 ms. Ifukebe (1982) described a system in which a variety of speech features were presented to a two by three array on the fingertip. Boothroyd (1985) described a

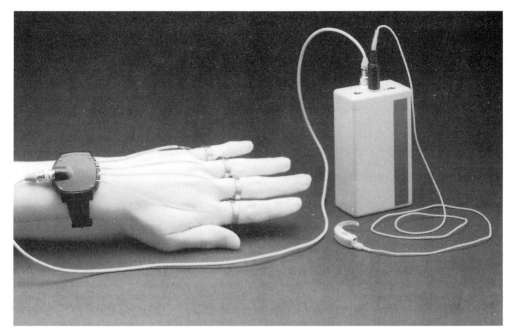

Figure 16.2 The Tickle Talker, a tactile hearing prosthesis which converts speech sounds to patterns of electrical stimulation sensed through digital nerve bundles on either side of the fingers on the non-dominant hand. (Courtesy of the Human Communication Research Centre, The University of Melbourne)

device where the logarithm of the F_0 frequency determines the location of the vibrotactile stimulation on the forearm using either eight or 16 channels. The Tactaid 7 is shown in Figure 16.3. The processing strategy used is that each channel is assigned to cover a frequency band within the first and second formants. A constant excitation frequency of 250 Hz is used. For a more detailed review, particularly of the processing strategies, the reader is referred to Mason and Frost (1992).

Despite the efforts of many workers over the last six decades, commercially manufactured tactile devices have only recently been available. Examples of these are the minifonator from Siemens PLC, the Tactaid 2 and 7 from Audiological Engineering Inc., and the Tactile Acoustic Monitor (TAM) from Summit. Compared to some of the devices described above, apart from the Tactaid 7, these devices use relatively simple coding of the acoustic signal into tactile stimulation. A comparative evaluation of four aids, including the minifonator, TAM and Tactaid 2 was carried out by Thornton and Philips (1992). As would be expected with three of the four devices being single channel and with the relatively simple coding, the benefit to speech-reading was limited. However, responses to the questionnaire showed that many of the users found the device of benefit for hearing environmental sounds and for voice control.

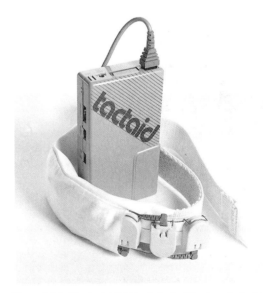

Figure 16.3 The tactaid 7 (Audiological Engineering) which uses seven vibrators in a flexible array which can be worn on various body sites

Clinical application

It is important to accept at the start that consideration of the clinical application of tactile aids will depend on many factors, such as whether the deafness is pre- or postlingual, the benefit obtained from hearing aids and the likely benefit that would be obtained from a cochlear implant. In the following discussion it is assumed that the deafness is of such a degree that the subject will obtain more benefit from an implant or tactile aid than from amplification by a hearing aid.

The first group to be considered is the *postlingually profoundly deafened adults*. Experience has shown that this category of patients does very well with multichannel cochlear implants, some having recognition of open set speech material without speech-reading. This level of communication has never been achieved with tactile device users, although, as described previously, the deaf-blind have achieved open set communication at reduced rates, suggesting that the capacity is there to achieve some assistance with a tactile device. Blamey and Cowan (1992) noted in their comparison of tactile aids with implants that, although the information carrying capacity of a tactile device for some users is comparable (as noted above), the technological investment has largely been in implants with tactile devices being seen as a 'second best'. They concluded, therefore, that part of this difference in performance in practice may be due to the lack of technological investment in tactile aids. However, compared with the currently available tactile devices, the cochlear implant remains the method of choice in this group and a tactile aid will only be considered where an implant is not fitted for a particular reason.

The second group to be considered is the *prelingually deafened adults*. Clark *et al.* (1987) have reported that cochlear implant users in this group obtain very little benefit. Two explanations given for this are their lack of auditory skills and their lack of motivation to learn a new method of communication given that they have developed non-auditory methods. There is therefore the possibility that this group can make use of their normally developed tactile sense, particularly in areas such as awareness of environmental sounds, which is not easily obtained in any other way.

The third group to be considered are *profoundly hearing impaired children*. Blamey and Cowan (1992) reported studies comparing results of the tickle talker and cochlear implants, each used by a different group of eight children. All the tickle talker group also wore hearing aids whereas only one implantee used a hearing aid in the non-implanted ear. The results suggested that the tickle talker group were performing at a higher level on a BKB sentence test. They concluded that tactile devices such as the tickle talker appear to offer an alternative for this category of the profoundly hearing impaired.

The last group to be considered are those whose hearing loss is not sufficient normally to consider an implant as being beneficial. Although the majority in this category are likely to benefit more from a hearing aid, the use of a tactile aid may provide a useful supplement, particularly where the aided thresholds with the hearing aid are high. The tactile aid could provide information on the quieter high frequency part of speech and useful information on environmental sounds. However, implants are now being used for the hearing impaired in this category and the application of tactile aids may well be reduced, if this proves successful, although the much lower cost of a tactile aid will weigh in its favour where an implant is not considered to be cost-effective.

Training programmes

A detailed description of suitable training programmes for tactile aids was given by Plant (1992). He stated that it is critical that a training programme should commence immediately after the tactile aid has been fitted. The programme will differ depending whether the hearing loss is congenital or acquired. The effect of training programmes on the acquisition of speech perception skills by tactile aid users has received little attention in the literature (Alcantara *et al.*, 1990a). Plant commented that this is surprising in that most tactile aids do not present speech information in a manner with which the subject is already familiar. For this reason he noted that it seems reasonable to assume that some formal training will be required in order to accelerate the level of perception of speech with the aid. As evidence for this he reported on work from an earlier study (Alcantara *et al.*, 1990b) which suggested that a group of subjects who received a combination of feature (analytic) and conversational (synthetic) training improved to a greater extent on feature-level recognition tests than did the group who received only conversational training. By contrast, the group who only had the conversational training did better on the conversational level tests.

Paediatric

Training programmes were established for the early vibrotactile aids as long ago as 1934 (Goodfellow). He emphasized the need to use the Gault Teletactor as an aid to speech-reading. Plant (1992) noted that this early work, in many ways resembled programmes currently provided to children. His own training programme, devised specifically for the Tactaid 2 (Plant, 1988), requires practice of pattern perception by carrying out exercises in four basic areas of sound detection, pattern perception, word syllable number and type, and high frequency detection. In general, the tasks are increased in complexity as the training proceeds. In addition, Plant noted that children fitted with tactile aids should be provided with exercises which provide the opportunity to practise using their tactile aids as a supplement to lip-reading. Again exercises start in a simple way by asking the child to identify single words by selecting between two or three pictures, the teacher then expanding the choice as the child is able to make more use of the tactile aid.

Adult

The main aim of training programmes in adults with acquired hearing loss is to enhance their communication skills. Plant (1992) described the commtram programme which he devised as a suitable method of training. The training includes both tactile alone and visual with tactile training, using both an analytic approach and a synthetic approach. Examples of tasks involved in the tactile only part of the training are identification of vowel and consonant contrasts and environmental sounds. For the visual plus tactile training, methods include the techniques of continuous discourse tracking (de Filippo and Scott, 1978), where the therapist reads from a prepared text section by section, the subject repeating the test as accurately as possible. The number of words correctly identified per minute is used as a measure of communication ability. Plant concluded that training should include both synthetic and analytic approaches using both the tactile alone and tactile plus visual training to achieve tactile integration with the visual (speech-reading) information. The training programme should be designed to suit the age of the subject, the nature of the hearing loss and the type of aid used and should be tailored to suit the individual needs of the subject.

Summary

In summary, tactile devices for the profoundly hearing impaired have not, as yet, offered the promise that data from psychophysical laboratory experiments would suggest. Although these data indicate that, in some cases, they offer an alternative to cochlear implantation, with comparable information transfer capacity in some subjects, performance in speech tests in practice for post-lingually deafened adults is much poorer. One theory for this is the unfamiliar nature of the tactile stimulation compared with the acoustic nature of implant stimulation. It is noted that this difference would be less in the case of prelingually deafened subjects.

The current application of tactile aids is largely in those patients who are unable to have a cochlear implant fitted for any reason. However, as the technology of tactile aids improves and starts to match the technology of implants, it may be that their application widens to include more of those who are not suitable for a cochlear implant and where the benefit obtained from hearing aids is marginal. For a more detailed review of the current literature the reader is referred to the recent book on tactile aids edited by Summers (1992).

References

ALCANTARA, J. I., WHITFORD L. A., BLAMEY, P. J., COWAN, R. S. C. and CLARK, G. M. (1990a) Speech feature recognition by profoundly hearing impaired children using a multiple-channel electrotactile speech processor and aided residual hearing. *Journal of the Acoustical Society of America*, **88**, 1260–1273

ALCANTARA, J. I., COWAN, R. S. C., BLAMEY, P. J. and CLARK, G. M. (1990b) A comparison of two training strategies for speech recognition with an electrotactile speech processor. *Journal of Speech and Hearing Research*, **33**, 195–204

ALCORN, S. (1932) The Tadoma method. *Volta Review*, **34**, 195–198

BLAMEY, P. J. and COWAN, R. S. C. (1992) The potential benefit and cost effectiveness of tactile devices in comparison to implants. In: *Tactile Aids for the Hearing Impaired*, edited by I. R. Summers. London, Whurr. pp.187–217

BLAMEY, P. J., COWAN, R. S. C., ALCANTARA, J. I. and CLARK, G. M. (1988) Phonetic information transmitted by a multichannel electrotactile speech processor. *Journal of Speech and Hearing Research*, **31**, 620–629

BOOTHROVD, A. (1985) A wearable tactile intonation display for the deaf. *IEEE Transactions in Acoustics Speech Signal Processing*, **33**, 111–117

BROOKS, P. L., FROST, B. J., MASON, J. L. and GIBSON, D. M. (1986) Continuing evaluation of the Queen's University tactile vocoder I: identification of open-set words. *Journal of Rehabilitation Research and Development*, **23**, 119–128

CLARK, G. M., BUSBY, P. A., ROBERTS, S. A., DOWELL, R. C., BLAMEY, P. J., MECKLENBURG, D. J. *et al.* (1987) Preliminary results for the Cochlear Corporation multielectrode intracochlear implant in six pre-lingually deaf patients. *American Journal of Otology*, **8**, 234–239

DE FILIPPO, C. L. and SCOTT, B. L. R. (1978) A method for training and evaluating the reception of ongoing speech. *Journal of the Acoustical Society of America*, **63**, 1186–1192

DODGSON, G. S., BROWN, B. H., FREESTON, I. L. and STEVENS, J. C. (1983) Electrical stimulation at the wrist as an aid for the profoundly deaf. *Clinical Physics and Physiological Measurement*, **4**, 403–416

GAULT, R. H. (1924) Progress in experiments on tactual interpretation of oral speech. *Journal of Abnormal and Social Psychology*, **19**, 155–159

GOFF, G. D. (1967) Differential discrimination of frequency of cutaneous mechanical vibration. *Journal of Experimental Psychology*, **74**, 294–299

GOODFELLOW, L. D. (1934) Experiments on the senses of touch and vibration. *Journal of the Acoustical Society of America*, **6**, 45–50

GUELKE, R. W. and HUYSSEN, R. M. J. (1959) Development of apparatus for the analysis of sound by the sense of touch. *Journal of the Acoustical Society of America*, **31**, 799–809

IFUKEBE, T. (1982) A cued tactual vocoder. In: *Uses of Computers in Aiding the Disabled*, edited by J. Ravin. Amsterdam: North Holland. pp. 197–215

KIRMAN, J. H. (1974) Tactile perception of computer-derived formant patterns from voiced speech. *Journal of the Acoustical Society of America*, **55**, 163–169

LINDNER, R. (1937) The physiological fundamentals of the electrical speech feeling and their application in the training of deaf mutes. *Z Sinnesphysiol.*, **67**, 114–144

MASON, J. L. and FROST, B. J. (1992) Signal processing strategies for multichannel systems. In: *Tactile Aids for the Hearing Impaired*, edited by I. R. Summers. London: Whurr. pp. 128–145

MASON, J. L., SCILLEY, P. L. and FROST, B. J. (1981) A vibrotactile auditory prosthetic device. *IEEE Conference Digest*, 104–106

MOWBRAY, G. H. and GEBHARD, J. W. (1957) Sensitivity of the skin to changes in the rate of intermittent mechanical stimuli. *Science*, **125**, 1297–1298

PLANT, G. (1988) *A Communication Training Programme for the Profoundly Deaf Adult*. National Acoustics Laboratory, Australia. NAL 122 no. 2142.8

PLANT, G. (1992) The selection and training of tactile users. In: *Tactile Aids for the Hearing Impaired*, edited by I. R. Summers. London: Whurr. pp. 146–166

REED, C. M., DURLACH, N. I. and DELHORNE, L. A. (1992) Natural methods of tactile communication. In: *Tactile Aids for the Hearing Impaired*, edited by I. R. Summers. London: Whurr. pp. 218–230

ROTHENBERG, M., VERRILLO, R. T., ZAHORIAN, S. A., BRACHMAN, M. L. and BOLANOWSKI, S. J. JR (1977) Vibrotactile frequency for encoding a speech parameter. *Journal of the Acoustical Society of America*, **62**, 1003–1012

SAUNDERS, F. A. (1973) Electrocutaneous displays. In: *Cutaneous Communications Systems and Devices*, edited by F. A. Geldard. Austin: The Psychonomic Society. pp. 20–26

SPARKS, D. W., KUHL, P. K., EDMONDS, A. E. and GRAY, G. P. (1979) Investigating the MESA: The transmission of connected discourse. *Journal of the Acoustical Society of America*, **65**, 810–815

SUMMERS, I. R. (ed.) (1992) *Tactile Aids for the Hearing Impaired*. London: Whurr

THORNTON, A. R. D. and PHILIPS, A. J. (1992) A comparative trial of four vibrotactile aids. In: *Tactile Aids for the Hearing Impaired*, edited by I. R. Summers. London: Whurr. pp. 231–252

TILLMAN, H. G. and PRIOTH, H. G. (1986) System for electrocutaneous stimulation. *Journal of the Acoustical Society of America*, **79**, (Suppl. 1)

VERRILLO, R. T. and GESCHEIDER, G. A. (1992) Perception via the sense of touch. In: *Tactile Aids for the Hearing Impaired*, edited by I. R. Summers. London: Whurr. pp. 1–36

WEINER, N. and WEISNER, J. (1949–1951) Felix (sensory replacement project). *Quarterly Progress Report*. RLE Cambridge: Massachusetts Institute of Technology

17

Central auditory dysfunction

Linda M. Luxon and Mazal Cohen

Central auditory dysfunction has generated growing interest over the last three decades for a number of reasons. Academically, there remains a challenge, as despite considerable progress in the understanding and management of 'peripheral' auditory dysfunction, the relationship between structure and function in the central auditory nervous system, in both health and disease, remains largely ill defined. Nonetheless, it has been demonstrated that early auditory deprivation may interfere with appropriate neuronal development of the central auditory nervous system and the important early role of development and maturation of central auditory processing in facilitating the development of language perception and production has been recognized. At the other end of the spectrum, the age-related changes that take place in the higher levels of the auditory perceptual system have been shown markedly to reduce the ability of aged listeners to understand speech under less than optimal listening conditions (Willott, 1991a). In addition, the pathogenesis of many types of hearing losses, once considered to be entirely peripheral, has now been shown to have a central auditory component, e.g. degeneration in the auditory pathways has been documented following exposure to noise (Willott, 1991a). Importantly, in the last decade, the structural resolution of MRI has allowed pathology in the central nervous system to be defined accurately and correlated with electrophysiological and/or psychophysical auditory tests.

The central auditory nervous system (Figure 17.1) is anatomically and physiologically complex. There are about 30 000 neural fibres in the auditory division of the VIIIth cranial nerve, but that number increases to some 250 000 in the auditory radiation between the nucleus of the medial geniculate body and the primary auditory cortex. In addition to this increase in neural substrate from the cochlea to the auditory cortex, there is an increase in the complexity of auditory processing, with a greater number of facets of auditory function, subserved at higher auditory levels, and multiple representations of each ear, on each side of the brain, at each level of the ascending auditory pathways.

These structural features of the central auditory nervous system result in a marked intrinsic redundancy, which results in a resistance of this system to exhibit deficits on standard auditory testing. Indeed, behavioural studies have shown that ablation of the auditory cortex does not lead to a complete loss of simple function, as, for example, in the visual system. In addition, many disorders which give rise to central auditory dysfunction are diffuse in nature and thus may affect more than one site in the central auditory nervous system, e.g. multiple sclerosis and vascular disease. Until the advent of MRI it had proved difficult to identify well-delineated lesions affecting the central auditory nervous system to allow correlation of abnormalities of structure and function. A further confounding factor is that a single neurological lesion may affect more than one site in the central auditory nervous system by interference with neural transmission, alteration of biochemical factors within the brain tissue, alteration of neurotransmitter function by pressure effects in the case of a tumour or reduction in blood flow. Thus, the precise association between central auditory dysfunction and site of lesion may be difficult to determine even in the face of excellent imaging techniques.

Not infrequently, the patient with pathology affecting the central auditory nervous system presents with neurological symptoms and signs unaccompanied by any complaint of hearing impairment. CT or MRI may define a structural abnormality in the brain stem, thalamus or cortex, while magnetic resonance angiography may identify a vascular deficit, but metabolic disease may defy such techniques (Spitzer and

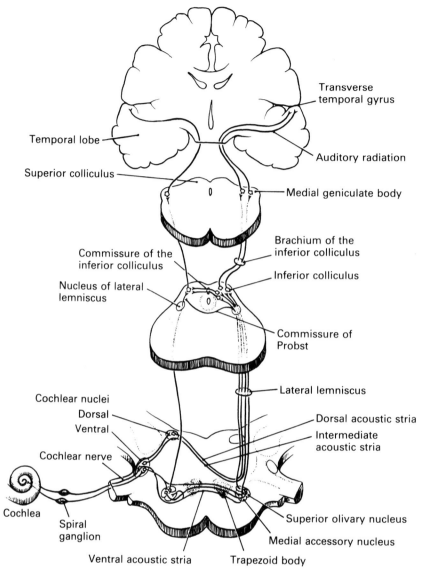

Figure 17.1 Diagram to illustrate the central auditory pathways. (From Benjamin, E. E. and Todd Troust, B. (1988) Central auditory disorders. In: *Otolaryngology 1*, edited by G. M. English. Philadelphia: J. B. Lippincott Co)

Ventry, 1980; Kustel *et al.*, 1993). Nonetheless, central auditory testing may highlight abnormalities of value in diagnosis. The aims of this chapter are therefore fourfold:

1 To outline briefly the anatomy and physiology of the central auditory system.
2 To highlight normal ageing changes in the central auditory nervous system.
3 To review psychophysical and electrophysiological tests which provide insight into central auditory dysfunction.

4 To review auditory disorders in brain stem and cortical pathology.

Anatomy and physiology

A brief review of the relevant anatomy (see Figure 17.1) and physiology of the central auditory nervous system facilitates a better understanding of central auditory tests that are used to define brain stem and cortical pathology.

The afferent auditory system

The central auditory nervous system begins at the neuroglia–neurolemma junction of the VIIIth cranial nerve within the internal auditory meatus. This junction separates central or glial derived myelin from peripheral or Schwann cell derived myelin. It is located 7–13 mm distal to the brain stem, usually being shorter in females and longer in males.

The central processes of the bipolar ganglion cells in the spiral ganglion form the myelinated cochlear portion of the VIIIth cranial nerve. There is a tonotopic arrangement of fibres within the nerve, with fibres subserving low frequency sounds, from the apex of the organ of Corti in the core of the nerve, while the basal fibres subserving high frequency sounds surround the apical fibres on the surface of the nerve (Sando, 1965).

The *cochlear nerve* enters the dorsolateral brain stem at the junction of the pons and medulla (Figure 17.2). The fibres divide into an ascending branch, which terminates on the anteroventral cochlear nucleus, and a descending fibre, which terminates either on the posteroventral nucleus or on the dorsal nucleus. The tonotopic organization of the auditory system is preserved at all levels of the central auditory nervous system and, within the cochlear nuclei, apical fibres terminate in the ventral part of the dorsal cochlear nucleus and in the ventral nucleus, while fibres from the basal portion of the cochlea terminate in the dorsal part of the dorsal cochlear nucleus (Carpenter, 1976).

Fibres from the *cochlear nuclei* project to both the ipsilateral and contralateral superior olivary nuclear complex, which lies in the lower pons but some fibres from the dorsal cochlear nucleus bypass the superior olivary complex and cross the median raphe via the dorsal acoustic stria and project directly in the contralateral lateral lemniscus to the inferior colliculus. The intermediate acoustic stria arises from the posterior portion of the ventral cochlear nucleus and passes medially through the reticular formation into the contralateral lateral lemniscus (Osen, 1972). The ventral acoustic stria arises from cells in the ventral cochlear nucleus and passes medially along the ventral border of the pontine tegmentum forming the trapezoid body. These fibres terminate in the reticular formation and the contralateral superior olivary complex.

The *superior olivary complex* is comprised of three nuclear groups: the medial and lateral superior olives and the nucleus of the trapezoid body. It is about 4 mm long and extends from the level of the facial nucleus in the pons to approximately the level of the motor nucleus of the trigeminal nerve. It is the first relay station both to receive and process binaural input from the organs of Corti. Thus, lesions at the level of the superior olivary complex or more rostrally in the central auditory nervous system do not give rise to unilateral hearing loss (Galambos, Schwartzkopff and Rupert, 1959).

The medial nucleus responds mainly to low frequency sounds, while the lateral nucleus responds to all auditory frequencies. Each of these nuclei is com-

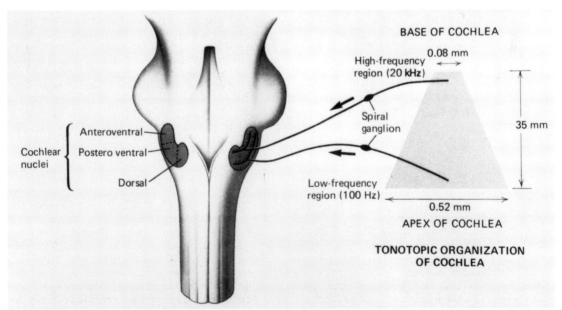

Figure 17.2 Diagram to illustrate the tonotopic projections of the fibres of the cochlear nerve from the basilar membrane of the cochlea to the cochlear nuclei. (From Noback, C. R. and Demarest, R. J. (1981) *The Human Nervous System.* 3rd edn. New York: McGrawhill, with permission)

posed of bipolar neurons, one pole of which receives neural input from the ipsilateral cochlear nuclei, while the other pole receives input from the contralateral cochlear nuclei. Thus, when a sound reaches one ear a fraction of a second prior to the other ear, the interaural time and intensity differences are conveyed to the bipolar neurons of the superior olivary nuclei, and thus allow interpretation of the localization of the source of the sound.

The *lateral lemniscus* is the principal ascending auditory pathway within the brain stem and lies within the lateral zone of the brain stem tegmentum. The nuclei of the lateral lemniscus, which are aggregations of cells within the tract of the lateral lemniscus, represent the next level of auditory function and, as at all levels within the central auditory nervous system, receive both ipsilateral and contralateral inputs. Projections from these cells run to the midbrain where they terminate in the inferior colliculus. Lemniscal fibres do not synapse within these nuclei but run uninterrupted to the inferior colliculus (Goldberg and Moore, 1967; Adams, 1979).

The *inferior colliculus* has been called the obligatory relay nuclear complex, as it serves as a relay station for all ascending and descending auditory fibres. It is divided into a central nucleus, the 'core', which is tonotopically organized in a laminated manner, and peripheral grey matter, which is known as the 'belt' and receives input from not only auditory stimuli, but also the spinothalamic tract and the medial lemniscus. The colliculi are joined by the commissure of the inferior colliculus. Interaural time-intensity comparisons occur at this level and so the inferior colliculus is also important in auditory localization. Animal work has demonstrated tonotopic organization within the central nucleus of the inferior colliculus, with low frequency fibres sited superficially and high frequency fibres in the deeper layers of the nucleus.

In addition to receiving ascending afferent fibres, the inferior colliculus receives descending projections from the ipsilateral medial geniculate body and the auditory cortex, both ipsilaterally and contralaterally.

Fibres project from the inferior colliculus to the *medial geniculate body*, which is on the caudal aspect of the thalamus (Figure 17.3) and is the final major relay centre for ascending auditory fibres before they reach the auditory cortex. In addition, the medial geniculate body receives projections from the spinothalamic tract, the medial lemniscus, the cerebellum and the superior colliculus. The structure is divided into a small-celled dorsal nucleus, known as the pars principalis, and a large-celled ventral nucleus. A tonotopic arrangement has been demonstrated in the medial geniculate body with low frequencies represented laterally and high frequencies located medially (Carpenter, 1976).

Physiological studies suggest that the brain stem

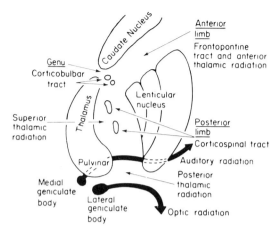

Figure 17.3 Diagram to show the relationships of the auditory pathway at the level of the medial geniculate body

auditory nuclei contribute to central auditory processing in a number of ways:

1 The integration of auditory inputs from the two ears.
2 The extraction of auditory signals from background noise over a wide range of stimulus intensity.
3 The processing of interaural intensity and timing differences.
4 The coding of the direction of sound in space.
5 The perception of frequency and amplitude modulated tones.

A number of auditory tests aimed at assessing brain stem function utilize the ability of the central auditory pathways to receive different auditory inputs from each ear and unify the information into a single recognizable and vocally reproducible event. Several studies have indicated that dichotic integration tasks appear more sensitive to brain stem lesions than dichotic separation tasks (see Tests of brain stem function).

Finally, fibres project in the auditory radiation from the medial geniculate body to the *primary auditory cortex*, Brodmann's areas 41 and 42 (Figure 17.4), which lies on the superior surface of the temporal lobe facing the lateral fissure. The primary auditory cortex known as the 'core', is tonotopically organized with the highest frequencies located caudomedially and the lowest frequencies located rostrolaterally. Brodmann's area 41 histologically resembles other primary cortical sensory regions known as koniocortex. However, Imig and Adrian (1977) have shown orthogonal organization of columns of cells from each ear perhaps related to stimulus location in space.

Surrounding the primary auditory cortex are several cortical fields or 'belt' regions, areas 52 and 22, which receive projections from the medial geniculate body and other thalamic groups. The audi-

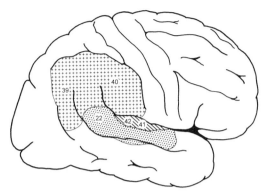

Figure 17.4 Diagram of the lateral aspect of the right cerebral hemisphere to show the primary auditory cortex (Brodmann areas 41 and 42) and the association area (area 22) together with the sensory speech areas (areas 39 and 40)

tory cortex therefore seems to continue the core and belt organization of the lower auditory nuclei. The 'belt' area is less specifically auditory than the 'core' area and has a greater proportion of multisensory input.

The auditory cortex has intrahemispheric connections which include area 8, the frontal eye fields and an area of multisensory cortex including areas 39, 40 and 22, in which auditory input is integrated with inputs from the visual and somatosensory cortices.

Each auditory cortical area is also reciprocally connected to a homeotypic area in the contralateral hemisphere via projections in the corpus callosum and the anterior commissure. The corpus callosum is a band of nerve fibres which serves as a channel through which synchronization of hemispheric function occurs and duplication, or competition of effort is prevented. In spite of these complex functions, split brain subjects do not have serious auditory problems and, even in callosal agenesis, auditory abnormalities are subtle (Temple, Jeeves and Vilarroya, 1989, 1990). This, in part, reflects that hemisphere disconnection is rarely complete and, in part, suggests that the role of the corpus callosum is perhaps more important in early life, but once the differences between the hemispheres have been established, the commissural role is not so critical.

Early electrophysiological work in animals has shown that an auditory stimulus has multiple representations in the cortex and, on the basis of observations on the auditory cortex of the monkey, there are five, or seven, or maybe even more, separate delineated representations in the cortex (Merzenich, 1982). It would appear that these are more than just expressions of tonotopic representations, and are of other perceptual dimensions, such as sound localization and distance of the vocalizing object from the listener.

It has therefore been concluded that the auditory cortex in man is important in the auditory processing of time, intensity and frequency parameters. On the basis of animal experiments, Pickles (1988) has identified a number of functions of the auditory cortex:

1 The cortex has a role in the analysis of complex sound such as speech and, indeed, electrophysiological experiments indicate that certain neurons are driven only by complex sounds.
2 The auditory cortex would appear to be necessary in the discrimination of auditory stimuli of short duration (less than 10 ms) as this task is impaired in brain-damaged people and lesioned animals. Moreover, the auditory cortex plays an important role in pattern discrimination when it is necessary to relate two or more stimuli separated in time.
3 It has been suggested that it is not possible to form the concept of auditory space without the auditory cortex and the primary auditory cortex is thought to subserve sound localization.
4 It would appear that difficult tasks are more easily affected by cortical lesions than are simple auditory tasks. In other words, it is not the difficulty of the task itself but the complexity of the strategy used by the animal in solving it, which determines whether a deficit results. One function of the auditory cortex may involve storing and utilizing strategies.
5 Ear selection and selective attention, in which it is possible to pay attention to stimuli in one ear, while ignoring stimuli presented simultaneously to the other ear, have been attributed to auditory cortical function. There is also anatomical and electrophysiological evidence to support the dominance of auditory projections to the contralateral hemisphere.

Penfield and Jasper (1954) demonstrated that electrical stimulation in the area of the primary auditory cortex produced a perception of elementary sound such as the noise of a cricket, ringing of a bell or the sound of a whistle. However, stimulation away from the fissure in the auditory association areas resulted in the perception of sound such as the barking of a dog or the perception of a human voice. Thus it would appear that the association areas are responsible for more complex interpretation of sound. This may in part explain why patients with lesions of the auditory cortex may have little difficulty perceiving pure tone sounds, but experience difficulty with degraded or masked speech.

The efferent auditory system

In addition to the ascending auditory system, there is a parallel descending system, although the role of this efferent pathway has not been fully clarified (Figure 17.5). The pathway arises from fibres in the

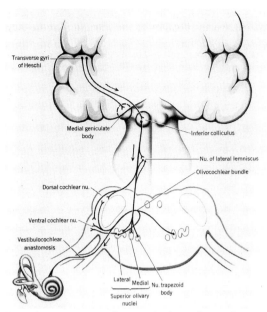

Figure 17.5 Diagram to illustrate the descending auditory pathways. The fibres of the olivocochlear bundle emerge from the medulla through the vestibular nerve and then pass via the vestibulocochlear anastomosis of the cochlear nerve. (From Noback, C. R. and Demarest, R. J. (1981) *The Human Nervous System*, 3rd edn. New York: McGrawhill, with permission)

auditory cortex, which pass via the medial geniculate body, the inferior colliculus, the superior olivary complex, and the nuclei of the lateral lemniscus, and thence directly from the lateral lemniscus and indirectly via the superior olivary complex to the cochlear nuclei. The main efferent pathway to the organ of Corti is known as the olivocochlear bundle which originates in the superior olivary complex bilaterally with both ipsilateral and contralateral projections. The more numerous crossed fibres (approximately 400) form the medial olivocochlear bundle which terminates exclusively on outer hair cells in the organ of Corti, while approximately 100 uncrossed fibres, forming the lateral olivocochlear bundle, terminate in the nerve plexus of the inner hair cells (Kimura and Wersall, 1962). Extensive investigation of the effect of sectioning the olivocochlear bundle in man has revealed only a marked improvement in the detection of unexpected signals in noise which was interpreted as reflecting impaired selective attention (Scharf *et al.*, 1994). The authors suggested that the major influence of the olivocochlear bundle may be developmental rather than intrinsically in processing auditory stimuli. Nonetheless, animal work has shown that electrical stimulation of the olivocochlear bundle in the floor of the IVth ventricle reduces

cochlear responses to contralateral acoustic stimuli (Galambos, 1956) and recent work has shown the failure of suppression of otoacoustic emissions following olivocochlear bundle section, as a consequence of vestibular neurectomy (Williams, Brookes and Prasher, 1994).

Ageing and the central auditory system

Age-related changes in the cochlear nucleus have not been clearly defined. Konigsmark and Murphy (1970, 1972) and Crace (1970) described a reduction in the 'volume' of the cochlear nuclei, but no significant change in the number of neurons with age. Degenerative changes within the cells, including an increase in lipofuscin, were noted. Similarly, Ferraro and Minckler (1977a) failed to identify a significant decrease in the size or number of neurons within the lateral lemniscus with age, although there was a significant decline in the total number of lateral lemniscal fibres. Assessing the inferior colliculus, the same authors found little evidence of loss of neurons or fibres (Ferraro and Minckler, 1977b).

Brody (1955), in his classic work on the cerebral cortex, assessed the auditory cortex in brains obtained from newborn to 95-year-old subjects. In comparison with other cortical areas, the superior temporal cortex had the greatest loss of cells and the strongest correlation coefficient (-0.99) with age. Cell size did not appear to be significantly affected by age, but thickness of the superior temporal gyrus decreased with age. Moreover, Hansen and Reske–Nielsen (1965) demonstrated gliosis and the accumulation of granules and amyloid in the cells of temporal lobes of the elderly, while Scheibel *et al.* (1975) documented a range of pathological changes in superior temporal cortical neurons and considered the progressive loss of horizontally orientated dendrites to be of particular importance, as they suggested that this led to the loss of synaptic interactions and subtle aspects of cortical function.

Thus, the limited evidence available on ageing changes in the central auditory nervous system in man shows most marked changes in the cochlear nuclei and the auditory cortex, although the functional significance of these changes remains uncertain as no study has assessed central auditory function prior to post-mortem histological examination. Moreover, there is little work available on the histopathology of the ageing central auditory nervous system in animals (Willott, 1991a), although on the basis of the studies available certain observations can be made. First, age-related changes appear to differ among neuron types. Second, significant genetic influences appear to be active with respect to age related histopathology. Third, there is very considerable individual variation of age-related histopathological changes (Willott, 1991a).

Physiologically, the effect of age-related changes in the central auditory nervous system has been studied in animals as techniques currently available to monitor the potentials of individual neurons in the brain cannot be used in humans. Willott (1991a) noted that while histopathological correlates of ageing in the central auditory nervous system are not greatly affected by peripheral pathology, this is not the case with respect to physiological responses. In mice, high frequency hearing loss causes a marked disruption of normal auditory responses, while ageing per se has a less pronounced effect on neuronal responses. He highlighted that 'sluggish' neurons become more common with ageing, although relatively normal response properties are the rule among surviving physiologically responsive neurons. Other age-related physiological changes include an increase in spontaneous neural activity in the cochlear nuclei, a reduction of the inhibitory gamma aminobutyric acid (GABA) system (in rats) and maintenance of energy metabolism in elderly auditory neurons. These facts would all be compatible with an increase in 'neural noise' in the elderly, but the functional significance of this in the central auditory nervous system remains unknown.

Two further changes that have been defined as a result of animal work have interesting implications (Willott, 1991b). First, tonotopic organization has been shown to be disrupted in the inferior colliculus with age and it would be expected that this would cause problems with the neural coding of frequency. Indeed, frequency discrimination and resolution are usually diminished in older people and the deficits are often not directly related to the degree of hearing loss, implying central pathology. Second, in C57 mice, it has been shown that the thresholds of neurons in the ventral cochlear nucleus are more severely affected by peripheral impairment than those in the dorsal cochlear nucleus. As different levels and parts of the central auditory system subserve different functions, it follows that peripheral pathology may affect various auditory functions in different ways. Thus, peripheral hearing loss may affect various perceptual functions in humans in a complex and multifaceted manner.

In conclusion, while the human and animal data on age related changes in the central auditory system are limited, it is clear that changes do occur and may seriously affect the perception of sound. Of relevance to this chapter, it cannot be overemphasized that tests of central auditory function must always be considered in the light of peripheral auditory activity and age.

Tests of central auditory function

As noted earlier, standard audiometric tests have proven ineffective in detecting the subtle deficits result-ing from pathology in the central auditory nervous system, partly because of the intrinsic redundancy within the central auditory nervous system and, partly, because of the extrinsic redundancy in both tonal and speech stimuli. Thus, a variety of tests have been designed in order to challenge the complexity of central auditory processing in the frequency, intensity and temporal domains. Clinical research in this area began some four decades ago with the classical studies of the Italian investigators, principally Bocca and Calearo and coworkers (Bocca, Calearo and Cassinari, 1954; Bocca et al., 1955) and a plethora of papers has been published since this time. Nonetheless, a standard central auditory test battery, which allows comparison of results from centre to centre has not been established. Thus, the correlation and interpretation of published results is hampered by the variability of test procedures, the variety and diffuse nature of pathologies studied, the difficulty in extrapolating animal work to man, the complexity of the central auditory nervous system and the unpredictable manifestations of factors such as age, sex, linguistic ability, intelligence and peripheral labyrinthine pathology (Katz, 1994) on test results in any given subject.

Central auditory tests can be divided into *behavioural* tests, which require patient cooperation in responding to a given stimulus, and *objective* tests, which do not require patient cooperation and provide recordable data in response to an acoustical stimulus. Objective tests include assessments of stapedial reflex thresholds, auditory brain stem responses and otoacoustic emission suppression with contralateral sound.

Objective tests are of particular value in assessing the brain stem. *Acoustic reflex threshold* measurements are directed at assessing the pathways of the acoustic reflex arc from the cochlea through the VIIIth nerve to the low brain stem; but they provide no useful application in detecting central auditory pathologies beyond these structures. *Electrophysiological test procedures*, particularly the auditory brain stem responses (ABR) and, to a lesser extent, the middle latency response and slow vertex potentials (SVR), have proved highly sensitive in detecting central auditory nervous system pathologies without the intersubject variability, which is so confounding in behavioural tests. Nonetheless, the correlation of the electrophysiological findings with auditory function is not entirely understood.

Behavioural tests (Table 17.1) are useful in the detection and localization of central auditory nervous system pathologies and have been used extensively in experiments designed to further our understanding of the pathophysiology of the central auditory nervous system, in that they provide a measure of the functional deficit resulting from a particular lesion. They may be grouped together into tests which share a common parameter, such as mode of presentation

Table 17.1 Behavioural tests of central auditory function

A   Monoaural tests
Degraded speech
Masked speech
Synthetic sentence identification with ipsilateral competing message

B   Binaural interaction tests
Congruent
    Dichotic digit
    Dichotic word
    Dichotic sentence identification
    Nonsense syllables
Non-congruent
    Binaural fusion
    Rapid alternating speech
    Interaural intensity difference
    Masking level difference
    Interaural timing

C   Binaural separation
Competing sentence
Threshold of interference

D   Sequencing tasks
Pitch pattern
Duration pattern
Intensity pattern
Psychoacoustic pattern discrimination

(e.g. monaural or binaural signals), or type of stimulus employed (e.g. tones or speech). In this chapter, to facilitate the application of such tests for the clinician, selected tests are described and grouped according to their sensitivity in detecting brain stem or cortical pathology. This approach is not without its limitations: first, most behavioural tests aimed at assessing the central auditory nervous system show deficits regardless of the level of the lesion affecting the auditory pathways. This is particularly true for tests directed at assessing cortical function, since the stimuli may be affected by peripheral and brain stem pathology, before reaching the cortex. Second, recent studies of the higher auditory system have reinforced the concept of parallel processing (Moore, 1987a). If a particular function is processed at more than one level or site, then inevitably deficits on certain tests will be observed regardless of the level of pathology. Furthermore, tests which are designed to target specific functions, thought to be subserved at a particular site, may in addition depend on the integration of circuits throughout the central auditory nervous system. Finally, the effect of peripheral cochlear pathology on central auditory nervous system test results needs to be quantified in a large number of controls to allow the distinction between 'peripheral' and 'central' effects. These limitations have to be understood if correct application and interpretation of central auditory nervous system testing are to be achieved.

However, in the last decade a combination of test procedures has evolved, which provide patterns of abnormality with a high sensitivity and specificity for pathology at the brain stem level. In addition, information regarding lateralization of unilateral brain stem lesions may also be obtained. Assessment of cortical pathology remains more difficult but, by assessing central auditory function with a battery of tests, the specificity of the tests of brain stem function can be employed either to confirm or refute a lesion at that level and thus indicate the possibility of a cortical lesion.

Tests of brain stem auditory function

Central behavioural tests allow us to study primary sensory function for diagnostic purposes, while electrophysiological procedures, impedence tests and imaging techniques (MRI, MRA, CT) are more effective in identifying and/or localizing pathology, but are unable to provide the clinician with information regarding the functional deficit resulting from the pathology.

The auditory brain stem is complex and compact so that a variety of central auditory effects have been defined, depending on the precise site and extent of pathology. The auditory brain stem response is probably the most specific and sensitive test for brain stem dysfunction, but its main application is in pontine lesions and thus to determine more rostral brain stem pathology other tests are required (Musiek *et al.*, 1988). Stapedial reflex threshold assessment has also proved of value in detecting brain stem lesions (Gelfand and Silman, 1982; Jerger *et al.*, 1986).

Objective tests

Acoustic reflex

Acoustic reflex threshold assessment is fully described in Chapter 12. The acoustic reflex arc is shown in Figure 17.6, and emphasizes the value of acoustic

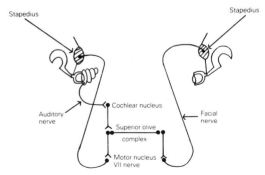

Figure 17.6 Diagram of the principal components of the ipsilateral and contralateral acoustic reflex

reflex threshold assessment in the identification and localization of brain stem auditory pathology (Griesen and Rasmussen, 1970; Borg, 1973; Jerger and Jerger, 1983). A variety of parameters of the acoustic reflex has been measured including threshold, latency, decay and amplitude. Neural auditory dysfunction characteristically increases reflex threshold, reduces reflex amplitude, prolongs latency and produces excessive (> 50%) decay. However, in order to interpret acoustic reflex threshold measurements accurately it is essential to define clearly the extent and type of any middle ear, cochlear and VIIIth nerve pathology. The application of criteria using both upper limits of acoustic reflex thresholds at adjacent frequencies and interaural differences has enabled acoustic reflexes to be used effectively to distinguish cochlear from retrocochlear pathology (Cohen and Prasher, 1992; Prasher and Cohen, 1993). This may be of value in defining whether a hearing loss with recruitment is of cochlear or central type (see Clinical presentations of brain stem hearing loss).

The application of acoustic reflex measurements in the identification of brain stem pathology has focused to a greater or lesser extent on a comparison of contralateral and ipsilateral reflex thresholds (Griesen and Rasmussen, 1970; Jerger and Jerger, 1983).

The absence of contralateral reflexes with preserved ipsilateral reflexes may be observed in patients with intrinsic axial brain stem pathology (Figure 17.7). These abnormalities are considered to be the result of the presence of a lesion in the area of the crossed brain stem pathways, while the uncrossed brain stem pathways remain intact (see Figure 17.6). Borg's (1982) detailed correlation of acoustic reflex abnormalities with carefully defined experimental lesions of brain stem auditory nuclei and pathways in rabbits has provided valuable information for the accurate interpretation of clinical reflex findings. He demonstrated that lesions in the ventral cochlear nucleus, but not the dorsal cochlear nucleus, i.e. in the vicinity of the VIIIth nerve root entry zone, produced findings indistinguishable from VIIIth nerve dysfunction with elevated ipsilateral reflex thresholds and excessive reflex threshold decay. In contrast, trapezoid body lesions spared the ipsilateral reflex activity but produced a modest increase in contralateral reflex thresholds with no decay, but pronounced latency and amplitude abnormalities. The medial portion of the superior olivary complex is a major structure in the crossed but not the uncrossed pathways, but involvement at this level may produce abnormalities on all recordings of acoustic reflex thresholds.

The acoustic reflex arc and the auditory brain stem responses share a common pathway from the cochlear nerve, cochlear nucleus to the superior olivary complex, but thereafter separate with the acoustic reflex pathway continuing to the facial motor nucleus and the auditory brain stem pathway continuing through the lateral lemniscus to the inferior colliculus. Thus, a number of studies (Hayes and Jerger, 1981; Hannley, Jerger and Rivera, 1983; Grenman *et al.*, 1984; Cohen and Prasher, 1988)

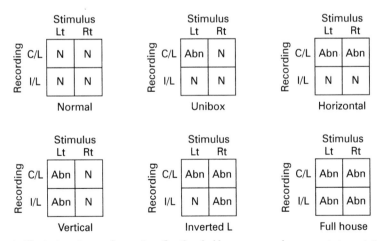

Figure 17.7 Diagram to illustrate patterns of acoustic reflex threshold responses and common interpretations. (Lt = left; Rt = right; C/L = contralateral;I/L = ipsilateral).
Unibox = small unilateral brain stem lesion medial to cochlear nucleus
Horizontal = midline brain stem lesion
Vertical = left VIIIth nerve lesion
Inverted L = intraxial brain stem lesion plus extension to the cochlear nucleus or VIIIth nerve on the affected side (NB: a conductive lesion may present in this way)
Full house = a midline brain stem lesion with extension to involve the cochlear nuclei and/or VIIIth nerves (NB: bilateral conductive disease requires exclusion)

have investigated the value of acoustic reflex threshold measurement together with auditory brain stem responses in order to determine more accurately the precise site of brain stem dysfunction.

Otoacoustic emissions

Otoacoustic emissions are considered fully in Chapter 12. Although there is no direct evidence, it is generally accepted that evoked otoacoustic emissions are generated by active mechanical processes in the cochlea, involving the outer hair cells (Figure 17.8). The crossed olivocochlear bundle innervates the outer hair cells in the organ of Corti. As noted earlier, animal work has shown that electrical stimulation of the olivocochlear bundle in the floor of the IVth ventricle reduces cochlear responses to contralateral acoustic stimuli (Galambos, 1956) and recent work has shown the failure of suppression of otoacoustic emissions following olivocochlear bundle section, as a consequence of vestibular neurectomy (Williams, Brookes and Prasher, 1994). A recent study has demonstrated absence of suppression of otoacoustic emissions with contralateral noise in the presence of intrinsic and extrinsic brain stem lesions (Prasher, Ryan and Luxon, 1994). The site and size of the lesion was shown to determine whether the suppression was affected unilaterally or bilaterally.

Auditory brain stem responses

This subject is considered in detail in Chapter 12 and this section will concentrate on the value of this technique in the diagnosis of brain stem pathology. As with the tests already discussed, conductive, cochlear and VIIIth nerve pathology may produce changes in the auditory brain stem response, which must be identified in order to define accurately any brain stem component. Notwithstanding this, auditory brain stem responses are established as an integral test in the evaluation of brain stem pathology.

A normal auditory brain stem response in man is shown in Figure 17.9 and demonstrates the characteristic waves I–V. Intracranial recording from the cochlear nerve in man (Møller and Jannetta, 1982a, b) has shown that the cochlear nerve is the generator of both waves I and II, while wave III is principally generated by the ipsilateral cochlear nucleus (Møller and Jannetta, 1983). Wave IV is considered to represent activity in the superior olivary complex, while wave V has a complex origin in both the lateral lemniscus and the inferior colliculus. A more precise understanding of the location of the generator sites of the components of the auditory brain stem response may be established by correlation of imaging of lesions in the brain stem with auditory brain stem response abnormalities. In evaluating the brain stem, auditory brain stem responses may provide information in three different areas. In certain diffuse neurological condi-

tions such as multiple sclerosis, an abnormal brain stem response may provide evidence of a 'silent lesion' and thus facilitate the diagnosis of lesions in more than one site. Second, auditory brain stem responses may be used in correlation with other techniques, e.g. imaging and behavioural tests, to define and increase our knowledge of central auditory function. Third, and in the context of this chapter most importantly, auditory brain stem responses may provide definitive evidence of auditory dysfunction in a patient with subtle auditory symptoms of unknown aetiology. Equally importantly, normal auditory brain stem responses may, as part of a test battery, help pinpoint a central auditory deficit arising in the cortex and auditory brain stem responses have been shown to be normal in cases of cortical deafness (Graham, Greenwood and Lecky, 1980; Ozdamar, Kraus and Currey, 1982).

In the differential diagnosis of VIIIth nerve and brain stem pathology, Antonelli, Bellotto and Grandori (1987) reported that auditory brain stem responses provided a 'fundamental contribution' in one-third to one-half of cases. These authors demonstrated frequent absence of wave I in VIIIth nerve lesions (12/15 cases) compared to presence of wave I in all 18 cases of intrinsic brain stem lesions. An abnormally prolonged I–II interpeak interval, with a normal III–IV interval is suggestive of VIIIth nerve pathology (Eggermont, Don and Brackmann, 1980). More recent work (Markand *et al.*, 1989) has defined auditory brain stem response abnormalities in 24 unilateral brain stem lesions, diagnosed using MRI. Pontine lesions demonstrated abnormalities in waves II and/or III, with prolongation of the I–III interpeak interval, while mesencephalic lesions produced abnormalities of the IV/V complex, with prolongation of the III–V interpeak interval. Lesions in the more rostral region of the pons were more likely to be associated with both ipsilateral and contralateral abnormalities. In another study using CT, Chu (1989) observed that wave V and the IV/V complex were not affected by lesions of the inferior colliculus, the central pons or the area dorsolateral to the aqueduct. However, waves IV and V were consistently abolished by lesions of the dorsal tegmentum of the midbrain–pontine junction and abnormalities were always ipsilateral to the side of monaural stimulation. Moreover, in a series of 20 cases of brain stem pathologies, Cohen and Prasher (1988) emphasized that 13 of 18 cases demonstrated bilateral auditory brain stem response abnormalities which were most commonly delay of wave V or unrepeatable responses (Figure 17.10). In contrast to Chu's (1989) findings, a well documented case of bilateral contusion of both inferior colliculi as demonstrated by MRI revealed bilateral sensorineural hearing loss and absent wave Vs on auditory brain stem response (Jani *et al.*, 1991).

Other work has emphasized the increase in amplitude of wave V of the auditory brain stem response

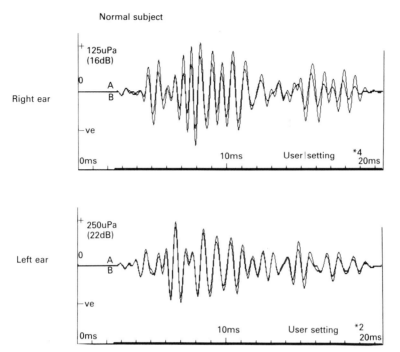

Figure 17.8 (*a*) Otoacoustic emissions recorded from each ear in a normal subject showing significant suppression as a result of the use of contralateral noise. (See difference between waveform A and B).

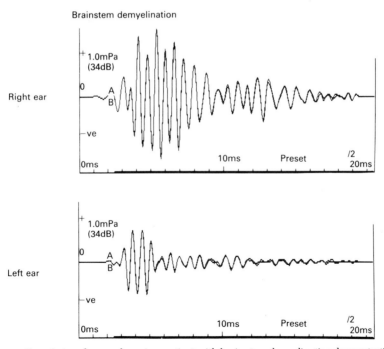

Figure 17.8 (*b*) Otoacoustic emissions from each ear in a patient with brain stem demyelination demonstrating absence of suppression of otoacoustic response with contralateral noise in each ear (i.e. almost exact superimposition of wave form A and B)

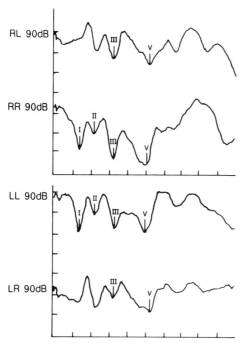

RL 90dB

RR 90dB

LL 90dB

LR 90dB

Figure 17.9 Diagram of a normal auditory brain stem response showing both ipsilateral (RR and LL) and contralateral (RL and LR) responses. (R = right, L = left.) (Scale: horizontal axis each mark represents 1 ms; vertical axis each mark represents 1 μV)

in response to binaural as opposed to monaural stimulation. This effect is attributed to binaural interaction at the level of the superior olivary complex and above, and has been demonstrated to be absent or impaired in brain stem pathology (Prasher, Sainz and Gibson, 1981). Earlier work had suggested that borderline auditory brain stem response abnormalities due to brain stem dysfunction might be accentuated by rapid presentation of test stimuli which would 'stress' the brain stem synaptic efficiency (Robinson and Rudge, 1977). However, Jacobsen and Newman (1989) failed to identify significant rate dependent wave V latency changes in patients with evidence of brain stem demyelination.

In conclusion, auditory brain stem responses have been used in the evaluation of a multiplicity of brain stem disorders including multiple sclerosis (Musiek *et al.*, 1989; Hendler, Squires and Emmerich, 1990; Drulovic *et al.*, 1994), vascular disease (Fisher *et al.*, 1982), metabolic disorders, trauma and tumours. Not surprisingly in diffuse multifocal pathology a multiplicity of results has been obtained and it cannot be overemphasized that in the evaluation of auditory brain stem responses in neurological conditions, the possibility of distant effects, as outlined above and/or additional undetected lesions must be borne in mind.

Behavioural tests

The strategy in constructing a test battery for brain

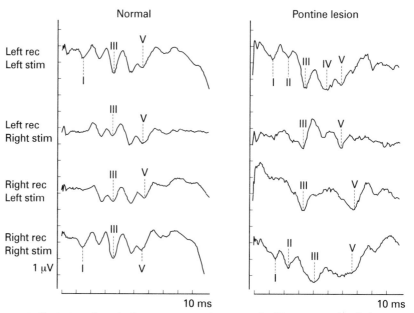

Figure 17.10 Diagram to illustrate auditory brain stem responses in a normal subject compared with the responses in a patient with a pontine lesion (note delay of waves III and V in the right ipsilateral recording and delay of wave V in the left contralateral recording – rec = recording; stim = stimulation)

stem dysfunction attempts to correlate physiological studies of brain stem function with specific auditory tasks. From anatomical studies, we know that the superior olivary complex is the first level in the auditory pathway where information from the two ears is received and can be integrated into one perceptual event. Physiological studies on animals (Pickles, 1988) suggest that the brain stem auditory nuclei contribute to central auditory processing in two main areas: the extraction of signals from a background of noise, which has led to the development of both monaural and binaural separation tests; and sound localization based on interaural intensity differences at high frequencies and interaural timing differences at low frequencies. Certain binaural integration tasks are aimed at assessing these facets of central auditory nervous system function. Tests of binaural interaction may use tones, noise or speech as the stimulus, while in monaural tests, the stimulus is degraded in some way, in order to overcome redundancy.

The behavioural tests, which have been suggested to be of particular value in the assessment of brain stem disorders, include the masked speech test, the synthetic sentence identification with ipsilateral competing message test (SSI-ICM), the masking level difference test (MLD) and the binaural fusion test. As with all tests, age/sex related normative data must be obtained in each laboratory in order to interpret results appropriately.

Monaural tests

In the majority of cases of lesions affecting the central auditory nervous system, conventional speech audiometry, such as the Boothroyd (AB) word lists, fail to show abnormal intelligibility scores. The reasons for this stem from the redundancy contained both in the stimulus and the neural pathways. In order to reduce this redundancy, monaural speech stimuli may be degraded electroacoustically by modifying the frequency, temporal or intensity characteristics of the undistorted signal, e.g. filtered speech, interrupted speech and time-compressed speech (Rintelmann, 1985). A wealth of literature on the value of such tests in the investigation of central auditory dysfunction has accumulated. Using low-pass and band-pass filtered speech (Calearo and Antonelli, 1963, 1968; Lynn and Gilroy, 1977) and interrupted speech (Korsan–Bengtsen, 1973), the consensus view is that these tests are sensitive for detecting both brain stem and temporal auditory cortex lesions, but are not of specific value in localizing central auditory nervous system lesions. However, time-compressed speech tests tend to be effective in detecting auditory cortex rather than brain stem pathology (Calearo and Antonelli, 1963, 1968; Korsan–Bengtsen, 1973; Kurdziel, Noffsinger and Olsen, 1976; Quaranta and Cervellera, 1977).

The monaural speech tests aimed at assessing brain stem dysfunction are based on the evidence that the brain stem nuclei play an important role in the extraction of signals from background noise. The presentation of a masker to the test ear, together with the signal, increases the difficulty of the task by decreasing the redundancy contained in the stimulus. The advantage of monaural tests is that they allow the assessment of each ear separately.

Masked speech

A large body of literature exists on the effects of white noise on the ability to perceive speech-in-noise, both in normal and hearing impaired subjects. In addition, a number of authors have investigated this technique in patients with known brain stem and cortical pathology (Dayal, Tarantino and Swisher, 1966; Morales-Garcia and Poole, 1972; Noffsinger *et al.*, 1972; Olsen, Noffsinger and Kurdziel, 1975).

Morales-Garcia and Poole (1972) proposed a test comprised of lists of 25 phonetically balanced, monosyllabic meaningful words, which are presented to the test ear at 50 dB sensation level (with respect to the average hearing level for the speech frequencies 0.5, 1 and 2 kHz) in the presence of white noise at various signal to noise ratios, ranging from −10 to +20 dB.

These workers applied the test to 21 control subjects and 15 patients with brain stem lesions. They found bilaterally reduced scores in 14 out of the 15 patients, indicating that it is an effective test of brain stem auditory function, requiring only basic audiological facilities. However, it was not possible to deduce the side of pathology in unilateral brain stem lesions. Moreover, contralateral ear deficits were also observed by the authors in unilateral temporal lobe lesions, indicating that the test is sensitive to central auditory pathology, but cannot be used to differentiate definitively brain stem from cortical pathology. A view also expressed by Olsen, Noffsinger and Kurdziel (1975) following their large study of patients with cochlear, VIIIth nerve, brain stem and cortical lesions.

Synthetic sentence identification with ipsilateral competing message (SSI-ICM)

This test was first developed in 1965 by Speaks and Jerger and represents another example of a test aimed at requiring the subjects to extract a primary stimulus from competing auditory information. It consists of 10 synthetic sentences of seven words each, representing a third-order approximation to actual English sentences, e.g. 'Go change your car colour is red' (Table 17.2). The sentences are presented as a closed set at an intensity level yielding 100% correct performance in both ears, which for most people is 50 dBSL.

The degradation of the stimulus is achieved by presenting it to the test ear, together with a continuous discourse at various message to competition ratios from +10 to −20 dB in 10 dB steps. In the English

Table 17.2 Synthetic sentences

1	Women view men with green paper should
2	Agree with him only to find out
3	Down by the time is real enough
4	Battle cry and be better than ever
5	That neighbour who said business is better
6	March around without a care in your
7	Forward march said the boy had a
8	Go change your car colour is red
9	Built the government with the force almost
10	Small boat with a picture has become

From Jerger, J., Speakes, C. and Trammell, J. (1968) and Katz, J. (1994).

version, this is achieved by the presentation of a continuous discourse concerning the life and diary of Queen Victoria (Figure 17.11). Normal performance ranges from 100% to 20% for the different message to competition ratios. Jerger and Jerger (1974) reported uniformly poor scores in a study of 11 patients with intrinsic brain stem lesions of varying aetiologies, compared with the controls. In a subsequent study, the same authors (1975) reported reduced SSI-ICM scores in 4 of 10 patients with brain stem lesions and observed that patients with cortical lesions usually obtained normal scores. Nonetheless, the side of the brain stem pathology could not be reliably correlated to the ear affected. Test results were found to be abnormal in both ears, the contralateral ear or the ipsilateral ear (Jerger and Jerger, 1975).

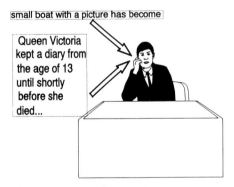

Figure 17.11 Diagram to illustrate the synthetic sentence identification–ipsilateral competing message test

The clinical application of the SSI-ICM test in differential diagnosis is further enhanced when it is applied and the results compared to those of a PB word list (Jerger and Hayes, 1977). A discrepancy in the maximum scores of the two tests and rollover exceeding 20% is suggestive of central pathology.

There are, however, two limitations of this test: it relies on the integrity of the visual system and thus cannot be used in visually impaired patients and

second, it is time-consuming, particularly if used as part of a comprehensive test battery.

Binaural interaction tests

Dichotic speech tests

Dichotic speech tests have been widely used in the detection of central auditory dysfunction (Kimura, 1961a; Berlin and McNeill, 1976) and may be divided into two main types:

Binaural interaction tasks, in which the subject is required to report information heard in both ears. This group of tests may be subdivided further into:

Congruent interaction tasks, in which competing auditory signals presented to each ear, are similar in onset time, intensity level, wave envelope and/ or linguistic structure and the subject is expected to report the information heard in both ears, e.g. dichotic digit (DD) test, dichotic word (DW) test and nonsense syllables (CV) test (See Section on Auditory Cortex Tests).

and

Binaural interaction tasks which rely on the ears effecting closure of *non-congruent* or non-competing auditory information (i.e. information separated by time, frequency or intensity factors presented to each ear), e.g. the binaural fusion test (BF), the rapidly alternating speech test (RASP), the interaural intensity difference test (IID) and masking level difference test (MLD).

Binaural separation tasks, in which the subject is required to report information heard in one ear and ignore competing information presented to the other ear.

Most of the literature on the use of dichotic auditory tests centres on the assessment of cortical/hemispheric evaluation and there is a relative paucity of information with respect to brain stem evaluation. Nonetheless, a series of reports has identified abnormalities in both binaural separation and congruent interaction tasks in patients with brain stem pathology (Pinheiro and Musiek, 1985). However, most of the behavioural tests aimed at assessing brain stem function rely on the ability of the brain stem nuclei to integrate noncongruent binaural stimuli. Different portions of auditory information are presented to each ear, and the subject is required to unify them into one perceptual event. As with monaural tests, the redundancy contained in the stimulus is reduced by manipulating the frequency, intensity and/or temporal components in order to make the task more difficult.

The *rapidly alternating speech perception test (RASP)* is an example of a binaural interaction task in which the *temporal* components of speech are manipulated (Bocca and Calearo, 1963; Lynn and Gilroy, 1977). The test consists of presenting alternating segments of sentences, of between 100–500 ms duration to each ear in turn and the subject is required to integrate the auditory information to identify the sentences correctly (Figure 17.12).

The red car raced down the street

LEFT EAR: T re   ar   ce   ow t   s ee

RIGHT EAR: he d c ra d d n he tr t

Figure 17.12 Diagram to illustrate the binaural alternating speech perception test

The *binaural fusion test* (Figure 17.13) is an example of a test in which there is manipulation of the frequency component of speech in order to degrade the stimulus. Matzker (1959) constructed a clinical test by filtering bi-syllable words into a low pass (500–800 Hz) component and a high pass component (1850–2500 Hz). The filtered portions of each word are presented simultaneously to the two ears. The information contained in each portion independently is not sufficient for the word to be discriminated accurately, but simultaneous presentation of the two portions in a normal subject allows integration of the auditory information and the word is identified correctly.

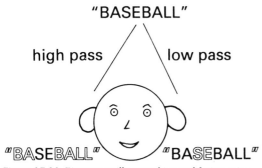

Figure 17.13 Diagram to illustrate binaural fusion using filtered words

Matzker (1959) proposed that the filtered words should be presented dichotically, then diotically (fused filtered portions presented simultaneously to the two ears) and then dichotically again. Controls scored similarly for the diotic and dichotic presentations, with a slight improvement for the second dichotic presentation, related to learning effect. Matzker hypothesized that patients with low brain stem lesions would show reduced scores in the dichotic mode, but good diotic recognition. His study proved that patients with pathological changes in the olivary region in the brain stem had reduced scores on this test, and he explained this on the basis of loss of synaptic function within the auditory centres of the brain stem.

A number of workers have subsequently repeated this work, with a variety of test modifications (Linden, 1964; Ivey, 1969; Smith and Resnick, 1972) which make the findings difficult to compare. Nonetheless, this technique would appear to be of merit in the behavioural assessment of brain stem lesions, particularly as Smith and Resnick (1972) showed that their modification of the test was essentially unaffected by cortical involvement. However, Katz (1994) has suggested that this may merely reflect poor sensitivity of the test. Thus, in conjunction with masking level difference, acoustic reflex thresholds and auditory brain stem responses, one version of this test (Ivey, 1969) has been incorporated into a standard battery of central tests used in the USA (Willeford, 1977).

Non-speech dichotic tests

The *interaural intensity difference* (IID) test is a task in which the intensity of the stimulus is manipulated. The procedure is to determine a threshold for noise bursts for each ear and then, presenting the bursts dichotically, a subjective midline is established. Gradually, the sound in one ear is then increased in 1 dB steps until lateralization occurs. Midline is re-established and the other ear tested; 10 dB is a normal IID for lateralization (Pinheiro and Tobin, 1971).

Interaural timing procedures

Interaural timing procedures have not been used routinely in the clinical assessment of central auditory nervous system dysfunction, but Musiek *et al.* (1988) have proposed their use in the assessment of brain stem function. Hausler and Levine (1980) studied interaural time discrimination in patients with multiple sclerosis using a two alternative forced choice paradigm in which patients were required to judge whether noise bursts were displaced to the left or right of a reference, as stimulus lead-lag times were varied in the two ears. More than half of the patients were shown to demonstrate abnormalities on this test, which were strongly correlated with auditory brain stem response abnormalities. Later work using this technique in another group of patients with multiple sclerosis suggested that this task was more sensitive than masking level difference tests, rapid alternating speech tests and auditory brain stem response for the detection of brain stem pathology (Matathias, Sohmer and Biton, 1985; Cranford, Boose and Moore, 1990).

Binaural masking level differences

The masking level difference is one of the simplest and most sensitive procedures for testing brain stem auditory function, achieved by manipulation of the phase relationship between a signal and a masker as originally described by Licklider (1948) and Hirsh (1948). The signal is usually a low frequency tone, although clicks or speech stimuli (Stubblefield and Goldstein 1977; Lynn *et al.*, 1981) can also be employed. The masker is a narrow band noise centred around the signal frequency.

In the tonal version of the test, the procedure is to find the threshold of a binaurally presented low frequency (usually a 500 Hz) tone referred to as the signal (S) in a background of noise (N) also presented to the two ears, and set at 60 dB hearing level (HL).

In the first condition, both the tone and the masker are in phase and this is referred to as the homophasic condition (S_0N_0). Once the threshold has been established the phase of the tone or the masker is changed by 180° in one ear only (S_0N_π or $S_\pi N_0$) and the threshold of the tone reassessed in the antiphasic condition (Figure 17.14). The masking level difference is the improvement in the threshold of the tone in the antiphasic condition compared to the homophasic condition, which for tones is in the order of 8–16 dB. Smaller masking level differences are obtained using speech stimuli.

Clinically, as in all central auditory tests, peripheral hearing impairment has been shown to exert a very significant effect on test results and may make the interpretation of masking level difference testing as a means of assessing the central auditory nervous system difficult or indeed impossible (Quaranta, Cassano and Cervellera, 1978). A number of studies of the masking level difference in neurological popula-

tions (Lynn *et al.*, 1981; Musiek *et al.*, 1989) has demonstrated that patients with brain stem lesions tend to have reduced masking level differences, while patients with cortical lesions have normal masking level differences. The clinical evidence implicates the brain stem and specifically the superior olivary complex as a processor for this phenomenon (Lynn and Gilroy, 1984). A recent study (Grose, Poth and Peters, 1994) has shown abnormal masking level difference test results in normally hearing elderly subjects compared with a young population and these authors have proposed that age-related degradation of binaural processing may contribute to the common problem in the elderly of difficulty understanding speech in a noisy environment.

Summary of brain stem assessment

No single auditory test provides all the information required by the clinician in terms of lesion detection (sensitivity), site and extent of involvement, specificity and functional deficit. The use of a battery approach has proved necessary in detecting pathologies at all levels of the auditory system, but particularly in pathologies affecting the central auditory nervous system (Lynn and Gilroy, 1984; Benjamin and Troost, 1988; Rodriguez, DiSarno and Hardiman, 1990). Musiek and Geurkink (1982) highlighted the efficacy of their central auditory test battery and auditory brain stem responses in defining dysfunction in 10 patients with brain stem pathology. Considering behavioural or electrophysiological tests separately, abnormalities in the whole group were not defined but,

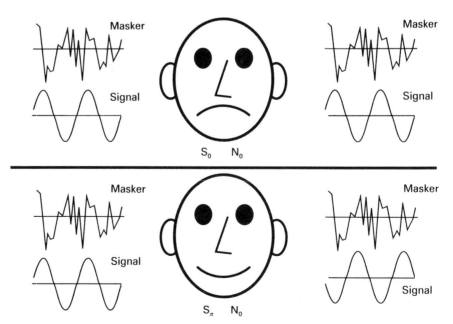

Figure 17.14 Diagram to illustrate the masking level difference test

combining the two types of test procedures all patients with brain stem pathology were identified. They therefore proposed that electrophysiological and psychophysical tests assess different auditory processes and thus the broader the range of tests conducted the better the probability of detecting subtle abnormal function within the brain stem.

Based on the authors' experience, the combination of tests which emerged as the most efficient in assessing these disorders consists of, in addition to the pure-tone audiogram, ipsilateral and contralateral acoustic reflex thresholds, auditory brain stem responses, masking level differences, suppression of transient evoked otoacoustic emissions and masked speech (Table 17.3). This suggested battery contains objective tests, which have been shown to be highly sensitive in detecting brain stem auditory function, together with behavioural procedures which, in addition to their diagnostic value, provide a measure of the functional deficit resulting from the lesion.

Table 17.3 'Brain stem' test battery

Acoustic reflex thresholds
Suppression of otoacoustic emissions
Auditory brain stem responses

Masking level difference

Masked speech
or
Synthetic sentence identification with ipsilateral competing message

---

Tests of auditory cortex function

Above the brain stem, the auditory pathways demonstrate to an even greater degree the characteristic features of tonotopicity, redundancy and bilateral representation. The complexity of the auditory neural substrate at the level of the auditory cortex is greater than within the compact brain stem. It is therefore possible for a lesion involving these pathways to remain undetected for long periods of time, without producing a significant sensory deficit.

The diagnosis requires sensitive and specific tests, based on the current understanding of the anatomy and physiology of the auditory cortex (see above). However, within the central auditory nervous system, acoustic signals are not necessarily processed in hierarchial order of task difficulty and parallel processing is known to occur (Moore, 1987a). This implies that tests which target specific functions, may not be linked with a unique anatomical site and may evoke activity in multiple locations. For example, sound localization tests, such as the interaural intensity difference (IID) test, can be physiologically correlated with both the superior olivary complex, and area A1

of the auditory cortex. Thus, test abnormalities may result from pathology at either or both sites.

Clinicians in audiology are rarely referred patients with suspected cortical pathology, partly because auditory deficits due to cortical lesions are subtle, and may be unnoticed by the patient and, partly, because significant cortical deafness due to bilateral temporal lobe pathology is very rare. Early diagnosis in cortical pathology is the primary objective and imaging techniques are the diagnostic test of choice. Moreover, the treatment of the underlying pathology is either surgical or medical and audiological rehabilitation is not available or useful in such cases. Nonetheless, electrophysiological and behavioural tests play a key role in three main areas:

1 *Diagnosis*: central auditory tests may identify abnormalities and indicate pathology undetected by imaging or radiological techniques (Jani *et al.*, 1991; Katz, 1994).
2 *Measurement of functional deficit*: while electrophysiological procedures and imaging techniques are efficient in identifying and/or localizing CNS pathology, the resultant functional deficits cannot be measured or understood unless behavioural tests are employed. This is of particular importance when surgery in the dominant hemisphere is considered.
3 *Rehabilitation*: the role of an intact auditory sensory system in the normal development and acquisition of language skills is gradually becoming apparent from research carried out in children with learning disabilities and developmental dysphasia (Tallal, Sainburg and Jernigan, 1991; Tallal, Miller and Fitch, 1993; Willeford, 1985). These findings are of relevance in developing a rehabilitative strategy for these children.

Electrophysiological tests

Middle latency response

The components of the middle latency evoked response occur within a time frame of 100 ms following the presentation of an effective auditory stimulus. Figure 17.15 demonstrates the response, which is characterized by a vertex positive peak (Pa) with a latency of about 30 ms and this is the most prominent and stable component of the response in adults. Between the auditory brain stem response and the middle latency response a small positive peak is often identified (P_0) with a latency of 12–15 ms and this is in part the result of activation of the postauricular muscle reflex (Kileny and Berry, 1983).

The generator sources of the middle latency response remain unidentified. A recent study revealed that bilateral lesions in the white matter, ventral and lateral to the posterior half of the putamen were associated with failure to identify Pa of the middle

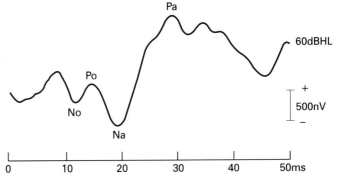

Figure 17.15 Tracing of a normal middle latency response with standard components marked

latency response, although the late cortical auditory evoked response was detected (Tanaka *et al.*, 1991). However, other studies have shown preservation of the Pa of the middle latency response in the absence of N1 of the late vertex response (Woods *et al.*, 1987; Bahls *et al.*, 1988). These studies suggest that the generator of N1 of the late vertex response is independent of that of Pa.

In case studies of patients with cortical lesions it would appear that the temporal lobe or thalamocortical projections are important in the generation of the Pa. In patients with *unilateral* temporal lobe lesions, the most consistent finding has been a reduction in wave Pa amplitude over the temporal lobe lesion, in comparison with the intact hemisphere (Pool *et al.*, 1989). In *bilateral* temporal lesions associated with cortical deafness, the Pa has been reported to be present (Bahls *et al.*, 1988) or completely absent (Graham, Greenwood and Lecky, 1980; Nakayama *et al.*, 1986). The presence or absence of wave Pa in bilateral temporal lobe lesions suggests that either the temporal lobe generators are only partially damaged or that the thalamus or projections from the thalamus may contribute significantly to the response. Animal work provides strong evidence for a generating system consisting of multiple contributions (Katz, 1994).

In conclusion, middle latency responses cannot be used specifically to define cortical auditory disorders, but may be a useful adjunct.

The slow vertex auditory evoked response

This occurs 50–500 ms after the presentation of an effective auditory stimulus, and is considered to be generated by the frontal association and/or the primary cortex (Picton *et al.*, 1974).

In an alert adult (Figure 17.16), the response consists of a vertex negative peak with a latency of 80–110 ms (N1) followed by a positive peak at 160–180 ms (P2).

Both these components are considered to be 'non-specific' components of the auditory evoked response

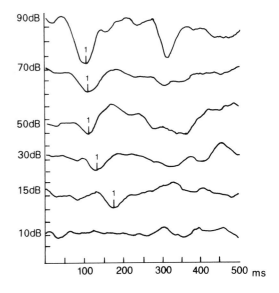

Figure 17.16 Tracings of cortical evoked responses recorded to threshold in a normal subject. (Scale: horizontal axis – each mark represents 50 ms; vertical axis – each mark represents 1 μv)

mediated by the reticular formation and sleep or drowsiness produces markedly diminished or absent N1 responses (Kevanishvili and Von Specht, 1979).

As noted above, a dissociation occurs between middle latency responses and slow vertex responses in patients with cortical deafness and auditory agnosia/word deafness. In the literature dealing with slow vertex responses in 'cortical deafness', the response varies from slightly elevated thresholds (Earnest, Monroe and Yarnell, 1977) to complete absence (Graham, Greenwood and Lecky, 1980; Bahls *et al.*, 1988). A discrepancy between auditory perception and cortical evoked response thresholds in cortical dysfunction has also been demonstrated in that a patient of Jerger *et al.* (1969) showed no slow auditory evoked response, although able to hear the test sound, whereas a patient of Earnest, Monroe and Yarnell (1977) showed responses at elevated thresholds, but was unable to hear the stimulus. Thus, slow vertex responses, like middle latency responses, do not seem to help in specifically defining 'cortical auditory disorders'.

Behavioural tests

Tests which employ tonal stimuli are infrequently used in clinical assessment of cortical function and the majority of the tests employ speech or speech-like stimuli.

Monaural speech tests

The clinical use of central auditory tests as a diagnostic tool began with the pioneering work of Bocca, Calearo and Cassinari on patients with unilateral cortical lesions. In a short report published in 1954, they described their findings of contralateral ear deficits in a patient with a right temporal lobe tumour, using low-pass filtered words. The pure-tone audiogram and a standard intelligibility score of words revealed no abnormality. A more extensive report, describing the pre- and postoperative results of standard and filtered speech tests on 18 patients with confirmed unilateral temporal lobe tumours, followed closely (Bocca *et al.*, 1955). Preoperatively most patients had deficits in the ear contralateral to the temporal lobe lesion, with either partial or full recovery postoperatively. The authors reported that there was no difference in behaviour between the right and left temporal lobe lesions that would justify claims of 'prevalence of one hemisphere for the reception and expression of speech'.

Monaurally degraded speech tests including masked speech and SSI-ICM have been described in the section devoted to tests of brain stem function and when applied to patients with cortical pathology reinforce the findings of Bocca *et al.* (Bocca, Calearo and Cassinari, 1954; Bocca *et al.*, 1955), of predominantly contralateral ear deficits in unilateral cortical pathology (Pinheiro and Musiek, 1985). The advantage afforded by this simple technique is that it allows each ear to be tested separately, and can lead to an efficient differentiation of brain stem from cortical pathology when performed in conjunction with 'objective', specific and sensitive tests such as auditory brain stem response and acoustic reflex threshold.

Dichotic tests

Dichotic tests (see Brain stem tests), where different stimuli are presented simultaneously to the two ears and the listener is required to respond to one or both stimuli, were first used by Broadbent in 1954. Over the years many different types of stimuli were used: digits, meaningful words, synthetic speech or nonsense syllables, but regardless of the type of stimulus, differences in performance of the two ears are frequently observed in normal listeners.

In 1961 Kimura studied the effect of unilateral cortical lesions on ear performance using Broadbent's dichotic paradigm with triple digits delivered to each ear (Kimura, 1961a,b). Seventy-one patients who had undergone surgery for focal cortical seizures, but who demonstrated normal hearing for speech, were selected. Kimura found significant auditory deficits in the ear contralateral to the lobectomy, with the most marked deterioration in contralateral ear performance in left hemisphere-damaged patients.

To explain her findings, using data obtained from animal experiments (Rosenzweig, 1951), Kimura proposed that the contralateral projections from each ear to the brain are more efficient than the ipsilateral projections. Further, she suggested that in the dichotic listening situation, the preference for the contralateral route is enhanced, while the ipsilateral route is suppressed. Thus, a stimulus presented to the left ear passes via the contralateral route to the right hemisphere, and then across the corpus callosum to the left hemisphere, which is thought to be specialized for processing verbal stimuli (Figure 17.17). The stimulus presented to the right ear arrives at the left hemisphere directly via the predominant contralateral route. This process is faster and the stimulus arrives in a 'better form' than that presented to the left ear. A right ear advantage may therefore emerge. Nonetheless, it should be emphasized that subsequent work has provided no evidence for 'suppression' of ipsilateral auditory pathways or 'degradation' of the auditory stimulus from the left ear.

In subsequent studies, Kimura used the dichotic listening technique to present musical chords to right-handed subjects; a task for which the right hemisphere is thought to be specialized, and demonstrated a left ear advantage (Kimura, 1964). Kimura's studies had a major impact on laterality and dichotic auditory research for several decades as her hypothesis was considered to show that dichotic presentation was a powerful method of determining hemispheric specialization of different types of auditory stimuli in the normal population.

Using this model, in unilateral temporal lesions the ear asymmetry is accentuated. Thus pathology involving the right temporal lobe and/or the corpus callosum would result in reduced scores in the signal presented to the left ear, but normal scores to the right. Left hemisphere lesions could result in bilaterally reduced scores which are more marked in the signal presented to the left ear since that signal (even under normal conditions) has a disadvantageous longer route.

However, Efron (1990) has presented a detailed analysis of the key publications in the field of laterality research both in the auditory and visual modali-

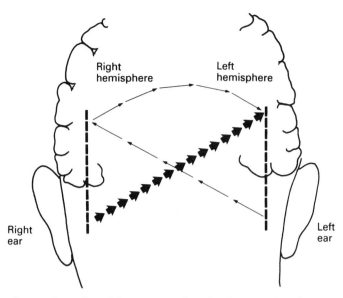

Figure 17.17 Diagram to illustrate Kimura's model. – – – – = ipsilateral pathway. ➡ ➡ = dominant contralateral pathway right ear to left hemisphere. → = contralateral pathway from left ear to right hemisphere to left hemisphere

ties, to question the validity of Kimura's hypotheses. His main points are:

1. Right ear advantage is observed not only for speech but for signals devoid of meaning such as nonsense syllables. These signals share a common complex spectral content, but cannot be categorized as verbal stimuli. In addition, there is an incongruity in the interpretation of *repetition* of digits, the auditory task presented to Kimura's patients, as a measure of understanding speech.
2. Underestimation of the incidence of left hemisphere dominance. Based on the incidence of aphasia in right hemisphere-damaged patients, only about 1–3% of right-handed subjects should have a left ear advantage on dichotic listening tests. However, depending on the various studies, up to 50% of right-handed people may exhibit a left ear advantage on dichotic tests (Speaks, Niccum and Carney, 1982).
3. The right ear advantage is weak, with large intra-subject variability, which is sometimes greater than the ear advantage itself.
4. Some dichotic tests using non-verbal stimuli showed a right ear advantage to pure tones.

The difficulty in understanding or inferring specialization of the left hemisphere for verbal material from dichotic speech tests is of no immediate interest to the clinician who is attempting to diagnose and lateralize cortical auditory pathology. However, it is important to appreciate the difficulties of interpretation of results of dichotic testing. Not only does the question of hemispheric asymmetry remain unre-solved, but it must be recalled that peripheral auditory dysfunction (even in the face of a normal pure tone audiogram) may give rise to asymmetry of dichotic results, as may asymmetries of earphone transducers, coupling between the earphones and the ear, pitch mechanisms and resonance characteristics of the external auditory meatus. Such variables must be considered if dichotic tests are to be accurately interpreted.

Notwithstanding these difficulties, dichotic tests can be extremely valuable and sensitive in detecting cortical pathology, provided the results are not over-interpreted. Nonetheless, lateralization of pathology is difficult, within the constraints of current knowledge regarding central processing of auditory signals. However, significantly reduced scores, either unilaterally or bilaterally, are observed in dichotic tests in patients with unilateral temporal lobe pathology, and their inclusion in a test battery aimed at assessing cortical function can be of great value.

A variety of stimuli has been used, including tones, nonsense syllables and sentences, which differ not only in duration and frequency spectrum, but also in extent of meaning and in redundancy of language cues. Differences also exist in the way each test is constructed: in some the onset alignment of the dichotic stimuli is critical; while the response required in different tests varies from repetition of the stimulus to selection of a response from an open set or a closed set to pointing, humming etc. As noted earlier, the variability in these factors and the lack of stand-ardization makes comparison between different studies impossible. Both congruent interaction and binaural separation tasks have been reported to be of particular value in the assessment of cortical function.

Binaural interaction tests

The dichotic digits test

Based on Kimura's early work (1961a,b) and others (Sparks and Geschwind, 1968; Sparks, Goodglass and Nickel, 1970), the dichotic digits test was reintroduced in a new form by Musiek in 1983. His test consists of dichotic presentation of 20 double pairs of naturally spoken digits from one to 10, excluding the number seven, at an intensity of 50 dB SL. The onset of the digits in each ear is synchronized. The subject is required to repeat the digits in any order (Figure 17.18).

In the preliminary study, the test was applied to 45 control subjects, 21 patients with high frequency hearing loss of cochlear origin and 21 patients with a variety of neurological diseases. A score of 90% in either ear was established as the lowest normal value, and scores below this were reported in 11 of 14 patients with brain stem or cortical pathology, despite normal thresholds for pure tones.

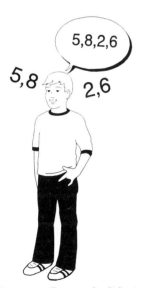

Figure 17.18 Diagram to illustrate the dichotic digit test

In patients with high frequency hearing loss of cochlear origin a lower limit of 80% score for either ear was found clearly to differentiate peripheral from central pathology (Musiek *et al.*, 1991).

The conclusions from these studies were that the dichotic digits test is relatively resistant to the effects of high frequency cochlear loss, and sensitive to central auditory nervous system pathology. The sensitivity of the test to brain stem and cortical pathology was equal, confirming earlier work (Stephens and

Thornton, 1976; Musiek and Guerkink, 1982). Thus this test is best employed as a screening test for central auditory nervous system pathology rather than in the clinical differentiation of brain stem from cortical pathology.

Dichotic sentence identification test

The test was devised by Fifer *et al.* (1983), and consists of dichotic presentation of randomly paired synthetic sentences that were originally constructed for the SSI-ICM test (Speaks and Jerger, 1965). Each of the sentences was edited to a duration of 2 seconds and the onset and offset of each pair were aligned with an accuracy of 100 μs.

Initially, the test consisted of 90 pairs of sentences, although in its present form only 30 test items are used following the presentation of practice items. The test items are presented to the listener at a comfortable level of 50 dB HL for normally hearing listeners. The gap between each presentation is set to 8 seconds, upon which the subject is required to identify the numbers of the two sentences that were heard from a closed set of six printed and numbered sentences (Figure 17.19). The test is applied to 14 normal hearing subjects, 28 subjects with a pure-tone average (re: 0.5, 1 and 2 kHz) of better than 50 dB in the poorer ear and a further 20 subjects whose pure-tone average in the poorer ear exceeded 50 dB. The purpose of this was to establish expected scores in normally hearing individuals and study the effect of cochlear impairment on those scores. Their results indicated that the dichotic sentence identification test is applicable for use in ears with a mean hearing level up to 49 dB. Six patients with suspected or confirmed retrocochlear lesions were also tested, all of whom had reduced scores, either unilaterally or bilaterally.

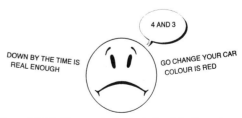

1. SMALL BOAT WITH A PICTURE HAS BECOME.
2. BUILT THE GOVERNMENT WITH A FORCE ALMOST.
3. GO CHANGE YOUR CAR COLOUR IS RED.
4. DOWN BY THE TIME IS REAL ENOUGH.
5. AGREE WITH HIM ONLY TO FIND OUT.
6. WOMEN VIEW MEN WITH GREEN PAPER SHOULD.

Figure 17.19 Diagram to illustrate the dichotic sentence identification test

Nonsense syllables

Consonant-vowels such as ba, da, ga, (voiced) and pa, ta and ka (unvoiced) have also been used as a dichotic test (Figure 17.20). Pairs of different syllables are presented simultaneously to the two ears, and are constructed from the six stop plosives and the vowel 'a'. The stimuli are counterbalanced such that each pair receives an identical number and type of syllable. Thirty pairs are presented at 50 dB HL or 30 dB above the speech reception threshold. Subjects are requested to mark the two syllables that are heard out of a closed set of six possibilities. The number of correct syllables reported for each ear is counted and a percentage score derived.

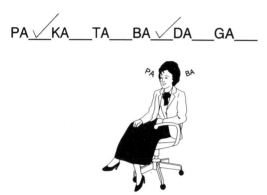

Figure 17.20 Diagram to illustrate the nonsense syllable test (i.e. dichotic consonant vowels)

Variations of this test have been widely used in patients with temporal lobe lesions and temporal lobectomies (Berlin *et al.*, 1972; Olsen, 1977; Niccum, Rubens and Speaks, 1981; Collard *et al.*, 1982). Abnormal results have been consistently found in the majority of patients with temporal lobe pathology, although both bilateral and unilateral abnormalities have been reported. Some studies suggest that the contralateral ear to the pathology is more likely to give abnormal results (Speaks *et al.*, 1975), but this is not invariably so (Olsen, 1977).

Staggered spondaic word test

This test was introduced by Katz in 1962 and has been widely used in central auditory testing since this time.

The staggered spondaic word test is composed of two spondees with a staggered onset. The last half of the first spondee and the first half of the second spondee are presented dichotically, while the remaining spondee segments are presented separately to opposite ears. An example of a test item is:

Left ear: foot ball
Right ear: door step

Forty test items are presented at 50 dB sensation level with respect to the speech reception threshold. The subject is required to repeat all the words presented. The scoring of this test is extremely compli-

cated (Brunt, 1978) and includes scoring errors in both the competing (dichotic) and non-competing (isolated) words, as well as comparing order effects, such as whether the lead spondee is reported first or second and adjusting the raw score for peripheral auditory deficits.

Despite these complications, up to 60% of subjects with brain stem disorders have been shown to demonstrate abnormal staggered spondaic word test results (Stephens and Thornton, 1976; Jerger and Jerger, 1975; Musiek and Guerkink, 1982; Musiek, 1983). The majority of patients with unilateral brain stem pathology showed ipsilateral or bilateral staggered spondaic word test abnormalities. This test has also been used widely in the assessment of temporal lobe pathology with a preponderance of abnormalities documented in the contralateral ear (Brunt, 1978; Lynn and Gilroy, 1977).

Binaural separation tasks

Binaural separation tasks constitute a variant of the dichotic paradigm, in which the subject is required to respond to a stimulus presented to a designated ear, and is instructed to ignore the simultaneously presented signal in the non-test ear.

The competing sentence test

The competing sentence test was developed by Willeford, but first described by Ivey in 1969, and is composed of simple English sentences. The test was specifically constructed to incorporate a competing signal of similar type (Table 17.4) and thus, the test resembles normal communication, in which competition between the two ears is more or less random. The two sentences are presented simultaneously, one to each ear and, although the two signals begin very nearly at the same time, no precise time matching was undertaken.

Ten competing sentence pairs were defined and the subject is instructed to listen and repeat the

Table 17.4 Selected examples of Willeford's competing sentences

(Weather)	a	I think we'll have rain today.
	b	There was frost on the ground.
(Time)	a	This watch keeps good time.
	b	I was late to work today.
(Family)	a	My mother is a good cook.
	b	Your brother is a tall boy.
(Food)	a	Please pass the salt and pepper.
	b	The roast beef is very good.
(Safety)	a	Fasten your seat belt.
	b	Get ready for take-off.

(From Katz, J. 1994).

'signal' message, which is presented at 35 dB sensation level, and ignore the 'competing' message, presented to the other ear, at 50 dB sensation level.

In a series of posterior temporal lobe tumours, Lynn and Gilroy (1975) demonstrated a marked degradation of the ability of the contralateral ear to repeat accurately the 'signal' message. However, there was a range in ear difference scores and Katz (1994) has emphasized that, while the competing sentence test is highly sensitive for posterior temporal lobe tumours, it is less sensitive for anterior temporal lobe tumours. Lynn and Gilroy (1975, 1976) have reported a variety of results in tumours in the parietal and frontal lobe indicating that the competing sentence test cannot be considered an effective tool for detecting lesions in these sites. However, Bergman, Hirsch and Solzi (1987), using the competing sentence test, identified a high incidence of central auditory dysfunction in patients with both cerebrocranial injuries and cerebrovascular accidents.

The results of competing sentence tests in brain stem lesions have been very variable. Musiek and Guerkink (1982) and Musiek (1983) reported abnormalities in approximately half of their subjects with brain stem lesions. In unilateral lesions the majority of abnormalities were ipsilateral. In isolated reports, a high brain stem lesion was shown to reveal no abnormality, while a low brain stem lesion revealed a zero score on the affected side and 100% score on the normal side (Rintelmann and Lynn, 1983). However, another study in a patient with a right pontine lesion reported a marked contralateral ear deficit (Pinheiro, Jacobson and Broller, 1982).

The threshold of interference test

This technique was introduced by Willeford (1976), who constructed a competing sentence test requiring attention and report only from a designated ear. The threshold of interference test (Bergman *et al.*, 1987) is based on Willeford's paradigm. The sentences employed in this test each contained three key words, each of which could be interchanged with the key words presented simultaneously to the competing ear, and remain meaningful (Figure 17.21).

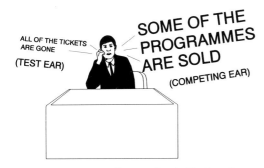

Figure 17.21 Diagram to illustrate threshold of interference test

The sentences are presented to the test ear at 20 dB SL (i.e. above the level at which two out of the three key words are repeated correctly). The level of the competing sentences is increased in 5 dB steps until the listener can no longer meet the performance criterion at the test ear. Bergman *et al.* (1987) applied the test to 15 control subjects (mean age 24 years). In a further 17 control subjects the test was applied using a transformed up-and-down threshold finding procedure, which is applied when a threshold of interference is not reached at the maximum level available in the competing ear. There were two experimental groups. The first consisted of nine patients (mean age 66.2 years) with focal cerebrovascular accidents in the right hemisphere, seven of whom showed left ear suppression. The second group consisted of 18 patients, with either left (*n* = 10) or right hemisphere damage (*n* = 8). Six of the 10 with left hemisphere damage had normal scores bilaterally and four had left ear suppression. CT scans were performed in this group, and the findings in three of the patients supported the possibility of a deep lesion involving the callosal fibres from the right side. Of the eight patients with right hemisphere damage, five showed either partial or complete left ear suppression and the rest had normal scores bilaterally. The authors recommended the test as an efficient and rapid procedure for exposing strong hemisphere suppression, particularly in right hemisphere damage. In the auditory cortex, the physiological correlate of this psychoacoustic phenomenon is that of ear selection and interaural attention.

Sequencing tasks

Sequencing or temporal ordering refers to tasks where a sequence of successive stimuli, which are separated in time, need to be identified. The ability to process a rapid succession of stimuli in a particular order is of particular relevance to language (Lashley, 1951; Neff, 1964; Hirsh, 1967), since words have meaning only when the different segments are combined in a particular order and sentences only become meaningful when the words are joined together in a specific way. The infero-temporal cortex in the left hemisphere is thought to contribute to the processing of this function.

The pitch pattern test

One of the more popular temporal ordering tests is the pitch pattern test (Pinheiro and Ptacek, 1971; Ptacek and Pinheiro, 1971). It consists of 120 sequences, each made up of three tone bursts of two different frequencies, arranged in six possible patterns (Figure 17.22). The high tone is 1122 Hz, and the low one is 880 Hz. Each sequence is 900 ms long, made up of three 200 ms long tone bursts separated

L = Low frequency (880 Hz)

H = High frequency (1122 Hz)

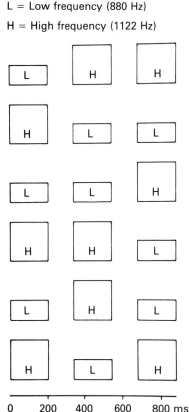

Figure 17.22 Diagram to illustrate pitch pattern test

by 150 ms gaps. The test items can be presented monaurally or binaurally, and verbal, manual and/or hummed responses are acceptable.

Patients with lesions of either hemisphere or of the interhemispheric pathways have been reported to experience difficulty in describing monaurally presented sequences (Musiek, Pinheiro, and Wison, 1980). However, lateralization of the pathology based on these results proved unreliable, since bilateral, ipsilateral and contralateral ear deficits were recorded following unilateral cortical pathology (Pinheiro and Musiek, 1985). In a subsequent study (Musiek and Pinheiro, 1987) the test was applied to 29 patients with cochlear hearing loss, 22 patients with brain stem lesions and 29 patients with unilateral cortical pathology. The test findings indicate high sensitivity and specificity in cerebral lesions (83% and 88.2% respectively). In brain stem lesions the sensitivity was considerably lower at 45%. In the cerebral group lateralization of the pathology based on the test findings was not possible. A small proportion of the patients with cochlear impairment had reduced pitch pattern scores. Based on these findings, and particularly the high specificity of the frequency patterns results in the cerebral group, the authors concluded

that the task could be useful in a battery of central auditory tests for the differential diagnosis of cortical lesions.

The paradigm and experimental design of the pitch pattern test has been used for two other sequencing tasks: the duration pattern test, in which the sequence is made up of a fixed frequency presented in two different durations, and the intensity pattern test, in which the frequency is also fixed and two different intensities are utilized.

Psychoacoustic pattern discrimination test

This test was developed by Blaettner, Scherg and Von Cramon (1989) with three aims: to devise a test which would detect unilateral telencephalic hearing disorders in patients, would not rely on speech material to avoid inherent perceptual deficits and would be relatively insensitive to peripheral auditory loss.

The procedure devised is comprised of noise bursts to assess discrimination changes in intensity and trains of clicks to test discrimination of changes in temporal structure. Using this test in patients with unilateral hemisphere lesions, the authors showed an increase in errors of discrimination in the ear opposite to the hemisphere lesion. Moreover, these workers showed that middle latency and slow vertex evoked potentials were abnormal in all cases with abnormal psychoacoustic pattern discrimination tests, although the converse correlation did not hold. The authors concluded that their test was relatively simple in comparison with other central auditory behavioural tests, appeared sensitive to temporal lobe lesions and insensitive to peripheral hearing loss. Thus, this may prove to be a valuable tool in the future.

Summary of cortical assessment

This brief review of tests of auditory cortical function highlights the difficulties in defining pathophysiology at this level of the auditory system. Much work remains to extend our understanding of the physiological mechanisms subserving higher auditory function which, in turn, will allow better interpretation of both the electrophysiological and behavioural tests available. Moreover, detailed correlation of well defined central nervous system lesions with high resolution MRI and angiography will undoubtedly enable much clearer conclusions to be drawn from case studies, which in the past have appeared to provide contradictory and confounding information.

A proposed central auditory test battery to define cortical dysfunction is more difficult to delineate than a similar schema for brain stem lesions. As noted in the text, peripheral and brain stem pathology affect auditory signals before they arrive at the auditory cortex and thus interpretation may be extremely difficult. Nonetheless, work has suggested that the dichotic digit test may be of value even in the presence of a significant cochlear hearing loss, as may the dichotic sentence identification test and the psychoacoustic pattern discrimination test. In terms of differentiating brain stem from cortical pathology, competing sentences and frequency pattern tests have been shown to be most efficient (Katz, 1994).

Clinical presentations of central auditory nervous system dysfunction

Brain stem hearing loss

The brain stem is a small compact structure comprised of cranial nerve nuclei, multiple afferent and efferent motor and sensory long tracts and the reticular formation. Any lesion which impinges on the auditory pathways is therefore almost certain to involve numerous adjacent structures, which may result in various combinations of motor weakness, ataxia, sensory loss and cranial nerve palsies. Not surprisingly damage to these vital structures may necessitate active medical intervention prior to any consideration of auditory symptoms.

Moreover, brain stem hearing loss is rarely encountered in clinical practice, because of the multiplicity of pathways and commissures beyond the point of decussation in the superior olivary complex and the symmetrical tonotopic organization subserved by the auditory nuclei at all levels (Moore, 1986, 1987b).

The audiometric configuration associated with a focal brain stem lesion is the subject of some debate. The most commonly reported configuration is a bilateral, symmetrical, high frequency, sloping configuration (Dix and Hood, 1973; Luxon, 1980). However, physiological studies on animals suggest that lesions affecting the medial superior olive bilaterally result in a low frequency loss, while reduced thresholds at high frequencies result if the lateral superior olives are bilaterally affected as well. In a recent study of well defined midline brain stem lesions, low frequency hearing loss was documented (Cohen, Luxon and Rudge, 1996).

At the level of the superior olivary complex, bilateral lesions involving the nuclei are required for a hearing loss to occur, but pathologies involving the cochlear nuclei often give rise to a unilateral hearing loss, which may be of any configuration, depending on the frequency columns that are involved.

In terms of clinical diagnosis, there is a number of problems in differentiating brain stem hearing loss from the more common cochlear pathologies. As noted, a bilateral, symmetrical, high frequency, sloping hearing loss, which is found in many cochlear pathologies, has been reported most commonly in brain stem disease. Furthermore, in the majority of these patients recruitment has been found. This phenomenon has historically been identified as a particular characteristic of cochlear damage, although some workers have suggested that it may also be a manifes-

tation of central auditory dysfunction (Dix and Hood, 1973; Luxon, 1980). Nonetheless, the high prevalence of recruitment associated with brain stem pathology raises the possibility of secondary involvement of the cochlea, either through pressure, as in the case of tumours; interference with the blood supply or involvement of the efferent olivocochlear bundle, which originates in the medial periolivary nuclei and synapses on the outer and inner hair cells of the cochlea. Dysfunction of the olivocochlear bundle may result in release of the outer hair cells on the basilar membrane from normal inhibitory influences, mediating recruitment via a central mechanism. As noted above, recent work has identified lack of suppression of transient evoked otoacoustic emissions with contralateral masking in brain stem lesions (Prasher, Ryan and Luxon, 1994).

The tests which are usually employed in diagnosing brain stem pathology, i.e. auditory brain stem responses, acoustic reflex threshold and masking level difference, are highly sensitive techniques in the absence of any peripheral auditory dysfunction. However, their application in defining characteristic features of brain stem hearing loss may be limited in the presence of significant 'peripheral' pathology, as these tests have been shown to exhibit abnormalities in the face of cochlear and/or VIIIth nerve pathology.

Moreover, speech tests exhibit large variability in scores when applied to patients with peripheral hearing impairment and are of limited value in this situation. In addition, the differentiation of cochlear from brain stem hearing loss based on recruitment, is open to question until further clarification of the physiological mechanisms subserving this phenomenon are defined more clearly.

Clinical research studies of hearing loss due to brain stem pathology should therefore concentrate on pathologies such as vascular events, where clearly defined and well circumscribed lesions may be identified. In addition, the cochlea and VIIIth nerve must be shown to be normal. Only a few cases of pure tone deficits of brain stem origin have been reported (Luxon, 1980), but without detailed imaging to allow definite clinical correlation of the pure tone deficit with the underlying brain stem pathology.

Lateralization of the deficit in unilateral brain stem lesions

Brain stem auditory pathologies are known to produce bilateral deficits most commonly on both auditory brain stem responses and acoustic reflex threshold measurements (Jerger and Jerger, 1974; Stockard and Rossiter, 1977; Musiek and Guerkink, 1982; Cohen and Prasher, 1988).

In unilateral brain stem pathology, the application of behavioural test results in correlating ear deficit with the side of the lesion is less predictable than that derived from the acoustic reflex threshold and auditory brain stem responses. The acoustic reflex threshold pattern of abnormality found in a particular case indicates a pathology involving a particular section of the reflex arc (Cohen and Prasher, 1988) and on the auditory brain stem responses, abnormally prolonged peak and/or interwave latencies are associated with involvement of the generator sites of the different peaks (Oh *et al.*, 1981) and may indicate the laterality of a lesion. However, the complexity of processing of speech signals with multiple relays running in parallel throughout the central auditory nervous system, make it extremely difficult on the basis of even monaural speech tests to identify the side of a focal lesion.

A number of studies has shown ipsilateral, contralateral and binaural audiological findings for definitely lateralized brain stem lesions (Bocca and Calearo, 1963; Calearo and Antonelli, 1968; Jerger and Jerger, 1974; Lynn and Gilroy, 1977). Inevitably, the precise findings will depend on the type, size and exact location of the lesion in the central auditory system and the presence or absence of any distant effects, e.g. pressure, oedema, ischaemia of the primary pathology. Notwithstanding this there is evidence to suggest that a lesion at the level of the cochlear nucleus or low brain stem is more likely to be associated with an ipsilateral deficit on both psychophysical and electrophysiological tests, while a unilateral lesion at the level of the superior olivary complex or higher may demonstrate ipsilateral, contralateral or binaural findings on both categories of testing (Gilroy and Lynn, 1978). Moreover, it should be emphasized that extra-axial brain stem lesions may result in more ipsilateral findings as a result of VIIIth nerve or cochlear nuclei compression whereas intra-axial pathology is more likely to show an array of abnormalities.

Cortical hearing impairment

Cortical hearing loss is a rare condition, which has most commonly been reported in association with vascular disease affecting both temporal lobes. Additional and often more dramatic neurological sequelae, including hemipareses and dysphasias are the rule.

The primary auditory cortex in man lies in the anterior and posterior transverse temporal gyri of Heschl. Each ear has bilateral representation in the cerebral cortex and it is possible to remove the nondominant hemisphere, in man, without significant effect on either the pure tone audiogram or the discrimination of distorted speech (Dandy, 1933). Both animal and clinical studies of cortical deafness have demonstrated that cortical lesions, which result in hearing impairment are bilateral and involve the temporal or temporoparietal lobes, including the primary auditory cortex (areas 41 and 42) on both transverse gyri of Heschl.

The auditory deficits resulting from purely cerebral lesions are various and have previously been divided into the *auditory agnosias* in which pure tone audiometry is normal or only minimally affected, while binaural speech discrimination tasks are markedly abnormal (Coslett, Brashaer and Heilman, 1984; Benjamin and Troost, 1988) and *cortical deafness*, in which a severe, if not total, hearing loss is present (Earnest, Monroe and Yarnell, 1977).

Auditory agnosia was originally defined by Freud (1891) as a selective disorder of sound recognition. 'I can hear you talking, but I can not translate it' (Jerger, Lovering and Wertz, 1972; Kanshepolosky, Kelley and Waggener, 1973). However, in the subsequent literature the term has been used to describe two different clinical presentations: patients who are unable to recognize all types of sound, (speech, music and environmental sounds) and patients who are unable to recognize non-verbal sounds only. Most cases reported in the literature correspond to the wider definition with impairment of all three domains of auditory function that are traditionally investigated (Lechevalier *et al.*, 1984).

Nonetheless, there are reports of verbal auditory agnosia, often referred to as 'word deafness' in which speech perception is severely impaired in distinction to other linguistic skills, while the recognition of non-verbal material such as musical tunes and environmental noises remains intact (Albert and Bear, 1974; Coslett, Brashear and Heilman, 1984; Metz–Lutz and Dahl, 1984; Takahashi *et al.*, 1992; Peretz *et al.*, 1995). In many cases of word deafness that have been reported, aphasic disturbances have accompanied the apparent auditory deficit (Goldstein, 1974; Buchman *et al.*, 1986). The possibility of a single deficit contributing to both disorders has been considered rarely (Praamstra *et al.*, 1991). Equally, there are cases of auditory agnosia in which there is impairment of recognition of non-verbal material while the recognition of speech remains intact (Spreen, Benton and Fincham, 1965; Lambert *et al.*, 1989; Fujii *et al.*, 1990). These reports would tend to suggest that the perception of speech and non-speech auditory signals are subserved by separate neural systems.

The recent report by Peretz *et al.* (1995) described two patients with fixed auditory deficits predominantly affecting the processing of music as opposed to any marked deficit of processing of speech or environmental sounds. Both patients were shown by MRI scanning to have bilateral lesions of the rostral, superior temporal gyri. Further studies of this type with detailed experimental measurements and *in vivo* imaging are necessary to advance knowledge of cortical auditory disorders and cerebral organization of higher auditory processing.

In some cases, the primary hearing deficit predominates and these cases have been described as true *cortical deafness* (Earnest, Monroe and Yarnell, 1977; Graham, Greenwood and Lecky, 1980; Ozdamar,

Kraus and Curry, 1982; Bahls *et al.*, 1988), although, this deafness may improve, leaving a residual agnosia for speech and other sounds with only a minor audiometric deficit (Jerger *et al.*, 1969; Goldstein, Brown and Hollander, 1975; Tanaka *et al.*, 1991). Thus, the relationship between auditory agnosia and cortical hearing loss may represent a continuum (Goldstein, 1974) dependent upon the precise site of pathology in the primary auditory cortex, the association areas, the optic radiation and the medial geniculate body. While further detailed assessments are necessary, this hypothesis would be supported by recent work in which word deafness has been reported in cases of bilateral infarction of the primary auditory cortex (Coslett, Brashear, and Heilman, 1984) and in association with bilateral damage to its underlying deep white matter (Brick *et al.*, 1985).

Goldstein (1927), in his discussion of the localization of word deafness, suggested that the middle portion of the superior temporal gyrus subserved this function. Thus the comprehension of verbal sounds has been attributed to pathways into and out of Heschl's gyrus, while the auditory cortex correlate for environmental sounds has been variously suggested to be sited in the upper bank of the Sylvian fissure and the inferior parietal lobe of the right hemisphere (Spreen, Benton and Fincham, 1965), bilateral temperoparietal cortices (Albert *et al.*, 1972) and more recently in the subcortical region adjoining the medial geniculate body bilaterally (Motomura *et al.*, 1986). These last authors again emphasized the continuum of clinical manifestations of auditory cortical lesions by describing a case with generalized auditory agnosia for verbal and environmental sounds, which, over a 2-month period resolved to a selective auditory agnosia for environmental sounds.

In a recent report in which a patient with pure word deafness was compared with two patients with profound cortical deafness, Tanaka *et al.* (1991) emphasized that the extent of bilateral damage to the white matter adjacent to the posterior half of the putamen, 'was crucial in determining the severity of the hearing loss'. They demonstrated that in two patients with severe hearing loss (i.e. 'cortical deafness') all or most of the white matter lateral to the posterior half of the putamen was involved in the temporoparietal infarction, while in their patient with auditory agnosia significant white matter lateral to the posterior half of the putamen on both sides was preserved. They concluded that bilateral lesions in the white matter ventral and lateral to the posterior half of the putamen, which interrupt *all* the projections from the medial geniculate body to the auditory related cortices are likely to result in severe persistent hearing disturbances.

Cortical sensory disturbances

Auditory hallucinations, including elementary sounds and complex sounds such as speech, music and voices, are well recognized in lesions of the temporal lobe including tumours, vascular events and temporal lobe epilepsy (Penfield and Rasmussen, 1950). In addition, elementary unformed auditory hallucinations have been reported in pontine lesions (Adams and Victor, 1981).

Paracusia have also been reported with temporal lobe lesions, in which sound volumes may be altered, changed in tone or timbre or may even sound strange or disagreeable (Adams and Victor, 1981). In both cortical deafness and word deafness unpleasant auditory sensations have been reported in association with bilateral temporal infarcts (Auerbach, 1981; Tanaka *et al.*, 1991).

Auditory extinction has been documented following acute hemispheric damage and may be demonstrated at the bedside by presenting two simultaneous auditory stimuli one to each ear (DeRenzi, Gentilini and Pattacine, 1984). This phenomenon is most evident immediately after an acute infarct and, in the majority of cases, improves over a period of 1 month.

Conclusions

In the majority of patients with central auditory nervous system disorders, pure tone audiometry is normal. At the brain stem level, there are only a few exceptions to this. Hearing loss due to cortical pathology is extremely rare and usually results from extensive bilateral ablation of the auditory cortices.

The fact that pure tone deficits due to central auditory nervous system pathology are rarely encountered facilitates the task of their identification, since the majority of the tests aimed at assessing the integrity of the central auditory nervous system are reliable only when the sensitivity to pure-tones is normal. When hearing loss is present, however, separation of the peripheral components from central mechanisms is a challenging task. In the elderly and in young children with middle ear disease, in whom peripheral deficits are prevalent, the strategy in developing a central auditory test battery aimed at these groups must include tests which are resistant to peripheral effects so that the clinical application of a central auditory test will not be restricted.

Considerable advances have been made in the clinical diagnosis of brain stem lesions with the introduction of auditory brain stem responses into neuro-otological assessment during the 1970s. Impedance measurements and behavioural tests complement the auditory brain stem responses and are used to enhance the sensitivity and specificity of the 'brain stem' test battery.

By contrast, little remains known about how the auditory brain functions, or the expected manifestations of lesions in the auditory cortex. A valuable contribution can be made by undertaking clinical studies of patients with unilateral focal lesions of the auditory cortex, supported by detailed imaging and behavioural auditory tests. If mistakes from the past have contributed anything at all to the field of laterality research, it is that the key principle which should be adopted is that all conclusions are based on sound scientific evidence of the data, rather than assumptions.

With the development of sophisticated imaging techniques, it may be expected that higher resolution brain mapping using positron emission tomography, magnetic resonance imaging and angiography and regional cerebral blood flow measurements, will enable a fuller understanding of structural and functional correlates of the central auditory nervous system.

References

ADAMS, J. C. (1979) Ascending projections to the inferior colliculus. *Journal of Comparative Neurology*, **183**, 519–538

ADAMS, R. D. and VICTOR, M. (1981) *Principles of Neurology*. New York: McGraw–Hill

ALBERT, M. L. and BEAR, D. (1974) Time to understand. A case study of word deafness with reference to the role of time in auditory comprehension. *Brain*, **97**, 373–384

ALBERT, M. L., SPARKS, R., VON STOCKERT, T. and SAX, D. (1972) A case study of auditory agnosia – linguistic and non-linguistic processing. *Cortex*, **8**, 427–443

ANTONELLI, A. R., BELLOTTO, R. and GRANDORI, F. (1987) Audiologic diagnosis of central versus eighth nerve and cochlear auditory impairment. *Audiology*, **26**, 209–226

AUERBACH, S. H. (1981) Central razzle: a central auditory pain syndrome? *Archives of Neurology*, **38**, 671

BAHLS, F. H., CHATRIAN, G. E., MESHER, R. A., SUMI, S. M. and RUFF, R. L. (1988) A case of persistent cortical deafness: clinical, neurophysiologic, and neuropathologic observations. *Neurology (Cleveland)*, **38**, 1490–1493

BENJAMIN, E. E. and TROOST, B. T. (1988) Central auditory disorders. In: *Otolaryngology*, edited by G. M. English. Philadelphia: J. B. Lippincott Co. pp. 1–33

BERGMAN, M., HIRSCH, S. and SOLZI, P. (1987) Interhemispheric suppression: a test of central auditory function. *Ear and Hearing*, **8**, 87–91

BERGMAN, M., HIRSCH, S., SOLZI, P. and MANKOWITZ, Z. (1987) The threshold of interference test: a new test of interhemispheric suppression in brain injury. *Ear and Hearing*, **8**, 147–150

BERLIN, C., LOWE-BELL, S., JANNETTA, P. and KLINE, D. (1972) Central auditory deficits after temporal lobectomy. *Archives of Otolaryngology*, **96**, 4–10

BERLIN, C. and MCNEIL, M. (1976) Dichotic listening. In: *Contemporary Issues in Experimental Phoetics*, edited by N. Lass. New York: Academic Press. pp. 327–388

BLAETTNER, U., SCHERG, M. and VON CRAMON, D. (1989) Diagnosis of unilateral telencephalic hearing disorders. *Brain*, **112**, 177–195

BOCCA, E. and CALEARO, C. (1963) Central hearing processes. In: *Modern Developments in Audiology*, edited by J. Jerger. New York: Academic Press. pp. 337–370

BOCCA, E., CALEARO, C. and CASSINARI, V. A. (1954) A new method for testing hearing in temporal lobe tumours: preliminary report. *Acta Otolaryngologica*, **44**, 219–221

BOCCA, E., CALEARO, C., CASSINARI, V. and MIGLIAVACCA, F. (1955) Testing 'cortical' hearing in temporal lobe tumours. *Acta Otolaryngologica*, **45**, 289–304

BORG, E. (1973) On the neuronal organization of the acoustic middle ear reflex. A physiological and anatomic study. *Brain Research*, **49**, 101–123

BORG, E. (1982) Dynamic properties of the intra-aural reflex in lesions of the lower auditory pathways: an experimental study in rabbits. *Acta Otolaryngologica*, **93**, 19–29

BRICK, J. F., FROST, J. L., SCHOCHET, S. S., GUTMANN, L. and CROSBY, T. W. (1985) Pure word deafness: CT localization of the pathology. *Neurology (Cleveland)*, **35**, 441–442

BROADBENT, D. E. (1954) The role of auditory localization in attention and memory span. *Journal of Experimental Psychology*, **47**, 191–196

BRODY, H. (1955) Organization of the cerebral cortex: III. A study of aging in the human cerebral cortex. *Journal of Comparative Neurology*, **102**, 511–556

BRUNT, M. (1978) The staggered spondaic word test. In: *Handbook of Clinical Audiology*, edited by J. Katz. Baltimore: Williams & Wilkins. pp. 262–275

BUCHMAN, A. S., GARRON, D. C., TROST-CARDAMONE, J. E., WICHTER, M. D. and SCHWARTZ, M. (1986) Word deafness: one hundred years later. *Journal of Neurology, Neurosurgery and Psychiatry*, **49**, 489–499

CALEARO, C. and ANTONELLI, A. R. (1963) 'Cortical' hearing tests and cerebral dominance. *Acta Otolaryngologica*, **56**, 17–26

CALEARO, C. and ANTONELLI, A. R. (1968) Audiometric findings in brainstem lesions. *Acta Otolaryngologica*, **66**, 305–319

CARPENTER, M. B. (1976) *Human Neuroanatomy*, 7th edn. Baltimore: Williams & Wilkins

CHU, N. S. (1989) Brainstem auditory evoked potentials: correlation between CT mid-brain-pontine lesion sites and abolition of wave V or the IV–V complex. *Journal of Neurological Sciences*, **91**, 165–177

COHEN, M. and PRASHER, D. K. (1988) The value of combining auditory brainstem responses and acoustic reflex threshold measurements in neuro-otological diagnosis. *Scandinavian Audiology*, **17**, 153–162

COHEN, M. and PRASHER, D. K. (1992) Defining the relationship between cochlear hearing loss and acoustic reflex thresholds. *Scandinavian Audiology*, **21**, 225–238

COHEN, M., LUXON, L. M. and RUDGE, P. (1996) Auditory deficits and hearing loss associated with focal brain stem haemorrhage. *Scandinavian Audiology*, **25**, 133–141

COLLARD, M., LESSER, R., LUEDERE, H., ROTHNER, A., ERENBERG, G., HAHN, J. *et al.* (1982) *Results of Four Dichotic Speech Tests for Temporal Lobectomy Candidates*, presented at Academy of Neurology, Washington DC, April 22

COSLETT, H. B., BRASHEAR, H. R. and HEILMAN, K. M. (1984) Pure word deafness after bilateral primary auditory cortex infarcts. *Neurology*, **34**, 347–352

CRACE, R. (1970) Morphologic alterations with age in the human cochlear nuclear complex. *PhD dissertation*. Ohio: Ohio University

CRANFORD, J., BOOSE, M. and MOORE, C. (1990) Tests of the precedence effect in sound localization reveal abnormalities in multiple sclerosis. *Ear and Hearing*, **11**, 282–288

DANDY, W. E. (1933) Physiological studies following extirpation of the right cerebral hemisphere in man. *Bulletin of Johns Hopkins Hospital*, **53**, 31–51

DAYAL, V. S., TARANTINO, L. and SWISHER, L. P. (1966) Neuro-otologic studies in multiple sclerosis. *Laryngoscope,* **76,** 1798–1809

DERENZI, E., GENTILINI, M. and PATTACINE, F. (1984) Auditory extinction following hemisphere damage. *Neuropsychologica,* **22,** 733–744

DIX, M. R. and HOOD, J. D. (1973) Symmetrical hearing loss in brain stem lesions. *Acta Otolaryngologica,* **75,** 165–177

DRULOVIC, B., RIBARIC–JANKES, K., KOSTIC, V. and STERNIC, N. (1994) Multiple sclerosis as the cause of sudden 'pontine' deafness. *Audiology,* **33,** 195–201

EARNEST, M. P., MONROE, P. A. and YARNELL, P. R. (1977) Cortical deafness – demonstrations of the pathologic anatomy by CT scan. *Neurology,* **27,** 1172–1175

EFRON, R. (1990) *The Decline and Fall of Hemisphere Specialization.* Hillsdale, New Jersey: Erlbaum Lawrence

EGGERMONT, J. J., DON, M. and BRACKMANN, D. E. (1980) Electrocochleography and auditory brainstem electric response in patients with pontine angle tumors. *Annals of Otology, Rhinology and Laryngology,* **89** (suppl. 75), 1–19

FERRARO, J. A. and MINCKLER, J. (1977a) The brachium of the inferior colliculus. *Brain and Language,* **4,** 156–164

FERRARO, J. A. and MINCKLER, J. (1977b) The human lateral lemniscus and its nuclei. *Brain and Language,* **4,** 277–294

FIFER, R. C., JERGER, J. F., BERLIN, C. I., TOBEY, E. A. and CAMPBELL, J. C. (1983) Development of a dichotic sentence identification test for hearing impaired adults. *Ear and Hearing,* **4,** 300–305

FISHER, C., MAUGUIERE, F., ECHALLIER, J. F. and COURJON, J. (1982) Contribution of brainstem auditory evoked potentials to diagnosis of tumours and vascular disease. *Advances in Neurology* **32,** 177–185

FREUD, S. (1891) *Zur Auffassung der Aphasien: eine Kritische Studie.* Vienna: Franz Deuticke

FUJII, T., FUKATSU, R., WATABE, S., OHNUMA, A., TERAMURA, K., KIMURA, I. *et al.* (1990) Auditory sound agnosia without aphasia following a right temporal lobe lesion (published erratum appears in *Cortex,* 1990; **26,** 672). *Cortex,* **26,** 263–268

GALAMBOS, R. (1956) Suppression of auditory nerve activity by stimulation of efferent fibers to cochlea. *Journal of Neurophysiology,* **19,** 424

GALAMBOS, R., SCHWARTZKOPFF, J. and RUPERT, A. (1959) Microelectrode study of superior olivary nuclei. *American Journal of Physiology,* **197,** 527–536

GELFAND, S. and SILMAN, S. (1982) Acoustic reflex thresholds in brain damaged patients. *Ear and Hearing,* **3,** 93–95

GILROY, J. and LYNN, G. E. (1978) Computerized tomography and auditory-evoked potentials. Use in the diagnosis of olivopontocerebellar degeneration. *Archives of Neurology,* **35,** 143–147

GOLDBERG, J. M. and MOORE, R. Y. (1967) Ascending projections of the lateral lemniscus in the cat and monkey. *Journal of Comparative Neurology,* **129,** 143–153

GOLDSTEIN, K. (1927) Die Lokalisation in der Grosshirnrinde. Nach den Erfahrungen an kranken Menschen. In: *Handbuch der Normalen und Pathologischen Physiologie,* edited by A. Bethe, G. V. Bergmann, G. Embden and A. Ellinger. Berlin: Springer. p. 600–842

GOLDSTEIN, M. N. (1974) Auditory agnosia for speech ('pure word deafness') – a historical review with current implications. *Brain and Language,* **1,** 195–204

GOLDSTEIN, M. N., BROWN, M. and HOLLANDER, J. (1975) Auditory agnosia and cortical deafness – analysis of a case with three year follow-up. *Brain and Language,* **2,** 324–332

GRAHAM, J., GREENWOOD, R. and LECKY, B. (1980) Cortical deafness. *Journal of the Neurological Sciences,* **48,** 35–49

GRENMAN, R., LANG, H., PANELIUS, M., SALMIVALLI, A., LAINE, H. and RINTAMAKI, J. (1984) Stapedius reflex and brainstem auditory evoked responses in multiple sclerosis patients. *Scandinavian Audiology,* **13,** 109–114

GRIESEN, O. and RASMUSSEN, P. (1970) Stapedius reflexes in otoneurological examination in brainstem tumors. *Acta Otolaryngologica,* **70,** 366–370

GROSE, J. H., POTH, E. A. and PETERS, R. W. (1994) Masking level differences for tones and speech in elderly listeners with relatively normal audiograms. *Journal of Speech and Hearing Research,* **37,** 422–428

HANNLEY, M., JERGER, J. and RIVERA, V. (1983) Relationship among auditory brainstem responses, masking level differences and the acoustic reflex in multiple sclerosis. *Audiology,* **22,** 20–33

HANSEN, C. C. and RESKE–NIELSEN, E. (1965) Pathological studies in presbycusis. *Archives of Otolaryngology,* **82,** 115–132

HAUSLER, R. and LEVINE, R. (1980) Brainstem auditory evoked potentials are related to interaural time discrimination in patients with multiple sclerosis. *Brain Research,* **191,** 589–594

HAYES, D. and JERGER, J. (1981) Patterns of acoustic reflex and auditory brainstem response abnormality. *Acta Otolaryngologica,* **92,** 199–209

HENDLER, T., SQUIRES, N. K. and EMMERICH, D. S. (1990) Psychophysical measures of central auditory dysfunction in multiple sclerosis: neurophysiological and neuroanatomical correlates. *Anatomy and Physiology,* **11,** 403–416

HIRSH, I. J. (1948) The influence of interaural phase on interaural summation and inhibition. *Journal of the Acoustical Society of America,* **20,** 536–544

HIRSH, I. J. (1967) Information processing in input channels for speech and language: the significance of serial order of stimuli. In: *Brain Mechanisms Underlying Speech and Language,* edited by C. H. Millikan and F. L. Darley. New York: Grune & Stratton. pp. 21–38

IMIG, T. J. and ADRIAN, H. O. (1977) Binaural columns in the primary field (A1) of cat. *Brain Research,* **13,** 338–359

IVEY, R. G. (1969) Tests of CNS auditory function. *Masters Thesis.* Fort Collins: Colorado State University

JACOBSEN, G. P. and NEWMAN, C. W. (1989) Absence of rate-dependent BAEP P5 latency changes in patients with definite multiple sclerosis: possible physiological mechanisms. *Electroencephalography and Clinical Neurophysiology,* **74,** 19–23

JANI, N. N., LAURENO, R., MARK, A. S. and BREWER, C. C. (1991) Deafness after bilateral midbrain contusion: a correlation of magnetic resonance imaging with auditory brainstem evoked responses. *Neurosurgery,* **29,** 106–109

JERGER, J. and HAYES, D. (1977) Diagnostic speech audiometry. *Archives of Otolaryngology,* **103,** 216–222

JERGER, J. and JERGER, S. (1974) Auditory findings in brainstem disorders. *Archives of Otolaryngology,* **99,** 324–350

JERGER, J., LOVERING, L. and WERTZ, M. (1972) Auditory disorder following bilateral temporal lobe insult – report of a case. *Journal of Speech and Hearing Disorders,* **37,** 523–535

JERGER, J., SPEAKES, C. and TRAMMEL, J. (1968) A new approach to speech and audiometry. *Journal of Speech and Hearing Disorders,* **33,** 318–328

JERGER, J., OLIVER, T., CHIMIEL, R. and RIVERA, V. (1986) Patterns of auditory abnormality in multiple sclerosis. *Audiology,* **25,** 193–209

JERGER, J., WEIKERS, N. J., SHARBROUGH F. W. and JERGER, S. (1969) Bilateral lesions of the temporal lobe. *Acta Otolaryngologica*, Suppl. 258, 1–57

JERGER, S. and JERGER, J. (1975) Extra and intra-axial brainstem auditory disorders. *Audiology*, 14, 93–117

JERGER, S. and JERGER, J. (1983) Neuroaudiologic findings in patients with central auditory disorders. *Seminar on Hearing*, 4, 133–159

KANSHEPOLSKY, J., KELLEY, J. J. and WAGGENER, J. D. (1973) A cortical auditory disorder – clinical, audiologic and pathologic implications. *Neurology*, 23, 699–705

KATZ, J. (1962) The use of staggered spondaic words for assessing the integrity of the central auditory system. *Journal of Audiological Research*, 2, 327–337

KATZ, J. (1994) *Handbook of Clinical Audiology*, 4th edn. Baltimore: Williams and Wilkins

KEVANISHVILI, Z. SH. and VON SPECHT, H. (1979) Human slow auditory evoked potentials during natural and drug-induced sleep. *Electroencephalography and Clinical Neurophysiology*, 47, 280–288

KILENY, P. and BERRY, D. A. (1983) Selective impairment of late vertex and middle latency auditory evoked responses in multiply handicapped infants and children. In: *The Multiply Handicapped Hearing Impaired Child*, edited by G. Mencher and S. Gerber. New York: Grune & Stratton. pp. 223–258

KIMURA, D. (1961a) Some effects of temporal-lobe damage on auditory perception. *Canadian Journal of Psychology*, 15, 156–165

KIMURA, D. (1961b) Cerebral dominance and the perception of verbal stimuli. *Canadian Journal of Psychology*, 15, 166–171

KIMURA, D. (1964) Left-right differences in the perception of melodies. *Quarterly Journal of Experimental Psychology*, 16, 355–358

KIMURA, R. and WERSALL, J. (1962) Termination of the olivocochlear bundle in relation to the outer hair cells of the organ of Corti in the guinea pig. *Acta Otolaryngologica*, 55, 11–32

KONIGSMARK, B. W. and MURPHY, E. A. (1970) Neuronal populations in the human brain. *Nature*, 228, 1335–1336

KONIGSMARK, B. W. and MURPHY, E. A. (1972) Volume of the ventral cochlear nucleus in man: its relationship to neuronal population and age. *Journal of Neuropathology and Experimental Neurology*, 31, 304–316

KORSAN–BENGTSEN, M. (1973) Distorted speech audiometry: a methodological and clinical study. *Acta Otolaryngologica*, Suppl. 310, 7–75

KURDZIEL, S., NOFFSINGER, D. and OLSEN, W. (1976) Performance by cortical lesion patients on 40% and 60% time-compressed materials. *Journal of the American Audiological Society*, 2, 3–7

KUSTEL, M., BUKI, B., GYIMESI, J., MAKO, J., KOMORA, V. and RIBARI, O. (1993) Auditory brainstem potentials in uraemia. *Otology, Rhinology and Laryngology*, 55, 89–92

LAMBERT, J., EUSTACHE, F., LECHEVALIER, B., ROSSA, Y. and ROSSA, Y. (1989) Auditory agnosia with relative sparing of speech perception. *Cortex*, 25, 71–82

LASHLEY, K. S. (1951) The problem of seriel order in behaviour. In: *Cerebral Mechanisms in Behaviour*, edited by L. A. Jeffress. New York: Wiley. pp. 112–136

LECHEVALIER, B., ROSSA, Y., EUSTACHE, F., SCHUPP, C., BONER, L. and BAZIN, C. (1984) Un cas de surdité corticale épargnant en partie la musique. *Revue de Neurologie (Paris)*, 140, 190–201

LICKLIDER, J. C. R. (1948) The influence of interaural phase relations upon the masking of speech by white noise. *Journal of the Acoustical Society of America*, 20, 150–159

LINDEN, A. (1964) Distorted speech and binaural speech resynthesis tests. *Acta Otolaryngologica*, 58, 32–48

LUXON, L. M. (1980) Hearing loss in brain stem disorders. *Journal of Neurology, Neurosurgery and Psychiatry*, 43, 510–515

LYNN, G. E. and GILROY, J. (1975) Effects of brain lesions on the perception of monotic and dichotic speech stimuli. *Proceedings of a Symposium on Central Auditory Processing Disorders*. Omaha: University of Nebraska Medical Centre. pp. 47–83

LYNN, G. E. and GILROY, J. (1976) Central aspects of audition. In: *Hearing Disorders*, edited by J. L. Northern. Boston: Little, Brown & Co. pp. 102–118

LYNN, G. E. and GILROY, J. (1977) Evaluation of central auditory dysfunction in patients with neurological disorders. In: *Central Auditory Dysfunction*, edited by R. W. Keith. New York: Grune and Stratton. pp. 117–221

LYNN, G. E. and GILROY, J. (1984) Detection and localization of central auditory disorders. In: *Hearing Disorders*, edited by J. L. Northern. Boston: Little, Brown & Co. p. 179

LYNN, G. E., GILROY, J., TAYLOR, P. C. and LEISER, R. P. (1981) Binaural masking-level differences in neurological disorders. *Archives of Otolaryngology*, 107, 357–362

MARKAND, O. N., FARLOW, M. R., STEVENS, J. C. and EDWARDS, M. K. (1989) Brainstem auditory evoked potential abnormalities with unilateral brainstem lesions demonstrated by magnetic resonance imaging. *Archives of Neurology*, 46, 295–299

MATATHIAS, H., SOHMER, H. and BITON, C. (1985) Central auditory tests and auditory nerve-brainstem evoked responses in multiple sclerosis. *Acta Otolaryngologica*, 99, 369–376

MATZKER, J. (1959) Two new methods for the assessment of central auditory functions in cases of brain disease. *Annals of Otology, Rhinology and Laryngology*, 68, 1188–1197

MERZENICH, M. M. (1982) Organization of primate sensory forebrain structures: a new perspective. In: *New Perspectives in Cerebral Localization*, edited by R. A. Thompson and S. R. Green. New York: Raven Press. pp. 47–62

METZ-LUTZ, M. N. and DAHL, E. (1984) Analysis of word comprehension in a case of pure word deafness. *Brain and Language*, 23, 13–25

MØLLER, A. R. and JANNETTA, P. J. (1982a) Evoked potentials from the inferior colliculus in man. *Electroencephalography and Clinical Neurophysiology*, 53, 612–620

MØLLER, A. R. and JANNETTA, P. J. (1982b) Auditory evoked potentials recorded intracranially from the brainstem in man. *Journal of Experimental Neurology*, 78, 144–157

MØLLER, A. R. and JANNETTA, P. J. (1983) Monitoring auditory functions during cranial nerve microvascular decompression operations by direct recording from the eighth nerve. *Journal of Neurosurgery*, 59, 493–499

MOORE, D. R. (1987a) Physiology of higher auditory system. In: *Hearing*, edited by M. P. Haggard and E. F. Evans. *British Medical Bulletin*, 43, 856–870

MOORE, J. K. (1986) Cochlear nuclei: relationship to the auditory nerve. In: *Neurobiology of Hearing: The Cochlea*, edited by R. A. Altschuler, D. W. Hoffman and R. P. Bobbin. New York: Raven Press. pp. 283–301

MOORE, J. K. (1987b) The human auditory brain stem: a comparative view. *Hearing Research*, 29, 1–32

MORALES-GARCIA, C. and POOLE, J. P. (1972) Masked speech audiometry in central deafness. *Acta Otolaryngologica*, **74**, 307–316

MOTOMURA, N., YAMADORI, A., MORI, E. and TAMARU, F. (1986) Auditory agnosia: analysis of a case with bilateral subcortical lesions. *Brain*, **109**, 379–391

MUSIEK, F. E. (1983) Assessment of central auditory dysfunction: the dichotic digit test revisited. *Ear and Hearing*, **4**, 79–83

MUSIEK, F. E. and GEURKINK, N. A. (1982) Auditory brain stem response and central auditory test findings for patients with brain stem lesions: a preliminary report. *Laryngoscope*, **92**, 891–900

MUSIEK, F. E. and PINHEIRO, M. L. (1987) Frequency patterns in cochlear, brainstem and cerebral lesions. *Audiology*, **26**, 79–88

MUSIEK, F. E., PINHEIRO, M. L. and WILSON, D. H. (1980) Auditory pattern perception in 'split brain' patients. *Archives of Otolaryngology*, **106**, 610–612

MUSIEK, F. E., GOLLEGLY, K. M., KIBBE, K. S. and REEVES, A. G. (1989) Electrophysiologic and behavioural auditory findings in multiple sclerosis. *American Journal of Otology*, **10**, 343–350

MUSIEK, F., GOLLEGLY, K., KIBBE, K. and VERKEST, S. (1988) Current concepts on the use of ABR and auditory psychophysical tests in the evaluation of brainstem lesions. *American Journal of Otolaryngology*, **9**, 25–35

MUSIEK, F. E., GOLLEGLY, K. M., KIBBE, K. S. and VERKEST–LENZ, S. B. (1991) Proposed screening test for central auditory disorders: follow-up on the dichotic digits test. *American Journal of Otology*, **12**, 109–113

NAKAYAMA, T., NOBUOKA, H., WADA, S. and MATSUKADO, Y. (1986) Cortical deafness following bilateral hypertensive putaminal haemorrhage. *Brain and Nerve, Tokyo*, **38**, 565–570

NEFF, W.D. (1964) Temporal pattern discrimination in lower animals and its relation to language perception in man. In: *Disorders of Language*, edited by A. V. S. de Rueck and M. O'Connor. Boston: Little Brown. pp. 183–199

NICCUM, N., RUBENS, A. and SPEAKS, C. (1981) Effects of stimulus material on the dichotic listening performance of aphasic patients. *Journal of Speech and Hearing Research*, **24**, 526–534

NOFFSINGER, D., OLSEN, W. O., CARHART, R., HART, C. W. and SAHGAL, V. (1972) Auditory and vestibular aberrations in multiple sclerosis. *Acta Otolaryngologica*, Suppl. 303, 1–63

OH, S. J., KUBA, T., SOYER, A., CHOI, I. S., BONIKOWSKI, F. P. and VITEK, J. (1981) Lateralization of brainstem lesions by brainstem auditory evoked potentials. *Neurology (New York)*, **31**, 14–18

OLSEN, W. O. (1977) Performance of temporal lobectomy patients with dichotic CV test materials. Presented at the *ASHA Convention*, Chicago. November

OLSEN, W. O., NOFFSINGER, D. and KURDZIEL, S. (1975) Speech discrimination in quiet and in white noise by patients with peripheral and central lesions. *Acta Otolaryngologica*, **80**, 375–382

OSEN, K. K. (1972) The projection of the cochlear nuclei to the inferior colliculus in the cat. *Journal of Comparative Neurology*, **144**, 355–369

OZDAMAR, O., KRAUS, N. and CURRY, F. (1982) Auditory brainstem and middle latency responses in a patient with cortical deafness. *Electroencephalography and Clinical Neurophysiology*, **53**, 224–230

PENFIELD, W. and JASPER, H. (1954) *Epilepsy and the Functional Anatomy of the Human Brain*. Boston: Little, Brown & Co.

PENFIELD, W. and RASMUSSEN, T. (1950) *The Cerebral Cortex of Man*. New York: The MacMillian Co.

PERETZ, I., BABAI, M., LUSSIER, I., HERBERT, S. and GAGNON, L. (1995) Corpus d'extraits Musicaux: indices relatifs à la familiarité, à l'age d'acquisition et aux evocations verbales. *Canadian Journal of Experimental Psychology* (In press)

PICKLES, J. O. (1988) *An Introduction to the Physiology of Hearing*. London: Academic Press

PICTON, T. W., HILLYARD, S. A., KRAUS, H. I. and GALAMBOS, R. (1974) Human auditory evoked potentials. I. Evaluation of components. *Electroencephalography and Clinical Neurophysiology*, **36**, 179–190

PINHEIRO, M., JACOBSON, G. and BROLLER, F. (1982) Auditory dysfunction following a gunshot wound of the pons. *Journal of Speech and Hearing Disorders* **47**, 296–300

PINHEIRO, M. L. and MUSIEK, F. E. (eds) (1985) Sequencing and temporal ordering in the auditory system. In: *Assessment of Central Auditory Dysfunction: Foundations and Clinical Correlates*. Baltimore: Williams & Wilkins. pp. 219–238

PINHEIRO, M. L. and PTACEK, P. H. (1971) Reversals in the perception of noise and tone patterns. *Journal of the Acoustical Society of America*, **49**, 1778–1782

PINHEIRO, M. L. and TOBIN, H. (1971) The interaural intensity difference as a diagnostic indicator. *Acta Otolaryngologica*, **71**, 326–328

POOL, K., FINITZO, T., CHI–TZONG–HONG, ROGERS, J. and PICKETT, R. B. (1989) Infarction of the superior temporal gyrus: a description of auditory evoked potential latency and amplitude topology. *Ear and Hearing*, **10**, 144–152

PRAAMSTRA, P., HAGOORT, P., MAASSEN, B. and CRUL, T. (1991) Word deafness and auditory cortical function. *Brain*, **114**, 1197–1225

PRASHER, D. K. and COHEN, M. (1993) Effectiveness of acoustic reflex threshold criteria in the diagnosis of retrocochlear pathology. *Scandinavian Audiology*, **22**, 11–18

PRASHER, D. K., RYAN, S. and LUXON, L. M. (1994) Contralateral suppression of transiently evoked otoacoustic emissions and neuro-otology. *British Journal of Audiology*, **28**, 247–254

PRASHER, D. K., SAINZ, M. and GIBSON, W. P. R. (1981) Binaural voltage summation of brainstem auditory evoked potentials: an adjunct to the diagnostic criteria for multiple sclerosis. *Annals of Neurology*, **11**, 86–91

PTACEK, P. H. and PINHEIRO, M. L. (1971) Pattern reversal in auditory perception. *Journal of the Acoustical Society of America*, **49**, 493–498

QUARANTA, A. and CERVELLERA, G. (1977) Masking level differences in central nervous system diseases. *Acta Otolaryngologica*, **103**, 482–484

QUARANTA, A., CASSANO, P. and CERVELLERA, G. (1978) Clinical value of the tonal masking level difference. *Audiology*, **17**, 232–238

RINTELMANN, W. F. (1985) Monaural speech tests in the detection of central auditory disordrs. In: *Assessment of Central Auditory Dysfunction*, edited by M. L. Pinheiro and F. E. Musiek. Baltimore: Williams & Wilkins. pp. 173–200

RINTELMANN, W. and LYNN, G. (1983) Speech stimuli for assessment of central auditory disorders. In: *Principles of Speech Audiometry*, edited by D. Konkle and W. Rintelmann. Baltimore: University Park Press

ROBINSON, C. and RUDGE, P. (1977) Abnormalities of the

auditory evoked potentials in patients with multiple sclerosis. *Brain*, **100**, 19–40

RODRIGUEZ, G. P., DISARNO, N. J. and HARDIMAN, C. J. (1990) Central auditory processing in normal-hearing elderly adults. *Audiology*, **29**, 85–92

ROSENZWEIG, M. R. (1951) Representations of the two ears at the auditory cortex. *American Journal of Physiology*, **167**, 147–158

SANDO, I. (1965) The anatomical interrelationships of the cochlear nerve fibre. *Acta Otolaryngologica*, **59**, 417–436

SCHARF, B., MAGNAN, J., COLLET, L., ULMER, E. and CHAYS, A. (1994) On the role of the olivocochlear bundle in hearing: a case study. *Hearing Research*, **75**, 11–26

SCHEIBEL, M. E., LINDSAY, R. D., TOMIYAN, U. and SCHEIBEL, A. B. (1975) Progressive dendritic changes in aging human cortex. *Experimental Neurology* **47**, 392–403

SMITH, B. B. and RESNICK, D. M. (1972) An auditory test for assessing brainstem integrity: preliminary report. *Laryngoscope*, **82**, 414–424

SPARKS, R. and GESCHWIND, N. (1968) Dichotic listening in man after section of neocortical commissures. *Cortex*, **4**, 3–16

SPARKS, R., GOODGLASS, H. and NICKEL, B. (1970) Ipsilateral versus contralateral extinction in dichotic listening resulting from hemisphere lesions. *Cortex*, **6**, 249–260

SPEAKS, C., GRAY, T., MILLER, J. and RUBENS, A. (1975) Central auditory deficits and temporal lobe lesions. *Journal of Speech and Hearing Disorders*, **40**, 192–205

SPEAKS, C. and JERGER, J. (1965) Method for measurement of speech identification. *Journal of Speech and Hearing Research*, **8**, 185–194

SPEAKS, C., NICCUM, N. and CARNEY, E. (1982) Statistical properties of responses to dichotic listening with CV nonsense syllables. *Journal of the Acoustical Society of America*, **72**, 1185–1194

SPITZER, J. B. and VENTRY, I. M. (1980) Central auditory dysfunction among chronic alcoholics. *Archives of Otolaryngology*, **106**, 224–229

SPREEN, O., BENTON, A. L. and FINCHAM, R. W. (1965) Auditory agnosia without aphasia. *Archives of Neurology*, **13**, 84–92

STEPHENS, S. and THORNTON, A. (1976) Subjective and electrophysiologic tests in brainstem lesions. *Archives of Otolaryngology*, **102**, 608–613

STOCKARD, J. J. and ROSSITER, V. S. (1977) Clinical and pathological correlates of brainstem auditory response abnormalities. *Neurology*, **27**, 316–325

STUBBLEFIELD, J. H. and GOLDSTEIN, D. P. (1977) A test-retest reliability study on clinical measurement of masking level differences. *Audiology*, **16**, 419–431

TAKAHASHI, N., KAWAMURA, M., SHINOTOU, H., HIRAYAMA, K., KAGA, K. and SHINDO, M. (1992) Pure word deafness due to left hemisphere damage. *Cortex*, **28**, 295–303

TALLAL, P., MILLER, S. and FITCH, R. H. (1993) Neurobiological basis of speech: a case for the prominence of temporal processing. *Annals of the New York Academy*, **682**, 27–47

TALLAL, P., SAINBURG, R. L. and JERNIGAN, T. (1991) The neuropathology of developmental dysphasia: behavioural, morphological and physiological evidence for the pervasive temporal processing disorder. *Reading and Writing: An interdisciplinary Journal*, **3**, 363–377

TANAKA, Y., KAMO, T., YOSHIDA, M. and YAMADORI, A. (1991) 'So-called Cortical Deafness'. *Brain*, **114**, 2385–2401

TEMPLE, C. M., JEEVES, M. A. and VILARROYA, O. O. (1989) Ten pen men: rhyming skills in two children with callosal agenesis. *Brain and Language*, **37**, 548–564

TEMPLE, C. M., JEEVES, M. A. and VILARROYA, O. O. (1990) Reading in callosal agenesis. *Brain and Language*, **39**, 235–253

WILLEFORD, J. A. (1976) Central auditory function in children with learning disabilities. *Audiology and Hearing Education*, **2**, 12–20

WILLEFORD, J. A. (1977) Assessing central auditory behaviour in children: a test battery approach. In: *Central Auditory Dysfunction*, edited by R. W. Keith. New York: Grune & Stratton. pp. 43–72

WILLEFORD, J. A. (1985) Assessment of central auditory disorders in children. In: *Assessment of Central Auditory Dysfunction: Foundations and Clinical Correlates*, edited by M. L. Pinheiro and F. Musiek. Baltimore: Williams & Wilkins. pp. 239–255

WILLIAMS, E. A., BROOKES, G. B. and PRASHER, D. K. (1994) Effects of olivocochlear bundle section on otoacoustic emissions in humans: efferent effects in comparison with control subjects. *Acta Otolaryngologica*, **114**, 121–129

WILLOTT, J. F. (1991a) *Aging and The Auditory System*. London: Whurr Publishers

WILLOTT, J. F. (1991b) Central physiological correlates of ageing and presbyacusis in mice. *Acta Otolaryngologica*, Suppl. **476**, 153–156

WOODS, D. L., CLAYWORTH, C. C., KNIGHT, R. T., SIMPSON, G. V. and NAESER, M. A. (1987) Generators of middle-and long-latency auditory evoked potentials: implications from studies of patients with bitemporal lesions. *Electroencephalography and Clinical Neurophysiology*, **68**, 132–148

18

Tinnitus

R. R. A. Coles

History

The first known writings on treatment of tinnitus appeared in the sixteenth century BC in Egyptian papyruses. The gradual development of concepts of tinnitus through Graeco-Roman times and the Middle Ages to the present century has been comprehensively reviewed by Stephens (1984), and the historical origins of tinnitus masking have been further elaborated by him in the introduction to a subsequent publication (Hazell *et al.*, 1985).

Definition

'Tinnitus' is a symptom rather than a specifiable disease state. Probably the best definition of tinnitus is an elaboration of that by McFadden (1982), by which it can be described as 'the conscious experience of a sound that originates in an involuntary manner in the head of its owner, or may appear to him to do so'. Note that this definition allows for the fact that in many tinnitus patients the sound may at first be thought by them to be coming from the environment: also for the occasional cases where the sound originates in the neck or chest, but is thought by the patient to be in the head.

Somato-sounds and 'objective tinnitus'

The term 'somato-sound' was coined at the Ciba Foundation Symposium (Anon, 1981a) for sounds emitted by the ear or body which might seem to be, and sometimes are, externally detectable correlates of tinnitus. The text reads as follows: 'In this definition, we wish to emphasise that the term *tinnitus* refers to the *sensation* and not to any externally detectable correlates. The term should not be used to describe the

acoustic vibration that can be detected by an observer as being emitted by the ear or elsewhere, including the phenomena formerly described as "objective tinnitus". These should be more appropriately referred to as "bruits" or "acoustic emissions", etc., which might be termed "somato-sounds" . . . We therefore regard the term "objective tinnitus" as a misnomer'.

This chapter therefore has no section on 'objective tinnitus' as such, since we are only concerned with auditory sensations which trouble patients.

Classification and mechanisms

There are at least two useful classifications of tinnitus: by aetiological diagnosis and by site of dysfunction.

Classification by diagnosis

This is purely a medical classification, helping in description and statistics, in counselling the patient and in defining the possibilities of treatment directed at the cause of the tinnitus. It depends on the 'probable' diagnosis. It has been suggested that the clinician should make a diagnosis only if the probability is assessed as being over 50% that a particular condition is causing the tinnitus (Anon, 1981a). On that criterion most cases of tinnitus would have to be classified as 'unknown', which is neither helpful in management nor likely to instil confidence or satisfaction in the patient. The other extreme, often used by clinicians, is to base diagnosis on what is considered to be the most likely single cause, however remote that possibility. Uncertainties intrinsic to the field of tinnitus call for a compromise approach that can be expressed verbally as 'the most likely, reasonably probable diagnosis'. In fact the diagnosis often has to be multiple, since most cases of tinnitus are associated with cochlear disorders and most of those have more than one cause.

Classification by site of auditory dysfunction

The presumed site of disorder and diagnosis of tinnitus are interwoven, and both are often indicated by the site of the hearing loss. However, whether or not tinnitus occurs in association with a cochlear disorder seems to depend not so much on the actual cause of the disorder as on its extent and rate of development. Thus, for the general understanding of tinnitus, for research on the subject, and for many aspects of management, it is more helpful to classify by the site of auditory dysfunction leading to the tinnitus. The scheme for this is shown in Figure 18.1.

Physiological

This covers the hearing of normal body sounds apparently arising from within the head. If people with normal hearing listen attentively in a very quiet environment, the vast majority of them will hear a sound within themselves, most commonly a humming, buzzing or ringing (Heller and Bergman, 1953). By the definition given here, this would be tinnitus; but only rarely will it amount to clinically significant tinnitus. Some of these sounds probably come from *circulatory hum* or *muscular tremor*, and perhaps even from *Brownian movement* of air at the tympanic membrane or of fluid within the cochlea. Other causes include the tinnitus associated with some minimal cochlear pathology, and possibly an auditory percept from normal ongoing auditory neuronal activity. Sometimes physiological tinnitus is pulsatile, for instance as a result of exercise or emotional arousal, or due to partial occlusion of arteries in the temporal or auricular region by externally applied pressure, e.g. when lying on a hard pillow.

Pathophysiological

This term is used here for tinnitus sounds that are either temporary in response to noise, damage or toxaemia and probably due to minor disorders of

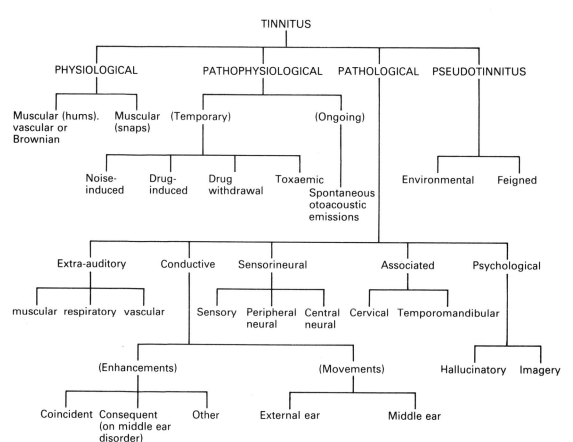

Figure 18.1 Classification by site of the auditory dysfunction (that is leading directly or indirectly to generation of tinnitus)

cochlear or brain-stem function without permanent structural or functional defect, or are ongoing and due to detection of spontaneous otoacoustic emissions.

Noise-induced

Loud sounds may, in some individuals, produce temporary tinnitus lasting for seconds up to days after the exposure. The duration of exposure needed to produce this effect varies between hours for 90 dB(A) noises to milliseconds for high level noises such as gunshots or explosions. The effect is supplementary to the dullness of hearing and sense of numbness of the ears often noticeable at the same time and the temporary threshold shift that may be measurable immediately after a noise exposure. Temporary noise-induced tinnitus and/or dullness of hearing should be taken as a warning that the causative noise exposure could be potentially hazardous to the hearing of the individual if repeated frequently and especially if tinnitus and/or dullness lasts for more than about 5 minutes. However, absence of or failure to recall such symptoms does not mean the noise is harmless for that individual.

The taking of a history of temporary noise-induced tinnitus and dullness of hearing can be of considerable help in evaluation of cases of noise-induced hearing loss for medicolegal purposes. This is particularly so in assessing the relative auditory risks where the individual has been exposed to more than one source of noise, and if the duration of tinnitus after noise exposure has gradually lengthened until eventually it becomes permanent.

Drug-induced

Probably the most commonly experienced temporary drug-induced tinnitus is from alcohol, although a few reports indicate that chronic severe alcoholism may be associated with permanent damage to hearing. On the other hand, in established cases of tinnitus, alcohol may sometimes bring about some reduction in the loudness of the tinnitus as well as a helpful element of sedation.

The most commonly used type of medicine that causes temporary tinnitus is the salicylate group including aspirin. Usually salicylate-induced hearing loss recovers completely, but permanent hearing damage may very occasionally result from prolonged high dosage or in combination with other ototoxic drugs or noise. Apart from the aminoglycosides and antitumour drugs (Griffin, 1988), the evidence for permanent effects of drugs on hearing is weak, there being no means of distinguishing an alleged drug effect from a coincidental unrelated hearing disorder. Even large-scale population studies have yielded equivocal results (Coles, 1984). Specially designed, difficult and carefully controlled studies would be needed to establish to what extent, if any, drugs such as the salicylates and other non-steroidal anti-inflammatory drugs, quinine, antidepressants and beta-blockers were associated with increased risk of permanent hearing loss and/or tinnitus.

Brown *et al.* (1981) listed a large number of drugs which may produce tinnitus; they distinguished two groups. The first has ototoxic effects as reflected in temporary or occasionally permanent tinnitus or hearing loss, e.g. salicylates and other non-steroidal anti-inflammatory drugs, quinine and the loop diuretics. Tinnitus arising from drugs of the severely ototoxic type (e.g. aminoglycosides and some antineoplastic drugs) should probably be taken as a warning of potential risk of permanent damage from prolonged administration. Drugs in the second group do not seem to cause damage to the ear, and probably would not normally cause permanent tinnitus, but may produce tinnitus temporarily because of their effect on biogenic amines in the central nervous system. Drugs in this group include some antidepressants and antihistamines, beta-blockers and caffeine.

Drug withdrawal

Tinnitus is occasionally a manifestation of the hyperexcitable state that can result from too rapid withdrawal from a sedative or addictive drug. Such tinnitus is usually only temporary if the patient maintains the withdrawal or, in the case of benzodiazepines, if the drug is partially reinstated and then very gradually withdrawn over several or many months.

Toxaemic

Probably some toxaemic states are capable of causing a slight but sufficient cochlear dysfunction to cause tinnitus, either temporarily or permanently, or to act as a triggering factor for tinnitus in an already defective cochlea.

Spontaneous otoacoustic emissions

Baskill, Coles and Lutman (unpublished data) have measured spontaneous otoacoustic emissions in about 75% (female) or 45% (male) normal or near-normal ears. It should be noted though that the apparent prevalence of spontaneous otoacoustic emissions depends heavily on the criteria used for their detection (Penner, Glotzbach and Huang, 1993), and on the sensitivity of the measuring equipment and the quietness of both patient and environment. Occasionally these emissions are audible and troublesome to their owners, accounting for about 1–2% of a tinnitus clinic caseload.

Spontaneous otoacoustic emission tinnitus could therefore be classified as physiological, being essentially a manifestation of normality. The factors distinguishing between audible and non-audible spontaneous otoacoustic emissions are as yet uncertain. In some cases, they may be a reduction in efferent inhibitory control of cochlear function, in others an element of instability in their intensity (Penner, 1992) preventing normal adaptation to these sounds. This suggests some pathological factor causing the instability. This notion is reinforced by our observation of five young patients with noise-induced tinnitus where the tinnitus itself was due to ongoing otoacoustic emissions – 'spontaneous' in the sense that at the time of measurement there had been no immediately preceding evoking stimulus. We had previously assumed that these persons had pre-existing spontaneous otoacoustic emissions which, as a result of the noise exposure, had become unstable, and thus audible. However, Penner (personal communication, 1993) has described how one of her laboratory staff had a similar experience following discotheque noise, but in his case the spontaneous otoacoustic emissions causing the tinnitus had definitely not been present previously and indeed, together with the tinnitus and a slight threshold shift, gradually reduced and disappeared over a few weeks.

Pathological

In this class, the tinnitus is associated with a definite disorder of physical or psychological type. It has five subdivisions.

Extra-auditory

This subdivision includes most of the relatively rare disorders associated with somato sounds. It is subdivided by type of source as follows.

Muscular

The most common abnormal muscular sound causing tinnitus is that of *palatal myoclonus* in which there is an irregular and often episodic twitching of the muscles of the soft palate, pharynx and probably of the tensor tympani muscle also. It causes unpleasant clicking sensations, which constitute the presenting symptom. The diagnosis is by means of the history, observation of synchronous twitching either in the soft palate, tympanic membrane or posterior pharyngeal wall, preferably viewed though a nasopharyngoscope to avoid possible inhibition of the twitching (Badia, Parikh and Brookes, 1994). The timing of the clicks can either be indicated by the patient by finger movements, heard through an auscultation tube or an intrameatal microphone and amplifier, or observed with an otoadmittance meter. The aetiology of the condition is not clear, but is presumably due to some neurological abnormality; the condition is said to be very occasionally associated with serious neurological disorder but frequently causes psychological disturbances. It often resolves

spontaneously. A tinnitus masker appears to help many of these patients (East and Hazell, 1987), perhaps by its soothing effect relieving the anxieties and annoyance caused by the condition and thereby bridging the gap to, or possibly even enhancing the tendency to, spontaneous remission. Alternatively, it may be abolished or reduced for several months at a time by injections of botulinus toxin into the palatal muscles (Saeed and Brookes, 1993).

Other forms of muscular tinnitus exist, but are even rarer. These include clicking sounds due to *middle-ear muscle myoclonus* occurring either spontaneously or with eyelid blinking, acoustic stimulation, cutaneous stimulation of the pinna area or phonation. In such cases division of the stapedius tendon may produce relief (Badia, Parikh and Brookes, 1994).

Another form of sound arising from the muscular movement which can cause distress is from the clicking sounds which can arise from a *temporomandibular joint abnormality* or a vibrational type of sound arising from *jaw clenching*. In some instances these can be alleviated totally or partially by appropriate orthodontic treatment.

Respiratory

The condition of *patulous eustachian tube* is associated with a form of tinnitus in which the patient complains of blowing sounds coincident with respiration. The patient may also or alternatively describe symptoms of autophony. The condition is most often associated with weight loss, and appears particularly in certain occupations such as diving and playing of wind or brass instruments. The diagnosis is made from the history especially if it disappears when bending or lying down, and the observation either of large slow fluctuations in otoadmittance coincidental with respiration or of visible tympanic membrane movements as the patient breathes through the nose. Various treatments have been used ranging from chemical or electrical cauterization of the eustachian tube orifice, to surgical closure or peritubular injection with such substances as paraffin, Teflon paste or gelatin sponge. O'Connor and Shea (1981) concluded that application of 20% silver nitrate is probably the best, being relatively simple to perform yet having good results with few side effects.

Vascular

Pulsatile tinnitus is not uncommon, but the border between physiological vascular sounds and pathological ones is ill-defined. It is often only intermittently present, and it may occur either as the only or main tinnitus sound or just as a pulsatile modulation of an ongoing sensorineural tinnitus. It is important in taking the history to ascertain the way and degree to which the pulsations are actually troublesome to the patient, as this will define the need for investigation and/or treatment of the pulsatility itself. Sometimes the pulsatility may not be troublesome, but is a symptom of some other disorder which itself needs investigation and treatment. All cases of pulsatile tinnitus should therefore be considered carefully and their examination should include the following: ascertainment of whether the pulsatility is synchronous with the heartbeat; measurement of pulse rate and rhythm and of the blood pressure; auscultation of both ears and both sides of the neck and head, first with the head central and then turned each way; compression of the jugular veins on each side to see if it reduces or abolishes the tinnitus. In some cases angiography may be required.

The most common cause of pulse-synchronous tinnitus is *arterial turbulence* caused, presumably, by atheromatous plaques or arteriosclerotic kinking of the arteries in the head or neck. This is particularly prominent where there is also hypertension, and may be much reduced or even abolished by antihypertensive therapy. Uncommon disorders causing pulsatile tinnitus are arterial aneurysms, arteriovenous fistulae and glomus jugulare tumours, or even abnormal and prominent cardiac sounds. If the tinnitus reduces when the head is turned to the side opposite that of the pulsating tinnitus, the diagnosis of *arteriovenous fistula* is suggested and surgical treatment comes into consideration. Further confirmation would come from compression of the jugular veins on the affected side which may also reduce or abolish the tinnitus. A jugular venous tie will then often abolish the tinnitus, but unfortunately it frequently recurs as other venous channels open up. Therapeutic embolization under angioradiographic control is a more effective but potentially more dangerous alternative.

Conductive

'Conductive tinnitus' is tinnitus associated with, exacerbated by, or just possibly created by, a middle-ear disorder and/or conductive hearing loss. In most cases, it arises by the revealing or enhancement of an underlying tinnitus of sensorineural or other type. A model of conductive tinnitus, illustrating the mechanisms involved in producing tinnitus in such disorders, is shown in Figure 18.2.

Much of the enhancement is probably due to reduction of the normal masking effect of ambient noise due to the conductive hearing loss. Sometimes the enhanced or revealed sounds are of *physiological* or *extra-auditory* type, but most often they are associated with a sensorineural hearing disorder. The latter may be due to a *coincident sensorineural* disorder that is independent of the middle-ear disorder causing the conductive hearing loss, or to a *consequent sensorineural* disorder arising from or in association with the middle-ear disorder, e.g. in mixed stapedial and

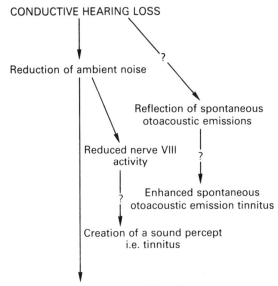

Figure 18.2 Model for 'conductive tinnitus'

cochlear otosclerosis and in cochlear involvement in otitis media.

When a patient with a sensorineural tinnitus comes back to the clinic complaining that the tinnitus has worsened, the cause is often an occlusion of the ear canal or damping of the tympanic membrane by accumulations of *wax* or debris adding a conductive hearing loss. This is particularly prone to happen where the patient makes daily use of a hearing aid, insertions of the earmould tending gradually to impact wax.

The reduction of masking by ambient noise does not seem to explain all cases of conductive tinnitus though. Sometimes the tinnitus persists in spite of use of a hearing aid or resolution of the conductive hearing loss. Possibly a prolonged auditory neuronal quietness becomes interpreted by the brain as an abnormal input from the ear, giving rise to an ongoing sound percept that persists long after return of normal sound conduction. Another possible and occasional cause of conductive tinnitus is the internal reflection, and possible amplification thereby, of spontaneous otoacoustic emissions (Kemp, 1981).

Only occasionally do disorders of the conductive mechanism themselves cause tinnitus. Such sounds result from *movements* within the external or middle ears. Patients may complain of noises in the ears due to movement of water in the external ear, particularly if retained there by wax or debris, or movement of a foreign body in the ear either passively as a result of the patient's movement or actively in the case of an animate foreign body. Likewise, movements of fluid in the middle ear or of bubbles in the fluid cause sounds which can trouble the patient. Clinical examination of the ear will usually reveal the nature of the disorder and the appropriate treatment.

Sensorineural

The majority of cases of tinnitus probably originate from a disorder within the cochlea, although other parts of the sensorineural pathways can sometimes be the primary site of disorder. In dealing with 'sensorineural tinnitus', the classification will be subdivided into sensory (cochlear), peripheral neural (VIIIth nerve) and central neural. This does not imply that a distinction between these can always be made easily or firmly, and in some cases there may be mixtures of peripheral, central and psychological elements in the tinnitus either from the outset or arising secondarily. Moreover, even when the initial site of disorder is in the cochlea, the actual sites of perception of the abnormal VIIIth nerve activity as a sound-like stimulus must lie somewhere in the central auditory nervous system, with its conscious perception and evaluation occurring at cortical level.

Sensory

The majority of cases of tinnitus in which a probable diagnosis can be made involve the cochlea. The most common diagnoses are age-associated hearing loss, noise-induced hearing loss, and head or ear trauma, disorders associated with endolymphatic hydrops and cochlear vascular deficiency or viral infection. The term age-associated hearing loss collectively embraces the progressive cochlear cellular degeneration which causes the steadily increasing sensory hearing loss that becomes measurable after the age of about 20 years, and the more rapid or stepwise and sometimes asymmetric hearing losses, often of uncertain causation, that occur with increasing frequency with advancing years. Certainly, in epidemiological studies (Coles, 1984), ageing and noise exposure are the main identifiable factors in determining prevalence of tinnitus in the general population.

The nature of the tinnitus sounds occurring in any particular cause of cochlear disorder varies widely and, in general terms, but with many individual exceptions, the tonal frequency to which the pitch of the tinnitus may be matchable is most commonly in or just before the frequency zone of the hearing impairment. For instance, in the study by Douek and Reid (1968) of 21 tinnitus patients diagnosed as having Menière's disorder, 20 had their main tinnitus at 500 Hz or below, although four of these had additional high-pitched whistles. In a study of patients with noise-induced hearing loss, Axelsson and

Sandh (1985) found a wide spread of tinnitus, from 250 Hz to over 10 kHz, although the majority of cases were in the 1.5–8 kHz region with the tinnitus pitch often at a slightly lower frequency than that of the greatest hearing loss.

There is much evidence relating the prevalence and severity of tinnitus to the amount of hearing loss. Coles, Smith and Davis (1990) reported an increasing prevalence of tinnitus as a function of high-tone hearing threshold level. Chung, Gannon and Mason (1984) showed an increasing prevalence of tinnitus in cases of noise-induced hearing loss as a function of hearing threshold level at 4 kHz in each of three age groups. They also showed that tinnitus was more common in the ear with the greater hearing loss, which is in keeping with general clinical experience. The reported loudness of tinnitus also increases with hearing threshold level (Hazell, 1981; Jakes *et al.*, 1986; Coles, Smith and Davis, 1990).

Peripheral neural

Tinnitus is sometimes the first symptom of vestibular schwannoma, such that cases of unexplained unilateral tinnitus, including patients with normal hearing thresholds, need further investigation to exclude that condition.

Nevertheless, tinnitus arising from VIIIth nerve disorders seems to be relatively uncommon in tinnitus patients as a whole, a finding supported by Graham (1981a) in his electrocochleographic analysis of 100 cases of sudden deafness: only 35% of the 23 retrocochlear cases had tinnitus compared with 70% of the 77 cochlear cases. There may also be a qualitative difference between sensory and peripheral neural tinnitus, the latter more often being described as a coarse buzzing type of sound.

The mechanism of production of tinnitus in VIIIth nerve lesions is not clear. It might be associated with demyelinization of the nerve fibres causing cross-talk between fibres (Møller, 1984) or due to variable degrees of slowing of conduction in the nerve fibres. Thus by distorting the resting state of discharge in auditory nerve fibres or by slowing conduction in specific fibres, abnormal nerve fibre firing patterns would reach the brain leading to a sound percept, tinnitus.

Central neural

It is reasonable to postulate that neurons at any level in the ascending nervous system fire spontaneously at other than usual rates, when deprived of the normal pattern of input from adjacent or lower level neurons. Such abnormal firing may itself become discounted by adaptation at higher levels but, on the other hand, may lead to an auditory sensation similar in character to the stimulus that would have caused that particular activity in those neurons. Thus, there is every reason to expect that disorders of the central auditory pathways would sometimes cause tinnitus. Some clinicians believe that when a patient describes his tinnitus as being 'in the head' this means the tinnitus is of central origin; but this does not necessarily follow for several reasons, not least the great difficulty many patients have in describing the character and location of their tinnitus.

Further evidence for tinnitus sometimes having a central site of generation comes from cases of persistence of tinnitus after labyrinthectomy or VIIIth nerve neurectomy. This may happen even where the initial or underlying pathology is peripheral, and sometimes the postoperative tinnitus is described as being exactly the same as preoperatively.

Many of the characteristics of tinnitus also support the concept of central neural generation, or at least central nervous influence through the efferent neural control of cochlear function. Onsets, offsets and fluctuations may occur for no apparent reason. Onset of tinnitus often occurs, with stress either as a precipitating or an aggravating factor, long after the onset of the original (peripheral) hearing disorder. Psychoacoustically, many forms of tinnitus behave quite unlike an external sound in several respects. For example, a unilateral tinnitus may be masked by another sound presented contralaterally at a level well below that which would cross-mask an externally presented signal at the tinnitus ear (Feldmann, 1971). Also the patterns of ipsilateral masking of tinnitus found in some patients with cochlear disorders are wholly different from the patterns of masking that occur with ordinary acoustic stimuli (Shailer, Tyler and Coles, 1981). These phenomena can only be explained by either a central generator or some central component in the tinnitus.

Associated

There are two types of chronic non-auditory disorder which may cause tinnitus by means of some ill-defined neurological mechanisms, namely temporomandibular joint and bite disorders (Rubinstein *et al.*, 1993), together with neck problems. Cervical spondylosis, previous cervical injury or even neck manipulation during intubation in anaesthesia may result in tinnitus, although vertebral arterial compression or spasm may be an alternative mechanism in some cases. These disorders are also associated with spasm of associated and nearby muscles, e.g. of the masseter and temporalis (often with bruxism), of the occipitofrontalis, or of the neck muscles. They can lead to tension headache and aggravation of tinnitus. Tinnitus can itself aggravate the muscular tension, and perhaps also cause tension in the intratympanic muscles leading to the otalgia that often accompanies distressing tinnitus. Whether or not these disorders can be a primary cause of tinnitus and of other otological symptoms is very uncertain, especially in cases of Costen's syndrome (Brookes, Maw and Coleman, 1980), but they certainly seem to aggravate tinnitus, either by increasing it or by decreasing the patient's ability to cope with it. Thus a check for these conditions and treatment of them is clinically worthwhile (Erlandsson, Rubinstein and Carlsson, 1991).

Psychological

This class of tinnitus has two variants, as described below.

Hallucinations

When the sounds heard are of highly organized type, such as the hearing of voices, and especially if what they say is accusatory or abusive, the 'tinnitus' is primarily hallucinatory and is likely to be a symptom of serious mental disorder requiring referral to a psychiatrist.

Imagery

More often, the tinnitus sounds of psychological origin are more benign both in their nature and in their implications. These sounds, such as of music or singing, have been termed 'auditory imagery' (Goodwin, 1980). They seem to be particularly common in elderly musicians or music lovers. In most cases they are probably a mental conversion of an ordinary tinnitus sound into a more musical sound; in some cases though, they are a mild form of psychosis or confusional state occurring in persons who also have tinnitus, the common factor increasing the chance of the two occurring together being age. In any event, they are relatively benign and psychiatric referral is not needed unless the images became very troublesome: treatment with flupenthixol has usually been helpful in such cases. In Goodwin's study, auditory imagery occurred in six (8%) out of 78 consecutive referrals to a tinnitus clinic; in the present author's own tinnitus clinic, it has been encountered in 1% (of nearly 2000 cases).

Pseudotinnitus

This is a tinnitus-like sound, but which does not comply with the definition of tinnitus. It has two main forms, described below.

Environmental

As already noted, a large proportion of tinnitus patients think at first that they are hearing some external sound, often asking others if they can hear the same sound and sometimes going to great lengths to discover the source of the sound. In a few cases, all the circumstantial and audiological evidence may point to the patient suffering from tinnitus, but it may take much effort to get the patient to accept this. Advice should be given on possible external noise sources on which to check, and how to get well-hearing relatives or friends to help in tracing or excluding them. If still convinced that there is some external sound causing this trouble, the patient may seek the help of the local environmental health officer. In instances where no sound source can be found, the environmental health officer's report may help to convince the patient that there is no external source for the noises causing the complaints.

Occasionally, there really is an external sound simulating tinnitus or additional to tinnitus. Examples are the ringing/humming from overhead wires and cables, hum from transformers or domestic machinery (e.g. a refrigerator), and rumbles from underground gas or water piping or from distant traffic or heavy machinery. Usually such a sound can be identified by careful history taking, noting in particular the fact that it is only heard in certain rooms or geographical locations and may be heard by others. These people usually have hearing within normal limits over at least some part of the normal audiometric range, and especially so at the frequencies relevant to the described pitch of the noise. Although further investigation and management may need the services of the local environmental health officer, such sounds are relevant to this textbook in that they may present as tinnitus, and they may constitute a considerable differential diagnostic problem. A recent review of 'hums' (Rice, 1994) elaborated many of these points.

Feigned

While some patients may tend to exaggerate their description of the severity of the tinnitus or of its effects on them for the purposes of gaining a greater amount of clinical attention, the majority of cases of feigned or exaggerated tinnitus arise in the medicolegal context where the motive is financial gain.

There is as yet no test that can tell us whether or not a patient has tinnitus, its degree of unpleasantness or the true extent of the effects it has on the patient. However, there are a number of observations and tests which can give some general pointers to the likelihood or otherwise of falsification or exaggeration in claims for noise-induced tinnitus. These are described below, but the wider aspects of assessment of tinnitus for compensation purposes can be found elsewhere (Coles, Smith and Davis, 1990; Axelsson and Coles, 1994).

General assessment

Apart from the general impressions given by the claimant as to the nature and effects of the tinnitus, enquiry should also be made as to whether the general practitioner has been consulted about the tinnitus. If not, unless further enquiry reveals some good reason, it is unlikely that the tinnitus is severe.

Audiological assessment

If a claimant fabricates or exaggerates tinnitus then it is likely that the same will be done in describing hearing difficulties and in performance during the audiological testing. However, their 'auditory honesty' can be checked. The use of audiological tests for indication of likelihood or proof of presence of non-organic hearing loss has been fully described elsewhere (Coles, 1982), as has the methodology and potentially high degree of accuracy of cortical electric response audiometry in medicolegal cases (Coles and Mason, 1984).

Tinnitus measurements

These are discussed in more detail later in this chapter. They can only give rather limited help in verification of tinnitus, in three ways. Pitch matching, provided the tinnitus is indicated as having some tonal element should, in most cases, indicate a pitch-match frequency in the region of, at the lower edge of, or just before any noise-induced high-tone hearing loss. In noise-induced hearing loss, the tinnitus loudness match when measured at the pitch-match frequency is rarely greater than 15 dB sensation level (i.e the number of decibels more intense than the threshold at that frequency). The results of repeat tests of the tinnitus loudness match or of minimal masking level should differ by not more than 5 dB.

Mechanisms of generation of tinnitus associated with cochlear lesions

It was noted earlier that the abnormal neuronal activity leading to tinnitus could be wholly or partly generated within the central nervous system even when the basic pathology is in the cochlea.

More traditionally such tinnitus is thought to be generated within the disordered cochlea. Indeed, some features of certain types of tinnitus would be difficult to explain other than by peripheral generator: examples are the 'triggering off' of tinnitus from an already disordered cochlea by such otherwise trivial and essentially peripheral occurrences as ear syringing or an otherwise innocuous noise exposure.

Model for 'cochlear tinnitus' (see Figure 18.3)

For a proper appreciation of such tinnitus, both for the clinician and the patient, it is necessary to look on the tinnitus as another manifestation of cochlear disorder in parallel with hearing impairments. The latter may, or in one-third of tinnitus patients may

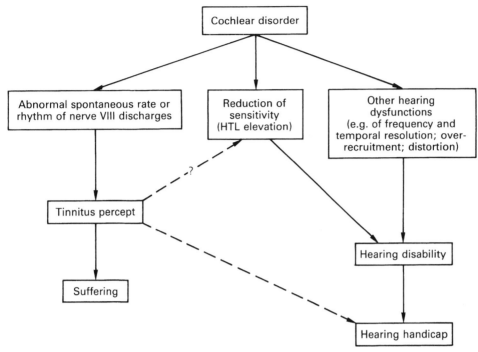

Figure 18.3 Model for 'cochlear tinnitus'

not, have been noticed by the patient, depending on its degree, the character of the patient, his auditory environment, and the amount of adaptation that has occurred where there is a slowly increasing impairment or expectation of hearing disorder with advancing age. The hearing impairment may be noticed earlier than, coincident with or later than the tinnitus.

Frequently the patient believes that hearing difficulties are a direct consequence of the tinnitus. In most cases this is probably a confusion between tinnitus and the effects of the coexisting hearing impairments. Whether tinnitus can actually contribute to hearing impairment by a masking-like effect is not certain, but the consensus of evidence is against this. It does not seem to interfere with hearing of speech either, Axelsson finding no more reduction of noise-masked speech identification ability in 100 ears with tinnitus (median score = 64%) than in 100 ears without tinnitus (median score = 60%), the ears being matched for age and sex and with similar sensorineural hearing losses (Axelsson and Coles, 1994). Nevertheless, tinnitus does sometimes increase the hearing disability by distraction of thought and mental concentration. Its main effect on the individual is, however, to cause the auditory equivalent of 'pain and suffering', loss of peace and quiet, an unpleasant sensation and a range of secondary symptoms in the psychological domain (and hence potentially reversible – an important consideration in its management).

The model implies that the tinnitus usually has the same fundamental cause(s) as the hearing impairment, and thus is related more to the functional abnormality than to the particular cause of the disorder. Indeed, it is logically economical to start aetiological considerations on the assumption that the tinnitus and sensorineural hearing loss have the same cause(s). Of course there can be exceptions, but the onus is on the clinician to justify the exception.

The model separates out the more familiar loss of hearing sensitivity that is measured by pure-tone audiometry from other more subtle hearing dysfunctions, such as frequency and temporal resolution, over-recruitment and distortion, and the occurrence of tinnitus. These usually accompany hearing loss of cochlear origin and may sometimes be more important than the loss of sensitivity in their effects on the patient, such as in the earliest stages of development of noise-induced hearing loss where audiometric impairments may be minimal.

Cochlear mechanisms of tinnitus generation

Cochlear disorders involve disturbances of the resting pattern of afferent nerve firing and this has the potential of being interpreted by the brain as a sound, i.e. tinnitus. The exact nature of the abnormal neural activity that results in a tinnitus percept is not yet known, with the result that there are currently a dozen or so theories as to the exact mechanism of generation of tinnitus. To describe these theories is outside the scope of this chapter, but conveniently they have recently been collected together into one volume by Vernon and Møller (1995). Probably it will eventually prove to be a question of not just one theory being right and the others wrong, but of one mechanism or mechanisms applying for some patients and different mechanisms for others. For the present purpose, it is sufficient to summarize the mechanisms of generation of 'cochlear tinnitus' as being due to the brain's interpretation of an abnormal spontaneous rate or rhythm of activity in the VIIIth cranial nerve.

Onset of tinnitus

Why does tinnitus develop at a particular stage in the progression of an auditory pathology? In slowly progressive cochlear disorders, the most common type of hearing disorder associated with tinnitus, there is an ever-present potential for the development of tinnitus. There is usually no apparent reason for onset of the symptom. Rather, some critical degree of abnormality appears to have been reached, the degree being highly particular to that individual or even to the particular ear. Indeed tinnitus can occur with little or no hearing loss, and may be absent in severe hearing loss.

Triggering factors

In a sizeable minority of cases with a cochlear disorder, the actual onset of tinnitus seems to have been precipitated by some triggering factor (Fowler, 1943). Some of these conjunctions, such as ear syringing, occur so frequently and are characterized by such obvious temporal coincidence that they simply cannot be attributed to chance. In the author's tinnitus clinic, a probable triggering factor has been noted in 26% of new patients. The most common apparent triggers were acute or increasing psychological stresses, either domestic, marital, occupational or bereavement; such stresses have previously been noted as tinnitus precipitators or aggravators (Fowler, 1943; Fowler and Fowler, 1948; Hallam, Rachman and Hinchcliffe, 1984). Next came ear syringing (without other mishap) or a noise exposure that would otherwise be regarded as trivial; indeed, ear syringing causes quite a loud noise in the ear and it may be that this noise is the tinnitus trigger (Jayarajan *et al.*, 1995). Many other factors have apparently precipitated or aggravated tinnitus, but could not be expected to have caused or increased the existing hearing loss. These include an intense, e.g. over 90 dB(A), noise exposure; mild head injury; jaw injury or acute temporomandibular joint disorder; acute neck injury, e.g. within about 4 weeks of a whiplash injury (although several other mechanisms have also been postulated in the delayed-onset cases);

changes in barometric pressures, in flying with or without barotrauma and in one case following tympanometry; surgical operations; myelography; drugs, especially salicylates and other non-steroidal anti-inflammatory drugs; acute rapidly resolving middle-ear infections; acute toxic states and metabolic disorders, e.g. thyrotoxicosis; too rapid withdrawal from a benzodiazepine or other dependency-forming drug; various affective disorders.

These triggering factors are interesting with respect to their possible mechanisms. While the influence of stress on the onset and severity of tinnitus could conceivably be mediated peripherally through changes in cochlear efferent activity, it seems far more likely that stress would exert its influence on the response of the central auditory system to an already abnormal input from the ear. Some of the other triggers seem more likely to have had a peripheral action. These would usually only have a temporary effect, but in some cases the associated anxiety then has the secondary effect of maintaining the tinnitus (see below).

Associations with psychological stress and with hyperacusis

The model of tinnitus generation shown in Figure 18.3 is restricted to a peripheral generator, i.e. an ear disorder leading to an abnormal neural input to the brain stem, and a central auditory perception and evaluation of this as a sound. But the model needs extending to explain a number of related phenomena: the frequent association of tinnitus with hyperacusis, the effect of low levels of wide-band noise in reducing or abolishing the tinnitus and hyperacusis as in retraining and desensitization therapies, the triggering effects of psychological stress and further aggravation of tinnitus by anxiety and tension, and the influence of the patient's psyche – probably the most important factor of all in terms of the degree of suffering that a tinnitus causes the individual. Figure 18.4 adds the required extensions.

How close the model may be to the truth is not yet known, but it complies well with the latest concepts of tinnitus generation, perception and evaluation (Jastreboff and Hazell, 1993). For the present time, at any rate, it seems to be a useful working model both for organization of thought on mechanisms and influences, and for clinical use in counselling on how a particular patient's hearing disorder is causing the tinnitus sensation, and often hyperacusis as well. It can also be helpful in explaining the mechanism of retraining and desensitization therapies with low-level noise, i.e. by increasing the neural input into the auditory brain stem. Further, it can be used to explain the crucial importance of combining prosthetic and psychological managements, notably in-depth and repeated counselling aimed at reducing the patient's fears and anxieties about the tinnitus.

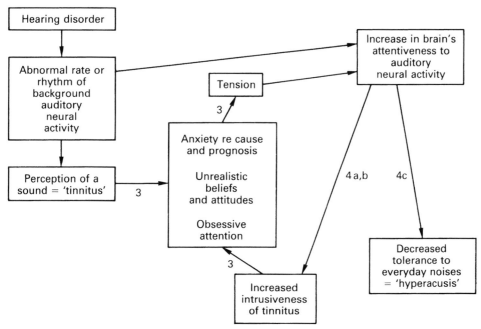

Figure 18.4 Association of tinnitus with psychological stress and with hyperacusis. (Note: numerals 3 and 4 refer to sites of possible psychological (3) and prosthetic (4) therapeutic interventions)

The reduced auditory neuronal activity associated with a hearing loss is believed to result in an attempt by the brain to compensate for the deficit. This leads to selective attention to sounds having components in the frequency range of the hearing loss, which frequently includes the tinnitus itself, as well as to an increased sensitivity to sounds in general, *hyperacusis*.

Strictly speaking, the term hyperacusis should mean abnormally acute hearing both at threshold and at suprathreshold levels. But in practice in all or most of its clinical presentations, including the most common – that associated with tinnitus and cochlear disorders – the oversensitivity is suprathreshold only and causes discomfort from everyday sounds that do not bother most other people. As such, it differs from recruitment in that it often occurs at frequencies where there is little or no hearing loss, and is generated at levels above the brain stem (Sood, Coles and Lutman, 1987; Sood and Coles, 1988), unlike recruitment which has a cochlear site of origin. It also has to be distinguished from phonophobia, an actual fear of or aversion to loud sounds, although the latter may develop secondarily to the hyperacusis or as a result of loud sounds causing temporarily increased loudness of tinnitus.

Hyperacusis can be defined by the onset of symptoms of loudness discomfort from everyday sounds that previously had not bothered the patient and/or uncomfortable loudness levels for pure tones in the 500–4000 Hz range of less than 70 dBHL. As such, it has been recorded in 43% of new patients, occasionally with the hyperacusis being more troublesome than the tinnitus. Previously, Hazell *et al.* (1985) found the mean uncomfortable loudness levels of 305 tinnitus patients to be 10–15 dB lower than expected in normal and cochlear-disordered people. The association has been further demonstrated epidemiologically (Sood and Coles, 1988), and therapeutically when Hazell and Sheldrake (1992) were the first to report resolution of a high proportion of cases of hyperacusis in tinnitus patients as a result of delivering a low level of wide-band noise to the affected ear(s) for about 6 hours a day over many months.

The model is not complete without including the psychological component. The trouble caused by the tinnitus is not so much the sound in itself, which in fact is seldom very loud (although sometimes perhaps having a very unpleasant character), but rather the anxiety it causes and the over-attention the patient gives to it. Both of these factors are heavily influenced by the patient's inherent psyche and his current attitude and psychological state. The tension resulting tends both to aggravate the tinnitus and to delay onset or return of sleep. The more the tinnitus is 'wound up' by tension, the more anxiety it causes – resulting in a vicious circle maintaining or increasing the tinnitus. Hence, careful counselling on the medical aspects and some form of further psychological management is needed in addition to any prosthetic treatment.

Epidemiology

The epidemiology of hearing deficits is presented in Chapter 3. With respect to tinnitus in adults, results from the National Study of Hearing have been presented in detail elsewhere (Coles, 1984; MRC Institute of Hearing Research, 1987; Coles, Smith and Davis, 1990) and are only summarized here.

Prevalence in the adult population

Estimate of tinnitus prevalence in industrialized countries based on the National Study of Hearing and other studies are as follows:

1 About 35% remember an experience of tinnitus of some type or duration at some time; while many of these are not troublesome, even the non-spontaneous and short-duration ones appear to be a nuisance to some of the people experiencing them
2 About 10% appear to have or to have experienced spontaneous tinnitus lasting over 5 minutes
3 At least 5% experience tinnitus causing interference with their getting to sleep, and/or moderate or severe annoyance; this would suggest about 2 million adults in the UK being so affected
4 0.5% experience tinnitus that has a severe effect on their ability to lead a normal life. This corresponds to about 200 000 persons in the UK.

Probably the most useful single statistic though is that 7% of the adult population of the UK have at some time been to see their family doctor about tinnitus. It is of interest also that, of adults with auditory complaints, over one-third were complaining of tinnitus.

Determinants of tinnitus prevalence

The significant determinants of reported tinnitus in the (UK) population are age, occupational noise exposure and socioeconomic group. However, these become non-significant when prior account is taken of the hearing threshold levels at high frequencies (Coles, Smith, and Davis, 1990). Thus, what matters is the degree of cochlear disorder, not its cause. In diagnostic or legal work this is useful as it supports the clinical dictum that 'whatever caused the hearing loss, probably caused the tinnitus too'.

Frequently the hearing loss has multiple causation, e.g. where the cochlea has been damaged by noise and is also subject to degenerative changes associated directly or indirectly with ageing. The noise exposure may even have ceased many years previously, yet the tinnitus may only have had a relatively recent onset. The actual onset is probably due to the extent of the cochlear disorder reaching a certain critical amount necessary for production of tinnitus, due to the combination of former noise damage with subsequent age-related deterioration.

Clinical aspects

Prevalence and features of tinnitus in clinical populations

Tinnitus is common in virtually all forms of otological disorder. Fowler (1944) reported its presence in 86% of 2000 consecutive patients with aural disease. Spoendlin (1987) estimated the frequency of occurrence of tinnitus in cochlear disorders to be as follows: 50% in sudden deafness, 70% in presbyacusis, 30–90% in intoxications, 50–90% in chronic acoustic trauma and 100% (by definition of course) in a Menière's attack. Because the fact of its occurrence has virtually no differential diagnostic significance, it tends to be overlooked as a symptom often requiring attention in its own right.

Considering the greater longevity of females and the increasing prevalence of tinnitus with age, one might expect that tinnitus clinics would show a female-to-male ratio of, perhaps, 3:2. This is not what actually happens. Over the period 1976–81 in the largest tinnitus clinic in the USA, 68% of the patients were male, with females outnumbering males only in the over-70 year age group (Meikle *et al.*, 1992). In a study of therapeutic masking based on three of the largest tinnitus clinics in the UK, of the 472 new patients entered into the study (mostly in 1981–82), 47% were male, with no apparent interaction between gender and age at first attendance (Hazell *et al.*, 1985) (Table 18.1). There are several possible causes of the different gender ratios in these two studies and for the higher proportion of male subjects in the American clinic, notably referral biases, economic factors, greater use of sporting guns in USA, and perhaps differences of attitude; these are discussed elsewhere (MRC Institute of Hearing Research, 1987). There is also a small but consistent tendency for a disproportionately higher attendance rate from the higher socioeconomic groups in the British clinics. The greatest first attendance rate is in the 51–60 and 61–70 years age groups, with 1–5 years as the most common interval between onset of tinnitus and clinic attendance.

Site of tinnitus

Clinical reports have indicated that tinnitus affects the left ear rather more commonly than the right, but only a marginally greater prevalence of tinnitus on the left side, and in males only, has been found in studies of the general population (Coles, 1984). The

Table 18.1 Age at first tinnitus clinic attendance

Meikle (1985)* (n = 1725)			Hazell et al. (1985)* (n = 472)		
Age band (years)	Percentage of sample	Male:female (%) (n = 1182:543)	Age band (years)	Percentage of sample	Male:female (%) (n = 223:249)
<21	3	66:34	<20	2	50:50
21–30	6	72:28	20–29	2	55:45
31–40	13	80:20	30–39	9	45:55
41–50	17	76:24	40–49	14	50:50
51–60	28	71:29	50–59	32	47:53
61–70	23	63:37	60–69	32	44:56
>70	10	45:55	>69	9	54:46
All	100	68:32	All	100	47:53

* After Meikle (1985) personal communication, and Hazell *et al.* (1985).

possible causes of this asymmetry have been discussed elsewhere (MRC Institute of Hearing Research, 1987; Meikle and Griest, 1992), but they do not seem to be associated with handedness nor, except in occasional cases, with asymmetrical noise exposure.

Pathological correlates

In the National Study of Hearing an attempt was made to tie down causal factors or correlated disease states by taking comprehensive clinical histories and a considerable number of measures of general health. Only somewhat borderline correlations with hearing threshold level or tinnitus, mostly with no aetiologically inviting interpretation, were found. These were for: history of cardiovascular disorder, systolic and diastolic blood pressure, and current use of beta-blocker drugs and loop diuretics. Of course those drugs are often taken because of cardiovascular disorders, which could themselves have contributed to the causation of the hearing disorder.

A range of haematological tests, liver, thyroid and renal function tests, general blood chemistry and serological tests for syphilis, were also carried out, but no correlation repeatable between phases was found between the results of these tests and either tinnitus or hearing threshold level. On the other hand, Browning, Gatehouse and Lowe (1986) have reported some further analyses of the National Study of Hearing data using the ratio between total protein and the albumin fraction, which provides an indirect measure of plasma viscosity. These analyses supported their conclusions from a separate study with otolaryngology clinic patients, which had suggested a substantial correlation of rheological properties of blood with degree of sensorineural hearing loss (and, by implication, with likelihood of developing tinnitus). An example of the clinical relevance of the null results is given by the syphilis serology tests. These

were only positive in nine out of 1171 persons so tested. Of the nine, seven had hearing within the range expected from their age, gender, noise exposure and socioeconomic status; the remaining two had middle ear pathology. Most clinicians faced with a patient with sensorineural hearing loss of unknown aetiology, on finding a positive syphilis serology would tend in most circumstances to attribute the hearing disorder to syphilis. On the present evidence this would not seem to be justified.

The lack of association of either tinnitus or hearing threshold level with the results of the various blood tests suggests that the conditions to which those tests are sensitive are not important determinants of tinnitus and/or hearing impairment in the population at large. Nevertheless, such blood tests continue to be useful investigations for particular patients with hearing disorders. A large literature suggests associations of hearing disorders with a wide variety of haematological disorders, hormonal disorders such as diabetes mellitus and hypothyroidism, bone disorders such as Paget's disease, and syphilis. Even if carefully controlled studies were eventually to show that these associations were marginal, the tests would still serve two other functions. They may indicate possible predisposing, synergistic or precipitating factors interacting with other known or unknown causes of hearing disorder. They may also identify conditions needing treatment in their own right. This, in turn, may lessen the handicapping or distressing effect of the coincident hearing disorder or tinnitus and improve the patient's ability to cope with these.

Tinnitus in children

There is no reason why hearing losses, at any rate the sensorineural ones, found in children should not be accompanied by tinnitus as often as they are in adults. Indeed, tinnitus has been shown in some studies to occur almost as frequently in hearing-impaired children as in hearing-impaired adults. Nodar and LeZak (1984) found it in 31 (56%) of 55 hearing-impaired children, although in only 35% of the 37 children with extreme-to-profound hearing impairment and only intermittently in all but two cases. Similar findings have been reported by Graham and Butler (1984), with tinnitus in 66% of 92 children in partially hearing units and in 29% of 66 children in schools for the deaf; again, in only two cases was the tinnitus continuous. However, while Nodar and LeZak stated that tinnitus 'does not seem to have the debilitating effect that it has had on many adults', 31% of a subsample of 78 in Graham and Butler's study reported high annoyance. Previously, Graham (1981b) described three forms of problem that tinnitus can produce in such children: confusion in audiometry, reluctance to wear a hearing aid which may exacerbate the tinnitus, and disturbances in concentration and behaviour.

In contrast, children or adults with congenital deafness are rarely seen in a tinnitus clinic. In general audiological/otological clinics they rarely present with tinnitus as a primary or troublesome complaint. The apparent discrepancy between the reported high prevalence of tinnitus in hearing-disordered children and their lack of complaint about it could be explained by a number of factors. If a child has experienced tinnitus for as long as can be remembered, it is likely to be regarded as something quite normal or not even be noticed. Children are also less liable to psychological overlay or anxiety about the medical significance of tinnitus, both of which are factors leading to tinnitus being troublesome to adults. There is, additionally, the likelihood that sometimes the child's complaint is ignored by adults, especially where it is of something as invisible and possibly related to imagination as tinnitus. On the other hand, the high prevalence rates may be an artefact of insufficiently rigorous study according to Stouffer *et al.* (1992), who found it in only 24–29% of hearing-impaired children. Nevertheless, tinnitus can cause problems in children, and the possibility of this should be considered carefully by those concerned with the welfare, education or medical management of deaf children.

The clinical relevance of tinnitus

Tinnitus as a symptom deserves clinical attention for four reasons:

1 Occasionally it can be the first indicator of some important pathology, e.g. an acoustic neuroma
2 It is often a symptom accompanying hearing impairment, which may be causing considerable disability but still not be recognized as such by the patient; on correction of this with a hearing aid, it is quite common to have delighted patients who had not previously realized the extent of their disability and its effects on their work and enjoyment of life
3 In other instances, the tinnitus may be a warning sign of developing impairment and risk of future disability, the most obvious and readily controllable example of which is damage by high sound levels in work or leisure
4 Finally, and most pressingly in practice, tinnitus is a symptom like pain which can cause much suffering and/or anxiety concerning its cause and its prognosis.

The effects of tinnitus

To document the consequences of tinnitus, Tyler and Baker (1983) investigated 97 people with tinnitus severe enough to lead them to join a local tinnitus self-help group. The patients wrote down all the difficulties caused by their tinnitus in order of importance. The average number of difficulties reported by the 72 respondents was 4.6, with a range of 1–13. There was no age or sex dependence, but those who reported having had their tinnitus longest reported slightly fewer difficulties. Table 18.2 shows their analyses of the particular complaints in terms of frequency of occurrence and importance weighting, subdivided into four categories.

These categories have essentially been confirmed by three subsequent more sophisticated investigations using factor analysis. The first (Jakes *et al.*, 1985) demonstrated that self-report of 'insomnia', 'intrusiveness' (its loudness and its distracting effects), 'emotional distress' due to tinnitus, interference with listening to certain sounds, and measurements of its loudness and maskability were all orthogonal. Hallam, Jakes and Hinchcliffe (1988) reported two later studies in which the 'insomnia' and 'distress' factors were replicated, although the 'intrusiveness' factor was less clear.

These analyses are fundamental to the development of practical clinical techniques in two respects:

1 They indicate the multiplicity of effects of tinnitus, and the need in history-taking to explore each category of effect in order to obtain a full understanding of the patient's problems.
2 They assist in evaluation of whether the patient's tinnitus needs any treatment additional to a full explanation of cause, nature, prognosis and therapeutic options; they also help to define the nature and vigour of any treatment that may be needed.

In order to obtain a comprehensive tinnitus history, it is best to explore the occurrence, severity and timing of effects under a series of headings. These could minimally be the four categories of effect shown in Table 18.2 or maximally the 15 most prominent effects listed, together with a fifth (or sixteenth) item 'Any other effects?'. It is probably better to question verbally from a schedule used as an interview prompt than to rely on an open-ended instruction such as 'list the effects that your tinnitus has on you'. A questionnaire saves clinical time, but has the disadvantage that a substantial proportion of tinnitus patients respond very incompletely or inaccurately.

It may be helpful to administer a personality inventory. However, although Stephens and Hallam (1985) have shown that tinnitus patients as a group show abnormally high general anxiety and depression scores, and somatic anxiety scores in the subgroup also reporting dizziness, the value of personality assessment is limited by an uncertainty of interpretation. The abnormal personality could lead the patient to habituate poorly and to seek help for tinnitus, as suggested by the lack of change in personality score as a result of (largely) successful therapy (Hazell *et al.*, 1985). Alternatively, the tinnitus could cause or contribute to change in the personality. Probably both processes are at work, in proportions that vary from individual to individual. Further discussion of the personality of the tinnitus patient is to be found in Chapter 4.

The 'severity' of tinnitus

Strictly the term 'severity' should be used to describe just the intrinsic unpleasantness of the tinnitus sound. However, patients find it difficult to distinguish this from the trouble that the tinnitus causes. For example, when a patient says the tinnitus has improved it may mean that the tinnitus sound itself has become less unpleasant in its character or loudness or that, for some reason which may not be very apparent, the patient's reaction to the sound has changed. Consequently, for the purposes of general or therapeutic assessment one has to regard tinnitus severity as an overall descriptor of the sound itself and of its effects on the patient. It is in the global sense of the word that the various components of severity are considered here.

Loudness

Loudness is the property of tinnitus that might be expected to correlate best with severity. It is difficult not only to measure it but also to interpret the measurements. Moreover, loudness and maskability measurements correlate very poorly with reported 'severity' (e.g. Jakes *et al.*, 1985, 1986). In fact, in the majority of cases the tinnitus sounds are not very loud (see Chapter 4) and have an annoying effect quite out of proportion to their loudness (Fowler, 1943). Thus, loudness as such does not appear to be the dominant factor in generating annoyance that it is often presumed to be. Of course, it is not unimportant either, as exampled by the patient's relief consequent on even a slight reduction in loudness achieved therapeutically.

Table 18.2 Fifteen most common difficulties attributed to tinnitus

Difficulty	Percentage of respondents	Importance weighting
A *Effects on hearing*	53	
Understanding speech	38	3.3
Understanding television	11	1.9
B *Effects on lifestyle*	93	
Getting to sleep	57	3.6
Persistence of tinnitus	49	3.6
Worse on awakening in morning	17	3.3
Avoid noisy situations	15	2.5
Withdraw, avoid friends	14	2.6
Avoid quiet situations	11	3.0
C *Effects on general health/health care*	56	
Dependence on drugs	24	2.5
Pain/headaches	18	3.0
Giddiness, balance, fuzzy head	14	3.0
D *Emotional problems*	69	
Despair, frustration, depression	36	2.7
Annoyance, irritation, inability to relax	35	2.6
Concentration, confusion	33	3.1
Insecurity, fear, worry	17	2.6

After Tyler and Baker (1983).

Quality

Patients find it difficult to describe tinnitus precisely, often because it differs from everyday sounds. It may have a tonal element, but this is often slight or absent. In any event, pitch matches with external signals are of limited value because the pitch match frequency can mimic only one aspect of the quality of the sound. Moreover, there appears to be no strict relationship between pitch of a sound and its unpleasantness, although, in general, high-pitched tinnitus seems to cause more trouble and a lowering in pitch as a result of treatment has been reported to be a beneficial change (Donaldson, 1978; Martin and Colman, 1980).

Thus, pitch matching tells us little about the actual tinnitus sound or about its unpleasantness. Matching of pitch is usually conducted with pure-tone signals. But it is possible to match to noise bands of various centre frequency and bandwidth, to more complex or distorted sounds, or to mixtures of tones and noise. This may take us closer to matching the tinnitus, but the interpretation of such sounds in terms of annoyance potential is still very uncertain. It is probable that some sounds are extremely unpleasant but defy measurement or definitive description due to their inherent subjectivity. It must therefore be accepted that the character of the tinnitus sound may sometimes be a very important but virtually unmeasurable contributor to its unpleasantness.

Temporal characteristics

By and large, a tinnitus that is continuous tends to be more troublesome than one that is intermittent. But there are many exceptions to this rule, particularly where the tinnitus fluctuates in loudness and/or quality, which causes some patients to live in fear of their bad spells. Likewise, a pulsatile element is sometimes the dominantly troublesome feature, although more often it causes little additional upset. Thus, while the temporal aspects may be important features determining the annoyance of tinnitus in some patients, their importance is very unpredictable both in degree and direction of effect.

Lateralization

Most patients regard their tinnitus as having worsened if it starts to affect both ears, having previously been confined to one ear. On the other hand, some with unilateral tinnitus report that it is unpleasant because it is always located on a particular side and this is unlike everyday sound. Thus, sidedness may sometimes be a factor in tinnitus severity, though again an unpredictable one.

Psychological reaction

This is probably the most important single component of severity as defined here, accounting for why some patients are very upset by tinnitus sounds that are not very loud in fact (Fowler, 1943). An analogy is the dripping tap or the next door baby's cry at night – sounds that are very faint in themselves but are very irritating and need much self-control to ignore. These aspects are discussed in depth in Chapter 4.

Associated stresses

The majority of tinnitus patients say that their tinnitus is worse when they are tired or tense. It is difficult to define whether the sound is actually changed at such times or whether it is their reaction to it which is changed. The stresses and/or tiredness may be due to external factors at work or at home, or be self-induced by worrying and over conscientiousness, or be due to tension and insomnia resulting from the tinnitus. These stresses and consequent tension and increased tinnitus set up vicious circles.

Assessment of severity

Despite the difficulties mentioned, tinnitus severity needs to be assessed for general clinical evaluation, in particular to decide if any treatment at all other than thorough counselling is required. In medicolegal settings, a rather more quantitative assessment may be requested but, for the reasons expressed earlier, much caution has to be used in interpreting the results of tinnitus measurements.

Another requirement for assessment of severity is in evaluation of the results of management either for clinical purposes or for research. There are frequently disparities between data from loudness matches or loudness scaling and the reported severity and effects. It is important therefore to include an array of tinnitus tests in the attempt to measure changes and, in the case of research studies, to characterize the patients included in a therapeutic trial. Subjective descriptors of the severity of tinnitus, both overall and also broken down into the various components described above, should also be included. A more complete discussion of the severity measures needed in therapeutic trials for tinnitus is to be found in Axelsson *et al.* (1993).

The prognosis for the tinnitus and its effects

The tendency towards habituation to tinnitus has often been noted (Fowler, 1944). More recently Hallam, Rachman and Hinchcliffe (1984) proposed a habituation model for the effects of tinnitus on the patient. The evidence for such a model is:

1 Epidemiological, in that the majority of people who have tinnitus do not complain of it (Coles, 1984)
2 The diminished number of problems caused by tinnitus as a function of time since onset (Tyler and Baker, 1983)
3 The lack of relationship between complaint behaviour and perceived loudness of tinnitus (see Chapter 4)
4 Anecdotal clinical evidence from many sources that tinnitus sufferers do indeed acquire tolerance.

The model is helpful in advising the patient about the prognosis and the process of habituation to the tinnitus. On its own, the statement 'you will have to learn to live with your tinnitus' is a bleak prospect. However, the empirical results enshrined in the model justify saying: 'The majority do in fact learn to live with their tinnitus', and 'Our aim is to help you to do this'.

Further information relevant to the prognosis has also been derived from the National Study of Hearing (MRC Institute of Hearing Research, 1987). The data support the habituation model. They further suggest that tinnitus that comes on suddenly seldom increases in loudness. Less reassuring is that in about one-third of the cases where it comes on gradually, it tends to go on increasing in loudness. On the other hand, paradoxically, this is frequently accompanied by a gradual reduction of annoyance. This agrees with general clinical experience of many patients learning to live with their tinnitus after an initial period of discomfort and anxiety. In contrast, the proportion of persons who experience sleep disturbance appears to remain much the same throughout; however, sleep disturbance has been shown to be a poor general index of severity (Coles *et al.*, 1992). The habituation model should not be overstated however, since in the majority of cases both loudness and annoyance remain at much the same levels. Moreover, any reduction in annoyance is usually only partial, to a reduced level of annoyance rather than to no annoyance at all.

In expressing the prognosis, the annoyance data are obviously the ones to be used, but should be referred to as 'severity' rather than annoyance, as many patients simply cannot believe that their present tinnitus could ever become less annoying and to suggest that it could do so may undermine the credibility of the rest of the counselling. Thus, from clinical observations and these epidemiological data, it seems justifiable to give the following sort of guarded reassurance to tinnitus patients, particularly to those where its onset was sudden: 'The general pattern of severity is unlikely to increase, and there is a good chance that it will gradually decrease. Sometimes the tinnitus gets softer and occasionally it disappears altogether: it does not often get markedly worse'.

If the tinnitus is still increasing when the patient is first seen, or begins to increase again, he can be reassured that: 'It is unlikely to go on and on increasing'. And if ageing has been mentioned as a factor in causation of the tinnitus, he can be reassured that: 'Although your hearing difficulties may slowly increase with advancing years, the evidence is that the severity of tinnitus usually does *not* increase'. Finally, it should be explained that this prognosis refers to untreated tinnitus. With treatment, the prognosis is better still.

Investigation of the patient complaining of tinnitus

History

Apart from the usual history to be taken in investigating the cause of any form of otological disorder, there are some additional features to explore in relation to tinnitus and its management. These include the following:

1 The time/'severity' course of the tinnitus, together with note of any apparent or suspected triggering or exacerbating factors, including starting or sudden stopping of drugs
2 The character and site of the most troublesome tinnitus sound, together with a brief description of any other troublesome sounds
3 The effects of tinnitus, perhaps under a series of headings as suggested earlier
4 Whether the tinnitus is a greater, equal or lesser problem to the patient than any hearing difficulty or hyperacusis that is being experienced (to avoid attention and treatment being mistakenly concentrated on the less important symptom)
5 The effect of environmental sound in masking or reducing the loudness of the tinnitus, an aspect which is often clarified by enquiring about the loudness of the tinnitus when it is quiet
6 The time(s) of day or night when the tinnitus is most troublesome.

For a patient referred primarily on account of tinnitus, extra time should be allocated to allow for the taking of a detailed history and for the careful professional counselling that all such patients need.

Clinical examination

Where tinnitus is the primary complaint, the ordinary otological examination would be supplemented by the following:

1 Checks and/or questions on general health, neurological function, neck mobility and temporomandibular joint function
2 Where there is pulsatility, check on pulse and

blood pressure, auscultate each side of the head and neck and the ears, and ascertain the effects on the tinnitus of neck turning and of jugular vein compression.

General investigations

Obviously a large number of other tests could be applied, but economy of time and expense usually dictates a conditional use of these. Nevertheless, account should be taken of the patient's expectations. The most useful further investigations are:

1 Radiological and/or MRI examination where there is any suspicion of infective, endocrine or neoplastic disorder of the ear or VIIIth nerve, or of relevant central neurological disorder.
2 A variety of blood tests (haematology and erythrocyte sedimentation rate, hepatic, renal and thyroid function tests, blood sugar, lipids, an immunological screen, and serological tests for syphilis), where there is suspicion of general ill health, if the tinnitus is of relatively recent and obscure origin, and especially if there is an unexplained progressive increase in hearing loss. Aetiological interpretation of the significance of many of these investigations has to be very careful however, as pointed out earlier.

Hearing testing

The purposes of audiological testing of a patient presenting with tinnitus are:

1 To assess the patient's hearing status for both diagnostic and rehabilitative purposes bearing in mind that few tinnitus patients have wholly normal hearing, that many need help with their hearing by means of a hearing aid, and that such help may be sufficient to enable the patient to cope with the tinnitus (either by increasing the therapeutic effects of ambient noise or by reducing auditory disability).
2 To provide a baseline for the tinnitus tests.
3 To measure the extent of any associated hyperacusis.

How much audiological testing is done will depend on time factors, but as a minimum it should comprise pure-tone threshold and uncomfortable loudness level measurement, noting any frequencies at which the test tones appear to be confused with the tinnitus. Tympanometry, with acoustic reflex threshold and decay measurements, and speech audiometry are sometimes useful in addition.

Tinnitus testing

Objectives

For patients in whom tinnitus is a major complaint, it is important to test the tinnitus itself for the following reasons:

1 To gain some appreciation of the pitch and loudness of the tinnitus, even though the quantitative significance of such measurements is limited and their interpretation has to be very guarded.
2 To provide quantitative data against which later changes occurring spontaneously or as a result of treatment may be compared, even though they may be only poorly correlated with severity.
3 To provide a more convincing background for the subsequent counselling of the patients and to meet their expectations of having their tinnitus properly assessed.

Many patients have more than one tinnitus sound. It is not necessary nor practicable to measure each of them; a brief description of the main ones as part of the history suffices for all but the *most troublesome tinnitus* sound. The first steps therefore are to agree upon the most troublesome tinnitus sound and to make it clear to the patient that the matching tests to follow apply to that sound only.

Pitch-match frequency

Since some patients misunderstand the word 'pitch', regarding it as a dimension of intensity or loudness (Coles, 1984), it may be necessary to supplement the test instructions with verbal or audiometric examples. The patient should then be asked not only to try to judge the pitch of the tinnitus, but also to indicate the degree to which there is any noticeable pitch at all; some tinnitus sounds simply do not have pitch. Pure tones should be used for pitch matching, as they give the purest representation of pitch and since the presentation levels of the pitch-matching stimuli have to be related to the audiogram. It should be explained to the patient that the tones will probably not sound anything like the tinnitus, but that they should select the tone which most closely matches the pitch of the most troublesome tinnitus sound – the 'pitch-match frequency'.

In view of the frequent unreliabilities (Penner, 1983; Tyler and Conrad-Armes, 1983a) and the very slight clinical importance of precise pitch-match frequency measurements, it seems quite unnecessary to use more than a small set of pure-tone frequencies. In a clinical setting, it is probably best to use a method which needs no special equipment and is not time consuming; i.e. using only the standard test frequencies delivered by an audiometer and an adaptive test procedure, and trying to keep the loudness of the matching tones constant across frequencies and at a low level, e.g. at 20 dB sensation level. Replications, if needed, are a better use of testing time than trying to achieve a fine degree of pitch definition in any one measurement.

Tinnitus loudness match

The patient's description of the loudness and annoyance of the tinnitus is the most relevant 'measurement'. However, quantification of the tinnitus loudness match level is also desirable to give a further appreciation of the actual loudness of the tinnitus, to provide a baseline against which to compare possible changes in the future, and to meet the patient's expectations.

The tinnitus loudness match is best obtained with a pure tone from an audiometer, often at the pitch-match frequency and in the ear with the troublesome tinnitus sound. In fact it is more useful for the patient to make judgements at the frequency (in either ear) that has the most sensitive hearing threshold level (Goodwin and Johnson, 1980). To avoid possible inhibition of the tinnitus, an ascending series of tone presentations should be used.

Where the threshold at the most sensitive frequency is normal or near-normal, the level of the loudness-matching tone can easily be appreciated. But where the threshold even at the most sensitive frequency is not normal, great caution has to be used. It may seem natural to express the result simply in terms of sensation level units, i.e. as the number of decibels above the threshold; but as this is likely to lead to a profound conceptual mistake if interpreted in terms of normal hearing sensation. In tinnitus patients, particularly at the pitch-match frequency, there is usually a sensory hearing loss and recruitment (Goodwin and Johnson, 1980; Tyler and Conrad-Armes, 1983b; Penner, 1984); thus a low sensation level value may in fact correspond to quite a loud sound.

The loudness can be estimated from the threshold and the tinnitus loudness match according to several methods. Of these, the least complicated for the user and the easiest to appreciate in terms of ordinary otological or audiological experience is the method of Matsuhira, Yamashita and Yasuda (1992) (Figure 18.5) or of Tyler, Aran and Dauman (1992).

Minimal masking level

The minimal masking level is measured by gradually increasing the level, usually in 5-dB steps, of the masking sound until the tinnitus is no longer audible. It may be delivered to one, each or both ears and the instructions should specify carefully whether the test refers to just the most troublesome tinnitus or to all the tinnitus sounds, and to just the ipsilateral ear or to both ears. If a range of pure tones or carefully calibrated narrow-band noises is used, this gives the tinnitus masking patterns along the lines first described by Feldmann in 1971. In practice, measure-

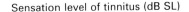
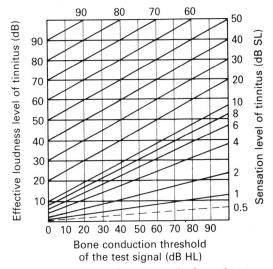

Figure 18.5 Nomogram for estimating loudness of tinnitus (adapted from Matsuhira, Yamashita and Yasuda, 1992). Enter the bone-conduction threshold if there is a substantial air-bone gap (if not, enter the air-conduction threshold) and the number of decibels by which the tinnitus loudness match is greater than the threshold, i.e. its sensation level. Then read off the effective loudness level, i.e. the loudness of the tinnitus as it would be to a normal-hearing person

ment of the masking patterns adds little diagnostic information over and above what is already available in the configuration of the audiogram and the patient's description of effects of everyday noises on the tinnitus.

The clinical importance of minimal masking level measurements has largely disappeared nowadays, since if therapeutic masking is to be used at all, most patients prefer masking noise levels below the minimal masking level, i.e. for partial masking or simply to remove the quiet in low environmental noise levels. Moreover, masking decay (Penner, Brauth, and Hood, 1981) occurs in about 50% of cases, which militates against both meaningful measurement of the minimal masking level and successful therapeutic use of complete masking.

A technique for measuring masking decay was described in the previous edition of this book, but is omitted here in view of its slender clinical relevance. The same goes for tests of residual inhibition, which only rarely occurs in practice and may simply be regarded as an additional bonus when it does. For details of how to carry out tests of pitch-match frequency, tinnitus loudness match, minimal masking level and residual inhibition, the most authoritative are those defined at the Ciba Symposium on Tinnitus (Anon, 1981b), subject to the modifying comments made above.

Testing sequence

Tinnitus can sometimes be abolished, reduced or increased by exposure to sounds, especially if prolonged or above threshold. It is therefore important to follow the sequence of tinnitus tests given above: pitch-match frequency, tinnitus loudness match, minimal masking level. It is also important to use where possible an ascending series of signal presentations. Ideally, the tinnitus tests should follow immediately after a basic air-conduction audiogram, which is needed anyway as a preliminary to the pitch-match frequency tests, before any masking procedures are carried out. The ideal may be difficult to achieve in practice though, and the full range of audiological tests may have to be done first. This is acceptable, provided that at the start of the tinnitus tests the patient is asked to compare the present loudness of his tinnitus to its usual loudness. If it is much softer or absent, the tinnitus tests will have to be done on a separate occasion.

Management of tinnitus

This section covers present day tinnitus management only, together with some pointers towards possible or likely future developments. For a historical perspective on the treatment of tinnitus, the reader is referred to Stephens' (1984) comprehensive review.

In fact, there are many helpful lines of management for tinnitus, but normally only a few of them are relevant to any particular patient. For both general clarification of the various possible managements and to assist in defining what is appropriate in the individual case, it is helpful to have a form of flow diagram. The one used by the author is a modification and extension of the diagram used a decade ago by Jakes (personal communication) to illustrate the effects of tinnitus and their potential reversibility. It is shown in Figure 18.6, together with the sites of effect and types of management options.

Tinnitus usually arises from within the auditory system, but in perhaps 3% of cases it is the hearing of an actual mechanoacoustic vibration elsewhere in the body. Clinical measurements of tinnitus tell us that the loudness of the sound is seldom very great, no louder than and usually much softer than most everyday sounds which we accept or ignore. Recent analysis of the author's patients, according to the methods of Matsuhira, Yamashita and Yasuda (Figure 18.5), showed the median tinnitus loudness to be equivalent to tones of only 21.6 dBHL (SD 14.6, range 0–65) as they would be heard by a normally hearing person. On the other hand, its character may be inherently unpleasant such as a screech or high-pitched whine, or intrusive such as with a vascular pulsing sound. But the unpleasant-ness of the sound, probably even in the most severe cases, does not compare with the unbearability of severe pain.

Thus, the tinnitus sound *per se* does not harm the individual, nor is it wholly intolerable. What makes it so upsetting to many patients is when they give undue attention to it – out of fear as to its possible cause and/or prognosis, unrealistic beliefs as to its effects on the person and his lifestyle, a sense of grievance as to its believed cause or of unfairness at being singled out to suffer from it, or such an obsession with it that it dominates their attention.

Just as there are many problems that tinnitus can cause, so there are many management options (see Figure 18.6), the choices of which for a particular patient depending greatly on the cause of the tinnitus and the nature and degree of trouble it is causing. For orderly description here, the classification shown beneath the figure will be followed. In this, for ease of memory, they were originally constrained into five headings each beginning with the letter P, but later this became inadequate and the three Ss were added. For clinical purposes on the other hand, there should be no question of simply following the order given in the classification or selecting one or more therapies at random, but rather of careful selection of the most appropriate management option(s) according to the answers to the following five questions.

1 Is there anything that can be done to prevent (management option 1) the tinnitus becoming worse?
2 Are there sufficient indications for further investigations, designed to uncover possible causes or aggravators that might need treatment in their own right, e.g. vestibular schwannoma, hypothyroidism, tertiary or congenital syphilis?
3 Is any treatment of the underlying pathological cause (management option 2) possible and likely to abolish or reduce the tinnitus?
4 What are the main troubles that the tinnitus is causing?
5 Is the tinnitus causing the patient enough trouble to justify any treatment additional to thorough professional counselling (management option 3a)? In answering this question, account should be taken of possible side effects, the tendency for most patients to habituate to tinnitus to some extent, the patient's lifestyle, and the counterproductive tendency for any active treatment to focus the patient's attention on his tinnitus.

Management option 1: preventive

Measures taken to prevent hearing loss due to such things as maternal rubella and excessive noise exposure will also reduce the incidence of tinnitus. But, of course, by the time a tinnitus patient reaches the

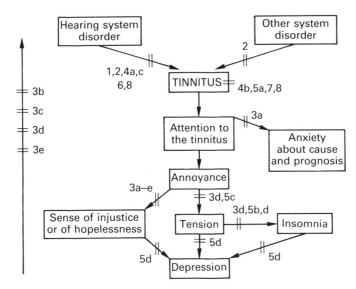

Figure 18.6 Effects of tinnitus (modified from Jakes, personal communication) and options (1–8) for its management

1 Preventive – e.g. rubella, noise-inducing hearing disorder
2 Pathological –   wax and other causes of conductive hearing loss; Menière's disorder; drug effects (e.g. quinine); benzodiazepine reinstatement and slow withdrawal; anaemia or hypertension; associated and intercurrent disorders
3 Psychological –   (3a) professional counselling literature, especially Robert Slater booklet and Nilsson leaflet
                    (3c) lay counselling, including information on BTA and local tinnitus groups and RNID's national telephone helpline
                    (3d) relaxation training therapy
                    (3e) psychological counselling and treatment
4 Prosthetic –   (4a) retraining therapy (with tinnitus masker or hearing aid)
                 (4b) masking (by hearing aid or tinnitus masker)
                 (4c) desensitization of hyperacusis (with tinnitus masker)
5 Pharmacological – to reduce the tinnitus:
                 (5a) clonazepam, carbamazepine, nimodipine, etc. to combat its effects
                 (5b) nocturnal sedatives
                 (5c) tranquillizers (may give nocturnal sedation too)
                 (5d) antidepressants (may give nocturnal sedation too)
6 Surgery (ablative)
7 Suppression (electrical, ?electromagnetic)
8 Suppression of spontaneous otoacoustic emissions

clinic, it is generally too late to be thinking of prevention. Nevertheless, even in the clinic, advice on noise limitation or ear protection and treatment of the cause of the underlying disorder (see management option 2) may reduce the risk of further hearing loss and increasing severity of tinnitus. Tinnitus is sometimes temporarily aggravated by noise exposure to such a degree that a change of job or early retirement may have to be considered: but, in considering the latter, account should be taken of the experience of some patients that with the relatively quiet and less busy life after retirement the tinnitus becomes more intrusive.

Management option 2: pathological

Contrary to popular understanding that tinnitus is 'incurable', in perhaps 5–10% of cases there is a cause for which treatment may result in abolition or reduction of tinnitus. In other instances tinnitus is a symptom of a more serious condition, e.g. a vestibular schwannoma, and needs treatment in the general health interests of the patient. Some of the more common examples of pathological treatment aimed at reducing the tinnitus are discussed below.

Conductive hearing loss

Anything which can be done to reduce conductive hearing loss will potentially help tinnitus, principally by restoring the normal masking and distracting effects of ambient noises. The most obvious example of this is conductive hearing loss due to acoustically-obstructing cerumen, which can, in the vast majority of cases, be removed without trouble. However, occasionally ear syringing seems to cause or aggravate tinnitus (Jayarajan *et al.*, 1995) and this forms another reason why wax is really better removed with a wax hook or by suction.

A more difficult question is whether middle-ear surgery is justifiable where reduction of tinnitus is the primary surgical objective. In the most contentious case, that of otosclerosis, the problem is that surgery that is successful with respect to improvement of hearing does not always succeed in reducing the tinnitus, and sometimes increases the tinnitus or results in a tinnitus that was not there before. Due to a sense of grievance at the surgeon or self-blame for having consented to the surgery, especially where the hearing also was not improved or was made worse, post-stapedectomy tinnitus is often particularly troublesome and resistant to treatment. It therefore seems doubtful if stapes surgery is justified as a treatment for tinnitus *per se*; and even where the surgical indication is to improve hearing, the small but finite risk of the operation resulting in tinnitus or increased tinnitus should be carefully explained to the patient beforehand.

At the other end of the scale, for tinnitus associated with middle-ear effusion, surgery would seem to be the correct line of treatment if the tinnitus continues to be very troublesome and the effusion is not resolving with time and medical treatment. In such surgery, the risk of damage to the internal ear and of increasing the tinnitus is minimal, while the surgery itself is minor in nature and usually effective.

Menière's disorder

While vertigo is usually the most distressing symptom of Menière's disorder, this is not always so, particularly in the later stages where the vestibular disorder may have largely 'burnt out' and constant tinnitus has developed. But even in the earlier reversible stages, attacks or exacerbations of tinnitus are sometimes the most distressing symptom.

Such attacks of tinnitus may be reduced in intensity, aborted or prevented by medical treatment, particularly if using a vigorous and comprehensive regimen. This, in the author's opinion, has up to five components and should be continued for a minimum of 3 months.

1 A cochlear vasodilator, preferably betahistine hydrochloride. This is usually recommended in 8 mg or 16 mg t.d.s. dosage, but Oosterveld (1987) has found in laboratory studies that higher doses are more effective in reducing vertigo and caused no side effects. For the last 5 years the author has used higher doses, 24 mg or 32 mg t.d.s., with seemingly increased success rate and seldom any side effects.
2 A diuretic, e.g. bendrofluazide 5 mg each morning
3 A reduced salt diet in order to reduce the hydrops. The value of reduction of fluid intake is debatable

though, and there may even be a case for increasing non-salty fluid intake.
4 Stress reduction, by counselling on limitation of self-inflicted stress and over-conscientious behaviour.
5 Relaxation training therapy.

Drugs, foods and liquids

Major ototoxic drugs, such as the aminoglycoside antibiotics and cytotoxic drugs, are liable to cause permanent hearing loss and tinnitus. Less liable to cause permanent damage, except from prolonged high dosage, are drugs such as quinine, the salicylates, and alcohol, but these may cause temporary tinnitus during and for a few days after their administration. Other drugs seem to do so as an occasional idiosyncratic effect. Thus, in evaluating a patient with tinnitus, the history taking should include enquiry as to the medication presently being taken, and in particular that started (or stopped) at about the time of the onset of tinnitus or of a major change in it. The most common culprit in this connection in the author's experience has been the taking of quinine to prevent muscle cramps, especially at night. In each case, the remedy is to try the effect of using a lower dose or none at all. In the case of quinine this may result in more cramps, often uncontrollable by other means: but at least the patient is then left with a choice, he understands his tinnitus and it is put into perspective in relation to the body as a whole.

Some foods, e.g. chocolate, certain cheeses and milk products, and liquids e.g. tea, coffee, red wines, ports, often of the type found in other patients to precipitate migraine, appear to exacerbate tinnitus. If this is suspected, the patient should keep a food, liquid and tinnitus diary, and then try a series of three successive withdrawals and rechallenges before deciding on a permanent or even intermittent abstinence from that particular food or liquid. The same goes for smoking and alcohol, with respect to their possible influence on tinnitus. Unfortunately some lay 'authorities' are apt to give dogmatic advice on these matters which, in most individuals, amounts to a useless further reduction in quality of life.

Benzodiazepine reinstatement

Too rapid withdrawal from addictive drugs is liable to result in a wide range of symptoms including restlessness, tension, anxiety, sensory oversensitivity and paraesthesias and also tinnitus. By far the most common drugs causing tinnitus in this way are the benzodiazepines. The possible connection between onset or exacerbation of tinnitus and drug withdrawal has to be detected from the patient's drug history. Quite often reinstatement of the drug followed by very gradual withdrawal results in much reduced or abolished tinnitus. But sometimes it fails to do so, especially where there is an underlying sensorineural hearing disorder. Then it seems likely that the drug withdrawal had triggered off the tinnitus from an ear disorder already predisposed to causing tinnitus.

Anaemia, hypertension and atherosclerosis

Either anaemia or hypertension may lead to pulsatile tinnitus, especially when combined with atherosclerosis in the carotid circulation which can lead to turbulent and thus noisy blood flow. With respect to pulsatility, it is necessary to define whether the tinnitus is wholly pulsatile or just a pulsatile modulation of an ongoing tinnitus and, if a pulsatile modulation, whether it is the pulsatility itself that is troubling the patient or, more commonly, the background tinnitus.

If the pulsatility is sufficiently troublesome, a blood count and a check on the blood pressure is indicated. Anaemia will deserve attention in its own right, and its correction may also result in reduced or abolished tinnitus. Likewise, with hypertension, but here the troublesome pulsation constitutes an indication for antihypertensive therapy at systolic pressure levels considerably lower, e.g. down to 150 mmHg, than would be regarded as needing treatment from the ordinary medical point of view. Occasionally, the carotid circulation may be so reduced, e.g. by over 80%, that endarterectomy may be justified for the tinnitus or indeed indicated in its own right in removing a potential threat to life.

Transient hypoglycaemia

Hypoglycaemia may be a factor in tinnitus that is worse immediately after sleep, especially on waking in the early morning. For such cases, the writer advises the 'Lucozade test' (a glucose-rich mineral drink) in which the patient has half a cup ready to drink by his bedside; when troubled by tinnitus on waking, the Lucozade is drunk with as little disturbance as possible. In about a quarter of such cases the tinnitus is reduced after 10–20 minutes, either permitting a return to sleep or seeming to start off a day less troubled by tinnitus than usual. The notion of worse tinnitus being related to hypoglycaemia is supported by the author's experience of four insulin-controlled diabetics whose most severe tinnitus occurred at times of impending hypoglycaemia and was immediately reducible by taking glucose.

Management option 3: psychological

The importance of psychological help for the tinnitus patient cannot be overemphasized, and its delivery should not be restricted to the psychologist or psychiatrist. Indeed, the otological and audiological professionals have the main responsibility for this, and can be most usefully reinforced and implemented by lay persons with tinnitus and tinnitus self-help organizations.

Professional counselling

The most important professional counsellor is the doctor, especially the otologist, either surgeon or physician. Not only is he best placed to provide the key ingredients, the probable diagnosis, prognosis and advice on the most relevant management, but he is also perceived by the patient to be the principal authority. If the doctor does not cover each of these points, and write them clearly into the case notes and letters so as to be readily available for the other professionals involved in the patient's management, the latter will be working at a major disadvantage both in their own particular work and in giving the further counselling which patients so often need.

Further counselling is needed because in the stress and haste of most medical consultations and from natural lapses of concentration or lack of understanding, much of the initial counselling, however carefully carried out, is not absorbed or remembered. Questions also arise in the mind of the patient at a later date. Consequently the counselling often has to be reinforced and elaborated by other members of staff, either otological at review or audiological when carrying out hearing-aid, tinnitus masker, lip-reading and other therapies. The same is true of any clinical psychologist who becomes involved, and effort must be put into their education too so that they understand tinnitus and are seen by the patient to do so.

To have the credibility it needs, professional counselling must start with listening carefully to the patient's complaints and obtaining all the relevant details, together with the necessary audiometric and tinnitus tests already discussed. This takes considerable time: but time is what the tinnitus patient needs, and sufficient time will usually not be available in an ordinary otolaryngological outpatient clinic. The comprehensive counselling needed may therefore have to be broken into two parts. First, a relatively brief one at the first attendance and given by the doctor to cover diagnosis, prognosis and decisions on management. Second, a special appointment allowing at least 15 minutes, preferably 30 or 45 minutes, for more detailed enquiry into the nature and degree of the patient's problems, for the rest of the counselling, and for discussion and decision on management. Provided the doctor has given the initial explanation and communicated its contents, the second part of the counselling can be delegated to one of the audiological staff having a special interest in tinnitus work.

The principal components of professional counselling are listed below:

1 Giving and explaining the most probable reasonable diagnosis. How can you really reassure some-

one, if you do not tell him what is wrong? It is so important to do this that usual diagnostic criteria need to be relaxed somewhat, provided this does not involve risk of hiding from further investigation or therapeutic attention a health-threatening condition.

To this end, a diagnosis of age-related hearing loss is often justified. While 'presbyacusis' would usually be reserved for the elderly, some losses of hearing at high frequencies becomes measurable by the age of 30 years and can be associated with tinnitus. Likewise small degrees of noise-induced hearing loss and minor genetic hearing losses causing dips or high-tone loss in the audiogram can be associated with tinnitus. Unexplained asymmetrical hearing loss associated with tinnitus can, after excluding investigations, be ascribed to viral or vascular disorders – better the former in the young and middle-aged patients in order to avoid causing anxiety about premature vascular disease.

With this approach, the author finds he can give a probable diagnosis of the likely cause of tinnitus in 90–95% of cases. Whether or not the diagnosis given is correct usually matters little, since it would not alter further management. What does matter is to make, and communicate, some positive diagnosis on which reassurance and further counselling can be based.

2 Once a relatively harmless diagnosis has been made, it is helpful to make a positive statement that the tinnitus is not due to cancer, brain tumour, impending madness or 'disease'. This should be done even if the patient does not voice such fears, as they are often present but hidden.

3 Many patients fear tinnitus as being a disease entity in itself. Its nature as a symptom, not a disease in itself, needs to be explained. Likening it to pain, e.g. as from arthritis, may help in this respect and is apt since there are many similarities between pain and tinnitus.

4 Any apparent trigger for onset or increase of the tinnitus needs comment. It is usually best to accept this as a possibility, rather than attempt to unseat any strong opinion held by the patient. Instead, explain the difference between the trigger and the underlying disorder, the latter being a condition liable to cause tinnitus at any time but sometimes needing a trigger to start the tinnitus.

5 Show the patient his audiogram as the starting point in explaining how the hearing disorder is causing tinnitus. This is particularly important in the one-third of tinnitus patients whose hearing losses are sufficiently small not to have caused noticeable hearing difficulty or who blame their hearing difficulties on the tinnitus.

6 Explain how the hearing disorder is generating the perception of a sound. The author often uses Figure 18.3 to illustrate this. Our brain has a perception of a sound when an actual sound causes changes in the firing rate in the auditory nerve. So if there is a reduction in the firing rate due to the hearing disorder, shown in the audiogram, this sooner or later is liable to be perceived by the brain as a sound, i.e. tinnitus.

7 The brain also tries to compensate for this deficiency in its auditory nerve input, by turning up its sensitivity. Unfortunately this tends to wind up the tinnitus and increase sensitivity to external sounds, thus explaining any hyperacusis present. Showing Figure 18.4 is useful in explaining this and reinforces the face-validity of the counselling. Likewise, the figure illustrates the importance of attention to the psychological aspects, and also the modes of action of prosthetic therapy.

8 Since most people with tinnitus tend to be shy about telling others about it, for fear of being thought to be going mad, there is a general lack of awareness of how common tinnitus is. The result is that many sufferers feel aggrieved at having been afflicted with what they perceive to be a rare condition. They need to be informed that in fact it is far from rare, e.g. that seven out of every 100 adults have been to see their doctor about it.

9 The generally favourable prognosis, even without any treatment, should be outlined.

10 Finally, if the patient seems to be looking for some cure, e.g. from surgery, a drug, alternative medicine, this may reflect an unwillingness to put effort into learning to live with tinnitus or into long-term prosthetic treatment. Prolonged searches for causes or palliatives should therefore be discouraged, as they merely serve to delay and make more difficult the process of coming to terms with the tinnitus and of reaping the potential benefits of psychological and prosthetic managements.

Counselling by literature

It is often helpful to reinforce professional counselling with suitable booklets, information sheets and suchlike. Lists of these can be obtained by patients or their professional advisors from the various sources of lay counselling (see below).

However, if specific printed materials are to be provided or recommended by the clinician, it is important that he has read the materials himself. He can then judge what is suitable and, equally important, what is not suitable for the particular patient. Strong preference should of course be given to the more positive, supportive and reassuring publications: some are too negative and gloomy and may need to be disadvised.

Lay counselling

Although much can be done by medical, audiological and psychological staff, their counselling always lacks a vital ingredient, the conviction of someone who has suffered from tinnitus. This is especially relevant to advice on how to live with tinnitus. It is better not to leave the patient quietly dissatisfied in this respect, but to meet the problem head on by admitting the deficiency and offering the following possible solutions.

Patients can be encouraged to join their national tinnitus association, by means of whose journals or newsletters they can keep informed about all aspects of and developments in tinnitus, and obtain comfort in the realization that they are far from being alone with their tinnitus and that most people do indeed gradually come to terms with it. The address of the British Tinnitus Association is: 14–18 West Bar Green, Sheffield S1 2DA. In the UK, there is also a national tinnitus helpline run by the Royal National Institute for Deaf People (tel: 0345 090210) which is charged at local rates. Information on other national tinnitus self-help organizations is available from the International Tinnitus Support Association, whose current address could be obtained from either of the above.

Local self-help groups are also useful sources of information on tinnitus, and additionally offer means of personal contact with other sufferers and their relatives. Their help in management of tinnitus patients can be very considerable, and is greatest where there is active collaboration between the otolaryngology department and the tinnitus group, and where the group has a positive and supportive attitude towards tinnitus.

Relaxation training therapy

The purpose of relaxation training therapy is to teach the patient to learn to recognize tension as it develops in the face of stressful events of all kinds, including tinnitus, and to reduce the effect of that stress (see Figure 18.4 and associated text). It is aimed at countering tension by relaxation as a way of life, and gradually, as this training is achieved, the need for recurrent relaxation training sessions reduces. Not all tinnitus patients are sufficiently tense to need relaxation training therapy, but for many it proves a great help. It is important to explain to the patient that the performance of relaxation exercises is not expected to have a direct or immediately noticeable effect on the loudness of their tinnitus; also that rigorous adherence to daily relaxation sessions is not necessary and indeed could be counterproductive in terms of inducing anxiety and stress if such adherence is difficult.

Relaxation training therapy is often best carried out on a group basis which, for most patients, is more effective due to the sharing of experiences and remedies between members of the group, which thereby becomes another, more supervised, form of lay counselling. Alternatively, relaxation training therapy can be carried out by means of a single counselling session, explanation of the importance and methods of relaxation and providing a training tape for use at home. Some patients need relaxation training therapy, but are unable to utilize local services on account of distance, immobility or time factors, or dislike the idea of group therapy; for these the author recommends purchase of tape recorded instructions, e.g. those available from the British Tinnitus Association. Patients who are too deaf to hear the tape or verbal instruction can get some benefit from written instructions, available from the author.

Psychological counselling and treatment

Since the manner and degree in which tinnitus causes suffering is dependent primarily on psychological factors, it is difficult to overemphasize the potential importance of the clinical psychologist in management of tinnitus patients. Effort should be made to develop a link with the local clinical psychological service and to ask for one or two members of its staff to take a special interest in tinnitus and balance disorders, and then to put some effort into educating them in these subjects.

It is important for the patient to understand that their referral is not a psychiatric one. If patients are carefully and explicitly told that there is no implication that tinnitus itself is psychological and they are not thought to be neurotic, most will readily accept such referral. Demonstration of Figure 18.4 in this respect can also help.

The actual methods and results of psychological counselling and treatment are dealt with in Chapter 4.

Management option 4: prosthetic

There are two main means of using prosthetic devices to help patients with tinnitus: *tinnitus retraining therapy* and *tinnitus masking*. In addition, the prostheses involved may help tinnitus patients in two other ways: by general *auditory rehabilitation* and, very occasionally, by post-stimulatory reduction of the tinnitus, i.e. by *residual inhibition*.

Tinnitus retraining therapy

The mechanism of this has already been outlined (see text relating to Figure 18.4). Its theoretical and evidential background has been described in some detail by Jastreboff and Hazell (1993). The retraining is a combination of prosthetic and psychological avenues. The latter is mainly in the form of in-depth and repeated professional counselling to counter the patient's tendency, often subsconscious, to regard it as a threat to health, working ability and enjoyment of life generally, and gradually to learn to develop the ability to ignore the tinnitus as a sound.

Long-term reduction in tinnitus intrusiveness is the aim. This is obviously more desirable than temporary, palliative use of masking and it also involves lower levels of therapeutic noise which are therefore less intrusive in themselves and less speech-interfering. The method also uses a constant low level of noise, which is largely independent of the tinnitus, so that its presence is soon forgotten. In contrast, with masking the patient tends to make frequent adjustments of level in order to try to maximize the effectiveness of the masking, a delicate balance between loudness of tinnitus and loudness of the masking noise: repeated listening to the tinnitus and readjustment of the masking level have the undesirable effect of drawing their attention to the tinnitus.

The first instrument to consider using for retraining therapy, or indeed any prosthetic treatment for tinnitus, is a *hearing aid* for one or both ears, or a hearing aid fitting modified to be more appropriate for tinnitus, e.g. by changing ear, changing to an open or more widely-vented earmould, or fitting binaurally even in a monaural tinnitus if one aid gave insufficient benefit.

Of course, the ear(s) to be aided have to be associated with some degree of hearing difficulty and/or hearing-loss, the lower limits for the latter being about 10 dB, more acute than might apply for aiding hearing alone. With minor hearing difficulties, the aid should be proffered primarily as a treatment for the tinnitus. Since one of its main likely benefits is achieved by providing a constant low level of amplified ambient noise, which is likely to have a retraining effect, the aid(s) should be worn for many hours a day, and particularly in the quieter periods.

In other cases the hearing loss is too small or too great for a hearing aid to be appropriate. Or hearing aids may have been tried but found to provide insufficient benefit or were strongly disliked for some other reason, e.g. recruitment or hyperacusis problems. Use of monaural or binaural *tinnitus maskers*, not for masking but as therapeutic noise generators, should then be tried.

These may be of ear-canal, in-the-ear or behind-the-ear type. In most cases, a low-power instrument is most suitable. Some ear-canal maskers are of standard shape and fit most ears. They are relatively inexpensive, do not need earmoulds, and can be worn at night. But they have to be loose in the ear so as not to occlude it, and therefore are not suitable for ears with very narrow canals or unusual shape or during periods of more than mild physical activity. For those cases, a behind-the-ear masker fitted to an *open earmould* (Hazell and Wood, 1981) is better. The rather wider spectrum of noise from these instruments is theoretically another advantage. However, this seems most uncertain in practice since the therapy is still successful in those who have who have high-frequency tinnitus associated with high-tone hearing loss, when the higher-frequency components of the noise would often not be heard anyway; and the treatment is also successful in those treated with less than wide-band noises, e.g. from a hearing aid or an ear-canal masker.

If compatible with the patient's lifestyle, the therapeutic noise should be applied for a minimum of six waking hours per day, preferably in the most acoustically quiet hours: it can be used in separate periods of 2 hours or more. It can also be used during sleep, but less effectively. This should be continued on all or most days over a minimum period of 12 months; however, sometimes the degree of benefit, in the form of lasting decrease in intrusiveness of tinnitus and of hyperacusis, may go on increasing over 24 or 36 months of treatment. If the condition relapses, as it occasionally does either spontaneously or as a result of psychological or acoustic stress, the treatment is repeatable.

Another uncertainty is whether or not it is sufficient to apply therapeutic noise to just one ear. Since the locus of the hyperacusis is above the auditory brain stem centres and we are trying to reduce the central auditory sensitivity to the tinnitus, it would seem that all that is needed is for the therapeutic noise to be audible. Certainly one instrument can be effective in masking bilateral tinnitus; but the benefits, even in a case of unilateral tinnitus, are sometimes much increased by use of two maskers or hearing aids. By analogy, this may be the case for retraining therapy also. Thus while a monaural instrument will often be sufficient, the likelihood of achieving benefit and its degree may be increased by binaural treatment.

The exact level to be used is another area of uncertainty and may need to be varied somewhat with each individual patient. Thus, it is difficult to specify a precise protocol suitable for everyone, but the following generalizations can be made. It is usually best to set the level in the quiet at the start of the day, and to leave it at that level. The starting level is one which is just clearly audible and less loud than the tinnitus. But if the lowest clearly audible noise level completely masks the tinnitus, then the instrument should simply be used as a masker, for comfort, as and when needed (see below). After a month, the level should be increased somewhat – to the loudest that is not unpleasant, speech-interfering, tinnitus-aggravating or completely masks out the tinnitus.

Certain events may happen later on in the day. Commonly the patient's thoughts keep turning towards tinnitus: he should be advised to make positive attempts to counter this, and at such times to concentrate on the therapeutic noise rather than the tinnitus. The tinnitus may become inaudible: if so, continue with the noise therapy for the intended number of hours, provided that the noise remains audible. The tinnitus may grow louder towards the end of the day: if so, a lower starting level should be tried on the next day, as the therapeutic noise may have been (temporarily) aggravating the tinnitus. The patient may move into a prolonged higher environmental noise level such that the therapeutic noise becomes inaudible; if so, the instrument should be taken out of the ear and its battery removed or disconnected, but its volume control left at its start-of-day setting so that the therapy can be continued at the same level when the environment becomes quiet enough. The higher noise levels will help in the retraining process especially if the tinnitus is still audible in it, but the greatest benefit from the therapy is likely to come when the environment is fairly quiet.

In spite of a commitment to 12 or more months of retraining therapy, the patient may additionally use the device as a masker for short periods, to reduce the discomfort of the tinnitus when it is being particularly troublesome or when trying to get to sleep.

It is too early in the history of retraining therapy to be able to quote formal studies and results. A large-scale controlled study is currently in progress (Hazell, personal communication, 1994). In the meantime, the study by Sheldrake and Hazell (1992) comes closest to providing data on the benefits resulting from this treatment. Their data show that after 1–2 years of retraining therapy, the tinnitus was having less effect on 16 (94 %) of 17 patients. And in the group of 36 patients after 2–4 years of therapy, tinnitus was worse in only one, the same in eight (22%), less in 15 (42%) and not noticed any longer in 12 (33%). The experience of the author, and that of Jastreboff (personal communication, 1993) in the USA, is similar.

The exact mechanism of benefit from retraining therapy is not at all certain, but seems likely to be due to a combination of extensive and repeated counselling, the prosthetic treatment itself and the normal tendency to habituate to tinnitus with time: the prolonged treatment certainly 'buys' 12–36 months of time in an easy non-intrusive way and in which the patient has a very positive involvement.

Hyperacusis desensitization therapy

If the hyperacusis is less troublesome than the tinnitus or equally troublesome, therapy should be directed at the tinnitus, as described above. The hyperacusis will often reduce as a result, its reduction often preceding that for the tinnitus and seeming then to constitute a hopeful prognostic indication. But if the patient finds the hyperacusis more disturbing than the tinnitus, and of course if there is hyperacusis without any tinnitus, then desensitization therapy for the hyperacusis becomes the priority. This utilizes the prosthetic part of retraining therapy but with some differences.

The starting level of therapeutic noise is selected much as before, although at a slightly higher level than just clearly audible and not influenced in any way by the relative loudness of any tinnitus present. This level is maintained for 6 or more hours a day. However, there will often be periods of uncomfortably loud environmental noise during the day: during such periods, the level of therapeutic noise should be

turned up slightly, to a level that begins to make the environmental noise less uncomfortable but not nearly enough to mask it. For occasional loud noise that cannot be dealt with by this means, earplugs can be used: but only while in such noise, as their use generally is counterproductive to the desensitization process. After a month, the level of noise is raised progressively, aiming to increase it gradually to higher and higher levels of tolerance – putting up with some discomfort, but not aggravating tinnitus.

Tinnitus masking

The first electronic approach to the masking of tinnitus appears to have been that of Jones and Knudsen (1928). However, the modern era of therapeutic masking only began when Vernon (1977) started to fit hearing aid-like devices designed to produce a noise in the ear.

In spite of the greater effectiveness and acceptability of retraining therapy, there is still some place for use of masking, which of course in many clinics has been for a decade or more the principal means of helping many tinnitus patients. It can, as already described, be used during retraining therapy as a temporary palliative in periods when the tinnitus is particularly troublesome. There are other patients whose tinnitus is only intermittently present or troublesome and who are sufficiently helped at these times by masking. Tinnitus masking can be used in two ways: *complete masking* and *partial masking*, that order being historical rather than of effectiveness and acceptability.

Complete masking

In this, masking noise is raised in level until the tinnitus becomes inaudible. The applicability of complete masking depends on several considerations. The minimal masking level for the masker noise should not be markedly louder than the loudness of the tinnitus. The noise has to have a more acceptable quality than the tinnitus, often described as 'more soothing'. At least, it has to be regarded by the patient as a welcome change of sound and one that is preferable since it is under his control and coming from outside the head. Most patients want the masker noise to be substantially different from the tinnitus sound(s); otherwise it is merely replacing one sound by a similar one, although occasionally that is what seems to be wanted. The effectiveness of the masking must also not decay appreciably with time, something that occurs in about 50% of cases.

Partial masking

In view of the various problems in complete masking, it is usually better to aim at partial masking. Nearly all patients will have noticed that their tinnitus is louder or more intrusive when the environment is quiet, usually in the evening, on going to bed or on waking in the morning. This observation can be utilized to illustrate to the patient the potential benefits of partial masking, that is to provide a background sound against which the loudness of the tinnitus is reduced. Alternatively, the masker can be turned up until its loudness is almost equal to that of the tinnitus, when the patient will often have to listen hard to hear the tinnitus at all.

Types of masker

The two main kinds of wearable masker have already been mentioned – the *ear-canal* and *behind-the-ear* instruments. Individually moulded *in-the-ear* maskers can also be provided, but are more expensive and less likely to be available from public-funded sources.

There is also the *combination instrument* – a hearing aid with a masker built into it, for those patients who need both amplification and masking. In practice though, these tend to be rather difficult to use and less than optimal in their hearing-aid performance. An alternative is to use separate instruments, either hearing aid(s) in communicating parts of the day and masker(s) at quiet times when the tinnitus is more troublesome, or an aid in one ear and a masker in the other.

In addition to the above wearable instruments, considerable help can be obtained from use of a variety of environmental noise sources. While some patients find out for themselves a variety of everyday sounds which cover up the tinnitus or distract them from it, others seem curiously unimaginative in this respect. Simple advice to try using a radio, cassette player, record player or TV can be very helpful, provided the material is not too intrusive or demanding. Some useful tape recordings, e.g. of seashore noise, are available. At night, more meaningless and continuous noise tends to be needed. A fan or a noisy clock can sometimes help; another quite popular solution is an FM radio turned off-station so that it emits a constant volume-controllable 'shsh'. For use in bed, an underpillow speaker of the kind available from most radio shops may add to acceptability of these methods. There are also available specially designed bedside maskers, but they are more expensive than a radio and have no other uses.

Auditory rehabilitation

A hearing aid used for many hours a day has a tinnitus retraining effect by feeding the auditory system with sound. The amplified ambient noise may also have a masking effect. But the benefits of hearing aids for tinnitus in patients with aidable hearing go further (Fowler, 1943), and include the following:

1 By improving the patient's hearing, something posi-

tive and helpful has been done – a psychological benefit.
2 It lessens the attention the patient gives to his hearing problems, including the tinnitus, and also reduces auditory stress.
3 The patient often believes it is the tinnitus which is causing the hearing difficulty, not realizing that the difficulty is due to the associated hearing impairments; if the hearing aid reduces the difficulty, then the patient may interpret this as the tinnitus being less troublesome.
4 The further counselling coincident with careful fitting of a hearing aid and follow up will also be beneficial.

These additional benefits can be further enhanced by associated methods of auditory rehabilitation – use of assistive listening devices, e.g. TV aids, and by instruction in listening tactics and lip reading. Thus, management of tinnitus should not be focused solely on the tinnitus, but should be part of an overall auditory rehabilitation programme.

Residual inhibition

Total or partial inhibition of tinnitus following acoustic stimulation was originally one of the main objectives in use of tinnitus maskers. It still is in some countries, but in the UK it has largely fallen into disuse. Residual inhibition is seldom achieved with the usual broad-band noise emitted by tinnitus maskers, such that when it occurs in practice it is regarded as little more than an unexpected bonus. It is also only poorly predicted by residual inhibition tests (Hazell *et al.*, 1985). Researchers have looked for the optimal noise spectrum and temporal characteristics for achieving residual inhibition but their findings have been more confusing than helpful. Vernon and Meikle (1981), based on their tinnitus clinic experience, believed that the best inhibitory noise is one like the tinnitus itself; but they also admitted that 'this proposition has not been formally tested'. In contrast, Terry *et al.* (1983) found that the frequency producing maximal residual inhibition is usually lower than the tinnitus frequency by as much as an octave, or two in some cases.

Management option 5: pharmacological

Pharmacological treatment of the underlying pathology and suppression of spontaneous otoacoustic emission-tinnitus is discussed elsewhere in this chapter. Drugs are also used sometimes in combatting the effects of tinnitus. They include *nocturnal sedatives* to help with sleep; *tranquillizers*, especially in an acute stage of tinnitus when the patient may be so distressed that he is incapable of listening to any detailed counselling and needs first to be calmed into a less desperate frame of mind; *antidepressants*, for management of depression and/or insomnia, when a sedating antidepressant such as amitriptyline or dothiepin can be particularly effective and also less habit-forming than a benzodiazepine.

Occasionally an antidepressant drug may seem to have aggravated the tinnitus, in which case a brief withdrawal or change to another drug can be tried. In other cases, the patient may have become so overmedicated generally that cessation or reduction of drug intake may improve the ability to enjoy life and cope with the tinnitus. On the other hand, there is an increasing tendency by doctors to avoid or minimize use of drugs, especially the benzodiazepines. Many patients also have a very understandable reluctance to take drugs in the fear of addiction or other undesirable effects. Certainly, with a persistent and non-curable symptom such as tinnitus, it is generally better for the patient to attempt to develop the ability to cope rather than resort to drugs. But sometimes the reluctance to use such drugs has to be overcome in order not to deny particular patients the very real potential benefits of these drugs either in short-term treatment or even in long-term use if an initial trial of up to a month has shown persisting benefit.

Drugs to reduce the tinnitus *per se*

The situation here is aptly summarized by Shea *et al.* (1981) who said: 'It is hard to find a remedy for the relief of tinnitus that has not been tried'. However, both the interest in and the rationalization of such treatments was much increased by the finding that intravenous injection of local anaesthetics can temporarily abolish or reduce tinnitus (Bárány, 1935; Fowler, 1953). Double-blind placebo-controlled cross-over trial has proved both the subjective and the objective effectiveness of intravenous *lignocaine* (Martin and Colman, 1980), the more objective changes being reductions in the pitch-match frequency and tinnitus loudness match. Over 50% experience at least 50% reduction of their tinnitus after intravenous injection of lignocaine (Melding, Goodey and Thorne, 1978; Martin and Colman, 1980). Unfortunately though, the relief is usually of too short a duration (up to a few hours) to be useful for a drug that has to be given by intravenous injection in order to obtain relief. Therefore, irrespective of their mode or site of action, a number of drugs with 'membrane-stabilizing' properties have been tried in the hope of finding one that is effective in suppressing tinnitus, and which can be taken by mouth and has no frequent, severe or hazardous side effects. These have included amylobarbitone sodium, carbamazepine, clonazepam, eperisone, flecainide, flunarizine, glutamic acid, mexiletine, nimodipine, oxazepam, phenytoin sodium, sodium valproate, tocainide and vigabatrin.

Results of the trials conducted so far are somewhat uncertain and difficult to interpret. They have previously been reviewed by Goodey (1981) and more recently by Murai *et al.* (1992), and by McKee (see Chapter 6), who indicate that these drugs are only occasionally if ever clinically useful, often at the cost of considerable side effects. None of them has been licensed (nor, therefore, advertised) in the UK for use on tinnitus. Consequently, 'antitinnitus' drugs have rather a small part to play in present day tinnitus management, their justification probably being limited to a last resort for those patients who are resistant to other lines of therapy and remain severely affected.

For those of the author's patients meriting drug treatment, clonazepam, carbamazepine and occasionally nimodipine are used. Tocainide involves risk of serious blood dyscrasias. Intravenous frusemide has also been tried, making possible use of its effect of reducing the endocochlear potential, but it does not appear to reduce tinnitus satisfactorily when given by mouth.

Clonazepam

This is considered to be the initial drug of choice, seeming to help in about one-third of cases by a self-reported reduction in either tinnitus severity or in tinnitus effects or both; it is uncertain if the drug has a direct effect on the tinnitus or reduces it by means of its tranquillizer effect, acting like relaxation training therapy by cutting into the vicious circle with tension (see Figure 18.4). The author's regimen is 0.5 mg o.n. for one week, increasing if not beneficial at that dosage to 0.5 mg b.d. or 1 mg o.n. for a week and finally to 1 mg b.d. for 2 weeks. If no benefit results the drug is stopped, withdrawal symptoms after such a short period of treatment being at most minimal. If benefit results the drug may be continued, subject to careful explanation and use of the lowest helpful dosage in order to minimize dependence.

Carbamazepine

In the author's hands, Goodey's (1981) regimen for carbamazepine has occasionally been successful. This is 100 mg o.n. for 1 week, building up in weekly 100 mg increments to a maximum dose of 200 mg t.d.s. Lack of success and/or prohibitive side effects are not infrequent, but perversely the patient sometimes reports favourably that at least something worse than tinnitus has been found!

Nimodipine

Nimodipine should be helpful according to the results of experimentation with an animal model of tinnitus (Jastreboff and Brennan, 1988), and occasionally does usefully reduce tinnitus in man according to Ewart Davies (personal communication, 1994). He has used it successfully with minimal side effects in a dose of 30 mg b.d. for 3 weeks and then increased, if needed, to 30 mg q.d.s. for a further 3 weeks or continuously if a worthwhile reduction in tinnitus is achieved.

Management option 6: surgery (ablative)

The surgical management of rare vascular abnormalities has been discussed earlier, as have considerations concerning middle-ear surgery. Surgery for Menière's disorder is not considered in this chapter, as tinnitus would hardly ever be a major indication for such treatment but, like middle-ear surgery, explanation and preoperative consideration needs to be given to the risk of surgery resulting in increased tinnitus. Perilymph leaks can cause troublesome tinnitus, although vestibular disturbances or progressive deafness are the usual reasons for surgical intervention.

There have been many analyses of the results of destructive operations on the internal ear, and of section of the VIIIth nerve for conditions often associated with tinnitus. The surgical indication has usually been vertigo, but occasionally in the case of VIIIth nerve surgery it has been for tinnitus. In a significant proportion of cases, the tinnitus has not been alleviated by surgery or has even been made worse (Barrs and Brackmann, 1984; Gardner, 1984; Baguley, Moffat and Hardy, 1992; Parving *et al.*, 1992). Tinnitus is sometimes due to pressure from a vascular loop around the auditory nerve; both its diagnosis and surgery are difficult, but good results have been achieved in expert hands (Møller *et al.*, 1993). It would therefore seem that, with very few exceptions, surgery is not advisable where tinnitus is the primary indication, a conclusion drawn previously by McFadden (1982).

Management option 7: suppression (electrical, magnetic and electromagnetic)

Electrical

Interest in this has been stimulated by reports of much reduced or abolished tinnitus when cochlear implants are switched on. Usually such implants have been carried out to help those with total or profound deafness, but on a small scale this application has been extended to treatment of tinnitus itself (House, 1984), with rather indifferent results. Investigatory electrical stimulation of the cochlea was also found to suppress tinnitus, partially or completely, in 60% of patients during stimulation with a round-window electrode and in 43% with a promontory electrode (Aran and Cazals, 1981), but only with positive currents. This was worrying since long-term use of DC currents carries with it a high risk of damage to the remaining neural structures in the cochlea. However, subsequent work by Hazell *et al.* (1993) has shown that a low-frequency, around 20 Hz, sinusoidal electrical stimulation through a round-window electrode can be useful: they achieved total suppression of tinnitus in seven out of nine patients, with three of them receiving permanent implants with long lasting benefit. Further work, in 91 patients in an eight-centre worldwide study (Staller *et al.*, 1994) using ear canal, promontory or round window stimulation, was rather less successful though – 26% achieving significant reduction of tinnitus from ear canal and/or promontory stimulation, and 33% from round window stimulation. These less promising results may have been due to less rigorous selection procedures than the acute electrical stimulation test used by Hazell *et al.*, or to not using a stimulation frequency below 50 Hz.

Electrical stimulation of the ear as a treatment for tinnitus remains a potential avenue of further development, although its most effective route, by a cochlear or round-window implant, may be limited to ears with total deafness. At the other extreme, external or remote stimulation rarely seems to confer useful benefit. Stimulation of the skin near the tympanic membrane may yet prove to be a useful compromise for the majority, whose tinnitus ears are not totally deaf.

Magnetic

In 1987, Takeda reported reduction of tinnitus in 37 of 56 ears by means of a small powerful magnet placed deep in the ear canal with its north (positive) pole oriented medially. However, in a subsequent study, Coles *et al.* (1991) reported no significant benefit in a double-blind placebo-controlled study. It would not seem that this form of cochlear stimulation is likely to achieve worthwhile clinical results.

Electromagnetic

Pulsed electromagnetic stimulation has been used in some British and American hospitals for treatment of musculoskeletal disorders. Its reputed mode of action was an increase in blood flow in the affected areas together with changes in the degree of polarization across cell membranes. Inevitably it came to be tried on tinnitus patients apparently with some benefit, such that Roland *et al.* (1993) set up a double-blind placebo-controlled study. They reported that 45% of the 54 (out of 58) patients who completed the trial improved on the active device, but only 9% on the placebo.

A further larger-scale study with 150 patients has recently been completed. Preliminary verbal reports (Roland, personal communication, 1994) again suggested some benefit for some patients. If the more detailed analysis being carried out confirms this, then a whole new area of therapeutic research may have been opened up.

In the meantime an instrument, the Therapak, is available by mail-order with a money-back guarantee if returned within 30 days. Some of the author's patients have tried this and a few of them have reported sufficient benefit from this or a new wide-band version that they have not returned the instrument. At the present juncture, it seems to be a harmless, sometimes helpful and relatively inexpensive therapy for patients with tinnitus resistant to other treatments to try for themselves.

Management option 8: suppression of spontaneous otoacoustic emission-tinnitus

Spontaneous otoacoustic emissions have already been discussed as a cause of tinnitus. They account for all or a significant part of the tinnitus in 1–2% of tinnitus clinic patients.

Most of these cases are satisfied therapeutically by the special investigations involved in their diagnosis, by graphic demonstration of the spontaneous otoacoustic emissions and by explanation of their essential relationship to normal or near-normal hearing. Those requiring further measures can usually obtain sufficient relief from masking, complete masking in this case since the sound is a real acoustic one and is easily masked, or by long-term retraining therapy. However, for a small minority more is needed and trial of pharmacological suppressive treatment becomes appropriate.

Aspirin is known to suppress spontaneous otoacoustic emissions (McFadden and Plattsmeir, 1984) and can be used to treat tinnitus due to these. Quinine is a possible alternative with fewer undesirable side effects than aspirin. Results in eight patients with spontaneous otoacoustic emission-tinnitus needing such treatment have been reported by Baskill and Coles (1992). In three cases, one reported in detail by Penner and Coles (1992), palliation was achieved without any drug-induced tinnitus intervening: they continued on this treatment (with enteric-coated aspirin up to 4.8 g daily) intermittently as needed. In the five other cases, severe but temporary drug-induced tinnitus prohibited further treatment.

Fringe medicine

Many fringe medical treatments have given reported benefit, usually only anecdotally. Some, such as meditation, some diets and vitamins, seem occasionally to help. Others are too nebulous to mention here: homeopathic pharmacopoeias mention tinnitus all too frequently. Nevertheless, they can help as a straw to be clutched by the desperate and, at a stage where all conventional medicine managements have been tried and have failed, should not be dismissed summarily. Two alternative medical treatments that have aroused particular interest in recent years are outlined below.

Acupuncture

In a large study (1001 patients) carried out in China, acupuncture was not found to change the hearing thresholds in sensorineural hearing loss (Quian, Yuan-cheng and Gui-zhen, 1982). This is hardly surprising given our understanding of the pathological basis of such disorders, but in view of the more somatopsychic nature of tinnitus it might be expected that acupuncture could sometimes be beneficial for this. Two double-blind cross-over (acupuncture and placebo-acupuncture) trials have been carried out. While Hansen, Hansen and Bentzen (1982) found no significant improvement with acupuncture in 17 patients, Marks, Emery and Onisiphorou (1984) found a slight temporary improvement in five out of 14 patients. The latter group's words summarize the present position on this line of treatment. 'It seems that for the general tinnitus sufferer, acupuncture probably does not have much to offer. However, we are reluctant to close the door on this harmless method of treatment and condemn it outright. There is a suggestion that a few patients might respond to courses of longer than two weeks.'

Finally, a more recent study by Nilsson, Axelsson and Li De (1992) with 56 carefully documented patients led to the same generally negative conclusions, but with a suggestion that it can sometimes help psychologically and in those patients who have associated muscle pain and tension headaches.

Ginkgo biloba extract

This vegetable extract, from the leaves of the maiden-hair tree, has been used for the last two decades in treatment of chronic cerebrovascular insufficiency and peripheral arterial disease, with some claims of success, including improvements in vertigo and tinnitus. It contains a range of flavonoids and terpenes having arterial vasodilatory, platelet-aggregation inhibitory and other effects. It has also been tried in retinopathies and in patients with various inner-ear disorders. Sprenger (1986) studied its effects on hearing and tinnitus, and reported improvement of 5–20 dB averaged across 500–3000 Hz in 59% of the 54 patients, abolition of tinnitus in 36% and reduced tinnitus in 15%. Although an uncontrolled study, the results are at least interesting, as are 10 other reported studies of the use of *Ginkgo biloba* extract in inner-ear disorders. Further studies, e.g. by Holgers, Axelsson and Pringle (1994), have had disappointing results though, and its clinical usefulness would seem to be slight.

References

ANON (1981a) Definition and classification of tinnitus. In: *Tinnitus: Ciba Foundation Symposium 85*, edited by D. Evered and G. Lawrenson, Appendix I. London: Pitman. pp. 300–302

ANON (1981b) Guidelines for recommended procedures in tinnitus testing. In: *Tinnitus: Ciba Foundation Symposium 85*, edited by D. Evered and G. Lawrenson, Appendix II. London: Pitman. pp. 303–306

ARAN, J-M. and CAZALS, Y. (1981) Electrical suppression of tinnitus. In: *Tinnitus: Ciba Foundation Symposium 85*, edited by D. Evered and G. Lawrenson. London: Pitman. pp. 217–231

AXELSSON, A. and COLES, R. R. A. (1994) Compensation for tinnitus in noise-induced hearing loss. In: *Proceedings of the Vth International Symposium on Effects of Noise on Hearing*, Gothenburg, May 12–14, 1994, edited by D. Henderson, R. J. Salvi and R. P. Hamernik. To be published.

AXELSSON, A. and SANDH, A. (1985) Tinnitus in noise-induced hearing loss. *British Journal of Audiology*, **19**, 271–276

AXELSSON, A., COLES, R., ERLANDSSON, S., MEIKLE, M. and VERNON, J. (1993) Evaluation of tinnitus treatment: methodological aspects. *Journal of Audiological Medicine*, **2**, 141–150

BADIA, L., PARIKH, A. and BROOKES, G. B. (1994) Management of middle ear myoclonus. *Journal of Laryngology and Otology*, **108**, 380–382

BAGULEY, D. M., MOFFAT, D. A. and HARDY, D. G. (1992) What is the effect of translabyrinthine acoustic schwannoma removal upon tinnitus? *Journal of Laryngology and Otology*, **106**, 329–331

BÁRÁNY, R. (1935) Die Beeinflussung des Ohrensausens durch intravenos injizierte Lokalanaesthetica. *Acta Oto-laryngologica*, **23**, 201–203

BARRS, D. M. and BRACKMANN, D. E. (1984) Translabyrinthine nerve section: effect on tinnitus. *Journal of Laryngology and Otology*, Suppl. 9, 287–293

BASKILL, J. L. and COLES, R. R. A. (1992) Current studies on spontaneous emissions and tinnitus. In: *Tinnitus 91: Proceedings of the Fourth International Tinnitus Seminar*, Bordeaux, 1991, edited by J-M. Aran and R. Dauman. Amsterdam: Kugler. pp. 79–83

BROOKES, G. B., MAW, A. R. and COLEMAN, M. J. (1980) 'Costen's syndrome' – correlation or coincidence: a review of 45 patients with temporomandibular joint dysfunction, otalgia and other aural symptoms. *Clinical Otolaryngology*, **5**, 25–36

BROWN, R. D. (1981) Discussion on Brown *et al.* (1981) In: *Tinnitus: Ciba Foundation Symposium, 85*, edited by D. Evered and G. Lawrenson. London: Pitman. pp. 166–167

BROWN, R. D., PENNY, J. E., HENLEY, C. M., HODGES, K. B., KUPETZ, S. A., GLENN, D. W. *et al.* (1981) Ototoxic drugs and noise. In: *Tinnitus: Ciba Foundation Symposium 85*, edited by D. Evered and G. Lawrenson. London: Pitman. pp. 151–171

BROWNING, G. G., GATEHOUSE, S. and LOWE, G. D. O. (1986) Blood viscosity as a factor in sensorineural hearing impairment. *Lancet*, i, 121–123

CHUNG, D. Y., GANNON, R. P. and MASON, K. (1984) Factors affecting the prevalence of tinnitus. *Audiology*, **23**, 441–452

COLES, R. R. A. (1982) Non-organic hearing loss. In: *Otolaryn-gology 1, Otology*, edited by A. G. Gibb and M. F. W. Smith, Chap. 10. London: Butterworths. pp. 150–176

COLES, R. R. A. (1984) Epidemiology of tinnitus: (1) prevalence, (2) demographic and clinical features. *Journal of Laryngology and Otology*, Suppl. 9, 7–15 and 195–202

COLES, R., BRADLEY, P., DONALDSON, I. and DINGLE, A. (1991) A trial of tinnitus therapy with ear-canal magnets. *Clinical Otolaryngology*, **16**, 371–372

COLES, R. R. A., LUTMAN, M. E., AXELSSON, A. and HAZELL, J. W. P. (1992) Tinnitus severity gradings: cross-sectional studies. In: *Tinnitus 91: Proceedings of the Fourth International Tinnitus Seminar*, Bordeaux, 1991, edited by J-M. Aran and R. Dauman. Amsterdam: Kugler. pp. 453–455

COLES, R. R. A. and MASON, S. M. (1984) The results of cortical electric response audiometry in medico-legal investigations. *British Journal of Audiology*, **18**, 71–78

COLES, R. R. A., SMITH, P. A. and DAVIS, A. C. (1990) The relationship between noise-induced hearing loss and tinnitus and its management. In: *Noise as a Public Health Problem, vol. 4, New Advances in Noise Research, part 1*, edited by B. Berglund and T. Lindvall. Stockholm: Swedish Council for Building Research. pp. 87–112. See also: Tinnitus: its epidemiology and management. In: *Presbyacusis: 14th Danavox Symposium*, edited by J. H. Jensen. Copenhagen: Danavox Jubilee Foundation. pp. 377–402

DONALDSON, I. (1978) Tinnitus: a theoretical view and a therapeutic study using amylobarbitone. *Journal of Laryngology and Otology*, **92**, 123–130

DOUEK, E. and REID, J. (1968) The diagnostic value of tinnitus pitch. *Journal of Laryngology and Otology*, **82**, 1039–1042

EAST, C. A. and HAZELL, J. W. P. (1987) The suppression of palatal (or intratympanic) myoclonus by tinnitus masking devices: a preliminary report. *Journal of Laryngology and Otology*, **101**, 1230–1234

ERLANDSSON, S. I., RUBINSTEIN, B. and CARLSSON, S. G. (1991) Tinnitus: evaluation of biofeedback and stomatognathic treatments. *British Journal of Audiology*, **25**, 151–161

FELDMANN, H. (1971) Homolateral and contralateral masking of tinnitus by noise-bands and by pure tones. *Audiology*, **10**, 138–144

FOWLER, E. P. (1943) Control of head noises: their illusions of loudness and of timbre. *Archives of Otolaryngology*, **37**, 391–398

FOWLER, E. P. (1944) Head noises in normal and in disordered ears: significance, measurement, differentiation and treatment. *Archives of Otolaryngology*, **39**, 498–503

FOWLER, E. P. (1953) Intravenous procaine in the treatment of Menière's disease. *Annals of Otology, Rhinology and Laryngology*, **62**, 1186–1200

FOWLER, E. P. and FOWLER, E. P. (1948) The emotional factor in tinnitus aurium. *Laryngoscope*, **58**, 145–154

GARDNER, G. (1984) Neurotologic surgery and tinnitus. *Journal of Laryngology and Otology*, Suppl. 9, 311–318

GOODEY, R. J. (1981) Drugs in the treatment of tinnitus. In: *Tinnitus: Ciba Foundation Symposium 85*, edited by D. Evered and G. Lawrenson. London: Pitman. pp. 263–278

GOODWIN, P. E. (1980) Tinnitus and auditory imagery. *American Journal of Otology*, **2**, 5–9

GOODWIN, P. E. and JOHNSON, R. M. (1980) The loudness of tinnitus. *Acta Oto-Laryngologica*, **90**, 353–359

GRAHAM, J. M. (1981a) Contribution to general discussion: a central or peripheral source of tinnitus? In: *Tinnitus: Ciba Foundation Symposium 85*, edited by D. Evered and G. Lawrenson. London: Pitman. pp. 283–284

GRAHAM, J. M. (1981b) Tinnitus in children with hearing

loss. In: *Tinnitus: Ciba Foundation Symposium 85*, edited by D. Evered and G. Lawrenson. London: Pitman. pp. 172–192

GRAHAM, J. M. and BUTLER, J. (1984) Tinnitus in children. *Journal of Laryngology and Otology*, Suppl. 9, 236–241

GRIFFIN, J. P. (1988) Drug-induced ototoxicity. *British Journal of Audiology*, **22**, 195–210

HALLAM, R. S., JAKES, S. C. and HINCHCLIFFE, R. (1988) Cognitive variables in tinnitus annoyance. *British Journal of Clinical Psychology*, **27**, 213–222

HALLAM, R. S., RACHMAN, S. and HINCHCLIFFE, R. (1984) Psychological aspects of tinnitus. In: *Contributions to Medical Psychology*, edited by S. Rachman, vol. 3, chapter 3. Oxford: Pergamon. pp. 31–53

HANSEN, P. E., HANSEN, J. H. and BENTZEN, O. (1982) Acupuncture treatment of chronic unilateral tinnitus – a double-blind cross-over trial. *Clinical Otolaryngology*, **7**, 325–329

HAZELL, J. W. P. (1981) Measurement of tinnitus in humans. In: *Tinnitus: Ciba Foundation Symposium 85*, edited by D. Evered and G. Lawrenson. London: Pitman. pp. 35–53

HAZELL, J. W. P., JASTREBOFF, P. J., MEERTON, L. E. and CONWAY, M. J. (1993) Electrical tinnitus suppression: frequency dependence of effects. *Audiology*, **32**, 68–77

HAZELL, J. W. P. and SHELDRAKE, J. B. (1992) Hyperacusis and tinnitus. In: *Tinnitus 91: Proceedings of the Fourth International Tinnitus Seminar, Bordeaux, 1991*, edited by J-M. Aran and R. Dauman. Amsterdam: Kugler. pp. 245–248

HAZELL, J. W. P. and WOOD, S. M. (1981) Tinnitus masking – a significant contribution to tinnitus management. *British Journal of Audiology*, **15**, 223–230

HAZELL, J. W. P., WOOD, S. M., COOPER, H. R., STEPHENS, S. D. G., CORCORAN, A. L., COLES, R. R. A. *et al.* (1985) A clinical study of tinnitus maskers. *British Journal of Audiology*, **19**, 65–146

HELLER, M. F. and BERGMAN, M. (1953) Tinnitus aurium in normally hearing persons. *Annals of Otology, Rhinology and Laryngology*, **62**, 72–83

HOLGERS, K-M., AXELSSON, A. and PRINGLE, I. (1994) Ginkgo biloba extract for the treatment of tinnitus. *Audiology*, **33**, 85–42

HOUSE, J. W. (1984) Effects of electrical stimulation on tinnitus. *Journal of Laryngology and Otology*, Suppl. 9, 139–140

JAKES, S. C., HALLAM, R. S., CHAMBERS, C. and HINCHCLIFFE, R. (1985) A factor analytical study of tinnitus complaint behaviour. *Audiology*, **24**, 195–206

JAKES, S. C., HALLAM, R. S., CHAMBERS, C. and HINCHCLIFFE, R. (1986) Matched and self-reported loudness of tinnitus: methods and sources of error. *Audiology*, **25**, 92–100

JASTREBOFF, P. J. and BRENNAN, J. F. (1988) Specific effects of nimodipine on the auditory system. *Annals of the New York Academy of Sciences*, **522**, 716–718

JASTREBOFF, P. J. and HAZELL, J. W. P. (1993) A neurophysiological approach to tinnitus: clinical implications. *British Journal of Audiology*, **27**, 7–17

JAYARAJAN, V., HARRIS, N. D., STEVENS, J. C. and COLES, R. R. A. (1995) Tinnitus following ear syringing. *Journal of Audiological Medicine*, **4**, 85–96

JONES, I. H. and KNUDSEN, V. O. (1928) Certain aspects of tinnitus, particularly treatment. *Laryngoscope*, **38**, 597–611

KEMP, D. T. (1981) Physiologically active cochlear micromechanics – one source of tinnitus. In: *Tinnitus: Ciba Foundation Symposium 85*, edited by D. Evered and G. Lawrenson. London: Pitman. pp 54–81

MCFADDEN, D. (1982) *Tinnitus: Facts, Theories and Treatments*. Washington, DC: National Academic Press

MCFADDEN, D. and PLATTSMIER, H. S. (1984) Aspirin abolishes spontaneous otoacoustic emissions. *Journal of the Acoustical Society of America*, **76**, 443–447

MARKS, N. J., EMERY, P. and ONISIPHOROU, C. (1984) A controlled trial of acupuncture in tinnitus. *Journal of Laryngology and Otology*, **98**, 1103–1109

MARTIN, F. W. and COLMAN, B. H. (1980) Tinnitus: a double-blind crossover controlled trial to evaluate the use of lignocaine. *Clinical Otolaryngology*, **5**, 3–11

MATSUHIRA, T., YAMASHITA, K. and YASUDA, M. (1992) Estimation of the loudness of tinnitus from matching tests. *British Journal of Audiology*, **26**, 387–395

MEIKLE, M. B. and GRIEST, S. E. (1992) Asymmetry in tinnitus perception: factors that may account for the higher prevalence of left-sided tinnitus. In: *Tinnitus 91: Proceedings of the Fourth International Tinnitus Seminar, Bordeaux, 1991*, edited by J-M. Aran and R. Dauman. Amsterdam: Kugler pp. 231–237

MEIKLE, M. B., GRIEST, S. E., PRESS, L. S. and STEWART, B. J. (1992) Relationships between tinnitus and audiometric variables in a large sample of tinnitus patients. In: *Tinnitus 91: Proceedings of the Fourth International Tinnitus Seminar, Bordeaux, 1991*, edited by J-M. Aran and R. Dauman. Amsterdam: Kugler pp. 27–34

MELDING, P. S., GOODEY, R. J. and THORNE, P. R. (1978) The use of intravenous lidocaine in the diagnosis and treatment of tinnitus. *Journal of Laryngology and Otology*, **92**, 115–121

MØLLER, A. R. (1984) Pathophysiology of tinnitus. *Annals of Otology, Rhinology and Laryngology*, **93**, 39–44

MØLLER, M. B., MØLLER, A. R., JANNETTA, P. J. and JHO, H. D. (1993) Vascular decompression surgery for severe tinnitus: selection criteria and results. *Laryngoscope*, **103**, 421–427

MRC INSTITUTE OF HEARING RESEARCH (1987) Epidemiology of tinnitus in adults. In: *Tinnitus*, edited by J. W. P. Hazell, chap. 3. Edinburgh: Churchill Livingstone. pp. 46–70

MURAI, K., TYLER, R. S., HARKER, L. A. and STOUFFER, J. L. (1992) Review of pharmacologic treatment of tinnitus. *American Journal of Otology*, **13**, 454–464

NILSSON, S., AXELSSON, A. and LI DE, G. (1992) Acupuncture for tinnitus management. *Scandinavian Audiology*, **21**, 245–251

NODAR, R. C. and LEZAK, M. H. W. (1984) Pediatric tinnitus (a thesis revisited). *Journal of Laryngology and Otology*, Suppl. 9, 234–235

O'CONNOR, A. F. and SHEA, J. J. (1981) Autophony and the patulous Eustachian tube. *Laryngoscope*, **91**, 1427–1435

OOSTERVELD, W. J. (1987) Effect of betahistine hydrochloride on induced vestibular nystagmus: a double blind study. *Clinical Otolaryngology*, **12**, 131–135

PARVING, A., TOS, M., THOMSEN, J., MOLLER, H. and BUCHWALD, C. (1992) Some aspects of life quality after surgery for acoustic neuroma. *Archives of Otolaryngology – Head and Neck Surgery*, **118**, 1061–1064

PENNER, M. J. (1983) Variability in matches to subjective tinnitus. *Journal of Speech and Hearing Research*, **27**, 274–279

PENNER, M. J. (1984) Equal-loudness contours using subjective tinnitus as the standard. *Journal of Speech and Hearing Research*, **27**, 274–279

PENNER, M. J. (1992) Linking spontaneous otoacoustic emissions and tinnitus. *British Journal of Audiology*, **26**, 115–123

PENNER, M. J., BRAUTH, S. and HOOD, L. (1981) The temporal course of the masking of tinnitus as a basis for inferring its origin. *Journal of Speech and Hearing Disorders*, **24**, 257–261

PENNER, M. J. and COLES, R. R. A. (1992) Indications for aspirin as a palliative for tinnitus caused by SOAEs: a case study. *British Journal of Audiology*, **26**, 91–96

PENNER, M. J., GLOTZBACH, A. and HUANG, T. (1993) Spontaneous otoacoustic emissions: measurement and data. *Hearing Research*, **8**, 229–237

QUIAN, L., YUAN-CHENG, D. and GUI-ZHEN, L. (1982) Evaluation of acupuncture treatment for sensorineural deafness and deaf mutism based on 20 years' experience. *Chinese Medical Journal*, **95**, 21–24

RICE, C. G. (1994) Annoyance due to low frequency hums. *British Medical Journal*, **308**, 355–356

ROLAND, N. J., HUGHES, J. B., DALEY, M. B., COOK, J. A., JONES, A. S. and MCCORMICK, M. S. (1993) Electromagnetic stimulation as a treatment of tinnitus: a pilot study. *Clinical Otolaryngology*, **18**, 278–281

RUBINSTEIN, B., ÖSTERBERG, T., ROSENHALL, U. and JOHANSSON, U. (1993) Tinnitus and craniomandibular disorders in an elderly population. *Journal of Audiological Medicine*, **2**, 97–113

SAEED, S. R. and BROOKES, G. B. (1993) The use of clostridium botulinum toxin in palatal myoclonus: a preliminary report. *Journal of Laryngology and Otology*, **107**, 208–210

SHAILER, M. J., TYLER, R. S. and COLES, R. R. A. (1981) Critical masking bands for sensorineural tinnitus. *Scandinavian Audiology*, **10**, 157–162

SHEA, J. J., EMMETT, J. R., MAYS, K., ORCHIK, D. J. and WEBB, W. (1981) Medical treatment of tinnitus. *Annals of Otology, Rhinology and Laryngology*, **90**, 601–606

SHELDRAKE, J. B. and HAZELL, J. W. P. (1992) Maskers *versus* hearing aids in the prosthetic management of tinnitus. In: *Tinnitus 91: Proceedings of the Fourth International Tinnitus Seminar*, Bordeaux, 1991, edited by J-M. Aran and R. Dauman. Amsterdam: Kugler. pp. 395–399

SOOD, S. K. and COLES, R. R. A. (1988) Hyperacusis and phonophobia in tinnitus patients. *British Journal of Audiology*, **22**, 228

SOOD, S. K., COLES, R. R. A. and LUTMAN, M. E. (1987) Relationship between equal loudness and minimal masking contours for tinnitus. In: *Proceedings of the Third International Tinnitus Seminar*, Munster, 1987, edited by H. Feldmann. Karlsruhe: Harsch Verlag. pp. 270–274

SPOENDLIN, H. (1987) Inner ear pathology and tinnitus. In: *Proceedings of the Third International Tinnitus Seminar*, Munster, 1987, edited by H. Feldmann. Karlsruhe: Harsch Verlag. pp. 42–51

SPRENGER, F-H. (1986) Innenohrschwerhörigkeit: gute therapieergebnisse mit Ginkgo biloba. *Arztliche Praxis*, **12**, 938–940

STALLER, S., DOBSON, C., AXELSSON, A., TJELLSTROM, A., EVANS, A., KECK, D. *et al.* (1994) Electrical tinnitus suppression in hearing and hearing-impaired subjects. In: *Advances in Cochlear Implantation, Proceedings of Third International Cochlear Implant Conference*, Innsbruck, 1993, edited by I. J. Hochmair-Desoyer and E. S. Hochmair. Vienna: Manz. pp. 457–461

STEPHENS, S. D. G. (1984) The treatment of tinnitus – a historical perspective. *Journal of Laryngology and Otology*, **98**, 963–972

STEPHENS, S. D. G. and HALLAM, R. S. (1985) The Crown-Crisp Experiential Index in patients complaining of tinnitus. *British Journal of Audiology*, **19**, 151–158

STOUFFER, J. L., TYLER, R. S., BOOTH, J. C. and BUCKRELL, B. (1992) Tinnitus in normal-hearing and hearing-impaired children. In: *Tinnitus 91: Proceedings of the Fourth International Tinnitus Seminar*, Bordeaux, 1991, edited by J-M. Aran and R. Dauman. Amsterdam: Kugler. pp. 255–258

TAKEDA, H. (1987) Magnetic therapy for tinnitus. *Otologia Fukuoka*, **33**, 700–706

TERRY, A. M. P., JONES, D. M., DAVIS, B. R. and SLATER, R. (1983) Parametric studies of tinnitus masking and residual inhibition. *British Journal of Audiology*, **17**, 245–256

TYLER, R. S., ARAN J-M. and DAUMAN, R. (1992) Recent advances in tinnitus. *American Journal of Audiology*, **1**, 36–44

TYLER, R. S. and BAKER, L. J. (1983) Difficulties experienced by tinnitus sufferers. *Journal of Speech and Hearing Disorders*, **48**, 150–154

TYLER, R. S. and CONRAD-ARMES, D. (1983a) Tinnitus pitch: a comparison of three measurement methods. *British Journal of Audiology*, **17**, 101–107

TYLER, R. S. and CONRAD-ARMES, D. (1983b) The determination of tinnitus loudness considering the effect of recruitment. *Journal of Speech and Hearing Research*, **26**, 59–72

VERNON, J. A. (1977) Attempts to relieve tinnitus. *Journal of the American Audiological Society*, **2**, 124–131

VERNON, J. A. and MEIKLE, M. B. (1981) Tinnitus masking: unresolved problems. In: *Tinnitus: Ciba Foundation Symposium 85*, edited by D. Evered and G. Lawrenson, London: Pitman. pp. 239–262

VERNON, J. A. and MØLLER, A. R. (eds) (1995) *Tinnitus Mechanisms*. Needham, MA: Allyn & Bacon.

Further general reading on tinnitus

ARAN, J-M. and DAUMAN, R. (eds) (1992) *Tinnitus 91: Proceedings of the Fourth International Tinnitus Seminar*, Bordeaux, 1991. Amsterdam: Kugler

EVERED, D. and LAWRENSON, G. (eds) (1981) *Tinnitus: Ciba Foundation Symposium 85*. London: Pitman

FELDMANN, H. (ed) (1987) *Proceedings of the Third International Tinnitus Seminar*, Munster, 1987. Karlsruhe: Harsch Verlag

HALLAM, R. S. (1989) *Living with Tinnitus: Dealing with Ringing in your Ears*. Wellingborough: Thorsons

HAZELL, J. W. P. (ed) (1987) *Tinnitus*. Edinburgh: Churchill Livingstone

MCFADDEN, D. (1982) *Tinnitus: Facts, Theories and Treatments*. Washington, DC: National Academic Press

SHULMAN, A. and BALLANTYNE, J. C. (eds) (1984) *Proceedings of the Second International Tinnitus Seminar*, New York, 1983. *Journal of Laryngology and Otology*, Suppl. 9

VERNON, J. A. and MØLLER, A. R. (eds) (1995) *Tinnitus Mechanisms*. Needham, MA: Allyn & Bacon

19

Overview of balance

Linda M. Luxon

Balance disorders span a breadth of conditions including vague dysequilibrium, attacks of vertigo/dizziness, chronic unsteadiness/ataxia and falls. Each year five out of every 1000 patients consult their general practitioner because of symptoms that are classified as vertigo and a further 10 in 1000 are seen for dizziness or giddiness (RCGP/OPCS, 1986). By late middle age, one in four people suffers from dizziness, which is even more common in the elderly population (Stephens, Hogan and Meredith, 1991). However, not only are symptoms of dysequilibrium very prevalent, but the morbidity associated with balance disorders is frequently overlooked. A recent study of 54 patients with peripheral vestibular disorders referred to a specialized neuro-otological centre, revealed that 35 developed a psychiatric illness as judged by the DSM IIIR criteria and most took time off work (an average of 9 months) (Eagger et al., 1992). Moreover, after head injury and whiplash injury, vestibular symptoms are one of the most likely sequelae to prevent rapid return to work (Luxon, 1995b). In addition, falls are recognized to be one of the important health problems of the elderly and represent the commonest cause of accidental death in the over 75 year olds (Downton, 1994). In the face of such statistics, it is perhaps surprising that balance disorders continue to be a low priority both in terms of medical education and in the current commercial market place of medicine. The lack of facilities for the diagnosis and management of balance disorders is even more surprising when one considers the plethora of diverse causes of dysequilibrium (Figure 19.1).

Man has developed a very sophisticated mechanism for maintaining balance, which relies upon visual, vestibular and proprioceptive inputs. These sensory inputs pass into the central nervous system, where they are integrated and modulated with activity from other neurological centres. Considering these complex interactions, it is not surprising that pathology in a wide variety of systems may give rise to symptoms of dysequilibrium (Figure 19.2) (see Chapter 20). Thus, there is an onus on the doctor, in almost all specialities, to acquire a basic understanding of the causes of balance disorders, together with a strategy for diagnosis and appropriate management. Notwithstanding this, the symptom of dysequilibrium is greeted with a sense of despair by the medical profession (Luxon, 1984) for a number of reasons. Dizziness is a vague symptom which does not instantly point to any specific pathology; second, despite the morbidity statistics cited above, it is a commonly held perception that this is a trivial symptom of no sinister significance and therefore time and scarce resources should not be wasted on its evaluation; third, it has not infrequently in the past been considered to be of 'neurotic' origin and fourth, it has been considered that there is little active intervention available for the management of dizziness. For all these reasons, most clinicians have adopted a rather negative approach in dealing with the patient complaining of imbalance. This brief review emphasizes that in the light of current knowledge and recent developments in effective management, a systematic approach to diagnosis and rehabilitation of balance disorders is to be encouraged, to provide an optimum outcome for every patient.

Good management relies upon accurate diagnosis and a single pathology can often be identified, but certain generalizations are worthy of note. Some pathologies may affect more than one site, e.g. cerebrovascular disease may give rise to an ischaemic labyrinthitis and brain stem dysfunction. Second, patients with peripheral vestibular disorders, e.g. viral

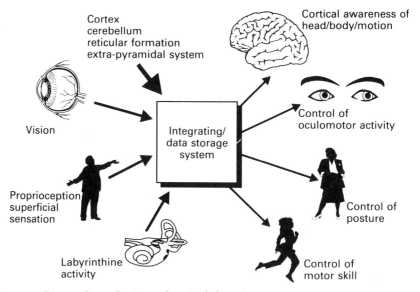

Figure 19.1 Diagram to illustrate the mechanisms subserving balance in man

labyrinthitis may make an initial excellent recovery, but subsequent psychological (redundancy, divorce, bereavement), or physical stress (e.g. a coincidental illness, which may be as minor as influenza) may precipitate decompensation with recurrence of symptoms. Thus, in some patients there may be a relapsing and remitting course of dysequilibrium on such a basis. Third, in the elderly patient, dysequilibrium may result from a multiplicity of pathologies in a variety of sites, e.g. there may be visual impairment due to a cataract, an alteration in proprioception due to cervical osteoarthritis and decompensation from a pre-existing and previously well compensated peripheral disorder. Superimposed upon such abnormalities, there may be age-related changes within the central nervous system in part due to degeneration and in part due to ischaemic changes, preventing adequate integration and meditation of the information required for balance.

Clinical assessment

The correct diagnosis of balance disorders relies heavily upon an accurate detailed history and clinical examination, including an assessment of the ears, eyes, central nervous system and cardiovascular systems. For the purposes of this brief review the following neuro-otological details are of particular relevance.

Character of complaint

In the first instance, non-specific lightheadedness, faintness and 'dizziness', which is commonly associated with general medical disorders, should be differentiated from vertigo, which is defined as an illusion or an hallucination of movement, and is a cardinal manifestation of a disordered vestibular system

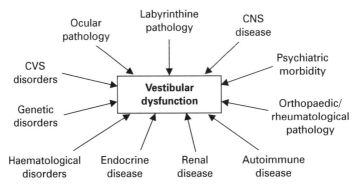

Figure 19.2 Diagram to illustrate the plethora of systems giving rise to dysequilibrium

ness of gait and a fear of falling, more commonly associated with neurological disease. Notwithstanding this, patients may have great difficulty describing their symptoms and will volunteer such bizarre complaints as, 'I feel my brain is sloshing around inside/lagging behind my head'; 'I feel as though I am in a goldfish bowl watching my life go by'; 'I feel as though I am standing outside myself' and 'I feel spaced out'. Such complaints are often accompanied by other unusual symptoms, such as difficulty in walking on a highly patterned carpet, a marked exacerbation of symptoms in supermarkets when scanning shelves or on escalators, and frequently leave the uninitiated clinician, at best, wondering how to proceed diagnostically and, at worst, assuming this patient requires a psychiatric referral without further objective investigation of the symptomatology. In dealing with balance disorders, it is enormously reassuring for patients to feel that they are communicating with a doctor who is familiar with such bizarre symptoms and who appreciates that they are having great difficulty in their description. Thus, it is helpful for the clinician to be alert to the possibility that symptoms of disorientation may manifest as a broad spectrum of unusual complaints.

Classically, vertigo of peripheral labyrinthine origin presents as acute, unprecipitated, short-lived episodes, associated with nausea and vomiting, while vertigo of central vestibular origin follows a more insidious and protracted course. Such complaints indicate the need for vestibular investigation, while symptoms of gait unsteadiness, stumbling and veering are significantly more common in neurological disease than in primary vestibular pathology.

A history of falls requires the evaluation of risk factors, such as drug intake, neurological conditions, cognitive function, general medical disorders and environmental factors, including uneven or slippery surfaces, poor lighting or an unfamiliar environment. Thus, potentially treatable predisposing factors can be identified and corrected. A patient who has suffered a single, uncomplicated fall, with no sequelae, may be reassured and discharged, but recurrent falls, with or without injury, require careful assessment and, in particular, a detailed assessment of balance. A valuable concept in considering falls is to consider the question 'why did this particular person fall at this particular time and in this particular place?'. For any particular fall, there is a 'liability' to fall factor and an 'opportunity' to fall factor (Downton, 1992).

Time course of the symptom

The time course of individual episodes of dysequilibrium and the overall time course of symptoms, identifying 'clusters' and periods of relapse and remission are of diagnostic value. Acute rotational vertigo of less than one minute's duration is most commonly associated with a diagnosis of benign positional vertigo of paroxysmal type, which is common following head injury and in association with vascular disease and ageing. Attacks frequently occur in clusters with periods of many weeks or months of freedom. Acute rotational vertigo of a few minutes' duration has been ascribed, particularly in the elderly, to recurrent vertebrobasilar insufficiency, but in the absence of other neurological symptoms and signs this diagnosis is almost certainly incorrect (Luxon, 1990).

Vertigo of several hours' duration is most commonly associated with Menière's disease and migraine. Both these conditions give rise to clusters of attacks with long periods of remission, and it should be recalled that in migraine, vertigo may occur with headache, but may also occur without. A single, acute episode of vertigo with gradual resolution over days or weeks would suggest peripheral vestibular pathology, such as viral or ischaemic labyrinthitis. A variety of mechanisms, generically known as 'cerebral plasticity', brings about compensation over a period of a few days to a few months. The crucial role of vision (Courjon *et al.*, 1977) and somatosensory input (Schaefer and Meyer, 1973) in the recovery of animals following labyrinthectomy has been well documented. The cerebellum is of primary importance in this recovery process, which includes central sensory substitution, together with spontaneous regeneration of vestibular activity in the affected side and physiological habituation (Ito, 1972).

Constant dysequilibrium may be identified in a poorly compensated peripheral vestibular disorder, but in the absence of an 'acute' onset, central vestibular pathology should be sought. In the presence of 'bobbing oscillopsia', vestibular failure should be considered (Rinne *et al.*, 1995).

Associated symptoms

Within the labyrinth and VIIIth nerve, the auditory and vestibular elements are in close proximity and thus auditory symptoms should always be specifically sought in any case of dysequilibrium. This is particularly important, as a gradual progressive hearing loss may not be noted and, moreover, in an elderly person it may be deemed by the patient that the hearing loss is only to be expected as a result of ageing, rather than appreciated that it is directly associated with the vestibular complaints. Moreover, neurological and general medical symptoms should be systematically sought.

Clinical examination

A full general medical examination is essential, with particular consideration of the fundi, visual fields, visual acuity, general neurological, cardiovascular and peripheral vascular systems. In all patients with dysequilibrium, it is essential to exclude active chronic middle ear disease by otoscopy.

A basic understanding of vestibular physiology and visuovestibular interaction, as outlined in Volume 1, Chapter 4, is essential if an informed assessment of vestibular function and an accurate interpretation of vestibular investigations are to be made. Most importantly, a detailed assessment of eye movements and particularly of spontaneous, positional and optokinetic nystagmus, is essential. An assessment of the Romberg test and gait testing is important in an overall assessment of balance, but it must be emphasized that these tests do not primarily assess vestibular function and should not be considered to be 'vestibular tests'. They rely on a variety of sensory inputs and good performance may only be achieved in the presence of normal motor function. Thus, each of these tests assesses a combination of sensorimotor skills.

Investigation

Apart from the clinical assessment outlined above, which may indicate the need for specialized general medical or neurological investigation, the main thrust of investigation of balance disorders is to define the presence (site and side) of vestibular pathology and provide information with respect to the aetiology. While in general the first requirement can be met with relative ease, there is no test which allows aetiological diagnosis.

Vestibular test procedures are hampered by some intrinsic difficulties in assessing the vestibular system and some extrinsic deficiencies primarily consequent upon the test procedures themselves (Table 19.1).

Table 19.1 Shortcomings of vestibular function tests

Only assess lateral semicircular canal function
Do not assess 'overall' balance
Do not assess balance strategies
Relatively insensitive
Lack of correlation with symptoms

As noted above a variety of pathologies can give rise to symptoms of dysequilibrium, but whatever the pathological process, damage to the vestibular apparatus brings about an asymmetry in vestibular activity,

which is interpreted by the brain as vertigo (see Volume 1, Chapter 4). Therefore, not surprisingly, a variety of different pathophysiological mechanisms may present with the same clinical picture, e.g. benign positional vertigo may result from head trauma, vascular disease or viral infection, which may damage the otolith organ. Equally, different conditions may involve the horizontal semicircular canal and give rise to a picture of 'acute labyrinthitis'. In essence, there is a 'final common pathway' in terms of vestibular symptoms, and while specific vestibular tests may identify damage at a particular site, they do not contribute to elucidating the aetiology causing that clinical presentation.

In the investigation of the dizzy patient, another important, but often overlooked fact, is that there is a marked discrepancy between symptoms of dysequilibrium and objective vestibular findings on investigation (Stephens, Hogan and Meredith, 1991; Yardley *et al.*, 1992). Thus, a patient with a minor canal paresis on caloric testing may be severely symptomatic, as in the case of Menière's disease, while a patient with a total canal paresis, e.g. in a case of vestibular schwannoma, may complain of little if any balance disorder. This is not surprising when it is appreciated that vestibular input is only one aspect of 'balance' but, if this concept is not embraced, this discrepancy between symptoms and signs can lead to the assumption that the patient is either elaborating his symptoms or being extremely stoic. It is important for the clinician to appreciate that impairment is not directly related to disability or handicap (Figure 19.3; Table 19.2) and to assess these important parameters for rehabilitation independently using specifically devised handicap and disability questionnaires (Jacobson and Newman, 1990; Yardley *et al.*, 1992).

Caloric test

In terms of identifying the presence of vestibular pathology, the caloric test, as conceived by Barany in 1906 and refined by Fitzgerald and Hallpike in 1942, has become the cornerstone of vestibular diagnosis, allowing identification of side and level of lesion. The test is simple and cheap, although it cannot be overemphasized that a significant level of skill and understanding of vestibular physiology is essential if reproducible and reliable results are to be obtained.

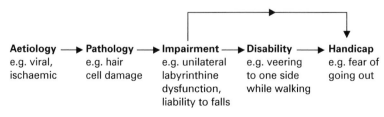

Figure 19.3 The relationship of impairment, disability and handicap

Table 19.2 Definitions of impairment, disability and handicap

Impairment	Implies deranged function
Disability	Refers to the balance problems as a result of the impairment
Handicap	Refers to the general effects on the individual's life arising indirectly from the vestibular dysfunction

Moreover, the clinician must be aware of the need to undertake full caloric testing with all four stimuli. 'Abbreviated' or 'shortened' caloric testing undertaken primarily in the interests of time and economy may be a valueless test, as in a combined pattern of responses normal nystagmic responses may be observed if only cold or indeed hot irrigations are undertaken, whereas when all four irrigations are undertaken it is observed that while at one temperature the two responses may be very similar, at the other temperature widely disparate responses are obtained.

Over the years, a multiplicity of criticisms of the caloric test has been raised. It is an unphysiological procedure, which most patients do not like and the need for careful, accurate explanation is essential if the anxiety of a vertiginous episode being precipitated by the procedure is to be allayed. Moreover, the correlation between stimulus and response is poorer than for rotation testing and the caloric test assesses only horizontal semicircular canal function. Thus, vestibular symptoms arising from the vertical canals or the otolith organs may be overlooked if it is not recalled that these structures are not routinely tested by either caloric or rotational procedures.

In addition, there is ongoing debate as to the manner in which the test should be conducted (Luxon, 1995a). Initially it was proposed that the duration parameter, as measured by direct observation of the nystagmic response should define caloric responses, but with the development of electronystagmography and the understandable preference for an objective recording, most centres now favour electronystagmographic recording of caloric induced nystagmus. However, this technique is not without its shortcomings. In order to obtain a large enough nystagmic response for recording purposes, it is necessary to conduct the test predominantly in the absence of optic fixation, but a short period of visual fixation is required if visuovestibular suppression is to be assessed. Inevitably, this requires light, which significantly affects the corneoretinal potential upon which electronystagmographic recordings are based. Errors may therefore be introduced. Moreover, studies have shown that while the slow component velocity may be a more physiological parameter to measure, there is greater variability than the duration parameter making the differentiation of

normal from abnormal more difficult. Importantly, the only major study comparing these two parameters in the same patient population found differing results (Vesterhauge, Zilstorff and Mansson, 1982), which would tend to suggest that these two techniques do not measure precisely the same physiological mechanism.

Further uncertainty centres on the exact physiological mechanism subserving the caloric response. Barany (1906) originally proposed that convection currents within the horizontal semicircular canal, as a result of the induced thermal gradient, brought about bending of the cupula and stimulation of the hair cells. Recent work in space has shown that other mechanisms must be important (Hood, 1989), e.g. direct thermal stimulation of the vestibular receptor organs.

Despite these criticisms, the caloric test is the most widely available vestibular test and when conducted in the standard manner by a skilled operator and with appropriate normative data, it is a valuable tool for assessment of the presence and severity of organic vestibular disease.

Rotation tests

Rotation testing with analysis of the resultant nystagmic response is invaluable if the expensive and sophisticated equipment together with appropriate technical and scientific expertise are available. This technique assesses both horizontal semicircular canals simultaneously and allows more accurate stimuli/response data to be obtained. Moreover, it is more acceptable to patients than the caloric test. For research purposes and for the assessment of visuovestibular interaction such equipment is essential, but in the current economic restraints it is most unlikely that many centres will be allowed the luxury of such facilities, which are not essential for routine vestibular assessment.

Galvanic tests

Galvanic testing is of particular value as it is the only vestibular test which allows differentiation of peripheral labyrinthine dysfunction from vestibular nerve damage, but in the past it has not gained acceptance as a clinical tool. Initially this was perhaps related to the fact that the current, which was required to be passed through the labyrinth in order to obtain a nystagmic response of sufficient magnitude to be observed, was uncomfortable. However, recent work in which body sway has been measured as a result of labyrinthine stimulation may prove to be a valuable tool in the future.

Posturography

In the last 50 years no new vestibular investigative technique has emerged. However, posturography, which was first used in the nineteenth century to assess balance (Snashall, 1994), has received much attention in the last decade.

A small amount of postural sway occurs normally and a variety of techniques has been used to measure this. The most common is the use of a force plate with a force transducer in each corner, that measures the centre of pressure of the body projected onto the plane of the force plate. However, as sway tends to be small when subjects stand on a stable platform, moving platforms have been developed in an attempt to increase sensitivity. This technique is known as dynamic posturography. The platform can be either tilted or linearly displaced and sway can be measured immediately after or during the movement. Moreover, in an attempt to assess the different sensory contributions to the maintenance of balance, systems have been developed which may selectively alter ankle proprioception and/or vision. With these devices, the angle of sway is fed back to a dynamic posture platform or to a movable visual surround so that the movement about the ankle joint or movement of the visual surround is sway referenced. Using this technique, early work suggested characteristic patterns of response in patients with vestibular disorders (Nashner and Peters, 1990). However, these early reports have not been reproduced and a recent statement on posturography by a panel of experts appointed by the American Academy of Neurology (1993) concluded that posturography, whether static or dynamic, does not help to localize lesions in the nervous system (including the vestibular apparatus) or to make a specific diagnosis. Notwithstanding this, the results of posturography, thus far, would suggest that it may prove an important clinical tool in the assessment of gait, falls and balance rehabilitation. In the evaluation of falls, it provides information about balance strategies, while in rehabilitation, it is of particular value in measuring the efficacy of physical rehabilitation programmes and in providing positive feedback to the patient.

Electro-oculography (electronystagmography)

Eye movement recordings provide a means of quantifying the ocular motor response to both visual and vestibular stimuli and are of paramount importance in identifying pathology at all levels within the vestibular apparatus. An ideal recording system would possess a number of features:

1 The ability to measure rotations of the globe in all three axes
2 Linearity over at least 90°
3 Sufficient sensitivity to record micromovements of a few seconds of arc
4 A band of arc widths of zero to a few hundred Hertz
5 The device must not interfere with vision
6 The response must be unaffected by head movement.

Not surprisingly no such system exists, but electro-oculography (electronystagmography) has the advantage of being the most simple and readily available method of recording eye movements. Other techniques include infrared recording, which provides a more sensitive clinical technique, albeit with a smaller range of linearity, while electromagnetic recording of eye movements is without doubt the most sensitive and accurate technique available, but limited for clinical application by the requirement of using a contact lens.

The principle of electro-oculography is based on the potential difference that exists between the cornea and retina (the corneoretinal potential). Electrodes are placed on either side of the eye with a ground electrode in a remote position. Displacement of the eye produces a difference in potential across the electrodes, which is amplified and used to produce a permanent record of the eye movement response. Standard vestibular assessment should include recording of pathological nystagmus, tests of vestibulo-ocular reflex function and tests of visual ocular control.

Management

A detailed history and clinical examination frequently enables general medical, neurological or otological balance disorders to be differentiated (see Figure 19.4). The specific management of general medical, cardiovascular and neurological disorders is undertaken following the appropriate referral. This review is confined to the management of central vestibular dysfunction, peripheral vestibular dysfunction (see Figure 19.4) and falls (Figure 19.5).

The management of central vestibular dysfunction remains poorly understood and is empirical in approach. Conditions associated with vertical nystagmus, such as the Arnold Chiari malformation and multiple sclerosis, frequently give rise to persistent oscillopsia with dysequilibrium and nausea. Such symptoms may be extremely distressing and are out of proportion to the clinical signs. In this situation, clonazepam, titrating the dose against sedative side effects, may be of value, as may baclofen, again titrating the dose against the side effect of muscular weakness. In patients with dizziness of central neurological origin, a trial of cinnarizine is occasionally effective, but failing this carbamazepine or clonazepam may be of help. Importantly, patients with instability associated with basal ganglion disorders and cerebellar disease may be greatly improved as a result of physiotherapy, teaching alternative gait and balancing strategies, as such an approach improves the patient's sense of confidence and ability to cope.

Patients with peripheral vestibular disorders fall into two main groups. Those with specific conditions

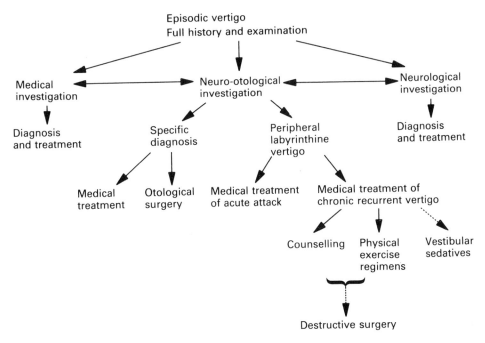

Figure 19.4 Flow diagram to illustrate the management of vertigo

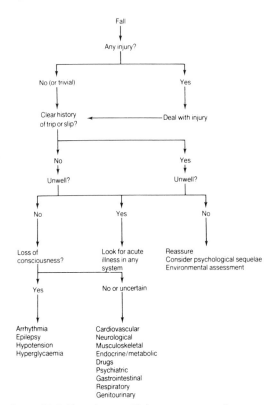

Figure 19.5 Flow chart to aid the assessment and management of falls. (From *Falls in the Elderly*, Downton, J. H., 1992 with kind permission)

for which there is a recognized treatment regimen and those in whom there is evidence of peripheral vestibular dysfunction on testing, but the precise underlying aetiology remains unresolved.

Certain specific peripheral vestibular disorders, such as Menière's disease, migraine, syphilitic labyrinthitis, vestibular schwannoma and perilymph fistula are well recognized. Benign paroxysmal positional vertigo is a condition which may be immediately diagnosed using the Hallpike manoeuvre and results from otolith dysfunction. Management is comprised of rehabilitative exercise regimens of which a number have been reported to be effective, including the Brandt Daroff regimen (Brandt and Daroff, 1980). However, more recently particle repositioning procedures such as the Semont manoeuvre (Semont, Freyss and Vitte, 1988) and the Epley manoeuvre (1992) have been reported to show an 80% recovery rate.

Acute vertigo associated with nausea and vomiting, requires immediate intervention and an antiemetic such as prochlorperazine, together with a vestibular sedative such as cinnarizine may be of value. However, it must be emphasized that while such drugs are useful in acute vertigo their use should be avoided in the treatment of chronic labyrinthine disease, as they may suppress vestibular activity which is crucial for vestibular compensation.

Chronic or recurrent vertigo due to poorly compensated vestibular pathology is a significant cause of morbidity, with restriction of both social and work activities. The primary symptoms of dizziness and/or vertigo are associated with secondary symptoms of psychological origin (anxiety, depression, phobic symptoms, malaise, fatigue and neck pain related to muscle tension as a result of conscious or subconscious limitation of head movements to reduce vertigo). As noted above, despite the prevalence of and the morbidity associated with balance disorders, the value of vestibular rehabilitation is not widely recognized and the availability of trained personnel and appropriate facilities is very limited both within and outside the National Health Service.

Physical exercise regimens

In 1946 Cawthorne, a renowned otolaryngologist, and Cooksey, an authority in rheumatology, reported the value of physiotherapy for patients with vestibular injuries secondary to head trauma or surgical intervention. They identified certain cases in whom post-traumatic vestibular disorders led to chronic invalidism, and identified that a graduated series of exercises aimed at encouraging head and eye movements improved recovery and lessened long-term sequelae. This empirical approach to a physical exercise regimen has been supported in more recent years by the animal experiments of Courjon and coworkers (1977) and Lacour, Roll and Appaix in 1976, outlined above.

Moreover, the work of Lacour and Xerri (1980) suggested that, following vestibular injury, there is a critical period of cerebral plasticity during which adapative changes induced by multisensory inputs are required, if full recovery is to be achieved. This has led to the current view that an active rehabilitation programme in which patients are encouraged to perform graded exercises to provoke their imbalance in a controlled and safe environment is highly effective in vestibular rehabilitation. Rarely, in patients who are extremely troubled by symptoms, it may be of value to cover the onset of exercises with a small dose of an antivertiginous drug such as cinnarizine, but such medication should be tailed off as soon as possible.

The Cawthorne Cooksey regimen of exercises has been shown to be effective in a number of studies, but recent workers have proposed that a customized, as opposed to a standardized, exercise regimen may be even more beneficial (Norré, 1987; Shepard *et al.*, 1993). As balance is dependent upon several sensory inputs, effective motor output and integration of these two systems, the rationale is that exercises specifically aimed at improving the deficient tasks in any given individual may be more effective in promoting recovery. However, to date there is no definitive evidence that such an approach is superior, but further work is required.

The rate and efficacy of vestibular compensation varies from one individual to another and the reasons for this are not fully understood. Impaired compensation may result from the nature or severity of the disorder, e.g. recurrent impairment of vestibular function, as seen in Menières' disease, and in continually changing vestibular input for which the central nervous system cannot compensate. Second, disorders which involve not only the peripheral vestibular apparatus, but also the central connections which are required for compensation, may preclude perfect recovery. Third, animal experiments have clearly shown that multiple sensory inputs are necessary for vestibular compensation to be effective. Thus, if the patient is immobilized or there is impairment of one of the other sensory systems, e.g. vision or proprioception, compensation is likely to be delayed or permanently impaired.

A common problem in patients with vestibular disorders is that they avoid moving the head to prevent dizziness. This imposes a strain on the neck muscles and neck pain develops. This in turn may be mismanaged by the use of a cervical collar, which further reduces neck movement and fails to allow the necessary input required for vestibular compensation to occur. The rationale for abandoning the neck collar and undertaking a physical exercise regimen must be clearly explained to the patient if compliance with the regimen is to be achieved.

Psychological support

Quite apart from any improvement in dysequilibrium that will be achieved as a result of the vestibular exercise regimen, significant psychological benefits accrue. In part because the detailed explanation of the regimen allows the patient to understand more fully the symptomatology and in part because the patients are actively encouraged to cope with their symptoms, rather than to avoid them (Yardley, Luxon and Haacke, 1994).

As noted above, patients with dysequilibrium develop psychological symptoms (Figure 19.6) particularly panic attacks, anxiety disorders and depression (Eagger *et al.*, 1992). In this study psychiatric symptoms occurred during the first 6 months after the onset of neuro-otological problems in two-thirds of the group. The commonest diagnoses were panic disorder, with or without agoraphobia, and phobic symptoms, including avoidance of crowds, enclosed

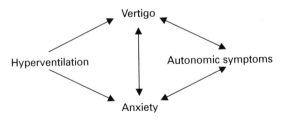

Figure 19.6 Diagram to illustrate relevant factors in vestibular disability and handicap

spaces such as underground trains, buses and cars, together with fear of going out alone, heights and the dark. Patients were fearful of being thought drunk and this led to an avoidance of social situations. In this context behavioural therapy is of considerable value in facilitating more rapid rehabilitation of such patients. No definitive study exists to assess the value of counselling in peripheral vestibular disorders, but it is the author's contention that a full and detailed explanation of the nature of the disorder, together with a structured plan of the rehabilitation pro-gramme to be followed is of great benefit in the long-term outcome of patients with balance disorders. This is particularly the case in patients with the type of bizarre symptoms noted at the beginning of this review as they find it hard to understand why visual symptoms, e.g walking on a striped carpet and the supermarket syndrome should result from an inner ear disturbance. This anxiety leads to preoccupations with sinister pathology such as brain tumours and equally importantly, patients frequently report that they feel 'as though they are going mad'. These views are of course reinforced when an inexperienced clinician dismisses their complaints as trivial or psychological in origin. Thus, rehabilitation with psychological support and an active physical exercise regimen with specific goals of returning to work and contining to undertake social activities, within realistic limits, should be defined.

Drug therapy

As noted above, vestibular sedative drugs have little role in the management of chronic vestibular disor-ders. Importantly, antiemetics such as prochlorpera-zine should not be prescribed long term as there is no evidence that they are effective in the managment of dysequilibrium and there is a danger of extrapyrami-dal side effects. Equally, psychotropic drugs should be avoided unless required for specific psychiatric indica-tions, as such drugs may interfere with vestibular compensation.

Surgical treatment

Surgical intervention in the treatment of episodic vertigo is indicated in three main situations:

1 The life-threatening complications of chronic middle ear disease
2 To improve the quality of life in a patient in whom all medical measures have failed
3 To exclude the presence of a perilymph fistula.

If destructive surgery is contemplated, detailed neuro-otological investigation *must* be undertaken to determine the exact site and severity of both auditory and vestibular function in each ear. Moreover, par-ticularly in an elderly person, vestibular compensa-tion may be prolonged or indeed incomplete as a consequence of age-related changes within the cen-tral nervous system. The concept that a subject will recover more efficiently from labyrinthine destruc-tion, than a partial deficit, is entirely misplaced. The risk of persisting imbalance must therefore be care-fully weighed against any possible advantage.

Conclusion

Balance disorders are prevalent in the general popula-tion and are associated with significant morbidity and mortality. Patients with dysequilibrium will present to many different specialities and it behoves the clinician to be familiar with a simple, but efficient management strategy. Active intervention based on a systematic diagnostic approach followed by aggres-sive rehabilitation will improve the quality of life in virtually all patients. In addition, significant econ-omic and social benefits will accrue to both the patient and society.

References

AMERICAN ACADEMY OF NEUROLOGY (1993) Report of the Therapeutic and Technology Assessment Subcommittee. Assessment: posturography. *Neurology*, **43**, 1261–1264

BARANY, R. (1906) Untesuchengen uber den vom Vestibu-larapparat des Ohres reflectorisch ausgelosten rhyth-mischen Nystagmus und seine Belgleiterscheinungen. *Monatschrift für Ohrenheilkunde*, **40**, 193–297

BRANDT, T. and DAROFF, R. B. (1980) Physical therapy for benign paroxysmal positional vertigo. *Archives of Otolaryn-gology*, **106**, 484–485

COURJON, J. H., JEANNEROD, M., OSSUZIO, I. and SCHMIDT, R. (1977) The role of vision in compensation of vestibulo-ocular reflex after hemilabyrinthectomy in the cat. *Experi-mental Brain Research*, **28**, 235–248

COOKSEY, F. S. (1946) Rehabilitation in vestibular injuries. *Proceedings of the Royal Society*, **39**, 273–275

DOWNTON, J. H. (1992) *Falls in the Elderly*. London: Edward Arnold

DOWNTON, J. H. (1994) Falls in the elderly – epidemiology, classification and causes. *Journal of Audiological Medicine*, **32**, iii–xiii

EAGGER, S., LUXON, L. M., DAVIES, R. A., COEHLO, A. and RON, M. A. (1992) Psychiatric morbidity in patients with periph-eral vestibular disorder: a clinical and neuro-otological study. *Journal of Neurology, Neurosurgery and Psychiatry*, **55**, 383–387

EPLEY, J. M. (1992) The canalith repositioning procedure: for treatment of benign paroxysmal positional vertigo. *Otolaryngology – Head and Neck Surgery*, **107**, 399–404

FITZGERALD, G. and HALLPIKE, C. S. (1942) Studies in human vestibular function. 1. Observations on the directional preponderance (Nystagmusbereitschaft) of caloric nystag-mus resulting from cerebral lesions. *Brain*, **65**, 115–137

HOOD, J. D. (1989) Evidence of direct thermal action upon the vestibular receptors in the caloric test. *Acta Otolaryngo-logica*, **107**, 161–165

ITO, M. (1972) Neural design of the cerebellar motor control system. *Brain Research*, **40**, 81–84

JACOBSON, G. P. and NEWMAN, C. W. (1990) The development of the dizziness handicap inventory. *Archives of Otolaryngology – Head and Neck Surgery*, **116**, 424–427

LACOUR, M., ROLL, J. P. and APPAIX, M. (1976) Modifications and development of spinal reflexes in the alert baboon (*Papio papio*) following a unilateral vestibular neurotomy. *Brain Research*, **113**, 255–269

LACOUR, M. and XERRI, C. (1980) Compensation of postural reactions to fall in the vestibular neuroectomized monkey. Role of the visual motion cues. *Experimental Brain Research*, **40**, 103–110

LUXON, L. M. (1984) A bit dizzy. *British Journal of Hospital Medicine*, **32**, 315–321

LUXON, L. M. (1990) Signs and symptoms of vertebrobasilar insufficiency. In: *Vascular Brainstem Diseases*, edited by B. Hofferberth. Basel: Karger. pp. 93–111

LUXON, L. M. (1995a) A comparison of measurement of duration (by examination) and slow phase velocity (by electronystagmography) of caloric nystagmus. *British Journal of Audiology*, **29**, 107–116

LUXON, L. M. (1995b) Post-traumatic Vertigo. In: *Handbook of Neuro-otology/Vestibular System*, edited by R. W. Baloh and M. Halmagyi. New York: Oxford University Press. (in press)

NASHNER, L. M. and PETERS, J. F. (1990) Dynamic posturography in neurotolgic diagnosis. *Neurologic Clinics*, **8**, 331–349

NORRE, M. E. (1987) Rationale of rehabilitation treatment for vertigo. *American Journal of Otolaryngology*, **8**, 31–35

RINNE, T., BRONSTEIN, A., RUDGE, P., GRESTY, M. and LUXON, L. M. (1995) Clinical findings in 53 patients with bilateral loss of vestibular function. (in press)

ROYAL COLLEGE OF GENERAL PRACTITIONERS and OFFICE OF POPULATION CENSUS AND SURVEYS (RCGP/OPCS) (1986) *Morbidity Statistics from General Practice*. London: HMSO

SCHAEFER, K. P. and MEYER, D. L. (1973) Compensatory mechanisms following labyrinthine lesions in the guinea pig. A simple model of learning. In: *Memory and Transfer of Information*, edited by H. P. Zippel. New York: Plenum. pp. 203–232

SEMONT, A., FREYSS, G. and VITTE, E. (1988) Curing the BPPV with a liberatory manoeuvre. *Advances in Otorhinolaryngology*, **42**, 290–293

SHEPARD, N. T., SMITH-WHEELOCK, M., TELIAN, S. A. and RAJ, A. (1993) Vestibular and balance rehabilitation therapy. *Annals of Otology, Rhinology, and Laryngology*, **102**, 198–204

SNASHALL, S. (1994) Nineteenth century posturography – the ataxiograph. *Journal of Audiological Medicine*, **3**, ii–iii

STEPHENS, S. D. G., HOGAN, S. and MEREDITH, R. (1991) The desynchrony between complaints and signs of vestibular disorders. *Acta Otolaryngologica*, **111**, 188–192

VESTERHAUGE, S., ZILSTORFF, K. and MANSSON, A. (1982) A comparision between caloric test, Hallpike-Fitzgerald and computer analysis of electronystagmographic data. *Acta Otolaryngologica*, Suppl. **386**, 228–230

YARDLEY, L., LUXON, L. M. and HAACKE, N. P. (1994) A longitudinal study of symptoms of anxiety and subjective well being in patients with vertigo. *Clinical Otolaryngology*, **19**, 109–116

YARDLEY, L., VERSCHUUR, C., MASSON, E., LUXON, L. M. and HAACKE, N. (1992) Somatic and psychological factors contributing to handicap in people with vertigo. *British Journal of Audiology*, **261**, 283–290

20

Causes of balance disorders

Cliodna F. O Mahoney and Linda M. Luxon

Man has developed a very sophisticated system by which perfect equilibrium is maintained. Sensory information from the eyes and the vestibular apparatus, together with proprioceptive information from the neck and the limbs, passes into the central nervous system where, at the level of the vestibular nuclei, it is integrated and modulated by activity arising in the cerebellum, the extrapyramidal system and the cortex. Pathways arising from the nuclei, connect with five main systems: the cerebral cortex, oculomotor nuclei, the motor part of the spinal cord, the cerebellum and the autonomic nervous system, resulting in static and dynamic spatial orientation, and control of locomotion and posture (Figure 20.1). Pathology affecting the cardiovascular system, the central nervous system, the eyes, the ears, the locomotor system, the blood and the endocrine glands may all alter this fine balance of neural information and result in dysequilibrium.

Despite the prevalence of such disorders, it is well recognized that most clinicians feel despondent when confronted with a patient complaining of a balance disorder; not least because the patient's complaints are often infuriatingly vague and non-specific. Some consideration of semantics is, therefore, of value. *Dizziness* is a lay term which encompasses a number of symptoms of dysequilibrium, including light-headedness, faintness, giddiness, sensations of 'swimming' or 'floating', imbalance, ataxia, minor episodes of mental confusion or loss of consciousness. In the Concise Oxford Dictionary, it is defined as a 'feeling of being dazed, or in a whirl, or as if about to fall'. In medical terms, it is of little value in identifying a precise underlying pathological process. In contradistinction, *vertigo* is a specific symptom related directly to dysfunction of the vestibular system. By definition, vertigo is 'an hallucination of movement' (Cawthorne, 1952) or 'disagreeable sensation of instability

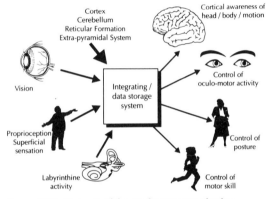

Figure 20.1 Diagram of the mechanisms involved in balance. (From Luxon, L. M. (1984) The anatomy and physiology of the vestibular system. In: *Vertigo*, edited by M. R. Dix and J. D. Hood. Chichester: John Wiley and Sons, with permission)

or disordered orientation in space' (Agate, 1963). However, it is unreasonable to expect a patient, alarmed and confused by unphysiological perceptions of movement, to define precisely the symptom of vertigo and it is often helpful to ask if the sensation is similar to that experienced on a roundabout. It must be emphasized, however, that rotation, either subjective or objective, is not a necessary component of vertigo and, indeed, many patients complain of a sensation of instability that is characterized by a rocking of the environment, or a feeling that the ground is not stable, e.g. as though they were on a boat.

A basic knowledge of vestibular function and the multiple connections of the vestibular system is essential if a systematic approach to balance disorders is to be undertaken. For a detailed explanation of the anatomy and physiology of the vestibular system, the reader is referred to Volume 1, Chapters 1 and 4. Briefly, the vestibular labyrinth is comprised of two parts: the semicircular canals, which respond to angular acceleration, and the otolith apparatus, which responds to linear acceleration. For practical purposes, the vestibular system may be considered in two halves, which are maintained in perfect balance, one with the other. Considering the semicircular canal system, upon turning the head, for example to the right, the right horizontal canal increases its firing rate, while activity of the left horizontal canal is reduced. It is the difference in activity between the functionally paired canals which is monitored by the central nervous system and allows awareness of head and body position in space, together with compensatory oculomotor and motor activity. During head movements, not only does vestibular input alter, but visual signals and the cervical proprioceptive input also vary. From birth, this information is integrated and stored in a data centre (Roberts, 1967), which is thought to be in the reticular formation of the brain stem. Afferent information is constantly compared with this data bank and, under normal circumstances, there is a perfect match between the visual, cervical proprioceptive and vestibular inputs. If one system is functioning inadequately, or the integrating ability of the brain stem is impaired, mismatch occurs between the information generated by one sensory modality and that of another. This mismatch may give rise to symptoms of dysequilibrium.

A common example of such a mismatch occurs in peripheral vestibular lesions, such as Menière's disorder, in which there is a change in the vestibular input to the central nervous system, but no change in the visual and proprioceptive inputs. Hence, a sense of vertigo is precipitated which is accompanied by spontaneous nystagmus. Alternatively, a sudden change in visual input, as occurs initially with the use of bifocal spectacles, may cause marked disorientation as a result of mismatch between visual signals and other sensory modalities required for balance. Although a derangement of one of the main sensory inputs may cause dysequilibrium, it is important to emphasize the multisensory deficit syndrome of dizziness identified by Drachman and Hart (1972). This is commonly seen in elderly patients and is associated with minor impairment in two or more of the systems required for equilibrium: visual dysfunction (not correctable), neuropathy, vestibular deficits, cervical spondylosis and orthopaedic disorders interfering with ambulation. Furthermore, in the elderly it must be recalled that loss of neurons in the central nervous system may impair modulation of sensory activity. In addition, other multiple pathologies, such as arthritis and cardiovascular disease, may result not only in dysfunction of the vestibular system itself, but also of the multiple central connections.

In healthy people, intersensory (e.g. visual versus vestibular) and intrasensory (e.g. semicircular canal versus otolith) mismatches may result from physiological stimuli which have not previously been encountered and/or not 'recognized' within the integrating centres, as in motion sickness and height vertigo (Brandt, 1991a).

Ageing of the vestibular system

Unfortunately, there is a common misconception that episodes of dizziness are to be expected as a part of old age. Hence, many elderly patients with dizziness are not given the benefit of proper medical investigation. This is compounded by the fact that, in the elderly, age-related effects upon the vestibular system are not well defined, with reports of both hypo-and hyperfunction.

Undoubtedly, the incidence of dysequilibrium is greater among the elderly, and is reported by Droller and Pemberton (1953) as being between 38% and 62%. Dizziness and vestibular abnormalities are reported to be a major risk factor predisposing to falls among the elderly (Svensson, Rundgren and Landahl, 1992; O'Loughlin *et al.*, 1993), the significance of which lies in the high morbidity, and indeed mortality, associated with falls occurring in this age group.

The finding of hyperexcitability of vestibular function has led to the hypothesis that the earliest signs of degenerative change in the vestibular system reflect a 'release of inhibition' by higher neuronal centres (Zelenka and Slaminova, 1964; Bruner and Norris, 1971). Thus, not surprisingly, compensatory recovery, which is dependent upon cerebral plasticity, is also slower and less complete in the elderly (Nadol and Schuknecht, 1990).

A number of findings may explain the presence of hypofunction. Degenerative changes have been described in the maculae (Johnsson and Hawkins, 1972), the cristae ampullaris (Rosenhall and Rubin, 1975) and in the vestibular nerve (Bergstrom, 1973). These include distortion and loss of hair cells (Rosenhall and Rubin, 1975; Engstrom, Ades and Engstrom, 1977), reduction in number and calibre of myelinated nerve fibres (Bergstrom, 1973) and alteration in supporting structures such as otoconia (Campos, Cazinares and Sanchez-Quevedo, 1990), walls of end organs and synaptic structures and afferent dendrites of the vestibular neurons (Engstrom, Ades and Engstrom, 1977). These changes usually occur symmetrically and do not give rise to an imbalance of afferent information arising from the vestibular end organs, which might result in vertigo. They are more likely to lead to a diminished efficiency in performing motor tasks, to which the elderly usually adapt by limiting their activities to what is appropriate and safe. However, asymmetrical degenerative changes have been reported which may result in initial severe vertigo and/or prolonged dysequilibrium (Nadol and Schuknecht, 1990).

It is more likely, however, that such symptoms are associated with simultaneous disorders in multiple systems normally involved in maintaining balance, i.e. the multisensory deficit syndrome (Nadol and Schuknecht, 1990) and/or related to age-dependent changes in other systems (Ahmed *et al.*, 1992; Baloh, 1992), e.g. the vascular tree (McIntosh, Da-Costa and Kenny, 1993), the cervical and other joint mechanoreceptors (Arnold and Harriman, 1970), perceptual deficiencies of cutaneous and visual modalities (Bender, 1975), and the central nervous system (Kuzuhara and Yoshimura, 1993). Norre, Forrez and Beckers (1987) demonstrated markedly increased postural sway in elderly patients with unilateral vestibular hypofunction when compared with younger patients also with vestibular hypofunction. This effect was more obvious with eyes closed. These findings suggested that central compensation became less effective with advancing age.

Clinical aspects

Dizziness is an extremely common symptom, which may be consequent to a diversity of pathologies. In approaching the diagnostic problem, it is helpful to ascertain whether the primary pathology is a vestibular, neurological or general medical disorder. To this end, a working knowledge of the differential diagnosis of dizziness is necessary (Table 20.1). It is essential to obtain a detailed and accurate history, to perform a full medical examination with special reference to the ears, eyes and neurological assessment, and to institute appropriate and specific special investigations. A simple diagnostic approach, as outlined in Figure 20.2, is of value. By considering the character of the complaint, the time course of the illness and the presence or absence of associated symptoms – cochlear, neurological or cardiovascular – it is often possible to gleen valuable information upon which to base further investigation. Certain generalizations may be made:

1 Vertigo is commonly associated with a vestibular disorder, whereas vague dizziness is more usually related to general medical disorders.

2 Classically, a peripheral vestibular disorder is characterized by sudden, unprecipitated, short-lived (less than 24 hours) episodes of vertigo, whereas central vestibular disorders are characterized by a gradual and insidious onset of continual imbalance. Anxious and depressed patients may also complain of constant dizziness, as may patients with bilateral vestibular failure. Notable exceptions to this generalization include temporal lobe epilepsy and vertebrobasilar ischaemia, which may give symptoms more typical of a peripheral vestibular lesion.

3 The duration of individual attacks is often a helpful diagnostic pointer: benign positional vertigo may last only 30–40 seconds, whereas vertigo associated with endolymphatic hydrops may last up to 24 hours and that secondary to labyrinthine failure may last for several days.

4 Lesions of the labyrinth, or VIIIth nerve may produce associated auditory symptoms such as hearing loss, tinnitus, a sensation of pressure, fullness or pain in the ear.

5 Vestibular symptoms and signs in the absence of cochlear abnormalities should indicate a careful search for other central nervous system abnormalities, with particular reference to oculomotor function.

6 A thorough cardiovascular assessment is essential, particularly if a history of angina, intermittent claudication or palpitations, suggestive of an underlying dysrhythmia, is elicited.

Table 20.1 Causes of dizziness/vertigo

General medical	Otological	Neurological	Miscellaneous
Haematological:	Trauma	Disorders affecting the VIIIth nerve	Cervical vertigo
anaemia	Infection	Brain stem disease	Ocular vertigo
polycythaemia	Vascular	Cerebellar disease	Iatrogenic
Cardiovascular:	Menière's disorder	Basal ganglia disease	
hypotension	Autoimmune disease	Cerebrovascular disease	
cardiac failure	Ototoxicity	Migraine	
dysrhythmia	Metabolic bone disease	Multiple sclerosis	
Metabolic:	Structural abnormalities	Trauma	
diabetes	of vestibular labyrinth	Infection	
hypoglycaemia		Epilepsy	
chronic renal failure			
alcohol			

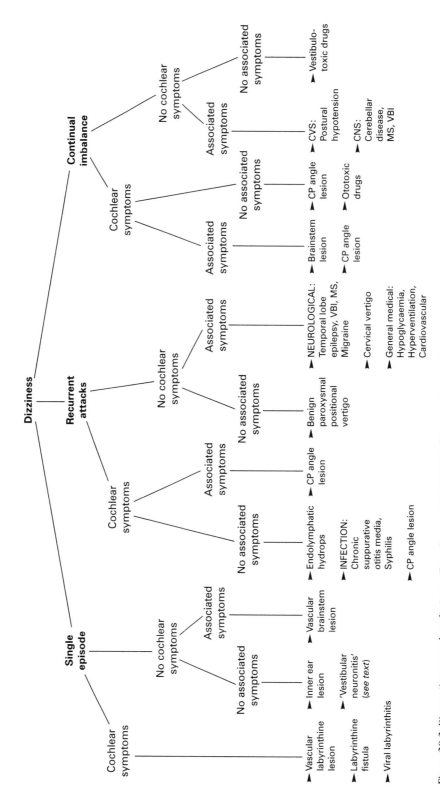

Figure 20.2 Diagnostic approach to dizziness. (From Luxon, L. M. (1984) All that rotates is not degenerative. *Current Practice*, **56**, 16–18 with permission)

General medical conditions

Cardiovascular disease

Cardiovascular disease may give rise to impaired cerebral perfusion resulting in dizziness and/or vertigo. Postural or systemic hypotension associated with impairment of reflex control of blood pressure or diminished cardiac output related to reduced intravascular blood volume, cardiac mechanical dysfunction or arrhythmias may all cause dizziness. In these situations dizziness may be a relatively minor complaint in comparison with chest pain, breathlessness, palpitations etc.

The most common underlying pathological process in cardiovascular disease is atherosclerosis which affects predominantly middle-sized arteries of the cerebral, myocardial and peripheral circulation.

Postural and systemic hypotension

Postural, or *orthostatic, hypotension* is a common medical cause of dizziness and is defined as a drop in blood pressure occurring on changing from a lying to an upright position. A commonly accepted criterion for a significant change is a decrease in the systolic blood pressure of 20 mmHg or more, and/or a drop of 10 mmHg or more in the diastolic pressure (Lipsitz, 1989). Postural hypotension occurs more commonly in the elderly and prevalences of between 5% and 30% have been quoted (Stumpf and Mitrzyk, 1994), although Mo, Omvik and Lund-Johansen (1994) have pointed out that an alerting reaction to sphygmomanometry causes the initial blood pressure recording (lying) to be spuriously high and thus the unwary may overdiagnose postural hypotension on the basis of a presumed excessive drop in pressure on subsequent measurement (standing). Postural hypotension is said to be commoner in patients also known to be hypertensive. This may support the suggestion of Kaplan (1992) that, in many cases, essential hypertension and postural hypotension are both manifestations of sympathetic nervous system dysfunction.

Associated symptoms, including dizziness, are thought to be due to cerebral hypoperfusion, although the correlation between the degree of change in blood pressure and the severity of symptoms is not always strong (Ensrud *et al.*, 1992). In addition, as both postural hypotension and dizziness are independently common in the elderly population and both are multifactorial in aetiology, caution must be exercised when assuming a cause–effect relationship between them.

The mechanisms whereby blood pressure is normally maintained in the face of gravity are complex and interrelated. The tendency of gravity to cause blood to pool in the legs leads to decreased venous return to the heart and a subsequent drop in cardiac output and pressure. These changes are detected by the arterial baroreceptors. Compensatory mechanisms include increased sympathetic arterial tone, increased cardiac contractility and heart rate, activation of the renin-angiotensin system and vasopressin release, leading to expansion of intravascular volume by water retention. Pathology in any of these compensatory systems may lead to a diminished ability to maintain blood pressure in the upright position, and thus it is not surprising that many different disorders may give rise to orthostatic hypotension (Table 20.2).

Stumpf and Mitrzyk (1994) have reviewed the causes of orthostatic hypotension in detail. Briefly, they divided them into autonomic and non-autonomic causes. Autonomic failure may be primary, such as idiopathic orthostatic hypotension, autosomal recessive familial dysautonomia (Riley Day syndrome), recently described postural hypotension caused by dopamine-B-hydroxylase deficiency (Robertson *et al.*, 1991; Gentric *et al.*, 1993), or it may occur as part of a more widespread central nervous system disorder such as multiple system atrophy. It used to be thought that the Shy-Drager syndrome was a separate disorder of autonomic function, but recent work (Quinn, 1989) has cast doubt on its existence as a distinct entity and suggests that the term should

Table 20.2 Causes of postural hypotension

Autonomic causes		*Non-autonomic causes*
Primary	*Secondary*	
Idiopathic	Diabetes mellitus	Dehydration
Familial (Riley Day syndrome)	Alcoholism	Haemorrhage
Multiple system atrophy	Vitamin B_1, B_{12} deficiency	Burns
Dopamine-B-hydroxylase deficiency	Parkinson's disease	Ageing
	Amyloidosis	Pregnancy
	Guillain Barré syndrome	Adrenal insufficiency
	Porphyria	Diabetes insipidus
	Tabes dorsalis	Drugs
	Syringomyelia	

be discarded. Some of the causes of secondary autonomic failure include diabetes mellitus, Guillain Barré syndrome, alcoholism, vitamin B_1 and B_{12} deficiencies among others. Non-autonomic causes of orthostatic hypotension include hypovolaemia due to haemorrhage, dehydration or burns. Very many commonly prescribed medications (e.g. diuretics, antihypertensives, antidepressants, phenothiazines, narcotics) may lead to orthostatic hypotension by a variety of mechanisms as outlined by Hugues, Munera and Le-Jeune (1992). Many other disorders such as Addison's disease, hypopituitarism, hypokalaemia, can cause postural hypotension. (For a more extensive list of causes, see Stumpf and Mitrzyk, 1994.) In severe cases these aetiological factors can give rise to persistent rather than just postural hypotension.

It is clear that many of these aetiological factors are more common in the elderly population. Ageing of the arterial baroreceptor reflex leading to decreased sensitivity (Gribben *et al.*, 1971), reduced cardiac contractility and decreased cerebral autoregulation (Wollner, 1978) may all contribute to a diminished ability to compensate for a drop in blood pressure. In addition, underlying factors such as renal disease, diabetes mellitus, vitamin deficiency and drug ingestion are all more common in the elderly, thus predisposing this age group to postural hypotension.

The diagnosis of postural hypotension depends on finding hypotension, in accordance with the above criteria, in association with symptoms of cerebral hypoperfusion. The differential diagnosis of primary or secondary autonomic failure from non-autonomic causes is usually possible clinically and is discussed by Stumpf and Mitrzyk (1994).

Mechanical cardiac dysfunction

Cardiac failure, either primarily right ventricular, such as that associated with chronic respiratory disease, or left ventricular usually due to myocardial ischaemia/infarction, causes a decrease in cardiac output and hence cerebral hypoperfusion and dizziness.

Other causes of reduced cardiac output include left ventricular outflow obstruction, such as occurs in aortic valve stenosis or hypertrophic obstructive cardiomyopathy. The former is more common in elderly men and, in the early stages, dizziness may be the sole symptom.

Hypertrophic obstructive cardiomyopathy first becomes symptomatic usually in late childhood or early adulthood. It presents with exertional angina, dyspnoea, fatigue, dizziness and syncope. It is a primary myocardial disease whose aetiology is uncertain. Recently a disorder of cardiac calcium metabolism has been postulated to play a role in the aetiology (Olbrich, Kaltenbach and Hopf, 1992).

Other disorders which should be considered, but in which dizziness may only be a minor manifestation, include primary atrial myxoma, myocarditis, pericarditis and ventricular hypokinesia.

Dysrhythmias

It is well established that cardiac dysrhythmias affect the cerebral circulation (Corday and Irving, 1960; Samet, 1973) and may result in dizziness and syncope. However some dysrhythmias may be asymptomatic and the relationship between a dysrhythmia and dizziness may not necessarily be causal. Other aetiologies need to be excluded, particularly if it is demonstrated by 24-hour ambulatory electrocardiographic monitoring for example, that the two are not always temporally related (Luxon *et al.*, 1980; Reig *et al.*, 1992).

The commonest cause of dysrhythmias in the Western world is *ischaemic heart disease* secondary to atherosclerosis. However thyroid disease, cardiomyopathies, intracranial pathology, drug-induced dysrhythmias and specific disorders of the cardiac conducting system, such as Wolff-Parkinson-White syndrome, need to be excluded.

A *hypersensitive carotid sinus reflex* is a known cause of dizziness and syncope in humans. Excessive sensitivity of the carotid sinus baroreceptors gives rise to vagal overstimulation of the heart and causes bradycardia and dizziness or, in extreme cases, cardiac arrest and syncope. Neck movement or even mild pressure on the carotid sinus may trigger these symptoms. Although it is quite rare, it usually occurs in association with atherosclerosis of the carotid sinus region. Because of the association of the symptoms with neck movement, an incorrect diagnosis of benign positional vertigo, or indeed vertebrobasilar insufficiency due to vertebral artery occlusion may be made. Diagnosis is confirmed by massaging the sinus while watching for the arrhythmia electrocardiographically.

The *sick sinus syndrome* occurs due to impairment of sinus node activity or failure of conduction of nodal impulses to the atria, giving rise to sinus bradycardia, sinus arrest or sinoatrial block. Escape tachycardias such as paroxysmal atrial fibrillation or flutter may occur. Tachycardia and bradycardia may alternate – the so-called *tachycardia-bradycardia syndrome*. Dizziness can be associated with either the tachycardia or the bradycardia (Bennett, 1990). This condition occurs most commonly in the elderly, due to idiopathic fibrosis of the node or ischaemic heart disease. It has also been associated with myocarditis and digoxin or quinine toxicity. Rarely it has been reported as a manifestation of cardiac haemochromatosis (Wang *et al.*, 1994) or as an early presentation of lymphoma (Bolis *et al.*, 1993).

Tachycardia, vertigo and/or syncope are presenting symptoms of the *Wolff-Parkinson White syndrome* (Woolf, 1992), for which favourable long-term results are reported following surgical or radio-frequency ablation of the offending accessory atrioventricular bundle (Deutsch *et al.*, 1993).

Haematological abnormalities

Anaemia and *polycythaemia* are the two commonest haematological causes of dizziness. Severe anaemia may present with throbbing headache, dizziness, visual disturbances and fainting. Polycythaemia rubra vera and other myeloproliferative disorders can give rise to dizziness/imbalance and vertigo in association with hearing loss, headache and visual problems, as part of the hyperviscosity syndrome (Andrews *et al.*, 1988; Lalanne *et al.*, 1992). The dizziness or vertigo are thought to be due to hypoxia of the vestibular labyrinth caused by obstruction of capillaries and venules by the excessively viscous blood (Andrews *et al.*, 1988). Secondary polycythaemia, for example in association with chronic respiratory disease, can give rise to similar symptoms.

Sensorineural hearing loss, most commonly a bilateral high frequency loss (Todd, Serjeant and Larson, 1973; Friedman *et al.*, 1980), in association with the various forms of sickle cell anaemia is thought to be caused either by hypoxia of the inner ear secondary to anaemia itself and/or by obstruction to blood flow due to the increased blood viscosity caused by the abnormally-shaped red blood cells. Though it seems both from clinical (Ogisi and Okafor, 1987; Ajulo, Osiname and Myatt, 1993) and histological reports (Morgenstein and Manace, 1969) that the hearing loss is generally cochlear in origin, retrocochlear pathology has been suggested (Orchik and Dunn, 1977) and bony encroachment on the internal acoustic meatus due to the expanded marrow of the temporal bone has been postulated as a mechanism. There are no reports specifically documenting vestibular function or histopathology in patients with sickle cell anaemia. However, Marcus and Lee (1976) described two sisters with sickle cell thalassaemia, both of whom complained of episodes of vertigo with or without hearing loss occurring after vigorous exercise.

Metabolic disease

Chronic dizziness is a common complaint in patients with *diabetes mellitus* and may result from the associated vascular pathology seen in these patients (Schuknecht, 1974). Thus the source of the dizziness may be in the peripheral labyrinth, VIIIth nerve or its central connections. However Myers *et al.* (1985) and Myers and Ross (1987) found pathological changes in the neuroepithelial and connective tissues of the utricle and saccule of rats with experimentally-induced diabetes mellitus, but no evidence of a vascular lesion.

Hypoglycaemia may cause acute dizziness and vertigo, and probably is the most frequent metabolic emergency (Binder and Bendtson, 1992). It usually results from inadvertent over-medication with insulin or oral hypoglycaemic agents. Much less common causes of hypoglycaemia include endocrine disorders, such as Addison's disease, hypopituitarism and rare insulin-producing tumours.

Chronic renal failure is also associated with hearing loss and dizziness. The pathogenesis is multifactorial relating to associated hypertension, serum sodium levels, ototoxic drugs and chronic anaemia among others. Whether or not improvement occurs after transplantation is controversial (Beaney, 1964; Mitschke *et al.*, 1977; Adler and Ritz, 1982; Gatland *et al.*, 1991). Histopathological changes have been reported in the peripheral vestibular labyrinth in chronic renal failure but are probably not specific to this condition (Naunton, Lindsay and Stein, 1973).

Alcohol intoxication, both acute and chronic, is associated with dizziness/vertigo. Within minutes of ingesting even quite moderate amounts of alcohol, positional vertigo may occur – probably due to the differential rates of diffusion of alcohol into the cupula and the endolymph of the semicircular canals (Money and Myles, 1974). More severe intoxication may cause dizziness due to cerebellar dysfunction and/or impaired function within the vestibular nuclei (Kashii *et al.*, 1984).

Chronic alcoholism, and its frequent concomitant malnutrition, in particular thiamine deficiency, is associated with ataxia. Pathological changes have been demonstrated in the vestibular nuclei of thiamine-deficient rats (Tellez and Terry, 1968), monkeys (Cogan, Witt and Goldman-Rakic, 1985) and humans (Victor, Adams and Collins, 1971). Similarly, cerebellar atrophy affecting mainly the vermis (Haubek and Lee, 1979) has been shown in chronic alcoholics, though again probably primarily caused by the associated malnutrition, including thiamine deficiency.

Otological conditions

Otological conditions must be excluded in all patients complaining of symptoms of vertigo, dizziness or disequilibrium. The large number of conditions to be considered may be divided into those involving:

1　The inner ear
2　The VIIIth nerve.

However, it must be remembered that at the current state of knowledge it is often not possible to establish the precise site of pathology and, in addition, many disorders may affect more than one site simultaneously.

Inner ear pathology

Congenital and hereditary lesions

Relatively little attention has been paid to vestibular disorders in association with hereditary disease. Between 1 and 2/1000 children born in the UK have sensorineural hearing loss. Up to one-half of these are of genetic origin, while probably over one-third represent a syndrome. Despite the size of the problem, there are few papers documenting the relationship between vestibular abnormalities and associated congenital or inherited hearing loss (Shambaugh, 1930; Lindenov, 1945; Arnvig, 1955; Sandberg and Terkildsen, 1965; Diepeveen and Jensen, 1968). The last two groups of workers reported a correlation between the degree of hearing impairment and vestibular pathology. Vestibular abnormalities were documented in 20% of subjects with a hearing loss of less than 90 dB, and in 80% of subjects with a hearing loss of more than 90 dB. Unfortunately, there was no clear information on the site of the vestibular abnormality with respect to the site of the auditory impairment.

Huygen and Verhagen (1994) have recently reviewed vestibular dysfunction in hereditary disorders. These disorders can be categorized into:

1 Those hereditary disorders where hearing loss is associated with other abnormalities
2 Hereditary hearing loss as an isolated disorder
3 Recently recognized entities of hereditary progressive vestibulocochlear dysfunction
4 Hereditary peripheral vestibular hypofunction without deafness.

Konigsmark and Gorlin (1976) listed over 150 separate syndromes associated with hereditary deafness. In certain of these syndromes, vestibular abnormalities are well documented.

Usher's syndrome is the association of retinitis pigmentosa and sensorineural hearing loss. Though some authors claim there are four separate clinical types, it is generally accepted that there are at least two. Type I is the more severe with the hearing loss probably congenital and visual symptoms occurring early in childhood. In type II the hearing loss is generally milder and of later onset and visual symptoms do not appear until late childhood or early adulthood. Vestibular hypofunction occurs in type I but not type II.

Some workers have shown normal vestibular function (Illum *et al.*, 1972) in *Pendred's syndrome* (sensorineural hearing loss associated with a goitre due to thyroid hormone dyshormogenesis) whereas others have reported decreased or absent function (Arnvig, 1955; Johnsen *et al.*, 1987).

In *Wildervanck's syndrome*, vestibular responses are often abnormal. Tomography may show the Mondini-Alexander type deformity, or a normal cochlea but with absent semicircular canals.

In *Waardenburg's syndrome*, Marcus (1968) has reported bilateral hyporeflexia in five of six patients with bilateral deafness and ipsilateral depressed caloric reflex in one case with unilateral deafness. Work by Hageman (1975) has supported a high incidence of vestibular dysfunction in this syndrome. A Mondini-Alexander dysplasia was found in one patient with deafness and vestibular areflexia (Marcus,

1968). Vestibular abnormalities have been found in some but not all patients with Waardenburg's syndrome. It is known that there are two clinical types of this syndrome. It is thought that type II is associated with vestibular dysfunction.

Branchio-otorenal syndrome is an autosomal dominant syndrome with sensorineural, conductive or mixed hearing loss, preauricular pits, branchial fistulae or cysts and renal anomalies. In twelve cases examined by Cremers *et al.* (1981) abnormal caloric reflexes were found in six and, on tomography, either unilateral or bilateral dysplasia of the horizontal semicircular canal in eight.

Patients with *albinism-deafness syndrome*, an X-linked recessive disorder consisting of sensorineural hearing loss and abnormal skin pigmentation (leopard skin), may have severe bilateral caloric hyporeflexia or areflexia.

Abnormal vestibular function has also been shown in *osteogenesis imperfecta type* I, *Albers-Schonberg disease* and the recently described *hyperostosis cranialis interna syndrome*.

In the various forms of isolated genetic hearing loss with no associated abnormalities in other systems, there are unfortunately few histopathological studies and little emphasis has been placed upon vestibular investigation. In general, the studies that have been carried out would suggest that vestibular function is normal, but investigations have often been rather crude, and in the absence of sufficient information, these results must be interpreted with some caution. Vestibular dysfunction has been shown in both congenital autosomal recessive and autosomal dominant sensorineural hearing loss (Muller, 1936; Konigsmark and Gorlin, 1976). Although, the lack of sufficient data and inadequate vestibular test procedures do not allow any definitive conclusions to be made at present, it has been suggested that adequate tests of vestibular function may help to separate various types of inherited deafness and allow characterization of specific subgroups.

The third category listed above includes three forms of *autosomal dominant progressive vestibulocochlear dysfunction* which have been recently described (Verhagen, Huygen and Joosten, 1988; Verhagen *et al.*, 1989; Verhagen, Huygen and Bles, 1992). The onset of vestibular and cochlear abnormalities was in the fourth and fifth decade and typically the vestibular disorder progressed to complete vestibular areflexia.

The fourth group includes hereditary vestibular failure in the absence of hearing loss or abnormality in any other system. Verhagen, Huygen and Horstink (1987) described an autosomal recessive form, while Baloh, Jacobson and Fife (1994) reported a series of three patients with bilateral vestibular loss, each with a similarly affected parent suggesting an autosomal dominant form of inheritance.

Developmental ear abnormalities are found in the rare trisomies of group D and E chromosomes: the auditory labyrinth is usually spared. Temporal bone studies in trisomy 13 and 18 have demonstrated vestibular abnormalities (Kos, Schuknecht and Singer, 1966).

In the last 10 years the relationship between hereditary disease and mitochondrial DNA has been recognized. The function of mitochondrial DNA is to code for 13 proteins, all of which are involved in oxidative phosphorylation (Harding, 1989) and thus ATP and energy production. Transmission of mitochondrial DNA is along the maternal line only. Disorders of mitochondrial DNA are most often associated with neurological and muscle disease, but increasingly other manifestations are being recognized. Tissues which are metabolically very active will be most vulnerable to the effects of abnormal oxidative phosphorylation. Involvement of the inner ear could be anticipated as the stria vascularis of the cochlea and the dark cell region of the vestibular system have high energy requirements in order to maintain the endolymphatic potential necessary for normal function.

Kearns-Sayre-syndrome is characterized by external ophthalmoplegia, pigmentary retinopathy, myopathy, ataxia, cardiac conduction defect and increased CSF protein (Shoffner and Wallace, 1990). It is probably part of a spectrum of diseases, including progressive external ophthalmoplegia alone, and Pearson's disease, all of which are associated with abnormal mitochondrial DNA. The deletion in the DNA probably occurs during embryogenesis, the earlier it occurs the more cells are affected and the more severe the manifestations are (Schoffner and Wallace, 1990). Deafness and vestibular disorders have been described.

Likewise a predisposition to aminoglycoside-induced deafness was found to be maternally inherited (Higashi, 1989; Hu *et al.*, 1991) and is probably attributable to an abnormality of mitochondrial DNA. A genetic susceptibility to the vestibular effects of aminoglycosides remains to be proven.

Congenital non-hereditary lesions

Congenital vestibular dysfunction may also be due to embryopathic factors such as *maternal rubella infection*. Barr and Lundstrom (1961) and Nishida, Ueda and Fung (1983) have described vestibular hypofunction in 30% of 80 children with the congenital rubella syndrome. Characteristically rubella infection can lead to the Scheibe deformity, a malformation affecting the cochleosaccular neuroepithelia and associated with atrophy of the VIIIth nerve but with sparing of the semicircular canal and utricular neuroepithelia. The occurrence of vestibular hypofunction unrelated to the degree of hearing loss has been described, and most cases show evidence of central compensation. Thalidomide taken during pregnancy can also lead to aplasias of the inner ear and VIIIth nerve (Phelps, 1983).

Trauma

In present day society, head injuries are extremely common as a result of simple falls, e.g. on ice, or downstairs; as a result of violent acts, e.g. muggings; and in road traffic accidents. Experimental work has demonstrated that post-traumatic petechial haemorrhages may be found in the labyrinth, the VIIIth nerve, the joints and nerves of the neck, the brain stem and the cerebral hemispheres. Hence it is not surprising that symptoms of dysequilibrium may result.

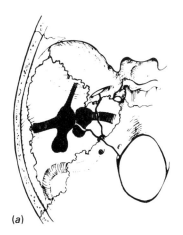 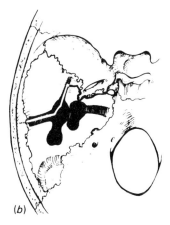

(a) (b)

Figure 20.3 Temporal bone fractures. (*a*) Transverse fracture, (*b*) longitudinal fracture. (From Hilger, P., Paparella, M. M. and Anderson, R. G. (1984) Conductive hearing loss. In: *Diagnosis and Management of Hearing Loss*, edited by W. L. Meyerhoff. Philadelphia: W. B. Saunders Company with permission)

Head injury

Occurrence of a post-traumatic syndrome, including dizziness and/or vertigo, after head and neck injuries is well recognized, and an organic vestibular basis for the dizziness, as opposed to a psychogenic aetiology, has been established. Confining the remarks in this section to the labyrinth, there are two main post-traumatic vestibular syndromes: vestibular failure and benign positional vertigo of paroxysmal type.

Severe trauma to the parietal region of the skull may give rise to fracture of the temporal bone (Figure 20.3). The more common type of fracture is a longitudinal fracture (i.e. parallel to the long axis of the petrous temporal bone), which usually does not involve the inner ear. Conductive hearing loss associated with a ruptured tympanum, ossicular dislocation or fracture, and middle ear haemorrhage may occur. The less common transverse fracture, however, usually damages the entire membranous labyrinth, giving rise to irreversible sensorineural hearing loss and acute vestibular symptoms. The VIIth and VIIIth nerves (both cochlear and vestibular divisions) may also be severed. Thus transverse fractures may give rise to severe vertigo, nausea and vomiting and these symptoms are associated with a loss of balance, a tendency to veer towards the affected side and the development of spontaneous nystagmus directed towards the normal side. Symptoms are most severe with the affected ear downwards and are aggravated by any movement. Over the first 3 or 4 days the symptoms gradually resolve, but it is 6–12 weeks before the patient becomes asymptomatic, due to the process of compensation, though the loss of both vestibular and cochlear function on that side is permanent. Compensation for the vestibular loss is likely to be slower or incomplete in the older patient. A fracture should be suspected if blood is present in the middle ear or in the external auditory meatus. The rare oblique fractures may also involve the labyrinth and the VIIIth nerve.

Severe head trauma, without temporal bone fracture, but usually with loss of consciousness, may give rise to cochlear and vestibular symptoms which may be reversible – so-called labyrinthine concussion.

Benign positional vertigo of paroxysmal type

The most common clinical syndrome after minor head injury is that of benign positional vertigo of paroxysmal type. The symptoms frequently develop after a symptom-free interval of some days or weeks. The patient then complains of brief, but severe, episodes of rotatory vertigo lasting less than a minute, upon sudden changes of head position, especially on lying down and turning towards the affected ear. The characteristic findings on Hallpike testing include a delay of 2–20 seconds (latent period) before the onset of vertigo/nystagmus, with or without nausea,

linear-rotatory nystagmus with the fast phase towards the undermost ear lasting less than 1 minute, reversal of the direction of nystagmus on sitting upright, and lessening or absence of symptoms and signs on repeated testing (fatiguability). The complaint may last for months or years, during which time the natural history of the disorder is that of relapses and remissions with eventual complete recovery in the otherwise healthy patient. Spencer-Harrison and Ozsahinoglu (1972) have made the observation that a delay in recovery, or indeed incomplete recovery from positional vertigo is much more likely in older patients.

In addition to accidental trauma, benign positional vertigo of paroxysmal type has been described by Andaz, Whittet and Ludman (1993), in association with surgery to remove a parietal lobe tumour. They attributed the vertigo to trauma secondary to use of the hammer and chisel during operation. Although trauma is the commonest known cause of benign positional vertigo of paroxysmal type, most cases are idiopathic (Baloh, Honrubia and Jacobson, 1987). It also frequently occurs in association with viral labyrinthitis, Menière's disease and vertebrobasilar insufficiency. Interestingly, Gyo (1988) described six cases of benign positional vertigo of paroxysmal type occurring after non-head-and-neck surgery. He postulated that prolonged postoperative bed rest facilitated the deposition of utricular otoconia onto the cupula of the posterior semicircular canal, and thus giving rise to the symptoms in accordance with Schuknecht's (1969) theory of 'cupulolithiasis' (see below).

It has been thought that the collection of symptoms and signs in benign positional vertigo of paroxysmal type arise from pathology in the posterior semicircular canal. Evidence supporting this view includes the nature of the nystagmus which is in keeping with the known ocular connections of the posterior semicircular canal, the response to sectioning of the singular nerve (posterior ampullary nerve) (Gacek, 1974) and plugging of the posterior semicircular canal (Parnes and McClure, 1990, 1991; Pace-Balzan and Rutka, 1991). However the exact pathology in the posterior semicircular canal remains unknown.

Schuknecht (1969) postulated that 'cupulolithiasis' was the underlying mechanism in this condition, though histopathological evidence is limited. He proposed that degeneration of the utricular otolithic membrane occurs secondary to trauma, ischaemia, infection, etc., and this gives rise to release of otoconia, which become deposited upon the cupula of the posterior semicircular canal, thereby altering the specific gravity of the cupula and converting it to a gravity receptor and thus provoking rotatory nystagmus on rapid change of head position. Brandt and Steddin (1993) suggested that all the features of benign positional vertigo of paroxysmal type are not explained on the basis of cupulolithiasis and themselves proposed 'canalolithiasis' as an alternative mechanism. According to them, otoconial debris, rather than becoming attached to the cupula (Schuknecht, 1969), forms a free-floating 'clot' in the posterior semicircular canal. Rapid changes of head position with respect to gravity then cause the clot to move downwards and induces endolymph flow, and thus cupular deflection. Gordon (1992) questioned the possibility of air bubbles in the endolymph having a role in the pathogenesis of benign positional vertigo of paroxysmal type. He suggested that a minor head injury could cause a rupture of the labyrinthine membrane window (round or oval) and allow air from the middle ear to enter the endolymph, and the subsequent movement of these air bubbles could account for the onset of vertigo. However, Brandt and Steddin (1992) claimed that the air bubble theory fails to explain all the features of benign positional vertigo of paroxysmal type.

The traditional thinking has been that benign positional vertigo of paroxysmal type arises from pathology in the posterior semicircular canal. However, some workers have reported cases of paroxysmal vertigo thought to arise from horizontal canal abnormalities, in that vertigo and horizontal nystagmus are provoked by rapid rolling from the supine position onto one side. Again Brandt and Steddin (1993) explained how these findings are consistent with canalolithiasis but not cupulolithiasis.

Whatever the exact pathogenic mechanism, paroxysmal vertigo and its associated paroxysmal nystagmus which conforms to the features described above (latency, fatiguability etc.) is very unlikely to suggest central nervous system disease. However classical benign positional vertigo of paroxysmal type must be distinguished from other forms of positional nystagmus. Nylen (1950) and Hallpike (1967) described a separate group in which nystagmus persisted as long as the critical head position was maintained, and Spencer-Harrison and Ozsahinoglu (1972) reported that 38% of patients with persistent positional nystagmus were found to have central nervous system pathology, compared with only 4% of those with paroxysmal positional nystagmus as defined above.

Whiplash injury

Dizziness/vertigo is reported to be one of the most frequent symptoms after whiplash injury. A variety of mechanisms has been proposed to account for its development, including disruption of the cervical input to the vestibular nuclei (Gray, 1956; Hinoki, 1985), ischaemia (Hyslop, 1952; Weeks and Travelli, 1955) and/or central nervous system dysfunction (Oosterveld *et al.*, 1991), and positional vertigo due to utricular otoconia being dislodged (Brandt and Daroff, 1980).

Cervical afferent input to the vestibular nuclei arises from the paravertebral joints and capsules and, to a lesser extent, from the paravertebral muscles (McCouch, Deering and Ling, 1951; Hikosaka and Maeda, 1973), with no input from the skin and superficial muscles. Thus soft tissue injury would be unlikely to give rise to vertigo. In addition, even the input from the paravertebral joints and muscles is minor in comparison to other inputs, and compensation has been shown to occur rapidly after lesions of the neck afferents, so it is difficult to explain persistent vertigo/dysequilibrium on the basis of disrupted cervical structures. Nonetheless, high cervical nerve damage has been documented after whiplash injury and it has been shown in experimental animals that anaesthesia of C2/C3 neural pathways can induce vertigo (de Jong *et al.*, 1977).

Compression of the vertebral artery against the transverse process of the seventh cervical vertebra by cervical fascia (Compere, 1968) has been proposed as a vascular cause of vertigo in whiplash injury, but in the absence of other vascular pathology or additional brain stem symptoms and signs, this would seem to be an unlikely explanation. However dissection of the extracranial vertebral artery has been reported following minor whiplash injury (Charles *et al.*, 1992)

Barotrauma

Vertigo or dizziness occurring as a result of changes in atmospheric pressure (increased pressure due to diving or decreased in association with aviation/space travel) have become more important due to recent increases in commercial, military and leisure diving/flying. The effects of these activities on the ear can be divided into those occurring due to the generalized condition of decompression sickness, and those affecting specifically the middle and inner ears (aural barotrauma). These two entities have been reviewed by Talmi, Finkelstein and Zohar (1991a,b) in relation to hearing loss. However, although the literature deals more extensively with the effects of pressure changes on hearing, vertigo/dizziness is also a recognized symptom of each of these conditions.

One per cent of divers experience decompression problems and approximately 5% of these suffer hearing or balance disturbances (Head, 1984). In decompression sickness, gas bubbles form in the body fluids when the pressure changes which occur are of such a degree that the gas can no longer remain in solution. This can lead to a myriad of symptoms (e.g. the familiar 'bends') including vertigo (Molvaer, 1991). Several mechanisms have been suggested to explain the effects of decompression sickness on the inner ear. These include gas bubble formation in the perilymph with or without inner ear membrane ruptures, vascular emboli, either gaseous, lipid or thrombotic which impair inner ear blood flow, and even fracture of the petrous temporal bone (Talmi, Finkelstein and Zohar, 1991a).

Aural barotrauma includes both middle ear and, the more serious, inner ear barotrauma. The former occurs when a subject is unable to equalize pressure on either side of the tympanic membrane due to poor eustachian tube dysfunction, and haemorrhage into the middle ear and/or tympanic membrane rupture may occur giving rise to a conductive hearing loss. Inner ear barotrauma may give rise to irreversible sensorineural hearing loss, tinnitus and vertigo/dizziness. The mechanisms proposed to explain inner ear barotrauma include rupture of the round/oval membranes, in particular the round window membrane, inner ear haemorrhage and rupture of internal inner ear membranes (Parell and Becker, 1993). Histological evidence in both animals and humans exists to support these mechanisms (Keleman, 1983; Parrell and Becker, 1993). Poor middle ear pressure equalization due to abnormal eustachian tube function predisposes to inner ear barotrauma. Other factors which may contribute to the occurrence of vertigo in association with changes in atmospheric pressure have been described by Molvaer (1991), and include sensory deprivation, optokinetic illusions, caloric stimulation of the vestibular apparatus by cold water during diving, high intensity noise affecting the peripheral vestibular apparatus, a 'high pressure neurological syndrome' giving rise to altered biochemical reactions in the nervous system, and a little recognized condition known as alternobaric vertigo (Wicks, 1989). This latter, is a transient form of vertigo, usually experienced by divers during ascent, and thought to be caused by asymmetrical eustachian tube dysfunction giving rise to a sudden pressure difference between both middle ears. It has also been reported among air crew but not in association with space travel.

Perilymphatic fistula

A perilymphatic fistula is an abnormal communication between the perilymph-filled inner ear and the air-filled middle ear. It is caused by rupture of one or both the delimiting membranes, i.e. oval and/or round window membranes, known as a labyrinthine membrane rupture. Perilymphatic fistula was first described in the early 1960s as a complication of stapes surgery. Since then, it has been described in association with various kinds of trauma-head injury (Fee, 1968) including minor head injury/barotrauma and 'spontaneous' fistulae (Stroud and Calcaterra, 1970) in relation to increased intracranial pressure such as may occur with coughing, sneezing, straining or lifting. Goodhill (1971) categorized perilymphatic fistula into two types – those which occur via an 'explosive' route and those occurring via an 'implosive' route. The former denotes labyrinthine membrane rupture caused by an increase in CSF pressure, which is then conducted via the cochlear aqueduct or the internal auditory meatus, to the perilymph and thus causing rupture. Labyrinthine membrane rupture caused by the implosive route occurs due to a sudden increase in pressure in the middle ear cavity such as may occur during a sudden forced Valsalva manoeuvre or while diving. Interestingly, increased middle ear pressure has been recorded in both animals (Matz, Rattenborg and Holaday, 1967) and humans (Thomsen, Terkildsen and Arnfred, 1965) in association with nitrous oxide anaesthesia. Labyrinthine membrane rupture, as a consequence of this increased pressure, has been postulated to be a probable cause of the sudden hearing loss and/or vertigo documented after nitrous oxide anaesthesia.

The symptoms of perilymphatic fistula include sudden, fluctuating or progressive sensorineural hearing loss, episodic vertigo or more vague disequilibrium, tinnitus and a feeling of pressure or fullness in the ear. Thus it can be very difficult to distinguish from Menière's disease. The actual mechanism whereby a perilymphatic fistula gives rise to these cochlear and vestibular symptoms is unclear. Simmons (1968) suggested that the sudden hearing loss was actually due to simultaneous rupture of Reissner's membrane. However Nishioka and Yanagihara (1986) demonstrated hearing loss in guinea-pigs with labyrinthine membrane rupture but with intact Reissner's membranes. They also reported the presence of air bubbles in the perilymph which had leaked in from the middle ear. They proposed that these air bubbles interfered with the normal pattern of the travelling wave along the cochlea and gave rise to sudden hearing loss. The subsequent resorption of these air bubbles could explain why the hearing loss of perilymphatic fistula sometimes resolves spontaneously. However, the vestibular symptoms are more difficult to explain. It is interesting too, that Gordon (1992) proposed an 'air bubble' theory to explain vertigo seen in benign positional vertigo of paroxysmal type, and though it is unlikely to explain all of the specific features of benign paroxysmal vertigo (Brandt and Steddin, 1992), it may explain at least some cases of vertigo occurring in association with perilymphatic fistula. Wall and Rauch (1994) proposed that perilymph flow caused by the leak directly stimulates the vestibular end organ and gives rise to the illusion of movement.

The preoperative diagnosis of perilymphatic fistula is notoriously difficult. Wall and Rauch (1994) in their review of perilymphatic fistula concluded that there is no reliable 'gold standard' for its diagnosis. Several workers have advocated the usefulness of various procedures including the 'fistula test', eye movement recording, caloric testing, vestibulo-ocular reflex testing, modified forms of electrocochleography (Gibson, 1992) and posturography (Black *et al.*, 1987), but the specificity and sensitivity of these tests have been disappointing. Even at tympanotomy the diagnosis of perilymphatic fistula can be impossible. Fluid in the middle ear may not necessarily imply a leak, but may be merely serum or indeed local anaesthetic. Bassiouny *et al.* (1992) have proposed that the finding of a substance known as B2 transferrin in the middle ear fluid would distinguish serum from CSF or perilymph as B2 transferrin is not found in serum but is present in the latter two fluids. If these results are verified then this could be a useful confirmatory test of perilymphatic fistula. However, at present, the preoperative diagnosis depends on the combination of a suggestive history in association with supportive investigative findings.

Traumatic otolith vertigo

This is a non-rotatory to and fro type of post-traumatic vertigo which is particularly associated with head acceleration and an unsteadiness of gait similar to walking on pillows. It has been postulated that it was caused by loosening of the otoliths, following head acceleration, resulting in an unequal load on the macula beds and a tonus imbalance between otolith organs. This condition may occur with or without concurrent benign paroxysmal positional vertigo. Gradual recovery, which occurs within a few days or weeks, is facilitated by exercise therapy and is believed to be due to central compensation.

Ylikoski (1988) among others has reported disturbances of balance following exposure to loud noise, but Hinchcliffe, Coles and King (1992) have concluded, following an extensive review of the literature, that there is no evidence for occupational noise-induced vestibular malfunction.

Infection

Viruses, bacteria, treponemes and fungi may give rise to infection of the inner ear.

Viral

The evidence that viruses cause damage to the vestibular labyrinth has increased over the years but, nevertheless, it is almost entirely circumstantial rather than definitive. Davis (1993) reviewed the body of evidence from various human studies – epidemiological, clinical and pathological – as well as animal studies. He emphasized that, ideally, to prove a causal role for a particular virus, the putative virus should be isolated from inner ear tissue or fluids of affected patients at the time of the acute infection. In addition, similar pathology should be demonstrable in experimental animals. Unfortunately only in very few instances is this kind of information available in humans. Westmore, Pickard and Stern (1979) reported the detection of mumps virus in the perilymph after sudden onset deafness. However, there is much clinical and serological evidence that vertigo occurs in association with various viruses – mumps, influenza A and B, Epstein-Barr, and herpes zoster – although in the last the pathology appears to be in

the vestibular nerve. Thomke and Hopf (1992) have reported a case of mumps presenting with unilateral vestibular paralysis as its sole manifestation.

There have been no temporal bone studies carried out on patients who died in the acute stages of the putative viral illness and thus findings at the time of post mortem, often years later, are necessarily less conclusive of a causal relationship. Nevertheless, temporal bone studies in patients who have developed sudden, sensorineural hearing loss during the course of a cold, pharyngitis, or other symptoms suggestive of a viral infection, have identified changes similar to those found in the labyrinths of patients with hearing loss related to measles, mumps and rubella. It has been postulated, therefore, that these inner ear lesions are of viral origin (Lindsay, 1973b; Sando *et al.*, 1977). In measles and rubella, changes have also been observed in the utricle and saccule of the vestibular system and it has been extrapolated, therefore, that acute episodes of vertigo may also be attributable to viral infection. It must be emphasized that clinical studies which employ serological titre rises or nasopharyngeal virus isolates should be interpreted with caution.

Animal studies have shown that mumps, rubeola, measles, cytomegalovirus, influenza A and B and herpes simplex viruses can all cause pathological changes in the vestibular labyrinth as well as the vestibular ganglion cells (Davis, 1993).

Viral infections may reach the inner ear via the blood stream, the meninges, the VIIIth nerve or the middle ear. Four viral infections are thought to affect the labyrinth by the blood-borne route – cytomegalovirus, mumps, measles and rubella. The virus of herpes zoster oticus enters the inner ear along the VIIth and VIIIth cranial nerves (Blackley, Friedman and Wright, 1967; Bance and Rutka, 1990).

Acquired immune deficiency syndrome (AIDS)

Since its first recognition in the early 1980s awareness of the otological manifestations of AIDS has increased. Sooy (1987) has suggested that between 41% and 71% of all manifestations of HIV are in the head and neck region, and include hearing loss, both conductive and sensorineural, vertigo and tinnitus. Clinical studies have demonstrated both central (Hart *et al.*, 1989; Hausler *et al.*, 1991) and peripheral (Hausler *et al.*, 1991) pathology in patients with cochleovestibular symptoms, and indeed in those whose pathology is subclinical. The pathophysiological mechanism of these symptoms is complex and probably involves many different causative agents, affecting both central and peripheral structures. Likely factors involved include direct damage to the inner ear or its central connections, caused by the HIV itself, or by the many opportunistic infections, such as *Pneumocystis carinii* (Breda *et al.*, 1988), tuberculosis, *Candida albicans* etc., to which patients with HIV are particularly susceptible. The difficulty of establishing an aetiological role of viral agents, especially those DNA viruses such as herpes, varicella, and Epstein-Barr viruses which may have long latent periods, in cochlear and vestibular disorders has been highlighted above. The situation becomes even more complex in the case of HIV-positive patients, as multiple viral/bacterial/fungal agents, as well as the HIV itself, may be involved simultaneously. In addition, ototoxicity secondary to drugs used in the treatment of these infections may give rise to cochleovestibular symptoms. Histopathological changes in eight temporal bones of HIV-positive patients have been reported by Chandrasekhar, Siverls and Sekhar (1992). Surprisingly, they found very little evidence of specific HIV damage to the cochlea. However, precipitates consisting of inflammatory cells were identified in both endolymph and perilymph, and changes in the otoconial membrane were also reported. These were thought to be important factors in the generation of cochlear and vestibular symptoms. No comment was made on the VIIIth nerve. Other studies, mentioned by Rarey (1990), also reported the presence of viral antigens and bacterial and fungal microorganisms in culture of inner ear tissue of HIV-positive patients. It appears that there can be both neuro-otological (Hausler *et al.*, 1991) and histological (Rarey, 1990) evidence of otological disease in HIV-positive patients who are otologically asymptomatic.

The involvement of the central auditory and vestibular systems in patients with AIDS syndrome is further discussed under the section on the neurological causes of balance disorders.

Bacterial

Vertigo, associated with bacterial infection of the middle ear cleft, is more commonly a result of chronic destructive middle ear disease progressing to affect the labyrinth, than of acute infection. Acute infective labyrinthitis is easily recognized by the development of severe rotational vertigo, together with sensorineural hearing loss.

A spontaneous fistula of the labyrinth is almost always the result of bone erosion by cholesteatoma, but rarely it may occur in syphilitic osteitis, tuberculous otitis media, chronic perilabyrinthine osteomyelitis or neoplasia, e.g. a glomus jugulare tumour.

Two bacterial infections, petrositis and malignant otitis externa, which may involve the inner ear and/or the VIIIth cranial nerve deserve special mention. Petrositis is the result of perilabyrinthine infection which extends into the apical portion of the petrous bone. It may present as Gradenigo's (1893) syndrome: otitis media with involvement of the trigeminal ganglion, giving rise to pain behind the ipsilateral eye and involvement of the abducens nerve, as it crosses the petrous bone, and consequent paralysis of

the ipsilateral lateral rectus muscle. The syndrome is often associated with vertigo and hearing loss, either as a result of labyrinthine or VIIIth cranial nerve involvement. Otitis externa is a common benign disorder but, in debilitated patients, particularly diabetics or those with the acquired immune deficiency syndrome, it may present in a more malignant form. An infection with *Pseudomonas aeruginosa* may invade the junction of the cartilaginous and osseous portions of the external auditory canal and spread through the adjacent bony structures, with consequent hearing loss and vertigo. Prolonged treatment with effective antibiotics, carbenicillin, gentamicin or ciprofloxacin, has improved the previously poor prognosis. Limanskii (1990) reported a case of sphenoiditis leading to a cochleovestibular dysfunction.

Spirochaetal

Syphilis, a chronic systemic infection caused by the spirochaete *Treponema pallidum*, can be either congenital or acquired. Both forms are associated with audiovestibular manifestations. The incidence of symptomatic acquired disease has increased in recent years, thought to be due, at least in part, to the emergence of HIV infection (Berry *et al.*, 1987; Johns, Tierney and Felsenstein, 1987; Smith and Canalis, 1989). They postulated that concurrent infection with HIV, by its effect on cell-mediated immunity, leads to reactivation of latent syphilis and thus may hasten the development of symptoms, including otosyphilis. Congenital syphilis with early onset hearing loss (before the age of 2 years) usually has no associated vestibular disorder (Darmstadt and Harris, 1989), although it may be that vestibular pathology is just not detected in this age group. However, late congenital syphilis may give rise to the first cochlear symptoms in adulthood and, in these cases, vertigo is more common. However, otological manifestations are rare in the absence of other signs of congenital syphilis (Steckelberg and McDonald, 1984; Darmstadt and Harris, 1989).

Acquired syphilis can be classified into primary and secondary syphilis (both included in so-called 'early' syphilis) and tertiary (late) syphilis. Late syphilis can be asymptomatic or symptomatic neurosyphilis, cardiovascular syphilis or involve the eye (optic atrophy). Audiovestibular complications of acquired syphilis have been reported mainly in relation to the late stage but also in some cases of early acquired syphilis. In the early phase they are thought to result either from basilar meningitis affecting the VIIIth nerve or from acute labyrinthitis. CSF changes are almost always seen, in the form of increased protein content, and pleocytosis with normal glucose level (Darmstadt and Harris, 1989). In general, the otological manifestations are similar in congenital syphilis presenting late and the late phase of acquired syphilis. There is no pathognomonic pattern of either the cochlear or vestibular disorder. The sensorineural hearing loss may be unilateral or bilateral, of sudden onset or gradually progressive affecting mainly high frequencies or causing a fluctuating low frequency loss. A conductive component to the hearing loss may occur secondary to osteitis of the ossicular chain. Episodic true vertigo, vague unsteadiness or the classic triad of Ménière's type symptoms may occur.

Wilson and Zoller (1981) reported electronystagmographic findings in 17 patients with otosyphilis, including both congenital and acquired forms. They concluded that the vestibular dysfunction was of peripheral rather than central origin, and that a greater degree of damage occurred in the congenital form. Kobayashi *et al.* (1991) also found predominantly peripheral vestibular pathology in patients with otosyphilis.

Histopathological findings in otosyphilis include obliterative endarteritis and infiltration of mononuclear inflammatory cells causing a reduction in blood supply and tissue necrosis (Karmody and Schuknecht, 1966). The effects include atrophy of the organ of Corti and stria vascularis and damage to the spiral ganglion and VIIIth nerve. Osteitis, both gummatous and non-gummatous, affecting the ossicles and the temporal bone, occurs, the latter giving rise to secondary damage to or even obliteration of the membranous labyrinth. Endolymphatic hydrops has also been documented (Karmody and Schuknecht, 1966) and is consistent with the recognized clinical finding of Ménière's-type symptoms and characteristic changes in the summating potentials seen on electrocochleography (Kobayashi *et al.*, 1991).

A presumed diagnosis of otosyphilis has relied on the presence of cochleovestibular disorder of no other known origin in association with positive syphilis serology. A high index of suspicion is necessary if the disorder is not to be missed (Luxon, Lees and Greenwood, 1979). Darmstadt and Harris (1989) reviewed the sensitivity and specificity of the various serological tests generally available and they, among others (e.g. Durham *et al.*, 1984), concluded that the most useful serological test for screening was the FTA-ABS (fluorescent treponemal antibody-absorbed) test, and that the technically more demanding and more expensive MHA-TP (microhaemagglutination test with *Treponema pallidum*) be reserved as a reliable confirmatory test. Birdsall, Baughn and Jenkins (1990) have proposed a new Western blot assay test which they claim eliminates the false-positive results sometimes seen with the FTA-ABS test, and distinguishes between autoimmune inner ear disease and otosyphilis and between active and inactive disease. Further evaluation is needed before the role of this test can be established.

Neoplasia of the temporal bone

Neoplasia of the temporal bone is not common but may cause audiovestibular symptoms. Primary malig-

nant neoplasms originating in the temporal bone such as rhabdomyosarcoma, osteogenic sarcoma, liposarcoma and fibrosarcoma are rare. Osteogenic sarcoma may occur in association with benign bony disease or after radiation to the head (Gertner, Podoshin and Fradis, 1983). Other head and neck tumours may spread locally from the middle ear or external auditory canal to involve the temporal bone (Michaels and Wells, 1980) or more rarely the labyrinth directly (Hiraide, Inouye and Ishii, 1983).

Schuknecht, Allam and Murakami (1968) reviewed the literature on metastatic spread to the temporal bone and concluded that its occurrence is under-recognized. They suggested that its incidence may be increasing as treatment for the primary tumour improves longevity and allows the development of intracranial metastases. Berlinger *et al.* (1980) reported four histological patterns of involvement of the temporal bone in metastatic and systemic malignancy. These included: isolated metastases from tumours of the kidney, lung, breast or thyroid; meningeal carcinomatosis affecting the pia/arachnoid membranes; spread to the temporal bone via the meninges; leukaemic infiltration. Symptoms of temporal bone involvement include hearing loss, vertigo and facial nerve deficits.

Vascular disease

The vertebrobasilar circulation supplies the peripheral labyrinth, VIIIth nerve and its central vestibular connections. The labyrinthine, or internal auditory artery, arises from the anterior inferior cerebellar artery or, more rarely, directly from the basilar artery (Sunderland, 1945) (Figure 20.4). It is an end artery, with no significant anastomoses with other arteries and so vascular disease, secondary to atheroma or more rarely meningovascular syphilis, hyperviscosity

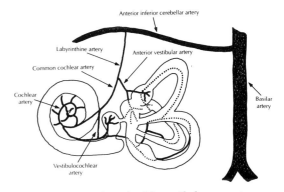

Figure 20.4 Arterial supply of the vestibular apparatus. (From Luxon, L. M. (1984) The anatomy and physiology of the vestibular system. In: *Vertigo*, edited by M. R. Dix and J. D. Hood. Chichester: John Wiley and Sons, with permission)

and hypercoagulability states, polyarteritis nodosa or giant cell arteritis, may precipitate profound ischaemia. Animal experiments and pathological examination of the cochlea in patients with hearing loss have demonstrated end organ necrosis associated with secondary neural degeneration (Gussen, 1976; Belal, 1980) and, indeed, Kimura and Perlman (1958) have shown primary vestibular epithelial changes following arterial destruction of the labyrinth. Kitamura and Berreby (1983) described severe degenerative changes in the cochlea, maculae and cristae of a patient who died 17 days after suffering occlusion of the right vertebral artery, basilar artery and most probably the right labyrinthine artery. In addition to the sensory epithelial changes, degeneration of the cochlear, superior and inferior vestibular nerves was documented. Most of Scarpa's ganglion cells were lost, particularly in the superior division. These findings concurred with those of Lindsay and Hemenway (1956), who reported a small group of patients with sudden severe vertigo, associated with nausea and vomiting, which gradually subsided over a number of weeks, but was replaced by the development of positional vertigo.

The majority of patients in whom a vascular cause of vertigo is suspected are over the age of 60 years and have a clear history of cardiovascular disease, hypertension or vertebrobasilar insufficiency. It must, of course, be emphasized that in the face of vertebrobasilar ischaemia (see below), it is often difficult clinically to determine the precise pathological site of the ischaemic lesion (labyrinth, VIIIth nerve or brain stem) giving rise to vertiginous symptoms. However, recent studies have reported a high incidence of peripheral and central vestibular abnormalities, diagnosed on the basis of caloric testing and electronystagmography, occurring both independently and together in patients with clear cut (Luxon, 1990) and presumed (Grad and Baloh, 1989) ischaemia in the vertebrobasilar territory.

Although the exact pathophysiological mechanism underlying migraine has not been fully elucidated, most authorities accept that vascular changes, either primary or secondary, play an important role. This is discussed in more detail below. A study by Kayan and Hood (1984) identified vestibular and/or cochlear symptoms of disabling severity, requiring medical intervention in 5% of 200 unselected patients with migraine. Full investigation of 80 migrainous subjects, referred because of vestibulocochlear symptoms, revealed that 77.5% had objective abnormalities – one-half indicating peripheral, and the other half indicating central pathology. It is likely that ischaemia of the peripheral or central vestibular pathways is the underlying mechanism of the audiovestibular symptoms. Migraine should therefore be considered in the differential diagnosis of peripheral vestibular disorders. It is of note that, in migraine, it would appear that the vertiginous episodes may precede or occur simultaneously with the headache, but may also occur during the headache-free periods (Kayan and Hood, 1984).

Drug-induced ototoxicity

Streptomycin was first isolated in 1944 (Waksman, Bugie and Schatz, 1944), and its effect on hearing and balance was reported soon after (Hinshaw and Feldman, 1945). The site of damage was localized to the peripheral labyrinthine structures by Causse (1949). In the search for less toxic alternatives, *gentamicin* was isolated in the 1960s and other related aminoglycosides over the next 10–15 years. Their usefulness lies in their activity against Gram-negative organisms, although the third generation cephalosporins have recently been introduced as alternatives.

All the aminoglycosides are ototoxic to varying degrees, some more cochleotoxic, (such as neomycin and kanamycin), while others are more vestibulotoxic (gentamicin and streptomycin). This difference is believed to be related to the number of free amino or methylamine groups present in the drug's structure. All this family of drugs has been shown to have a delayed toxicity, i.e. the inner ear defect progresses despite withdrawal of the drug. In the past it was thought that the specific ototoxic effect of aminoglycoside antibiotics was best explained by the high concentration of drug which accumulates in the inner ear fluid, and the prolonged half-life of the aminoglycoside antibiotics in perilymph compared with other body fluids. In addition, it was thought that aminoglycosides were almost totally excreted unchanged via the kidney. However, both these theories have recently been challenged and current thinking reviewed by Schacht (1993). It is known that renal failure decreases the rate of excretion of aminoglycosides and potentiates their toxicity. As they are also nephrotoxic themselves, this further compounds the situation.

The histopathological findings in the aminoglycoside-damaged vestibular system include damage, in the early stages, to the type I hair cells and so the changes are seen at the crest of the cristae and the striolar region of the maculae. In the later stages type II cells are also affected. Lindeman (1969) documented clear regional differences in vulnerability to vestibular damage. The sensory epithelia of the cristae ampullaris of the semicircular canals are more vulnerable than the utricular macula, which in turn is more susceptible than the saccular macula.

The biochemical basis of aminoglycoside toxicity has been a subject of controversy and has been reviewed in detail by Schacht (1993). There appear to be two stages, an acute and potentially reversible stage (thus supporting reports of clinical reversibility of hearing loss, e.g. Brummet and Fox, 1989) and a chronic irreversible stage. The acute stage may be related to competitive blocking of calcium channels at the cell membrane and thus interference with normal transduction process, while the chronic toxicity is associated with energy-dependent entry of the drug into the hair cells and subsequent compromise of intracellular metabolism. As mentioned above, it was believed that the aminoglycosides themselves were the toxic agents, but it may be that one or more metabolites are the culprits, thus explaining many features of aminoglycoside toxicity including delayed toxicity. It may also explain why the ototoxic effects do not correlate well with the serum or tissue levels of the aminoglycoside. Although much of the research has been performed on hair cells from the cochlea, it is likely that similar mechanisms apply to the vestibular hair cells.

A typical history of vestibular ototoxicity is of a gravely ill patient in bed, who, upon remobilization, begins to notice a balance problem, and often complains of movement of the environment in association with head movements. This is known as 'bobbing oscillopsia' and is the result of a failure of vestibular activity to generate a normal compensatory eye movement in response to head movement. The tragedy of this situation is that a patient who was gravely ill makes an excellent medical recovery, only to find himself a vestibular invalid. With the passage of time, the patient may adapt by using visual and proprioceptive information to maintain his balance. However, in elderly subjects, the symptoms are particularly intractable and the patient may be crippled by vestibular failure.

Clinically, vestibular toxicity is probably underdiagnosed for several reasons. Patients receiving aminoglycosides are often severely ill and complaints of dizziness may be ascribed to general debility or the effects of other centrally acting sedating drugs. In addition, due to a process of compensation, the symptomatic manifestations of the peripheral vestibular deficits will often resolve. Thirdly, tests of otolith function are not routinely available clinically and thus objective assessment of toxic damage to the maculae is difficult. Indeed, vestibular testing in general, in a severely ill patient may not always be feasible, though specific bedside vestibular test procedures have been developed (Longridge and Mallinson, 1987; Halmagyi and Curthoys, 1988; O'Leary and Davis, 1990).

The risk factors for developing aminoglycoside toxicity include, the dose of drug, presence of renal and hepatic failure, simultaneous administration of diuretics or other ototoxic agents including noise, extremes of age and the presence of pre-existing vestibular damage. It has been shown that albino guinea-pigs have increased susceptibility to the toxic effects of aminoglycosides compared to pigmented species (Conlee *et al.*, 1991) although a similar effect has not been demonstrated in humans. In addition it has recently been reported that a familial predisposition to streptomycin ototoxicity exists, transmitted maternally via the mitochondrial genome (Higashi, 1989; Hu *et al.*, 1991). This has not yet been proven for other aminoglycosides.

Although the ototoxicity of the aminoglycosides is usually reported with respect to parenteral administration, several animal experiments suggest neomycin and gentamicin are ototoxic when applied topically. However, Gyde (1976) found no evidence of ototoxicity in 300 patients with tympanic membrane perforation, treated with topical gentamicin. Dose-dependent toxicity has been reported in guinea-pigs and baboons in which neomycin was instilled into the middle ear. (For a detailed review of topical agents associated with ototoxicity see Rohn, Meyerhoff and Wright, 1993.)

Transplacental aminoglycoside ototoxicity has also been described in both animals and humans (reviewed by Henley and Rybak, 1993).

Many other drugs, apart from aminoglycosides, such as cis-platinum, diuretics, salicylates, vancomycin and others, have been shown to be ototoxic, and presumably as new drugs appear the list will continue to grow. However, most of the reports refer to cochleotoxicity. Myers, Blakley and Schwan (1993) found no clear evidence of vestibulotoxicity in 34 patients undergoing cis-platinum therapy. Schweitzer (1993) reviewed the evidence for cis-platinum-induced vestibular toxicity, and concluded that there was little functional or histopathological evidence in animals or humans of vestibular disorder. Similarly, Elidan, Lin and Honrubia (1986) reported minimal if any effect of loop diuretics on the vestibular labyrinth.

There is no evidence of salicylates causing vestibular dysfunction. Transient positional abnormalities due to quinine ingestion have been reported by Zajtchuk *et al.* (1984) in three out of four subjects. Vertigo has been described in association with the tetracycline, *minocycline*. Gould and Brookler (1972) reported vertigo occurring in six out of a series of 20 patients receiving minocycline for meningococcal prophylaxis, and Williams, Laughlin and Lee (1974) found vertigo, ataxia, nausea and vomiting within 24–48 hours of initiation of therapy, in 17 of 19 patients. They postulated a vestibular aetiology though no vestibular testing was undertaken. Drew *et al.* (1976) published a series of 80 patients treated with minocycline, 78% of whom developed vestibular symptoms. However, at the much lower doses used for treatment of acne vulgaris, Cullen and Cohen (1976) reported no vestibular symptoms. Lim (1984) postulated that otoconial abnormalities may lead to disorders of balance and orientation, and as Balsamo, De Vincentiis and Marmo (1969) showed that tetracycline can affect otoconial development, it is possible that the observed vestibular effect may be related to changes in the otoconia. However, it would be difficult to explain how minocycline would give rise to symptoms so soon after starting the drug if the effect were mediated via otoconial changes.

There have been several reports of hearing loss,

usually, but not always, reversible in association with *erythromycin*. Only one report of vestibular disorder has been documented (Agusti *et al.*, 1991). They reported vestibular hyporeflexia, on the basis of electronystagmography, persisting over a period of 7 months after treatment with erythromycin. These changes were deemed by the authors to be indicative of permanent vestibular damage.

Menière's disease

As Menière's disease is discussed in detail in Volume 3, Chapter 19, only brief general comments will be made here.

Although the literature abounds with controversy on all aspects of this disorder, most clinicians agree that fluctuating hearing loss, tinnitus and vertigo, often with associated fullness of the ear, are the cardinal features. In 60% of those affected, both vestibular and cochlear symptoms have developed within 6 months of the onset of the disease. The disorder can affect all age groups and in the majority of cases the aetiology remains unknown, although viral labyrinthitis, autoimmune disease, endocrine and genetic factors have all been implicated. Bilateral involvement is reported to occur in as few as 10% (Cawthorne, 1969) or as many as 60% (Morrison, 1986) of cases, this discrepancy probably reflecting variation in the criteria used for diagnosis. The pathological correlate of Menière's disease is known to be endolymphatic hydrops, although the pathophysiological mechanisms remain poorly understood (Figure 20.5). Paparella (1991) suggested that the final common pathway, through which many different aetiologies may act, could be endolymphatic absorptive dysfunction, predisposed to by abnormalities of the endolymphatic sac either developmental and/or acquired; the latter due for example, to infective or immunological reactions.

Clinical variants of classical Menière's disease have been described. 'Vestibular Menière's' refers to the episodic occurrence of vestibular symptoms in the absence of cochlear symptoms. Though there is some histological evidence in support of the possibility of endolymphatic hydrops occurring in the vestibular system alone, most authorities suggest that vestibular Menière's is not a separate entity but could be merely episodic vertigo due to some other cause such as that associated with migraine. It is obviously important that the distinction be clearly made as appropriate treatment for the two conditions is very different.

Delayed endolymphatic hydrops is a Menière-like syndrome which develops in a patient in whom there has been total, or subtotal, cochlear damage many years previously, e.g. post meningitis (Rosenhall and Kankunen, 1981; Schuknecht, Suzuka and Zimmermann, 1990). Such cases are relatively common and are identified by the presence of a previous history of long-standing unilateral hearing loss.

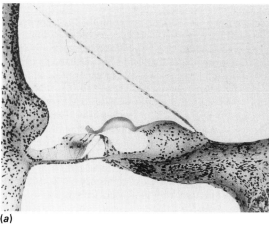

(a)

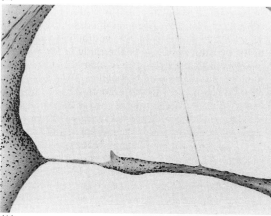

(b)

Figure 20.5 (*a*) Normal organ of Corti. (*b*) Organ of Corti destroyed by endolymphatic hydrops, with marked displacement of Reissner's membrane. (Reproduced with the kind permission of Duphar)

Otosclerosis

Otosclerosis is a primary disease of bone derived from the otic capsule. It is seen histologically in 10% (Guild, 1944) of the white population but clinically in only 1%. It is much rarer in black populations. It is generally thought to be autosomal dominantly inherited with incomplete penetrance. However, in 1989, Gordon reviewed the genetics of otosclerosis and suggested that clinical and histological otosclerosis may be the phenotypic expression of a genetically heterogeneous group of disorders.

The commonest manifestation of otosclerosis is conductive hearing loss due to involvement of the oval window area, but for over 80 years it has been suggested that sensorineural hearing loss is also associated with otosclerosis and many subsequent reports have confirmed this. However, the mechanism is still uncertain, and controversy exists as to whether otosclerosis of the cochlea occurs in the absence of stapedial otosclerosis, so-called 'cochlear otosclerosis'. The prevalence of vestibular involvement in otosclerosis has been quoted to be in the region of 20% to 30% (Cawthorne, 1955; Meurman, Aantaa and Virolainen, 1969). Morales–Garcia (1972) reported a higher incidence of vestibular dysfunction in patients with otosclerosis associated with sensorineural hearing loss, although the vestibular and cochlear symptoms can occur independently. Morrison (1984) has documented that 4% of patients with otosclerosis demonstrated benign positional vertigo of paroxysmal type and 1% of patients gave a history of paroxysmal attacks of vertigo, similar to Menière's disease.

Several mechanisms have been proposed to explain the association of otosclerosis and vertigo. An otosclerotic focus affecting the labyrinth may release toxic substances into the inner ear fluids and cause the degenerative changes in the vestibular end-organs noted by Gussen in 1973. Alternatively biochemical changes in the perilymph may alter vestibular function (Sando, Hemenway and Miller, 1974; Ghorayeb and Linthicum, 1978). In addition, it has been suggested that otosclerosis may cause endolymphatic hydrops and thus give rise to vertigo. Although the association of endolymphatic hydrops and otosclerosis has been documented in the past (Black *et al.*, 1969; Igarashi *et al.*, 1982) it has been considered rare and merely coincidental. Liston *et al.* (1984) suggested that capsular otosclerosis can cause endolymphatic hydrops particularly if there is otosclerotic involvement around the endolymphatic duct and sac. The findings of Li, Schachern and Paparella (1994) support this view in that they found extensive otosclerosis involving the round and oval windows, bony cochlear labyrinth, vestibule, vestibular aqueduct, semicircular canals and the internal auditory meatus in association with endolymphatic hydrops. Yoon *et al.* (1990) reported otosclerosis involving the vestibular aqueduct with fibrosis of the endolymphatic duct and sac associated with endolymphatic hydrops. The presence of a conductive hearing loss in a patient with dysequilibrium should raise the possibility of a diagnosis of otosclerosis. The diagnosis is confirmed radiologically. As the labyrinthine capsule is normally the densest bone in the body, Phelps and Lloyd (1990a) pointed out that increased radio-opacity is not possible and thus inactive inner ear otosclerosis can only be demonstrated by showing thickening of the bone with distortion of the labyrinthine cavity. However, the active phase of bone remodelling is shown by areas of rarefaction seen with high resolution CT scanning. Phelps and Lloyd (1990a) stressed the usefulness of densitometry readings in order to detect areas of rarefaction which are too subtle to be easily apparent on direct inspection, and also the need to monitor changes over time, for example as a result of progression of the disease or the response to treatment.

Metabolic disease affecting the inner ear

Diabetes mellitus

The relationship between audiovestibular symptoms and diabetes mellitus is still a subject of controversy. Some authors have shown an increased incidence of sensorineural hearing loss (Friedman, Schulma and Weiss, 1975; Kurien, Thomas and Bhanu, 1989) while others report no difference between diabetics and controls (Axelsson, Sigroth and Vertes, 1978; Gibbon and Davis, 1981; Parving, 1991). Jorgensen and Buch (1961) reported an association between diabetes and auditory and vestibular disorders while Harner (1981) refuted this association. This unresolved contradiction probably arises because the population with diabetes mellitus is not homogeneous. Traditionally diabetes mellitus has been divided into insulin-dependent and non-insulin-dependent diabetics, but even within these groups the clinical condition of diabetes may be the final common pathway of many different pathological processes, some of which affect the ear and others which do not. A case in point is the recently recognized role of mitochondrial DNA in some forms of diabetes mellitus. There is little doubt that diabetes occurring as a result of mitochondrial DNA abnormalities, is associated with sensorineural hearing loss, the pathogenic mechanism being disruption of energy production which thus compromises tissues with high metabolic requirements (Harding, 1989).

Few studies have investigated the possibility of an association between diabetes mellitus and vestibular changes. Aantaa and Lehtonen (1981) showed mainly peripheral vestibular abnormalities in approximately half of a series of 24 young adults with insulin-dependent diabetes, none of whom complained of vertigo. The incidence of vestibular dysfunction increased with the duration of the disease but did not correlate with other diabetic complications. Biurrun *et al.* (1991) showed depressed caloric responses in 21.8% of a series of 46 children and young adults with type I diabetes. As in Aantaa and Lehtonen's (1981) report, no patient complained of vertigo/dizziness and no correlation was found between vestibular dysfunction and any other diabetic complication or between vestibular and cochlear abnormalities.

Vestibular function in the subgroup of diabetics with abnormalities of mitochondrial DNA mentioned above, has been poorly described. Reardon *et al.* (1992) reported normal vestibular function in three cases with mitochondrially determined diabetes mellitus and deafness.

It is likely that many pathogenic mechanisms, occurring individually or simultaneously, give rise to the audiovestibular symptoms in diabetes. Some authors have suggested that the hearing loss is a form of diabetic neuropathy, while others suggest that it is related to diabetic microangiopathy affecting the laby rinth. In those patients with abnormal mitochondrial DNA, a basic defect in cellular metabolism occurs which could compromise high energy-dependent tissues such as the labyrinth. Wackym and Linthicum (1986) reported microangiopathic changes in the basilar membrane and endolymphatic sac of temporal bones from diabetics when compared with normal bones. Vascular changes affecting the cochlea had previously been noted by several authors including Jorgensen and Buch (1961), and Makishima and Tanaka (1971). However, these findings were not confirmed by Naufal and Schuknecht (1972). In addition Myers *et al.* (1985) and Myers and Ross (1987) examined, histologically, the saccule and utricle of diabetic rats and found no evidence of diabetic microangiopathic changes in these structures, but did find pathological changes in the connective and neuroepithelial tissues.

Renal disease

The development of inner ear symptoms in patients with renal disease was emphasized by Beaney (1964), when he identified six patients with auditory and/or vestibular symptoms in a series of 262 chronically haemodialysed patients. However, prior to this, the association of hereditary renal disease and sensorineural hearing loss had been recognized in Alport's syndrome. There have been many subsequent reports of sensorineural hearing loss associated with chronic renal disease (Bergstrom *et al.*, 1973; Adler and Ritz, 1982; Gatland *et al.*, 1991), but the underlying pathogenic mechanism has proved difficult to elucidate, as in any one patient so many factors exist which may be contributory to the hearing loss that it has been difficult to incriminate any one independently of the others. Some of the relevant factors are: the underlying disease which caused the renal failure, such as diabetes or autoimmune disease, the uraemia itself or other toxic products of renal dysfunction causing damage to the cochlea, or the effects of various treatments such as antibiotics for intercurrent infection, diuretics, the chelating agent desferroxamine, haemodialysis or transplantation. In fact some authors (Bergstrom *et al.*, 1973; Booth, 1982) suggested that all the hearing loss seen in patients with renal failure may be explicable on the basis of the treatment they received. However, other authors have stressed the physiological, antigenic, and ultrastructural similarities (Quick, Fish and Brown, 1973) between the cochlea and the nephron and hypothesized that renal disease itself, and not only its treatment, is associated with inner ear disease. Yassin, Safwat and Fatt-hi (1966) suggested that the hearing loss may be due to a central effect of uraemia, but in 1970, Yassin, Badry and Fatt-hi proposed that it correlated with hyponatraemia of renal failure, though this has been disputed by others.

There is also much controversy about the effect of haemodialysis and transplantation on hearing. Some workers have documented an improvement in hearing thresholds (Mitschke *et al.*, 1977; Gatland *et al.*, 1991) or vestibular symptoms (Beaney, 1964) after dialysis or transplantation, whereas others have found no improvement (Adler and Ritz, 1982) or have actually implicated these treatments, or complications thereof, as the cause of the hearing loss (Oda, 1974; Rizvi and Holmes, 1980; Kligerman *et al.*, 1981). The suggested mechanisms of the hearing loss reported with haemodialysis include marked changes in osmotic gradients due to the rapid lowering of serum urea, deranged calcium and phosphate metabolism, or hypotension and embolism giving rise to ischaemia of the inner ear.

Few reports have specifically mentioned vestibular symptoms, although Bergstrom *et al.* (1973) reported one patient with hearing loss and episodic vertigo and another with a sudden hearing loss and absent response to caloric testing. Oda (1974) reported dizziness in one case and vertigo in a second of a series of eight patients with chronic renal failure.

Temporal bone studies in patients with uraemia treated with transplantation and/or haemodialysis have failed to show any change specific to renal disease. Oda (1974) showed blue strial concretions, sometimes associated with strial degeneration, in the temporal bone of eight patients with chronic renal failure treated with dialysis or transplantation. He found similar concretions in the subepithelial layer of the saccule and posterior semicircular canal. However these are not specific to inner ear disease associated with renal disease, and may be non-specific changes occurring secondary to degeneration from any cause (Naunton, Lindsay and Stein, 1973). Oedema of the supporting cells of the cochlea, stria vascularis, saccule, utricle and cristae (Rizvi and Holmes, 1980), as well as endolymphatic hydrops (Bergstrom *et al.*, 1973) have also been reported, in keeping with the finding of Gatland *et al.* (1991) of fluctuating hearing loss, and possibly supporting the hypothesis of fluid changes being an important cause of audiovestibular dysfunction in patients with chronic renal failure.

Paget's disease

Paget's disease (osteitis deformans) is a metabolic bone disorder of unknown aetiology, characterized by abnormal bony resorption and deposition, affecting mainly the middle aged and elderly. In the presence of characteristic skeletal changes (Figure 20.6) (enlarged skull, short stature, kyphosis, bowing of the legs), the diagnosis is obvious, but osteitis deformans may be symptomless. Skull radiographs displaying the characteristic demineralization, together with an elevated serum alkaline phosphatase and increased total urinary hydroxyproline confirm the diag-

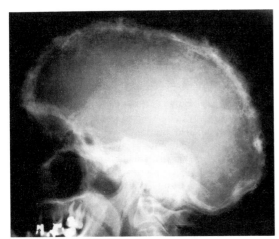

Figure 20.6 Radiograph of the skull of a 63-year-old man presenting with drop attacks, episodes of dizziness and sensorineural hearing loss, showing gross Paget's disease of the skull with temporal bone involvement

nosis. It has been reported that up to 50% of people with Paget's disease have hearing loss – predominantly sensorineural or mixed – and up to 25–30% (Clemis *et al.*, 1967; Nager, 1975) complain of vertigo. The hearing loss is specifically related to involvement of the temporal bone in the pagetic process.

Histopathological studies on temporal bones have shown many changes in the inner ear in Paget's disease such as loss of cochlear outer hair cells, strial atrophy, cochlear neuronal degeneration, narrowing of the internal auditory meatus causing compression of the VIIIth nerve, microfractures involving the vestibule, semicircular canals and margins of the round and oval windows as well as microfibromas of the vestibular portion of the VIIIth nerve. Postulated mechanisms of the vertigo include the liberation of toxic substances from the active pagetic bone causing damage to inner ear structures, distortion of the labyrinthine lumen due to bony overgrowth, perilymphatic leaks cause by microfractures of the bony margins of the round and oval windows, compression of the VIIIth nerve by the pagetic bone of the internal auditory meatus (Applebaum and Clemis, 1977) or involvement of the VIIIth nerve by microfibromas. However, there are very few reports of neurovestibular testing in the literature. Clemis *et al.* (1967) found abnormal caloric responses in only one of a series of 17 patients with Paget's disease, although six of them had symptoms attributed to vestibular dysfunction. Four of these six had involvement of the semicircular canal by pagetic bone demonstrated radiographically. Proops, Bayley and Hawke (1985) documented central vestibular pathology in the one patient of a series of three who had vestibular tests. They hypothesized that this was of vascular origin as

this patient had platybasia with basilar invagination. However, Khetarpal and Schuknecht (1990) questioned the relationship of the above histological findings to Paget's disease, and suggested that most of these changes could be merely the effects of ageing. In their study of 26 temporal bones, they found no specific pathological correlate for sensorineural hearing loss or vertigo in patients with Paget's disease, and concluded that inner ear symptoms may be caused by functional changes due to alterations in the density, mass and form of the inner ear bony structures.

As Paget's disease is common in the middle-aged and elderly population, and as sensorineural hearing loss, usually bilateral, is a common, or indeed the only, complication, skull radiography is indicated in the investigation of bilateral sensorineural hearing loss of unknown origin in this age group. Phelps and Lloyd (1990b) recommended thin section, high-resolution CT scanning of the skull base to show the 'cotton wool' appearance of the pagetic bone and to demonstrate encroachment on the labyrinthine capsule.

Hypophosphataemic rickets

Hypophosphataemic (vitamin D resistant) rickets/osteomalacia is generally thought to be an X-linked dominant disorder, although Stamp and Baker (1976) postulated an autosomal recessive inheritance pattern in one family. Davis, Kane and Valentine (1984) reported the association of hearing loss, both conductive and sensorineural, with X-linked hypophosphataemic rickets. Investigations showed the latter to be a cochlear loss often with a hydropic type picture. This was further corroborated by O'Malley *et al.* (1985). Proposed causes for the cochlear loss include spiral ligament or basilar membrane calcification or overgrowth of the bony cochlea, although biochemical factors may also play a role. Stamp and Baker (1976), however, suggested that the hearing loss seen in their patients was as a result of bony overgrowth of the internal auditory meatus encroaching on the VIIIth nerve. However, this was based solely on radiological findings and no audiometric investigations were available. There is little documentation of vestibular status in hypophosphataemic rickets. In a study by Davis, Kane and Valentine (1984) 10 of 18 patients with both hearing loss and hypophosphataemic rickets showed abnormal responses on caloric testing. Boneh *et al.* (1987) postulated that there are two subtypes of the condition encoded by separate genes, one of which shows cochlear hearing loss and peripheral vestibular dysfunction, and the other without inner ear abnormalities. They further suggested that these were the human counterparts of the 'Gy' and 'Hyp' mouse mutations respectively. The work of Lyon *et al.* (1986) further supported the theory of Boneh *et al.* (1987) by showing that labyrinthine abnormalities, both vestibular and cochlear, were seen histologically in the 'Gy' but not the 'Hyp' mouse mutant. Thus, if there are two separate types of X-linked hypophosphataemic rickets in humans, it may be possible to distinguish them on the basis of audiovestibular symptoms and signs.

Autoimmune disorders

Autoimmunity is defined as the state in which immune reactions of the host are directed against his own antigenic structures. Such immune reactions are mediated by sensitized lymphocytes and/or antibodies and can lead to destruction of the antigens involved, and consequently to disease. Autoimmunity is being increasingly recognized as a probable cause of cochleovestibular symptoms which were previously of unknown aetiology, though often ascribed to unproven viral or vascular pathologies.

In broad terms, two possible pathogenetic mechanisms could account for the association between autoimmunity and inner ear symptoms. First, the ear may be one of many organs involved in what is essentially a multisystem autoimmune disease, such as systemic lupus erythematosus. Alternatively immune reactions may be directed specifically against inner ear antigens and this may give rise to an organ-specific disease akin to autoimmune thyroiditis. In the past it was thought that the inner ear was immunologically isolated, and neither mounted an immune response itself, nor released antigens into the general circulation. However, a large body of both experimental and clinical evidence to the contrary has evolved. Hariri (1993) has reviewed the experimental evidence that the inner ear does react immunologically and that the result of these immune reactions leads to inner ear symptoms and signs.

Clinical evidence for an autoimmune aetiology for cochleovestibular symptoms dates back to 1958, when Lehnhardt found autoantibodies in patients suffering from sudden deafness and proposed an autoimmune aetiology. Kikuchi (1959) and subsequently Harris, Low and House (1985), reported cases of 'sympathetic otitis', whereby surgery on one ear was associated with a sudden hearing loss in the other. They proposed an immune mechanism to explain their findings.

In 1979 McCabe hypothesized a new disease entity called *autoimmune sensorineural hearing loss*. He reported 18 patients with cochleovestibular symptoms demonstrating immunological findings and suggesting an autoimmune phenomenon. All patients responded to long-term cortisone and cyclophosphamide therapy. By 1985, McCabe had added a further 38 patients to his series and reported that vestibular spells or crises were not a feature of the disease, but ataxia in the dark was a feature of all patients who had moderate to severe disease. In addition, he noted that vestibular symptoms and caloric test results gen-

erally paralleled the hearing loss. Furthermore, in patients with severe to profound hearing loss, all ocular counter-rolling is lost and he therefore suggested that the autoimmune process involves not only the cochlea, but the entire membranous labyrinth including the otolith organs.

In 1982, Stephens, Luxon and Hinchcliffe found a high incidence of cochleovestibular symptoms in patients suffering from a variety of autoimmune disorders including autoantibody-mediated disease such as the Vogt–Koyanagi–Harada syndrome and immune-complex-mediated disease, such as systemic lupus erythematosus, polyarteritis nodosa, Wegener's granulomatosis, Cogan's syndrome and Behçet's syndrome.

In the *Vogt–Koyanagi–Harada syndrome* (bilateral inflammation of the eye with granulomatous uveitis and pigmentary disturbances), meningitic symptoms and sensorineural hearing loss, vertigo and vestibular hypofunction are common findings (Maxwell, 1963; Seals and Rise, 1967).

Bowman *et al.* (1986) described two cases of sensorineural hearing loss associated with *systemic lupus erythematosus*, but no mention was made of vestibular symptoms or signs. McCrae and O'Reilly (1957) reported vertigo in four out of a series of 55 patients with systemic lupus erythematosus. The site of vestibular dysfunction was not identified. Caldarelli, Rejowslei and Corey (1984) described sudden onset bilateral profound hearing loss and unsteadiness, with absent caloric responses, as the initial presentation of systemic lupus erythematosus. Trune *et al.* (1989) suggested that the stria vascularis was the primary site of autoimmune damage. Though the latter reported the vestibular end organs as being 'normal', no specific mention was made of the dark cell regions – thought to have similar function in the vestibular system as the stria vascularis has in the auditory system. Vyse, Luxon and Walport (1994) reported acute audiovestibular failure in two patients with high titres of antiphospholipid antibodies, one of whom had systemic lupus erythematosus and the other the primary phospholipid syndrome. The cause of the audiovestibular symptoms was presumed to be thrombotic in nature. The site of the lesion in the case with systemic lupus erythematosus was found to be the brain stem, whereas in the case with primary phospholipid syndrome it was considered to be peripheral.

Sensorineural hearing loss has been described in association with *ulcerative colitis* (Summers and Harker, 1982; Weber, Jenkins and Cohen, 1984; Herdman, Hariri and Ramsden, 1991) and in association with ulcerative colitis and *giant cell arteritis* together (Jacob et al., 1990) and an immune mechanism has been proposed as a unifying aetiology. In the report by Herdman, Hariri and Ramsden (1991), acute vestibular symptoms were described in their two cases in association with the hearing loss, considered to be of peripheral origin.

Row–Jones, Macallan and Sorooshian (1990) reported a case of a woman, whose initial presentation of *polyarteritis nodosa* was bilateral acute cochleovestibular failure. A temporal bone study in a patient with polyarteritis nodosa (Gussen, 1977) revealed hydropic changes in the cochlea. Jenkins, Pollak and Fisch (1981) confirmed the finding of endolymphatic hydrops, with additional changes in the organ of Corti and stria vascularis in another patient with polyarteritis nodosa. Similar changes of hydrops together with ossification in the scala vestibuli have been reported on histological examination of the temporal bones in patients with *Cogan's syndrome* (Wolff *et al.*, 1965; Zechner, 1980), consistent with the symptoms of vertigo, tinnitus and hearing loss described by Cogan in 1948.

In *Behçet's syndrome* there are a number of reports of vestibular involvement (Brama and Fainaru, 1980; Gemignani *et al.*, 1991; Yoshio *et al.*, 1991). In Brama and Fainaru's study, on the basis of audiometric and vestibular examinations, the site of involvement was identified as the labyrinth, whereas Gemignani *et al.* found evidence of peripheral as well as central vestibular lesions – the latter possibly being the first indication of the development of neuro-Behçet's syndrome.

Autoimmunity of the inner ear is now recognized as a cause of endolymphatic hydrops (Hughes *et al.*, 1985). Yoo *et al.* (1982) found an increased collagen antibody titre in patients with Menière's disease, and in 1982, Shea and Yoo reported a good response to cortisone treatment in patients with both Menière's disease and immunopositive findings.

The entity of cochleovestibular dysfunction on an autoimmune basis appears to be well established, although it should be emphasized that different authors have adopted various criteria for confirming the diagnosis of autoimmune ear disease. A presumptive diagnosis of autoimmune disorder based on a response to steroid treatment must be regarded with extreme caution as the therapeutic effects of steroids are by no means specific to autoimmunity. Reports where positive antigen specific tests, such as lymphocyte transformation or migration inhibition tests using inner ear antigens, are documented are more convincing as evidence of autoimmune inner ear disease.

VIIIth cranial nerve pathology

In the last 20 years, the introduction of electrophysiological investigations, including electrocochleography and auditory brain stem responses, has facilitated the clinical feasibility of diagnosing VIIIth nerve lesions with confidence. The clinical problem of differentiating cochlear from VIIIth nerve pathology is compounded by the unusual pathophysiological degenerative changes exhibited by the cochleovestibular nerve.

In the auditory division, sensory and neural degeneration are interdependent (Johnsson, 1974; Dupont, Guilhaume and Aran, 1993), whereas the vestibular nerve behaves rather differently. Following labyrinthectomy in the cat, monkey and man, it has been shown that vestibular neurons in Scarpa's ganglion may survive (Cass, Davidson and Goshgarian, 1989) certainly for longer than the spiral ganglion cells (Dupont, Guilhaume and Aran, 1993). Their peripheral processes may atrophy, but the central axons have been shown to remain intact in the cat (Cass, Davidson and Goshgarian, 1989) and other experimental animals, thus with the possibility of retaining their functional synaptic connections in the brain stem.

It is of value to consider those pathologies which have been identified as probably affecting primarily the VIIIth cranial nerve.

Congenital and hereditary disorders

The VIIIth nerve may be affected in many congenital and inherited disorders. There may or may not be associated abnormalities of the peripheral vestibular organs.

Complete failure of development of the bony labyrinth or VIIIth nerve as described by Michel in 1863, or arrested development at the primitive otocyst stage are associated with no cochlear/vestibular function (Phelps, 1983). The Michel anomaly has been associated with thalidomide toxicity (Phelps, 1983), but most are of unknown aetiology.

Abnormality of the cochlear and saccular neuroepithelia associated with atrophy of the vestibular and cochlear nerves was first described by Scheibe (1892) in congenitally deaf patients, and is known as cochleosaccular dysplasia. *Rubella* embryopathy has been associated with the Scheibe abnormality but, in most cases, the cause is unknown. Although it generally occurs sporadically, two cases with probable autosomal dominant inheritance and one with autosomal recessive inheritance (Walby and Schuknecht, 1984) have been described. Similar changes have been described in association with chromosomal abnormalities (Nadol and Burgess, 1982). When similar pathology occurs later in life, it is known as cochleosaccular degeneration. It has been suggested that the degenerative form may in some cases, also be genetically determined, and cochleosaccular degeneration has been described in association with *Refsum's disease*, *Kearns–Sayre syndrome* and as occurring in three sisters with progressive sensorineural hearing loss, absent gastric motility, small bowel diverticula and sensory neuropathy (reviewed by Nadol and Burgess, 1982). Although saccular function is not assessed in routine clinical vestibular testing, the involvement of the vestibular nerve can lead to clinically detectable vestibular abnormalities.

Cochleovestibular nerve aplasia may occur in the

presence of a normal cochlear and vestibular labyrinth (Phelps, 1983), but will, of course, be incompatible with any audiovestibular function. Narrowed internal acoustic meatus containing only the facial nerve will be seen radiographically. Shelton *et al.* (1989) reported three children with congenital deafness and no vestibular response to rotation, who failed to respond to electrical stimulation of their cochlear implants. All three children had narrowed internal acoustic meatuses, but had normal cochleae, semicircular canals and middle ears. One of these children, and two other children, also with deafness, absent vestibular function and narrowed internal auditory meatus had diabetic mothers. They postulated that as maternal diabetes can cause optic nerve hypoplasia (Nelson, Lessell and Sadun, 1986), it may have caused the aplasia of the VIIIth nerve seen in these children. The facial nerve, which embryologically develops separately, was intact.

The VIIIth nerve is involved bilaterally in *neurofibromatosis type 2*. This has recently been reported to have a prevalence in the UK of between 1 in 33 000 and 1 in 40 000 (Evans *et al.*, 1992a).

The condition is autosomal dominant with complete penetrance, the gene for which has been localized to chromosome 22. Approximately 50% of cases represent new mutations. There is evidence of the possible existence of two subgroups of neurofibromatosis type 2, a more severe form with early onset of bilateral vestibular schwannomas and multiple other tumours (meningiomas, gliomas), and a milder form with later onset of bilateral VIIIth nerve tumours only. The age of onset and age at death appear to be earlier in cases which are maternally inherited. According to Evans *et al.* (1992b), since the recommendations of the NIH consensus conference on acoustic neuroma (1991), the clinical distinction between type 1 and type 2 neurofibromatosis should not pose much of a problem. Type 2 has relatively few peripheral features with the brunt of the condition falling on the nervous system. On the other hand, type 1 can give complications in almost any system (Huson, Harper and Compston, 1988). In patients with neurofibromatosis type 2 there are rarely more than five café au lait patches greater than 0.5 cm in diameter before puberty or greater than 1.5 cm after puberty. In addition skin tumours are less numerous and recent histology reports suggest that they are schwannomas and not neurofibromas, as is the case in type 1. Caution needs to be exerted when interpreting CT scans. Widened internal acoustic meatus may suggest bilateral vestibular schwannomas and a diagnosis of neurofibromatosis type 2. However, very wide meatus (with other skull base deformities) may occur in type 1 mimicking bilateral VIIIth nerve tumours, but in reality caused by bony dysplasia.

Atrophy of the VIIIth nerve may also occur in inherited conditions in which there are associated skeletal abnormalities such as anencephaly (Lindsay, 1973a), Treacher-Collins syndrome (Lindsay, 1973a), branchio-otorenal syndrome (Fitch, Lindsay and Srolovitz, 1976) and Wildervanck's (1963) syndrome.

The VIIIth nerve may be involved in the congenital malformation of the hind-brain, the *Arnold-Chiari malformation*. The more frequent and severe form manifests itself within the first few months of life and is associated with hydrocephalus and other malformations of the CNS. The less common type I malformation may not present until adulthood and between 10% and 20% will have audiovestibular symptoms. It has been postulated that these symptoms may be the result of stretching of the VIIIth cranial nerve, with changes in brain stem position with age, or may be the result of compression of the VIIIth nerve as it is bent over the edge of the porus acusticus. There are no pathological data to confirm or refute these hypotheses.

Involvement of the VIIIth nerve occurs in association with many widespread degenerative neural disorders. *Friedreich's ataxia*, the most commonly encountered of the spinocerebellar degenerations, is inherited as an autosomal recessive disorder localized to chromosome 9. It is characterized by progressive ataxia, dysarthria, loss of joint position and vibration sense, scoliosis, pes cavus and cardiac abnormalities. Vestibular hypofunction has been reported in between 30% and 100% (Verhagen and Huygen, 1994) of cases. Histologically, Spoendlin (1974) found degeneration of both branches of the VIIIth nerves as well as involvement of the vestibular nuclei in two sisters with Friedreich's ataxia.

Charcot-Marie-Tooth disease, a hereditary motor and sensory neuropathy, is divided into two types, I and II. The clinical differentiation of these two conditions can be difficult, but type I appears to be the more severe. Measurement of motor nerve conduction velocity is helpful, being normal or near normal in type II but reduced in type I. Both are usually autosomal dominantly inherited, though recessive pedigrees have been described. Ataxia of unknown origin has been reported in type I disease, and described as being of a severity not explicable by the peripheral neuropathy alone. No mention of vestibular function was made (Baraitser, 1990). Verhagen and Huygen (1994) cited reports of three patients with sensorineural hearing loss in association with type I disease, and the caloric responses were reported as being bilaterally absent in one.

Dysfunction of the VIIIth nerve is also reported in *progressive external ophthalmoplegia* (Verhagen and Huygen, 1994), a mitochondrially determined disorder which clinically and genetically may overlap with Kearns-Sayre syndrome (Reardon and Harding, 1995).

The vestibular nerve is affected in many other inherited conditions and these are reviewed in detail by Huygen and Verhagen (1994) and Verhagen and Huygen (1994).

Trauma

Blunt trauma to the parietal region of the skull may give rise to fractures of the temporal bone. These fractures may be longitudinal, transverse or rarely oblique. Longitudinal fractures are by far the commonest, and involve the middle ear, but usually do not involve the labyrinth or VIIIth nerve. Transverse fractures comprise 10–30% of temporal bone fractures (Tos, 1971) and involve the VIIth and/or VIIIth cranial nerves in about 50% of cases. The rare oblique fracture may also involve the VIIIth nerve. The prognosis depends not only upon damage to the vestibular nerve, but also upon damage to the peripheral vestibular labyrinth and any other central nervous system sequelae. In the case of complete unilateral vestibular failure with normal neurological function, gradual improvement of vestibular function occurs over 6–12 weeks, during which time central compensation occurs reducing the patient's symptoms of dysequilibrium.

Penetrating injuries, most commonly gunshot wounds, may involve the labyrinth and/or VIIIth nerve and cause irreversible vestibular damage (Kerr and Smyth, 1987).

Infection

Bacterial, mycotic and viral infections are important causes of VIIIth nerve pathology. Damage to the nerves usually occurs by direct invasion by the organism along the nerves and vessels of the internal auditory canal as a consequence of meningoencephalitis.

Viral infection

As discussed previously in the section on infection affecting the inner ear, definitive proof of a causal role for viruses in inner ear disease is lacking though much circumstantial evidence exists (Davis, 1993). Similarly, conclusive evidence of viruses causing VIIIth nerve pathology is also lacking. Lindsay (1973b) has demonstrated marked infiltration of the VIIIth cranial nerve neural remnants in the modiolus of the cochlea, and branches of the vestibular nerve by lymphocytes and histiocytes and attributed these findings to viral infection of the VIIIth nerve. Nonetheless, the aetiological role remains unproven.

The clinical syndrome of *Ramsay Hunt* (facial palsy, auricular herpetic rash and hearing loss) is often associated with vertigo. Devriese (1968) described vestibular symptoms in 72% of 32 patients with Ramsay Hunt syndrome, while Abramovich and Prasher (1986) reported vertigo in 85% of their series. Yagi, Yamaguchi and Nonaka (1988) reported positional nystagmus in 69% and hypofunction on caloric test in 52% of 25 patients with this condition. As discussed above there is histological evidence of inflammation of the vestibular division of the VIIIth nerve in association with viral infection. Moreover, Blackley, Friedman and Wright (1967) described histological changes in both neural tissue and in the organ of Corti itself, while Proctor *et al.* (1979) reported vestibular dysfunction associated with labyrinthine destruction in one patient. However, Wilson (1986) has postulated viral labyrinthitis, ganglionitis or cranial neuropathy as the pathophysiological mechanisms of inner ear dysfunction in herpes infections.

Clinically, the site of lesion in the Ramsay Hunt syndrome has been assessed using both auditory and vestibular investigations, but the results are equally inconclusive. In one series electrophysiological auditory tests suggested both cochlear and retrocochlear dysfunction (Abramovich and Prasher, 1986), while other workers concluded that the primary lesion was cochlear using similar electrophysiological tests (Kusakari *et al.*, 1988). In contrast, a vestibular study based on galvanic responses in both Bell's palsy and the Ramsay Hunt syndrome identified retrocochlear dysfunction (Watanabe *et al.*, 1993). This diversity of findings would suggest that both sites may be involved, perhaps dependent on such factors as the severity of infection, host response and the association of anterograde/retrograde neural degeneration with cochlear/vestibular damage, as mentioned in the introduction to VIIIth nerve disorders.

Vestibular dysfunction has been described in *Bell's palsy*, or idiopathic facial palsy, by several authors (Koizuka *et al.*, 1988; Yagi, Yamaguchi and Nonaka, 1988) and an incidence of between 20 and 92% has been quoted. The wide variation in these figures could arise from differing intervals between the onset of the palsy and vestibular testing as it has been shown that abnormal vestibular function resolves within a period of weeks. Despite the high occurrence of vestibular abnormalities, there is general agreement that the presence of vestibular abnormalities is not of significant value prognostically (Adour and Doty, 1973; Uri and Schuchman, 1986). Many mechanisms for this vestibular involvement have been postulated including compression of the VIIIth nerve by the oedematous VIIth nerve, and involvement of both VIIth and VIIIth cranial nerves in the same disease process.

In addition, there is evidence that the pathology in Bell's palsy is not limited to ipsilateral VIIth and VIIIth cranial nerves. Adour and Doty (1973) found reduced caloric responses on the side contralateral to the palsy, and Safman (1971) reported subclinical involvement of the opposite side, as judged by electromyography and nerve conduction studies, in 75% of cases with Bell's palsy. Adour and colleagues (1980) have postulated that Bell's palsy is one expression of a cranial polyneuritis associated with the herpes simplex virus. In this respect, it is known that rheovirus, herpes simplex virus and rubeola virus may infect the ganglion cells of the vestibular ganglia. Uri,

Schuchman and Pratt (1984) found abnormalities of the auditory brain stem response in 25% of patients with Bell's palsy, characteristically, prolongation of brain stem conduction time which was not specifically related to the side of the palsy. Koizuka *et al.* (1988) reported abnormalities of optic fixation on electronystagmography, suggestive of central pathology. It has thus been suggested that, rather than being a mononeuropathy limited to the facial nerve, Bell's palsy may be a clinical sign of a diffuse central nervous system disorder.

Although the above description has dealt with the Ramsay Hunt syndrome and Bell's palsy separately, the demarcation line between these two entities is becoming increasingly blurred. Up to recent years it was thought that the Ramsay Hunt syndrome was synonymous with herpes zoster oticus. However, Lewis (1958) reported clinical Ramsay Hunt syndrome, but without evidence of herpes zoster infection, and Wayman *et al.* (1990) were able to confirm virologically herpes zoster in only 25% of their cases of Ramsay Hunt syndrome.

Conversely, other workers (Pietersen and Anderson, 1967; Djupesland *et al.*, 1975) found evidence of herpes zoster infection in patients thought to have idiopathic facial palsy, i.e. Bell's palsy, further pointing to the conclusion that the distinction may be purely a descriptive one and not based on truly different aetiologies. Nor has it been possible to differentiate the two conditions on the basis of viral serology, neuro-otological investigation (Yagi, Yamaguchi and Nonaka, 1988), galvanic body sway tests (Watanabe *et al.*, 1993) or gadolinium enhanced MRI scanning (Tada *et al.*, 1994). Thus the current thinking is that the separation of Ramsay Hunt and Bell's palsy is spurious and that there is much overlap in their aetiology or aetiologies, and indeed that both clinical entities may be accompanied by evidence of more widespread subclinical pathology in the central nervous system (Koizuka *et al.*, 1988; Wayman *et al.*, 1990).

The role of the *HIV* in causing dizziness is discussed in more detail in the sections on viral infections of the inner ear and of the central nervous system. Abnormalities of both central and vestibular dysfunction have been described both clinically (Hart *et al.*, 1989; Hausler *et al.*, 1991) and histopathologically (Hart *et al.*, 1989; Chandrasekhar, Siverls and Sekhar, 1992). No specific mention was made of the histology of the VIIIth nerve. However, as it is thought that the HIV virus is neurotropic, and it is known that it causes polyneuropathy, it would not be surprising if VIIIth nerve pathology contributed to the symptoms of dizziness/vertigo associated with HIV infection.

No discussion of the viral pathology of the VIIIth nerve is complete without some consideration of the controversial subject of *vestibular neuronitis*. The precise diagnosis and underlying pathology of vestibular neuronitis remains as elusive today as when the vestibular syndrome was initially outlined by Ruttin in 1909. The term vestibular neuronitis was first coined in 1949 and the first series, of 100 cases, published by Dix and Hallpike in 1952. Diagnostic criteria described in the classical paper consisted of an acute onset of vestibular symptoms, with decreased or absent caloric response, in the absence of cochlear or neurological deficits. These authors postulated that focal sepsis produced toxic damage to the VIIIth cranial nerve.

However, controversy exists about almost every aspect of this condition, many of which are summarized by Silvoniemi (1988) and Ryu (1993). Even the nomenclature is confusing and several terms have been used apparently interchangeably by different authors including vestibular neuritis, acute vestibular failure, vestibuloneuropathy among others.

The supposed absence of associated cochlear and CNS signs has been questioned. High frequency hearing losses have been documented (Aantaa and Virolainen, 1979; Rahko and Karma, 1986). Abnormalities of eye movements (Wennmo and Pyykkö, 1982), auditory brain stem responses (Rosenhall *et al.*, 1984) and EEG tracings all suggest more extensive CNS disease.

The number of aetiological agents postulated to cause vestibular neuronitis is legion, and include infections due to viruses, spirochaetes and toxoplasma, vascular disease and diabetes. Histopathological studies are few and inconclusive. Thus, not surprisingly, the clinical course is variable and unpredictable. In addition, contrary to previous beliefs, it is now recognized that the prognosis for so called vestibular neuronitis is not necessarily as favourable as was presumed (Matsuo and Sekitani, 1985; Okinaka *et al.*, 1993). Indeed many patients initially thought to have relatively trivial 'vestibular neuronitis' subsequently required revision of the diagnosis to disorders such as benign positional vertigo, Menière's disease or cerebellar infarct (Wallace and Barber, 1983; Magnusson and Norrving, 1993) with the obvious therapeutic and prognostic implications.

Thus, as a diagnosis of vestibular neuronitis has no value in terms of aetiology, management or prognosis, it is an unhelpful term to use as once such a label is attached it may be felt that further investigation is unnecessary and a favourable prognosis can be anticipated. On the contrary, full neuro-otological investigation is warranted and perhaps in this way it will be possible in the course of time to identify characteristics of the different aetiologies which at present are included under the umbrella term of vestibular neuronitis.

Bacterial and mycotic infections

Bacterial meningitis is an important cause of acquired hearing loss, usually in childhood. Approximately

5% of children with bacterial meningitis will go on to have severe or profound deafness. The site of the lesion is unclear. It is thought that suppurative labyrinthitis (Kay, 1991) is important aetiologically but the VIIIth nerve may also be involved (Harada *et al.*, 1988). The incidence of vestibular disturbance as a result of bacterial meningitis is less well documented. Rasmussen, Johnsen and Bohr (1991) reported that of 94 survivors, nine patients with vertigo and 13 with vestibular areflexia were identified between 4 and 16 years after pneumococcal meningitis. Naess *et al.* (1994) found audiovestibular complications in 13 of a series of 93 patients 1 year after meningococcal disease. Clinically, Aust (1994) found peripheral vestibular lesions in 60 of 106 labyrinths from 53 children examined. He also reported 29 cases of central vestibular dysfunction.

The most common organisms causing bacterial meningitis are *Streptococcus pneumoniae*, *Meningococcus* and *Haemophilus influenzae*. Although the immediate mortality is greatest with meningococcal meningitis, cranial nerve involvement is more common in survivors of pneumococcal meningitis, due to involvement of the basal meninges.

Other causes of basilar meningitis include tuberculosis, cryptococcosis, and coccidioidomycosis and these may affect multiple cranial nerves, including the VIIIth (Maslan, Graham and Flood, 1985; Baloh and Honrubia, 1990a). Igarashi and co-workers (1975) reported a marked reduction in the cochlear and vestibular nerve fibres within the internal auditory meatus, and damage to the auditory and vestibular receptor organs in the temporal bones of a young woman who died of cryptococcal meningitis, whereas McGill (1978) identified neuronal loss but with good preservation of the hair cells. Although the latter organisms are still relatively rare causes of meningitis in the Western world, their incidence has increased in recent years particularly with the advent of the human immunodeficiency virus (HIV), and its attendant immunodeficient state.

Two other bacterial infections, petrositis and malignant otitis externa, may affect the VIIIth nerve as well as the labyrinth, and have previously been discussed in the section on infections of the inner ear.

Syphilitic labyrinthitis has been discussed above. It was estimated by Jerger and Jerger in 1981 that VIIIth nerve involvement secondary to syphilitic meningitis occurred in only about 0.2% of patients with syphilis. However, Smith and Canalis (1989) and Dreier *et al.* (1993) have suggested that concomitant infection with the HIV virus, even without any clinical manifestations, may alter the natural history of syphilis and hasten the development of otosyphilis. Thus HIV infection should be considered in every patient with otosyphilis and conversely syphilis sought in patients, known to be HIV positive, who have unexplained otological symptoms.

Another spirochaete, *Borrelia burgdorferi*, causes the multisystem condition known as *Lyme disease*. The spirochaete infects humans by way of a tick bite. The initial manifestation is usually of the skin, erythema chronicum migrans, often in association with an influenza-like illness. Within 2 weeks to 2 years acute systemic illness may occur, affecting the heart and joints. Infection of the nervous system (neuroborreliosis) occurs within 6 months to 2 years, giving rise to abnormalities of both the central and peripheral nervous systems (Halperin *et al.*, 1989, 1990). Otolaryngological manifestations, including sensorineural hearing loss, tinnitus and vertigo have been described (Rosenhall, Hanner and Kaijser, 1988; Hanner *et al.*, 1989; Lesser, Dort and Simen, 1990). Lesser, Dort and Simen (1990) found that dizziness affects 12% of patients with Lyme disease. Rosenhall, Hanner and Kaijser (1988) studied 73 patients with a primary complaint of vertigo and found that 10 (14%) had serological evidence of borreliosis, although a cause–effect relationship cannot be presumed. Takahashi (1993) urged caution in making the assumption of a causal relationship between the serological findings and the vertigo and pointed out the absence of any pathological study confirming the presence of the organism in nervous tissue.

Ishizaki, Pyykko and Nozue (1993) reported 350 patients who presented with symptoms of vertigo, sensorineural hearing loss or facial nerve paresis and who were tested for antibodies against *Borrelia burgdorferi*. They found 12 patients with elevated levels of antibody on ELISA testing of serum and in six the CSF was positive on ELISA testing. In nine of these the major symptom was vertigo. Both central and peripheral vestibular abnormalities were documented which they attributed to the neuroborreliosis affecting central vestibular connections and the VIIIth nerve respectively. Rosenhall, Hanner and Kaijser (1988) found positional vertigo, both central and peripheral in nature, in all 10 patients who had vertigo and serological evidence of *Borrelia* infection.

Neuroborreliosis appears to affect the white matter of the nervous system, but the exact pathogenesis still remains unclear. It had been thought that it was a demyelinating disorder and parallels had been drawn between it and multiple sclerosis, not least of all because both conditions can give rise to such widespread lesions of the nervous system. However, Halperin *et al.* (1990) suggested, from electrophysiological studies on peripheral nerves, that demyelination is rarely if ever the pathology seen in Lyme disease and that the occasionally reported association between the diagnosis of multiple sclerosis and infection with *Borrelia burgdorferi* is purely coincidental and not causal. Two other reports (Schmutzhard, Pohl and Stanek, 1988; Coyle, 1989) also refute the association between multiple sclerosis and Lyme disease. It may be that axonal damage is a more likely mechanism of nerve dysfunction, possibly caused by a vascular neuropathy or by autoimmune damage.

The diagnosis of neuroborreliosis is important and must be considered particularly as reversal of both the peripheral and central nervous system symptoms with appropriate antibiotic treatment is well documented (Halperin *et al.*, 1989, 1990). In addition, Ishizaki, Pyykko and Nozue (1993) reported that their patients with vertigo, thought to be caused by *Borrelia*, responded to treatment with intravenous cephalosporin, further evidence that Lyme disease was the cause of the vertigo.

Vascular disease

The vertebrobasilar circulation supplies the VIIIth cranial nerve, as well as the peripheral labyrinth and the brain stem. Ischaemia of the nerve may occur but precise definition of the site of pathology may prove impossible clinically (Luxon, 1980). This is compounded by the fact that the majority of patients in whom vascular disease is suspected are over 60 years of age, and present with histories of previous cardiovascular disease, hypertension, or vertebrobasilar insufficiency. Morrison (1975) has reported a case of sudden unilateral VIIIth nerve dysfunction in a patient with heart block and a history of two previous cerebrovascular episodes. Other less common causes of arterial occlusion which may affect the VIIIth nerve include the subclavian steal syndrome, polycythaemia, emboli, including those associated with cardiopulmonary bypass (Kessler and Patterson, 1970), arteritis and the hyperviscosity syndrome.

Amarenco and Hauwe (1990) have reported auditory and/or vestibular symptoms and/or signs in eight out of 13 patients with infarction of the anterior inferior cerebellar artery. Histologically half of these patients had involvement of the VIIIth nerve, and in one this was the only manifestation. The internal auditory artery arises from the anterior inferior cerebellar artery in 83% of people, and thus this finding is not unexpected. Therefore, anterior inferior cerebellar artery infarction may cause occlusion of the internal auditory artery, ischaemia of the VIIIth nerve fibres in the lateral pontine area and damage at the level of the vestibular nuclei or the flocculus and its connections. In all but one, there were multiple cranial nerve palsies.

Lindsay and Hemenway (1956) reported on a small group of patients with sudden severe vertigo associated with nausea and vomiting, which subsided after a few days and was replaced by a positional vertigo. The temporal bone of one of these patients showed degeneration of part of Scarpa's ganglion with severe atrophy of the superior division of the vestibular nerve and its associated macula and cristae. Although a mass of convoluted vessels in the internal auditory meatus suggested a vascular aetiology for these findings, Schuknecht and Kitamura (1981) postulated that these changes could alternatively, be in keeping with a viral aetiology.

The anterior inferior cerebellar artery forms a loop before it supplies the pons and cerebellum and this loop lies inside the internal meatus in 40% of people, at the porus in 27%, and in the cerebellopontine angle in 33% (Mazzoni, 1969). Thus it is not surprising that aneurysms (Porter and Eyster, 1973; Mori, Miyazaki and Ono, 1978) and large vascular loops (Mafee *et al.*, 1985) of the anterior inferior cerebellar artery may compress the VIIIth cranial nerve and give rise to vestibular and auditory symptoms, clinically indistinguishable from other cerebellopontine angle lesions. Applebaum and Valvassori (1984) documented ipsilateral hearing loss in 10 patients with large vascular loops and McCabe and Harker (1983) suggested such vascular loops to be a cause of episodic vertigo in their eight patients. Phelps and Lloyd (1990c) demonstrated a double loop of the anterior inferior cerebellar artery in a patient with vertigo. Compression of the VIIth and VIIIth nerves by an anomalous vertebral artery has also been reported (Ohashi *et al.*, 1992). The correct diagnosis is made at angiography, air meatography (Phelps and Lloyd, 1982) or using magnetic resonance (Mosley, 1988).

Neoplasia

As in all sites, neoplasia may be divided into malignant and benign tumours. Malignant disorders, involving the VIIIth cranial nerve, are rarely of temporal bone origin and are more usually the result of secondaries (see above) which may either arise from contiguous areas and compress the nerve, or metastases arising from a remote site.

Vestibular schwannoma

Acoustic neuromas, or more correctly, vestibular schwannomas, are discussed separately in Volume 3 Chapter 21, and will be dealt with only briefly in this section.

The majority are said to arise within the internal acoustic meatus from the Schwann cells of the superior division of the vestibular part of the VIIIth nerve. However, Clemis *et al.* (1986) suggested that many more than were previously thought may arise from the inferior division of the vestibular nerve or from the cochlear division. Vestibular schwannomas account for 8–10% of intracranial neoplasms and 70–80% of cerebellopontine angle tumours. Bilateral tumours are characteristically associated with the autosomal dominant condition neurofibromatosis type 2 discussed earlier.

Although unilateral high frequency hearing loss is the most common presenting symptom, hearing loss of any configuration, tinnitus and vertigo/dizziness/unsteadiness may all occur in any combination. Although symptoms are typically constant and progressive, Morrison (1984) reported that 5% of patients with VIIIth nerve tumours suffer paroxysmal attacks of vertigo, which may mimic Menière's disease, while 16% suffer momentary vertigo or dizziness on sudden head movements and 8% may suffer acute vestibular failure with or without hearing loss during the course of the disorder. Other clinical symptoms and signs include involvement of the Vth and VIIth cranial nerves, encroachment upon the cerebellum, displacement of the brain stem and raised intracranial pressure.

Although gadolinium enhanced MRI scanning is the single most sensitive test for the diagnosis of vestibular schwannoma, with only few false-positive (Von Glass *et al.*, 1991) and no false-negative results reported, several problems may arise. As there is a discrepancy between the incidence of clinically significant tumours (1:100 000/year) and those found at post mortem (0.03–2.4%), and it has been shown that small tumours do not invariably enlarge with time (Bederson *et al.*, 1991), the high sensitivity of MRI scanning may mean that clinically insignificant tumours may be detected, thus causing unnecessary anxiety and leading to an excessive number of potentially dangerous and costly operations. This has to be balanced against the significantly decreased mortality/morbidity associated with surgery for smaller tumours.

Thus, in addition to merely establishing the presence or absence of a vestibular schwannoma, audiovestibular investigations will yield information about the clinical significance as well as the exact site of the tumour, which may influence the subsequent surgical approach taken, and the prognosis for the preservation of hearing (Wilson *et al.*, 1992). The last factor has important implications for preoperative counselling.

Tumours other than vestibular schwannomas account for 25% of all cerebellopontine angle tumours, and include meningiomas, epidermoid cysts, neuromas of the Vth and VIIth cranial nerves and brain stem gliomas. Prasher *et al.* (1991) have reported that patients with cerebellopontine angle tumours other than vestibular schwannomas are more likely to have normal hearing, no stapedial reflex decay, normal caloric tests, bilateral abnormalities on auditory brain stem responses and central abnormalities on electronystagmography including broken pursuit, abnormal optokinetic nystagmus and saccades. In addition, meningiomas are identifiable on angiography as vascular tumours with major feeding vessels arising from the external carotid circulation. Epidermoid cysts, which classically cause erosion of the petrous apex visible on routine skull radiographs, also show a characteristic scalloped surface contour on posterior fossa myelography.

Paraneoplastic syndromes

Additionally, audiovestibular symptoms can occur as manifestation of a paraneoplastic syndrome. A para-neoplastic syndrome is the occurrence of signs and symptoms in association with a malignant tumour, but not directly related to the site of the tumour or its metastases. The pathophysiological mechanism of neurological paraneoplastic syndrome is not proven, though autoimmune mechanisms have been postulated (Gulya, 1993). McGill (1976) described sudden onset hearing loss and vertigo associated with degeneration of the cochlear and both divisions of the vestibular nerve in a patient with oat-cell carcinoma of the lung. The vestibular nuclei were normal. Gulya (1993) described a case with very similar symptoms and pathological findings. A 56-year-old woman with advanced oat-cell carcinoma of the lung, developed sudden unilateral hearing loss, tinnitus and vertigo. At autopsy the cochlea, maculae and cristae were normal but there was an almost complete loss of vestibular and cochlear afferent neurons and demyelination of the VIIIth nerve. Loss of neuronal cells in the cochlear nuclei was seen, but the vestibular nuclei were normal. Further neuropathological examination revealed neuronal loss in the brain stem and cervical cord. A diagnosis of paraneoplastic encephalomyelitis was made.

Though paraneoplastic syndromes are rare, occurring in less than 1% of patients with cancer (Anderson, Cunningham and Posner, 1987), their identification is of importance in that the recognition of this syndrome affects the management and prognosis of the patient. In addition, the symptoms of neurological paraneoplastic syndromes may predate those of the underlying malignancy in almost two-thirds of cases (Croft and Wilkinson, 1969) and if recognized as such could lead to earlier diagnosis with improvement of outcome.

Carcinomatous meningitis

Carcinomatous meningitis, secondary to systemic cancer, is a well documented cause of both hearing impairment and vestibular symptomatology. Symptoms of the VIIIth nerve have been reported in 10% of patients with this condition (Alberts and Terrence, 1978). The hallmark of carcinomatous meningitis is the simultaneous occurrence of symptoms and signs in more than one area of the neuraxis. Olson, Chernik and Posner (1974) emphasized that neurological signs are much more prominent than the symptoms. The clinical diagnosis is confirmed by the presence of malignant cells in the cerebrospinal fluid. In addition, Paparella *et al.* (1973) have reported that temporal bone examination of 11 of a series of 25 patients with various forms of leukaemia revealed infiltration of the VIIIth cranial nerve.

Metabolic disorders affecting the VIIIth nerve

Although the main otological pathology associated with *diabetes mellitus* appears to be in the labyrinth,

Kovar (1973) has described thickening of the walls of the vasa nervorum of the VIIIth nerve with demyelination and axonal beading.

In acquired *renal disease* audiovestibular symptoms are undoubtedly multifactorial in aetiology; coincidental ear disease, infection, inflammatory disorders, immunosuppression, uraemia, electrolyte disturbances, ototoxic drugs and genetic factors all playing a part in individual cases. Although the main histological findings reported involve the membranous labyrinth, degeneration of the VIIIth nerve has been documented and the question of the contribution of uraemic polyneuropathy has been raised (Bergstrom *et al.*, 1973).

The occurrence of vestibular symptoms in *otosclerosis* has been discussed previously. Sando, Hemenway and Miller (1974) studied the temporal bones of two patients with otosclerosis with vertiginous symptoms. They documented otosclerotic foci, in apposition to the superior vestibular nerve, with distal neural degeneration by encroachment upon the VIIIth cranial nerve in the internal auditory meatus.

Auditory and vestibular symptoms are well recognized in *Paget's disease*. However, the site of pathology or the mechanism of these symptoms remains controversial, as discussed in the section on metabolic bone disease affecting the inner ear. Vestibular symptoms usually take the form of progressive unsteadiness, but rarely, episodic vertigo has been described. It has been reported that the VIIIth nerve may be compressed by pagetic involvement of the bone of the internal auditory meatus (Applebaum and Clemis, 1977) or by microfibromas of the VIIIth nerve, but Khetarpal and Schuknecht (1990) found no correlation between vestibular symptoms and such histopathological findings in 26 temporal bones. It is most likely that vestibular symptoms may be multifactorial in aetiology, including damage to the neuroepithelia of the labyrinthine organs, fractures of the labyrinth, perilymphatic leaks as well as VIIIth nerve pathology.

Hypophosphataemic rickets, discussed in detail in the section on inner ear disease, is associated with deafness but very little work has been done on its possible vestibular manifestations. Though most of the literature on the deafness associated with the condition suggests that the primary defect is in the cochlea, the VIIIth nerve may be affected due to overgrowth of the bony internal auditory meatus compressing the nerve (Stamp and Baker, 1976).

Bone dysplasias affecting the VIIIth nerve

Fibrous dysplasia is a moderately common disorder of unknown aetiology in which skeletal aberrations are associated with endocrinopathies and pigmentary disturbance. The disorder has a predilection for the craniofacial skeleton, and the temporal bone may be affected, causing compression of the VIIIth nerve (Nager, Kennedy and Kopstein, 1982).

The *osteopetroses* are a group of uncommon genetic disorders characterized by increased skeletal density and abnormalities of bone modelling. Miyamoto, House and Brackmann (1980) reported that symptoms of VIIth and VIIIth nerve dysfunction may be the first indication of one of these diseases. Both auditory and vestibular nerves may be affected.

Hyperostosis cranialis interna is an autosomal dominant disorder giving rise to hyperostosis of the skull base. Presenting symptoms include recurrent facial nerve palsy, and impairment of vision, smell, hearing and vestibular function, probably due to the encroachment of the hyperostotic bone into neural foramina and entrapment of the cranial nerves (Manni *et al.*, 1990).

Cammurati-Engelmann's disease or progressive diaphyseal dysplasia is a congenital hyperostotic skeletal dysplasia. A rare, progressive autosomal dominant bony disorder, it is characterized by deposition of sclerotic bone along the endosteal and periosteal surfaces of the diaphyses of long bones, base of skull and clavicle. Miyamoto, House and Brackmann (1980) have reported narrowing of cranial nerve foramina in 13% of patients, due to skull base involvement with resultant compression of the nerves or their vascular supply. The optic, facial and vestibulocochlear nerves are the first to be affected (Miyamoto, House and Brackmann, 1980). Vestibular symptoms may vary from persistent dizziness or dysequilibrium to episodic vertigo. Computed tomography and MRI scanning revealed marked flask-shaped narrowing of the internal auditory meatus in addition to the gross thickening of the entire skull base (Miyamoto, House and Brackmann, 1980). Conservative treatment with steroids has been reported partially to restore the associated sensorineural hearing loss. Surgical decompression of the nerve may also give partial and temporary relief of audiovestibular and facial symptoms (Miyamoto, House and Brackmann, 1980).

Toxic disorders

Thalidomide has been documented to produce aplasia of the VIIIth cranial nerve (Jorgenson, Kristensen and Buch, 1964; Phelps, 1983) with or without dysplasia of the labyrinth. As a consequence of the teratogenic effects of thalidomide its use has been severely curtailed in the last 30 years. However, recently it has proved successful in the treatment of many disorders, including erythema nodosum leprosum (Sampaio *et al.*, 1993), Behçet's disease, primary biliary cirrhosis (Rhoton, 1993), recurrent giant aphthous ulceration (Menni *et al.*, 1993) and persistent aphthous ulceration in HIV-positive patients (Ghigliotti *et al.*, 1993).

Poisoning with both lead and mercury is known to produce auditory and vestibular symptoms, but the pathophysiological mechanisms of these symptoms are poorly understood (Mizukoshi *et al.*, 1975).

Animal studies in *lead poisoning* have been controversial, with 75% of young guinea-pigs showing extensive segmental demyelination and axonal degeneration of the VIIIth cranial nerve following weekly intraperitoneal injections of 1% lead (Gozdzik–Zolnierkiewicz and Moszynski, 1969), while adult squirrel monkeys were unaffected (Wilpizeski, 1974). This discrepancy may be due to reduced susceptibility of the adult nervous system to lead toxicity. No human studies have been reported.

While a high incidence of auditory and vestibular abnormalities has been described following *mercury poisoning* no temporal bone or VIIIth nerve studies are available to identify the pathological site of dysfunction (Mizukoshi *et al.*, 1975).

Immunological disorders

There is a number of reports in the literature of retrocochlear hearing loss consequent upon immunological disorders, but reports of vestibular symptoms are rare. Morrison (1975) reported the case of a 17-year-old girl who developed retrocochlear deafness with vertigo after a hypersensitivity reaction to ampicillin. A good recovery was made following treatment with corticosteroids and it was postulated that an autoimmune mechanism was responsible.

Auditory and vestibular abnormalities are well documented in many autoimmune disorders, as outlined above, but there is no evidence of vestibular nerve involvement. In most forms of autoimmune disease such as polyarteritis nodosa (Gussen, 1977), Wegener's granulomatosis (Watanuki, Kawamoto and Kakizaki, 1975), Cogan's syndrome (Zechner, 1980) or Behçet's syndrome (Brama and Fainaru, 1980), the primary pathological lesion seems to be end organ dysfunction with secondary neural degeneration. However, in Hashimoto's disease (Stephens, 1970) and rheumatoid arthritis, primary neural degeneration has been described.

Five per cent of patients with sarcoidosis develop a granulomatous meningitis which directly infiltrates the cranial nerves. The VIIIth nerve is the fourth most frequently affected cranial nerve, and the resultant vestibular symptoms may be the first manifestation of neurosarcoidosis (Jahrsdoerfer *et al.*, 1981). Steroid therapy may improve the audiovestibular symptoms in sarcoidosis providing therapy is commenced early before irreversible changes have occurred in the VIIIth nerve and/or inner ear (Brihaye and Halama, 1993).

Neurological conditions

A particular concern for the otologist is the differentiation of peripheral vestibular disorders from central nervous system disease. A clear understanding of central vestibular physiology is necessary if the correct interpretation of vestibular signs and investigations is to allow this differentiation to be made. An examination of the ocular movements, as part of the neuro-otological examination, is invaluable in locating vestibular pathology. The examination and tests are described in Chapter 21.

Cerebrovascular disease

The cerebral vessels are a site of predilection for atherosclerosis, together with the myocardial and peripheral vasculature. The specific risk factors identified with cerebral ischaemia are diabetes mellitus, an elevated haematocrit and hypertension.

Vertebrobasilar ischaemia

Vertebrobasilar insufficiency is defined as a state of transient decrease in the cerebral blood flow, without actual infarction, resulting in transient inability to meet the metabolic requirements of the brain. As it is a transient ischaemic episode, by definition, no fixed deficit should persist beyond 24 hours.

As the vertebrobasilar circulation supplies the vestibular labyrinth, VIIIth nerve, and brain stem (as well as the cerebellum and occipital lobes) vertebrobasilar ischaemia may give rise to end organ or VIIIth nerve dysfunction as described previously, but vestibular symptoms frequently arise as a result of ischaemia of the vestibular nuclei (and their connections), which occupy a large area in the lateral zone of the brain stem (Gillilan, 1964) and are particularly susceptible to a reduction in the blood flow in the vertebrobasilar system.

The pathophysiology of brain stem ischaemia has been reviewed by Caplan (1990). Atherosclerotic occlusion of the intra- and extracranial part of the vertebrobasilar system is the most common cause. Other causes of vascular events include embolism (from atherosclerotic plaques of proximal arteries or from a cardiac source), vasospasm, vertebral artery anomalies (Sheehan, Bauer and Meyer, 1960; Beaujeux *et al.*, 1992), rupture of aneurysms of the posterior circulation or vertebral artery dissection. The latter may be either spontaneous or traumatic. Fibromuscular dysplasia, a non-inflammatory, non-atheromatous arteriopathy of unknown cause may affect the vertebral artery and give rise to spontaneous dissection and/or occlusion. It is seen particularly in young people after cervical trauma or rotatory movements of the neck and is associated with cervical pain and vertebrobasilar signs and symptoms. Factors which decrease cardiac output (cardiac failure, aortic valve stenosis), postural/systemic hypotension and haematological disorders such as anaemia and hyperviscosity syndrome will also increase the risk of vertebrobasilar ischaemia.

Rarely, syphilitic endarteritis and the autoimmune

vasculitides, such as systemic lupus erythematosus, giant cell arteritis and polyarteritis nodosa, may give rise to transient ischaemic episodes in the vertebrobasilar territory.

Williams and Wilson (1962) reported vertigo as the first symptom in 48% of patients with vertebrobasilar insufficiency and subsequently Williams (1964) commented that vertigo occurred in almost two-thirds of patients with vertebrobasilar insufficiency, vertigo and visual changes being the two most frequent symptoms. Fisher (1967) reported that vertebrobasilar ischaemia gives rise to the following symptoms in order of frequency: dizziness and/or vertigo, dysarthria, numbness of the face, hemiparesis, headache and diplopia. Similarly, Luxon (1990), in a series of 40 patients with vertebrobasilar insufficiency, found that vertigo occurred in 75%, more than double the next most frequent symptoms of sensory disturbance, visual loss and dysarthria. Other common, although less frequently encountered, symptoms include oscillopsia, dimness of vision, visual field defects, transient blindness, dysphasia, drop attacks, alternating weakness of opposite sides of the body, dysaesthesia and cerebellar ataxia. The diversity of symptoms and signs reflects the close proximity of cranial nerve nuclei with motor and sensory tracts within the small confines of the brain stem. As both Fisher (1967) and Luxon (1990) stressed, vertigo in the absence or other brain stem signs or symptoms should not be diagnosed as being due to vertebrobasilar ischaemia.

Transient ischaemic attacks vary in duration but, by definition, must be less than 24 hours. Classical symptoms as outlined above do not present a diagnostic dilemma, but isolated episodes of vertigo, particularly in an elderly patient with other cardiovascular symptoms and signs, may give rise to diagnostic difficulties.

In differentiating peripheral vestibular dysfunction from vertebrobasilar episodes, tinnitus and deafness are unusual manifestations of vertebrobasilar ischaemia and, if present, are almost always accompanied by other symptoms and signs of brain stem involvement. However, although no patient complained of auditory symptoms in Luxon's (1990) series of 40 patients, one was found to have a unilateral high frequency sensorineural hearing loss without evidence of peripheral vestibular pathology and five others had bilateral symmetrical high frequency sensorineural hearing loss of greater degree than would be expected for their age. These auditory findings were consistent with Luxon's (1980) previous finding of such a hearing loss being the most common type in brain stem disorders. Huang *et al.* (1993) reported seven patients (from a series of 503) with vertebrobasilar occlusive disease whose presenting symptoms included a sudden bilateral sensorineural hearing impairment and tinnitus, in addition to vertigo, and these authors pointed out that hearing loss may not be as uncommon as was previously thought, and that it may carry a grave prognosis.

The diagnosis of vertebrobasilar ischaemia is usually based on eliciting a history of a combination of symptoms associated with the vertebrobasilar circulation in a patient over 50 years of age with relevant risk factors. By definition episodes are short lived and between attacks neurological examination is normal. Soft neuro-otological signs, indicative of both peripheral and central vestibular pathology, may be seen and further support the clinical impression of disease in the vertebrobasilar circulation. However, no characteristic pattern of neuro-otological findings has emerged in this disorder (Corvera *et al.*, 1980; Luxon, 1990).

In vertebrobasilar ischaemia conventional MRI scanning will be normal, unless a previous infarct has occurred. In recent years magnetic resonance angiography, although still in the experimental stages, has been shown to be of probable benefit in providing information on vascular anatomy and blood flow (Sartor, 1990). Kikuchi *et al.* (1993) reported a significantly greater incidence of slow blood flow as shown by MRI in elderly patients with vertigo and dizziness than in elderly patients without these symptoms. They further suggested that finding slow blood flow on MRI correlated with a high risk of further episodes of vertebrobasilar ischaemia and hypothesized that this may be due to a persistent narrowing of the vertebrobasilar system, rather than just vasospasm, and thus may have prognostic as well as diagnostic implications.

Although the risk of subsequent stroke in patients with vertebrobasilar transient ischaemic attacks is less than that of patients suffering carotid artery transient ischaemic attacks, great emphasis has been placed upon the early diagnosis of vertebrobasilar disease, on the assumption that intervention reduces this risk.

The *subclavian steal syndrome* is found in 3% of patients with vertebrobasilar symptoms. There is occlusion of the subclavian artery such that use of the involved upper limb causes reversal of blood flow in the vertebral artery on that side, so that it acts as a collateral to the upper limb. Blood is syphoned from the vertebrobasilar system into the distal subclavian artery (Figure 20.7). This diagnosis should be considered when claudication or fatigue of the upper limb is accompanied by vertebrobasilar symptoms. A systolic bruit in the supraclavicular fossa with a disparity of blood pressure between the two arms is the characteristic sign of this disorder.

Completed strokes

Cerebrovascular accidents of the posterior circulation, affecting the brain stem, such as the lateral and medial medullary syndromes, are commonly associated with dizziness and vertigo. These are discussed

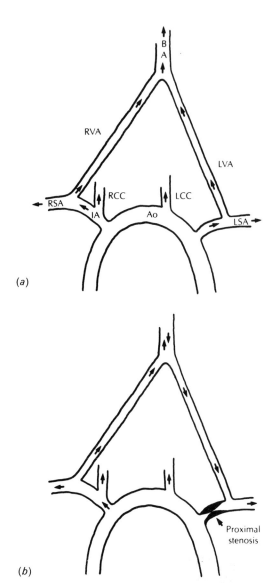

(a)

(b)

Figure 20.7 Subclavian steal syndrome. (*a*) Diagram to illustrate the flow of blood in the normal posterior circulation and (*b*) in a patient with a proximal stenosis in the left subclavian artery giving rise to the subclavian steal syndrome. BA: basilar artery; VA; vertebral artery; SA; subclavian artery; CC: common carotid artery; IA: innominate artery; Ao: Aorta; R: right; L: left. (From Luxon, L. M. (1984) Vertigo in old age. In: *Vertigo*, edited by M. R. Dix and J. D. Hood. Chichester: John Wiley and Sons Limited, with permission)

in detail in the section on brain stem disorders. Likewise cerebellar infarcts are discussed in the section on cerebellar disease.

Cerebrovascular disease affecting the internal carotid and middle cerebral artery system also, although

less often, gives rise to dizziness or vertigo. Fisher (1967) reported dizziness in 8% of patients with hemiplegic stroke or recurrent transient ischaemic attacks, most commonly in those with lesions of the non-dominant hemisphere. A recent large study of predictors of major vascular events following transient ischaemic attacks, has shown that the occurrence of rotatory vertigo in these patients is a protective predictor (The Dutch TIA study group, 1993). Although vestibulo-ocular function depends mainly on infratentorial structures it is also modified by the cerebral hemispheres (Leigh and Zee, 1991a).

Dysequilibrium after *hemispheric stroke* has usually been presumed to result from unilateral weakness and disordered proprioception and/or vision. Recently Catz *et al.* (1993, 1994) have shown abnormalities of the vestibulo-ocular reflex and vestibulo-ocular reflex suppression after infarcts affecting the internal capsule, parietal lobe, temporoparietal or frontoparietal areas of the cerebral hemispheres. They postulated that as impairment of the vestibulo-ocular integration occurs similar abnormalities of vestibulospinal activity may arise, thus contributing, at least to some degree, to the impairment of equilibrium seen after such strokes. These findings may have important implications in the rehabilitation of patients following strokes.

By far the commonest cause of strokes is atheromatous disease. However, *fibromuscular dysplasia* is a non-atheromatous, non-inflammatory, segmental arteriopathy of unknown aetiology, affecting mainly the tunica media. Symptoms and signs are caused either by occlusion of the affected artery or by spontaneous dissection. The condition has a predilection for the renal and carotid arteries, and when affecting the latter can give rise to vertigo, recurrent transient ischaemic attacks, and cerebral infarcts, in the same way as atheromatous occlusive disease described above (Sandmann *et al.*, 1992). Fibromuscular dysplasia can also affect the vertebral artery system, causing occlusion and giving rise to sudden onset dizziness. The diagnosis of fibromuscular dysplasia is based on the angiographic findings of beaded and tubular stenoses of the affected artery. The prognosis is generally good and treatment usually conservative. In a few cases angioplasty may be necessary. Sandmann *et al.* (1992) reported that of 15 patients, 13 made a good recovery and of these seven had no residual neurological deficit.

Migraine

Migrainous headache has been recognized throughout history, and its association with balance disorders and auditory symptoms was documented by Aretaeus (cited by Olsson, 1991) almost 2000 years ago. It is the most commonly encountered neurological disorder in the UK, affecting 5–10% of the population. It can be usefully classified into classic migraine, common migraine (or 'sick' headache) and complicated migraine. Classic migraine is preceded by neurological symptoms (the aura), such as flashing lights or scotomas, followed by unilateral throbbing headache associated with vomiting, photophobia and phonophobia. In 'sick headache' type migraine there is no aura, the throbbing headache is more often bilateral, but is associated with nausea and vomiting and photophobia. Complicated migraine implies that the neurological symptoms persist when the headache has subsided, such as occurs in hemiplegic or ophthalmoplegic migraine. Basilar artery migraine, first described by Bickerstaff in 1961, is a form of migraine particularly common in adolescent girls and closely related to the menstrual cycle. The aura lasts 2–45 minutes and consists of vertigo, ataxia, dysarthria, tinnitus and sensory disturbance in the distal limbs and around the lips, along with visual disturbances. The headache is more often occipital than hemicranial, but vertigo can be the most prominent symptom to such a degree that headache may not be mentioned unless specific enquiry is made. The specific symptoms described in basilar artery migraine are thought to be due to the disturbance being in the territory supplied by the vertebrobasilar rather than the carotid circulation (see below).

Parker (1991) reviewed the literature looking at the relationship between dizziness and vertigo in patients with migraine and concluded that there is a strong association between migraine and vertigo. The various studies reported that between 25% and 42% of patients with migraine also had episodic vertigo, and 43–54% of those with recurrent episodes of vertigo/dysequilibrium had a history of migraine. Episodes of vertigo and dizziness may occur as part of the aura of migraine, may accompany the headache, occur paroxysmally during headache-free periods, occur as part of the 'migraine syndrome' but without headache being a symptom, i.e. as a migraine equivalent, or as a precursor of migraine in a patient with no history of headache when first presenting with vertigo, but who subsequently develops migrainous headaches months or even years later.

Although the aetiology of migraine remains poorly understood, it used to be thought that vascular disturbances played a key role. However, the theory that vasoconstriction of intracranial blood vessels gives rise to the symptoms of the aura and subsequent vasodilation causes the headache is probably an oversimplification. Results of blood flow studies performed during the phases of migraine, quoted by Parker (1991), show that the correlation between the hypoperfused or hyperperfused areas of the central nervous system and the symptoms was poor. Thus the situation is probably more complex, and inflammatory processes, the generation of vasoactive substances and autoregulatory mechanisms may be involved. Alternative, although not necessarily mutually exclusive, theories of the genesis of migraine, including a neural theory, have been discussed by Olsson (1991). The neural theory suggests that the primary disorder is in the brain itself and that vascular changes are secondary. The nature of the neural disorder is unknown but may be related to changes in spontaneous neural activity with associated changes in intraneuronal metabolism altering local blood flow. A combination of both theories is possible. Cutrer and Baloh (1992) proposed two separate pathophysiological mechanisms to explain the dizziness: short duration vertiginous attacks lasting from a few minutes to 2 hours, temporarily associated with the headache, due to transient vasospasm and/ or a spreading wave of depression of spontaneous neural activity, and longer duration attacks of vertigo and motion sickness with or without a headache, lasting days, due to the release of vasoactive peptides into the peripheral and central vestibular structures, and causing an increased baseline firing of primary afferent neurons and increased sensitivity to motion. Of relevance to these theories, Olesen (1990) reported that calcium antagonists with primarily vasoactive properties were less efficacious for migraine prophylaxis than those thought to act via a neural mechanism, thus supporting a neural role in the generation of migraine.

Whatever the pathophysiological mechanism, familial factors also appear to be important in the aetiology of migraine. Patients with migraine were quoted in Parker's review (1991) to have a positive family history of migraine in 55–65% of cases. Likewise over 50% of patients primarily complaining of recurrent vertigo had a family history of migraine. Interestingly, Baloh, Jacobson and Fife (1994) found a strong history of migraine in other family members of patients with a newly described dominantly inherited familial vestibulopathy syndrome. Although a relationship between migraine and Menière's disease has often been claimed (Hinchcliffe, 1967; Kayan and Hood, 1984) there is not universal agreement on this issue. Rassekh and Harker (1992) suggested that there is no such aetiological relationship, and that in addition, the increase in prevalence of migraine which they reported in patients with so called 'vestibular Menière's' was because these patients' vertigo was a form of migraine equivalent and not Menière's disease in the first place. In fact they questioned the existence of 'vestibular Menière's' as a separate entity and suggested that it was not a valid diagnostic group at all!

Parker (1991) suggested that the site of the pathology giving rise to vertigo in migraine – whether it be due to neural, vascular, or other pathology – may be cortical, brain stem or the peripheral vestibular endorgan. Olsson (1991) concluded that the vertigo occurring in association with basilar artery migraine is usually due to central dysfunction but that in a small percentage of cases the peripheral end organ is affected.

Thus the strong association of vertigo/dizziness with migraine, underlines the importance of establishing a personal or family history of migraine or migraine equivalents, in any patient with paroxysmal vertigo (Harker and Rassekh, 1988), especially as antimigrainous medication may prevent the distressing symptoms.

Multiple sclerosis

Multiple sclerosis is a demyelinating disease of uncertain aetiology which usually affects young and middle-aged adults. It follows a relapsing remitting course in most, though a malignant and rapidly progressive course in 5–10%. It is one of the most commonly encountered conditions in neurological practice. Multiple sclerosis is characterized by lesions of demyelination which occur randomly in time and space. The diagnosis is usually based on clinical criteria (e.g. of Schumacher *et al.*, 1965 or Rose *et al.*, 1976), supplemented by characteristic investigative findings on examination of the cerebrospinal fluid (elevated protein, lymphocyte count and the presence of oligoclonal bands), abnormalities of electrophysiological potentials (visual evoked potentials, auditory brain stem responses, and somatosensory responses) and magnetic resonance imaging.

Vertigo and dizziness are common complaints at some time during the course of the disease in patients who have definite multiple sclerosis (Rudge, 1983), and vertigo is the initial symptom in approximately 5–10% of cases. It has been reported that vertigo, as an onset symptom, was a poor prognostic indicator for life expectancy (Riise *et al.*, 1988). Neurologically, as the disease is characterized by disseminated lesions, the presentation is infinitely variable, but certain features deserve special mention because of the consistency of their occurrence. Retrobulbar neuritis, with blurring and/or loss of vision and pain in or behind the eye, is associated with demyelination of the optic nerve and is an initial presenting symptom in approximately 20% of cases. Diplopia, limb weakness, sensory disturbances and ataxia also occur early in the course of the disease and are due to an intranuclear ophthalmoplegia resulting from lesions of the medial longitudinal fasciculus in the pons and mesencephalon (Rivera, 1990). In longstanding cases, examination frequently reveals involvement of the pyramidal tracts, with hyperreflexia and extensor plantar responses; cerebellar signs of intention tremor, dysdiadochokinesia, ataxia and dysarthria; sensory involvement and visual disturbance. Psychological changes are also common (Rivera, 1990).

Neuro-otologically, multiple sclerosis is characterized by derangement of eye movements. Pursuit has been reported to be almost always deranged and a high incidence of saccadic abnormalities has also been reported. Spontaneous nystagmus occurs in many patients with multiple sclerosis, over the age of 40 years, and positional nystagmus of the central type is also commonly seen (Katsarkas, 1982; Rosenhall, 1988). Grenman (1985) examined 70 patients, all of whom fulfilled Schumacher's criteria for definitive multiple sclerosis. Only one patient exhibited normal results on all neuro-otological tests used. Abnormalities of smooth pursuit occurred in 96%, of saccadic eye movement in 76%, of optokinetic nystagmus in 53%, of visual suppression in 43% and of caloric testing in 40%. He concluded that a completely normal otoneurological and audiological assessment is so atypical of multiple sclerosis as to suggest strongly that an alternative diagnosis should be considered.

Acquired pendular nystagmus and dissociated nystagmus are particularly valuable diagnostic pointers in multiple sclerosis, as they are relatively unusual findings in other disease processes. Vertical nystagmus is another frequent finding, in particular upbeat nystagmus. Cerebellar and brain stem lesions may result in abnormalities of nystagmus induced by rotation or caloric testing. Caloric responses in the presence of optic fixation are commonly symmetrically enhanced (Huygen, 1983; Grenman, 1985) and, characteristically, removal of optic fixation does not enhance the vestibular response. This is mostly probably the result of disruption of the cerebellar pathways to the vestibular nuclei. Brain stem involvement at the level of the vestibular nuclei may give rise to a canal paresis, with or without a directional preponderance.

Many authors stress the importance of multimodal electrophysiological testing, (including visual, somatosensory and auditory evoked potentials) an audiovestibular test battery (Grenman, 1985) including both objective and subjective audiological tests (Protti-Patterson and Young, 1985) in the detection of lesions especially in the face of negative MRI scan results, and in monitoring responses to drug therapy (Herrera, 1990; Jacobson and Jacobson, 1990). Many authors acknowledge the importance of imaging techniques especially MRI scanning with gadolinium enhancement, in the detection of scattered/multiple CNS lesions in this condition. However, Grenman *et al.* (1988) reported that otoneurological findings using electronystagmography were the most sensitive indicators of lesions in the brain stem or cerebellum, even superior to MRI.

Trauma

Closed head injury, most commonly due to sudden deceleration, may give rise to dizziness. Even quite minor injuries can cause petechial haemorrhages in the brain stem and vestibular nuclei. However, Mitchell and Adams (1973) emphasized that isolated brain stem involvement is uncommon and is generally associated with other CNS damage. Symptoms such as headache, emotional lability, insomnia and poor concentration and information processing skills, usually coexist. Vertigo in isolation should not be attributed to brain stem injury, but may arise from damage to the VIIIth nerve.

Infection

Viral infection

Viral encephalitis may involve the vestibular nuclei, as well as the nerve roots. The clinical history and findings on examination may suggest the diagnosis, which is confirmed by examination of the cerebrospinal fluid.

Acquired immune deficiency syndrome has been previously discussed in the section on inner ear disorders. Many of the manifestations of AIDS are related to opportunistic infections caused by the immunodeficient state. However, the CNS appears to be directly infected by the HIV virus itself (Carne and Adler, 1986), causing subacute encephalitis and dementia with associated myelopathy and polyneuropathy. Hart *et al.* (1989) found vestibular dysfunction of central origin in one patient with AIDS. These clinical findings were in keeping with pathological changes found at autopsy, in the cerebrum, cerebellum and brain stem. Hausler *et al.* (1991) examined 43 patients with HIV infection, and found a high incidence of central audiovestibular abnormalities in those with stage IV disease. Two patients had concomitant peripheral vestibular deficits. In addition, more than one-third of the asymptomatic HIV-positive patients had signs of CNS involvement on neuro-otological testing. These observations are in keeping with the report of Koenig *et al.* (1986) of neurological dysfunction being clinically evident in only one-third of patients with AIDS, whereas post-mortem neuropathological examination reveals disease of the central nervous system in over 75% of cases. Thus it may be that neuro-otological investigation may be a useful tool in detecting subtle changes in patients with early disease and monitoring the effect of therapy. On the other hand, HIV infection should be considered in patients with unexplained audiovestibular abnormalities, even if clinically there are no other symptoms of HIV infection.

Bacterial/mycotic infection

Bacterial meningitis can give rise to dizziness/vertigo, probably due to involvement of the VIIIth nerve. This is particularly so with infections such as tuberculosis, cryptococcidiosis and coccidioidomycosis which cause a basilar meningitis.

Intracranial complications of middle ear infection are rare in the western world, since the advent of effective antibiotics for acute otitis media. However, they have not completely disappeared. Extradural abscess, subdural abscess, lateral sinus thrombosis, cerebral abscess or meningitis may occur. Usually other symptoms such as fever, headache, vomiting or fits take precedence over complaints of imbalance. In the case of a cerebellar abscess, ataxia may be prominent, though may be difficult to elicit if the patient is examined on the bed only and the lesion affects the midline giving rise to truncal ataxia without limb ataxia. Asymmetric gaze evoked nystagmus may be seen.

Lyme disease, caused by the spirochaete, *Borrelia burgdorferi*, affecting the VIIIth nerve has already been discussed. As well as its effect on peripheral and cranial nerves, involvement of the central nervous system giving rise to meningitis is also well recognized. In addition, Halperin *et al.* (1989) described an encephalopathy in association with this infection. They attributed this to active CNS disease on the basis of intrathecal antibody production against *Borrelia burgdorferi*, and MRI evidence of multifocal inflammatory lesions, which resolved with adequate antispirochaetal therapy. On neuro-otological examination Rosenhall, Hanner and Kaijser (1988) found evidence of both peripheral and central vestibular abnormalities in 10 patients with vertigo and borrelia infection. Ishizaki, Pyykko and Nozue (1993) also reported mild abnormalities of saccades, again suggestive of CNS pathology. These findings are in keeping with subsequent reporting of both peripheral and central nervous system manifestations (Halperin *et al.*, 1989, 1990) of this disease.

Basal ganglion disorders

Imbalance, alterations in gait, and postural abnormalities are commonplace in *Parkinson's disease*, which is one of the most common neurological disorders, occurring in about 1 in every 200 of the population over the age of 50 years. The disease is characterized by rigidity, akinesia and 4 Hz pill-rolling tremor, which is present at rest. The aetiology of Parkinson's disease is unknown. Current theories have been reviewed by Langston (1989), and include the role of ageing, free radical production, neuromelanin accumulation and other toxic agents in causing neuronal damage. A genetic vulnerability to the toxic effects of these agents is discussed, but twin studies do not support this view. Schapira (1994) discussed the very strong evidence for the existence of a defect in the mitochondrial respiratory chain in Parkinson's disease and its possible relevance to the pathogenesis of the disorder. He also discussed the possibility of this respiratory chain defect being related to an abnormality of mitochondrial DNA, though a recent report by Maraganore, Harding and Marsden (1991) showed little evidence in favour of the maternal transmission pattern expected of a mitochondrial DNA abnormality.

There are many reports in the literature of vestibular and oculomotor disorders in Parkinson's disease but much of the work is contradictory. Many of the inconsistencies may arise because the group of patients labelled Parkinson's disease clinically, may not be a pathologically homogeneous group, as other akinetic-rigid syndromes exist which may be misdiagnosed as Parkinson's disease. As discussed below it may be that neuro-otological investigation can contribute to the correct differentiation of these entities.

In the past, abnormal eye movements including convergence and gaze palsies (Corin, Elizon and Bender, 1972) and 'multiple step' type saccades (Cipparrone *et al.*, 1988) have been reported in patients thought to have Parkinson's disease. However, more recent reports suggest that patients with such abnormalities do not have idiopathic Parkinson's disease, but a different akinetic-rigid syndrome, e.g. multiple system atrophy. Similarly, vestibulo-ocular reflex suppression has been reported to be abnormal by some authors, but Rascol *et al.* (1993) found no statistically significant difference in the vestibulo-ocular reflex or suppression between normal subjects and patients with Parkinson's disease, when evaluated as a group. However 10% of patients with Parkinson's disease did show abnormalities of vestibulo-ocular reflex suppression and the authors questioned whether these patients may have a different extrapyramidal disease, rather than true Parkinson's disease.

Thus, Parkinson's disease must be differentiated from other akinetic-rigid syndromes, e.g. that of cerebrovascular disease, which is often accompanied by pyramidal signs and dementia but, in contrast to Parkinson's disease, tremor is almost never present. Demented patients with *Alzheimer's disease* may develop frank signs of basal ganglia dysfunction with akinesia, rigidity and instability late in the natural course of the disorder (Pearce, 1974). The relatively recently described *multiple system atrophy* is a degenerative disease of the central nervous system affecting many different structures including the pyramidal, extrapyramidal, cerebellar and autonomic systems. The pattern of involvement and thus the clinical signs may vary from patient to patient, and over time in any one patient. In addition, there is confusion about terminology as features of autonomic dysfunction in association with atypical Parkinson's disease, also occur in the so-called *Shy-Drager syndrome*. However, Quinn (1989) proposed that the Shy-Drager syndrome is not a separate entity in itself and the term should not be used. Multiple system atrophy is said to account for up to 10% of patients previously diagnosed as having parkinsonism (Quinn, 1989). Differential diagnosis is important as multiple system atrophy has a poorer prognosis than Parkinson's disease with no, or only transient, response to dopaminergic drugs. Indeed, dopaminergic drugs

often give rise to severe nausea and vomiting in patients with multiple system atrophy.

No one investigation will distinguish the two conditions and Quinn (1989) emphasized the need to look at the overall clinical picture in conjunction with a battery of investigations. Plasma noradrenalin levels, MRI scanning, positron emission tomography and nerve conduction studies have all been advocated as being useful for the differential diagnosis of Parkinson's disease and multiple system atrophy. Neuro-otological investigations may also be of use in this respect. Prasher and Bannister (1986) showed abnormalities of latency and of the ratio of the amplitude of wave V to wave I on testing the brain stem auditory evoked responses in patients with multiple system atrophy. However, Quinn (1989) suggested that these findings are only specific in the late stages of the disease. Rascol *et al.* (1993) found a significant reduction in vestibulo-ocular reflex suppression in patients with multiple system atrophy compared with both normal subjects and those with Parkinson's disease. This was particularly so if the patients showed clinical evidence of cerebellar dysfunction, but some patients with multiple system atrophy and abnormal vestibulo-ocular reflex suppression had no clinical evidence of a cerebellar lesion. They proposed that the abnormal vestibulo-ocular reflex suppression was evidence of subclinical cerebellar pathology but that the associated akinesia and rigidity masked the clinical features of cerebellar dysfunction, making the differential diagnosis more difficult clinically. Thus, the authors suggested that eye movement recording, by demonstrating abnormalities of visuovestibular interaction, may be of value to distinguish Parkinson's disease from multiple system atrophy.

The *Steele–Richardson–Olszewski* (1964) syndrome, whose aetiology remains unknown, may superficially resemble Parkinson's disease. It is characterized by marked axial rigidity, expressionless facies, mild dementia and a supranuclear palsy, while the combination of absence of tremor and relatively normal tone in the limbs may help in the differentiation of the two conditions. MRI scans show midbrain atrophy early in the course of the disease, with subsequent atrophy of the pons and frontal and temporal lobes. Histologically, it is characterized by the presence of neurofibrillary tangles, pathology being predominantly seen in the brain stem (Gibb, 1992). Although Lewy bodies are sometimes seen in this condition, they are thought to represent coincidental Parkinson's disease (Gibb and Lees, 1989). Vertical eye movements are affected before horizontal gaze, and voluntary eye movements before pursuit. Frequently, downgaze is more involved than upgaze and saccadic velocities are reduced (Dix, Harrison and Lewis, 1971). This disorder usually presents in the sixth decade of life, or later, and is progressive, with death occurring within 7 years of the first symptom. As in multiple system atrophy there is little response to conventional antiparkinsonian therapy.

The introduction of L-dopa has done much to alleviate the symptoms of idiopathic Parkinson's disease, a dramatic motor response almost always occurring. The opposite is true for patients with multiple system atrophy and other extrapyramidal disorders, who exhibit only a poor transient response to L-dopa, or even, in some cases, experience exacerbation of symptoms. In terms of management and prognosis, accurate diagnosis is therefore essential and idiopathic Parkinson's disease must be differentiated from drug-induced (phenothiazine and butyrophenones) Parkinson's syndrome, postencephalitic Parkinson's disease, benign essential tremor and other disorders of the basal ganglia as discussed above. The incidence of drug-induced parkinsonism increases with age (Ayd, 1961), as does idiopathic Parkinson's disease. Following withdrawal of a causative drug, it may take as long as 18 months for recovery to occur.

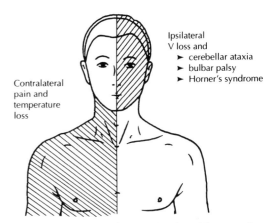

Figure 20.8 Diagram to illustrate the clinical features of Wallenberg's syndrome. (From Luxon, L. M. (1984) Vertigo in old age. In: *Vertigo*, edited by M. R. Dix and J. D. Hood. Chichester: John Wiley and Sons Limited, with permission)

Brain stem disease

Many disorders such as ischaemia (either occlusive or haemorrhagic), neoplasia, demyelinating disease, can affect the brain stem. Dizziness or vertigo are common symptoms of brain stem lesions. Neuro-otological assessment can be of great benefit in determining the site of pathology.

This association between vertigo and vertebrobasilar transient ischaemic attacks has been discussed above. Likewise in completed brain stem strokes, vertigo with oculomotor dysfunction is seen. The *Wallenberg (lateral medullary) syndrome* is one of the most widely recognized brain stem syndromes, usually caused by occlusion of the ipsilateral posterior inferior cerebellar artery, the vertebral artery, or occasionally by multiple sclerosis affecting that region. Characteristic features include ipsilateral dissociated sensory loss in the distribution of the facial nerve, contralateral truncal loss of pain and temperature sensation along with ipsilateral Horner's syndrome, bulbar palsy and limb ataxia (Figure 20.8).

One study (Kim *et al.*, 1994) reported that 91% of 33 patients with Wallenberg's syndrome complained of vertigo or dizziness, this being more marked with more caudal lesions. A second study, also of 33 patients found these symptoms in only 51% of patients (Sacco *et al.*, 1993). Typical neuro-otological findings include spontaneous nystagmus which may be horizontal with the fast phase away from the side of the lesion, upbeat nystagmus or a mixed pattern. Smooth pursuit is also impaired when tracking away from the side of the lesion. Saccade dysmetria with overshoot towards the side of the lesion and undershoot away from that side (ocular lateropulsion) has also been described (Benjamin, Zimmerman and Troost, 1986; Leigh and Zee, 1991b).

Medullary haemorrhage is far less common than infarction due to ischaemia as described above. Possible aetiologies include rupture of a vascular malformation, hypertension or anticoagulant therapy, but often the cause remains unknown. Nevertheless, vertigo is one of the most common presenting features (Mazagri, Shuaib and Denath, 1992; Barinagarrementeria and Cantu, 1994).

Pathology affecting the pontine region causes pursuit to the affected side to be impaired due to involvement of the parapontine reticular formation which is important for generating horizontal pursuit eye movements. However, such abnormalities are not specific to the pons since, as mentioned elsewhere, smooth pursuit is also impaired in medullary and cerebellar lesions or as a result of certain drugs. Indeed spontaneous nystagmus occurring in an acute peripheral vestibular pathology may intrude on the normal pursuit pattern and cause broken horizontal pursuit, though the gain remains normal, but with no central nervous system pathology. In addition, impaired velocity of saccades, though with preservation of accuracy, occurs in pontine lesions.

'Ocular bobbing', a disorder of vertical ocular movement, also occurs in pontine infarcts (Troost, 1990). The medial longitudinal bundle can be affected in the pons or midbrain, often caused by multiple sclerosis, and classically gives rise to internuclear ophthalmoplegia.

Midbrain lesions, commonly due to infarction, pineal tumours or multiple sclerosis, cause abnormalities of saccades and optokinetic nystagmus in the vertical plane, but with preservation of pursuit.

Primary *brain stem gliomas* (Figure 20.9) are unusual in adults but metastases, pineal tumours, haemangiomas and haemangioblastomas may occur. Diz-

In the figure labels:
Ipsilateral V loss and
► cerebellar ataxia
► bulbar palsy
► Horner's syndrome

Contralateral pain and temperature loss

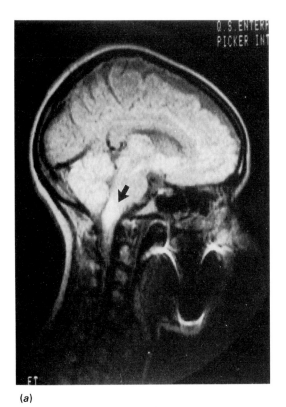

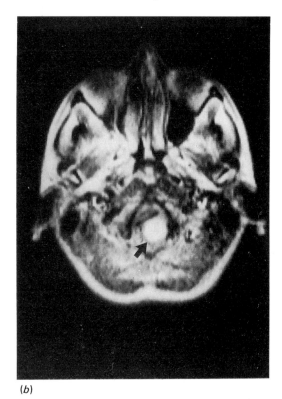

Figure 20.9 Magnetic resonance scans of patient with brain stem glioma (arrowed)

ziness or vertigo occurs early in the course of the disease in 25% of cases. Other features include progressive development of cranial nerve palsies associated with long tract signs. In addition to eye movement abnormalities, auditory tests may also have a role diagnostically. Bilateral symmetrical hearing loss has been described by Luxon (1980) and stapedial reflex (Jerger, Neely and Jerger, 1980) and auditory brain stem response measurements (Prasher, 1981) have been shown to be of value in brain stem neoplasia.

The *Arnold Chiari* malformation is a congenital deformity associated with hydrocephalus and other central nervous system malformations, such as syringomyelia and its extension into the medulla and pons known as syringobulbia. It is a malformation of the hindbrain and may involve the caudal cerebellum and caudal medulla. A variety of eye movement abnormalities in addition to auditory dysfunction may occur. The former include, downbeat nystagmus, gaze evoked, positional (central type), and rebound nystagmus. Smooth pursuit is impaired and saccadic dysmetria occurs. The gain of the vestibulo-ocular reflex is increased.

Although characteristically the caloric test is normal in brain stem pathology this is not always so. Francis *et al.* (1992) compared 10 patients with

canal paresis of central origin (lesions of the vestibular nuclei and fascicle) with 10 who had canal paresis due to peripheral vestibular pathology. In the central group the degree of paresis was less and no enhancement of nystagmus occurred with removal of optic fixation.

Brandt and Dieterich (1993) and Dieterich and Brandt (1993) reported that ocular torsion, and tilt of the subjective visual vertical plane were sensitive signs of brain stem pathology capable of both lateralizing the lesion and localizing it within the brain stem.

Cerebellar disease

Many different disorders affect the cerebellum, e.g. infection, neoplasia (direct involvement, metastases or paraneoplastic cerebellar degeneration), demyelinating disease, degenerative conditions (including many inherited conditions, myxoedema, alcoholism and phenytoin intoxication) (Figure 20.10), toxic disorders and Arnold–Chiari malformation, among others. The cerebellum may be affected in isolation or as part of a more widespread central nervous system disease.

Cerebellar disease typically presents with persistent symptoms of imbalance and unsteadiness, particularly on changes of head position, and less often with

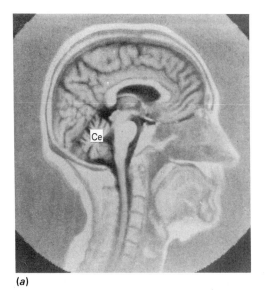
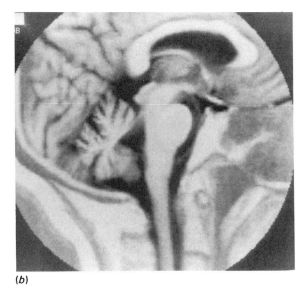

(a)   (b)

Figure 20.10 Magnetic resonance scans illustrating marked cerebellar atrophy with widening of the cerebellar sulci

rotatory vertigo. Episodic symptoms are unusual, except in inherited periodic ataxia. In 1922, Holmes described the classic cerebellar syndrome comprising gait and limb ataxia, hypotonia, disordered eye movements and slurred speech. However, midline cerebellar lesions may produce truncal ataxia as the only sign and, to the untrained eye, this may be misinterpreted as a hysterical gait disorder, particularly as the routine neurological examination carried out with the patient on the bed will fail to reveal any abnormality. Futhermore, lesions of the vermis may only manifest as an oculomotor disorder.

As equilibrium is normally maintained by integration of information from the visual, vestibular and proprioceptive systems, damage to this integrative function may lead to disequilibrium. The cerebellum has been shown to play a major role in this function both in animals (Ritchie, 1976) and man, although the precise mechanisms subserved by the cerebellum are not fully understood and probably vary between species. The literature on neuro-otological manifestations in cerebellar disease is confusing perhaps for two reasons. In the first place, many CNS disorders affect structures other than the cerebellum, thus making it difficult to ascribe findings to cerebellar dysfunction alone. Second, different areas of the cerebellum may have different effects on visuovestibular interaction. Baloh, Yee and Honrubia (1986) documented the oculographic features in 10 patients with pure cerebellar atrophy, (based on clinical examination in conjunction with CT and/or MRI scanning), affecting predominantly the midline region. Gaze evoked nystagmus with abnormalities of smooth pursuit and vestibulo-ocular reflex suppression were consistently found. Saccade dysmetria, particularly hyper-

metria, was found in three of the 10 patients, possibly related to involvement of the deep nuclei as well as the cerebellar cortex in these cases. Optokinetic nystagmus elicited using a drum was impaired at certain frequencies though full field optokinetic nystagmus was normal, implying that only foveal pursuit was affected. These findings were in keeping with previous studies of patients with familial and sporadic cerebellar atrophy (Baloh, Konrad and Honrubia, 1975; Zee *et al.*, 1976), and similar to findings reported by Gulya (1993) in one patient with paraneoplastic cerebellar degeneration associated with ovarian carcinoma.

It is thought that the Purkinje cells in the cerebellum have an inhibitory effect on the vestibulo-ocular reflex, this being a possible explanation for the increase in vestibulo-ocular reflex gain reported by Baloh and Demer (1993) in cases of cerebellar atrophy. However Baloh, Yee and Honrubia (1986) found vestibulo-ocular reflex gain relatively unaffected in their series of 10 patients with pure cerebellar atrophy. Kattah, Kolsky and Luessenhop (1984) reported a patient with lower and posterior vermis haematomas in whom abnormal pursuit, dysmetric saccades and positional downbeating nystagmus, but with normal vestibulo-ocular reflex suppression were found. These apparent contradictions may reflect the differences in the exact site and extent of involvement of the cerebellum in the various studies, as well as species variation.

Although it is not fully clarified, the effect of the cerebellum on visuovestibular interaction is nevertheless important diagnostically. As was pointed out above, acute vertigo, while unusual, may be the first presentation of cerebellar dysfunction, particularly if the aetiology is vascular or demyelination. Masson *et al.* (1992) and Garin *et al.* (1992) reported acute vertigo as the first presentation of cerebellar infarctions, but with normal peripheral vestibular function on testing. Likewise Magnusson and Norrving (1993) found deranged pursuit in patients with acute vertigo, initially thought to have 'vestibular neuronitis', but subsequently found to have cerebellar infarctions. These reports emphasize the importance of neuro-otological assessment to exclude central pathology, even in acute vertigo.

Cerebellar dysfunction also occurs as part of more extensive syndromes of the CNS such as Friedreich's ataxia, olivopontocerebellar atrophy and cerebello-olivary atrophy. Moschner, Perlman and Baloh (1994) compared the oculomotor findings in these conditions and concluded that the different patterns of abnormality seen in these three syndromes suggested that oculomotor testing was useful in their differential diagnosis. On the other hand, Fetter *et al.* (1994) were unable to distinguish between patients with cerebellar lesions alone from those known to have both cerebellar and extracerebellar pathology as diagnosed by MRI scanning.

The hereditary neuropathies, which may be associated with vestibular dysfunction, include a large number of disorders which are usually classified on the basis of the clinical presentation and pattern of inheritance. Certain of these conditions, such as *Refsum's disease*, have been biochemically identified, but the majority have not. The importance of diagnosing Refsum's disease, by measuring the serum level of phytanic acid, is that progression of the disease can be halted by exclusion of phytanic acid from the diet. The occurrence of neuro-otological abnormalities in this group of patients is rare, but the diagnosis should be considered in a patient with dysequilibrium and a family history of neuropathy.

Verhagen and Huygen (1994) have reviewed the vestibular and oculomotor findings in 35 hereditary disorders affecting the CNS, many of which are known to cause cerebellar pathology.

Frontal lobe lesions

Frontal lobe lesions may lead to gait apraxia (loss of ability to use the lower limbs appropriately, which cannot be accounted for by any demonstrable sensory or motor impairment) and balance disturbances (Meyer and Barron, 1960). True ataxia, produced by a frontal lobe lesion, has been attributed to compressions of corticocerebellar connections (Frazier, 1936). However, as discussed in the section on strokes affecting the carotid/middle cerebral circulation, the cerebral cortex has a modifying influence on vestibular function and this also could contribute to ataxia/imbalance. In this regard, Catz *et al.* (1993, 1994) demonstrated abnormalities of the vestibulo-ocular reflex in patients with infarcts of the frontoparietal cortex, and postulated that similar abnormalities of the vestibulospinal reflexes probably occur.

Associated frontal lobe signs include grasp reflexes, gegenhalten gait and difficulty in copying movements, such as kicking a ball.

Hydrocephalus

Both communicating and non-communicating hydrocephalus may give rise to a gait disturbance associated with loss of sphincter control and cognitive impairment, leading to dementia. Scanning may provide the diagnosis and, in appropriate cases, benefit is derived from ventricular shunting.

Epilepsy

The association of vertigo and epilepsy has been considered rare, although this is not necessarily correct (Kogeorgeos, Scott and Swash, 1981). Vertigo may be a manifestation of an aura, or part of a temporal lobe seizure, but has also been identified with other forms of epilepsy (Lennox, 1960; Schneider, Calhoun and Crosby, 1968). In 1907, Gowers reported dysequilibrium in 90 of a series of 505 cases of epilepsy. Smith and Docherty (1982) reported a patient with temporal lobe epilepsy who complained of oscillopsia and demonstrated nystagmus, and more recently Furman, Crumrine and Reinmuth (1990) described a woman with episodic vertigo and nystagmus, in association with EEG changes in the temporoparietal region.

Epilepsy is associated with ataxia in many of the so-called mitochondrial myopathies (Reardon and Harding, 1995). The cause of the ataxia in these conditions may be cerebellar or vestibular in origin, although in many cases it is unidentified.

Toxic disorders

Acute exposure to *industrial solvents*, usually hydrocarbon compounds, may give rise to nausea, vomiting, headache and vertigo. Symptoms of chronic exposure include fatigue, mood changes, poor concentration and dysequilibrium. After many years chronic toxic encephalopathy, previously known as psycho-organic syndrome, develops, the main features of which are personality and intellectual changes in addition to those described above. It seems that different solvents may have different toxic potential (Odkvist *et al.*, 1983), possibly related to their being aromatic or aliphatic compounds. Further clarification of this is needed.

Neuro-otological tests on animals have suggested that the cerebellum is an important site of predilection of the toxic damage (Odkvist *et al.*, 1980) as evidenced by increased nystagmic response to rotation and poor vestibulo-ocular reflex suppression. Similarly humans exposed to industrial solvents (Odkvist *et al.*, 1983) showed evidence of cerebellar damage, both clinically and neuro-otologically, abnormalities of the visual suppression test being one of the more sensitive tests. Subsequent studies confirmed the cerebellar site of damage and further suggested concomitant cortical dysfunction on the basis of abnormalities of central auditory processing (Odkvist *et al.*, 1987). While these workers found no evidence of brain stem involvement on the basis of auditory brain stem response in one study, Odkvist, Moller and Thuomas (1992) reported pathological pursuit, suggestive of brain stem dysfunction, in all patients of a group of 18 exposed to styrene. The latter study further reported on the usefulness of dynamic posturography and MRI scanning in the diagnosis of CNS effects of solvents.

The mechanism of damage of CNS structures by these solvents is as yet unproven, but it has been postulated that they block the normal inhibitory mechanisms arising from the cerebellum probably by interfering with the function of the neurotransmitter gamma-amino-butyric acid.

As it is thought that even changes due to chronic exposure, may be reversible, early diagnosis is of importance. With that in mind, neuro-otological evaluation, and in particular assessment of vestibulo-ocular interaction should form part of the diagnostic test battery in conjunction with neurological and psychometric tests.

Carbon monoxide poisoning is the commonest single cause of fatal poisoning in the UK, and dizziness is among its early clinical symptoms. Early diagnosis is largely circumstantial but important, as hyperbaric oxygen therapy produces dramatic results (Thomson *et al.*, 1992).

Vestibular symptoms have also recently been reported following exposure to *industrial chemicals* such as sulphur trioxide (Stueven, Cogan and Valley, 1993), carbon disulphide (Vanhoorne *et al.*, 1992) and nickel-cadmium (Bar-sela *et al.*, 1992), among others. While the underlying pathophysiological mechanisms have not yet been identified, in some instances (Vanhoorne *et al.*, 1992) it may be due to potentiation of the side effects of other pharmaceuticals consumed by the victim. Agricultural chemicals including pesticides (Lessenger, 1992) may have similar effects.

The adverse effects on the central nervous system of other toxic substances such as *heavy metals* has been discussed by Sandsdead (1986), but further work is required to document specific vestibular effects, and to identify the site or sites of pathology.

Cervical vertigo

Cervical vertigo is defined as 'vertigo occurring in association with neck disease, the vertigo being in-

duced by changes of position of the neck, in relation to the body'. Opinion varies as to the incidence of this entity in humans. Reports range from it being the commonest cause of vertigo to being almost non-existent.

In experimental animals, ataxia, gait disorder and positional nystagmus have been described in association with unilateral anaesthesia of the deep neck muscles (i.e. those muscles which have proprioceptive muscle spindles), thought to arise because of decreased cervical afferent proprioceptive input. Similarly in man, experimental anaesthesia of the deep cervical muscles gives rise to vague 'floating' sensations and disorientation rather than true vertigo. In addition, 'unsteadiness' is commoner than rotatory vertigo in patients diagnosed as having 'cervical vertigo', consistent with the above experimental findings (Alund *et al.*, 1993).

The underlying pathophysiological mechanism whereby vertigo occurs in association with disease of the neck is poorly understood.

One proposed mechanism relates to deranged somatosensory input from the cervical kinaesthetic receptors (Wyke, 1979). Loss of cervical articular mechanoreceptors due to age–related degeneration (Arnold and Harriman, 1970) or arthritis, and/or damage to the proprioceptive muscle spindles (e.g. whiplash injury) in the deep cervical muscles could compromise normal equilibrium. But, although the cervico-ocular reflex plays a significant role in maintaining gaze stability and equilibrium in lower animals, its functional role in normal humans is generally thought to be minimal (Dichgans *et al.*, 1973; Bronstein and Hood, 1986). However, in patients with bilateral vestibular loss, the cervico-ocular reflex becomes important in re-establishing equilibrium (Bronstein and Hood, 1986) assuming there is intact cerebellar and smooth pursuit/optokinetic pathways to allow compensation to occur (Bronstein, Mossman and Luxon, 1991).

Thus, while dizziness/unsteadiness is well recognized in association with whiplash and other neck injuries, the assumption that the association is one of cause–effect may not be well founded. Factors other than the neck pathology itself may account for the symptoms. Stell *et al.* (1991) emphasized this point in their work on one specific disorder of the neck, spasmodic torticollis. While it may be presumed that the asymmetry of the vestibulo-ocular reflex reported in spasmodic torticollis (Bronstein and Rudge, 1986; Stell, Bronstein and Marsden, 1989) was caused by abnormal cervical proprioceptive input impinging on the central vestibular pathways, Stell *et al.* (1991) found no evidence of abnormal cervicovestibular interaction and suggested that the observed vestibulo-ocular reflex asymmetry may be due to a primary vestibular disorder. Similarly, dizziness in a patient also complaining of neck pain may be wrongly attributed to cervical spondylitis on the basis of radiographic evidence of degenerative changes in the cervical spine, as 75% of people over the age of 50 years show osteoarthritic spurs, or other degenerative changes in the cervical vertebrae which are not directly related to symptomatology (Pallis, Jones and Spillane, 1954).

Other proposed mechanisms of cervical vertigo include:

1 Chronic irritation of the sympathetic plexus giving rise to circulatory dysfunction resulting in ischaemia in the vertebrobasilar territory (Barre, 1926) and so giving rise to cochleovestibular symptoms
2 Intermittent vertebral artery compression by osteophytes, caused by cervical spondylosis (Sheehan, Bauer and Meyer, 1960).

In relation to the second of these mechanisms, a widely held belief, particularly about the elderly, is that vertigo and nystagmus are the result of vertebrobasilar ischaemia, secondary to compression of the blood vessels of the posterior circulation, by arthritic changes in the neck. It must, however, be noted that unilateral, or indeed bilateral compression of the vertebral arteries, in the presence of a normal circle of Willis and internal carotid arteries, produces only minimal brain stem ischaemia. In addition, as discussed in the section on vertebrobasilar insufficiency, vertigo or dizziness alone is unusual in this condition and other brain stem symptoms such as diplopia, dysarthria etc. usually occur.

Much work is still needed to clarify the mechanisms involved in the aetiology of cervical vertigo and, as Pfaltz and Richter (1958) postulated, cervical vertigo is probably not the result of a single pathophysiological mechanism, but of multifactorial aetiology.

Kuilman (1959), Jongkees (1969) and Pfaltz (1984) have outlined the symptomatology associated with cervical vertigo. Classically, neck and/or occipital pain occurring particularly in the morning is associated with signs of cervical root compression: paraesthesiae in the arms, muscle weakness and wasting, corresponding depression of reflexes and reduction of posterior column sensation. In Kuilman's (1959) series, approximately one-third of patients complained of tinnitus and approximately one-fifth of balance disorders. Jongkees (1969) described a number of patients with classical Menière's syndrome on the basis of cervical vertigo, but vestibular symptomatology was more prominent than cochlear symptoms.

One of the reasons why the existence of the condition 'cervical vertigo' has been disputed was that available neuro-otological tests were normal in patients suspected of having the condition. No specific test existed to objectively document the disorder. Recently, Alund *et al.* (1993) documented significantly more abnormalities of dynamic posturography in patients with neck disorders associated with vertigo/unsteadiness as compared with two other age and sex matched groups, one with neck symp-

toms but no dizziness, and the other a healthy control group. Other otoneurological tests failed to distinguish the group with presumed cervical vertigo from the other two groups. It may be that as further specific tests are developed the condition of cervical vertigo will be more accurately characterized and its pathophysiology clarified.

Ocular vertigo

In 1794, Erasmus Darwin (cited in Brandt, 1991b) wrote: 'many people, when they arrive at 50 or 60 years of age, are affected by slight vertigo; which is generally ascribed to indigestion, but in reality arises from the beginning of a defect of their sight. These people do not see objects so distinctly as formerly and by exerting their eyes more than usual, they perceive the apparent motion of objects, and confound this with the real motion of objects, and, therefore cannot accurately balance themselves to preserve their perpendicularity'. As maintenance of equilibrium depends on the integrated input from the visual, vestibular and proprioceptive systems, a defect in visual input will give rise to a mismatch between the information from these systems and cause unsteadiness or disorientation – ocular vertigo.

Physiological visual vertigo may be induced by optokinetic stimulation, or by a critical distance between the subject and the closest stationary visible landmark, as for example in height vertigo. Changes in refraction due, for example, to presbyopia usually develop gradually, and thus allow compensation to occur. However, correction of such errors of refraction by the wearing of spectacles may initially be accompanied by dizziness or disorientation. Not only may this result in 'expected' versus 'real' image mismatch, but it may also disturb an individual's meridional magnification and aniseikonia (inequality in size of retinal images). This generally resolves spontaneously. However, correction of severe visual impairment such as by cataract extraction with lens implant may give rise to more persistent dizziness (Baloh and Honrubia, 1990b) especially in the elderly in whom the ability to compensate is poorer. Pathological visual vertigo may also be secondary to a mismatch between the true and expected eye position in the head, as may occur with an acute extraocular muscle paresis (Brandt, 1991b).

Iatrogenic dizziness

Iatrogenic dizziness may be either surgical or medical in origin. It is well established that otological surgery carries a risk of inducing dizziness/vertigo postoperatively. With the decrease in the incidence of chronic otitis media and improved surgical techniques, vestibular disturbance following middle ear surgery for otitis media or otosclerosis has fallen dramatically. Various forms of labyrinthine/VIIIth nerve surgery have been advocated for management of intractable vertigo such as those discussed in the sections on Menière's disease or benign positional vertigo of paroxysmal type. While a temporary increase in dizziness is to be expected after such an operation, persistent postoperative dizziness may occur if the side of the lesion is incorrectly identified, or if for example in Menière's disease, the condition is bilateral. Incomplete sectioning of the VIIIth nerve or failure to remove totally the vestibular epithelium will also lead to persistent dizziness. Similarly, in patients with coexistent additional pathology which impairs their ability to compensate from vestibular disturbance, (a point of particular relevance in the elderly), long-term dizziness may occur after labyrinthine surgery.

Vestibular disturbance after non-otological surgery has been described by Johnson *et al.* (1985), Gyo (1988) and Andaz, Whitlet and Ludman (1993). Recently a series of 12 patients has been reported by O Mahoney, Gatland and Luxon (1995) in whom unilateral or bilateral peripheral vestibular dysfunction, benign positional paroxysmal vertigo and central vestibular disorder occurred immediately after non-otological surgery. Various mechanisms have been postulated to explain the vestibular disturbance, including effects of nitrous oxide anaesthesia, ischaemia secondary to emboli or peroperative hypotension, CSF leakage to mention but a few.

MacArthur, Lewis and Knox (1992) reported a 2% incidence of dizziness during epidural analgesia, and suggested that this was caused by a drop in systemic blood pressure during the procedure.

Many, if not all drugs may produce dizziness by a wide variety of mechanisms (Ballantyne and Ajodhia, 1984) (Table 20.3). The situation is even more complex in the elderly. Older patients are more likely to have multiple pathologies which may themselves contribute to dizziness and dysequilibrium, be on multiple drugs with the potential risks of adverse drug interactions or poor compliance, have diminished renal and hepatic function or changes in protein binding capacity which may alter the pharmacodynamics of drugs (Macphee and Brodie, 1988).

From the preceding sections in this chapter it is clear that dizziness can be the end result of many different pathological mechanisms. Ototoxic drugs which directly damage the vestibular labyrinth have been discussed above. Drugs which cause anaemia, cardiac mechanical dysfunction or arrhythmias, induce postural or systemic hypotension by various means, or give rise to metabolic disturbances such as hypoglycaemia, may all lead to dizziness. Psychotropic drugs such as the major and minor tranquillizers, and centrally-acting analgesics such as morphine derivatives may cause dizziness by impairing oculomotor function and central integrative functions necessary to maintain perfect balance. Anticonvulsants

Table 20.3 Drugs causing dizziness/vertigo

Central nervous system

Antidepressants	Tricylics, tetracyclics, MAOIs
Tranquillizers	Phenothiazines, benzodiazepines
Anticonvulsants	Phenobarbitone, phenytoin, carbamazepine
Analgesics	Paracetamol, acetylsalicylate, non-steroidal, anti-inflammatory drugs, opiates
Anaesthetics	Nitrous oxide, halothane
Antihypertensives	Diuretics (thiazides and loop), beta-blockers, captopril, calcium channel blockers, methyldopa, hydralazine
Anti-arrhythmic	Verapamil, amiodarone, disopyramide, mexiletine, flecanide
Anti-angina	Glyceryl trinitrate, isosorbide dinitrate, nifedipine, verapamil

Antimicrobials
Aminoglycosides, minocycline, isoniazid, rifampicin, chloroquine, erythromycin

Anti-allergic
Chlorpheniramine, cyproheptadine, ephedrine, promethazine

Endocrine
Hypoglycaemics, corticosteroids

Chemotherapeutic
Cis-platinum, busulphan, vinblastine

exert a toxic effect on the central vestibular pathways producing severe imbalance and nystagmus and also cause ataxia secondary to cerebellar dysfunction. A more complete discussion of drug induced vertigo can be found in Brandt (1991c).

A number of other diagnostic/therapeutic procedures have been reported to cause dizziness, including hepatitis B vaccination (McMahon *et al.*, 1992), (though it was thought that the association may be coincidental) and external irradiation of the head and neck (Gabriele *et al.*, 1992). In the latter case peripheral vestibular dysfunction was demonstrated in 10 out of 20 patients being treated with radiotherapy, the vestibular abnormalities first appearing weeks to months after cessation of therapy. Lumbar puncture and myelography have been reported to cause auditory dysfunction, possibly secondary to leakage of CSF, though Mizuno, Yamasoba and Nomura (1992) postulated that dizziness in two patients occurring after myelography may have been caused by direct irritation of the vestibular nerve by the oily contrast medium (Pantopaque) used.

Conclusions

This account of balance disorders provides the clinician faced with a dizzy patient with a working knowledge of the differential diagnosis. Priority must be given to determining whether the balance disorder is primarily of vestibular, neurological or general medical origin. The possibility of multiple sensory deficits should be considered as being one of the commoner causes of dizziness, particularly in the elderly. The main abnormalities reported by Drachman and Hart (1972) in patients with multiple sensory deficit syndrome were peripheral neuropathy (85%), cervical spondylosis (71%), vestibular abnormalities, as shown by inadequate labyrinthine responses (64%) and visual loss, secondary to cataracts (35%). It is clear that only by a thorough general medical examination are the multiple components of dizziness likely to be identified. On the basis of a detailed history and examination, specific investigative procedures may be required. Certain identifiable vertiginous syndromes, e.g. syphilitic labyrinthitis, vestibular schwannomas, benign paroxysmal positional vertigo and temporal lobe epilepsy, may require precise therapeutic regimens. However, in general, the pathophysiology of many vestibular disorders is poorly understood, and it is therefore impossible to consider specific therapy. Symptomatic treatment may be surgical, physical, pharmacological or psychological. In general terms, surgical intervention is indicated only for one of three main reasons:

1 To treat potentially life-threatening disease, e.g. the complications of otitis media
2 To confirm/exclude a perilymph fistula
3 To improve the quality of life in a patient suffering from severe rotational vertigo in whom all medical measures have failed.

The non-surgical management of vertigo is discussed fully in Chapters 6 and 22 and may be summarized as comprising counselling, which is of the utmost importance, together with vestibular rehabilitation and appropriate vestibular sedatives.

References

AANTAA, E. and LEHTONEN, A. (1981) Electronystagmographic findings in insulin-dependent diabetics. *Acta Otolaryngologica*, **91**, 15–18

AANTAA, E. and VIROLAINEN, E. (1979) Vestibular neuronitis; a follow-up study. *Acta Otorhinolaryngologica Belgica*, **33**, 401–404

ABRAMOVICH, S. and PRASHER, D.K. (1986) Electrocochleography and brainstem potentials in Ramsay Hunt syndrome. *Archives of Otolaryngology – Head and Neck Surgery*, **112**, 925–928

ADLER, D. and RITZ, E. (1982) Terminal renal failure and hearing loss. *Archives of Otorhinolaryngology*, **235**, 587–590

ADOUR, K. K. and DOTY, H. E. (1973) Electronystagmographic comparison of acute idiopathic and herpes zoster facial paralysis. *Laryngoscope*, **83**, 2029–2034

ADOUR, K. K., HILSINGER, R. L. and BYL, F. M. (1980) Herpes simplex polyganglionitis. *Otolaryngology – Head and Neck Surgery*, **88**, 270–274

AGATE, J. (1963) In: *The Practice of Geriatrics*. London: Heinemann. p. 91

AGUSTI, C., FERRAN, F., GEA, J. and PICADO, C. (1991) Ototoxic reaction to erythromycin. *Archives of Internal Medicine*, **151**, 380

AHMED, N., WILSON, J. A., BARR–HAMILTON, R. M., KEAN, D. M. and MACLENNAN, W. J. (1992) The evaluation of dizziness in elderly patients. *Postgraduate Medical Journal*, **68**, 558–561

AJULO, S. O., OSINAME, A. I. and MYATT, H. M. (1993) Sensorineural hearing loss in sickle cell anaemia – a United Kingdom study. *Journal of Laryngology and Otology*, **107**, 790–794

ALBERTS, M. C. and TERRENCE, C. F. (1978) Hearing loss in cases of carcinomatous meningitis. *Journal of Laryngology and Otology*, **92**, 233–241

ALUND, M., LEDIN, T., ODKVIST, L. and LARSSON, S. E. (1993) Dynamic posturography among patients with common neck disorders. A study of 15 cases with suspected cervical vertigo. *Journal of Vestibular Research*, **3**, 383–389

AMARENCO, P. and HAUWE, J. J. (1990) Cerebellar infarction in the territory of the anterior and inferior cerebellar artery. A clinicopathological study of 20 cases. *Brain*, **113**, 139

ANDAZ, C., WHITTET, H. B. and LUDMAN, H. (1993) An unusual cause of benign paroxysmal positional vertigo. *Journal of Laryngology and Otology*, **107**, 1153–1154

ANDERSON, N. E., CUNNINGHAM, J. M. and POSNER, J. B. (1987) Autoimmune pathogenesis of paraneoplastic neurological syndromes. *Critical Reviews in Neurobiology*, **3**, 245–299

ANDREWS, J. C., HOOVER, L. A., LEE, R. S. and HONRUBIA, V. (1988) Vertigo in the hyperviscosity syndrome. *Otolaryngology – Head and Neck Surgery*, **98**, 144–149

APPLEBAUM, E. L. and CLEMIS, J. D. (1977) Temporal bone histopathology of Paget's disease with sensorineural hearing loss and narrowing of the internal auditory canal. *Laryngoscope*, **87**, 1753–1759

APPLEBAUM, E. L. and VALVASSORI, G. E. (1984) Auditory and vestibular system findings in patients with vascular loops in the internal auditory canal. *Annals of Otology, Rhinology and Laryngology*, **112** (suppl.), 63–70

ARNOLD, N. and HARRIMAN, D. G. (1970) The incidence of abnormality in control of human peripheral nerves studied by single axon dissection. *Journal of Neurology, Neurosurgery and Psychiatry*, **33**, 55–61

ARNVIG, J. (1955) Vestibular function in deafness and severe hardness of hearing. *Acta Otolaryngologica*, **45**, 283–288

AUST, G. (1994) Early and late damage to the auditory and vestibular area after meningitis in chilhood and adolescence. *Hals, Nase, Ohren*, **42**, 14–21

AXELSSON, A., SIGROTH, K. and VERTES, D. (1978) Hearing in diabetics. *Acta Otolaryngologica Supplementum*, **356**, 3–23

AYD, F. J. (1961) A survey of drug-induced extrapyramidal reactions. *Journal of the American Medical Association*, **175**, 1054–1060

BALLANTYNE, J. and AJODHIA, J. M. (1984) Iatrogenic dizziness. In: *Vertigo*, edited by M. R. Dix and J. D. Hood. Chichester: John Wiley and Sons Ltd. pp. 217–248

BALOH, R. W. (1992) Dizziness in older people. *Journal of the American Geriatric Society*, **40**, 713–721

BALOH, R. W. and DEMER, J. L. (1993) Optokinetic–vestibular interaction in patients with increased gain of the vestibulo-ocular reflex. *Experimental Brain Research*, **97**, 334–342

BALOH, R. W. and HONRUBIA, V. (1990a) Infectious disorders. In: *Clinical Neurophysiology of the Vestibular System*, edited by F. Plum. Philadelphia: F. A. Davis. p. 206

BALOH, R. W. and HONRUBIA, V. (1990b) The history in the dizzy patient – ocular dizziness. In: *Clinical Neurophysiology of the Vestibular System*, edited by F. Plum. Philadelphia: F. A. Davis. p. 103

BALOH, R. W., JACOBSON, K. and FIFE, T. (1994) Familial vestibulopathy: a new dominantly inherited syndrome. *Neurology*, **44**, 20–25

BALOH, R. W., KONRAD, H. R. and HONRUBIA, V. (1975) Vestibulo-ocular function in patients with cerebellar atrophy. *Neurology (Minneapolis)*, **25**, 160–168

BALOH, R. W., YEE, R. D. and HONRUBIA, V. (1986) Late cortical cerebellar atrophy. Clinical and oculographic features. *Brain*, **109**, 159–180

BALOH, R. W., HONRUBIA, V. and JACOBSON, K. (1987) Benign positional vertigo: clinical and oculographic features in 240 cases. *Neurology*, **37**, 371–378

BALSAMO, G., DE VINCENTIIS, M. and MARMO, F. (1969) The effect of tetracycline on the processes of calcification of the otoliths in the developing chick embryo. *Journal of Embryological and Experimental Morphology*, **22**, 327–332

BANCE, M. and RUTKA, J. (1990) Speculation into the etiologic role of viruses in the development of Bell's palsy and disorders of inner ear dysfunction: a case history and review of the literature. *Journal of Otolaryngology*, **19**, 46–49

BARAITSER, M. (1990) Hereditary motor and sensory neuropathy (HMSM). In: *Genetics of Neurological disease*, 2nd edn. Oxford Monographs on Medical Genetics, no. **18**. Oxford: Oxford University Press

BARINAGARREMENTERIA, F. and CANTU, C. (1994) Primary medulla haemorrhage. Report of four cases and review of the literature. *Stroke*, **25**, 1684–1687

BARR, B. and LUNDSTROM, R. (1961) Deafness following maternal rubella. *Acta Otolaryngologica*, **53**, 413

BARRÉ, J. A. (1926) Sur un syndrome sympathique cervical posterieure et sa cause fréquente l'arthrite cervicale. *Revue de Neurologie*, **33**, 1246–1252

BAR–SELA, S., LEVY, M., WESTLIN, J. B., LASTER, R. and RICHTER, E. D. (1992) Medical findings in nickel–cadmium battery workers. *Israeli Journal of Medical–Science*, **28**, 578–583

BASSIOUNY, M., HIRSCH, B. E., KELLY R. H., KAMERER, D. B. and CASS, S. P. (1992) Beta 2 transferrin application in otology. *American Journal of Otology*, **13**, 552–555

BEANEY, G. P. E. (1964) Otolaryngeal problems arising during the management of severe renal failure. *Journal of Laryngology and Otology*, **78**, 507–515

BEAUJEUX, R. L., REIZINE, D. C., CASASCO, A., AYMARD, A., RUFENACHT, D., KHAYAT, M. H. *et al.* (1992) Endovascular treatment of vertebral arteriovenous fistula. *Radiology*, **183**, 361–367

BEDERSON, J. B., VON AMMON, K., WICHMANN, W. W. and YASARGIL, M. G. (1991) Conservative treatment of patients with acoustic tumours. *Neurosurgery*, **28**, 646–651

BELAL, A. (1980) Pathology of vascular sensorineural hearing impairment. *Laryngoscope*, **90**, 1831–1839

BENDER, M. (1975) The incidence and type of perceptual deficiencies in the aged. In: *Neurological and Sensory Disorders in the Elderly*. New York: Stratton. pp. 15–31

BENJAMIN, E., ZIMMERMAN, C. and TROOST, B. (1986) Latero-

pulsion and upbeat nystagmus are manifestations of central vestibular dysfunction. *Archives of Neurology*, **43**, 962–964

BENNETT, D. H. (1990) Cardiac arrhythmias. In: *Oxford Textbook of Medicine*, 2nd edn, edited by D. J. Weatherall, J. G. G. Ledingham and D. A. Warrell. Oxford: Oxford Medical Publications. pp. 13, 117–13, 132

BERGSTROM, B. (1973) Morphology of the vestibular nerve. *Acta Otolaryngologica*, **76**, 173–179, 331–338

BERGSTROM, L. V., JENKINS, P., SANDO, I. and ENGLISH, G. M. (1973) Hearing loss in renal disease: clinical and pathological studies. *Annals of Otology, Rhinology and Laryngology*, **82**, 555–576

BERLINGER, N. T., KOUTROUPAS, S., ADAMS, G. and MAISEL, R. (1980) Patterns of involvement of the temporal bone in metastatic and systemic malignancy. *Laryngoscope*, **90**, 619–627

BERRY, C. D., HOOTON, T. M., COLLIER, A. C. and LUKEHART, S. A. (1987) Neurologic relapse after benzathine penicillin therapy for secondary syphilis in a patient with HIV infection. *New England Journal of Medicine*, **316**, 1587–1589

BICKERSTAFF, E. R. (1961) Basilar artery migraine. *Lancet*, i, 15–17

BINDER, C. and BENDTSON, I. (1992) Endocrine emergencies. Hypoglycemia. *Baillière's Clinical Endocrinology and Metabolism*, **6**, 23–39

BIRDSALL, H. H., BAUGHN, R. E. and JENKINS, H. A. (1990) The diagnostic dilemma of otosyphilis. A new western blot assay. *Archives of Otolaryngology – Head and Neck Surgery*, **116**, 617–621

BIURRUN, O., FERRER, J. P., LORENTE, J., DE ESPANA, R., GOMIS, R. and TRASERRA, J. (1991) Asymptomatic electronystagmographic abnormalities in patients with type I diabetes mellitus. *Oto-Rhino-Laryngology*, **53**, 335–338

BLACK, F. D., SANDO, I., HILDYARD, V. H. and HEMENWAY, W. G. (1969) Bilateral multiple otosclerotic foci and endolymphatic hydrops: histological case report. *Annals of Otology, Rhinology and Laryngology*, **78**, 1062–1073

BLACK, F. O., LILLY, D. J., NASHNER, L. M., PEETERKA, R. J. and PESZNECKER, S. C. (1987) Quantitative diagnostic test for perilymph fistulas. *Otolaryngology, Head and Neck Surgery*, **96**, 125–134

BLACKLEY, B., FRIEDMAN, I. and WRIGHT, L. (1967) Herpes zoster auris with facial nerve palsy and auditory nerve symptoms. A case report with histological findings. *Acta Otolaryngologica*, **63**, 553–560

BOLIS, S., BREGANI, E.R., ROSSINI, F., SCHIAVINA, R. and POGLIANI, E. M. (1993) Atrial flutter followed by sick sinus syndrome as presenting symptoms of B-cell malignant non-Hodgkin lymphoma involving the heart. *Haematologica*, **78**, 332–334

BONEH, A., READE, T. M., SCRIVER, C. R. and RISHIKOF, E. (1987) Audiometric evidence for two forms of X-linked hypophosphatemia in humans, apparent counterparts of 'Hyp' and 'Gy' mutations in mouse. *American Journal of Medical Genetics*, **27**, 997–1003

BOOTH, J. B. (1982) Medical management of sensorineural hearing loss. Part I. *Journal of Laryngology and Otology*, **96**, 673–684

BOWMAN, C. A., LINTHICUM, F. H. JR, NELSON, R. A., MIKAMI, K. and QUISMORIO, F. (1986) Sensorineural hearing loss associated with systemic lupus erythematosus. *Otolaryngology Head and Neck Surgery*, **94**, 197–204

BRAMA, L. and FAINARU, M. (1980) Inner ear involvement

in Behcet's disease. *Archives of Otolaryngology*, **106**, 215–217

BRANDT, T. H. (1991a) Physiological vertigo. In: *Vertigo and its Multisensory Systems*, edited by M. Swash. London: Springer Verlag. pp. 307–320

BRANDT, T. H. (1991b) Visual vertigo and acrophobia. In: *Vertigo and its Multisensory Systems*, edited by M. Swash. London: Springer Verlag., pp. 233–275

BRANDT, T. H. (1991c) Drugs and vertigo. In: *Vertigo and its Multisensory Systems*, edited by M. Swash. London: Springer Verlag. pp. 215–225

BRANDT, T. and DAROFF, R. B. (1980) Physical therapy for benign paroxysmal positional vertigo. *Archives of Otolaryngology*, **106**, 484

BRANDT, T. and DIETERICH, M. (1993) Skew deviation with ocular torsion: a vestibular brainstem sign of topographic diagnostic value. *Annals of Neurology*, **33**, 528–534

BRANDT, T. and STEDDIN, S. (1992) Reply to the letter by Gordon 'Benign paroxysmal postional vertigo (BPPV) or bubble provoked positional vertigo'? *Journal of the Neurological Sciences*, **111**, 231–233

BRANDT, T. and STEDDIN, S. (1993) Current view of the mechanism of benign paroxysmal positioning vertigo: cupulolithiasis or canalolithiasis? *Journal of Vestibular Research*, **3**, 373–382

BREDA, S. D., HAMMERSCHLAG, P. E., GIGLIOTTIE, F. and SCHINELLA, R. (1988) *Pneumocystis carnii* in the temporal bone as a primary manifestation of the acquired immunodeficiency syndrome. *Annals of Otology, Rhinology, and Laryngology*, **97**, 427–431

BRIHAYE, P. and HALAMA, A. R. (1993) Fluctuating hearing loss in sarcoidosis. *Acta Otorhinolaryngologica Belgica*, **47**, 23–26

BRONSTEIN, A. M. and HOOD, J. D. (1986) The cervico-ocular reflex in normal subjects and patients with absent vestibular function. *Brain Research, Amsterdam*, **373**, 399–408

BRONSTEIN, A. M. and RUDGE, P. (1986) Vestibular involvement in spasmodic torticollis. *Journal of Neurology, Neurosurgery and Psychiatry*, **49**, 290–295

BRONSTEIN, A. M., MOSSMAN, S. and LUXON, L. M. (1991) The neck-eye reflex in patients with reduced vestibular and optokinetic function. *Brain*, **114**, 1–11

BRUMMETT, R. E. and FOX, K. E. (1989) Aminoglycoside-induced hearing loss in humans. *Antimicrobial Agents and Chemotherapeutics*, **33**, 797

BRUNER, A. and NORRIS, T. W. (1971) Age related changes in caloric nystagmus. *Acta Otolaryngologica*, Suppl. 282, 1–24

CALDERELLI, D. D., REJOWSLEI, J. E. and COREY, J. P. (1984) Sensorineural hearing loss in lupus erythematosus. *American Journal of Otology*, **7**, 210–213

CAMPOS, A., CAZINARES, F. J. and SANCHEZ–QUEVEDO, M. C. (1990) Otoconial degeneration in the aged utricle and saccule. *Advances in Oto-Rhino-Laryngology*, **45**, 143–153

CAPLAN, L. R. (1990) Pathobiology of vascular brain stem diseases. In: *Vascular Brain Stem Disease*, edited by B. Hofferberth, G. G. Brune, G. Sitzer and H-D Weger. Basel: Karger. pp. 25–36

CARNE, C. A. and ADLER, M. W. (1986) Neurological manifestations of human immunodeficiency infection. *British Medical Journal*, **293**, 462–463

CASS, S. P., DAVIDSON, P. and GOSHGARIAN, H. (1989) Survival of the vestibular nerve after labyrinthectomy in the cat. *Otolaryngology, Head and Neck Surgery*, **101**, 459–465

CATZ, A., RON, S., SOLZI, P. and KORCZYN, A. D. (1993)

Vestibulo-ocular reflex suppression following hemispheric stroke. *Scandinavian Journal of Rehabilitation Medicine*, **25**, 149–152

CATZ, A., RON, S., SOLZI, P. and KORCZYN, A. D. (1994) The vestibulo-ocular reflex and dysequilibrium after hemispheric stroke. *American Journal of Physical Medicine and Rehabilitation*, **73**, 36–39

CAUSSE, R. (1949) Action toxique vestibulaire et cochleaire de la streptomycin du point de vue experimental. *Annales d'Otolaryngologie (Paris)*, **66**, 518–538

CAWTHORNE T. (1952) Vertigo. *British Medical Journal*, **2**, 931–933

CAWTHORNE, T. (1955) Otosclerosis. *Journal of Laryngology and Otology*, **69**, 437–456

CAWTHORNE, T. (1969) Choice of labyrinthine surgery for hydrops. *Archives of Otolaryngology*, **89**, 108–111

CHANDRASEKHAR, S. S., SIVERLS, V. and SEKHAR, H. K. C. (1992) Histopathologic and ultrastructural changes in the temporal bones of HIV-infected human adults. *American Journal of Otology*, **13**, 207–214

CHARLES, N., FROMENT, C., RODE, G., VIGHETTO, A., TURJMAN, F., TRILLET, M. *et al.* (1992) Vertigo and upside down vision due to an infarct in the territory of the medial branch of the posterior inferior cerebellar artery caused by dissection of a vertebral artery. *Journal of Neurology, Neurosurgery and Psychiatry*, **55**, 188–189

CIPPARRONE, L., GINANNESCHI, A., DEGL'INNOCENTI, F., PORZIO, P., PAGNINI, P. and MARINI, P. (1988) Electro-oculographic routine examination in Parkinson's disease. *Acta Neurologica Scandinavica*, **77**, 6–11

CLEMIS, J. D., BOYLES, J., HARFORD, E. R. and PETASNICK, J. P. (1967) The clinical diagnosis of Paget's disease of the temporal bone. *Annals of Otology*, **76**, 611–623

CLEMIS, J. D., BALLAD, W. J., BAGGOT, P. J. and LYON, S. T. (1986) Relative frequency of inferior vestibular schwannoma. *Archives of Otolaryngology – Head and Neck Surgery*, **112**, 190–194

COGAN, D. G. (1948) Syndrome of non-syphilitic interstitial keratitis and vestibulo-audiometry symptoms. *Archives of Ophthalmology*, **33**, 144–149

COGAN, D. G., WITT, E. D. and GOLDMAN–RAKIC, P. S. (1985) Ocular signs in thiamine-deficient monkeys and in Wernicke's disease in humans. *Archives of Ophthalmology*, **103**, 1212

COMPERE, W. E. JR (1968) Electronystagmographic findings in patients with 'whiplash' injuries. *Laryngoscope*, **78**, 1226–1233

CONLEE, J. W., JENSEN, R. P., PARKS, T. N. and CREEL, D. J. (1991) Turn-specific and pigment dependent differences in the stria vascularis of normal and gentamicin-treated albino and pigmented guinea pigs. *Hearing Research*, **55**, 57–69

CORDAY, E. and IRVING, D. W. (1960) Effect of cardiac arrhythmia on the cerebral circulation. *American Journal of Cardiology*, **6**, 803–808

CORIN, M. S., ELIZON, T. S. and BENDER, M. B. (1972) Oculomotor function in patients with Parkinson's disease. *Journal of Neurophysiology*, **15**, 251–265

CORVERA, J., BENITEZ, L. D., LOPEZ-RIOS, G. and RABIELA, M. T. (1980) Vestibular and oculomotor abnormalities in vertebrobasilar insufficiency. *Annals of Otology, Rhinology and Laryngology*, **89**, 370–376

COYLE, P. K. (1989) *Borrelia burgdorferi* antibodies in multiple sclerosis patients. *Neurology*, **39**, 760–761

CREMERS, C. W., THIJSSEN, H. O., FISCHER, A. J. and MARRES, E.

H. (1981) Otological aspects of the earpit-deafness syndrome. *ORL* **43**, 223–239

CROFT, P. B. and WILKINSON, M. (1969) The course and prognosis in some types of carcinomatous neuromyopathy. *Brain*, **92**, 1–8

CULLEN, S. I. and COHEN, R. H. (1976) Minocycline therapy in acne vulgaris. *Cutis*, **17**, 1208–1210

CUTRER, F. M., and BALOH, R. W. (1992) Migraine-associated dizziness. *Headache*, **32**, 300–304

DARMSTADT, G. L. and HARRIS, J. P. (1989) Luetic hearing loss: clinical presentation, diagnosis and treatment. *American Journal of Otolaryngology*, **10**, 410–421

DAVIS, L. E. (1993) Viruses and vestibular neuritis: review of human and animal studies. *Acta Otolaryngologica*, Suppl. 503, 70–73

DAVIS, M., KANE, R. and VALENTINE, J. (1984) Impaired hearing in X-linked hypophosphataemic (vitamin-D-resistant) osteomalacia. *Annals of Internal Medicine*, **100**, 230–232

DE JONG, P. T. V. M., DE JONG, J. M. B. V., COHEN, B. and JONGKEES, L. B. (1977) Ataxia and nystagmus induced by injection of local anesthetics in the neck. *Annals of Neurology*, **1**, 240–246

DEUTSCH, M., GLOOR, H. O., CANDINAS, R., AMANN, F. W., VON SEGESSER, L. and TURINA, M. (1993) Clinical late results following surgical ablation of an accessory atrioventricular connection in Wolff–Parkinson White syndrome. *Schweizerische Rundschau fur Medizin Praxis*, **82**, 220–225

DEVRIESE, P. P. (1968) Facial paralysis in cephalic herpes zoster. *Annals of Otology, Rhinology and Laryngology*, **77**, 1101–1119

DICHGANS, J., BIZZI, E., MORASSO, P. and TAGLIASCO, V. (1973) Mechanisms underlying recovery of eye-head coordination following bilateral labyrinthectomy in monkeys. *Experimental Brain Research*, **18**, 548–562

DIEPEVEEN, J. E. and JENSEN, J. (1968) Differential caloric reactions in deaf children. *Acta Otolaryngologica*, **65**, 570–574

DIETERICH, M. and BRANDT, T. (1993) Ocular torsion and tilt of subjective visual vertical are sensitive brainstem signs. *Annals of Neurology*, **33**, 292–299

DIX, M. R. and HALLPIKE, C. S. (1952) The pathology, symptomatology and diagnosis of certain common disorders of the vestibular system. *Annals of Otology, Rhingology and Laryngology*, **61**, 987–1016

DIX, M. R., HARRISON, M. J. G. and LEWIS, P. D. (1971) Progressive supranuclear palsy (the Steele Richardson Olszewski syndrome). *Journal of Neurological Science*, **13**, 237–256

DJUPESLAND, G., BERDAL, T., JOHANESSEN, T. A., DEGRE, M., STEIN, R. and STREDE, S. (1975) The role of viral infection in acute peripheral facial palsy. *Acta Otolaryngologica*, **79**, 221–227

DRACHMAN, D. A. and HART, C. (1972) A new approach to the dizzy patient. *Neurology*, **22**, 323–334

DREIER, A., MARTINEZ, V., JIMENEZ, M. L., ORUS, C., JURGENS, A. and AMESTI, C. (1993) Sudden bilateral deafness of luetic origin in an HIV positive patient. *Acta Otorinolaringologica Espana*, **44**, 315–317

DREW, T. M., ALTMAN, R., BLACK, K. and GOLDFIELD, M. (1976) Minocycline for prophylaxis of infection with *Neisseria meningitidis*: high rate of side effect in recipients. *Journal of Infectious Diseases*, **133**, 194–198

DROLLER, H. and PEMBERTON, J. (1953) Vertigo in a random sample of elderly people living in their homes. *Journal of Laryngology and Otology*, **67**, 689–695

DUPONT, J., GUILHAUME, A. and ARAN, J. M. (1993) Neuronal degeneration of primary cochlear and vestibular innervations after local injection of sisomicin in the guinea pig. *Hearing Research*, **68**, 217–228

DURHAM, J. S., LONGRIDGE, N. S., SMITH, J. M., and JONES, H. (1984) Clinical manifestations of otological syphilis. *Journal of Otolaryngology*, **13**, 175–179

THE DUTCH TIA STUDY GROUP (1993) Predictors of major vascular events in patients with a transient ischemic attack or nondisabling stroke. *Stroke*, **24**, 527–531

ELIDAN, J., LIN, J. and HONRUBIA, V. (1986) The effect of loop diuretics on the vestibular system. Assessment by recording the vestibular evoked response. *Archives of Otolaryngology – Head and Neck Surgery*, **112**, 836–839

ENGSTROM, H., ADES, H. W. and ENGSTROM, M. B. (1977) Changes in the vestibular epithelia in elderly monkeys and humans. *Advances in Otorhinolaryngology*, **22**, 93–110

ENSRUD, K. E., NEVITT, M. C., YUNIS, C., HULLEY, S. B., GRIMM, R. H. and CUMMINGS, S. R. (1992) Postural hypotension and postural dizziness in elderly women. The study of osteoporotic fractures. *Archives of Internal Medicine*, **152**, 1058–1064

EVANS, D. G. R., HUSON, S. M., DONNAI, D., NEARY, W., BLAIR, V., TEARE, D. *et al.* (1992a) A genetic study of type 2 neurofibromatosis in the United Kingdom, I. Prevalence, mutation rate, fitness, and confirmation of maternal transmission effect on severity. *Journal of Medical Genetics*, **29**, 841–846

EVANS, D. G. R., HUSON, S. M., DONNAI, D., NEARY, W., BLAIR, V., NEWTON, V. *et al.* (1992b) A genetic study of type 2 neurofibromatosis in the United Kingdom. II. Guidelines for genetic counselling. *Journal of Medical Genetics*, **29**, 847–852

FEE, G. A. (1968) Traumatic perilymph fistulas. *Archives of Otolaryngology*, **88**, 477–480

FETTER, M., KLOCKGETHER, T., SCHULZ, J. B., FAISS, J., KOENIG, E. and DICHGANS, J. (1994) Oculomotor abnormalities and MRI findings in idiopathic cerebellar ataxia. *Journal of Neurology*, **241**, 234–241

FISHER, C. M. (1967) Vertigo in cerebrovascular disease. *Archives of Otolaryngology*, **85**, 529–534

FITCH, N., LINDSAY, J. R. and SROLOVITZ, H. (1976) Temporal bone in the preauricular pit, cervical fistula, hearing loss syndrome. *Annals of Otology, Rhinology and Laryngology*, **85**, 268–275

FRANCIS, D. A., BRONSTEIN, A. M., RUDGE, P. and DU BOULAY, E. (1992) The site of brainstem lesions causing semicircular canal paresis: and MRI study. *Journal of Neurology*, **55**, 446–449

FRAZIER, C. H. (1936) Tumour involving the frontal lobe alone. *Archives of Neurology and Psychiatry*, **35**, 525–575

FRIEDMAN, S. A., SCHULMA, R. H. and WEISS, S. (1975) Hearing and diabetic neuropathy. *Archives of Internal Medicine*, **135**, 573–576

FRIEDMAN, E. M., LUBAN, N. L. C., HERER, G. R. and WILLIAMS, I. (1980) Sickle cell anaemia and hearing. *Annals of Otology, Rhinology and Laryngology*, **89**, 342–347

FURMAN, J. M., CRUMRINE, P. K. and REINMUTH, O. M. (1990) Epileptic nystagmus. *Annals of Neurology*, **27**, 686–688

GABRIELE, P., ORECCHIA, R., MAGNANO, M., ALBERA, R. and SANNAZZARI, G. L. (1992) Vestibular apparatus disorders after external radiation therapy for head and neck cancers. *Radiotherapy – Oncology*, **25**, 25–30

GACEK, R. R. (1974) Transection of the posterior ampullary nerve for the relief of benign paroxysmal positional vertigo. *Annals of Otology, Rhinology and Laryngology*, **83**, 596–605

GARIN, P., DEGGOUJ, N., DECAT, M. and GERSDORFF, M. (1992) Acute vertigo caused by cerebellar vascular accident. *Revue de Laryngologie, Otologie et Rhinologie (Bordeaux)*, **113**, 87–90

GATLAND, D., TUCKER, B., CHALSTREY, S., KEENE, M. and BAKER, L. (1991) Hearing loss in chronic renal failure – hearing threshold changes following haemodialysis. *Journal of the Royal Society of Medicine*, **84**, 587–589

GEMIGNANI, G., BERRETTINI, S., BRUSCHINI, P., SELLARI-FRANCE-SCHINE, S., FUSARI, P., PIRAGINE, F. *et al.* (1991) Hearing and vestibular disturbances in Behcet's syndrome. *Annals of Otology, Rhinology and Laryngology*, **100**, 459–463

GENTRIC, A., FOUILHOUX, A., CAROFF, M., MOTTIER, D. and JOUQUAN, J. (1993) Dopamine B hydroxylase deficiency responsible for severe dysautonomic orthostatic hypotension in an elderly patient. *Journal of the American Geriatric Society*, **41**, 550–551

GERTNER, R., PODOSHIN, L. and FRADIS, M. (1983) Osteogenic sarcoma of the temporal bone. *Journal of Laryngology and Otology*, **97**, 627–631

GHIGLIOTTI, G., REPETTO, T., FARRIS, A., ROY, M. T. and DE MARCHI, R. (1993) Thalidomide: treatment of choice for aphthous ulcers in patients seropositive for human immunodeficiency virus. *Journal of the American Academy of Dermatology*, **28**, 271–272

GHORAYEB, B. Y. and LINTHICUM F. H. JR (1978) Otosclerotic inner ear syndrome. *Annals of Otology, Rhinology and Laryngology*, **87**, 85–90

GIBB, W. R. (1992) Neuropathology of Parkinson's disease and related syndromes. *Neurologic Clinics*, **10**, 361–376

GIBB, W. R. and LEES, A. J. (1989) The significance of the Lewy body in the diagnosis of idiopathic Parkinson's disease. *Neuropathology and Applied Neurobiology*, **15**, 27–44

GIBBON, K. P. and DAVIS, C. G. (1981) A hearing survey in diabetes mellitus. *Clinical Otolaryngology*, **6**, 345–350

GIBSON, W. P. R. (1992) Electrocochleography in the diagnosis of perilymphatic fistula: intraoperative observations and assessment of a new diagnostic office procedure. *American Journal of Otology*, **13**, 146–151

GILLILAN, L. A. (1964) The correlation of the blood supply to the human brainstem with clinical brainstem lesions. *Journal of Neuropathology and Experimental Neurology*, **23**, 78–108

GOODHILL, V. (1971) Sudden deafness and round window rupture. Presidential address at the 74th annual meeting of the American Laryngological Rhinological and Otological Society, San Francisco, California. May 25–27. *Laryngoscope*, **81**, 1462–1474

GORDON, A. G. (1992) Benign paroxysmal positional vertigo (BPPV) or bubble provoked positional vertigo. *Journal of the Neurological Sciences*, **111**, 229–230

GORDON, M. A. (1989) The genetics of otosclerosis: a review. *American Journal of Otology*, **10**, 426–438

GOULD, W. J. and BROOKLER, K. H. (1972) Minocycline therapy. *Archives of Otolaryngology*, **96**, 291

GOWERS, W. R. (1907) *Epilepsy and Other Chronic Convulsive Diseases: their Causes, Symptoms and Treatment*. New York: Dover Publications Incoroporation, 1964

GOZDZIK-ZOLNIERKIEWICZ, T. and MOSZYNSKI, B. (1969) VIIIth nerve in experimental lead poisoning. *Acta Otolaryngologica*, **68**, 85–89

GRAD, A. and BALOH, R. W. (1989) Vertigo of vascular origin. Clinical and elctronystagmographic features in 84 cases. *Archives of Neurology*, **46**, 281–284

GRADENIGO, G. (1893) On the clinical signs of affections of the auditory nerve. *Archives of Otolaryngology*, **22**, 213–230

GRAY, L. B. (1956) Extra-labyrinthine vertigo due to cervical muscle lesions. *Journal of Laryngology and Otology*, **70**, 352–361

GRENMAN, R. (1985) Involvement of the audiovestibular system in multiple sclerosis. An otoneurologic and audiologic study. *Acta Otolaryngologica*, Suppl. 420, 1–95

GRENMAN, R., AANTAA, E., KALEVIKATEVUO, V., KORMANO, M. and PANELIUS, M. (1988) Otoneurological and ultra low field MRI findings in multiple sclerosis patients. *Acta Otolaryngologica*, **449**, 78–83

GRIBBEN, B., PICKERING, T. G., SLEIGHT, P. and PETO, R. (1971) Effect of age and high blood pressure on baroreflex sensitivity in man. *Circulation Research*, **29**, 424–431

GUILD, S. (1944) Histologic otosclerosis. *Annals of Otology, Rhinology and Laryngology*, **53**, 246–266

GULYA, A. J. (1993) Neurologic paraneoplastic syndromes with neurotologic manifestations. *Laryngoscope*, **103**, 754–761

GUSSEN, R. (1973) Otosclerosis and vestibular degeneration. *Archives of Otolaryngology*, **97**, 484–487

GUSSEN, R. (1976) Sudden deafness of vascular origin: a human temporal bone study. *Annals of Otology, Rhinology and Laryngology*, **85**, 94–100

GUSSEN, R. (1977) Polyarteritis nodosa and deafness. A human temporal bone study. *Archives of Otology, Rhinology and Laryngology*, **217**, 263–271

GYDE, M. C. (1976) When the weeping stopped. An otologist reviews otorrhea and gentamicin. *Archives of Otolaryngology*, **102**, 542

GYO, K. (1988) Benign paroxysmal positional vertigo as a complication of postoperative bedrest. *Laryngoscope*, **98**, 332–333

HAGEMAN, M. J. (1975) Het syndroom van Waardenburg. Naarden: Los

HALLGREN, V. (1959) Retinitis pigmentosa combined with congenital deafness; with vestibulo-cerebellar ataxia and mental abnormality in a proportion of cases. A clinical and geneticostatistical study. *Acta Psychiatrica Scandinavica Supplementum*, **138**, 1–101

HALLPIKE, C. S. (1967) Some types of ocular nystagmus and their neurological mechanism. *Proccedings of the Royal Society of Medicine*, **60**, 1043–1054

HALMAGYI, G. M. and CURTHOYS, I. S. (1988) A clinical sign of canal paresis. *Archives of Neurology*, **45**, 737

HALPERIN, J., LUFT, B. J., ANAND, A. K., ROQUE, C. T., ALVAREZ, O., VOLKMAN, D. J. *et al.* (1989) Lyme neuroborreliosis: Central nervous system manifestations. *Neurology*, **39**, 753–758

HALPERIN, J., LUFT, B. J., VOLKMAN, D. J. and DATTWYLER, R. J. (1990) Lyme neuroborreliosis: peripheral nervous system manifestations. *Brain*, **113**, 1207–1221

HANNER, P., ROSENHALL, U., ENGSTROM, S. and KAIJSER, B. (1989) Hearing impairment in patients with antibody production against *Borrelia burgdorferi* antigen. *Lancet*, i, 13–15

HARADA, T., SEMBA, T., SUZUKI, M., KIKUCHI, S. and MUROFUSHI, T. (1988) Audiological characteristics of hearing loss following meningitis. *Acta Otolaryngologica*, Suppl. 456, 61–67

HARDING, A. E. (1989) The mitochondrial genome – breaking the magic circle. *New England Journal of Medicine*, **320**, 1341

HARIRI, M. A. (1993) Autoimmune inner-ear disease. Review Paper. *Journal of Audiological Medicine*, **2**, 41–52

HARKER, L. A. and RASSEKH, C. (1988) Migraine equivalent as a cause of episodic vertigo. *Laryngoscope*, **98**, 160–164

HARNER, S. G. (1981) Hearing in adult onset diabetes mellitus. *Otolaryngology, Head and Neck Surgery*, **89**, 322–327

HARRIS, J. P., LOW, N. C. and HOUSE, W. F. (1985) Contralateral hearing loss following inner ear injury; sympathetic cochleolabyrinthitis. *American Journal of Otology*, **6**, 175–180

HART, C. W., COKELY, C. G., SCHUPBACH, J., DAL CANTO, M. C. and COPPLESON, L. W. (1989) Neurotologic findings of a patient with acquired immune deficiency syndrome. *Ear and Hearing*, **10**, 68–76

HAUBEK, A. and LEE, K. (1979) Computed tomography in alcoholic cerebellar atrophy. *Neuroradiology*, **18**, 77

HAUSLER, R., VIBERT, D., KORALNIK, I. J. and HIRSCHEL B. (1991) Neurotological manifestations in different stages of HIV infection. *Acta Otolaryngologica*, Suppl. 481, 515–521

HEAD, P. W. (1984) Vertigo and barotrauma. In: *Vertigo*, edited by M. R. Dix and J. D. Hood. Chichester: John Wiley and Sons Limited. pp. 199–216

HENLEY, C. M. and RYBAK, L. P. (1993) Developmental ototoxicity. *Otolaryngology Clinics of North America*, **26**, 857–871

HERDMAN, R. C. D., HARIRI, M. and RAMSDEN, R. T. (1991) Autoimmune inner ear disease and ulcerative colitis. *Journal of Laryngology and Otology*, **105**, 330–331

HERRERA, W. G. (1990) Vestibular and other balance disorders in multiple sclerosis. *Neurologic Clinics*, **8**, 407–420

HIGASHI, K. (1989) Unique inheritance of streptomycin-induced deafness. *Clinical Genetics*, **35**, 433–436

HIKOSAKA, O. and MAEDA, M. (1973) Cervical effects on abducens motoneurons and their interaction with vestibulo-ocular reflex. *Experimental Brain Research*, **18**, 512–530

HINCHCLIFFE, R. (1967) Headache and Menière's disease. *Acta Otolaryngologica*, **63**, 384–390

HINCHCLIFFE, R., COLES, R. R. A. and KING, P. F. (1992) Occupational noise induced vestibular malfunction? *British Journal of Industrial Medicine*, **49**, 63–65

HINOKI, M. (1985) Vertigo due to whiplash injury: a neurotological approach. *Acta Otolaryngologica*, Suppl. 419, 9–29

HINSHAW, H. C. and FELDMAN, W. H. (1945) Streptomycin in the treatment of tuberculosis: a preliminary report. *Proceedings of the Mayo Clinic*, **20**, 313–318

HIRAIDE, F., INOUYE, T. and ISHII, T. (1983) Primary squamous cell carcinoma of the middle ear invading the cochlea. A histopathological case report. *Annals of Otology, Rhinology and Laryngology*, **92**, 290–294

HOLMES, G. (1922) The clinical symptoms of cerebellar disease and their interpretation. Croonian lectures. *Lancet*, i, 1177, 1231; ii, 59, 111

HU, D. N., QIU, W. Q., WU, B. T., FANG, L. Z., ZHOU, F., GU, Y. P. *et al.* (1991) Genetic aspects of antibiotic induced deafness: mitochondrial inheritance. *Journal of Medical Genetics*, **28**, 79–83

HUANG, M. H., NUANG, C. C., RYU, S. J. and CHU, N. S. (1993) Sudden bilateral hearing impairment in vertebrobasilar occlusive disease. *Stroke*, **24**, 132–137

HUGHES, G. B., KINNEY, S. E., BARNA, B. P. and CALABRESE, L. H. (1985) Autoimmune Meniere's syndrome. Immunobiology, autoimmunity and transplantation in otorhinolaryngology. *Proceedings of the First International Conference*, Utrecht, The Netherlands. Amsterdam: Kugler Publications. pp. 119–129

HUGUES, F. C., MUNERA, Y. and LE-JEUNNE, C. (1992) Drug induced orthostatic hypotension. *Revue de Medecin Interne*, **13**, 465–470

HUSON, S. M., HARPER, P. S. and COMPSTON, D. A. S. (1988) Von Recklinghausen neurofibromatosis: a clinical and population study in south east Wales. *Brain*, **111**, 1355–1381

HUYGEN, P. L. M. (1983) Vestibular hyperactivity in patients with multiple sclerosis. *Advances in Otolaryngology*, **30**, 141–149

HUYGEN, P. L. M. and VERHAGEN, W. I. M. (1994) Peripheral vestibular and vestibulo-cochlear dysfunction in hereditary disorders. *Journal of Vestibular Research*, **4**, 81–104

HYSLOP, G. (1952) Intra-cranial circulatory complication of injuries to the neck. *Bulletin of the New York Academy of Medicine*, **28**, 729–733

IGARASHI, M., JERGER, S., O-UCHI, T. and ALFORD, B. R. (1982) Fluctuating hearing loss and recurrent vertigo in otosclerosis: an audiologic and temporal bone study. *Archives of Otorhinolaryngology*, **236**, 161–171

IGARASHI, M., WEBER, S. C., ALFORD, B. R., COATS, A. C. and JERGER, J. (1975) Temporal bone findings in cryptococcal meningitis. *Archives of Otolaryngology*, **101**, 577–583

ILLUM, P., KIAER, H. W., HVIDBERG-HANSEN, J. and SONDERGAARD, G. (1972) Fifteen cases of Pendred's syndrome. Congenital deafness and sporadic goitre. *Archives of Otolaryngology*, **96**, 297

ISHIZAKI, H., PYYKKO, I. and NOZUE, N. (1993) Neuroborreliosis in the etiology of vestibular neuronitis. *Acta Otolaryngologica*, Suppl. 503, 67–69

JACOBS, A., LEDINGHAM, J. G., KERR, A. I. and FORD, M. J. (1990) Ulcerative colitis and giant cell arteritis associated with sensorineural deafness. *Journal of Laryngology and Otology*, **104**, 889–890

JACOBSON, J. T. and JACOBSON, G. P. (1990) The auditory brainstem response in multiple sclerosis. *Seminars in Hearing*, **11**, 248–263

JAHRSDOERFER, R. A., THOMPSON, E. G., JOHNS, M. M. and CANTRELL, R. W. (1981) Sarcoidosis and fluctuating Hearing loss. *Annals of Otology, Rhinology and Laryngology*, **90**, 161–163

JENKINS, H. A., POLLAK, A. M. and FISCH, U. (1981) Polyarteritis nodosa as a cause of sudden deafness. A human temporal bone study. *American Journal of Otolaryngology*, **2**, 99–107

JERGER, J. and JERGER, S. (1981) *Auditory Disorders*. Boston: Little, Brown and Company

JERGER, J., NEELY, G. G. and JERGER, S. (1980) Speech impedance and auditory brainstem response audiometry in brainstem tumours. *Archives of Otolaryngology*, **106**, 218–223

JOHNS, D. R., TIERNEY, M. and FELSENSTEIN, D. (1987) Alteration in the natural history of neurosyphilis by concurrent infection with the human immunodeficiency virus. *New England Journal of Medicine*, **316**, 1569–1572

JOHNSEN, T., LARSEN, C., FRIIS, J. and HOUGAARD-JENSEN, F. (1987) Pendred's syndrome. Acoustic, vestibular and radiological findings in 17 unrelated patients. *Journal of Laryngology and Otology*, **101**, 1187–1192

JOHNSON, J. T., WALL, C., BARNEY, S. A. and THEARLE, P. B. (1985) Postoperative vestibular dysfunction following head and neck surgery. *Acta Otolaryngologica*, **100**, 316–320

JOHNSSON, L. G. (1974) Sequence of degeneration of Corti's organ and its first order neurons. *Annals of Otology, Rhinology and Laryngology*, **83**, 294

JOHNSSON, L. G. and HAWKINS, J. E. (1972) Sensory and neural degeneration with aging as seen in microdissections of the human inner ear. *Annals of Otology, Rhinology and Laryngology*, **81**, 179–193

JONGKEES, L. B. W. (1969) Cervical vertigo. *Laryngoscope*, **79**, 1473–1484

JORGENSEN, M. and BUCH, N. (1961) Studies on inner ear function and cranial nerves in diabetes. *Acta Otolaryngologica*, **53**, 350–364

JORGENSEN, M., KRISTENSEN, H. K. and BUCH, N. (1964) Thalidomide-induced aplasia of the inner ear. *Journal of Laryngology and Otology*, **78**, 1095–1101

KAPLAN, N. M. (1992) Two faces of sympathetic nervous activity – hypotension and hypertension. *American Journal of Medical Science*, **303**, 271–279

KARMODY, C. S. and SCHUKNECHT, H. F. (1966) Deafness in congenital syphilis. *Archives of Otolaryngology*, **83**, 18–27

KASHII, S., ITO, J., MATSUOKA, I., SASA, M. and TAKAORI, S. (1984) Effects of ethanol applied by electrosmosis on neurons in the lateral and medial vestibular nuclei. *Japanese Journal of Pharmacology*, **36**, 153

KATSARKAS, A. (1982) Positional nystagmus of the 'central type' as an early sign of multiple sclerosis. *Journal of Otolaryngology*, **11**, 91–93

KATTAH, J. C., KOLSKY, M. P. and LUESSENHOP, A. J. (1984) Positional vertigo and the cerebellar vermis. *Neurology*, **34**, 527–529

KAY, R. (1991) The site of the lesion causing hearing loss in bacterial meningitis – a study of experimental streptococcal meningitis in guinea-pigs. *Neuropathology, Applied Neurobiology*, **17**, 485–493

KAYAN, A. and HOOD, J. D. (1984) Neuro-otological manifestations of migraine. *Brain*, **197**, 1123–1142

KELEMAN, G. (1983) Temporal bone findings in cases of salt water drownings. *Annals of Otology, Rhinology and Laryngology*, **92**, 134–136

KERR, A. G. and SMYTH, G. D. L. (1987) Ear trauma. In: *Scott Brown's Otolaryngology*, 5th edn, edited by A. G. Kerr, Vol. 3, *Otology*, edited by J. B. Booth. London: Butterworths. pp. 172–184

KESSLER, J. and PATTERSON, R. H. JR. (1970) The production of microemboli by various blood oxygenators. *Annals of Thoracic Surgery*, **9**, 221–228

KHETARPAL, U. and SCHUKNECHT, H. F. (1990) In search of pathologic correlates for hearing loss and vertigo in Paget's disease. *Annals of Otology, Rhinology and Laryngology*, Suppl. 145, 1–16

KIKUCHI, M. (1959) On the sympathetic otitis. *Zibi Rinosyo Kyoto*, **37**, 1–16

KIKUCHI, S., KIMITAKA, K., YAMASOBA, T., HIGO, R., OUCHI, T. and TOKUMARU, A. (1993) Slow blood flow of the vertebrobasilar system in patients with dizziness and vertigo. *Acta Otolaryngologica*, **113**, 257–260

KIM, J. S., LEE, J. H., SUH, D. C. and LEE, M. C. (1994) Spectrum of lateral medullary syndrome. Correlation between clinical findings and magnetic resonance imaging in 33 subjects. *Stroke*, **25**, 1405–1410

KIMURA, R. and PERLMAN, H. B. (1958) Arterial obstruction of the labyrinth. (1) Cochlear changes. (II) Vestibular changes. *Annals of Otology, Rhinology and Laryngology*, **67**, 5–25

KITAMURA, K. and BERREBY, M. (1983) Temporal bone histopathology associated with occlusion of vertebrobasilar arteries. *Annals of Otology, Rhinology and Laryngology*, **92**, 33–38

KLIGERMAN, A. B., SOLANGI, K. B., VENTRY, I. M., GOODMAN, A. I. and WESELEY, S. A. (1981) Hearing impairment associated with chronic renal failure. *Laryngoscope*, **91**, 583–592

KOBAYASHI, H., MIZUKOSHI, K., WATANABE, Y., NAGASAKI, T., ITO, M. and ASO, S. (1991) Otoneurological findings in inner ear syphilis. *Acta Otolaryngologica*, Suppl. **481**, 551–555

KOENIG, S., GENDELMAN, H. E., ORENSTEIN, J. M., DAL CANTO, M. C., PEZESHKPOUR, G. H., YUNGBLUTH, M. *et al.* (1986) Detection of AIDS virus in macrophages in brain tissue from AIDS patients with encephalopathy. *Science*, **5**, 1089–1094

KOGEORGEOS, J., SCOTT, D. F. and SWASH, M. (1981) Epileptic dizziness. *British Medical Journal*, **282**, 687–689

KOIZUKA, I., GOTO, K., OKADA, M., KUBO, T. and MATSUNAGA, T. (1988) ENG findings in patients with bell's palsy. *Acta Otolaryngologica*, **446**, 85–92

KONIGSMARK, B. W. and GORLIN, R. J. (1976) *Genetic and Metabolic Deafness*. Philadelphia: W. B. Saunders Company

KOS, A.O., SCHUKNECHT, H. F. and SINGER, A. J. (1966) Temporal bone studies in 13–15 and 18 trisomy syndrome. *Archives of Otolaryngology*, **83**, 439–445

KOVAR, M. (1973) The inner ear in diabetes mellitus. *Journal of Otolaryngology and Related Specialties*, **35**, 42

KUILMAN, J. (1959) The importance of the cervical syndrome in otology. *Practica Oto-rhino-laryngology*, **21**, 174–185

KURIEN, M., THOMAS, K. and BHANU, T. S. (1989) Hearing thresholds in patients with diabetes mellitus. *Journal of Laryngology and Otology*, **103**, 164–168

KUSAKARI, J., TAKEYAMA, M., KAWASE, T., TAKAHASHI, K. SASAKI, Y. and TAKASAKA, T. (1988) Studies with electrocochleography and auditory brainstem response in Ramsay Hunt syndrome. *Acta Otolaryngologica*, **446**, 81–84

KUZUHARA, S. and YOSHIMURA, M. (1993), Clinical and neuropathological aspects of diffuse Lewy body disease in the elderly. *Advances in Neurology*, **60**, 464–469

LALANNE, M. C., DOUTREMEPUICH, C., BOJ, F., TRAISSAC, L. and QUICHAUD, F. (1992) Some hemostatic and hemorheological disorders in auditory and vestibular impairments. *Thrombosis Research*, **66**, 787–791

LANGSTON, J. W. (1989) Current theories on the cause of Parkinson's disease. *Journal of Neurology, Neurosurgery and Psychiatry*, Special Suppl., 13–17

LEHNHARDT, E. (1958) Plotzliche Horstorungen, auf beiden Seiten gleichzeitig oder nacheinander aufgetreten. *Zeitschrift für Laryngologie, Rhinologie, Otologie und ihre Grenzgebiete*, **37**, 1–16

LEIGH, R. J. and ZEE, D. S. (1991a) Synthesis of the commands for conjugate eye movements. In: *The Neurology of Eye Movements*, edited by F. Plum. Philadelphia: Davis Company. p. 208

LEIGH, R. J. and ZEE, D. S. (1991b) Diagnosis of central disorders of ocular motility. In: *The Neurology of Eye Movements*, edited by F. Plum. Philadelphia: Davis Company. p. 423

LENNOX, L. G. (1960) *Epilepsy and Related Disorders*. Boston: Little Brown and Company

LESSENGER, H. E. (1992) Five office workers inadvertently

exposed to cypermethrin. *Journal of Toxicology and Environmental Health*, **35**, 261–267

LESSER, T. H. J., DORT, J. C. and SIMMEN, D. P. B. (1990) Ear nose and throat manifestations of Lyme disease. *Journal of Laryngology and Otology*, **104**, 301–304

LEWIS, G. W. (1958) Zoster sine herpete. *British Medical Journal*, **5093**, 418–421.

LI, W., SCHACHERN, P. A. and PAPARELLA, M. M. (1994) Extensive otosclerosis and endolymphatic hydrops: histopathologic study of temporal bones. *American Journal of Otolaryngology*, **15**, 158–161

LIM, D. J. (1984) Otoconia in health and disease. A review. *Annals of Otology, Rhinology and Laryngology*, Suppl. 112, 17–24

LIMANSKII, S. S. (1990) Kokhleovestibuliarnyi sindrom vsledstvie sfecnokita. (Cochleovestibular syndrome caused by sphenoiditis). *Vestnik Otorinolaringolosii (Moskva)*, **1**, 66–67

LINDEMAN, H. H. (1969) Regional differences in sensitivity of the vestibular sensory epithelia to oto-toxic antibiotics. *Acta Otolaryngologica*, **67**, 177–189

LINDENOV, H. (1945) *The Aetiology of Deaf – Mutism*. Copenhagen: Einar Munksguard

LINDSAY, J. R. (1973a) Profound childhood deafness. Inner ear pathology. *Annals of Otology, Rhinology and Laryngology*, **82**, (Suppl. 5), 5–121

LINDSAY, J. R. (1973b) Histopathology of deafness due to postnatal viral disease. *Archives of Otolaryngology*, **98**, 258–264

LINDSAY, J. R. and HEMENWAY, W. G. (1956) Postural vertigo due to unilateral sudden partial loss of vestibular functions. *Annals of Otology, Rhinology and Laryngology*, **65**, 692–708

LIPSITZ, L. A. (1989) Orthostatic hypotension in the elderly. *New England Journal of Medicine*, **321**, 952–957

LISTON, S. L., PAPARELLA, M. M., MANCINI, F. and ANDERSON, J. H. (1984) Otosclerosis and endolymphatic hydrops. *Laryngoscope*, **94**, 1003–1007

LONGRIDGE, N. S. and MALLINSON, A. I. (1987) The dynamic illegible E (DIE) test: a simple technique for assessing the ability of the vestibulo-ocular reflex to overcome vestibular pathology. *Journal of Otolaryngology*, **16**, 97

LUXON, L. M. (1980) Hearing loss in brainstem disorders. *Journal of Neurology, Neurosurgery and Psychiatry*, **43**, 510–515

LUXON, L. M. (1990) Signs and symptoms of vertebrobasilar insufficiency. In: *Vascular Brain Stem Diseases*, edited by B. Hofferberth, G. G. Brune, G. Sitzer and H. D. Weger. Basel: Karger. pp. 93–111

LUXON, L. M., LEES, A. J. and GREENWOOD, R. J. (1979) Neurosyphilis today. *Lancet*, **i**, 90–93

LUXON, L. M., CROWTHER, A., HARRISON, M. J. G. and COLTART, D. J. (1980) Controlled study of 24 hour ambulatory electrocardiographic monitoring in patients with transient neurological symptoms. *Journal of Neurology, Neurosurgery and Psychiatry*, **43**, 37–41

LYON, M. F., SCRIVER, C. R., BAKER, L. R. I., TENENHOUSE, H. S., KRONICK, J. and MANDLA, S. (1986) The 'Gy' mutation: another cause of X-Linked hypophosphatemia in mouse. *Proceedings of the National Academy of Sciences USA*, **83**, 4866–4903

MACARTHUR, C., LEWIS, M. and KNOX, E. G. (1992) Investigation of long term problems after obstetric epidural anaesthesia. *British Medical Journal*, **304**, 1279–1282

MCCABE, B. F. (1979) Autoimmune sensorineural hearing loss

Annals of Otology, Rhinology and Laryngology, **88**, 585–589

MCCABE, B. F. (1985) Autoimmune inner ear disease. Immunobiology, autoimmunity and transplantation in otorhinolaryngology. *Proceedings of the 1st International Conference*, Utrecht, The Netherlands. Amsterdam: Kugler Publications. pp. 107–110

MCCABE, B. F. and HARKER, L. A. (1983) Vascular loop as a cause of vertigo. *Annals of Otology, Rhinology and Laryngology*, **92**, 542–543

MCCOUCH, G. P., DEERING, I. D. and LING, T. H. (1951) Location of receptors for tonic neck reflexes. *Journal of Neurophysiology*, **14**, 191–195

MCCRAE, D. and O'REILLY, S. (1957) On some neuro-oto-ophthalmological manifestations of systemic lupus erythematosus and polyarteritis nodosa. *Eye, Ear, Nose and Throat Monthly*, **36**, 721–726

MCGILL, T. (1976) Carcinomatous encephalomyelitis with auditory and vestibular manifestations. *Annals of Otology, Rhinology and Laryngology*, **85**, 120–126

MCGILL, T. (1978) Mycotic infections of the temporal bone. *Archives of Otolaryngology*, **104**, 140

MCINTOSH, S., DA-COSTA, D. and KENNY, R. A. (1993) Outcome of an integrated approach to the evaluation of dizziness, falls and syncope in elderly patients referred to a syncope clinic. *Age and Ageing*, **22**, 53–58

MACMAHON, B. J., HELMINIAK, C., WAINWRIGHT, R. B., BULKOW, L., TRIMBLE, B. A. and WAINWRIGHT, K. (1992) Frequency of adverse reactions to hepatitis B vaccine in 43,618 persons. *American Journal of Medicine*, **293**, 254–256

MACPHEE, J. A. and BRODIE, M. (1988) Drugs in the elderly. *Medicine International*. *Clinical Pharmacology*, **59**, 2441–2446

MAFEE, M. F., KUMAR, A., VALVASSORI, G. E., DOBBEN, G. D. and MAYER, D. (1985) Diagnostic potential of CT in neuro-otological disorders. *Laryngoscope*, **95**, 505

MAGNUSSON, M. and NORRVING, B. (1993) Cerebellar infarctions as the cause of 'vestibular neuritis'. *Acta Otolaryngologica*, Suppl. 503, 64–66

MAKISHIMA, K. and TANAKA, K. (1971) Pathological changes of the inner ear and central auditory pathways in diabetes. *Annals of Otology, Rhinology and Laryngology*, **80**, 218–228

MANNI, J. J., SCAF, I. J., HUYGEN, P. L. M., CRUYSBERG, J. R. and VERHAGEN, W. I. (1990) Hyperostosis cranialis interna: a new hereditary syndrome with cranial nerve entrapment. *New England Journal of Medicine*, **322**, 450

MARAGANORE, D. M., HARDING, A. E. and MARSDEN, C. D. (1991) A clinical and genetic study of familial Parkinson's disease. *Movement Disorders*, **6**, 205–211

MARCUS, R. E. (1968) Vestibular function and additional findings in Waardenburg's syndrome. *Acta Otolaryngologica*, Suppl. 229, 5–30

MARCUS, R. E. and LEE, Y. M. (1976) Inner ear disorders in a family with sickle cell thalassaemia. *Archives of Otolaryngology*, **102**, 703–705

MARSDEN, C. D. (1990) In: *Oxford Textbook of Medicine*, 2nd edn, edited by Weatherall, Ledingham and Warrell

MASLAN, M. J., GRAHAM, M. D. and FLOOD, L. M. (1985) Cryptococcal meningitis: presentation of sudden deafness. *American Journal of Otology*, **6**, 435–437

MASSON, C., STERKERS, O., CHAIGNE, P., COLOMBANI, J. M. and MASSON, M. (1992) Isolated vertigo disclosing infarction in the area of the posterior and inferior cerebellar arteries. *Annales d'Otolaringologie et de Chirurgie cervico-faciale*, **109**, 80–86

MATSUO, R. and SEKITANI, T. (1985) Vestibular neuronitis: neurotological findings and progress. *Otorhinolaryngology,* 47, 199–206

MATZ, G. J., RATTENBORG, C. G. and HOLADAY, D. A. (1967) Effects of nitrous oxide on middle ear pressure. *Anesthesiology,* 28, 948–950

MAXWELL, O. N. (1963) Hearing loss in uveitis. *Archives of Otolaryngology,* 78, 138–142

MAZAGRI, R., SHUAIB, A. and DENATH, F. M. (1992) Medullary haemorrhage causing vertigo and gaze nystagmus. *Ear, Nose and Throat Journal,* 71, 402–403

MAZZONI, A. (1969) Internal auditory canal arterial relations at the porus acousticus. *Annals of Otology, Rhinology and Laryngology,* 78, 797–814

MENNI, S., IMONDI, D., BRANCALEONE, W. and CROCI, S. (1993) Recurrent giant aphthous ulcers in a child: protracted treatment with thalidomide. *Pediatric Dermatology,* 10, 283–285

MEURMAN, O. H., AANTAA, E. and VIROLAINEN, E. (1969) Vestibular disturbances in clinical otosclerosis. *Archives of Otolaryngology,* 90, 756–768

MEYER, J. S. and BARRON, D. W. (1960) Apraxia of gait: a clinico–physiological study. *Brain,* 83, 261–284

MICHAELS, L. and WELLS, M. (1980) Squamous carcinoma of the middle ear. *Clinical Otolaryngology,* 5, 235–248

MICHEL, M. (1863) Memoire sur les anomalies congenitals de l'oreille interne. *Gazette medicale de Strasbourg,* 4, 55–58

MITCHELL, D. E. and ADAMS, J. H. (1973) Primary focal impact damage to the brain stem in blunt head injuries. Does it exist? *Lancet,* ii, 215

MITSCHKE, H., SCHMIDT, P., ZAZGORNIK, J., KOPSA, H. and PILS, P. (1977) Effect of renal transplantation on uremic deafness; a longterm study. *Audiology,* 16, 530–534

MIYAMOTO, R. T., HOUSE, W. F. and BRACKMANN, D. E. (1980) Neurotologic manifestations of the osteopetroses. *Archives of Otolaryngology,* 106, 210–214

MIZUKOSHI, K. M., OHNO, Y., ISKIKAWA, K., AOYAGI, M., WATANABE, Y., KATO, I. et al. (1975) Neuro-otological studies upon intoxication by organic mercury compounds. *ORL,* 37, 74–87

MIZUNO, M., YAMASOBA, T. and NOMURA, Y. (1992) Vestibular disturbance after myelography. Contrast media in the internal auditory canal. *ORL,* 54, 113–115

MO, R., OMVIK, P. and LUND-JOHANSEN, P. (1994) The Bergen blood pressure study estimated prevalence of postural hypotension is influenced by the alerting reaction to blood pressure measurement. *Journal of Human Hypertension,* 8, 171–176

MOLVAER, O. I. (1991) Vestibular problems in diving and space. *Scandanavian Audiology,* Suppl. 34, 163–170

MONEY, K. E. and MYLES, W. S. (1974) Heavy water nystagmus and effects of alcohol. *Nature,* 247, 404–405

MORALES-GARCIA, C. (1972) Cochleovestibular involvement in otosclerosis. *Acta Otolaryngologica,* 73, 484–492

MORGENSTEIN, K. M. and MANACE, E. D. (1969) Temporal bone histopathology in sickle cell disease. *Laryngoscope,* 79, 2172–2180

MORI, K., MIYAZAKI, H. and ONO, H. (1978) Aneurysm of the anterior inferior cerebellar artery at the internal auditory meatus. *Surgical Neurology,* 10, 297–300

MORRISON, A. W. (1975) In: *Management of Sensorineural Deafness.* London: Butterworths.

MORRISON, A. W. (1984) Meniere's disease. In: *Vertigo,* edited by M. R. Dix and J. D. Hood. Chichester: John Wiley & Sons Limited. pp. 133–152

MORRISON, A. W. (1986) Predictive tests for Meniere's disease. *American Journal of Otology,* 7, 5–10

MOSCHNER, C., PERLMAN, S. and BALOH, R. W. (1994) Comparison of oculomotor findings in the progressive ataxia syndromes. *Brain,* 117, 15–25

MOSLEY, L. (1988) In: *Magnetic Resonance Imaging in Disorders of the Nervous System.* Blackwell, Oxford.

MULLER, E. (1936) Vestibularisstorungen bei erblicher Taubheit. *Archiv für Ohren, Nasen und Kehlkopfheilkunde,* 142, 156–163

MYERS, S. F. and ROSS, M. D. (1987) Morphological evidence of vestibular pathology in long-term experimental diabetes mellitus. *Acta Otolaryngologica,* 104, 40–49

MYERS, S. F., BLAKLEY, B. W. and SCHWAN, S. (1993) Is cisplatinum vestibulotoxic? *Otolaryngology, Head and Neck Surgery,* 108, 322–328

MYERS, S. F., ROSS, M. D., JOKELAINEN, P., GRAHAM, M. D. and MCCLATCHEY, K. D. (1985) Morphological evidence of vestibular pathology in long-term experimental diabetes mellitus. *Acta Otolaryngologica,* 100, 351–364

NADOL, J. B. and BURGESS, B. (1982) Cochleosaccular degeneration of the inner ear and progressive cataracts inherited as an autosomal dominant trait. *Laryngoscope,* 92, 1028–1037

NADOL, J. B. and SCHUKNECHT, H. F. (1990) Pathology of peripheral vestibular disorders in the elderly. *American Journal of Otolaryngology,* 11, 213–227

NAESS, A., HALSTENSEN, A., NYLAND, H., PEDERSEN, S. H., MOLLER, P., BORGMANN, R. et al. (1994) Sequelae one year after meningococcal disease. *Acta Neurologica Scandinavica,* 89, 139

NAGER, G. T. (1975) Paget's disease of the temporal bone. *Annals of Otology, Rhinology and Laryngology,* 84 (Suppl. 22), 1–32

NAGER, G. T., KENNEDY D. W. and KOPSTEIN, E. (1982) Fibrous dysplasia: a review of the disease and its manifestations in the temporal bone. *Annals of Otology, Rhinology and Laryngology,* 91 (Suppl. 92), 5–52

NAUFAL, P. M. and SCHUKNECHT, H. F. (1972) Vestibular, facial and oculomotor neuropathy in diabetes mellitus. *Archives of Otolaryngology,* 96, 468

NAUNTON, R. F., LINDSAY, J. R. and STEIN, L. K. (1973) Concretions in the stria vascularis. *Archives of Otolaryngology,* 97, 376–380

NELSON, M., LESSELL, S. and SADUN, A. A. (1986) Optic nerve hypoplasia and maternal diabetes mellitus. *Archives of Neurology,* 43, 20–25

NIH CONSENSUS DEVELOPMENT CONFERENCE. (1991) Consensus Statement. *Acoustic Neuroma,* 9, 1–24

NISHIDA, Y., UEDA, K. and FUNG, K. (1983) Congenital rubella syndrome: function of equilibrium of 80 cases with deafness. *Laryngoscope,* 93, 938–940

NISHIOKA, I. and YANAGIHARA, N. (1986) Role of air bubbles in the perilymph as a cause of sudden deafness. *American Journal of Otology,* 7, 430–438

NORRE, M. E., FORREZ, G. and BECKERS, A. (1987) Vestibular dysfunction causing instability in aged patients. *Acta Otolaryngologica,* 104, 50–55

NYLEN, C. O. (1950) Positional nystagmus. A review and future prospects. *Journal of Laryngology and Otology,* 64, 295–318

ODA, M. (1974) Labyrinthine pathology of chronic renal failure patients treated with haemodialysis and kidney transplantation. *Laryngoscope,* 84, 1489–1506

ODKVIST, L. M., MOLLER, C. and THUOMAS, K.A. (1992)

Otoneurologic disturbances caused by solvent pollution. *Otolaryngology, Head and Neck Surgery*, **106**, 687–692

ODKVIST, L. M., LARSBY, B., FREDRICKSON, J. M., LIEDGREN, S. R. C. and THAM, R. (1980) Vestibular and oculomotor disturbances caused by industrial solvents. *Journal of Otolaryngology*, **9**, 53–59

ODKVIST, L., LARSBY, B., THAM, R. and HYDEN, D. (1983) Vestibulo-oculomotor disturbances caused by industrial solvents. *Otolaryngology, Head and Neck Surgery*, **91**, 537–539

ODKVIST, L. M., ARLINGER, S. D., EDLING, C., LARSBY, B. and BERGHOLTZ, L. M. (1987) Audiological and vestibulo-oculomotor findings in workers exposed to solvents and jet fuel. *Scandinavian Audiology*, **16**, 75–81

OGISI, F. O. and OKAFOR, L. A. (1987) Assessment of auditory function in sickle cell anaemia patients in Nigeria. *Tropical Geographic Medicine*, **39**, 28–31

OHASHI, N., YASAMURA, S., NAKAGAWA, H., MIZUKOSHI, K. and KUZE, S. (1992) Vascular cross-compression of the VIIth and VIIIth cranial nerves. *Journal of Laryngology and Otology*, **106**, 436–439

OKINAKA, Y., SEKITANI, T., OKAZAKI, H., MIURA, M. and TAHARA, T. (1993) Progress of caloric response in vestibular neuronitis. *Acta Otolaryngologica*, Suppl. 503, 18–22

OLBRICH, H. G., KALTENBACH, M. and HOPF, R. (1992) Ventricular function in hypertrophic cardiomyopathy. Systolic and diastolic ventricular function. *Fortschritte der Medizin*, **110**, 481–484

O'LEARY, D. P. and DAVIS, L. L. (1990) High frequency autorotational testing of the vestibulo-ocular reflex. *Neurology Clinics*, **8**, 297

OLESEN, J. (1990) Calcium antagonists in migraine and vertigo. Possible mechanisms of action and review of clinical trials. *European Neurology*, 30 (Suppl.), 31–34

O'LOUGHLIN, J. L., ROBITAILLE, Y., BOIVIN, J. F. and SUISSA, S. (1993) Incidence of and risk factors for falls and injurious falls among the community dwelling elderly. *American Journal of Epidemiology*, **1**, 342–354

OLSON, M. E., CHERNIK, N. L. and POSNER, J. B. (1974) Infiltration of the leptomeninges by systemic cancer. A clinical and pathologic study. *Archives of Neurology*, **30**, 122–137

OLSSON, J. E. (1991) Neurotologic findings in basilar migraine. *Laryngoscope*, **101**, 1–41

O MAHONEY, C. F., GATLAND, D. J. and LUXON, L. M. (1995) Audiovestibular complications of non-otological surgery. *Clinical Otolaryngology*, (in press)

O'MALLEY, S., RAMSDEN, R. T., LATIF, A., KANE, R. and DAVIES, M. (1985) Electrocochleographic changes in the hearing loss associated with X-linked hypophosphataemic osteomalacia. *Acta Otolaryngologica*, **100**, 13–18

OOSTERVELD, W. J., KORTSCHOT, H. W., KINGMA, G. G., DE JOHN, H. A. A. and SAATCI, M. R. (1991) Electronystagmographic findings following cervical whiplash injuries. *Acta Otolaryngologica*, **111**, 201–205

ORCHIK, D. J. and DUNN, J. W. (1977) Sickle cell anaemia and sudden deafness. *Archives of Otolaryngology*, **103**, 369–370

PACE–BALZAN, A. and RUTKA, J. A. (1991) Non-ampullary plugging of the posterior semicircular canal for benign paroxysmal positional vertigo. *Journal of Laryngology and Otology*, **105**, 901–906

PALLIS, C., JONES, A. M. and SPILLANE, J.-D. (1954) Cervical spondylosis. *Brain*, **77**, 274–289

PAPARELLA, M. M. (1991) Pathogenesis and pathophysiology of Menière's disease. *Acta Otolaryngologica*, Suppl. 485, 26–35

PAPARELLA, M., BERLINGER, N. T., ODA, M. and FIKY, F. E. (1973) Otological manifestations of leukaemia. *Laryngoscope*, **83**, 1510–1526

PARELL, G. J. and BECKER, G. D. (1993) Inner ear barotrauma in scuba divers: a long-term follow up after continued diving. *Archives of Otolaryngology – Head and Neck Surgery*, **119**, 455–457

PARKER, W. (1991) Migraine and the vestibular system in adults. *American Journal of Otology*, **12**, 25–34

PARNES, L. S. and MCCLURE, J. A. (1990) Posterior semicircular canal occlusion for intractable benign paroxysmal positional vertigo. *Annals of Otology, Rhinology and Laryngology*, **99**, 330–334

PARNES, L. S. and MCCLURE, J. A. (1991) Posterior semicircular canal occlusion in the normal hearing ear. *Otolaryngology, Head and Neck Surgery*, **104**, 52–57

PARVING, A. (1991) Hearing problems and hormonal disturbances in the elderly. *Acta Otolaryngologica*, Suppl. **476**, 44–53

PEARCE, J. (1974) The extrapyramidal disorder of Alzheimer's disease. *European Neurology*, **12**, 94–103

PFALTZ, C. R. (1984) Vertigo in disorders of the neck. In: *Vertigo*, edited by M. R. Dix and J. D. Hood. Chichester: John Wiley & Sons Limited. pp. 179–198

PFALTZ, C. R. and RICHTER, H. (1958) Die cochleovestibulare symptomatologie des cervicalsyndrome. *Archiv für Ohren–Nasen und Kehlkopfheilkunde*, **172**, 519–534

PHELPS, P. D. (1983) Congenital malformations of the ear – a radiological study with clinical and pathological correlation. *MD Thesis*, University of London

PHELPS, P. D. and LLOYD, G. A. S. (1982) High resolution air CT meatography: the demonstration of normal and abnormal structures in the cerebello-pontine cistern and internal auditory meatus. *British Journal of Radiology*, **55**, 19–22

PHELPS, P. D. and LLOYD, G. A. S. (1990a) Otosclerosis and bony dysplasia. In: *Diagnostic Imaging of the Ear*, 2nd edn. London: Springer Verlag. pp. 203–209

PHELPS, P. D. and LLOYD, G. A. S. (1990b) Otosclerosis and bony dysplasias. In: *Diagnostic Imaging of the Ear*, 2nd edn. London: Springer Verlag. pp. 209–210

PHELPS, P. D. and LLOYD, G. A. S. (1990c) Lesions of the internal acoustic meatus and posterior cranial fossa. In: *Diagnostic Imaging of the Ear*, 2nd edn. London: Springer Verlag. p. 180

PIETERSEN, E. and ANDERSON, P. (1967) Spontaneous cause of 220 non-traumatic facial palsies. *Acta Otolaryngologica*, Suppl. 224, 296–300

PORTER, R. J. and EYSTER, E. (1973) Aneurysm in the anterior inferior cerebellar artery at the internal acoustic meatus: a report of a case. *Surgical Neurology*, **1**, 27–28

PRASHER, D. (1981) Studies of early auditory evoked potentials and their clinical applications. *PhD Thesis*, University of London

PRASHER, D. and BANNISTER, R. (1986) Brain stem auditory evoked potentials in patients with multiple system atrophy with progressive autonomic failure (Shy-Drager syndrome). *Journal of Neurology, Neurosurgery and Psychiatry*, **49**, 278–279

PRASHER, D., COELHO, A., NADKARNI, J. and LUXON, L. (1991) Differentiating an acoustic neuroma from other cerebello-pontine angle lesions. In: *Acoustic Neuroma*. Proceedings of the first international conference on acoustic neuroma, Copenhagen, Denmark, August 1991, edited by M. Tos and J. Thomsen. Kugler Publications. pp. 953–956

PROCTOR, L., PERLMAN, H., LINDSAY, J. and MATZ, G. (1979) Acute vestibular paralysis in herpes zoster oticus. *Annals of Otology, Rhinology and Laryngology*, **88**, 303–310

PROOPS, D., BAYLEY, D. and HAWKE, M. (1985) Paget's disease of the temporal bone – a clinical and histopathological review of six temporal bones. *Journal of Otolaryngology*, **14**, 20–29

PROTTI-PATTERSON, E. and YOUNG, M. L. (1985) The use of subjective and objective audiologic test procedures in the diagnosis of multiple sclerosis. *Otolaryngologic Clinics of North America*, **18**, 241–255

QUICK, C. A., FISH, A. and BROWN, C. (1973) The relationship between cochlea and kidney. *Laryngoscope*, **83**, 1469–1482

QUINN, N. (1989) Multiple system atrophy – the nature of the beast. *Journal of Neurology, Neurosurgery and Psychiatry*, Special Suppl., 78–89

RAHKO, T. and KARMA, P. (1986) New clinical finding in vestibular neuritis: high-frequency audiometry hearing loss in the affected ear. *Laryngoscope*, **96**, 198–199

RAREY, K. E. (1990) Otologic pathophysiology in patients with human immunodeficiency virus. *American Journal of Otolaryngology*, **11**, 366–369

RASCOL, O. J., CLANET, M., SENARD, J. M., MONTASTRUC, J. L. and RASCOL, A. (1993) Vestibulo-ocular reflex in Parkinson's disease and multiple system atrophy. *Advances in Neurology*, **60**, 395–397

RASMUSSEN, N., JOHNSEN, N. J. and BOHR, V. A. (1991) Otologic sequelae after pneumococcal meningitis: a survey of 164 consecutive cases with a follow-up of 94 survivors. *Laryngoscope*, **101**, 876–882

RASSEKH, C. and HARKER, L. A. (1992) The prevalence of migraine in Meniere's disease. *Laryngoscope*, **102**, 135–138

REARDON, W. and HARDING A. E. (1995) Mitochondrial genetics and deafness. *Journal of Audiological Medicine*, (in press)

REARDON, W., ROSS, R. J. M., SWEENEY, M. G., LUXON L. M., PEMBREY, M. E., HARDING, A. E. *et al.* (1992) Diabetes mellitus associated with a pathogenic point mutation in mitochondrial DNA. *Lancet*, ii, 1376–1379

REIG, J., DOMINGO, E., REGUANT, J. and CORRONS, J. (1992) Orthostatic and exercise induced advanced atrioventricular block. *Chest*, **102**, 970–972

RHOTON, A. J. (1993) Role for thalidomide in primary biliary cirrhosis treatment? *Gastroenterology*, **105**, 956

RIISE, T., GRONNING, M., AARLI, J. A., NYLAND, H., LARSEN, J. P. and EDLAND, A. (1988) Prognostic factors for life expectancy in multiple sclerosis analysed by Cox-models. *Journal of Clinical Epidemiology*, **41**, 1031–1036

RITCHIE, L. (1976) Effects of cerebellar lesions on saccadic eye movements. *Journal of Neurophysiology*, **39**, 1246–1256

RIVERA, V. M. (1990) The nature of multiple sclerosis. *Seminars in Hearing*, **11**, 207–219

RIZVI, S. S. and HOLMES, R. A. (1980) Hearing loss from hemodialysis. *Archives of Otolaryngology*, **106**, 751–756

ROBERTS, T. D. M. (1967) *Neurophysiology of Postural Mechanisms*. New York: Plenum Press

ROBERTSON, D., HAILE, V., PERRY, S. E., ROBERTSON, R. M., PHILLIPS, J. A. and BIAGGIONI, I. (1991) Dopamine B hydroxylase deficiency. A genetic disorder of cardiovascular regulation. *Hypertension*, **18**, 1–8

ROHN, G. N., MEYERHOFF, W. L. and WRIGHT, C. G. (1993) Ototoxicity of topical agents. *Otolaryngologic Clinics of North America*, **26**, 747–758

ROSE, A. S., ELISON, G. W., MYERS, L. W. and TOURTELOTTE, W. W. (1976) Criteria for clinical diagnosis of multiple sclerosis. *Neurology*, **26**, 20–22

ROSENHALL, U. (1988) Positional nystagmus. *Acta Otolaryngologica*, Suppl. 455, 17–20

ROSENHALL, U. and KANKUNEN, A. (1981) Hearing alterations following meningitis, 2. Variable Hearing. *Ear and Hearing*, **2**, 170–176

ROSENHALL, U. and RUBIN, W. (1975) Degenerative changes in the human vestibular sensory epithelium. *Acta Otolaryngologica*, **79**, 67–85

ROSENHALL, U., HANNER, P. and KAIJSER, B. (1988) Borrelia infection and vertigo. *Acta Otolaryngologica*, **106**, 111–116

ROSENHALL, U., PEDERSEN, K., JOHANSSON, E. and KALL, A. (1984) Auditory brain stem responses in patients with vertigo. *Clinical Otolaryngology*, **9**, 149–154

ROW-JONES, J. M., MACALLAN, D. C. and SOROOSHIAN, M. (1990) Polyarteritis nodosa presenting as bilateral sudden onset of cochleovestibular failure in a young woman. *Journal of Laryngology and Otology*, **104**, 562–564

RUDGE, P. (1983) Other conditions: multiple sclerosis. In: *Clinical Neuro-otology*. London: Churchill Livingstone. pp. 273–280

RUTTIN, B. (1909) Zur differentialdiagnose der labyrinthu. Hornerverkrankungen. *Zeitschrift für Ohrenheilkunde*, **57**, 327–331

RYU, J. H. (1993) Vestibular neuritis: an overview using a classical case. *Acta Otolaryngologica*, Suppl. 503, 25–30

SACCO, R. L., FREDDO, L., BELLO, J. A., ODEL, J. G., ONESTI, S. T. and MOHR, J. P. (1993) Wallenberg's lateral medullary syndrome. Clinical-magnetic resonance imaging correlations. *Archives of Neurology*, **50**, 609–614

SAFMAN, B. L. (1971) Bilateral pathology in Bell's palsy. *Archives of Otolaryngology*, **93**, 55–57

SAMET, P. (1973) Haemodynamic sequelae of cardiac arrhythmias. *Circulation*, **47**, 399–407

SAMPAIO, E. P., KAPLAN, G., MIRANDA, A., NERY, J. A., MIGUEL, C. P., VIANA, S. M. *et al.* (1993) The influence of thalidomide on the clinical and immunologic manifestations of erythema nodosum leprosum. *Journal of Infectious Diseases*, **168**, 408–414

SANDBERG, L. E. and TERKILDSEN, K. (1965) Caloric tests in deaf children. *Archives of Otolaryngology*, **81**, 350–354

SANDMANN, J., HOJER, G., BEWERMEYER, H., BAMBORSCHKE, S. and NEUFANG, K. F. (1992) Fibromuscular dysplasia as a cause of cerebral infarct. *Nervenarzt (Berlin)*, **63**, 335–340

SANDO, I., HEMENWAY, W. G. and MILLER, D. R. (1974) Vestibular pathology in otosclerosis: temporal bone histopathological report. *Laryngoscope*, **84**, 593–595

SANDO, I., HARDA, T., LOEHR, A. and SOBEL, J. H. (1977) Sudden deafness. Histopathologic correlation in temporal bone. *Annals of Otology, Rhinology and Laryngology*, **86**, 269–279

SANDSDEAD, H. (1986) A brief history of the influence of trace elements on brain function. *American Journal of Clinical Nutrition*, **43**, 293–298

SARTOR, K. (1990) Radiologic methods in vascular brain stem diseases. In: *Vascular Brain Stem Diseases*, edited by B. Hofferberth, G. G. Brune, G. Sitzer, and H.-D. Weger. Basel: Karger

SCHACHT, J. (1993) Biochemical basis of aminoglycoside ototoxicity. *Otolaryngologic Clinics of North America*, **26**, 845–856

SCHAPIRA, A. H. V. (1994) Evidence for mitochondrial dysfunction in Parkinson's disease – a critical approach. *Movement Disorders*, **9**, 125–138

SCHEIBE, A. (1892) A case of deaf-mutism, with auditory atrophy and anomalies of development in the membranous labyrinth of both ears. *Archives of Otolaryngology*, **21**, 12–22

SCHMUTZHARD, E., POHL, P. and STANEK, G. (1988) Borrelia burgdorferi antibodies in patients with relapsing/remitting form and chronic progressive form of multiple sclerosis. *Journal of Neurology, Neurosurgery and Psychiatry*, **51**, 1215–1218

SCHNEIDER, R. C., CALHOUN, H. D. and CROSBY, E. C. (1968) Vertigo and rotational movement in cortical and subcortical lesions. *Journal of the Neurological Sciences*, **6**, 493–516

SCHUKNECHT, H. F. (1969) Cupulolithiasis. *Archives of Otolaryngology*, **90**, 113–126

SCHUKNECHT, H. F. (1974) In: *Pathology of the Ear*, Cambridge, Massachusetts: Harvard University Press. pp. 336; 386–388

SCHUKNECHT, H. F. (1984) The pathophysiology of Meniere's disease. *American Journal of Otology*, **5**, 526–527

SCHUKNECHT, H., ALLAM, A. and MURAKAMI, Y. (1968) Pathology of secondary malignant tumours of the temporal bone. *Annals of Otology, Rhinology and Laryngology*, **77**, 5

SCHUKNECHT, H. F. and KITAMURA, K. (1981) Vestibular neuritis. *Annals of Otology, Rhinology and Laryngology*, **90** (Suppl. 48), 1–19

SCHUKNECHT, H. F., SUZUKA, Y. and ZIMMERMANN, C. (1990) Delayed endolymphatic hydrops and its relationship to Menière's disease. *Annals of Otology, Rhinology and Laryngology*, **99**, 843–853

SCHUMACHER, G. A., BEEBE, G., KIBLER, R. E., KURLAND, L. T., KURTZKE, J. F., MCDOWE, H. F. *et al.* (1965) Problems of experimental trials in multiple sclerosis: report by the panel on evaluation of experimental trials of therapy in multiple sclerosis. *Annals of the New York Academy of Sciences*, **122**, 552–568

SCHWEITZER, V. G. (1993) Ototoxicity of chemotherapeutic agents. *Otolaryngologic Clinics of North America*, **26**, 759–789

SEALS, R. L. and RISE, E. N. (1967) Vogt-Koyanagi-Harada syndrome. *Archives of Otolaryngology*, **86**, 419–423

SHAMBAUGH, G. E. (1930) Statistical studies of children in public schools for the deaf: additional report of committee, division of medical sciences, national research council. *Archives of Otolaryngology*, **12**, 190–194

SHEA, J. J. and YOO, T. J. (1982) Dexamethasone treatment of Menieres disease. *Eighth extraordinary meeting of the Barany Society*, Basle, paper number 55.

SHEEHAN, S., BAUER, R. B. and MEYER, J. S. (1960) Vertebral artery compression in cervical spondylosis. *Neurology*, **10**, 968–986

SHELTON, C., LUXFORD, W. M., TONOKAWA, L. L., LO, W. W. M. and HOUSE, W. F. (1989) The narrow internal auditory canal in children: a contraindication to cochlear implants. *Otolaryngology, Head and Neck Surgery*, **100**, 227–231

SHOFFNER, J. M. and WALLACE, D. C. (1990) Oxidative phosphorylation diseases. Disorders of two genomes. *Advances in Human Genetics*, **19**, 267–330

SILVONIEMI, P. (1988) Vestibular neuronitis, an otoneurological evaluation. *Acta Otolaryngologica*, Suppl. 453, 2–72

SIMMONS, F. B. (1968) Theory of membrane breaks in sudden hearing loss. *Archives of Otolaryngology*, **88**, 41–48

SMITH, M. E. and CANALIS, R. F. (1989) Otologic manifestations of AIDS: the otosyphilis connection. *Laryngoscope*, **99**, 365–372

SMITH, N. J., and DOCHERTY, T. B. (1982) Case report. Nystagmus: an unusual manifestation of temporal lobe epilepsy. *Journal of Electrophysiological Technology*, **8**, 7–13

SOOY, C. D. (1987) The impact of AIDS on otolaryngology – head and neck surgery. *Otolaryngology, Head and Neck Surgery*, **1**, 1–28

SPENCER-HARRISON, M. and OZSAHINOGLU, C. (1972) Positional vertigo: aetiology and clinical significance. *Brain*, **95**, 369–372

SPOENDLIN, H. H. (1974) Optic and cochleovestibular degenerations in hereditary ataxias. Temporal bone pathology in two cases of Friedreich's ataxia with vestibulo-cochlear disorders. *Brain*, **97**, 41–48

STAMP, T. C. B. and BAKER, I. (1976) Recessive hypophosphataemic rickets, and possible aetiology of the 'vitamin D-resistant' syndrome. *Archives of Disease in Childhood*, **51**, 360–365

STECKELBERG, J. M. and MCDONALD, T. S. (1984) Otologic involvement in late syphilis. *Laryngoscope*, **94**, 753–757

STEELE, J. C., RICHARDSON, J. C. and OLSZEWSKI, J. (1964) Progressive supranuclear palsy. *Archives of Neurology*, **10**, 333–359

STELL, R., BRONSTEIN, A. M. and MARSDEN, C. D. (1989) Vestibulo-ocular abnormalities in spasmodic torticollis before and after botulinum toxin injections. *Journal of Neurology, Neurosurgery and Psychiatry*, **52**, 57–62

STELL, R., GRESTY, M., METCALFE, T. and BRONSTEIN, A. M. (1991) Cervico-ocular function in patients with spasmodic torticollis. *Journal of Neurology, Neurosurgery and Psychiatry*, **54**, 39–41

STEPHENS, S. D. G. (1970) Temporary threshold shift in myxoedema. *Jounral of Laryngology and Otology*, **84**, 317

STEPHENS, S. D. G., LUXON, L. M. and HINCHCLIFFE, R. (1982) Immunological disorders and auditory lesions. *Audiology*, **21**, 128–148

STROUD, M. H. and CALCATERRA, T. C. (1970) Spontaneous perilymph fistulas. *Laryngoscope*, **80**, 479–487

STUEVEN, H. A., COGAN, P. and VALLEY, V. (1993) A hazardous material episode: sulfur trioxide. *Veterinary and Human Toxicology*, **35**, 37–38

STUMPF, J. L. and MITRZYK, B. (1994) Management of orthostatic hypotension. *American Journal of Hospital Pharmacology*, **51**, 648–660

SUMMERS, R. W. and HARKER, L. (1982) Ulcerative colitis and sensorineural hearing loss: is there a relationship? *Journal of Clinical Gastroenterology*, **4**, 251–252

SUNDERLAND, S. (1945) The arterial relations of the internal auditory meatus. *Brain*, **68**, 23–27

SVENSSON, M. L., RUNDGREN, A. and LANDAHL, S. (1992) Falls in 84 to 85 year old people living at home. *Accident Analysis and Prevention*, **24**, 527–537

TADA, Y., AOYAGI, M., TOJIMA, H., INAMURA, H., SAITO, O., MAEYAMA, H. *et al.* (1994) Gd-DTPA enhanced MRI in Ramsay Hunt syndrome. *Acta Otolaryngologica*, Suppl. 511, 170–174

TAKAHASHI, A. (1993) Lyme disease with neurological complications in Japan. *Acta Otolaryngologica*, Suppl. 503, 96

TALMI, Y. P., FINKELSTEIN, Y. and ZOHAR, Y. (1991a) Decompression sickness induced hearing loss. A review. *Scandinavian Audiology*, **20**, 25–28

TALMI, Y. P., FINKELSTEIN, Y. and ZOHAR, Y. (1991b) Barotrauma induces hearing loss. Review article. *Scandinavian Audiology*, **20**, 1–9

TELLEZ, I. and TERRY, R. D. (1968) Fine structure of the early changes in the vestibular nuclei of the thiamine-deficient rat. *American Journal of Pathology*, **52**, 777

THOMKE, F. and HOPF, H. C. (1992) Unilateral vestibular paralysis as the sole manifestation of mumps. *Journal of Neurology, Neurosurgery and Psychiatry*, **55**, 858–859

THOMSEN, K. A., TERKILDSEN, K. and ARNFRED, I. (1965) Middle ear pressure variations during anesthesia. *Archives of Otolaryngology*, **82**, 609–611

THOMSON, L. F., MARDEL, S. N., JACK, A. and SHIELDS, T. G. (1992) Management of the moribund carbon monoxide victim. *Archives of Emergency Medicine*, **9**, 208–213

THORNTON, A. R. D., FARRELL, G. and HAACKE, N. P. (1991) A non-invasive, objective test of endolymphatic hydrops. *Acta Otolaryngologica*, Suppl. 485, 35–43

TODD, G. B., SERJEANT, G. R. and LARSON, M. R. (1973) Sensorineural hearing loss in Jamaicans with SS disease. *Acta Otolaryngologica*, **76**, 268–272

TOS, M. (1971) Fractures of the temporal bone. The course and sequelae of 248 fractures of the petrous temporal bone. *Ugeskrift for Laeger*, **133**, 1449–1456

TROOST, B. T. (1990) Signs and symptoms of stroke syndromes of the brain stem. In: *Vascular Brain Stem Diseases*, edited by B. Hofferberth, G. G. Brune, G. Sitzer and H. D. Weger. Basel: Karger. pp. 112–124

TRUNE, D. R., CRAVEN, J. P., MORTON, J. I. and MITCHELL, C. (1989) Autoimmune disease and cochlear pathology in the C3H/1pr strain mouse. *Hearing Research*, **38**, 57–66

URI, N., SCHUCHMAN, G. and PRATT, H. (1984) Auditory brainstem evoked potentials in Bell's palsy. *Archives of Otolaryngology*, **110**, 301–304

URI, N. and SCHUCHMAN, G. (1986) Vestibular abnormalities in patients with Bell's palsy. *Journal of Laryngology and Otology*, **100**, 1125–1128

VANHOORNE, M., BLANCKE, V., DE-BACQUER, D., DEPOORTER, A. M. and BOGAERT, M. (1992) Use of pharmaceuticals in industrial workers – possible implications for epidemiological studies. *International Archives of Occupational and Environmental Health (Berlin)*, **64**, 25–30

VERHAGEN, W. I. M. and HUYGEN, P. L. M. (1994) Central vestibular, vestibulo-acoustic and oculomotor dysfunction in hereditary disorders. A review of the literature and a report on some additional findings. *Journal of Vestibular Research*, **4**, 105–135

VERHAGEN, W. I. M., HUYGEN, P. L. M. and BLES, W. (1992) A new autosomal dominant syndrome of idiopathic progressive vestibulo-cochlear dysfunction with middle-age onset. *Acta Otolaryngologica*, **112**, 899–906

VERGHAN, W. I. M., HUYGEN, P. L. M. and HORSTINK, N. W. I. M. (1987) Familial congenital vestibular areflexia. *Journal of Neurology, Neurosurgery and Psychiatry*, **50**, 933–935

VERHAGEN, W. I. M., HUYGEN, P. L. M. and JOOSTEN, E. M. G. (1988) Familial progressive vestibulocochlear dysfunction. *Archives of Neurology*, **45**, 766–768

VERHAGEN, W. I. M., HUYGEN, P. L. M., THEUNISSEN, E. J. J. M. and JOOSTEN, E. M. G. (1989) Hereditary vestibulo-cochlear dysfunction and vascular disorders. *Journal of Neurological Sciences*, **92**, 55–63

VICTOR, M., ADAMS, R. D. and COLLINS, C. H. (1971) *The Wernicke–Korsakoff Syndrome*. Philadelphia: FA Davis

VON GLASS, W., HAID, C., CIDLINSKY, K., STENGLEIN, C. and

CHRIST, P. (1991) False-positive MR imaging in the diagnosis of acoustic neurinomas. *Otolaryngology, Head and Neck Surgery*, **104**, 863–867

VYSE, R., LUXON, L. M. and WALPORT, M. J. (1994) Audiovestibular manifestations of the antiphospholipid syndrome. *Journal of Laryngology and Otology*, **108**, 57–59

WACKYM, P. A. and LINTHICUM, F. H. (1986) Diabetes mellitus and hearing loss: clinical and histopathological relationship. *American Journal of Otolaryngology*, **7**, 176–182

WAKSMAN, S. A., BUGIE, E. and SCHATZ, A. (1944) Isolation of antibiotic substances from soil microorganisms with special reference to streptothricin and streptomycin. *Proceedings of Staff meeting, Mayo Clinic*, **19**, 537

WALBY, A. P. and SCHUKNECHT, H. F. (1984) Concomitant occurrence of cochleosaccular dysplasia and Down's syndrome. *Archives of Otolaryngology*, **110**, 477–479

WALL, C. and RAUCH S. D. (1996) Perilymphatic fistula. In: *Handbook of Neurotology*. Oxford: Oxford Press

WALLACE, I. R. and BARBER, H. O. (1983) Recurrent vestibulopathy. *Journal of Otolaryngology*, **12**, 61–63

WANG, T. L., CHEN, W. J., LIAU, C. S. and LEE, Y. T. (1994) Sick sinus syndrome as the early manifestation of cardiac haemochromatosis. *Journal of Electrocardiology*, **27**, 91–96

WATANABE, Y., ASO, S., YASUMURA, S., KOBAYASHI, H. and MIZUKOSHI, K. (1993) Retro-labyrinthine disorder in cases with peripheral facial palsy. *Acta Otolaryngologica*, Suppl. 503, 202–204

WATANUKI, K., KAWAMOTO, K. and KAKIZAKI, L., (1975) Pathological findings of the temporal bone. *Otologia*, **21**, 601

WAYMAN, D. M., PHAM, H. N., BYL, E. M. and ADOUR, K. K. (1990) Audiological manifestations of Ramsay Hunt syndrome. *Journal of Laryngology and Otology*, **104**, 104–108

WEBER, R. S., JENKINS, H. A. and COHEN, N. J. (1984) Sensorineural hearing loss associated with ulcerative colitis. *Archives of Otolaryngology*, **110**, 810–812

WEEKS, V. and TRAVELLI, J. (1955) Postural vertigo due to trigger areas in sternocleidomastoid muscle. *Journal of Paediatrics*, **47**, 315–327

WENNMO, C. and PYYKKÖ, I. (1982) Vestibular neuronitis. *Acta Otolaryngologica*, **94**, 507–515

WESTMORE, C. A., PICKARD, B. H. and STERN, H. (1979) Isolation of mumps virus from the inner ear after sudden deafness. *British Medical Journal*, **655**, 14–15

WICKS, R. E. (1989) Alternobaric vertigo: an aeromedical review. *Aviation Space Environment Medicine*, **60**, 67–72

WILDERVANCK, L. G. (1963) Perceptive deafness associated with split-hand and foot syndrome: a new syndrome? *Acta Genetica, Basel*, **13**, 161–169

WILLIAMS, D. (1964) Vertebrobasilar ischaemia. *British Medical Journal*, **1**, 84–86

WILLIAMS, D. and WILSON, G. (1962) The diagnosis of the major and minor syndromes of basilar insufficiency. *Brain*, **85**, 741–774

WILLIAMS, D. N., LAUGHLIN, L. W. and LEE, Y. H. (1974) Minocycline: possible vestibular side-effects. *Lancet*, ii, 744–746

WILPIZESKI, C. (1974) Effects of lead on the vestibular system: preliminary findings. *Laryngoscope*, **84**, 821–832

WILSON, D. F., HODGSON, R. S., GUSTAFSON, M. F., HOGUE, S. and MILLS, L. (1992) The sensitivity of auditory brainstem response testing in small acoustic neuromas. *Laryngoscope*, **102**, 961–964

WILSON, W. R. (1986) The relationship of the herpes virus

family to sudden hearing loss: a prospective clinical study and literature review. *Laryngoscope*, **96**, 870–877

WILSON, W. R. and ZOLLER, M. (1981) Electronystagmography in congenital and acquired syphilitic otitis. *Annals of Otology*, **90**, 21–24

WOLFF, D., BERNHARD, W. G., TSUTSUMI, S., ROSS, I. S. and NUSSBAUM, H. E. (1965) The pathology of Cogan's syndrome causing profound deafness. *Annals of Otology, Rhinology and Laryngology*, **74**, 507–520

WOLLNER, L. (1978) Postural hypotension in the elderly. *Age and Ageing*, Suppl. 7, 112–117

WOOLF, P. K. (1992) A 15 year old with palpitations and dizziness. *Paeditric Emergency Care*, **8**, 59–60

WYKE, B. (1979) Cervical articular contributions to posture and gait: their relation to senile disequilibrium. *Age and Ageing*, **8**, 251–258

YAGI, T., YAMAGUCHI, J. and NONAKA, M. (1988) Neurotological findings in Bell's palsy and Hunt's syndrome. *Acta Otolaryngologica*, Suppl. 446, 97–100

YASSIN, A., BADRY, A. and FATT-HI, A. (1970) The relationship between electrolyte balance and cochlea disturbances in cases of renal failure. *Journal of Laryngology and Otology*, **84**, 429–436

YASSIN, A., SAFWAT, F. and FATT-HI, A. (1966) Ear, nose and throat manifestations in cases of renal failure treated by dialysis. *Annals of Otology, Rhinology and Laryngology*, **75**, 192

YLIKOSKI, J. (1988) Delayed endolymphatic hydrops syndrome after heavy exposure to impulse noise. *American Journal of Otology*, **9**, 282–285

YOO, T. J., STUART, J. M., KANG, A. H., TOWNES, A. S. and TOMODA, K. (1982) Collagen autoimmunity as a cause of otosclerosis and Menière's disease. In: *Abstracts of the Fifth Mid-winter Research Meeting*, St. Petersburg, Florida.

YOON, T. H., PAPARELLA, M. M. and SCHACHERN, P. A. (1990) Otosclerosis involving the vestibular aqueduct and Menière's disease. *Otolaryngology, Head and Neck Surgery*, **103**, 107–112

YOSHIO, S., TOKUMASU, K., FUJINO, A., NAGANUMA, H., NOGUTI, H., NITTA, K. *et al.* (1991) Neuro-otological study on Behçet's disease. *Nippon–Jibiinkoka Gakkai Kaiho*, **94**, 1716–1726

ZAJTCHUK, J. T., MIHAIL, R., JEWELL, J. S., DUNNE, M. J. and CHADWICH, S. G. (1984) Electronystagmographic findings in long-term low-dose quinine ingestion. A preliminary report. *Archives of Otolaryngology*, **110**, 788–791

ZECHNER, G. (1980) The Cogan syndrome. *Acta Otolaryngologica*, **89**, 310–316

ZEE, D. S., YEE, R. D., COGAN, D. G., ROBINSON, D. A. and ENGELS, W. K. (1976) Oculomotor abnormalities in hereditary ataxia. *Brain*, **99**, 207–234

ZELENKA, J. AND SLAMINOVA, B. (1964) Changes of labyrinth function due to age. *Cesk Otolaryngologica*, **13**, 21–26

21

Diagnostic testing of the vestibular system

Rosalyn A. Davies and Peter A. Savundra

The assessment of the giddy patient or the patient with a neuro-otological problem is a complex task which needs to be approached in an organized manner. For some conditions, most notably a vestibular schwannoma, a specific investigation (here a gadolinium-enhanced MRI scan) can offer a definitive diagnosis, but the lack of facilities and cost factors require that only selected cases are referred for such investigations. The difficulty, therefore, is knowing how to select the right cases from the many patients presenting with similar complaints of dizziness or imbalance. The problem can be addressed by the collection of a comprehensive history, by a physical examination which is directed towards detecting subtle abnormalities of eye movements, but which is mindful of those factors which can compromise the value of the signs elicited, and the collection of confirmatory data with the use of those investigatory tools which are readily available. On the other hand, the majority of patients presenting with neuro-otological symptoms do not have a space-occupying lesion and the over-reliance on imaging techniques would miss more common conditions such as benign paroxysmal positional vertigo or the failure to compensate following an acute unilateral labyrinthine event.

Whatever methods are chosen, the role of the neuro-otologist is to identify the site of the lesion, and gather information which may lead to an aetiological diagnosis and from there to formulate a method of management.

Balance information is integrated within the brain, in the central vestibular structures which include the vestibular nuclei of the brain stem, the cerebellum, the reticular formation, the extrapyramidal system and the cerebral cortex. These projections process information from the vestibular, visual and proprioceptive systems. The vestibular nuclei receive projections from the velocity and acceleration receptors of the peripheral vestibular apparatus and also projections from the central vestibular areas, including the cerebellum, and a direct visual input (Waespe and Henn, 1977). Collaterals from the vestibular nuclei pass to the cerebellum, in particular the flocculonodular lobe and the vermis. The cerebellum also receives inputs from the visual system via the accessory olivary tract and from the proprioceptive system via the posterior columns. Therefore, any derangement of the structure or function of central vestibular structures is likely to cause balance disorders and it is important that the assessment of the patient with a balance disorder includes a careful neurological assessment.

Although the exclusion of otological pathology is essential in any balance disorder, many conditions will elude diagnosis if balance is equated purely with a disorder of audiovestibular function. For example, Drachman and Hart (1972) have emphasized the importance of multisensory deficits, particularly in the elderly, and have postulated a syndrome, producing dizziness, when two or more of the following conditions are present: visual impairment (not correctable), neuropathy, vestibular deficits, cervical spondylosis and orthopaedic disorders which interfere with ambulation. An appreciation and understanding of the concept that disequilibrium may be consequent upon multiple pathologies is essential if appropriate investigation and interpretation of the data are to be achieved. As the primary pathology may lie outside the vestibular system, for example it may be cardiac valvular disease or a blood dyscrasia, a full and comprehensive history is essential, together with a complete general medical examination, with particular attention to the eyes, the ears, the central nervous system, the cardiovascular system and the locomotor system. The use of appropriate general medical investigations should also be considered.

History

The history is taken to elicit those symptoms which can lead to a site of lesion diagnosis, give information on the possible aetiology and highlight those investigations which are required to confirm the diagnosis. The history should also assist in gaining a better understanding of the psychological status of the patient, highlight those factors which will influence the interpretation of the signs elicited and give information on how the management of the patient will be tailored to his needs.

Symptoms

The symptoms reported by patients can vary from the highly specific description of 'vertigo', i.e. an illusion of movement, or a loss of balance, to much more vague complaints of dizziness, disequilibrium, anxiety, difficulty thinking in certain environments or panic, faintness, giddiness, sensations of swimminess or floating, and unexpected falls with no sequelae. It is the task of the physician to interpret the patient's complaints and represent them in terminology of more precise definition.

Vertigo, dizziness, oscillopsia

The term *vertigo* is usually defined as an illusion of movement (Ludman, 1979) or the disagreeable sensation of instability or disordered orientation in space (Agate, 1963). Cawthorne (1952) defined vertigo as an hallucination of movement highlighting the reality of the perception of some sufferers, while Ludman's use of the word illusion suggests the understanding by some sufferers that they and their environment are not actually moving. The lay term *dizziness* can be used to cover the less specific synonyms noted above. Other patients have *oscillopsia* (Bender, 1965), an illusion of horizontal or vertical oscillation of the visual world or bobbing of vision exacerbated by head movements.

Sensory inputs are normally combined to provide an accurate model of the physical world. Symptoms can arise when there is an unusual combination of sensory inputs triggered by exposure to visual stimuli, such as rapidly changing images on a television screen, striped material or fast-moving traffic and crowds. This is termed *visual vertigo* and is the result of a mismatch of visual and vestibular inputs. Such symptoms can occur in the absence of demonstrable vestibular disease. Roberts (1967) has suggested a hypothesis to explain this phenomenon. From birth, the information required for balance is integrated and stored in data centres within different sites in the brain. New information is constantly compared with learned data and under normal circumstances 'immediate recognition' of sensory patterns enables ves-

tibular activity to occur at a subconscious level, but new data patterns which are not immediately recognized will precipitate the perception of vestibular activity.

The false perception of motion of self and/or external objects may be provoked by visual, vestibular or neurological disease, by the presentation of unphysiological stimuli, or by the removal or distortion of the stimuli. A common manifestation is the feeling of imbalance caused by the wearing of new spectacles or bifocal lenses. The loss of the sense of turning in normal subjects flying in cloud is well-known (Benson and Burchard, 1973). In the motorist's vestibular disorientation syndrome (Page and Gresty, 1985) patients with vestibular disease develop an illusion of turning and make inappropriate postural or steering adjustments when travelling at speed, particularly in the dark or on open featureless roads. Symptoms of imbalance can arise if the driver suddenly loses his expected environmental cues, as when overtaking high-sided vehicles. Vertigo can be triggered in supermarkets by lines of shelves under featureless, shadowless fluorescent lighting.

The resulting misleading sense of movement and disorientation may be associated with somatic symptoms, such as nausea and sweating and feelings of panic, anxiety and inadequacy (Brandt and Daroff, 1980). Similar symptoms have been described in space phobia (Marks, 1981) and the importance of defining the presence or absence of a vestibular or visual disturbance is crucial in order to institute appropriate treatment.

Whether the symptoms are *spontaneous* or *provoked* should be determined. If provoked, questions should be asked on the nature of precipitating factors, whether the vertigo is aggravated by head or eye movements and whether it is triggered by visual stimuli, such as patterns, stripes, fast moving TV images, escalators, the tread of stairs, shelves and the lighting in department stores. If head movements trigger vertigo it is important to determine whether laying back in bed or tilting the head back, for example to hang out the washing or look at overflying aircraft, will trigger vertigo, as this may be suggestive of benign paroxysmal positional vertigo and indicate that the Hallpike positioning manoeuvre must be a mandatory part of the clinical examination.

Ascertaining which other symptoms are coincident with the vestibular symptoms is helpful in determining the site of lesion. Auditory symptoms of tinnitus, otalgia and hearing loss suggest cochlear involvement, while diplopia, swallowing difficulties, sensory symptoms, motor weakness and altered levels of consciousness suggest neurological disease. While teichopsia and field defects suggest migraine, chest pain and palpitations indicate that cardiac disease should be investigated.

Knowledge of the duration of the illness, the duration of each attack and whether the attacks occur in clusters may also be helpful. The vertigo of benign paroxysmal positional vertigo is of the order of a few seconds to a minute, although there may be longer lasting mild symptoms. The vertigo of Menière's syndrome resolves within a few hours. The duration of the vertigo of an acute peripheral vestibular disturbance is of the order of several days. The picture of a failure subsequently to compensate takes the nature of clusters of bouts of milder attacks occurring at irregular intervals over a period of months and years.

A detailed description of the first attack and any coincident history may be of immense value. Acute unilateral lesions of a labyrinth cause a typical picture (Magnus, 1924) with the development of nystagmus with the fast component directed away from the side of the lesion, the head rotating to keep the affected ear lowermost, the trunk curling with the concavity on the contralateral side and the contralateral limbs extending. Following an acute labyrinthine lesion, there is usually a rapid recovery over a few days. In some patients less severe symptoms recur usually aggravated by changes of head position.

Falls

Falls are common in the elderly. Community studies indicate that over one-third of the population over the age of 65 years and nearly half of those over the age of 80 had suffered one or more falls in the previous year (Campbell *et al.*, 1981; Perry, 1982). Dizziness in the elderly is also common, and was reported by 47% of men and 61% of women over the age of 70 (Droller and Pemberton, 1953). However, the falls may be abrupt without warning and present as drop attacks. While it is mandatory to assess the elderly fallers for visual and proprioceptive loss, cardiovascular factors (particularly aortic stenosis and dysrhythmias), musculoskeletal disorder, and foot deformities (Gibson *et al.*, 1987), vestibular dysfunction, itself, is a common factor (Belal and Glorig, 1986; McClure, 1986; Norre, Forrez and Beckers, 1987).

Symptoms due to otolith dysfunction

A feature of vestibular dysfunction is that patients can present with symptoms which may appear bizarre. This is particularly true where the otolith organs are involved. As the otolith organs mediate gravitational acceleration, dysfunction can lead to symptoms of false feelings of falling, or lateropulsion (being pushed to the side), of the ground appearing to rise or fall, or of difficulty finding the visual vertical (aligning objects to the vertical) (Halmagyi, Gresty and Gibson, 1979). The effect of otolith dysfunction is to cause the eyes and head to skew in the vertical and oblique directions (the *ocular tilt reaction*), so patients may complain of diplopia and have a head tilt. For example, destruction of the left labyrinth may cause leftward head tilting, leftward ocular counter-rolling and the right eye to be higher than the left – a right-over-left skew deviation (Halmagyi, Gresty and Gibson, 1979). They may experience oscillopsia or vertigo when straining, coughing or sneezing (Healy, Strong and Sampogna, 1974). Their heads may tilt in response to loud sounds (Dieterich, Brandt and Fries, 1989) or they may have more obviously organic-sounding symptoms such as postural imbalance, oscillopsia, display ataxia (Brandt and Daroff, 1980) or positional vertigo (Schuknecht and Ruby, 1973).

Pressure vertigo

Some patients may complain of transient disturbances of balance and vertigo, even in the absence of aural pathology, when exposed to changes in ambient pressure. This has been recorded in airmen (van Wulfften Palthe, 1922; Jones, 1957; Lundgren and Malm, 1966) and divers (Lundgren, 1973). As these symptoms are more likely to occur where there are problems opening the eustachian tubes (Merica, 1942; Ingelstedt, Ivarsson and Tjernstrom, 1974), questions should be asked about upper respiratory tract symptoms and allergies.

Patients should be asked if they develop vertigo when exposed to loud sounds, i.e. *Tullio's phenomenon* (Tullio, 1929) or by sneezing and coughing (Goodhill, 1981). These symptoms should be distinguished from *hyperekplexia*, the loss of consciousness or falls when startled and *cataplexy*, the loss of voluntary movement and collapse precipitated by emotion or startle.

Motion sickness

Motion sickness is a normal physiological response to certain types of real or apparent motion. Motion sickness is characterized by nausea, vomiting, pallor and cold sweating, and may occur during sea, air, car, space and camel travel and it can be encountered on swings, on fun fair rides and aircraft simulators.

Central vertigo

Lesions of the vestibular root entry zone (Uemura and Cohen, 1973), vestibular nuclei and midbrain also cause balance problems and vertigo. Lesions of the low brain stem are likely to cause severe vertigo accompanied by vomiting. The patient falls or veers towards the side of the lesion. The involvement of central otolith pathways causes difficulty judging visual vertical. Sometimes patients report blurring of vision and the carers report seeing abnormalities of eye movements. This may be due to nystagmus. Lesions of the tegmentum of the pontomedullary and pontomesencephalic junctions cause upbeat vertical nystagmus. Patients may report double vision due to an internuclear ophthalmoparesis or a gaze paresis. Patients may report a difficulty looking upwards.

This may be due to cervical dystonia secondary to extrapyramidal disorders. Mesencephalic lesions can cause a supranuclear gaze palsy, in which there is a loss of volitional gaze, with vertical movements lost before horizontal.

Lesions involving the cerebellum may occasionally cause vertigo. More usually the patients complain of unsteadiness and clumsiness and describe symptoms due to intention tremor. They may have blurring of vision due to nystagmus and have difficulty with communication due to dysarthria.

Epileptogenic lesions of the cerebral cortex can cause vertigo. Currie *et al.* (1971) reported that 16% of patients with temporal lobe epilepsy had vertigo as an aura preceding an attack. Therefore, the patients should be asked if their balance disorder is accompanied by alterations of consciousness or motor, sensory, uncinate or visual hallucinations.

Cervical vertigo

Vertigo can be precipitated by loss of cervical joint proprioception. de Jong *et al.* (1977) infiltrated the cervical apophyseal joints with local anaesthetic and caused the subject to feel vertiginous and fall towards the side of the injection. There are also hypotheses that head movements can cause vertigo due to compression of the vertebrobasilar arteries (Sheehan, Bauer and Meyer, 1960) or irritation of the cervical sympathetic plexus (Barre, 1926). It is important therefore to elicit symptoms of neck pain and stiffness and if the possibility of vertebrobasilar insufficiency is to be entertained, that questions are asked about coincident symptoms of loss of consciousness, diplopia, visual loss, swallowing difficulties, sensory and motor loss.

Clinical examination of eye movements
General examination of the eye
Visual acuity

A rapid assessment of visual acuities, using the Snellen chart at 6 metres, is required to confirm that the patient is capable of seeing the visual targets presented as part of the eye movement examination.

In patients complaining of oscillopsia, i.e. symptoms of blurred vision on walking, with the world appearing to bob or move around, there may be a loss of dynamic visual acuity, i.e. visual acuity with head movement. This can be detected by asking the patient to rotate his head from side to side (horizontal rotation of the head through a vertical axis) at approximately 2 Hz, while attempting to read the Snellen chart. Loss of dynamic visual acuity occurs because of either hypo- or hyperactivity of the vestibulo-ocular reflex. A drop in the dynamic visual acuity of more than one line on the Snellen chart

suggests such an impairment of the vestibulo-ocular reflex, though the exact site of lesion is not revealed.

Visual fields

The visual fields should be checked by conventional confrontation examination techniques to exclude central scotoma or peripheral field defects. An inability to see visual targets would clearly cause abnormalities of pursuit and saccadic eye movements and optokinetic nystagmus, compromising the interpretation of tests of vestibular function.

Examination of the eye movements
Cover test for squint

The presence of a manifest or a latent squint (i.e. strabismus) needs to be determined as either can cause an abnormal eye movement examination because of the changing optic fixation from one fovea to the other. Where one eye has become amblyopic, the other eye should be assessed for the purposes of the clinical eye movement examination and for ENG (electronystagmographic) recordings of all components of the rotary chair protocol (see below).

To perform the cover test, each eye is covered in turn either with the hand or a piece of card held close to the eye (to obscure vision but also to prevent optic fixation with the covered eye) and the patient asked to fixate on a visual target held by the examiner in front of the patient's eyes at approximately his focal point, i.e. > 3 cm away. The covered eye should then be observed as the cover is taken away. A divergent strabismus arising from the covered eye will result in the covered eye moving inwards as the cover is removed and a convergent strabimus will cause the covered eye to move outwards as refixation occurs.

Range of eye movements

Each eye should be tested separately for the range of eye movements in all directions and together for convergence and conjugate gaze. When there is a restriction in the range of eye movements bilaterally in one or more directions, the lesion is likely to be due to a *gaze paresis*, implying a central lesion, and where there is a dissociation of eye movements, there is likely to be an *ocular paresis*, which implies a lesion at the level of or peripheral to the oculomotor nuclei.

A gaze palsy may be nuclear or supranuclear with reference to the oculomotor nuclei within the brain stem. Lesions of the *frontal eye fields* in the cortex may result in a contralateral horizontal gaze paresis, whereas lesions of the tegmentum of the *pontomedullary* and *pontomesencephalic junctions* may cause an ipsilateral gaze paresis. *Mesencephalic lesions* can cause a supranuclear gaze palsy, in which there is a loss of volitional gaze, with vertical movements lost before horizontal ones. A *supranuclear gaze palsy* is identified by the finding of a full range of eye movements in response to rotational and caloric stimulation of the vestibulo-ocular reflex, while in a nuclear palsy or an ocular paresis, the eye movements remain limited.

An ocular paresis may be due to a retro-orbital space-occupying lesion or due to involvement of the extraocular muscles (e.g. in *thyroid eye disease* or *mitochondrial cytopathy*). *Myasthenia gravis* causes a fluctuating unpredictable and variable ocular palsy. Lesions of the IIIrd, IVth and VIth cranial nerves or their nuclei cause a paresis in the direction of pull of the muscles they innervate. A lesion of the IIIrd cranial nerve causes the eye to be 'down and out'. There may be an associated *ptosis* and dilated pupil if the lesion involves the circumferential fibres (e.g. due to compression from a space-occupying lesion). A lesion of the IVth cranial nerve causes the eye to be slightly elevated. This increases on adduction and the head may tilt away from the side of the lesion to reduce diplopia. A lesion of the VIth cranial nerve causes a loss of abduction. A VIth nerve lesion may cause the head to be rotated towards the side of the lesion to reduce diplopia.

Ocular stabilizing systems

There are three visually controlled systems producing eye movements which stabilize gaze (Waespe and Henn, 1977): the *saccadic* system, the *smooth pursuit* system and the *optokinetic* system. The saccadic system responds to error in the direction of gaze by initiating a rapid eye movement to correct 'retinal position error'; the smooth pursuit system is responsible for maintaining gaze on a moving target by keeping the target within the foveal visual field; and the optokinetic system is thought to be a more primitive form of smooth pursuit involving the whole retina instead of the fovea alone. Each of the systems is discussed with reference to its anatomy and physiology as part of the eye movement examination.

Saccades

A saccade is a fast eye movement with a velocity between 350–600°/s, increasing with increased amplitude of eye movement (Robinson, 1964). Saccades can be voluntary or involuntary. Voluntary saccades are used to move the eyes between visual targets in the shortest possible time whereas the purpose of the involuntary saccadic system is to maintain the target on the fovea when there has been a slip of the retinal image.

With visually triggered saccades, the direction of the saccade is such as to move the globe rapidly towards targets already moving towards the fovea, i.e. the saccade resets the fovea on the target. If the subject is within an optokinetic drum rotating from the subject's left to right, the new target is coming from the left, so the saccade is to the left. While the saccade may be visually triggered, as in optokinetic nystagmus, it can also be of vestibular (Melville Jones, 1964; Barnes, 1979) or cervical origin (Bronstein and Hood, 1986), when the fast phase of nystagmus shifts the eyes in the direction of the ongoing head movement, before there is a slow phase compensatory drift.

Normal subjects are accurate up to a target jump of 20°, above which a small corrective saccade is required to bring the fovea on target. Overshoots are rare. The normal saccadic latency before a new saccade can be generated is 200 ms. For predicted saccades, the reaction time is less and the saccade may anticipate the target jump. During a saccade there is no useful visual perception (Gresty, Trinder and Leech, 1976).

Anatomy

The saccade is generated by groups of 'burst' neurons in the paramedian pontine reticular formation and pretectal region of the brain stem, the former generating horizontal saccades and the latter generating vertical saccades (Hoyt and Daroff, 1971). The pretectal areas for downward saccades are distinct from those for upward saccades. The eye position is maintained by 'tonic' cells which continue to fire after the saccade is complete (Cohen and Henn, 1972).

The ability to make saccades depends on the integrity of projections between the frontal eye fields, caudate nucleus, substantia nigra reticulata and the deep and intermediate layers of the superior colliculus (Zee, 1984; Bronstein and Kennard, 1987). Projections are to the paramedian pontine reticular formation and from here to the ipsilateral abducens nerve nucleus, and by the median longitudinal bundle to the contralateral oculomotor nucleus of the medial rectus. The pretectal neurons also project to the oculomotor nuclei, both sets of neurons connecting to the vestibular nuclei.

Clinical assessment

Saccadic eye movements are assessed by asking the patient to look back and forth between two targets in front of him sited approximately 30° to the right and to the left of the midline respectively. Increasing the distance between the targets beyond 30° increases the chance of detecting a hypometric saccade, while reducing the distance between targets increases the chance of detecting a hypermetric saccade (Zee *et al.*, 1976).

Abnormalities of saccadic eye movements

Three variables are examined: saccadic reaction time (latency), saccadic velocity and saccadic accuracy.

Abnormalities of any of these features may be due to CNS pathology or ocular myopathy, i.e. myasthenia (Henriksson *et al.*, 1981). Peripheral vestibular pathology does *not* cause abnormal saccadic eye movements.

Unilateral lesions of the *parapontine reticular formation* cause loss of all types of rapid ipsilateral movement and the eyes move to the contralateral visual field. During contralateral optokinetic nystagmus or ipsilateral rotation, the eyes display a tonic contralateral deviation with a loss of the fast phase of the nystagmic response. With ipsilateral optokinetic nystagmus or contralateral rotation, there is a normal ipsilateral slow wave response and a normal contralateral saccade (Dix, Harrison and Lewis, 1971).

Internuclear ophthalmoparesis

An internuclear ophthalmoparesis may present as ataxic nystagmus, whereby adducting saccades away from the side of the lesion are slower than abducting saccades. Subtle early lesions can be revealed by ENG with slowing of the adducting saccade away from the side of the lesion with a normal velocity but hypermetric abducting saccade. An explanation for the signs seen in internuclear ophthalmoparesis was offered by Pola and Robinson (1976): the horizontal saccade is generated by a pulse-step in neural activity, part of which excites medial rectus motoneurons of the fibres of the median longitudinal bundle. The median longitudinal bundle is thought to carry excitatory fibres to the ipsilateral medial rectus and inhibitory fibres to the contralateral medial rectus. Therefore, a median longitudinal bundle lesion will result in slowing and inaccuracy of adduction of the ipsilateral eye and overshoot of the contralateral abducting eye and there will be in consequence a derangement of conjugate contralateral gaze (Figure 21.1).

With more extensive brain stem pathology affecting the ipsilateral paramedian pontine reticular formation and both median longitudinal bundles (Pierrott–Deseilligny *et al.*, 1981), the *one and a half syndrome* can result with a failure of conjugate gaze in one direction and a bilateral internuclear ophthalmoparesis (Fischer, 1967).

The pathways subserving vertical and horizontal saccades are independent, such that in general, vertical saccades are unimpaired by lesions of the paramedian pontine reticular formation while lesions of the mesencephalic reticular formation affect vertical saccades (Buettner, Buettner–Ennever and Henn, 1977). The relationship between the mesencephalic reticular formation and the paramedian pontine reticular formation is not entirely clear, but vertical saccades can be abolished by stimulation of units in the paramedian pontine reticular formation (Keller, 1974).

In *cerebellar pathology*, the accuracy of the saccades may be impaired with undershooting (hypometria)

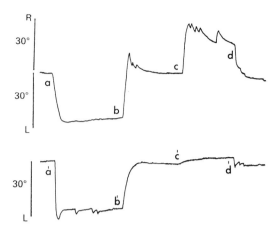

Figure 21.1 Internuclear ophthalmoplegia (INO). ENG recordings of separate eye saccades showing an INO: the upper trace documents movements of the right eye and the lower trace those of the left eye. At point a/a', the eyes are looking straight ahead, at b/b' the eyes are looking out at 30° to the left, at c/c' the eyes are again looking straight ahead, and at d/d' the eyes are attempting to look out at 30° to the right. This patient has a left INO, with failure of the left eye to adduct (c') and nystagmus in the abducting right eye (c). There is also a suggestion of a mild right INO with some slowing of the adducting right eye saccade and nystagmus in the abducted left eye, i.e. at b/b'

and/or overshooting (hypermetria) ipsilateral to the lesion (Zee *et al.*, 1976), followed by compensatory saccades (Figure 21.2). Hypermetria rarely occurs in normal subjects and its presence is therefore strongly suggestive of CNS pathology. Hypermetria is more common in cerebellar lesions than hypometria, while in intrinsic brain stem lesions, due to vertebrobasilar insufficiency, multiple sclerosis, or infiltrating tumours, hypometria is more likely (Goebel *et al.*, 1971).

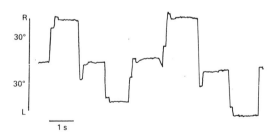

Figure 21.2 Saccadic dysmetria. Bitemporal ENG recordings of saccadic eye movements in a patient with cerebellar dysmetria. The patient has been asked to look to his right at a 30° target (deflection upwards) then to recentre, and then to look out to the left at a 30° target (deflection downwards), and to recentre. This is then repeated. The trace shows examples of both undershooting (hypometria) and overshooting (hypermetria)

In *supranuclear degeneration*, multiple system atrophy (Steele-Richardson-Olazewski syndrome, Shy–Drager syndrome, progressive supranuclear palsy and Huntington's chorea), saccade reaction time is prolonged. In these conditions, hypometria can also occur. In supranuclear lesions, vertical eye movements are usually affected before horizontal, initially with upgaze often more involved than downgaze (Dix, Harrison and Lewis, 1971) and saccades more affected than pursuit. The velocity of the saccades is usually reduced before the amplitude (Pasik, Pasik, and Bender, 1969; Kompfe *et al.*, 1979). The pathological process involves the burst neurons associated with saccades (Newman *et al.*, 1970). The reciprocal innervation of the lateral and medial recti is preserved, but there is a failure of this in the inferior rectus muscle on attempted upgaze (Pinhas *et al.*, 1978).

With *frontal pathology*, there may be hypometria or loss of horizontal saccades contralateral to the side of the lesion (Baloh, Honrubia and Sills, 1977), while vertical saccades are not affected. However, frontal lesions affect voluntary antisaccades. Normal subjects can direct a saccade in the opposite direction to an illuminated fixation target in the periphery. Subjects with frontal lesions tend to make an involuntary saccade to the target before the antisaccade.

In *ocular myasthenia*, the saccades may be normal at the start of testing, but with repeated testing, there may develop a deficiency of acetylcholine and the saccades will slow. Intravenous edrophonium may reverse this deterioration. Fatigue, alcohol and benzodiazepines will also cause slowing but saccadic movements are less impaired than smooth pursuit (Ajodhia and Dix, 1975).

It is important to distinguish ocular myasthenia (with the effect of intravenous edrophonium) from an internuclear ophthalmoparesis (by measuring the different velocities and amplitudes of abducting and adducting saccades), ocular palsies (by their classical presentations), and supranuclear gaze palsies (by the increase in eye movements on stimulation of the vestibulo-ocular reflex by head movements, rotation and caloric stimulation).

Smooth pursuit

In humans, the smooth pursuit system is responsible for maintaining gaze on a moving target, so that the target is stabilized on the fovea (Dodge, 1903). It compares and then matches target and eye velocities. In the absence of a target, pursuit eye movements cannot occur and the attempt to move the eye, even slowly, results in a saccade, although subjects can pursue *apparent* target motion in the absence of a target moving across the retina (Steinbach, 1976). While one stimulus, therefore, is the presence of a target moving across the retina, other factors appear to drive the system, including perhaps retinal posi-

tion, retinal velocity error and perceived target motion (Pola and Wyatt, 1980).

The degree of match between eye and target movement is given by the gain:

$$\text{gain} = \text{eye velocity/target velocity}$$

In normal subjects, the gain of the pursuit system approaches unity at peak velocities of 30°/s or sinusoidal rotation at 0.1 Hz (Baloh *et al.*, 1988). Above a peak velocity of 60°/s or sinusoidal rotation at 1 Hz, the gain falls off rapidly and catch-up saccades are required (Young and Stark, 1963). In man, the gain during sinusoidal oscillation at these levels in the dark (to stimulate the vestibulo-ocular reflex alone) is only 0.4, while, at 1–4 Hz and velocities greater than 100°/s, the gain is near unity (Barnes, 1979). Therefore, the smooth pursuit and the vestibulo-ocular reflex systems are complementary in stabilizing the retinal image with the pursuit system efficient at low target velocities and the vestibulo-ocular system efficient at high input velocities.

The smooth pursuit system is of particular clinical importance as it is considered to be intimately related with the mechanisms by which the vestibulo-ocular reflex is suppressed by optic fixation and this is of the utmost importance in differentiating peripheral from central vestibular pathology.

Lesions of the fovea, calcarine cortex (Yee *et al.*, 1982), parieto-occipital cortex (Lynch and McLaren, 1983), parietotemporal region, dorsolateral pontine nucleus and the cerebellar flocculus result in an impairment of smooth pursuit eye movements (Zee *et al.*, 1981; May, Keller and Suzuki, 1988). A pursuit pathway originates in Brodmann areas 19 and 39 and descends to the brain stem through the posterior limb of the internal capsule (Morrow and Sharpe, 1990).

Abnormalities of the smooth pursuit system

The smooth pursuit system can be examined clinically by moving a target (i.e. the examiner's finger) slowly back and forth in a sinusoidal fashion, initially in the horizontal and then in the vertical plane, in front of the patient's eyes. In chronic peripheral vestibular disorders, pursuit is normal.

In *acute peripheral vestibular disorders*, contralateral pursuit may be impaired. In *vestibular schwannomas*, pursuit movements are usually not impaired until brain stem compression has occurred. In *pretectal* and *basal ganglia lesions*, vertical pursuit is frequently impaired. There is ipsilateral derangement in *cerebellar, pontine* and *parieto-occipital lesions* (Schalen, Henriksson and Pyykko, 1982). *Low brain stem* lesions can cause derangement of downwards pursuit eye movements.

Pursuit eye movements are symmetrically affected by age, psychotropic medication, alcohol, anticonvulsants and vestibular and CNS sedatives (Ajodhia and Dix, 1975).

Optokinetic nystagmus

Optokinetic nystagmus is the name given to the rhythmical series of slow then rapid eye movements of the kind induced in a person looking at the scenery from a moving vehicle. The function of the optokinetic response is thought to stabilize the eyes relative to space during slow head movements in the low frequency range which are ill-served by the vestibulo-ocular reflex (Robinson, 1977).

Optokinetic nystagmus has a similar character to vestibular nystagmus as it is saw-toothed, and this gave rise to the original belief that the two reflexes involved a common neurological mechanism. Extracellular recordings from the vestibular nuclei of the monkey show a striking similarity between the response to both rotational and full-field optokinetic stimuli (Waespe and Henn, 1977), including algebraic summation of the two responses, indicating that the vestibular nuclei are incapable of distinguishing one stimulus from the other and in keeping with other studies demonstrating clear sensory convergence.

In fact, the pathways subserving optokinetic nystagmus are entirely independent of those subserving the slow component of vestibular nystagmus, although there are common neurological pathways subserving conjugate voluntary gaze and the fast components of optokinetic and vestibular nystagmus. The optokinetic system includes the peripheral retina, the accessory optic tract, the vestibular nuclei (Yee *et al.*, 1982) and the reticular formation. While there is no doubt that the neural pathway of optokinetic nystagmus in man is complex and that it is possible that more than one subcortical route exists (Hood, 1967), the abnormalities observed on testing patients with lesions at different levels in the nervous system are a useful aid to neuro-otological diagnosis.

Clinically, Barany introduced tests of optokinetic nystagmus, as part of the neuro-otological examination as early as 1922. A qualitative assessment of the optokinetic response may be undertaken at the bedside, or in the outpatient department, using either a hand-held or preferably mechanically driven rotating striped drum (Figure 21.3). The small drum consists of a cylinder, 30 cm in diameter, which can be rotated through 90° to elicit nystagmus in either the vertical or the horizontal plane, at speeds of 72, 180 and 360°/s. It is preferable not to ask the patient actively to follow the movement of the drum by counting each stripe as it appears as this evokes the pursuit and not the optokinetic nystagmus response.

For quantitative, diagnostic purposes, more precise and reproducible stimulus parameters are obtained by seating a patient inside a large, striped, rotating drum and stimulating the entire visual field (Figure 21.4).

Alternatively, a moving field of parallel bars, projected on to a surface covering approximately 60° of

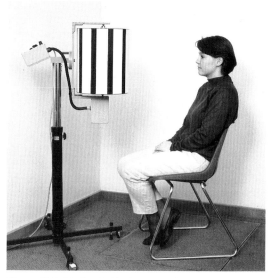

Figure 21.3 Mechanically-driven optokinetic nystagmus drum. The patient is seated 30 cm from a mechanically-driven optokinetic nystagmus drum which can be rotated either through a vertical or a horizontal axis at speeds of 72°, 180° or 360°/second. The tester stands behind the drum to observe the patient's optokinetic nystagmus response to horizontal and vertical optokinetic nystagmus stimuli, respectively

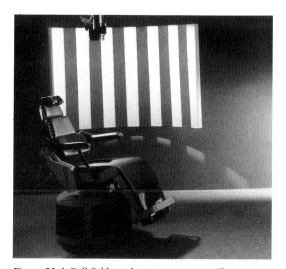

Figure 21.4 Full-field optokinetic nystagmus. The patient is seated in front of a moving field of parallel bars (projected from a source above the patient's head onto a surface subtending 60° of visual angle). The stripes are rotated to both right and left, reversing direction every 9 seconds, initially at 40°/s and then at 60°/s. (Reproduced with permission of Jaeger Toennies, Wurzberg, Germany)

visual angle, may be used. A striped tape can be used for bedside examination.

Although there are many aspects to be documented, two types of optokinetic nystagmus are recognized:

1 Cortical optokinetic nystagmus of the 'active' or 'look' type; this is induced more through foveal input and by using a small drum as well as a large full field one
2 Subcortical optokinetic nystagmus of the 'passive' or 'stare' type in which it is believed that the peripheral retina is involved without participation of the cerebral cortex.

Although the two types of optokinetic nystagmus responses are similar, the slow component velocity in the passive situation is consistently less than drum velocity, whereas in the active type, providing the subject can maintain his attention, eye velocity matches drum velocity. In addition, with reversal of drum direction, the direction of eye deviation is in the direction of the fast component when the subcortical system (i.e. passive type) is stimulated, when the subject is merely gazing at the drum and not trying to follow the passing stripes (Hood and Leech, 1974) and the deviation of the eyes occurs in the direction of the slow component of the nystagmus when the cortical system (or active type) predominates, the subject actively following the stripes on the drum.

In general, optokinetic nystagmus occurs in the opposite direction to that of the rotation of the drum – the exception being patients with congenital nystagmus who often exhibit reversed optokinetic nystagmus.

Clinical abnormalities seen with the small optokinetic nystagmus drum

Peripheral lesions

The imbalance of vestibular tone resulting from lesions of the labyrinth and VIIIth nerve can give rise with the small optokinetic nystagmus drum to a directional preponderance of the optokinetic nystagmus response (Baloh, Honrubia and Sills, 1977). The preponderance is clearest on direct inspection of the eyes with repeated abrupt reversal of drum direction. It is thought that optokinetic nystagmus can summate with the vestibular nystagmus and the preponderance tends to occur in the direction contralateral to the lesion, but occasionally exceptions occur with irritative lesions of the labyrinth.

Central lesions

As a general rule, abnormalities of optokinetic nystagmus slow components parallel abnormalities in smooth pursuit, and abnormalities of fast components correlate with abnormalities of voluntary saccades. Symmetrically decreased slow component velocity is produced by diffuse disease of the cortex, midbrain, brain stem and cerebellum. Focal lateralized disease of the parietal occipital region, brain stem and cerebellum results in impared optokinetic nystagmus when the stimulus moves toward the damaged side.

Brain stem lesions

Because the optomotor pathways lie in close anatomical proximity to the medial longitudinal bundle on either side of the midline, both the right and left pathways are liable to be involved synchronously by disease. Thus brain stem lesions usually cause bilateral optokinetic nystagmus depression resulting in a grossly deranged optokinetic nystagmus waveform which is readily identifiable.

Other abnormalities include sluggish or absent responses. Optokinetic nystagmus abnormalities may be seen with internuclear ophthalmalgia, particularly when nystagmus is not a prominent feature of the condition. The optokinetic nystagmus response is greater in the eye to which the fast component is directed. In cerebellopontine angle lesions optokinetic nystagmus asymmetry suggests considerable brain stem compression.

Congenital nystagmus

Reversal of optokinetic nystagmus is a characteristic feature of a significant proportion of cases of congenital nystagmus. In this situation the nystagmus beats paradoxically in the opposite direction to that anticipated from movement of the drum. It is thought that the waveform of this type of nystagmus is strongly influenced by movement of the drum so that when the direction of movement of the eye coincides with the direction of movement of the drum, the eye velocity will be enhanced and appear as a fast component (Halmagyi, Gresty and Leech, 1980) (Figure 21.5).

Tests of optokinetic nystagmus in the vertical plane help in revealing retraction nystagmus (i.e. with the drum rotating downwards, the eyes jerk irregularly backwards into the orbits) due to upward gaze paralysis caused by midbrain lesions, and can be a significant diagnostic feature in lesions involving the lower brain stem and in particular the craniocervical junction as in the Arnold–Chiari malformation.

Cerebellar lesions

Various abnormalities can be found in cerebellar disease and usually occur in association with smooth pursuit abnormalities (Baloh, Honrubia and Sills, 1977). In cerebellar atrophy, there is bilateral hypomobility and irregularities of waveform. Unilateral cerebellar lesions cause a directional preponderance of the optokinetic nystagmus towards the pathological side (Westheimer and Blair, 1973). Lesions of the flocculus also cause a reduction in slow phase velocity of optokinetic nystagmus (from about 100°/s to 40°/

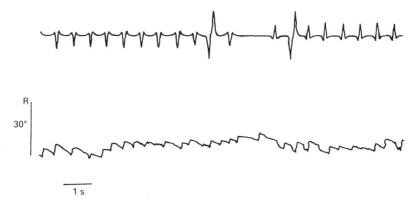

Figure 21.5 Congenital nystagmus and reversal of optokinetic nystagmus. When the drum reverses direction (as indicated by the change in direction of the spikes on the upper, target trace) the nystagmus continues beating to the right, i.e. the change in direction of the optokinetic stimulus is not paralleled by a reversal in the direction of the nystagmus

s) which distinguish them from lesions of the cerebellar hemispheres and paraflocculus which do not have this effect.

Cortical and subcortical lesions

Examination of the optokinetic nystagmus is of great value in the localization of some supratentorial lesions. With unilateral lesions deep in the parietal lobe, occipital lesions extending forwards into the corpus callosum and subcortical forebrain lesions, there is an ipsilateral directional preponderance, i.e. when the stimulus moves towards the affected side, optokinetic nystagmus is depressed or absent (Cogan, 1956; Baloh, Honrubia and Sills, 1977). The localizing value is strengthened when the optokinetic nystagmus asymmetry is associated with contralateral upper quadrant hemianopia and spasticity of conjugate gaze.

ENG abnormalities with full-field optokinetic nystagmus

Peripheral vestibular abnormalities of the labyrinth or VIIIth nerve rarely give rise to optokinetic derangements (Abel and Barber, 1981; Yee *et al.*, 1982) when tested with full-field optokinetic nystagmus. Full-field optokinetic nystagmus is, therefore, of great clinical value in distinguishing peripheral from central vestibular disorders.

Disorders affecting saccadic eye movements, or smooth eye movement, may result in derangements of optokinetic nystagmus. Neurological disease involving either the brain stem, cerebellum or IIIrd and

VIth cranial nerves may result in derangement of the fast saccadic components. The slow component may be deranged by lesions of the afferent visual pathways, or lesions of the efferent motor pathways, within the central nervous system. Lesions at every level from the brain stem, basal ganglia, cerebellum and cortex have been shown to cause derangement of the slow component velocity of the optokinetic response. A directional preponderance towards the side of the lesion occurs with cortical and subcortical lesions.

Assessment of nystagmus

Nystagmus is a combination of alternating slow phase and fast phase eye movements in opposite directions. For clinical purposes, the direction of nystagmus is defined by the fast phase. Nystagmus can be physiological or pathological – pathological nystagmus can be congenital or acquired.

Physiological vestibular nystagmus

The semicircular canal-ocular reflexes produce eye movements that compensate for head rotations. If a small rotational head movement is made, a slow compensatory eye movement occurs in the direction opposite to rotation, which serves to stabilize the gaze. If a larger stimulus is applied, i.e. such that the compensatory eye movement cannot be contained within the confines of the orbit, the slow vestibular-induced eye deviation is interrupted by a fast eye movement in the opposite direction, generating *physiological nystagmus*. The slow phase is generated by the vestibular nuclei of the opposite side of the brain stem and the fast phase is an involuntary saccadic eye movement, generated by neurons in the parapontine reticular formation on the same side (Raphan and Cohen, 1978). Neurons in the parapontine reticular formation monitor vestibulo-ocular signals and intermittently discharge to produce corrective fast components based on certain features of the vestibulo-ocular signal.

Physiological nystagmus can also be generated by extremes of eye deviation, i.e. more than 30° laterally from the primary position (*physiological end-point nystagmus*) as well as by rotational, caloric and visual stimulation (see below).

A relationship between the magnitude of induced nystagmus and the state of *arousal* in human subjects receiving vestibular stimulation has been noted (Collins, 1974a), i.e. if the subject was instructed to relax and day-dream, the velocity was less than when the subject was instructed to perform continuous mental arithmetic. However, if a subject is continuously rotated at low sinusoidal frequencies, there is a gradual decrease in gain, i.e. slow phase velocity, an effect known as *habituation* (Baloh *et al.*, 1982). Subjects experiencing repeated angular accelerations, e.g. ice-skaters and dancers, may display permanent habituation with a reduction or loss of nystagmus in response to vestibular stimulation (Collins, 1974b).

Physiological nystagmus may also be modified by optic fixation (Hood, 1968), by other sensory stimuli, i.e. auditory, tactile or cervical information (Baloh and Honrubia, 1979), by age (Tibbling, 1969), and by drugs (Nozue, Mizuno and Kaga, 1973).

Pathological vestibular nystagmus (or spontaneous vestibular nystagmus)

Spontaneous nystagmus results from an imbalance of tonic signals arriving at the oculomotor neurons. Because the vestibular system is the main source of oculomotor tonus, it is the driving force of most types of spontaneous nystagmus.

Spontaneous vestibular nystagmus, i.e. resulting from an imbalance of vestibular tone, results in a constant drift of the eyes in one direction interrupted by fast corrective components in the opposite direction. It may originate from a labyrinthine, vestibular nerve or vestibular nuclei lesion.

Experimental lesions at different levels of the vestibulo-ocular pathways in animals have allowed documentation of the induced nystagmus. Damage to one labyrinth results in spontaneous nystagmus, the slow component of which is directed towards the side of the lesion, the tonic input from the intact side being no longer balanced by input from the damaged side. Spontaneous nystagmus produced by sectioning of the vestibular nerve duplicates that resulting from labyrinthectomy. If both labyrinths are equally damaged however, spontaneous nystagmus does not result as there is no imbalance of vestibular afferent information, demonstrating that for production of nystagmus, the relative balance of input is more important than the absolute magnitude of input.

The direction of the spontaneous nystagmus generated by lesions of the vestibular nuclei is less predictable and depends on the location and extent of the lesion, imbalance produced between inhibitory and excitatory secondary vestibular neurons dictating the direction of the nystagmus (Uemura and Cohen, 1973). Lesions of the vestibulo-ocular pathways in the brain stem may affect either the slow vestibular component of the nystagmus, the fast saccadic component or both phases of nystagmus.

Lesions involving the peripheral vestibular pathways (i.e. vestibular end-organ and nerve) affect nystagmus in both eyes equally because the central pathways are symmetrically connected. Central lesions lying anywhere from the vestibular nuclei to the oculomotor neurons often produce dysconjugate nystagmus because the pathways to the eye muscles diverge beginning at the vestibular nuclei, proximally.

Clinical assessment

Spontaneous nystagmus is an invaluable sign in siting vestibular and neurological disease (Rudge, 1983). If maximal diagnostic information is to be obtained, alterations in the nystagmic response produced by change of eye position (30° right and left from midposition of gaze) or presence and absence of optic fixation, need to be documented.

Nystagmus is graded by its presence in different directions of resting eye position (Alexander's law). If it is only observed in the resting position ipsilateral to the fast phase, it is *first degree*; if it is also seen in the primary position, it is *second degree*; if it is seen in the resting position, contralateral to the fast phase, it is *third degree*.

With labyrinthine and vestibular nerve lesions, nystagmus is usually in the direction contralateral to the lesion because of vestibular hypofunction, but in the presence of an irritative lesion, as for example in the acute phase of Menière's syndrome, the nystagmus may be directed towards the affected ear. If the lesion is small or compensation has occurred, nystagmus may only be elicited with the removal of optic fixation. This is an important criterion to identify nystagmus due to peripheral pathology; the nystagmus usually displays an increase of amplitude with a reduction of slow phase velocity with the removal of optic fixation (Dix and Hallpike, 1966; Korres, 1978). The nystagmus may be detected in the dark by electronystagmography or by direct observation with either an infrared viewer or Frenzel's glasses.

Gaze-evoked nystagmus

Patients with gaze-evoked nystagmus are unable to maintain stable conjugate eye deviation away from the primary position. The eyes drift backward towards the centre with an exponentially decreasing waveform. Corrective saccades constantly reset the eye in the desired position, thus gaze-evoked nystagmus is always in the direction of gaze and as the angle of gaze increases, so the amplitude of nystagmus increases. Furthermore, in the absence of optic fixation, although the amplitude of gaze paretic nystagmus increases, the frequency and slow component velocity decrease. The underlying abnormality is a failure of gaze maintenance, which may be secondary to a lesion anywhere from the neuromuscular junction to the multiple brain centres controlling conjugate gaze. Dysfunction of the oculomotor integrator may be a common mechanism for several types of gaze-evoked nystagmus. Gaze paretic nystagmus should be distinguished from vestibular nystagmus.

Symmetrical gaze paretic nystagmus is commonly observed in association with deranged pursuit following the use of anticonvulsants, in particular phenytoin and phenobarbitone, ingestion of psychotropic drugs and alcohol. Asymmetrical horizontal gaze paretic nystagmus is likely to indicate a structural brain lesion and, in the case of cerebellar or cerebellopontine angle disease, the nystagmus is of larger amplitude towards the side of the lesion (*Brun's nystagmus*). Cerebellar lesions cause profound abnormalities of eye movements with an inability to maintain ipsilateral eccentric gaze (Westheimer and Blair, 1973).

Positional nystagmus

Nystagmus can be elicited by critical head postures in certain pathological states. *Positional nystagmus* is present if the nystagmus occurs while the head is stationary in the critical position. *Positioning nystagmus* is present if the nystagmus begins while the head is still moving. Positional nystagmus is due to the position itself and the effect of the gravity vector while positioning nystagmus is due to linear and angular acceleration forces.

The *Hallpike manoeuvre* (Dix and Hallpike, 1952) is a valuable test in such patients and, indeed, is the only method of diagnosing benign paroxysmal positional nystagmus, central positional nystagmus and atypical positional nystagmus. It consists of moving the sitting patient with the head turned 45° towards the examiner, rapidly into the lying position with the head extended 30° over the back of the couch. In this way, the posterior semicircular canal of the undermost ear is moved directly through its plane of orientation. The patient should feel relaxed in the physician's hands needing little support from his own nuchal musculature. The manoeuvre is repeated for both the right and left ears undermost positions.

The patient is told not to close his eyes and to keep his gaze centred on the examiner's forehead and he should be warned that he may feel very dizzy. Before the manoeuvre the patient's spectacles should be removed. Many physicians carry out this test with Frenzel's glasses to eliminate fixation. The clinical value of this is uncertain as positional nystagmus under these conditions occurs in as many as 30% of asymptomatic patients (Stahle and Terrins, 1965).

Benign paroxysmal positional vertigo was described by Barany (1921). In this condition, the patients give a history of positional vertigo – vertigo typically triggered by particular head movements. They may give a history of a preceding head injury (Barber, 1964), migraine, hypertension or vascular event. In patients with benign paroxysmal positional vertigo, with the pathological ear undermost, the Hallpike manoeuvre may produce a cluster of classical signs. There is a latent period to onset of nystagmus of 2–30 seconds, followed by the development of rotational nystagmus, with the fast phase towards the ground (geotropic) and accompanied by vertigo. The vertigo and nystagmus adapt, but on sitting up, the nystagmus may reverse and is again accompanied by vertigo. Both the symptoms and signs fatigue on retesting.

Less common than benign paroxysmal positional vertigo is *central positional nystagmus*. If the positional nystagmus is not accompanied by vertigo or if it takes another form, the aetiology may lie centrally, e.g. in the cerebellum (Riesco, 1957; Fernandez, Alzate and Lindsay, 1959; Harrison and Ozsahinoglu, 1972) or around the floor of the fourth ventricle (Hallpike, 1967). In such cases, there is usually, though not invariably, no latency before the onset of nystagmus, often no vertigo, no adaptation and no fatiguability. The direction of nystagmus may be towards the uppermost ear, or may be upbeat or downbeat. In essence, although some of the diagnostic characteristics of benign paroxysmal positional vertigo may be met, others are absent, raising the suspicion of central pathology. While the patients may have a history of intracranial tumours, multiple sclerosis, Arnold–Chiari malformation or cerebrovascular disease, occasionally central positional nystagmus may be the only sign of posterior fossa pathology.

It should be noted that occasionally patients with the typical features of paroxysmal positional vertigo have central pathology. Warning clues are a history of neurological symptoms, i.e. choking or swallowing difficulties, and/or cranial nerve, brain stem or cerebellar signs.

The Hallpike manoeuvre involves three nystagmogenic factors: the cervical factor, the movement factor (the positioning effect) and final resting position (the positional effect). It is important to assess the contribution of each component. The cervical factor, which may also include the effect of kinking of the vertebral arteries, can be assessed by tilting back the head with the patient sitting. The head can be kept in this position for sufficiently long to exclude kinking of the vertebral arteries as a cause of the patient's symptoms. The patient should be asked to report what he experiences and complaints of syncopal or neurological symptoms should abort the test. Clearly this manoeuvre has to be carried out by a competent physician. The positioning and positional effects are distinguished by the presence or absence of a latent period between the time of onset of vertigo and nystagmus. A latent period after the head has achieved the test position indicates the response was positional rather than positioning.

Benign paroxysmal positional vertigo is unlikely to be the result of a single lesion. Various mechanisms have been postulated, but the most widely accepted hypothesis is the *cupulolithiasis* model, according to which degenerated dense material from the utricular macula becomes attached to the cupula of the posterior semicircular canal leading to the utriculofugal deflection of the cupula stimulation of the posterior semicircular canal when it is undermost (Schuknecht and Ruby, 1973). In support of this model is the specificity of the direction of stimulation required to produce the clinical picture, with the head inclined in the angle which would maximally stimulate the ampulla of the posterior semicircular canal and the effect of denervation of the posterior semicircular canal ampulla by section of its nerve (Gacek, 1978). While these observations would support the role of the posterior semicircular canal, the 'heavy cupula' concept has been called into question by the results of experiments where a heavy cupula is created by alcohol or deuterium ingestion, when the resulting nystagmus in a particular head position is sustained for long periods of time, rather than the classic picture in benign paroxysmal positional vertigo of transient nystagmus (Money, Johnson and Carlett, 1970; Money and Myles, 1974). Alternative hypotheses include the *canalolithiasis* model which suggests that the dense debris is localized in the long arm of the posterior semicircular canal (Hall, Ruby and McClure, 1979; Epley, 1980; Parnes and McClure, 1992), and hypotheses that there is a single calcified mass (Vyslonzil, 1963) or that there is a non-homogeneous layering of endolymph (McClure, 1985).

The main points of difference between benign paroxysmal positional vertigo and central positional nystagmus are summarized in Table 21.1.

Atypical positional nystagmus

Atypical positional nystagmus has some features which do not readily match either the benign paroxysmal positional vertigo or central positional nystagmus category. This type is associated with subjective vertigo but there may be no latent period, or no adaptation, or the nystagmus is not directed towards the downmost ear. Atypical positional nystagmus has been reported in patients with tumours affecting the cerebellar vermis (Riesco, 1957) and it may also be associated with plaques of multiple sclerosis or it may be an atypical presentation of benign paroxysmal positional vertigo.

Vertical nystagmus

Vertical nystagmus invariably implies central nervous system disease (Bogousslavsky, Regli and Hunberbuhler, 1980; Fisher *et al.*, 1983). Downbeat nystagmus is commonly associated with an intra-axial lesion at the level of the foramen magnum and is well recognized in association with the Arnold–Chiari malformation (Cogan and Burrows, 1954). The patient complains of oscillopsia; clues to the site of lesion may be given by a history of swallowing difficulties or choking when laying down and in such patients MRI scanning is indicated even in the presence of the classical picture of benign paroxysmal positional vertigo in the Hallpike manoeuvre.

Rebound nystagmus

Rebound nystagmus is characteristic of cerebellar dysfunction. It manifests itself as gaze evoked nystagmus, which disappears, or reverses, as the direction of gaze is held and, on recentring, a burst of nystagmus is initiated in the direction of the return saccade (Hood, Kayan and Leech, 1973; Baloh, Konrad and Honrubia, 1975).

Table 21.1 Differences between benign positional nystagmus (BPN) and central positional nystagmus (CPN)

	BPN	CPN
Latent period	2–30 s	None
Adaptation	Within 30 s	Persists
Fatiguability	Disappears on repetition	Persists
Vertigo	Present and may be severe	Usually absent or very mild
Direction of nystagmus	Rotatory towards downmost ear	Any
Incidence	Common	Rare

Dysconjugate nystagmus

Dysconjugate nystagmus is commonly due to central nervous system disease. Ataxic nystagmus, associated with an internuclear ophthalmoplegia, is the most well-recognized variety. It is the result of a lesion in the median longitudinal bundle (Cogan, Kubik and Smith, 1950) and most commonly occurs in multiple sclerosis. *Monocular nystagmus*, by definition, is dysconjugate, and has been reported in a number of ophthalmological and neurological conditions (Nathansan, Bergman and Berker, 1955; Donin, 1967). *See-saw nystagmus* is rare but is associated with lesions near the optic chiasma (Arnott and Miller, 1970; Williams *et al.*, 1982).

Periodic alternating nystagmus

Periodic alternating nystagmus changes direction with a change of head or eye position. Patients complain of oscillopsia. The cycle length varies from 1 to 6 minutes with null periods of 2–20 seconds. The precise site of the lesion is unknown, but both the cerebellum (Baloh, Honrubia and Konrad, 1976; Rudge and Leech, 1976; Furman and Wall, 1990) and the caudal brain stem (Keane, 1974) have been implicated. There is an abnormality of central vestibular function: the horizontal semicircular canal-ocular reflex during sinusoidal rotation displays an abnormal gain and phase with a variable rate of decay of the post-rotatory responses, canal-otolith interaction is abnormal and the otolith-ocular response displays an enlarged modulation component (Furman and Wall, 1990), suggesting that there is an abnormality of central velocity storage.

Head shaking nystagmus

In the absence of rotation tests, head shaking nystagmus is a candidate as a screening test for vestibular pathology. The test should be applied with caution in the elderly, in those with significant cervical pathology, and is contraindicated in those with raised intracranial pressure or a history of retinal detachments.

Nystagmus which appears after rapid horizontal head shaking is termed head shaking nystagmus and is attributed to a lesion in the vestibular system (Kamei *et al.*, 1964; Hain, Fetter and Zee, 1987). The test involves shaking the head from side to side $\pm 30°$ at a frequency of > 1.5 Hz (peak velocity $> 280°/s$ for 10–20 seconds and then suddenly stopping. Spontaneous nystagmus is abnormal and indicates an asymmetry in the vestibular system.

The response follows the physiological directional asymmetry in vestibular responses described in Ewald's second law (1892), i.e. the differential effects of ampullofugal versus ampullopetal endolymph flow – excitatory inputs versus inhibitory inputs. Normally in head shaking the directional asymmetries balance, but with a unilateral peripheral lesion, there is an asymmetry which is revealed by the nystagmus with the slow phase in the direction of the pathological side.

The direction of the nystagmus is not always that predicted by Ewald's second law (Takahashi *et al.*, 1990). It has been suggested that head shaking nystagmus is a function of the directional preponderance of peripheral vestibular asymmetry and also of the amount of velocity storage (Hain, Fetter and Zee, 1987). For the nystagmus to appear after the head shaking has stopped, the directional asymmetry must have been stored. Some storage would be the result of cupula-endolymph mechanics, but the importance of central velocity storage is reflected by the loss of head shaking nystagmus in the acute phase after unilateral labyrinthectomy (Fetter *et al.*, 1990). Furthermore, if there is a direction specific asymmetry in the central velocity storage mechanism, the direction of the head shaking nystagmus may not be as predicted according to Ewald's law (Demer, 1985).

Nystagmography

Although a good examination of eye movements can be made by direct observation, recording techniques, including *electronystagmography*, *photoelectric* or *video recording* and *scleral coil recording in a magnetic field* (Collewijn, van der Mark and Jansen, 1975), allow a more detailed evaluation and provide a permanent record for comparative purposes. There are two methods of recording the eye movements electrically which are commonly used.

The photoelectric method

A beam of light is focused onto the sclera of the subject and the reflection is measured. This method is often difficult to use as random eye movements may seriously interfere with the test. Nystagmus cannot be recorded with the eyes closed. The only real use of the photoelectric method is during galvanic testing.

Electronystagmography

Principle of ENG

Electronystagmography is the simplest and most readily available system for recording eye movements. In theory, this test should be named 'electro-oculography' to conform with the nomenclature of other electrical tests, i.e. electrocardiography, but when used for evaluating vestibular function, the term electronystagmography is used and is interchangeable with the term electro-oculography.

The technique depends on the potential difference

between the cornea and retina, created by the retinal pigmentary epithelium. The pigmented layer of the retina maintains a negative potential with respect to the rest of the eye by means of active ion transport. The eyeball behaves as a dipole with its axis coinciding with the optical axis of the eye. An electrode placed lateral to the eye becomes more positive when the eye rotates towards it and more negative when it rotates away, with reference to an electrode at a more remote location. The voltage change represents the change in eye position as only small angular movements are involved in nystagmus and the relationship between voltage change and the eye movement is virtually linear at these small degrees of arc.

Recordings are usually made with a three electrode system, using two 'active' electrodes placed lateral to each eye, and a 'ground' electrode is placed somewhere remote from the eye, normally on the forehead. The potential difference between the two active electrodes is amplified and used to control the displacement of the pen recorder or similar device to produce a permanent record. Because the differential amplifiers monitor the difference in voltage between the two active electrodes, remote electrical signals, i.e. of electrocardiographic or electroencephalographic origin, arrive at the electrodes with approximately equal amplitude and phase and will be cancelled out. The polarity of the recording is arranged so that a deflection of the eye to the left causes a downward deflection of the pen, and a deflection of the eye to the right causes an upward deflection of the pen (Figure 21.6).

The recording instrument commonly consists of a preamplifier, amplifier and galvanometer to enable the pen to deflect on paper moving with a set speed, thereby registering the eye position against time. Recording using AC amplifiers causes substantial amplitude loss depending on the time constant used, whereas in DC recording, no amplitude loss takes place and the pen deflection is an accurate reflection of the eye position (Hood, 1968). This confers a considerable advantage in recordings with the eyes closed and in darkness. In AC amplification, gaze deviations to the right and left are denoted by no more than transient shifts of the baseline (Figure 21.7).

This form of amplification, therefore would be adequate for ENG recording of caloric or rotationally induced nystagmus where knowledge of the eye position is of less importance, but can be very misleading when direction of gaze deviation determines the type of nystagmus. By contrast, in DC amplification, the tracings provide a complete description of the nystagmus. It does however require the use of electrodes which are relatively free of the drift caused by electrochemical potentials generated at the skin–electrode interface and the only real advantage of an AC machine is that it is easier to obtain electrode stability.

The sensitivity of the ENG with well-designed amplification can consistently record eye rotations of 0.5°. This sensitivity is less than that of direct visual inspection which is approximately 0.1°.

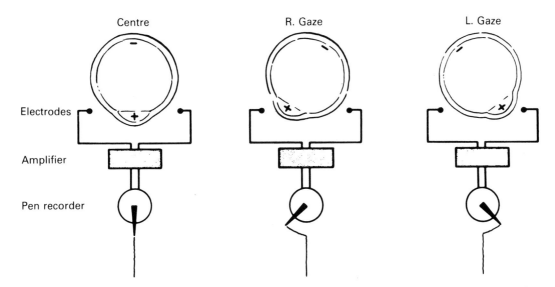

Figure 21.6 Corneoretinal potential. The electrode lateral to the eye becomes more positive when the eye rotates towards it, and more negative when the eye rotates away. The voltage change represents the change in eye position. (Adapted from Baloh and Honrubia, 1990; with permission from Professor Bob Baloh)

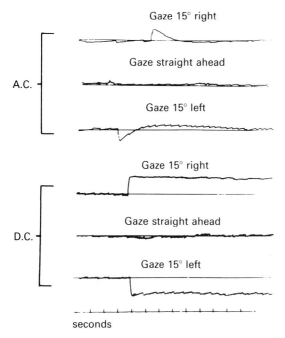

Gaze 15° right

Gaze straight ahead

A.C.

Gaze 15° left

Gaze 15° right

Gaze straight ahead

D.C.

Gaze 15° left

seconds

Figure 21.7 AC versus DC amplification. ENG recordings from the same patient using AC and DC amplification. With AC recordings, deviations of gaze are represented by transient shifts of the base-line, whereas DC recordings are an accurate representation of the eye position. (From Dix and Hood, 1984; reproduced with permission from Dr Derrick Hood)

Electrodes and electrode placement

The plane of the recording electrodes defines the plane of recorded eye movement. Electrodes attached medial and lateral to the eye will record the horizontal components of eye movement; those above and below the eye, the vertical components. A single channel ENG machine summates the horizontal movements of both eyes from bitemporal recordings onto the same trace. This has the advantage of improving the signal to noise ratio but disguises dysconjugate eye movements. The vertically aligned electrodes sense the voltage associated with both eye and eyelid movement, summing the two movements. For this reason the vertical ENG cannot be used for quantitative analysis of vertical eye movements, although it can provide a valuable monitor of eye blinks.

Simultaneous and separate recording of horizontal and vertical movements of both eyes requires multi-channel recording facilities.

A two-channel ENG machine can record the movement of each eye separately (monocular recordings) and provides a sensitive means of detecting dysconjugate eye movements. A four channel machine can, in addition, simultaneously record the vertical movements of each eye and allows a separate assessment of the vertical components of nystagmus.

A paper speed of 10 mm/s is frequently used for routine clinical testing of eye movements. For separate eye recordings to examine saccade accuracy and velocity, and to examine nystagmus fast phase velocity, 100 mm/s or an even faster speed may be necessary. To demonstrate the overall pattern or duration of induced nystagmus, i.e. post-caloric or post-rotatory nystagmus very slow paper speeds can be used.

Signal and noise

Artefacts can cause interference with the genuine eye movement signal and can be electrical or bioelectrical. High frequency, uniform oscillation can be caused by poor electrode contact due to a loose electrode, poorly prepared skin or insufficient electrode gel.

Insufficient shielding of the recording instrument or the presence of other electronic instruments in the vicinity may result in 50 Hz mains electricity artefacts.

The commonest bioelectrical artefacts are blinks and muscle activity. Muscle activity tends to occur in unrelaxed patients and presents typical electromyographic patterns of irregular high frequency spike activity. EEG patterns (7–20 Hz low amplitude oscillations) may also be picked up. Drowsiness may cause slow sinusoidal oscillations of the tracing. Some patients may show constant lid flutter with eye closure that looks like nystagmus, and for this reason recordings should always be made with eyes open in the dark.

Calibration

In order to interpret ENG recordings, calibration must be performed so that a standard angle of eye deviation is represented by a known amplitude of pen deflection. The patient is asked to look straight ahead and then at a series of lights or fixation points 10°, 20° or 30° away from the midline on each side of, above and below the central fixation point directly in front of him (the angle used for the fixation target is a matter of choice). This is repeated several times to ensure that the eye movements are precise and that the amount of pen deflection is constant. A convenient calibration is to adjust the amplifier to obtain 10 mm pen deflection per 10°.

Once the chosen relationship is established, the amplitude, duration and velocity of recorded eye movements can be easily calculated. By convention, the recording electrode arrangement is adjusted to obtain an upward pen deflection for eye movement to the right and a downward pen deflection for pen movement to the left. For vertical recordings, upward and downward eye movements produce upward and downward deflections respectively. A typical beat of vestibular nystagmus as recorded with ENG is shown in Figure 21.8.

The fast component moves to the left, so by convention, the nystagmus is to the left. A 10° fast component would have an average velocity (i.e. a/fd) of 100°/s. The slow component velocity (i.e. a/sd) is usually much slower, in this case 10°/s. Digital computers are well suited to calculating the slow component velocity from the product of the amplitude and frequency so long as the fast duration is long compared to the slow duration. After analogue to digital conversion of the data, a digital computer using an algorithm calculates the amplitude, duration and velocity of each of the slow and fast components.

As the corneoretinal potential varies with the amount of light striking the retina, the ENG signal must be calibrated frequently and major shifts in the room lighting avoided (n.b. the maximum light-adapted potential is approximately twice the dark adapted-potential). If any alteration has occurred, the gain of the recorder should be adjusted.

Clinical relevance of ENG

The main advantage of ENG is that some patients reveal nystagmus which is not readily visible on naked eye examination. ENG recordings also allow for quantification and the provision of a permanent record of nystagmus. The clinical applications are best considered by describing particular findings under various circumstances.

Peripheral vestibular disorders

Unless acute, these lesions are unlikely to be associated with nystagmus in the presence of optic fixation, but the nystagmus is revealed or increased in amplitude in darkness. The nystagmus is unidirectional with the largest amplitude on horizontal gaze towards the direction of the fast component, i.e. away from the side of the lesion.

Vestibular nuclei lesions

Nystagmus is reduced or abolished by eye-closure. In darkness, the amplitude of the nystagmus may hardly alter but the velocity of the slow phase may be decreased. Often the nystagmus is bidirectional.

Cerebellar lesions

These may be associated with multiple *square waves*, i.e. with a duration of < 200 ms. Another highly characteristic abnormality which can only be detected in DC ENG recordings is the failure to maintain lateral gaze (Figure 21.9) either in darkness or with eye-closure, and slow drifting movements of the eyes in the absence of fixation (Leech *et al.*, 1977). Centripetal nystagmus, in which the fast phase of the nystagmus beats towards the position of primary gaze on eye-closure or in darkness, and rebound nystagmus (Hood, Kayan and Leech, 1973) are common in cerebellar disease but are also encountered in a vari-

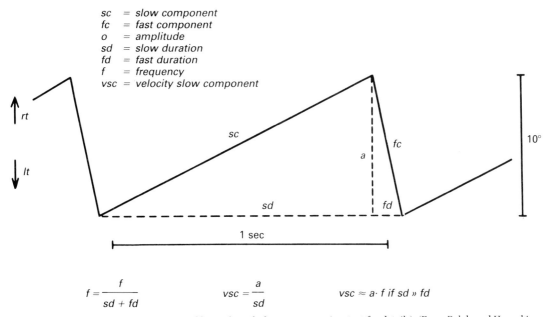

sc = slow component
fc = fast component
o   = amplitude
sd = slow duration
fd = fast duration
f   = frequency
vsc = velocity slow component

$$f = \frac{f}{sd + fd} \qquad vsc = \frac{a}{sd} \qquad vsc \approx a \cdot f \text{ if } sd \gg fd$$

Figure 21.8 Vestibular nystagmus. A typical beat of vestibular nystagmus (see text for details). (From Baloh and Honrubia, 1990; reproduced by permission of Professor Bob Baloh)

ety of other conditions including peripheral vestibular disorders, drug intoxication and congenital abnormalities. *Rebound nystagmus*, i.e. nystagmus to the right, is evident on gaze deviation to the right, but unlike brain stem nystagmus it is transitory and only persists for some 20 s; at the end of this period the eyes are returned to the primary position of gaze, a transitory nystagmus to the left, not present initially, makes its appearance. Next, gaze deviation to the left brings about transitory nystagmus to the left, and on returning the eyes to the primary position a nystagmus now beating to the right is produced.

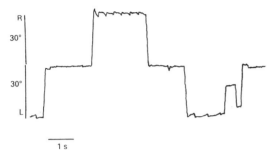

Figure 21.9 Gaze-evoked nystagmus. Bitemporal ENG recordings of a patient with bidirectional gaze-evoked nystagmus due to phenytoin toxicity. Gaze at 30° to the right provoked fine right-beating nystagmus, and gaze at 30° to the left provoked fine left-beating nystagmus

Patients with cerebellar disease may also have difficulties in executing command saccadic eye movements. When they are asked to turn their gaze laterally quickly, they overshoot the target. This abnormality is known as ocular *dysmetria* (Orzechowski, 1927). If present, it may be easily detected on ENG recordings.

Supranuclear lesions

These lesions may exhibit a nystagmus which is reduced or more often abolished both by eye-closure and by darkness. The nystagmus may be disassociated. Optokinetic ENG recording usually reveals broken up, sluggish responses. Saccadic velocities are slowed. This can be readily demonstrated by ENG. The ENG recordings are taken from both eyes separately (dual channel recording) using DC coupling and with a fast paper speed. Normal eye velocities fall within the range 450–600°/s and adduction is normally faster than abduction. In an internuclear ophthalmoparesis velocities are reduced with adduction usually affected first.

Congenital nystagmus

This generally has a pendular character although saw-toothed (similar to vestibular) nystagmus may be supra-added on lateral gaze. Congenital nystagmus

is usually unaffected by removal of optic fixation. The optokinetic responses are always abnormal and are often reversed (see above).

Standard protocol for visuovestibular stimulation

Recording for pathological nystagmus

- Calibration: centre, right 30°, recentre, left 30° (repeat)
- Centre gaze: fixation at mid-position, with eyes open and then in dark for 20 s, i.e. fixation inhibited (n.b. with constant mental alerting)
- Gaze held at 30° right for 10 s, then 20 s in the dark
- Gaze held at 30° left for 10 s, then 20 s in the dark
- Gaze held at 30° up and then 30° down each with and without optic fixation

Visual tests (i.e. laser visual target)

- Saccades: 5–30°, target can be series of dots or lights
- Separate eye saccades: recordings taken from both eyes separately paper speed 10 × normal, i.e. 100 mm/s 30°R, 0°, 30°L, 0° (repeat)
- Smooth pursuit: at 0.1, 0.2, 0.3, 0.4 Hz target displacement + 15° to − 15°
- OKN nystagmus: curtain speed/stripe velocity 40 and 60°/s (reverse direction after 9 seconds, 2 ×) OKN slow build-up: 20 s run to R then L

Rotary chair tests

- Impulsive rotational testing: acceleration rise time of < 1 s constant velocity of 60°/s
- Sinusoidal vestibulo-ocular reflex testing: at 0.1, 0.2, 0.3, 0.4 Hz maximal velocity 40°/s
- Vestibulo-ocular reflex suppression: at 0.1, 0.2, 0.3, 0.4 Hz maximal velocity 40°/s

The use of a *laser target* allows quantification of smooth pursuit eye movements. The patient is asked to follow the movement of a laser as it moves horizontally from side to side at 0.1 m before his eyes at different frequencies as above. The advantage of a laser target is that its size remains constant with distance from its source unlike conventional light sources and an infinite number of computerized projection paradigms are possible for different test and research purposes.

Tests of semicircular canal dysfunction

The investigation of disordered vestibular function includes audiometric tests, in particular recording the pure tone audiogram, otoadmittance, the ipsilateral and contralateral stapedius reflex thresholds, otoacoustic emissions and auditory brain stem responses. This discussion is confined to the vestibular investigations.

Investigations of vestibular function
(Table 21.2)

While every physician should perform the vestibular tests included in the clinical examination, the investigations described in the next section may only be available at certain sites. Caloric testing should be available to all clinicians. It is of immense value to have access to DC-ENG chart recording techniques to document nystagmus, pursuit eye movements and saccades and to obtain data in the dark in the absence of optic fixation. Rotational testing and a large optokinetic stimulus should be available at tertiary referral sites, though a thorough clinical examination and the application of the other techniques should reduce their importance.

Table 21.2 Investigations (outline)

Audiometry	Pure-tone audiogram (including bone conduction thresholds if necessary)
	Otoadmittance testing
	Acoustic reflex thresholds
if indicated	Auditory brain stem responses
	Click-evoked otoacoustic emissions
	Speech audiometry
	Electrocochleography
Vestibular tests	Bithermal caloric tests
	Electronystagmography
	Rotational tests
if indicated	Sono-ocular test
	Galvanic tests
	Posturography
Imaging if indicated	Gadolinium enhanced MRI scan
Blood investigations	Full blood picture (haemoglobin, white blood cell count, ESR), Serology including fluorescent treponemal antibody-absorption (FTA abs), thyroid stimulating hormone (TSH)

Other specific tests as clinically indicated

The role of vestibular tests

A careful history and general, neurological and neuro-otological clinical examination, particularly of eye movements will contribute greatly towards the making of the final diagnosis and, as a result, the value of vestibular tests in clinical medicine has been questioned. In addition, in positional and positioning nystagmus, the clinical examination and, where indicated imaging studies, are of more value than rotational and caloric tests. On the other hand, a variety of eye movement recording techniques can be used to examine eye movements in the absence of optic fixation and offer the advantage of providing objective, permanent records of nystagmus enabling measurements of slow phase velocities and durations, and the documentation of other disordered eye movements. Electronystagmography is the most widely available technique for recording eye movements and offers great advantages in the recording of responses to both visual and vestibular stimuli, i.e. gaze testing with and without optic fixation, saccadic and pursuit eye movements, optokinetic responses, and caloric and rotational stimuli with and without suppression of the vestibulo-ocular reflex. It should be appreciated that ENG recordings of eye movements are less sensitive than direct observation of the eyes and that they are of little quantitative value if the response has a significant element in the vertical plane.

Frenzel's glasses, although helpful in the absence of a dark room, are less efficient than electronystagmography, as they do not adequately eliminate optic fixation and the blurred image can cause artefactual eye movements. Moreover, no documentation for purposes of measurement or comparison can be obtained.

Caloric testing

The caloric test is the most widely available of all the vestibular tests and is the cornerstone of vestibular diagnosis. There are two major reasons for this: it allows each labyrinth to be tested separately; and the stimulus is easy to apply with inexpensive methodology. Caloric abnormalities have been documented in a large range of vestibular and neurological conditions, and the caloric test remains unrivalled as a method of demonstrating an organic cause of vertigo.

Principle of caloric testing

When the ear is irrigated with water above and below body temperature, a temperature gradient is set up across the labyrinth. If during the irrigation the patient is reclined on a couch with his head at 30° to the horizontal, the plane of the horizontal semicircular canal becomes vertical and the temperature gradient is established from one side of the canal to the other.

The endolymph is thought to circulate because of the difference in its specific gravity on the two sides of the canal. With the warm water stimulus the column of endolymph nearest the middle ear rises because of its decreased density, resulting in cupula deflection towards the utricle (ampullopetal flow). Cupula deflection results in activation of the vestibulo-ocular reflex leading to a sensation of vertigo and inducing horizontal nystagmus directed towards the stimulated ear.

However, the above convection theory, proposed by Barany (1906), has been questioned after the clear observation of caloric nystagmus under microgravity conditions and in space, where convection currents cannot explain the findings (Baumgarten, Benson and Berthoz, 1984; Scherer *et al.*, 1986). It has also been noted that the duration of nystagmus (McNally *et al.*, 1947) and the maximum slow-phase velocities (Coats and Smith, 1967) are greater in the face-up than face down positions. Coats and Smith have suggested that one component of caloric nystagmus was a direct thermal stimulation of the vestibular sensory epithelium and the ampullary nerve endings. Their explanation was that warming would increase neural discharge and would produce nystagmus towards the irrigated ear, regardless of body position. This would add to the convection effect in the face-up position, but would subtract from the convection effect in the face-down position. Further support for this hypothesis came from the re-interpretation of the Coats and Smith data by Hood (1989).

The Fitzgerald–Hallpike bithermal caloric test

Of the various test procedures available, the bithermal caloric test of Fitzgerald and Hallpike (1942) remains the best method of assessing the integrity of each labyrinth and its central nervous system connections. The subject lies supine on a couch with the head inclined at 30° to bring the horizontal canals into the vertical plane. Each ear is irrigated in turn for periods of 40 seconds with water at 7° below and then 7° above body temperature, i.e. at 30° and 44° respectively. A minimum of 5 minutes should be allowed between each irrigation to avoid cumulative effects. A severe caloric reaction may occasionally occur and in this situation, irrigation for a briefer period should be considered, e.g. if, after 20 seconds the patient becomes very distressed, the irrigation period should be limited to 30 seconds. It is important that before irrigation, otoscopy should be performed to exclude otitis externa, acute otitis media and perforations of the tympanic membrane – aural conditions which preclude water irrigation.

It is essential that the ears are correctly irrigated: the meatus should be free of any wax, it should be straightened and the water introduced with a flow-rate of betwen 350 and 500 ml/minute. After warm irrigation, the tympanic membrane should be inspected to check the presence of a red flush upon its surface.

Cold irrigations cause a slow deviation of the eyes towards the irrigated ear, with the fast saccadic phase directed away from the irrigated ear. The converse situation occurs for hot irrigations leading to the mnemonic 'cows': *c*old irrigation causing nystagmus to the *o*pposite side, *w*arm irrigation causing nystagmus directed towards the *s*ame side. (NB: if both meatus are irrigated simultaneously with cold water, under normal circumstances the effect within both horizontal semicircular canals is equal and self-cancelling; eventually, the cold water stimulates the vertical canals and causes a downward deflection of the eyes with an up-beating vertical nystagmus ('cud', *c*old-*u*pward nystagmus).

Direct observation of the eyes allows the end-point of the nystagmic reation to be measured. During the procedure the patient is asked to direct his gaze at a fixation point on the ceiling above his head, making the end point easier to determine, and then, by switching off the light and observing the eyes with Frenzel's glasses or an infrared viewer, the effect of removing optic fixation on the end-point of nystagmus can be measured. The endpoints of each test are graphically recorded (Figure 21.10).

Quantitative analysis

In a normal caloric response, nystagmus with fixation ceases between 90 and 140 seconds after the onset of the irrigation and returns for a further 30–60 seconds following the removal of optic fixation. Dysfunction gives rise to two characteristic patterns of response which may appear separately or in combination.

A complete loss of labyrinthine function in one ear is demonstrated by the total absence of nystagmus following both 30° and 44° irrigations even in the absence of optic fixation, i.e. canal areflexia or *canal paresis*. It should be confirmed that irrigation had been performed correctly and if so the test should be repeated using cold water at 20° for 60 seconds to ensure that there is indeed no reaction. A canal paresis is due to an ipsilateral lesion of the labyrinth, the vestibular nerve or the vestibular nuclei within the brain stem, and may be partial.

Directional preponderance occurs when the responses to the different thermal irrigations produce an excess of nystagmus in one direction, i.e. towards either the right or left. It typically occurs in association with a canal paresis (i.e. a combined pattern) with the direction of preponderance being towards the unaffected ear. It indicates an imbalance of tone arriving at the oculomotor nuclei resulting from an imbalance of vestibular tonus between the two halves of the vestibular system. Tonic discharges from a number of sources normally keep the two halves in equilibrium. Lesions of the labyrinth, the vestibular nerve, the vestibular nuclei, the cerebellum, or the corticofugal fibres deep in the temporal lobe will result in imbalance of tone between the vestibular inputs and hence give a directional preponderance. With more pronounced degrees of vestibular tone imbalance, spontaneous nystagmus appears (Figure 21.11).

Figures for duration of the nystagmic responses in seconds can be entered into Jongkees formula (Jongkees, Maas and Philipzoon, 1962) which allows calculation of a percentage figure expressing the degree of canal paresis or directional preponderance:

% canal paresis

$$= \frac{(R30° + R44°) - (L30° + L44°)}{(R30° + R44° + L30° + L44°)} \times 100$$

% directional preponderance

$$= \frac{(L30° + R44°) - (L44° + R30°)}{(L30° + R44° + L44° + R30°)} \times 100$$

The *optic fixation index* is calculated by dividing the summed durations in the light by the summed durations in the dark. When the caloric responses are prolonged with no enhancement in the absence of optic fixation, i.e. an optic fixation index of 1, the cause may be a lesion of the cerebellum or of the tracts which connect the cerebellum to the vestibular

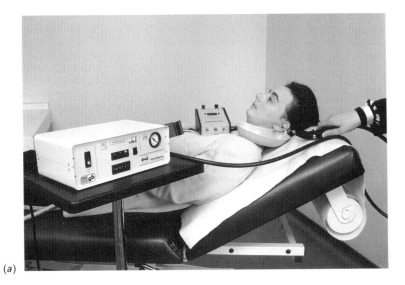

(a)

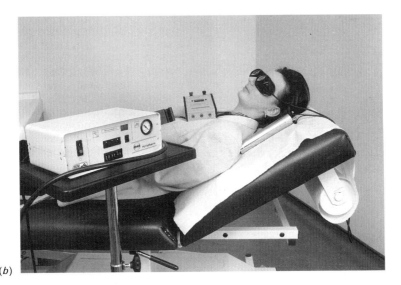

(b)

Figure 21.10 (a) Patient undergoing caloric testing. The patient's head is inclined at 30° to bring the horizontal canals into the vertical plane (see text for further details). (b) Use of Frenzel's glasses during caloric testing. The effect of removing optic fixation on the end-point of nystagmus duration can be observed in a darkenend room using Frenzel's glasses once nystagmus has disappeared with optic fixation

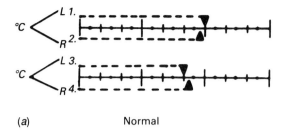

(a)   Normal

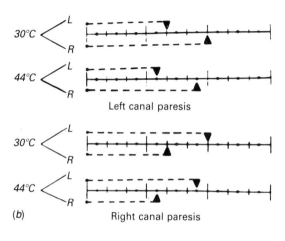

Left canal paresis

Right canal paresis

(b)

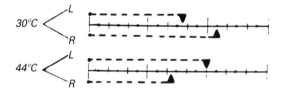

Directional preponderance to left

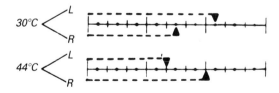

(c)   Directional preponderance to right

Figure 21.11 Caloric test abnormalities. (*a*) A graphic record of a set of normal responses to caloric irrigations as described in the text; (*b*) two sets of caloric responses recording a partial left and a partial right canal paresis, respectively; (*c*) two sets of caloric responses recording a left and a right directional preponderance, respectively

nuclei, or the corticofugal fibres deep in the temporal lobe (Hood and Korres, 1979).

Bilaterally decreased caloric responses may indicate bilateral vestibular impairment or may be the result of *vestibular habituation*. For example, professional acrobats, ice-skaters and ballet dancers, can suppress vestibular nystagmus following bodily rotation about the vertical axis provided that vision is unimpeded (Collins, 1966; Dix and Hood, 1969). Anxious patients with long-standing vestibular impairments may also learn to suppress their vestibular responses. It is thought that the instability of the eyes resulting from vestibular disorders will give rise to visual symptoms compounding dizziness and suppression of these eye movements has a valuable role in adaptation. The removal of optic fixation causes nystagmus of normal duration if the cause is vestibular habituation, i.e. with optic fixation indices of < 0.5.

Some patients with central vestibular disorders, i.e. cerebellar atrophy, may show no difference in caloric-induced nystagmus with or without optic fixation, i.e. they will have an optic fixation index of 1.0. When measured with fixation, the responses in these patients will appear hyperactive when compared with normal subjects.

ENG caloric recordings

There are both advantages and disadvantages associated with the use of ENG in caloric testing. It provides a permanent record of the caloric response in both light and dark, allowing individual features of the nystagmus, i.e. the slow component velocity, the interbeat frequency and the amplitude, to be analysed and stored for further reference. However, it is difficult to detect the endpoint of the nystagmus either with or without optic fixation, the eye detecting finer nystagmus beats than the ENG technology. Recording the caloric nystagmus with the eyes closed is compromised by Bell's phenomenon. Eye-closure causes an unpredictable ocular response, usually the eyes roll upwards, but often the eye deviates towards the side of the slow component and these movements inhibit nystagmus. It is recommended that caloric testing is performed with the eyes open in darkness. However, the subject must undergo a period of dark adaptation before recordings are taken, as the corneoretinal potential does not reach a constant figure for about 10 minutes. This requirement has disadvantages in a busy clinic. Hood and Korres (1979) provided a clear demonstration of how the caloric induced nystagmus is much enhanced by eye closure in the case of normal and peripheral lesions, but appreciably less so or even inhibited in the case of central lesions.

Other electronystagmographic measures of caloric nystagmus include the amplitude, the interbeat interval as well as the velocity of the slow or fast phase, which can all be calculated from the ENG printout.

Figure 21.12 shows the ENG tracing of a subject undergoing a warm caloric irrigation into the left ear, plus the plots of slow component velocity, slow component amplitude and beat frequency analysed by the digital computer. Each measurement shows beat-beat variability, but of the measurements performed, the slow phase velocity shows least variability.

Henriksson (1956) made a direct comparison of the maximum slow component velocity and the durations of the four caloric responses in 25 normal subjects. He found that whereas the durations were relatively stable, the slow component velocities in any one subject showed considerable variations. Hood (1977) also found that the test/retest unreliability of the slow component velocity was unacceptably high. Direct visual observation has the advantage that the endpoint of the nystagmus can be estimated more reliably both with and without optic fixation, and also, that abnormalities in the character of the nystagmus, such as rotatory movements or movements in the vertical plane can easily be detected. It does however rely on an experienced observer if the full value of the test is to be realized.

Closed circuit and air caloric testing

Several commercial systems allow warming and cooling of the water with closed irrigation systems.

The air caloric test has the advantages of not wetting the patient and also being applicable to patients with tympanic membrane perforations. There are two problems, however. First, the temperature of the air in the external meatus must be known accurately as air cools rapidly. This difficulty is overcome by modern technology as the air temperature can be accurately monitored at the probe tip. Second, the specific heat of air is much lower than that of water, which means that a greater temperature difference is needed to alter the temperature within the labyrinth by the same amount compared to water. Coats, Herbert and Atwood (1976) advised a flow rate of 13 l/min through a 3 mm probe tip. An air temperature of 45.5° corresponds to a water irrigation of 44°, and an air temperature of 17.5° corresponds to a water temperature of 30°, but the air irrigation must last 100 s compared with the 40 s of water irrigation. There are further difficulties as the amount of bone lying over the lateral canal varies between subjects. The other major disadvantage lies with the high cost of the equipment.

The hot caloric test

This is probably the best caloric screening test (Barber, Wright and DeManuele, 1971). If use is made of the optic fixation index, many of the abnormalities present on bithermal testing can be detected and the clinician can save valuable time. Mistakes may be made in long-standing cases of vestibular dysfunction. In this test only warm irrigation is performed.

Clinical value of caloric testing

Caloric testing is an essential part of the evaluation of the dizzy patient. It tests both labyrinths

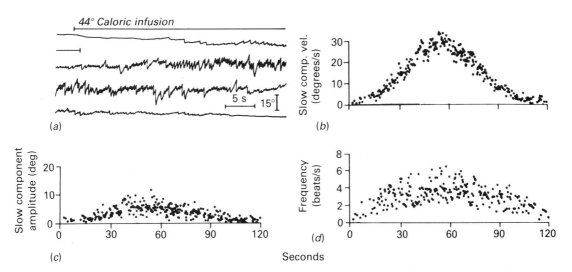

Figure 21.12 Caloric nystagmus parameters. (*a*) ENG tracings of a subject undergoing a warm caloric irrigation; (*b*) the plots of slow component velocity; (*c*) slow component amplitude; (*d*) beat to beat frequency versus time. (From Baloh and Honrubia, 1990; reproduced with permission from Professor Bob Baloh)

individually and does not require sophisticated instrumentation when water irrigation is used, and the difficulties in testing patients with perforated tympanic membranes has, in part, been overcome by introducing air irrigators.

The quantification and normal values of the measured parameters of the caloric-induced nystagmus have been well established. The calculation of relative values for induced nystagmus using Jongkees formula to identify percentage canal paresis and directional preponderance, minimize intersubject variability, due for example to variability of the heat transfer across the temporal bone. These help greatly in distinguishing normal from abnormal vestibular responses, helping both to lateralize the lesion and to localize it to either the peripheral or central nervous system.

Rotational testing

Principle of rotational testing

Vestibulo-ocular reflexes act during all natural head movements in life in coordination with visuo- and cervico-ocular reflexes, to provide the most appropriate eye position and eye stability during head movement. The vestibulo-ocular reflex specifically facilitates the stability of the eyes during head movements by driving compensatory eye movements in the direction opposite to head movement, in virtually the same range as that of the head.

In response to horizontal angular acceleratory/deceleratory forces, the two cupulae of the paired horizontal semicircular canals are deflected in the direction opposite to acceleration. The combined excitatory effect of utriculopetal deflection on one side and inhibitory effect of ampullofugal deflection on the other, results in slow conjugate, deviation of the eyes in the direction opposite to rotation (Figure 21.13).

If the range of angular acceleration of the head is so large that the eyes can no longer move in the opposite direction within the orbit because of soft tissue constraints, they are quickly brought back towards the midline by a corrective fast saccade, generating jerk nystagmus. This nystagmus is not seen in daily life with natural head movements because vision has a powerful suppressive effect on the vestibular nystagmus when the slow phase eye movement has a greater velocity than that of the smooth pursuit eye movement tracking the desired visual target. The nystagmus can be seen however by watching the eyes behind Frenzel's glasses or recording eye movements using ENG, during natural head movements. Rotating chairs have been developed to produce various forms of acceleratory/deceleratory movements of the head together with the body in a way whereby the strength of the stimulus can be closely controlled and the eye movement response can be measured.

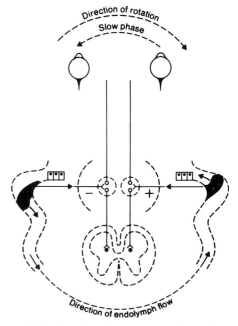

Figure 21.13 The effect of clockwise angular acceleration. There is utriculopetal deviation of the cupula of the right horizontal ampulla and an increase in the tonus of the corresponding ampullary nerve. In the left horizontal ampulla the cupula moves ampullofugally resulting in a decrease in the tonic activity of the corresponding nerve. (From Henriksson *et al.*, 1972; reproduced by permission of Dr Nils Henriksson)

Cupulometry

Much of our present knowledge of the vestibular system is based upon results of rotational testing. The slow component velocity of rotational-induced nystagmus should be proportional to the deviation of the cupula, which is in turn proportional to the intensity of stimulation.

Ewald, in 1892, established the relationship between the planes of the semicircular canals, the direction of endolymph flow and the direction of induced head and eye movements. He is credited with the observations that utriculopetal endolymph flow in the horizontal canal caused a greater reponse than ampullofugal flow, and the opposite for the vertical canals, i.e. ampullofugal flow caused a greater response than utriculopetal flow. Steinhausen (1931) and later Dohlman (1938), by injecting India ink into the semicircular canals of fish, visualized the movement of the cupula during endolymph flow. From the similarity between cupular movement and that of a pendulum in a viscous medium, Steinhausen proposed a model for the cupular kinematics known as the pendulum model (1931).

In 1907, Barany introduced an impulsive rotational test during which the chair, in which the patient was seated, was manually rotated 10 times in 20 seconds and then suddenly stopped with the patient facing the observer. The function of the horizontal canals was assessed by measuring the duration of the nystagmic response to clockwise and anticlockwise rotations and the preponderance of one over the other taken as evidence of vestibular pathology. Not only was the stimulus imprecise, but it produced such severe responses that the test did not gain general acceptance. Van Egmond, Groen and Jongkees (1948) devised a more scientific approach to impulsive rotational testing by slowly bringing the subject to different constant velocities, allowing a sufficient period of rotation for the cupula to return to its resting position, before abruptly bringing the patient to rest, monitoring the duration of the resultant vertigo and nystagmus. They introduced the term 'cupulogram' to describe the graphical representation of these responses. The cupula responds only to angular acceleration or deceleration and the period at constant rotation is necessary to allow the cupula to return to its rest position before the impulsive deceleration. For the range of impulses used, the duration of post-rotatory nystagmus was proportional to the log of the impulse intensity (Figure 21.14).

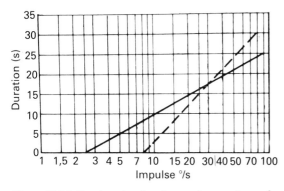

Figure 21.14 Cupulometry. Cupulogram for sensation and nystagmus derived from 50 normal subjects (see text for details). —— Normal average sensation cupulogram; – – – – normal average nystagmus cupulogram. (From Van Egmond, Groen and Jongkees (1948), reproduced by permission of *Journal of Laryngology and Otology*)

Further studies in patient populations with peripheral and central disorders using cupulometry revealed normal and pathological cupulometric patterns. The concepts of vestibular recruitment and hyperexcitability were also introduced (Van Egmond, Groen and Jongkees, 1948). However, cupulometry is time consuming, its responses extremely variable and impaired by habituation effects whereby each preceding stimulus exerts an effect upon the responses to subsequent stimuli, and has never become part of routine vestibular testing. Nonetheless, Barany's chair and cupulometry retain their importance, with contemporary techniques, which employ high precision rotary chairs, ENG and computational analyses, basing their design on the same elementary principles.

Stimulus response relationships

With modern rotating chairs, accelerational stimuli can be precisely controlled and responses accurately documented and analysed by computer. Three types of rotational stimuli are commonly applied. (In each situation, the subject is rotated in the plane of the horizontal semicircular canals with the eyes open in complete darkness while he is asked to perform continuous mental arithmetic to maintain mental alertness.)

Impulsive (or step-velocity) rotational stimuli

Constant velocities such as 40, 60, 80 and 120°/second are attained with an abrupt acceleration of the chair within 1 second to a constant velocity rotation for up to 2 minutes. The chair is suddenly brought to rest with the same rate of deceleration. Baloh and Honrubia (1979) established the normal limits of nystagmus intensity values. The induced nystagmus adapts and gradually disappears, the duration following the cupular time constant. A secondary nystagmus of lower intensity appears consistently following constant velocity values > 120°/s.

The main advantage of impulsive rotational testing is that it provides a rapid assessment of the gain (peak slow component velocity / change in chair velocity) and the time constant (time for the slow component velocity to fall to 37% of its initial value) of the canal reflex independently in each direction.

Sinusoidal rotational stimuli

These are achieved by to and fro swinging movements of the chair around its vertical axis with variable stimulus parameters – frequency, i.e. duration of each cycle, and amplitude. The commonest measure in use is the frequency 0.05 Hz. The amplitude can be adjusted to between 5° and 360°. The normal subjective threshold for the sensation of turning is about $0.5°/s^2$. The threshold for recordable nystagmus, defined as the angular acceleration, which maintained for 20 seconds will produce nystagmus, is $0.15°/s^2$ in the absence of optic fixation. With optic fixation, the nystagmus threshold is raised and is normally about $1°/s^2$.

Vestibulo-ocular reflex suppression with sinusoidal stimuli

Rotational testing is normally performed in darkness (i.e. without optic fixation) but sinusoidal rotation can also be performed with the eyes focused on a target, just in front of the eyes, which revolves with the patient, for the purpose of assessing vestibulo-ocular reflex suppression. This is an important test of central vestibular function as the visual suppression of the vestibulo-ocular reflex is mediated via cerebellar vestibular pathways, and at certain chair frequencies and velocities the vestibulo-ocular reflex is completely suppressed.

Trapezoidal stimulation

Angular acceleration is applied at different rates followed by a constant velocity for a period exceeding the cupular time constant. The rotation is then terminated either by the same deceleration as the initial acceleration or by sudden deceleration in one second (step velocity). 1, 2 and 4°/s² acceleration for 30 seconds is followed by 30°, 60° and 120°/s constant velocity for 2 or 3 minutes and then the rotation is brought to rest by an abrupt deceleration (Montandon, 1954). The tests are carried out consecutively in clockwise and couterclockwise stimulation (Figure 21.15).

A directional preponderance expressed as a percentage is analagous to that derived in caloric testing and can be calculated from the formula:

% Directional preponderance

$$= \frac{(\text{clockwise} - \text{counterclockwise})}{(\text{clockwise} + \text{counterclockwise})} \times 100$$

Greater than 20% asymmetry on this normalized difference formula is considered abnormal.

In subjects accustomed to rotational stimuli, such as ballet dancers and gymnasts, the threshold with optic fixation is higher, sometimes reaching 7°/s², but the nystagmus threshold in darkness remains normal, demonstrating that the mechanism for vestibular habituation in these subjects is due to an enhancement of the optic fixation mechanism. Sometimes a similar vestibular habituation is encountered on testing patients suffering from anxiety states.

Clinical relevance of rotary chair testing

Impulsive stimuli can be used to demonstrate a directional preponderance as determined by the ratio of the duration of nystagmus following the onset of acceleration to that following deceleration. A disadvantage of rotational testing is that both labyrinths are tested simultaneously and thus a unilateral dysfunction may be difficult to identify when the lesion is chronic and the patient has become well compensated. However, in unilateral vestibular dysfunction, an asymmetrical response to rotatory stimuli may be observed because of the difference in excitation and inhibition between utriculopetal and ampullofugal stimulation of the labyrinth. This asymmetry is most pronounced after high intensity stimuli, but is consistent only in identifying complete unilateral, peripheral, vestibular paralysis (Honrubia *et al.*, 1980).

Rotational testing is of particular value in certain

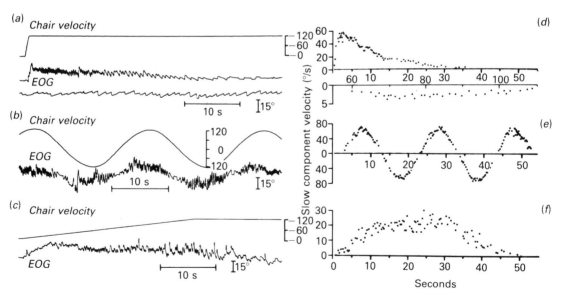

Figure 21.15 Types of rotating chair stimuli. On the left side of the figures, the nystagmic response (EOG) to three types of angular acceleration resulting in a maximum velocity of 120°/s is seen: (*a*) impulsive or step velocity stimulus (acceleration 140°/s²): (*b*) sinusoidal stimulus (at 0.005Hz): (*c*) constant acceleration stimulus (4°/s² for 30 s). On the right the slow velocity component of the nystagmic response to each of the three types of angular acceleration is seen. (From Baloh and Honrubia, 1990; with permission from Professor Bob Baloh)

situations. If the caloric test reveals no observable response, high frequency oscillation or high intensity acceleration may provide evidence of some *residual vestibular function*. Vestibular thresholds may be identified by applying minimal angular accelerations; it may therefore be possible to identify ototoxic damage, e.g. before total vestibular failure supervenes. Rotational testing allows the possibility of detecting unilateral *vestibular recruitment* (Matsuhira *et al.*, 1991). If recruitment is present, the directional preponderance would be greatest at the threshold of the affected ear and the asymmetry would lessen as the damaged end-organ displays recruitment. Rotational testing also permits the investigation of *visuovestibular interactions* (Baloh *et al.*, 1982). The failure to suppress the vestibulo-ocular reflex with fixation is evidence of central vestibular dysfunction.

One of the advantages of rotational testing is that the precise physical force applied to the labyrinths can be calculated. With computerized analysis of responses to rotary chair testing, results can be depicted in a quadrantic fashion following the sequence of start/stop stimuli in a clockwise, and then anticlockwise fashion. These displays include mathematical computation of directional preponderance using slow-phase velocity as well as durational criteria and the presence of 'background' second degree nystagmus can be identified (see below) (Figure 21.16).

Limitations of caloric and rotary chair tests

It should be emphasized that neither rotary chair tests nor caloric tests can distinguish between pathology of the end-organ and the vestibular nerve. A further limitation of both tests is that the function of the entire vestibule is not examined. In monaural caloric irrigation, only the ipsilateral horizontal canal, its ampullary nerve and its central connections are tested, while in binaural irrigation, only both sets of vertical canals, their ampullary nerves and central connections are tested (in the absence of caloric asymmetry of the horizontal canals). Caloric testing does not elicit responses from the utricle and saccule and rotary chair tests examine only the horizontal canals. Although, rotational tests with the head eccentric may elicit otolith responses, the value of this in clinical practice is uncertain (Barratt, Bronstein and Gresty, 1987) as the abnormalities can be readily detected clinically by the Hallpike manoeuvre.

Comparing the two test protocols, the rotary chair provides well-controlled vestibular stimulation closer to natural stimuli but, nonetheless, allows use of a wide variety of stimulus intensities and frequencies. Test–retest variability is considerably lower with rotary chair testing than with caloric tests, and the test is well tolerated with no unpleasant effects. In bilaterally reduced vestibular function rotary tests are more reliable than caloric tests but unilateral vestibular impairment may remain undetected with

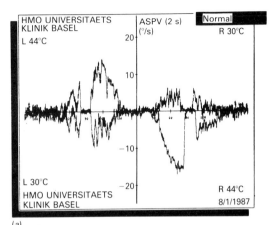

(a)

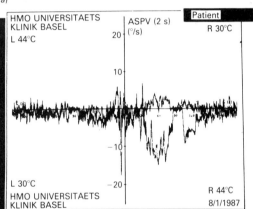

(b)

Figure 21.16 Four quadrant display of caloric nystagmus. Following consecutive irrigations of each ear at 30° and 44°C respectively on-line ENG analysis computes a four quadrant display of the average slow phase velocity (ASPV) over 2 s of the caloric induced nystagmus. Caloric testing is performed in darkness, but with a 10 s fixation period after 90 s. (*a*) The results in a normal subject; (*b*) the analysis of a patient with a left canal paresis. (From Toennies Computer-Assisted Diagnostic Systems, with permission of Professor Michael Allum, Basel, Switzerland and Jaeger Toennies, Wurzberg, Germany)

rotary chair testing if the lesion is well compensated. Central nervous system pathology is indicated in both test conditions by failure of vestibulo-ocular reflex suppression, and in caloric tests by perversion of the induced nystagmus.

Balance testing

It is well established that alterations in vestibular function may profoundly affect posture (Magnus, 1924). In animal experiments as early as 1892, Ewald was able to demonstrate the effect of vestibular stimulation on posture by rotating animals on a turn-table; when rotation ceased, the tendency of the animal to fall in the direction of rotation was counteracted by a reflex increase in extensor tone in the antigravity muscles of the limb on the side towards which the animal was falling, and a reduction in extensor tone in the contralateral limb, thereby allowing the animal to maintain its balance.

Similarly, in man, postural control is a vital physiological function if we are to continue any of our daily activities such as standing, sitting, walking or lying and remain well-balanced. Postural control is determined by a complex sensorimotor feedback system dependent on a variety of coordinated reflexes which include vestibular, proprioceptive and visual postural reflexes.

An understanding of the complexity of the organization of the vestibulospinal postural reflexes helps to illustrate why man's postural control system has been so difficult to probe. Until a decade ago assessment of the patient with loss of balance or falls, was essentially a clinical skill, as no controlled stimulus response measures were possible and no direct inference can be drawn between the state of the vision-stabilizing system (i.e. as assessed with tests of the vestibulo-ocular reflex) and the vestibulomodulated postural mechanisms.

The vestibulospinal postural reflexes

The vestibulospinal system plays an important role in maintaining upright bipedal posture within the gravitational field. Vestibulospinal tracts relay sensory information from the vestibular labyrinth (predominantly from the otolith organs) to the lateral vestibular nucleus on the floor of the IVth ventricle and from there to the spinal and lower extremity antigravity muscles. These antigravity muscles are the extensors of the neck, trunk and extremity muscles. It is of note that the vestibulospinal reflexes are mediated by a push-pull mechanism controlling the balance between the extensor and flexor skeletal muscles, similar to the mechanism controlling the extraocular muscles mediating the vestibulo-ocular reflexes.

The vestibular apparatus exerts an influence on the control of posture by way of the myotactic reflex (the deep tendon reflex), which is the elementary unit for control of tone in the trunk and extremity skeletal muscles. The myotactic reflexes of the antigravity muscles are under the combined excitatory and inhibitory influence of multiple supraspinal neural centres (Bard, 1961). In the cat, there are thought to be two main facilitatory centres (the lateral vestibular nucleus and the rostral reticular formation), and four inhibitory centres (frontal cortex, basal ganglia, cerebellum and caudal reticular formation), exerting influence on the myotactic reflex arc via the vestibulospinal and reticulospinal tracts, and the corticobulbar-reticular, caudatospinal, cerebelloreticular and reticulospinal tracts, respectively.

The balance of input from these different centres determines the degree of tone in the antigravity muscles, i.e. mid-brain section results in decerebrate rigidity by removing the inhibitory influence of the basal ganglia and the frontal cortex which results in hyperactive deep tendon reflexes in the extensor antigravity muscles; and unilateral labyrinthine destruction removes facilitatory tone leading to an ipsilateral loss of tone to such an extent that the ipsilateral vestibulospinal tract is considered to be the main excitatory input to the anterior horn cells (Fulton, Liddell and Rioch, 1930).

Thus the vestibulospinal reflex interacts with the spinal and supraspinal long-loop reflexes to allow for accurate adaptation to changes in bodily orientation in relation to gravity and to changes in the support surface as detected by ankle-joint and musculotendinous stretch receptors. Finally these reflexes are compared within the CNS against visual world motion to produce the most appropriate postural response under all combinations of body, visual surround and support-surface perturbation.

Complexity of the vestibulospinal reflexes

One of the main reasons for the neglect of the vestibulospinal system has been the difficulty of isolating the vestibulospinal reflex from the other afferent systems, i.e. the proprioceptive and visual postural reflexes.

The influence of vestibular activity on postural muscles is more difficult to define and less clearly understood than the vestibular control of eye movements (Anderson, Soechting and Terzuolo, 1979). This can be explained partly by the fact that the vestibular system is only one of many afferent inputs to a complex multisensory postural control system, and partly by the fact that vestibular activity produces postural change only after it has been processed and monitored in the light of other learned responses.

Furthermore, vestibular activity affects neck muscles in a different manner to that of the rest of the somatic musculature. Jones and Milsum (1965) have proposed that the vestibular-neck orientation system can be considered as a closed-loop, negative feedback control system, in contrast to the vestibular-limb/torso system where changes in vestibular activity cannot be used directly to detect error or deviations in limb position. Similarly, afferent fibres from the extraocular muscles appear to exert little or no direct effect on the oculomotor response and have no direct representation within the vestibular nuclei. Thus the oculomotor reflex is also essentially an open-loop system.

Clinical tests of the vestibulospinal system

Vestibulospinal function is assessed clinically by examination of stance and gait. These clinical tests of postural stability are relatively crude and demonstrate both low specificity and low sensitivity, i.e. they depend upon the normal functioning of a variety of sensory and motor systems as well as the vestibular system. Abnormal postural sway may be seen in vestibular, neurological, musculoskeletal and orthopaedic conditions and a patient may have considerable loss of peripheral vestibular function unilaterally without showing abnormalities on any of the following tests.

Nonetheless, in specific instances these tests make an invaluable contribution to the clinical assessment of patients with balance disorders and an understanding of the tests and their limitations is important if that contribution is to be fully realized.

Romberg test

Traditionally, the Romberg test (Romberg, 1846) has been used to assess postural stability. The subject stands feet together, hands by the side, first with the eyes open and then with eyes closed. A positive test is recorded if the patient demonstrates an increased sway or falls when the eyes are closed.

Romberg first described his test after he was impressed by the destabilizing effect of eye closure in patients with gross sensory ataxia due to tabes dorsalis. In these 'deafferented' patients the additional loss of the stabilizing sensory information provided by vision results in gross loss of balance.

Patients with vestibular disorders may fall or sway towards the side of the lesion. However instability may also be due to other sensory, motor or cerebellar causes and the localizing value of the Romberg test in subacute or chronic vestibular conditions is not always clear-cut. Patients with cerebellar lesions also tend to fall towards the pathological side but with little enhancement with eye closure. Patients with central disorders often sway in different directions on repeated testing. Patients with extrapyramidal disorders may fall forwards or backwards. Falling straight backwards like a wooden soldier suggests a non-organic disorder.

Unterberger's or stepping test

If the patient is stable on Romberg testing, further information can sometimes be gained by using the stepping test. This test was first described by Unterberger (1938) and later refined by Fukuda (1959). The test studies the tendency of vestibular stimulation or unilateral vestibular lesions to induce blindfolded subjects to turn in the earth's vertical axis when walking. The patient is asked to clasp the palms of both hands together and to stretch his arms out in front of him. He then is asked to step up and down on the same spot with his eyes closed. Visual and auditory directional cues should be minimized. The patient's angular deviation from his initial to his final position is taken as a measure of his vestibular imbalance. There is marked variability in the rotational angle from one subject to another and in the same subject on repeated testing.

Gait testing

In this test the patient is asked to walk a straight line quickly between two points 3–4 m apart, first with eyes open and then with eyes closed. Patients with unilateral vestibular lesions tend to deviate towards the affected side with eyes closed. Patients with bilateral vestibular failure (i.e. from streptomycin intoxication) may be able to walk relatively easily with their eyes open but become very unstable on eye-closure, and when asked to walk over a length of soft rubber mattress with eyes closed, will fall, being deprived of all reliable sensory information. These patients should be cautioned about walking over soft or uneven surfaces in the dark and warned not to swim underwater.

The sensitivity of gait testing can be increased by asking the patient to tandem walk, i.e. placing the heel of the leading foot directly in front of the toe of the other. When performed with eyes open, tandem gait is primarily a test of cerebellar function, because vision will compensate for a chronic vestibular or proprioceptive deficit. Tandem walking with the eyes closed provides a better test of vestibular function so long as proprioceptive and cerebellar functions are intact. Most normal subjects can make a minimum of 10 accurate tandem steps in three trials.

Gait testing can provide information about the many other systems which give rise to imbalance. Loss of proprioception, as seen in the dorsal column pathology of tabes dorsalis, and to a lesser extent in sensory neuropathy, results in a characteristic high-stepping, foot-slapping gait. A hemiplegic gait, with dragging of the leg and flexion of the affected arm, indicates pyramidal tract pathology such as is seen in patients following a stroke. The shuffling small-stepping gait of the parkinsonian patient, who walks with the head bowed and back bent, with little arm swing on the affected side is also characteristic. Midline cerebellar dysfunction tends to give rise to a broad-based, ataxic gait, while unilateral, cerebellar hemisphere pathology, like unilateral peripheral vestibular pathology, causes a tendency to veer to the affected side. The stiff painful gait of the patient with arthritis, or the waddle, i.e. rotation of the pelvis from side to side with every step, is seen in the patient with myopathy of the limb girdle muscles. A hysterical gait is recognized by bizarre features which do not conform to any specific organic disease pattern.

Biomechanics of balance

During normal standing, the body is in continuous motion, even when attempting to remain still. This is an active process whereby any loss of balance is compensated by movement of the body's *centre of gravity*. These movements result in visually detectable sway movements (i.e. physiological postural sway or spontaneous sway) which maintain the body's centre of gravity vertically over the base of support.

The state of a person's balance is best described in terms of angular displacement of the centre of gravity from the gravitational vertical. The centre of gravity sway angle is the angle between a vertical line projecting upwards from the centre of the area of foot support, and a second line projecting from the same point to the subject's centre of gravity (Figure 21.17).

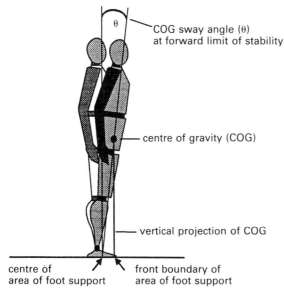

Figure 21.17 Centre of gravity, centre of gravity sway angle and stability limits (see text for further details). (Reproduced with permission from NeuroCom International Inc., USA)

The *limit of stability* is the maximal possible sway angle as a function of sway direction away from the centre position. It depends on the placement of the feet and the base of support. The limit of stability perimeter is best described as an ellipse of 12.5° from back to front. This tends to be the same for people of various heights as the height of the centre of gravity and the foot-length co-vary. The limit of stability also depends on the centre of gravity sway frequency, i.e. for the average adult, centre of gravity movements within the full range of the limit of stability are possible when sway oscillation lasts 2 to 3 seconds or more, but when the sway frequency is increased to 1 Hz the limit of stability contracts to approximately 3°.

The limits of spontaneous sway while standing still

(i.e. the periodic corrections to the centre of gravity which serve to overcome the destabilizing influence of gravity) depend on sensory conditions as well as the configuration of the base of support. The *limits of sway*, i.e. the sway envelope, are well within the limits of stability (Figure 21.18).

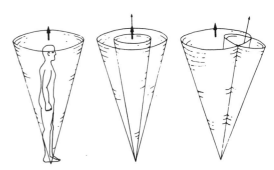

Figure 21.18 Relations between the limit of stability, sway envelope and centre of gravity alignment. The middle figure shows the centre of gravity alignment centred within the limit of stability. The right figure shows the centre of gravity aligned forward relative to the centre (see text for further details). (Reproduced with permission from NeuroCom International Inc., USA)

Centre of gravity alignment determines the maximum limit of sway such that if the centre of gravity is over the centre of the base of support, the limits of sway may be as large as the limits of stability.

Sensing the position of the centre of gravity relative to gravity and the base of support requires a combination of visual, vestibular and proprioceptive inputs. Vision measures the orientation of the eyes and head in relation to the surrounding objects. Proprioceptive information measures the orientation of the body parts relative to one another and to the support surface. The vestibular system measures gravitational, linear and angular acceleration of the head in relation to inertial space.

During situations of *sensory conflict*, i.e. when one or more of the senses provides information that is misleading or inaccurate, the brain must quickly select the sensory input providing accurate orienting information and ignore the misleading ones. The selection and integration of appropriate sensory information is called *sensory organization*.

Posturography

A simple method of measuring body sway was used by Sheldon (1963) in studying the effect of ageing on falls in the elderly. He used a method consisting of a pen attached to the forehead of a person standing comfortably with legs apart. The pen made a tracing on squared paper, and the number of squares covered by the tracing gave the amount of lateral sway. He showed that postural stability gradually became established before 20 years of age and remained at this level until a gradual deterioration began at the age of 40 years. Overstall *et al.* (1977), studying the liability of the elderly to fall, used Wright's ataxiometer to register anteroposterior sway movements, by a fine wire attached to a belt around the subject's waist, the wire operating a ratchet mechanism to document sway.

Static forceplate posturography

With forceplate technology, the use of so-called 'static' posturography has expanded Romberg's original concept by enabling examiners to acquire more quantitative measurement and analysis of the patient's postural sway (Kapteyn and de Wit, 1972; Jansen, Larsen and Olesen, 1982; Trieson *et al.*, 1982). The typical forceplate consists of a flat, rigid surface supported on three or more points by independent force measuring devices. As the patient stands on the forceplate surface, the vertical forces recorded by the measuring devices are used to calculate the position of the centre of the vertical forces exerted on the forceplate over time, providing an indirect measurement of postural sway. When the height and weight of the patient on the forceplate are known, a computer model of body dynamics can be used to derive the centre of gravity sway angle over time from the centre of vertical force movements.

The forceplate can also be used to measure the horizontal shear forces exerted by the patient's feet against the support surface. Horizontal shear forces measure the accelerations of the body's centre of gravity in the anteroposterior and lateral directions. These small accelerations increase dramatically as the frequency of centre of gravity motion increases, identifying the pattern of body motion being used to produce centre of gravity.

Forceplate posturography has confirmed the following observations (Nashner, 1973; Barigant, Merlet and Orfait, 1972):

1 The centre of gravity of the erect whole body mass plumbs to a point on the ground a few centimetres in front of the transverse ankle axis from a point in the centre pelvis immediately below the level of the umbilicus
2 Postural sway activity along the anteroposterior (*x*) axis is generally much more prominent than along the transverse body (*y*) axis because of the greater *x* axis instability of the ankle joint
3 Postural control is modulated by local regulation from spinal reflexes commanded by information from muscle spindle and tendon stretch receptors, and by extraspinal feedback from the visual and vestibular systems
4 Frequency analyses of oscillations on a moving

platform have shown that 1.5–2.5 Hz oscillations are increased by eye-closure, while slower oscillations (0.5–1 Hz) are decreased. The faster oscillations could be attenuated with the feet apart or by splinting the ankles, suggesting involvement of the ankle joint. On the other hand, slow oscillations were increased with the feet apart. Begbie (1967) has suggested that these slower oscillations are the result of reflexes generated by the vestibular system.

However, despite providing objective measurement of body sway and increasing the understanding of the biomechanics of balance, forceplate posturography has had limited clinical applications for the assessment of postural control. This is mainly because it does not allow for controlled stimulus-response measurements, i.e. it represents the equivalent of assessing the vestibulo-ocular reflex by monitoring eye position in the absence of vestibular stimulation.

Moving platform posturography

As balance is a complex process involving the integrated activity of multiple sensory and biomechanical components, it follows that to assess objectively any one component, the other components must be kept constant. Moving-force platforms have been designed to overcome the limitations of static force platforms by controlling the relative contributions of the visual, somatosensory and vestibular inputs that are normally used to maintain upright posture, and by incorporating stimulus response measurements.

Nashner and colleagues introduced the concept of computerized dynamic posturography (CDP) in the early 1980s with a prototype platform that measured sway using a hip-mounted potentiometer (Nashner, Black and Wall, 1982). From these early experiments, a commercially available apparatus was produced that calculated body sway based on changes in horizontally (shear) and vertically oriented (torque) strain guages mounted within the support surface (Equitest, NeuroCom, Inc., Clackamas, Oregon) (Figure 21.19). Both the support surface and a visual surround could be modulated in phase with the patient's own body sway, i.e. *sway-referencing*. This 'coupling' of either the platform or the visual surround to the sway of the subject allows the angle between the foot and lower leg to be maintained at a constant value, i.e. minimizing somatosensory input, and visual input to remain constant despite the subject's sway. Six conditions were developed where sway was analysed as the visual surround and support-surface conditions were altered – *sensory organization testing*.

The sensory organization testing component of computerized dynamic posturography exposes the standing patient to six sensory conditions of increasing difficulty. The conditions include all combinations of normal standing, standing with eyes closed, with the platform sway-referenced, and the vision sway-

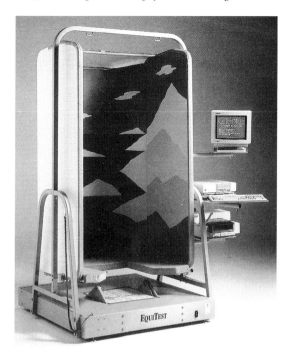

Figure 21.19 Equitest balance platform. Computerized dynamic posturography allows sway-referencing of both the support surface and the visual surround (see text for further details). (Reproduced with permission from NeuroCom International Inc., USA)

referenced. The purpose of testing is to isolate each of the three principal balance senses: vision, vestibular and somatosensory, and to determine the function of each and, by further comparisons, to assess the sensory preference of the individual (Figure 21.20).

The *movement coordination test* component of computerized dynamic posturography exposes the standing patient to a sequence of unexpected and brief displacements of the support surface. Displacements include backward, forward, toes up and toes down tilts. The latency and amplitude of reflex muscle contractions during these sudden unpredictable platform translation or rotations are quantified and the properties of patients reflex postural reactions to external challenges analysed.

The sensory organization testing and movement coordination test batteries address both the patient's ability to integrate visual, vestibular and somatosensory cues under varying degrees of sensory conflict and to react via the long-loop motor reflexes to support surface change.

Clinical relevance of posturography

Age-related changes

Various studies using forceplate posturography have demonstrated the degradation of postural stability that accompanies age (Sheldon, 1963; Corso, 1975; Black *et al.*, 1977) and the greater loss of postural stability resulting from vestibular loss in the elderly than in the young (Norre, Forrez and Beckers, 1987).

Wolfson *et al.* (1992), in a large computerized dynamic posturography study of balance in the elderly has shown a diminished capacity of the elderly to process conflicting sensory input as well as a narrowing of the limit of stability. This was thought to be a result of biomechanical or central processing changes rather than because of diminished sensory or vestibular input, and that impairment of balance was the result of age-related disease rather than an inevitable consequence of ageing.

Standardization of postural sway measures

Different investigators have used different measures of postural sway – sway area (Sheldon, 1963), sway frequency (Seliktar *et al.*, 1978), total sway path (Diener *et al.*, 1984; Taguchi and Tada, 1988), sway velocity (Taguchi and Tada, 1988), power spectral density (Diener *et al.*, 1984) and mean squared displacement (Black, 1982) – in part because different equipment has different sensitivities. While intra-subject reproducibility has been reported as good (Thyssen *et al.*, 1982), there may be a significant learning effect (Holliday and Fermie, 1979).

Strong evidence of reproducibility has been provided by the pre-and post-flight computerized dynamic posturography test results of the NASA astronauts (Paloski *et al.*, 1992), who demonstrated identical baseline and seven-day post-flight posturographic patterns.

Posturography as a diagnostic tool

Posturographic patterns using forceplate measurements are not well defined and have not been shown to be diagnostically useful for vestibular pathology. This is for reasons described above, i.e. the multisensory inputs for postural control cannot be individually tested with these systems, and hence the site of pathology cannot be detected.

However, these types of studies may have a role in differentiating basal ganglia disorders, cerebellar dysfunction and incipient ataxia: in cerebellar disorders, there is a peak in the frequency spectrum between 2 and 4 Hz, and in anterior lobe atrophy due to alcoholic cerebellar degeneration, an additional superimposed 3 Hz tremor has been recorded during anteroposterior sway oscillations (Dichgans *et al.*, 1976; Diener *et al.*, 1984). In patients with bilateral vestibular hypofunction, an increase in anteroposterior sway at 0.4 Hz has been recorded (Tokita, Maeda and Miyata, 1981) and Kapteyn and de Wit (1972) have suggested that a low frequency peak of 0.2 Hz is of vestibular origin.

Dynamic posturography has allowed other study paradigms to be tested, such as the effect of moving

SENSORY ANALYSIS

RATIO NAME	TEST CONDITIONS	RATIO PAIR	SIGNIFICANCE
SOM Somatosensory	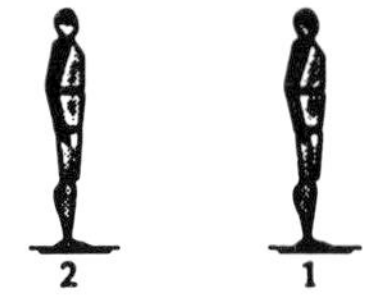 2 1	Condition 2 / Condition 1	**Question:** Does sway increase when visual cues are removed? **Low scores:** Patient makes poor use of somatosensory references.
VIS Visual	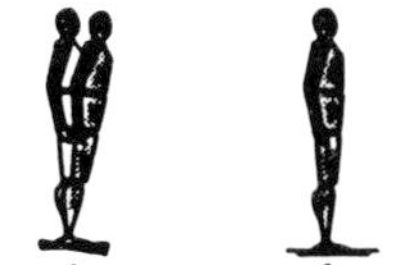 4 1	Condition 4 / Condition 1	**Question:** Does sway increase when somatosensory cues are inaccurate? **Low scores:** Patient makes poor use of visual references.
VEST Vestibular	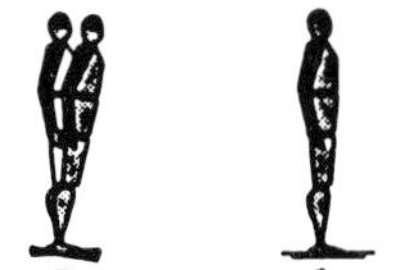 5 1	Condition 5 / Condition 1	**Question:** Does sway increase when visual cues are removed and somatosensory cues are inaccurate? **Low scores:** Patient makes poor use of vestibular cues, or vestibular cues unavailable.
PREF Visual Preference	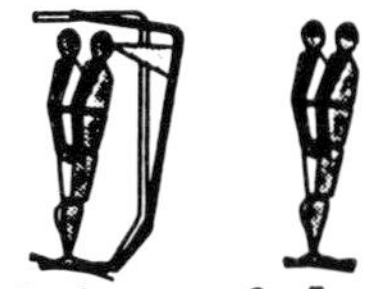 3 + 6 2 + 5	Condition 3 + 6 / Condition 2 + 5	**Question:** Do inaccurate visual cues result in increased sway compared to no visual cues? **Low scores:** Patient relies on visual cues even when they are inaccurate.

Figure 21.20 Sensory analysis. In the sensory analysis of computerized dynamic posturography, the six sensory conditions are compared in the manner shown to assess the sensory preference of the individual. (Reproduced with permission from NeuroCom International Inc., USA)

or stationary visual fields and platforms (Black and Nashner, 1984) giving more physiological and pathophysiological information.

It has been claimed that vestibular abnormalities could be detected earlier than with other vestibular tests (Kapteyn and de Wit, 1972) but more recent work has not supported this claim. For example, Voorhees (1989) obtained abnormal posturographic scores in only 45% of patients with peripheral vestibular disease and 72% of patients with central vestibular disease. Although by adding head extension and a more complex calculation involving sway energy, Jackson, Epstein and Boyete (1991) increased the sensitivity to 68%, posturography is probably redundant as a diagnostic tool.

Clinical use of computerized dynamic posturography and its role in vestibular rehabilitation

From computerized dynamic posturography studies of a variety of vestibular, brain stem, cerebellar and traumatic disorders, certain clinical patterns have emerged which tend to correlate with some disorders of balance rather than others (Goebel, 1992). The sensory organization test battery has identified abnormal patterns of postural control not adequately as-

sessed by studies of the vestibulo-ocular reflex alone. This was done by examining the utilization and integration of visual and somatosensory inputs with vestibular information, especially under conditions of sensory conflict.

This information is helpful in the development of individualized rehabilitation programmes, and use of computerized dynamic posturography in assessment of postural control strategies and as an outcome measure has been well reported (Norre and Forrez, 1986; Horak, Nashner and Diener, 1990; Shepard *et al.*, 1993). It remains to be seen whether generalized or customized rehabilitation programmes are more effective for some subgroups of patients.

Computerized dynamic posturography has been used to monitor the effects of vestibular neurectomy (Cass and Goshgarien, 1991) and orbital space flight (Paloski *et al.*, 1993) on postural stability. Both trials included serial computerized dynamic posturography measurements, including baseline, immediately post-perturbation and long-term posturography outcomes. In both studies, significant effects on balance as measured by computerized dynamic posturography were noticed in the short-term posturography measurements. These results demonstrate some of the research applications of computerized dynamic posturography, and the study on vestibular neurectomy patients suggests potential clinical applications.

Thus posturography should be considered as an additional quantitative measure of postural control mechanisms and not as a site of lesion test. Any pattern observed in isolation could be easily misinterpreted without knowledge of other physical findings, i.e. neurological disease, musculoskeletal deformity; test results (ENG, rotary chair, magnetic resonance imaging, CSF findings) and psychological factors. Nonetheless, it allows a functional view of the patient's balance disorder and may help in devising successful rehabilitation strategies to hasten recovery and maximize function in daily life.

Miscellaneous tests
Galvanic testing

Galvanic stimulation may be obtained by placing saline pads on the tragus, external ear canal, or over the mastoid, with a further electrode attached to the sternum. Stimulation can be bilateral or unilateral and the cathode is excitatory. At a threshold of 1–2 mA, in the dark, in healthy volunteers, the body sways away from the cathode and nystagmus is produced with the fast phase towards the cathode. Cessation of stimulation produces a reversed response, although this can be uncomfortable if sudden. Pfaltz (1969) described similar thresholds in most of his subjects with Menière's disorder, but absent responses with ipsilateral vestibular schwannoma. With body sway platforms, the normal threshold for detection of a response is 0.25–1 mA (Baron, 1978).

Galvanic stimulation of the vestibular system can cause vertigo and activate the vestibulo-ocular reflex. This has been used to differentiate between labyrinthine and retrolabyrinthine pathology (Pfaltz, 1969) as the response depends on the integrity of Scarpa's ganglion and the central vestibular connections (Huizinga, 1931; Dohlman, 1938). However, the thresholds are raised in vestibular neuronitis and long-standing Menière's disease, where it has been presumed the lesion is at the end-organ level (Dix and Hallpike, 1952).

The early difficulty with galvanic testing lay in the discomfort felt when the thresholds for nystagmus were raised to 7–10 mA. Moreover, electronystagmography may be complicated due to electrical artefacts, but the markedly lower currents required for posturographic sway measurements have overcome these shortcomings (Kapteyn and de Wit, 1972; Watanabe *et al.*, 1983).

Vestibular evoked responses

The recording of vestibular evoked responses is a research technique. It is not possible to record near-field vestibular neuronal responses non-invasively. Therefore evoked responses have been considered. The criteria necessary to record evoked responses include the need for the response to have resolved before the next stimulus is delivered, and sufficient stimulus-response data to have been collected to obtain a sufficiently high signal to noise ratio for a response to be recognized. The particular difficulties of recording vestibular evoked responses include the long time constants of the mechanics of the vestibular system and therefore the recording of vestibular evoked responses is complicated.

A further problem, which has complicated the interpretation of the results of previous studies (e.g. Greiner *et al.*, 1967; Salami *et al.*, 1975) is that the stimulus has to be refined to be specific to the vestibular end-organs and not involve cervical proprioceptive, visual or somatosensory receptors and the response itself can be contaminated by corneoretinal potentials. Hood and Kayan (1985) attempted to resolve the difficulties and determined an evoked response in subjects with vestibular function and none in subjects with absent vestibular function.

Sono-ocular test

This test, if positive, can localize the pathology to the vestibular end-organ.

The test is based on the Tullio phenomenon (Tullio, 1929). Classically, the Tullio phenomenon occurs if there is more than one mobile window on the vestibular side of the vestibular membrane and it was commonly noted in the days of fenestration operations. The phenomenon also occurs in other conditions such as congenital hearing loss, direct vestibular trauma, endolymphatic hydrops and after stapedectomy (Stephens and Ballam, 1974).

The sono-ocular test quantifies the Tullio phenomenon. Loud sounds are introduced into the ear (usually 2 pulses/s at 110 dBHL at frequencies between 500 and 4000 Hz, and at 120 dB at 250 Hz). Any resulting nystagmus is measured using electronystagmography.

The test can also be performed during posturography.

Judgement of visual vertical
(Friedmann, 1970)

There are various versions of this test. In one method, the subject is seated 2 m from a screen on which is projected an illuminated rod, 0.5 m in length, which he can rotate with a joystick. Initially he judges the horizontal and vertical with the lights switched on, and then he repeats the test several times in darkness.

Normal subjects can judge the horizontal and vertical with an error of less than 2°. Most patients with peripheral vestibular disorders can judge the horizontal and vertical within normal limits. Immediately after labyrinthectomy some patients misplace the vertical towards the side of the lesion. No abnormality can be detected in most patients with cerebellar and cortical lesions. Patients with large VIIIth nerve tumours which are compressing the brain stem and patients with brain stem lesions often deviate in their judgement of the vertical towards the side of the lesion.

The limitations of vestibular tests

A major disadvantage of all types of vestibular test is that the normative data are not universal, and the normative data have to be collected for each set of equipment before it can be used for clinical diagnosis. The equipment for rotational tests, posturography and evoked responses is expensive. Space and completely darkened rooms are required. The rotating chair and the target have to be properly set up. Trained personnel are required. Despite the reservations, the use of posturography and rotation testing is becoming more widespread (Honrubia *et al.*, 1980; Rubin, 1981). The main advantages are the access to hard copy data for more detailed analysis, to test the patient in different paradigms, for documentation purposes, to assist rehabilitation and to contribute to research.

References

ABEL, S. and BARBER, H. O. (1981) Measurement of optokinetic nystagmus for otoneurological diagnosis. *Annals of Otorhinolaryngology*, **90**, 1–12

AGATE, J. (1963) *The Practice of Geriatrics*. London; Heinemann. p. 91

AJODHIA, J. M. and DIX, M. R. (1975) Ototoxic effects of drugs. *Minerva Otorhinolaringologica*, **25**, 117–131

ANDERSON, J. H., SOECHTING, J. F. and TERZUOLO, C. A. (1979) Role of vestibular inputs in the organization of motor output to the forelimb extensors. *Progress in Brain Research*, **50**, 582–596

ARNOTT, F. J. and MILLER, S. J. H. (1970) Seesaw nystagmus. *Transactions of the Ophthalmological Society of the UK*, **84**, 251–257

BALOH, R. W. and HONRUBIA, V. (1979) *Clinical Neurophysiology of the Vestibular System*. Philadelphia: F. A. Davis Company

BALOH, R. W. and HONRUBIA, V. (eds) (1990) *Clinical Neurophysiology of the Vestibular System*. Philadelphia: F. A. Davis Company

BALOH, R. W., HONRUBIA, V. and KONRAD, H. R. (1976) Periodic alternating nystagmus. *Brain*, **99**, 11–26

BALOH, R. W., HONRUBIA, V. and SILLS, A. (1977) Eye tracking and optokinetic nystagmus: results of quantitative testing in patients with well-defined nervous system lesions. *Annals of Otology, Rhinology and Laryngology*, **86**, 108–114

BALOH, R. W., KONRAD, H. R. and HONRUBIA, V. (1975) Vestibulo-ocular function in patients with cerebellar atrophy. *Neurology*, **25**, 160–168

BALOH, R. W., YEE, R. D., HONRUBIA, V. and JACOBSON, K.
(1988) A comparison of the dynamics of horizontal and vertical smooth pursuit in normal human subjects. *Aviation Space and Environmental Medicine*, **59**, 121–124

BALOH, R. W., YEE, R. D., JENKINS, H. A. and HONRUBIA, V. (1982) Quantitative assessment of visual-vestibular interaction using sinusoidal rotatory stimuli. In: *Nystagmus and Vertigo: Clinical Approaches to the Patient with Dizziness*, edited by V. Honrubia and M. A. B. Brazier. New York: Academic Press. pp. 231–239

BARANY, R. VON (1906) Untersuchungen uber den vom Vestibularapparat des Ohres reflektorisch ausgelosten rhythmischen Nystagmus und seine Begleiterscheinungen. *Monatschrift für Ohrenheilkunde*, **40**, 193–297

BARANY, R. VON (1907) Die Untersuchungen der reflektorischen vestibularen und optischen Augenbewegungen und ihre Bedeutung fur die topische Diagnostik der Augenmuskellahmungen. *Munchener medizinische Wochenschrift*, **54**, 1072–1074, 1132–1135

BARANY, R. VON (1921) Diagnose von Krankheitser-scheinungen im Bereiche des Otolithenapparates. *Acta Otolaryngologica*, **2**, 434–437

BARANY, R. VON (1922) Zur Klinik und Theorie des Eisenbahn-nystagmus. *Acta Otolaryngologica*, **3**, 260–265

BARBER, H. O. (1964) Positional nystagmus, especially after head injury. *Laryngoscope*, **74**, 891–894

BARBER, H. O., WRIGHT, C. W. and DEMANUELE, F. (1971) The hot caloric test as a clinical device. *Archives of Otolaryngology*, **94**, 335–337

BARD, P. (ed.) (1961) Postural coordination and locomotion and their central control. In: *Medical Physiology*, 11th edn. St Louis: C. V. Mosby

BARIGANT, P., MERLET, P. and ORFAIT, J. (1972) New design of ELA statokinestiometer. *Aggressologie*, **13C**, 69–74

BARNES, G. R. (1979) Vestibulo-ocular function during coordinated head and eye movements to acquire visual targets. *Journal of Physiology*, **287**, 127–147

BARON, J. B. (1978) Statokinesimetrie. *Les Feuillets du practicien*, **45**, 1246–1253

BARRATT, H., BRONSTEIN, A. M. and GRESTY, M. A. (1987) Testing the vestibular-ocular reflexes: abnormalities of the otolith contribution in patients with neuro-otological disease. *Journal of Neurology, Neurosurgery and Neuropsychiatry*, **50**, 1029–1035

BARRE, J. A. (1926) Sur un syndrome sympathique cervical posterieur et sa cause frequente: l'arthrite cervicale. *Revue de Neurologie*, **45**, 1246–1253

BAUMGARTEN, R. VON, BENSON, A. and BERTHOZ, A (1984) Effects of rectilinear acceleration and optokinetic and caloric stimulations in space. *Science*, **225**, 208–212

BEGBIE, G. H. (1967) Some problems of postural sway. In: *Myotactic Kinesthetic and Vestibular Mechanisms*, edited by A. V. S. de Reuck and J. Knight. Boston: Little Brown & Co. pp. 80–92

BELAL, A. and GLORIG, A. (1986) Disequilibrium of aging (presbyastasis). *Journal of Laryngology and Otology*, **100**, 1037–1041

BENDER, M. B. (1965) Oscillopsia. *Archives of Neurology*, **13**, 204–213

BENSON, A. J. and BURCHARD, E. (1973) Spatial disorientation in flight. *NATO AGARD-AG*, **170**

BLACK, F. O. (1982) Vestibular function assessment in patients with Meniere's disease: the vestibulo-spinal system. *Laryngoscope*, **92**, 1419–1435

BLACK, F. O. and NASHNER, L. M. (1984) Vestibulospinal control differs in patients with reduced versus distorted vestibular function. *Acta Otolaryngologica Supplementum*, **404**, 110–114

BLACK, F. O., O'LEARY, D. P., WALL, C. and FURMAN, J. (1977) The vestibulo-spinal stability test: normal limits. *Transamerican Academy of Ophthalmology and Otolaryngology*, **84**, 549–560

BOGOUSSLAVSKY, J., REGLI, F. and HUNBERBUHLER, J. P. (1980) Downbeat nystagmus. *Neuro-ophthalmology*, **1**, 137–143

BRANDT, T. and DAROFF, R. B. (1980) The multisensory physiological and pathological vertigo syndromes. *Annals of Neurology*, **7**, 195–203

BRONSTEIN, A. M. and HOOD, J. D. (1986) The cervico-ocular reflex in normal subjects and patients with absent vestibular function. *Brain Research*, **373**, 399–408

BRONSTEIN, A. M. and KENNARD, C. (1987) Predictive eye saccades are different from visually triggered saccades. *Vision Research*, **27**, 517–520

BUETTNER, U., BUETTNER–ENNEVER, J. A. and HENN, V. (1977) Vertical eye movements related to unit activity in the rostral mesencephalic reticular formation of the alert monkey. *Brain Research*, **130**, 234–252

CAMPBELL, A. J., REINKEN, J., ALLAN, B. C. and MARTINEZ, G. S. (1981) Falls in old age: a study of frequency and related clinical factors. *Age and Ageing*, **10**, 264–270

CASS, S. P. and GOSHGARIAN, H. G. (1991) Vestibular compensation after labyrinthectomy and vestibular neurectomy in cats. *Otolaryngology – Head and Neck Surgery*, **104**, 14–19

CAWTHORNE, T. E. (1952) Vertigo. *British Medical Journal*, **2**, 931–933

COATS, A. C. and SMITH Y. (1967) Body position and the intensity of caloric nystagmus. *Acta Otolaryngologica*, **63**, 515–532

COATS, A. C., HERBERT, F. and ATWOOD, G. R. (1976) The air caloric test. A parametric study. *Archives of Otolaryngology*, **102**, 343–354

COGAN, D. G. (1956) *Neurology of the Ocular Muscles*. Springfield: Charles C. Thomas

COGAN, D. G. and BURROWS, L. J. (1954) Platybasia and the Arnold-Chiari malformation. *Archives of Ophthalmology*, **52**, 13–29

COGAN, D. G., KUBIK, C. S. and SMITH, W. L. (1950) Unilateral internuclear ophthalmoplegia: report on 8 clinical cases with post-mortem study. *Archives of Ophthalmology*, **44**, 783–796

COHEN, B. and HENN, V. (1972) Unit activity of the pontine reticular formation associated with eye movements. *Brain Research*, **46**, 403–410

COLLEWIJN, H. F., VAN DER MARK, F. and JANSEN, T. C. (1975) Precise recording of human eye movements. *Vision Research*, **15**, 447–450

COLLINS, W. E. (1966) Vestibular responses from figure skaters. *Aerospace Medicine*, **37**, 1098–1104

COLLINS, W. E. (1974a) Arousal and vestibular habituation. In: *Handbook of Sensory Physiology: The Vestibular System*, edited by H. H. Kornhuber. New York: Springer-Verlag. Vol. VI, pp. 361–368

COLLINS, W. E. (1974b) Habituation of vestibular responses with and without visual stimulation. In: *Handbook of Sensory Physiology: The Vestibular System*, edited by H. H. Kornhuber. New York: Springer-Verlag. Vol. VI, pp. 369–388

CORSO, J. F. (1975) Sensory processes in man during maturity and senescence. In: *Neurobiology of Ageing: An Interdisciplinary Life-span Approach*, edited by J. M. Ordy and K. R. Brizzee. New York: Plenum Press. pp. 119–145

CURRIE, S., HEATHFIELD, K. W. G., HENSON, R. A. and SCOTT, D. F. (1971) Clinical course and prognosis of temporal lobe epilepsy. *Brain*, **94**, 173–190

DE JONG, P. I. V. M., DE JONG, J. M. V. B., COHEN, B. and JONGKEES, L. B. W. (1977) Ataxia and nystagmus induced by injection of local anaesthetic in the neck. *Annals of Neurology*, **1**, 240–246

DEMER, J. L. (1985) Hypothetical mechanisms of head-shaking nystagmus (HSN) in man: asymmetrical velocity storage. *Society of Neuroscience, Abstracts*, **11**, 1038

DICHGANS, J., MAURITZ, K. H., ALLUM, J. H. J. and BRANDT, T. (1976) Postural sway in normals and ataxic patients: stabilising and destabilising effects of vision. *Aggressology*, **17**, 15–24

DIENER, H. C., DICHGANS, J., BACHER, M. and GOMPF, B. (1984) Quantification of postural sway in normals and patients with cerebellar diseases. *Electroencephalography and Clinical Neurophysiology*, **57**, 134–142

DIETERICH, M., BRANDT, T. and FRIES, W. (1989) Otolith function in man: results from a case of otolith Tullio phenomenon. *Brain*, **112**, 1377–1392

DIX, M. R. and HALLPIKE, C. S. (1952) The pathology, symptomatology, and diagnosis in certain disorders of the vestibular system. *Proceedings of the Royal Society of Medicine*, **45**, 341–354

DIX, M. R. and HALLPIKE, C. S. (1966) Observations on the clinical features and neurological mechanisms of spontaneous nystagmus resulting from unilateral neurofibromata. *Acta Otolaryngologica*, **61**, 1–22

DIX, M. R., HARRISON, M. J. G. and LEWIS, P. D. (1971) Progressive supranuclear palsy (the Steele Richardson–Olszewski syndrome): a report of 9 cases with particular reference to the mechanism of the oculomotor disorder. *Journal of Neurological Sciences*, **13**, 237–256

DIX, M. R. and HOOD, J. D. (1969) Observations upon the nervous mechanism of vestibular habituation. *Acta Otolaryngologica*, **67**, 310–381

DIX, M. R. and HOOD, J. D. (eds) (1984) *Vertigo*. Chichester: Wiley

DODGE, R. (1903) Five types of eye movements in the horizontal meridian plane of the field of regard. *American Journal of Physiology*, **8**, 307–329

DOHLMAN, G. (1938) On the mechanism of transmission into nystagmus on stimulation of the semicircular canals. *Acta Otolaryngologica*, **26**, 425–442

DONIN, J. F. (1967) Acquired monocular nystagmus in children. *Canadian Journal of Ophthalmology*, **2**, 212–215

DRACHMAN, D. A. and HART, C. (1972) An approach to the dizzy patient. *Neurology*, **22**, 323–334

DROLLER, H. and PEMBERTON, J. (1953) Vertigo in a random sample of elderly people living in their homes. *Journal of Laryngology and Otology*, **67**, 689–695

EPLEY, J. M. (1980) New dimensions of benign paroxysmal positional vertigo. *Otolaryngology – Head and Neck Surgery*, **88**, 599–605

EWALD, J. R. (1892) *Physiologische Untersuchungen uber das Endorgan des Nervus Octavus*. Wiesbaden: Bergmann

FERNANDEZ, C. A. R., ALZATE, R. and LINDSAY, J. R. (1959) Experimental observations on positional nystagmus in the cat. *Annals of Otology, Rhinology and Laryngology*, **68**, 816–829

FETTER, M., ZEE, D. S., KOENIG, E. and DICHGANS, J. (1990) Head-shaking nystagmus during vestibular compensation in humans and Rhesus monkeys. *Acta Otolaryngologica*, **110**, 175–181

FISHER, A., GRESTY, M. A., CHAMBERS, B. and RUDGE, P. (1983) Primary position upbeating nystagmus. *Brain*, 106, 949–964

FISCHER, C. M. (1967) Some neuro-otological observations. *Journal of Neurology, Neurosurgery and Neuropsychiatry*, 30, 383–392

FITZGERALD, G. and HALLPIKE, C. S. (1942) Studies in human vestibular function: 1. Observations on the directional preponderance ('Nystagmusbereitschaft') of caloric nystagmus resulting from cerebral lesions. *Brain*, 65, 115–137

FRIEDMANN, G. (1970) The judgement of visual vertical and horizontal with peripheral and central vestibular lesions. *Brain*, 93, 313–328

FULTON, J. F., LIDDELL, E. G. T. and RIOCH, D. M. (1930) The influence of unilateral destruction of the vestibular nuclei upon posture and the knee jerk. *Brain*, 53, 327–343

FUKUDA, T. (1959) Vertical writing with eyes covered: a new test of vestibulospinal reaction. *Acta Otolaryngologica*, 50, 26

FURMAN, J. and WALL, C. (1990) Vestibular function in periodic alternating nystagmus. *Brain*, 1425–1439

GACEK, R. (1978) Further observations of posterior ampullary nerve transection for positional vertigo. *Annals of Otology, Rhinology and Laryngology*, 87, 300–305

GIBSON, M. J., ANDRES, R. O., ISAACS, B., RADEBURGH, T. and WORM–PETERSEN, J. (1987) The prevention of falls in later life. *Danish Medical Bulletin*, 34 (suppl. 4), 1–24

GOEBEL, H. H., KOMATSUZAKI, A., BENDER, M. B. and COHEN, B. (1971) Lesions of the pontine tegmentum and conjugate gaze paralysis. *Archives of Neurology*, 24, 431–440

GOEBEL, J. A. (1992) Contemporary diagnostic update: clinical utility of computerized oculomotor and posture testing. *Americal Journal of Otology*, 13, 591–597

GOODHILL, V. (1981) Ben H. Senturia lecture. Leaking labyrinth lesions, deafness, tinnitus and dizziness. *Annals of Otorhinology and Laryngology*, 90, 99–106

GREINER, G. F., COLLARD, M., CONRAUX, C., PICART, P. and ROHMER, F. (1967) Recherche des potentials évoqués d'origine vestibulaire chez l'homme. *Acta Otolaryngologica*, 63, 320–329

GRESTY, M. A., TRINDER, E. and LEECH, J. (1976) Perception of everyday visual environments during saccadic eye movements. *Aviation Space and Environmental Medicine*, 47, 991–992

HAIN, T. C., FETTER, M. and ZEE, D. S. (1987) Head-shaking nystagmus in patients with unilateral peripheral vestibular lesions. *American Journal of Otolaryngology*, 8, 36–47

HALL, S. F., RUBY, R. R. F. and MCCLURE, J. A. (1979) The mechanics of benign paroxysmal vertigo. *Journal of Otolaryngology*, 8, 151–158

HALLPIKE, C. S. (1967) Some types of ocular nystagmus and their neurological mechanisms. *Proceedings of the Royal Society of Medicine*, 60, 1–12

HALMAGYI, G. M., GRESTY, M. A. and GIBSON, W. P. R. (1979) Ocular tilt reaction with peripheral vestibular lesion. *Annals of Neurology*, 6, 80–83

HALMAGYI, G. M., GRESTY, M. A. and LEECH, J. (1980) Reversed optokinetic nystagmus, mechanism and clinical significance. *Annals of Neurology*, 7, 429–435

HARRISON, M. S. and OZSAHINOGLU, C. (1972) Positional vertigo: aetiology and clinical significance. *Brain*, 95, 369–372

HEALY, G. B., STRONG, M. S. and SAMPOGNA, D. (1974) Ataxia, vertigo, and hearing loss. A result of rupture of the inner ear window. *Archives of Otolaryngology*, 100, 130–135

HENRIKSSON, N. G. (1956) Speed of the slow component and duration in caloric nystagmus. *Acta Otolaryngologica*, Suppl. 125, 1–29

HENRIKSSON, N. G., HINDFELT, B., PYYKKO, I. and SCHALEN, L. (1981) Rapid eye movements reflecting neurological disorders. *Clinical Otolaryngology*, 6, 111–119

HENRIKSSON, N. G., PFALTZ, C. R., TOROK, N. and RUBIN, W. (1972) In: *A Synopsis of the Vestibular System*. The Barany Society

HOLLIDAY, P. J. and FERMIE, G. R. (1979) Changes in measurement of postural sway resulting from repeated testing. *Aggressologie*, 20, 225–228

HONRUBIA, V., BALOH, R. W., YEE, R. D. and JENKINS, H. A. (1980) Identification of the location of vestibular lesions on the basis of vestibulo-ocular reflex measurements. *American Journal of Otolaryngology*, 1, 291–301

HOOD, J. D. (1967) Observations upon the neurological mechanism of optokinetic nystagmus with special reference to the contribution of peripheral vision. *Acta Otolaryngologica*, 63, 208–215

HOOD, J. D. (1968) Electronystagmography. *Journal of Laryngology and Otology*, 82, 167–183

HOOD, J. D. (1977) Whither vestibular tests? *Proceedings of the Royal Society of Medicine*, 70, 675–676

HOOD, J. D. (1989) Evidence of direct thermal action upon the vestibular receptors in the caloric test. *Acta Otolaryngologica*, 107, 161–165

HOOD, J. D. and KAYAN, A. (1985) Observations upon the evoked responses to natural vestibular stimulation. *Electroencephalography and Clinical Neurophysiology*, 62, 266–276

HOOD, J. D. and KORRES, S. (1979) Vestibular suppression in peripheral and central vestibular disorders of the brain. *Brain*, 102, 785–804

HOOD, J. D. and LEECH, J. (1974) The significance of peripheral vision in the perception of movement. *Acta Otolaryngologica*, 77, 72–79

HOOD, J. D., KAYAN, A. and LEECH, J. (1973) Rebound nystagmus. *Brain*, 96, 507–526

HORAK, F. B., NASHNER, L. M. and DIENER, H. C. (1990) Postural strategies associated with somatosensory and vestibular loss. *Experimental Brain Research*, 82, 167–177

HOYT, W. F. and DAROFF, F. R. B. (1971) Supranuclear disorders of ocular control in man. In: *The Control of Eye Movements*, edited by P. Bach-Y-Rita, C. C. Collins and J. E. Hyde. New York: Academic Press. pp. 175–263

HUIZINGA, E. (1931) De la reaction galvanique de l'appareil vestibulaire. *Acta Otolaryngologica*, 15, 451–468

INGELSTEDT, S., IVARSSON, A. and TJERNSTROM, O. (1974) Vertigo due to relative overpressure in the middle ear. *Acta Otolaryngologica*, 78, 1–14

JACKSON, R. T., EPSTEIN, C. M. and BOYETE, J. E. (1991) Enhancement of posturography testing with head tilt and energy measurements. *American Journal of Otology*, 12, 420–425

JANSEN, C., LARSEN, R. E. and OLESON, M. B. (1982) Quantitative Romberg's test. *Acta Neurologica Scandinavica*, 66, 93–99

JONES, G. M. (1957) A study of current problems associated with disorientation in man-controlled flight. *Flying Personnel Research Committee Report*, no. 1006. London: Air Ministry

JONES, G. M. and MILSUM, J. H. (1965) Spatial and dynamic aspects of visual fixation. *IEEE Transactions on Biomedical Engineering*, 12, 54–62

JONGKEES, L. B. W., MAAS, J. P. M. and PHILIPZOON, A. J. (1962) Clinical nystagmography. *Practica Otolaryngologica*, **24**, 65–93

KAMEI, T., KIMURA, K., KANEKO, H. and NORO, K. (1964) Revaluation of the head-shaking test as a method of nystagmus provocation. Part 1. Its nystagmus eliciting effect. *Japanese Journal of Otolaryngology*, **67**, 1530–1534

KAPTEYN, T. S. and DE WIT, G. (1972) Posturography as an auxiliary in vestibular investigations. *Acta Otolaryngologica*, **73**, 104–111

KEANE, J. R. (1974) Periodic alternating nystagmus with downbeating nystagmus: a clinical anatomical case study of multiple sclerosis. *Archives of Neurology*, **30**, 399–402

KELLER, E. L. (1974) Participation of median pontine reticular formation in eye movement generation in monkey. *Journal of Neurophysiology*, **37**, 316–332

KOMPFE, D., PASIK, T., PASIK, P. and BENDER, M. B. (1979) Downward gaze in monkeys: stimulation and lesion studies. *Brain*, **102**, 527–558

KORRES, S. (1978) Electronystagmographic criteria in neuro-otological diagnosis. 2: Central nervous system lesions. *Journal of Neurology, Neurosurgery and Psychiatry*, **41**, 254–264

LEECH, J., GRESTY, M., HESS, K. and RUDGE, P. (1977) Gaze failure, drifting eye movements, and centripetal nystagmus in cerebellar disease. *British Journal of Ophthalmology*, **61**, 774–782

LUDMAN, H. (1979) Vestibular function. In: *Diseases of the Ear*, 4th edn, edited by S. R. Mawson and H. Ludman. London: Edward Arnold. p. 195

LUNDGREN, G. E. C. (1973) On alternobaric vertigo – epidemiological aspects. *Forsvarsmedicin*, **9**, 406–409

LUNDGREN, G. E.`C. and MALM, L. U. (1966) Alternobaric vertigo among pilots. *Aerospace Medicine*, **37**, 178–180

LYNCH, J. C. and MCLAREN, J. W. (1983) Optokinetic nystagmus deficits following parieto-occipital cortex lesions in monkeys. *Experimental Brain Research*, **49**, 125–130

MCCLURE, J. A. (1985) Horizontal canal BPV. *Journal of Otolaryngology*, **14**, 30–35

MCCLURE, J. A. (1986) Vertigo and imbalance in the elderly. *Journal of Otolaryngology*, **15**, 248–252

MCNALLY, W. J., STUART, E. A., JAMIESON, J. S. and GAULTON, G. (1947) Some experiments with caloric stimulation of the human labyrinth to study the relative values of ampullopetal and ampullo-fugal endolymphatic flow (Ewald's laws). *Transactions of the American Academy of Ophthalmology and Otolaryngology*, **52**, 513–541

MAGNUS, R. (1924) *Korperstellung*. Berlin: Springer

MARKS, I. M. (1981) Space 'phobia': a pseudo-agoraphobic syndrome. *Journal of Neurology, Neurosurgery and Neuropsychiatry*, **44**, 387–391

MATSUHIRA, T., YAMASHITA, K., YASUDA, M. and OHKUBO, J. (1991) Detection of the unilateral vestibular recruitment phenomenon using the rotation test. *Acta Otolaryngologica*, Suppl. 481, 486–489

MAY, J. G., KELLER, E. L. and SUZUKI, D. A. (1988) Smooth-pursuit eye movement deficits with chemical lesions in the dorsolateral pontine nucleus of the monkey. *Journal of Neurophysiology*, **59**, 952–977

MELVILLE JONES, G. (1964) Predominance of anti-compensatory oculomotor response during rapid head rotation. *Aerospace Medicine*, **35**, 965–968

MERICA, F. W. (1942) Vertigo due to obstruction of the Eustachian tubes. *Journal of the American Medical Association*, **118**, 1282–1284

MONEY, K. E. and MYLES, W. S. (1974) Heavy water nystagmus and effects of alcohol. *Nature*, **247**, 404–405

MONEY, K. E., JOHNSON, W. H. and CARLETT, B. A. (1970) Role of semicircular canals in positional alcohol nystagmus. *American Journal of Physiology*, **208**, 1065–1070

MONTANDON, A. (1954) A new technique for vestibular investigation. *Acta Otolaryngologica*, **44**, 594–596

MORROW, M. J. and SHARPE, J. A. (1990) Cerebral hemispheric localization of smooth pursuit asymmetry. *Neurology*, **40**, 284–292

NASHNER, L. M. (1973) Vestibular and reflex control in normal standing. In: *Control of Posture and Locomotion*, edited by R. B. Stein and K. G. Pearson. New York: Plenum Press. pp. 291–308

NASHNER, L. M., BLACK, F. O. and WALL, C. (1982) Adaptation to altered support and visual conditions during stance: patients with vestibular deficits. *Journal of Neuroscience*, **2**, 536–544

NATHANSON, M., BERGMAN, T. S. and BERKER, M. B. (1955) Monocular nystagmus. *American Journal of Ophthalmology*, **40**, 685–692

NEWMAN, N., GAY, A. J., STROUD, M. H. and BROOKS, J. (1970) Defective rapid eye movements in progressive supranuclear palsy. *Brain*, **93**, 775–784

NORRE, M. E. and FORREZ, G. (1986) Vestibulospinal function in otoneurology. *Journal for Oto-Rhino-Laryngology and its Allied Specialities*, **48**, 37–44

NORRE, M. E., FORREZ, G. and BECKERS, A. (1987) Vestibular dysfunction causing instability in aged patients. *Acta Otolaryngologica*, **104**, 50–55

NOZUE, N., MIZUNO, M. and KAGA, K. (1973) Neuro-otological findings in diphenylhydantoin intoxications. *Annals of Otology*, **82**, 389–394

ORZECHOWSKI, K. (1927) De l'ataxie dysmetrique des yeux: remarques sur l'ataxie des yeux dite myoclonique (opsoclonie, opsochorie). *Journal für Psychologie und Neurologie*, **35**, 1–18

OVERSTALL, P. W., EXTON–SMITH, A. N., IMMS, F. J. and JOHNSON, A. L. (1977) Falls in the elderly related to postural imbalance. *British Medical Journal*, **1**, 261–264

PAGE, N. G. R. and GRESTY, M. A. (1985) Motorist's vestibular disorientation syndrome. *Journal of Neurology, Neurosurgery and Neuropsychiatry*, **48**, 729–735

PALOSKI, W. H., BLACK, F. O., RESCHKE, M. F., CALKINS, D. S. and SHUPERT, C. (1993) Vestibular ataxia following shuttle flights: effects of microgravity on otolith-mediated sensorimotor control of posture. *American Journal of Otology*, **14**, 9–17

PALOSKI, W. H., RESCHKE, M. F., DOXEY, D. D. and BLACK, F. O. (1992) Neurosensory adaptation associated with postural ataxia following spaceflight. In: *Posture and Gait: Control Mechanisms*, vol I, edited by M. Woollacott and F. Horak. Eugene: University of Oregon Books. pp. 311–314

PARNES, L. S. and MCCLURE, J. A. (1992) Free-floating endolymph particles: a new operative finding during posterior canal occlusion. *Laryngoscope*, **102**, 988–992

PASIK, T., PASIK, P. and BENDER, M. B. (1969) The pretectal syndrome in monkeys. *Brain*, **92**, 871–884

PERRY, B. C. (1982) Falls among the aged living in a high rise apartment. *Journal of Family Practice*, **14**, 1069–1073

PFALTZ, C. R. (1969) The diagnostic importance of galvanic test in neuro-otology. *Practica Oto-Rhino-Laryngologica*, **31**, 193–203

PIERROTT–DESEILLIGNY, C., CHAIN, F., SERARA, M., GRAY, F. and L'HERMITTE, F. (1981) The 'One and a half' syndrome:

electro-oculographic analyses of five cases with deductions about physiological mechanisms of lateral gaze. *Brain*, 104, 665–700

PINHAS, I., PINHAS, A., GOLDHAMMER, Y. and BRAHAM, J. (1978) Progressive supranuclear palsy: EMG examination of eye muscles. *Acta Neurologica Scandinavica*, 58, 304–308

POLA, J. and ROBINSON, D. A. (1976) An explanation of eye movements seen in internuclear ophthalmoparesis. *Archives of Neurology*, 33, 447–452

POLA, J. and WYATT, H. J. (1980) Target position and velocity: the stimuli for smooth pursuit eye movements. *Vision Research*, 20, 523–534

RAPHAN, T. and COHEN, B. (1978) Brainstem mechanisms for rapid and slow eye movements. *Annual Review of Physiology*, 40, 527–552

RIESCO, J. S. (1957) Es el vertigo aural de origen exclusivemente periferico. *Revista Oto-Rhino-Laryngologica*, 17, 42–54

ROBERTS, T. D. M. (1967) *Neurophysiology of Postural Mechanisms*. New York: Plenum Press

ROBINSON, D. A. (1964) The mechanics of human saccadic eye movement. *Journal of Physiology*, 174, 245–264

ROBINSON, D. A. (1977) Vestibular and optokinetic symbiosis: an example of explaining by modelling. In: *Control of Gaze by Brain Stem Neurons*, edited by R. Baker and A. Berthoz. Amsterdam: Elsevier/North Holland. pp. 49–58

ROMBERG, M. H. (1846) *Lehrbuch der Nerven Krankheiten des Menschen*. Berlin: A. Duncker

RUBIN, W. (1981) Sinusoidal harmonic acceleration test in clinical practice. *Annals of Otology, Rhinology and Laryngology*, 90 (suppl. 86), 18–25

RUDGE, P. (1983) *Clinical Neuro-otology*. Edinburgh: Churchill Livingstone

RUDGE, P. and LEECH, J. (1976) Analysis of a case of periodic alternating nystagmus. *Journal of Neurology, Neurosurgery and Psychiatry*, 39, 314–319

SALAMI, J., POTVIN, A., JONES, K. and LANDRETH, J. (1975) Cortical evoked responses to labyrinthine stimulation in man. *Psychophysiology*, 2, 55–61

SCHALEN, L., HENRIKSSON, N. G. and PYYKKO, I. (1982) Quantification of tracking eye movements in patients with neurological disorders. *Acta Otolaryngologica*, 93, 387–395

SCHERER, H., BRANDT, U., CLARKE, A. H., MERBOLD, U. and PARKE, R. (1986) European vestibular experiments on the Spacelab-I mission 3. Caloric nystagmus in microgravity. *Experimental Brain Research*, 64, 255–263

SCHUKNECHT, H. F. and RUBY, R. F. (1973) Cupulolithiasis. *Advances in Oto-rhino-laryngology*, 20, 434–443

SELIKTAR, R., SUSAK, Z., NAJENSON, T. and SOLZI, P. (1978) Dynamic features of standing and their correlation with neurological disorders. *Scandinavian Journal of Rehabilitation Medicine*, 10, 59–64

SHEEHAN, S., BAUER, R. B. and MEYER, J. S. (1960) Vertebral artery compression in cervical spondylosis. *Neurology*, 10, 968–986

SHELDON, J. H. (1963) The effect of age on the control of body sway. *Gerontology Clinics*, 5, 129–138

SHEPARD, N. T., TELIAN, S. A., SMITH-WHEELOCK, M. and ANIL, R. (1993) Vestibular and balance rehabilitation therapy. *Annals of Otology, Rhinology and Laryngology*, 102, 198–205

STAHLE, J. T. and TERRINS, J. (1965) Paroxysmal positional nystagmus. *Annals of Otology, Rhinology and Laryngology*, 74, 69–83

STEINBACH, M. J. (1976) Pursuing the perceptual rather than the retinal stimulus. *Vision Research*, 16, 1371–1376

STEINHAUSEN, W. (1931) Uber den Nachweis der Bewegung der Cupula in der intaken Bogengangsampulle des Labyrinthes bei der naturlichen rotatorishen und calorishen Reizung. *Pflugers Archiv für die Gesamte Physiologie des Menschen und der Tiere*, 228, 322–328

STEPHENS, S. D. G. and BALLAM, H. M. (1974) The sono-ocular test. *Journal of Laryngology and Otology*, 88, 1049–1059

TAGUCHI, K. and TADA, C. (1988) Change of body sway with growth of children in posture and gait. Development, adaptation and modulation. *Amsterdam International Congress Series*, 812, 59–66

TAKAHASHI, S., FETTER, M., KOENIG, E. and DICHGANS, J. (1990) The clinical significance of head-shaking nystagmus in the dizzy patient. *Acta Otolaryngologica*, 109, 8–14

THYSSEN, H. H., BRYNSKOV, J., JANSEN, E. C. and MUNSTER–SWENDSEN, J. (1982) Normal ranges and reproducibility for the quantitative Romberg's test. *Acta Neurologica Scandinavica*, 66, 100–104

TIBBLING, L. (1969) The rotatory nystagmus response in children. *Acta Otolaryngologica*, 68, 459–467

TOKITA, T., MAEDA, M. and MIYATA, H. (1981) The role of the labyrinth in standing posture control. *Acta Otolaryngologica*, 91, 521–527

TRIESON, H. H., BRINSCOMBE, J., JANSEN, E. and SWENSON, J. M. (1982) Normal ranges in the reproducibility for the quantitative Romberg's test. *Acta Neurologica*, 66, 100–104

TULLIO, P. (1929) *Das Ohr und die Enstenhung der Sprahe und Schrift*. Berlin, Vienna: Schwartzenberg

UEMURA, T. and COHEN, B. (1973) Effects of vestibular nuclei lesions on vestibulo-ocular reflexes and posture in monkeys. *Acta Otolaryngologica Supplementum*, 315, 1–71

UNTERBERGER, S. (1938) Neue objective registrierbare Vestibularis-Korperdrehreaktion erhalter duch Treten auf der Stelle. Der Tretversuch. *Archiv für Ohren, Nasen und Kehlkopfheilkunde*, 179, 273–282

VAN EGMOND, A. A. J., GROEN, J. J. and JONGKEES, L. B. W. (1948) The turning test with small regulable stimuli. *Journal of Laryngology and Otology*, 62, 63–69

VAN WULFFTEN PALTHE, P. M. (1922) Function of the deeper sensibility and of the vestibular organs in flying. *Acta Otolaryngologica*, 4, 415–448

VOORHEES, R. L. (1989) The role of dynamic posturography in neuro-otologic diagnosis. *Laryngoscope*, 99, 995–1001

VYSLONZIL, E. (1963) Uber eine umschriebene anasmmlung von Otokien in hinteren hautigen Bogengange. *Monatsschriftliche Ohrenheilkunde*, 97, 63

WAESPE, W. and HENN, V. (1977) Neuronal activity in the vestibular nuclei of the alert monkey during vestibular and optokinetic stimulation. *Experimental Brain Research*, 27, 523–538

WATANABE, K., OHI, H., SAWA, M., OHASHI, N., KOBAYASHI, H. and MIZOKOSHI, K. (1983) Clinical findings of galvanic body sway test in cases of vestibular disorders. In: *Vestibular and Visual Control on Posture and Locomotor Equilibrium*, edited by M. Igarashi and F. O. Black. Basel: Karger. pp. 322–330

WESTHEIMER, G. and BLAIR, S. M. (1973) Oculo-motor defects in cerebellectomised monkeys. *Investigative Ophthalmology*, 12, 618–621

WILLIAMS, I. M., DICKINSON, P., RAMSAY, R. J. and THOMAS, L. (1982) Seesaw nystagmus. *Australian Journal of Ophthalmology*, 10, 19–25

WOLFSON, L., WHIPPLE, R., DERBY, C. A. AMERMAN, P., MURPHY, T., TOBIN, J. N. and NASHNER, L. (1992) A dynamic posturography study of balance in healthy elderly. *Neurology*, **42**, 2069–2075

YEE, R. D., BALOH, R. W., HONRUBIA, V. and JENKINS, H. A. (1982) Pathophysiology of optokinetic nystagmus. In: *Nystagmus and Vertigo. Clinical Approaches to the Patient with Dizziness*, edited by V. Honrubia and M. Brazier. New York: Academic Press. pp. 251–296

YOUNG, L. R. and STARK, L. (1963) Variable feedback experiments testing a sample data model for eye tracking movements. *IEEE Transactions Human Factors in Electronics HFE-4*, 38–51

ZEE, D. S. (1984) Ocular motor control: the cerebral control of saccadic eye movements. In: *Neuro-ophthalmology 1984*, edited by S. Lessel and J. T. W. van Dalen. Amsterdam: Elsevier. pp. 141–156

ZEE, D. S., YAMAZAKI, A., BUTLER, P. H. and GUCER, G. (1981) Effects of ablation of flocculus and paraflocculus on eye movements in primate. *Journal of Neurophysiology*, **46**, 878–899

ZEE, D. S., YEE, R. D., COGAN, D. G., ROBINSON, D. A. and ENGLE, W. K. (1976) Oculomotor abnormalities in hereditary cerebellar ataxia. *Brain*, **99**, 207–234

Rehabilitation of balance disorders

Johanna Beyts

Since Hecker, Haug and Herndon (1974) reported an 85% rate of improvement by simply counselling chronic dizzy patients on how to do Cawthorne and Cooksey exercises there has been a number of major developments in the field of balance rehabilitation. One of the major changes has been the introduction of computerized dynamic posturography which now makes it possible to measure objectively how the patient achieves the process of balancing in a number of diverse ways. However, while this new technology greatly increases the range and complexity of potential objective measurements of how a given patient fares during treatment, vestibular compensation can also be measured objectively in simpler or less expensive ways. Hence both low cost, low technology and high technology means of assessment will be reviewed.

The seminal work of Margaret Dix (1974, 1979, 1984, 1985) in this field is briefly reviewed. She attempted to define, on the basis of her years of clinical experience, which diagnostic groups would and would not benefit from vestibular rehabilitation. Her approach remains unique in that it attempts to relate diagnostic category to physiotherapeutic management in a very comprehensive system. Hence, despite the lack of controlled clinical trials with each diagnostic group, as a body of observations they remain relatively unchallenged. Shepard, Telian and Smith-Wheelock (1990), however, have treated some cases of central imbalance caused by multiple sclerosis with their team's approach to balance therapy, and thus challenge Dix's proposition that it is not likely that these 'central' patients will benefit from balance rehabilitation. Their teams's approach is discussed later. This assertion on Dix's part was presumably motivated by the desire to avoid raising false hopes in cases where there is a chronic progressive neurological condition, which may or may not go into remission during the course of treatment. This concern also applies to Menière's disorder, and Dix recommended treating this. The compromise between these two positions of either treating or not treating conditions with a marked central component might be simply to adopt a management approach best described as an 'equal collaborative partnership' with the patient; inform the patient as to the estimated prognosis, and leave the decision to him, making it clear that a high level of commitment to a regimen of exercise is required. For example, in peripheral vestibular disorders with a small central element, the treatments may vary between requiring a few days (Norré, 1984), to 6 weeks (Horak et al., 1992) to 14 weeks (Shepard et al., 1993a,b) to 2 years (Hamid, 1992) according to the severity of the symptoms. Nevertheless, peripheral disorders, even with mixed lesions, seem to take only about 16 weeks with an individually tailored rehabilitation programme of the type described by Smith-Wheelock et al. (1991) and Shepard et al. (1993a,b). However, ultimately the issue of prognosis in cases where CNS pathology may have caused lesions in the central vestibular system or the vestibular nuclei, is one where the time course may well remain uncertain as these may cause vertigo that does not respond to retraining exercises (see Rudge and Chambers, 1982). This does not mean that other coping strategies cannot be suggested for non-compensatible lesions (Overstall, 1983; Kataria and Das, 1985; Squires and Bayliss, 1985; Black, Maki and Fernie, 1993) that have not responded to balance retraining.

A study by Fiebert and Brown (1979), who subjected stroke patients to rotatory stimulation prior to conventional balance physiotherapy, found that their ambulation scores improved. Therefore this central group benefitted from vestibular habituation applied with a rotating chair. The central effects of the cardiovascular accidents may well have been diverse throughout this population of patients, as the effects of head injury are often diverse in terms of their central effects. It is therefore of interest that Dix (1984) recommended Cawthorne and Cooksey exercises for patients with head injuries which is generally a group with central lesions. Furthermore, in Shepard *et al.* (1993a), the effects of mixed central and peripheral lesions or central lesions on the time needed in treatment were relatively similar (see Figure 22.8), although the exact definition of how their group with central lesions was selected is unclear. However, they do point out that the group with a history of head injury took slightly longer, and had a poorer overall outcome. This may be because this group already had an established disability pension which may have affected their motivational levels or reporting of symptoms. This area is discussed in more detail later.

Due to the close association between anxiety of diverse kinds and the problems of chronic imbalance, this literature will be briefly reviewed, particularly in relation to the recent studies which report a high level of audiovestibular abnormalities in patients classified as having panic disorder which is, after all, an extreme form of anxiety. This American work uses a definition of panic disorder offered by the DSM III system of psychiatric classification which is routinely used in the USA. As the symptoms of vertigo, imbalance, or dizziness usually generate three potential areas of investigation in the astute general practitioner (Yardley *et al.*, 1992b), some of which require referral to specialist services, i.e. neuro-otological, neurological or psychological (or psychiatric), this important area will be reviewed. Some suggestions will be given on management both of simple cases of imbalance and complex cases where either the acute vertiginous episodes or the chronic balance problem are complicated by hyperventilation syndrome or panic attacks.

There have been developments in the field of biofeedback for treating vasospasm, as in the treatment of migraine (Blanchard *et al.*, 1982) and in the treatment of congenital nystagmus (Abadi, Carden and Simpson, 1980), which could benefit certain patients. The reader is referred to the original texts as these approaches lie beyond the scope of this chapter. Recent studies of new techniques such as Semont's liberatory manoeuvre (Semont, Freyss and Vitte, 1988) and also Epley's (1992) canalith repositioning procedure will be discussed, as these approaches seem to promise very effective management techniques for benign paroxysmal positional vertigo.

Vestibular compensation

The art of maintaining balance occurs largely unconsciously in the fit person, so the sense of balance is not one that the normal individual is aware of until

it goes wrong, either through alcohol abuse or some pathology or injury. It is also not a unitary 'sense' as might be suggested by the words used, in that the vestibular compensation can be defined as a multifactorial process of physiological changes, involving the central reintegration by the brain of three sensory inputs. These are proprioception, vision, and vestibular information. Vestibular information is also multifactorial containing elements of tilt information, linear acceleration and sensitivity to gravity (which is also sensitivity to linear acceleration). As the studies involving computerized dynamic posturography have shown, the 'righting' reflexes or 'strategies' used to correct imbalance, such as the hip, ankle and stepping strategies (Figure 22.1) occur at latencies which make it unlikely that voluntary control is exercised consciously with any degree of elaboration. However, this does not mean that it is not possible for the patient to try to influence deliberately or fake results when undergoing this form of objective testing, but this tends to generate physiologically inconsistent data and so is easily detectable. This area will be discussed in more detail later. Hence the interaction of voluntary and involuntary components to the act of balancing is complex. This in turn implies that the interaction between higher order processes (e.g. voluntary control) and involuntary reflexes is complex.

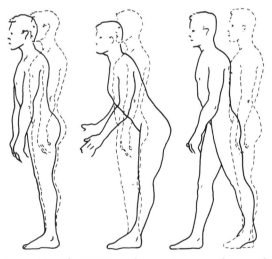

Figure 22.1 Three strategies for correcting perturbations of balance (from Shumway-Cook and Horak, 1989. Reprinted with permission from *Seminars in Hearing*, **10**, 196–209, 1989 Thieme Medical Publishers, Inc)

The process of vestibular compensation was historically objectively assessed by tests such as the Unterberger's stepping test (1962), the Romberg test, or even a battery of tests such as those provided by Fregly and Graybiel (1968). In terms of the initial diagnosis the use of electro-oculography, while relevant to the task of localizing the lesion to the vestibular system in the process of differential diagnosis, did not yield information that necessarily related causally to the rate of vestibular compensation as, for example, a canal paresis remains long after the patient has compensated, although the direction of the nystagmus (the directional preponderance) will change. This desynchrony between those measurements specific to the vestibular ocular reflex (electronystagmography and vestibular ocular reflex measures) and the process of compensation as demonstrated clearly by Norré (1984), is not ultimately surprising (Hallam, Beyts and Jakes, 1988; Stephens, Hogan and Meredith, 1991). This is because the process of vestibular compensation not only involves three different sensory systems (vision, proprioception and the vestibular inputs) but also (importantly) a voluntary decision on the part of the patient to make himself dizzy or light-headed in the course of the treatment needed to utilize the natural recovery processes (McCabe, 1970). Hence the patient who arrives at the clinic with chronic neck stiffness and dizziness on turning his head from side to side may well have made a conscious or semiconscious decision to restrict his own head movements in the interests of avoiding the noxious sensation of dizziness or avoiding physical danger. Thus previously (Beyts, 1987), a vicious circle model was proposed (Figure 22.2) where three types of anxious thought were depicted as generating reasons why head movements (or indeed a range of other

movements) might be avoided in the untreated patient, simply through fearing a number of possible aversive outcomes.

It was further proposed in the context of this model that these anxieties, through elevating central arousal levels, would lead to increased nystagmus, as Collins (1969) demonstrated in his habituation studies. (See Jacob *et al.*, 1988 for a more extensive review of this literature connecting the experimental manipulation of anxiety with nystagmus.) This anxiety about the meaning of the dizzy sensation was also seen as leading to the avoidance of the very movements that were necessary to retrain the sense of balance (McCabe, 1970: Lacour, Roll and Appaix, 1976). Therefore Hecker, Haug and Herndon (1974) deliberately clarified the reasons why movement which induced dizziness was needed to retrain the sense of balance when attempting to motivate their patients to do the Cawthorne and Cooksey's head and balance exercises. They used a computer analogy in their counselling session, which referred to the brain as type of balance computer which needed the 'error messages' of dizziness or imbalance to trigger the 'reprogramming' of the sense of balance, i.e. sensory reintegration. McCabe's (1970) rather amusing attempts to motivate his patients included attempts to change their interpretations of the meanings of the dizzy sensations. This technique (as we shall see later) has been adopted formally as an important component of treatment in the psychological management of panic attacks (Salkovskis and Clark, 1986).

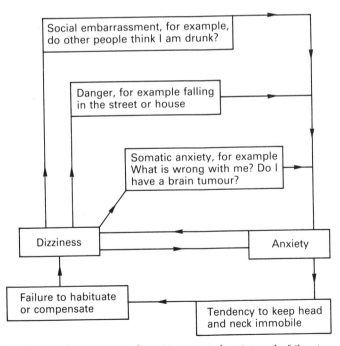

Figure 22.2 The vicious circle showing the interaction of cognitions, central anxiety and a failure to compensate

In McCabe's case he suggested saying to the patient, 'see the dizziness as your friend; the more often you meet it, the better you will be'. Clark, Salkovskis and Chalkley's (1985) methods to change the meaning of sensations caused by hyperventilation syndrome (which included the sensation of dizziness) relied on explaining the physiology of the hyperventilation syndrome and are therefore rather more formal. These authors also used a vicious circle model to explain how the behaviour of stress-induced changes in breathing rate causes respiratory alkalosis, and potentially induces a range of diverse sensations (see Table 22.6). These are then interpreted by the patient as pathological signs, that is 'symptoms' rather than 'sensations' which, in turn, increase the anxiety levels which again increases the respiration rate, thus exacerbating the situation. They proposed that it is relatively 'catastrophic' interpretations of these sensations which leads to the development of a panic attack. It is this cognitive interpretation of autonomic nervous system sensations (or as the patient sees it, symptoms) caused by respiratory alkalosis which is proposed as the crucial causal factor in the aetiology of the panic attacks (see Figure 22.12). As hyperventilation syndrome is a common secondary problem in patients with diverse medical conditions, including vertigo (Drachman and Hart, 1972; Cluff, 1984; Pilgrim, 1986; Theunissen, Huygen and Folgering, 1986) this area will be discussed in more detail below.

Vestibular compensation was traditionally defined as it related to electronystagmographic measures (Igarashi, 1989), to posturographic measures (Norré, 1988) or to the habituation of sensations (Norré, 1984; Beyts, 1987). However, because achieving compensation also often involves motivating the patient to comply with physiotherapy (namely stimulating a higher order purposive activity), methods of counselling the dizzy patient will also be discussed. Furthermore, the precise nature of the relationship between mind and body in this field remains a very complex area (Stephens, 1975; O'Connor *et al.*, 1988; Hallam and Hinchcliffe, 1991; Yardley, 1991, Yardley and Putman, 1992; Yardley *et al.*, 1992a, b). Hence, as the factor of anxiety may also contribute to decompensation, the area of hyperventilation management and the role of anxiety will be discussed in more detail in a later section.

Those investigators who deliberately set out to examine the relationship between subjective complaint and objective measures (or measures of 'mind' and 'body') do nevertheless report some interesting desynchrony and some interesting correlations between measures of handicap, distress, symptoms and autonomic nervous system 'signs' of activity. In the next sections I shall review their separate evolution in the field of subjective measures, and later, objective measures, in addition to discussing the recent advances in physiotherapeutic management.

Subjective complaint measures

The recent studies by Yardley and her collaborators (Yardley and Putman, 1992; Yardley, Gresty and Bronstein, 1992; Yardley *et al.*, 1992, a, b) set out to develop validated questionnaire measures of the complaint behaviour of vertiginous patients. Hence, this body of work greatly extends the scope of potential measures of subjective complaints about vertigo, imbalance and the distress or handicap it causes, which can provide valuable insights into the psychological effects of the disease process in addition to providing an inexpensive method of evaluating progress through treatment. The World Health Organization's definition of handicap is given below. Handicap, 'is characterised by a discordance between the individual's performance or status and the expectation of the individual himself or the particular group of which he is a member' (WHO, 1980).

Interestingly, this is a definition which relies in part on the person's subjective assessment of their social or socioeconomic position. Hence, measuring the patient's subjective assessment of the limitations imposed by their imbalance or dizziness is an important part of understanding the whole picture of how the frequently invisible symptoms like 'a persistent sense of imbalance', can greatly reduce a patient's freedom to enjoy life or attain life goals. So, while there have historically been a number of references to the enormous problems inherent in classifying the sheer variety and complexity of subjective complaints with which dizzy patients have presented (Kerr, 1983), it would seem that this World Health Organization definition of handicap would make measurement of subjective complaints an important component of any clinician's assessment. Furthermore, it is not uncommon to find that the fear of vertigo exerts a profoundly limiting effect on a patient's life, despite there being clear evidence that a patient has compensated to a range of different movements. Hence the power of these subjective factors and belief systems should not be underestimated. The most dramatic demonstration of these was found in the study of placebo surgery in Menière's patients which showed that 77% of the group receiving placebo surgery reported significant improvements in their dizziness after 3 years (Thompsen *et al.*, 1981, 1983). This was a marginally better improvement than that reported by the group who received 'real' surgery.

Assessing subjective complaints

The assessment of subjective complaints can be done in a variety of ways, the choice varying according to practical constraints such as the availability of time, or ancillary staff available to the clinician. One simple method of assessment is to classify the severity of vertigo attacks and sensations informally, perhaps along the lines suggested by Kerr (1983), where a distinction is made between the true rotatory vertigo of the major attacks, and a more vague sense of imbalance. O'Connor *et al.* (1988) devised a list of sensations when investigating the characteristics of major episodes of vertigo, and these included visual symptoms (indicative of a migraine component (Kayan, 1984; Kayan and Derrick–Hood, 1984)), autonomic sensations like sweating or pallor etc., and signs of anxiety or hyperventilation such as 'difficulty in breathing'.

In terms of placing these different types of sensations or symptoms into some theoretical framework, the authors (O'Connor *et al.*, 1988) suggested that a distinction be made between sensations arising from sympathetic and parasympathetic nervous system activity (Hinoki, 1985), the truly audiovestibular sensations or symptoms (tinnitus increasing, vertigo, light-headedness) and migrainous visual symptoms (flashing lights, spots before the eyes). Hence, this questioning of patients presenting to a neuro-otology clinic about which sensations occurred during a major attack yielded a definition of a major attack as consisting of over 38 sensations. So it is not surprising that Dix referred to the way that a clinician's heart can sink when listening to a dizzy patient describing his symptoms, if only because of their sheer complexity.

While it is possible to reduce the time spent on history taking by simply asking patients to fill in questionnaires assessing these factors, the clinician clearly needs to decide on what level of complexity is needed to be able thoroughly to assess the patient for the purposes of clinical management. For example, assessing the major attacks of vertigo in great detail in terms of 38 sensations may not be as relevant to the clinical management decisions as simply ascertaining whether drug management is effective in reducing the overall severity or frequency of major attacks, and differentiating these from the positional components. Norré (1984) made a very useful distinction between major attacks and positional components, suggesting that positional components are defined as movements which reliably induce dizziness. Major attacks are seen as totally unpredictable and associated with dizziness or vegetative symptoms such as nausea, which last longer than 20 minutes. If patients have positional components and also suffer from an additional problem of the hyperventilation syndrome, it often presents as a semicontinual sense of imbalance (rather than vertigo) which is described as being made worse by movements or any exertion, which may induce additional excessive breathlessness. Hence these definitions may well be crucial to certain management decisions for physiotherapists, or other clinical staff involved in the management, or indeed the patients as they acquire self-management skills in the process of rehabilitation. This proposal that a continual sense of dizziness may be caused by

the hyperventilation syndrome implies that this complaint is not always 'functional', as might be assumed by some authors (Tiwari and Bakris, 1981), but rather the physiological consequence of respiratory alkalosis (Gibson, 1979).

Norré further suggested (1984) that it was very important, in the early stages of rehabilitation, to make the patient's expectations of treatment as realistic as possible and to offer treatment including physiotherapy in an optimistic way. He therefore advocated emphasizing that the Cawthorne and Cooksey exercises were directed at treating the positional components rather than completely 'curing' the major episodes of vertigo. Hence clarifying this distinction between the positional components that are *reliably* caused by movements, from the major episodes of dizziness (that only rarely *seem* to be caused by movements) from clusters of attacks, is seen to be an integral part of his system of rehabilitation. Norré recommended that when the dizziness induced by movements lasted longer than 20 minutes during physiotherapeutic treatment the patient should stop exercising for that day and resume treatment the following day.

This type of management approach is helpful for those patients who appear to be going through an active phase of their endolymphatic hydrops or Menière's disease, when vertiginous episodes are occurring fairly frequently. Often, these kinds of distinctions are left to the patient to deduce or to the physiotherapist to explain, so one way of ensuring a consistent explanation of the treatment rationale, in this confusing area of subjective description, is to develop booklets which embody these definitions, and further explain the rationale of treatment, particularly how the exercises help to retrain the sense of balance. It also helps to have a clear distinction drawn between the dizziness caused by the pathological process (i.e. paroxysmal attacks), dizziness which is part of the recovery process which occurs as part of the process of vestibular compensation, i.e. positional components, and dizziness which may be caused by hyperventilation. This is clearly an integral aspect of counselling patients. The types of subjective measures that could be used for such an approach as applied to Cawthorne and Cooksey exercises are given below (Table 22.1).

This explanation, namely that the effects of making repetitive movements cause habituation in positional components, is seen by Norré as the vital initiation of the rehabilitation process, as the clinician breaks into a vicious circle of anxiety and behavioural restriction. This is an important intervention because not all dizziness need necessarily cause such acute anxiety as would a major paroxysmal attack. So teaching this kind of distinction between 'recovery dizziness', that needs 'retraining' as in the positional components, and the dizziness which is generally reflective of the underlying pathological process (namely major

Table 22.1 Exercise check list for levels 1 and 2 (see text for explanation)

Name:
No. of exercise session:
Description of exercise

	Eye exercise level 1				Head exercise level 2				Date
	1 (i) Look up and down	1 (ii) Look from side to side	1 (iii) Move finger towards you and back	1 (iv) Move finger from side to side	2 (i) Move head forwards and backwards	2 (ii) Move head side to side	2 (iii) Head forwards and backwards eyes closed	2 (iv) Head side to side eyes closed	
Time taken for dizziness/ imbalance to go									
Lightheaded or dizzy rating									
Number of movements completed									
Comments e.g. easy, very easy, hard, very hard									
Target no. of movements	20	20	20	20	20	20	20	20	
Scales to rate effects of exercises									
	No lightheadedness L0	Slight l/headedness L1	Moderate l/headedness L2		Bad l/headedness L3		Very bad l/headedness L4		
	No dizziness D0	Slight dizziness D1	Moderate dizziness D2		Bad dizziness D3		Very bad dizziness and nausea D4		

attacks) will not only help motivate the patient to persevere with the physiotherapy aimed at inducing habituation to the movement related dizziness, but will also (by making the overall complaint less confusing) make 'the dizziness' less anxiogenic. One further effect of teaching this distinction is that it will help to ensure that the patient's expectations of what physiotherapy is likely to achieve are realistic, namely consisting of a gradual habituation to the movements rather than a total or instant 'cure' for major attacks. Furthermore, this reinterpretation of some of the causes of the dizzy sensations is an important cognitive manipulation (analogous to the reinterpretation of sensations used in the cognitive management of panic disorder), which effectively makes it possible for the patient to habituate by reducing the secondary anxiety about positional components. The danger of just giving the over simplified advice that 'these exercises will make the dizziness better' is that the patient will give up if he has another major vertigo attack, on the grounds that the exercises made 'the dizziness worse'. If he has realistic expectations of the effects that the exercises are likely to have, both in terms of generating noxious sensations, and how long they are likely to take to effect improvement, a patient is more likely to comply with treatment.

However, as Yardley *et al.* (Yardley and Putman, 1992; Yardley, Gresty, Bronstein and Beyts, 1996; Yardley *et al.*, 1992 a, b) pointed out, complaint behaviour about dizziness (both positional components and major attacks), degree of disability, handicap and emotional distress, can be complex. Typically (Beyts, 1991; Yardley *et al.*, 1992a), patients describe being able to maintain one activity, e.g. holding down a part time job, at the 'cost' of giving up other activities, e.g. housework or socializing. Some patients make quite complex analyses of the costs and benefits of persevering with certain behaviours or activities, many of which are based on the core assumption that their dizziness will not go away. Some patients do (of course) independently manage to progress through vestibular compensation despite their disabling symptoms. This group frequently report reasons or justifications to persevere with the activities, despite the initial dizziness induced by the activities. They then report a psychological benefit from returning to a normal life, so persist, and maintain their improvement. Such patients who independently learn coping strategies constitute an under-examined area in studies of subjective complaint behaviour. An example of such a coping strategy would be that of staring at a fixed point when travelling on an escalator to reduce the 'optokinetic' effects of passing advertisement hoardings. This can be seen as a form of training the vestibular ocular reflex suppression that Hood (1970, 1975) observed to be so highly developed in ballet dancers.

Yardley *et al.* (Yardley and Putman, 1992; Yardley, Gresty, Bronstein and Beyts, 1996; Yardley *et al.*,

1992 a, b) have developed well-validated questionnaires to measure various aspects of subjective complaint. They gave good examples of the decision-making processes surrounding the development of behaviours which ultimately cause the dizzy patient to develop a complaint that superficially seems similar to agoraphobia. Yardley *et al.* (1992a) interviewed 23 individuals with vertigo of various types generating over 2000 statements about the complaint, which were then condensed into four tables with summary statements representing the prevalent reactions. They discussed the effect of the symptoms in great detail, both on the relationships the patient had with his family or spouse, and the perceived effects of the stigma surrounding the illness on the family and close friends. They summarized the sometimes elaborate emotional effects of these frequently 'invisible' complaints like persistent dizziness or nausea. They discussed the internal contradictions that occur in some patients' descriptions, such as those patients who attempted to conceal the vertigo in order to avoid the stigmatization of being ill, but who became continually anxious because they fear that at any time they might be 'discovered' as being disabled, or socially discredited. They quoted one patient, 'You can't ever be confident ... that something is going to work out right'. Others, wishing to cope independently, expressed a sense of inadequacy or guilt at having to rely on others, 'You can't restrict people all the time, because that's what you're doing. You are saying, "Don't leave me on my own", or you are saying, "Please come out with me". It's very, very difficult'. Active attempts to cope with vertigo are described as being 'often enshrined in self-generated rules designed either to avoid provoking vertigo or to prevent public exposure', and these rules can themselves become a cause of secondary anxiety or depression. This was considered to happen, 'insofar as they exerted unwanted constraints upon behaviour, often far more extensive than the direct effects of vertigo itself'. In various accounts of cognitive therapy, this type of 'over-generalized behavioural rule' is seen as a common logical error and a common source of psychological distress (Beck, 1976; Beck *et al.*, 1979; Fennel, 1989).

The authors proposed 'the result can be an apparently insoluble dilemma in which subjects are torn between the fear of invoking vertigo and the desire to escape a depressingly simple lifestyle' and then proceeded to form a conceptual model of the various processes but acknowledged that in each individual there may be various 'vicious circles of escalating handicap and distress'. They distinguished between the long-term adaptation effects related to loss of confidence, depression, and the 'psychophysiological' processes that maintain symptom severity. If fact, as each patient is unique they will have their own variants on the thought patterns described, but these are useful general models, based on actual data.

The vicious circle model shown earlier (Figure 22.2) differs in that it is a psychophysiological model (Beyts, 1987) whereby the cognitive activity related to social embarrassment, fear of nausea, or of physical danger is seen as maintaining a high level of autonomic arousal, which in turn contributes to a failure to habituate (Lader and Wing, 1964; Lader, Gelder and Marks, 1967) to the sensation of dizziness. Within the context of this model it is arguable that predictable dizziness caused by the patient's own movements should be less stressful than unpredictable paroxysmal major attacks, because people habituate more readily to predictable noxious stimuli than to unpredictable ones (Katz, 1982). The work of Yardley *et al.* gives an understanding of why not all patients spontaneously compensate. They take into account the whole patient, i.e. the mental activity that he chooses to engage in order to try to make his life less dangerous, more manageable, and more predictable.

The degree to which people can accurately report on internal physiological processes varies considerably from person to person, and may well depend on diverse factors such as a knowledge of basic physiological concepts, or certain personality characteristics such as the degree of introspection that the patient engages in (Nisbett and DeCamp Wilson, 1977). Therefore it is probable that this awareness of the internal processes involved in movement, dizziness and habituation is a differential conditioning task (as is found in several biofeedback studies), so is highly responsive to training, of which counselling and explanation form one category. Needless to say, the kinds of complex intellectual activity described by the patients in the Yardley *et al.* (1992a) study, and their internal debates about dependency on family and friends, their need to avoid being stigmatized, or the level of physical danger with which they decide to cope, understandably directs their attention away from trying to determine whether an attack of dizziness is predictable or not. In fact it seems that, in chronic illness, this type of analytical activity is sometimes abandoned as a fruitless exercise, particularly in cases where symptoms are frequent or severe, or where the patient is depressed. Nevertheless,

this work provides a useful general model of cognitive activity, shown in Figure 22.3.

In the second study of subjective complaint, Yardley and Putman (1992) devised a further questionnaire based loosely on this earlier work, called the vertigo handicap questionnaire comprising 46 statements. They found no significant relationship between the total handicap scores and age, sex or time since the onset of the vertigo. Diagnostic category was, however, related to the handicap score ($P < 0.03$) (Table 22.2).

Patients with episodic (recurrent) and positional vertigo had the highest scores, and those with residual dizziness following a single vestibular episode scored lowest. This provides some validity for the scale in that most clinicians familiar with these patients would expect that those who had experienced only one episode of dizziness would be considerably less handicapped than those who had experienced several. The questionnaire was completed six months later by 27 of the original subjects who were also asked three further questions about whether they thought their condition had improved or not. Those who thought it had improved showed reduced handicap scores.

Multiple regression analyses on the data from 84 subjects was carried out to identify those elements of disability and handicap that contributed to patient distress. Five factors were identified. The first was described as relating to *restriction of activity*, which included items describing interference with social plans, travelling, going out alone, moving around quickly, and walking long distances. Factor two was labelled *social anxieties* and was characterized by concern that colleagues and friends might not understand or sympathize with the vertigo. Factor three grouped together *fears about vertigo* incorporating both the immediate fear inspired by an attack and anxiety about a possible sinister cause of the vertigo. The fourth factor was dominated by two items assessing the reported *severity of vertigo* attacks.

A repeat regression analysis indicated that restriction of activities was one of the most distressing aspects of the total handicap score. However, after

Table 22.2 The relationship of vertigo handicap scores with diagnostic category

Category	No. subjects	Mean handicap	
		%	s.d.
Episodic rotatory vertigo	16	52	15
Single episode rotatory vertigo (with residual dizziness)	6	31	14
Positioning vertigo	15	52	16
Neck positional vertigo	8	47	12
Non-rotatory vertigo (unsteadiness, 'wooziness')	15	38	14
Miscellaneous	24	48	

From Yardley and Putman, 1992 with permission

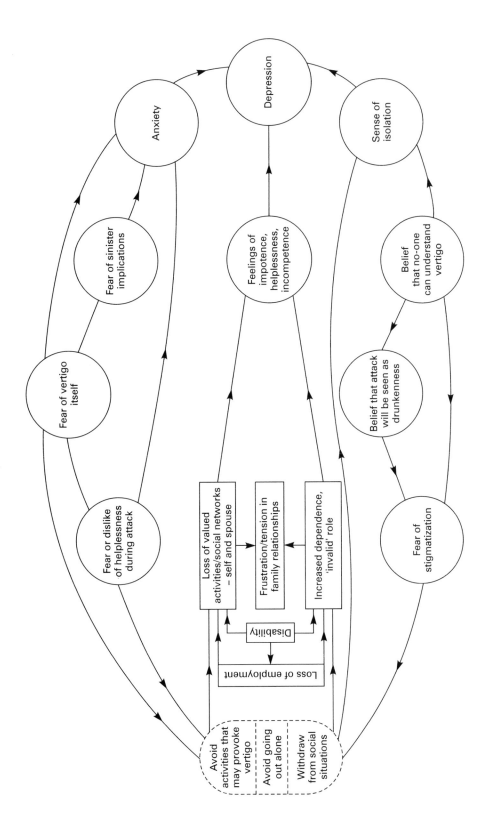

Figure 22.3 Model illustrating common responses to and consequences of vertigo, and some of the hypothesized principal interconnections. Self-generated rules are enclosed in broken lines, beliefs and emotional responses are presented in circles, and consequences appear in solid rectangles. (From Yardley *et al.*, 1992a, by kind permission of the authors)

further analysis the authors concluded, 'Social anxieties, fears about vertigo, and behavioural restriction accounted for roughly equivalent proportions of the variance in emotional distress'. From the somatopsychic perspective this indicates that these three factors contribute approximately equally to patient distress, and show a similarity to the proposals in the Beyts model (1987), although the psychosomatic effects of previous psychological traits predisposing the patient to develop problems cannot be ruled out. The severity and the frequency of attacks appeared to contribute little to behavioural or emotional responses to vertigo in this sample, once mediating psychological and behavioural factors were taken into account. On the other hand, fears about vertigo contributed to distress not only directly but also by causing alterations in lifestyle. This work thus helps to clarify the interactions between cognitive activity and behaviour which lead to increases in handicap over time.

The incidence of fears about vertigo was high despite having received thorough investigation and routine reassurance on a minimum of two occasions prior to completing the questionnaire. Whether this is due to an inability to process complex medical information when the patient is anxious, educational or memory factors is unclear, but certainly corresponds with the author's own clinical experience. Patients occasionally seem initially to be unable to process or understand what has been ruled out as a result of the diagnostic process in terms of potentially sinister causes for vertigo. However, the factors affecting medical communications are many and varied and the reader is referred to Salkovskis (1989a) for a review of the relevant literature as this lies beyond the scope of the present chapter. Salkovskis, in particular, suggested that health anxiety can lead to biases in what is taken in during medical consultations, which can complicate management.

Yardley and Putman (1992) concluded that, 'since fears about vertigo are apparently widespread, persistent and central to handicap in vertiginous patients it seems likely that in-depth counselling and reassurance might be able to bring about significant reductions in patient distress even in those cases where the actual vertigo cannot be controlled'.

Yardley *et al.* (1992b) further developed a vertigo symptom scale which consisted of four subscales. The two subscales measuring vertigo of long and short duration were sensitive to diagnostic category, but completely uncorrelated with a measure of somatic anxiety so, in the authors' words, 'provide a valid new method of evaluating the level of functional impairment caused by vertigo'.

They proposed that these statistically validated scales will overcome the interactions of confounding variables within the field of subjective complaint. This study therefore set out to examine the way in which 'enduring personality characteristics (trait anxiety), current emotional disturbance (anxiety and depression) and reported symptomatology affected disability', handicap and distress. All these dependent variables were also measured with questionnaire scales rather than, for example, behavioural observation (Yardley *et al.*, 1992b).

Women were found to have slightly higher vertigo handicap questionnaire scores than men, and reported worse acute vertigo (*P* = 0.003), disability (*P* = 0.01) and autonomic/anxiety symptoms (*P* = 0.02). Although handicap and emotional distress were unrelated to age, disability was slightly greater in the older patients (*P* = 0.02). Duration of vertigo was found to be correlated to handicap measures, and disability measures, but not with distress. The standard audiovestibular tests were performed on this sample (where possible) and results were found to be 'uncorrelated with any other variable measured in this study including diagnostic category and reported disability handicap or distress'. Once again this can be seen as illustrative of desynchrony between physiological and psychological measures, similar to that observed by O'Connor *et al.* (1988).

The main relationships between somatic and psychological factors are shown in Figure 22.4. The factors which were found to predict disability were quite different from those which predicted emotional distress. Reported disability was most clearly related to indices of physical status such as vertigo severity, its duration, and the patient's age. In contrast, levels of anxiety and depression were unrelated to the illness characteristics, except inasmuch as these factors contributed to handicap. The authors further proposed that these results extend those of Yardley and Putman (1992) which suggested that

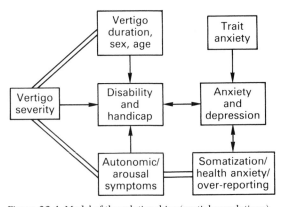

Figure 22.4 Model of the relationships (partial correlations) between symptoms, handicap and distress. The principal associations with disability, handicap, anxiety and depression (revealed by the multiple regression analyses) are shown as solid arrows. The open lines represent those additional associations between elements in the model which reached significance after controlling for other variables

the causes of emotional distress are fear of vertigo and consequent restriction of activity, although these variables in turn were affected by illness severity. Handicap scores were associated with a mixture of somatic and psychological variables. This pattern of relationships was deemed consistent with the authors' expectations of this scale since 'the impact of illness upon lifestyle is affected by both disability and psychosocial status'.

Since anxiety-prone individuals were not unusually prevalent in this population, the authors suggested that, 'the correlation between state anxiety with disability and handicap can best be explained in terms of somatopsychic processes'. This was given partial support by the fact that almost double the number of patients were sent to a psychiatrist after being diagnosed as suffering from dizziness compared to the number who were referred beforehand.

The authors went on to suggest that, 'the findings that different variables predicted different aspects of patient status had implications for patient management'. They suggested that, 'medical treatment and physiotherapy would seem the most suitable method of reducing disability' since this is determined mainly by physical factors. Handicap might be further alleviated by providing control of autonomic symptoms which can be achieved by means of reassurance, or breathing or relaxation techniques (Beyts, 1987). Furthermore, more extensive counselling and behavioural therapy might be required in order to prevent the development of secondary emotional problems in patients who are prone to anxiety (McKenna, Hallam and Hinchcliffe, 1991).

Hence, subjective complaint about the effects of vertigo and imbalance on patients' lives can be broken down into a number of factors. First, there is the severity of the actual vertigo attacks, and how complex they are. While some authors advocated a simple dichotomy between attacks characterized by rotatory and non-rotatory vertigo, O'Connor *et al.* identified 38 possible sensations that could occur during major attacks. Yardley *et al.* (Yardley and Putman, 1992; Yardley *et al.*, 1992a, b; Yardley, 1994) have identified a number of factors relating to aspects of handicap or disability through the statistical analysis of subjective questionnaire data resulting in scales measuring somatization, restriction, the vertigo severity scale, and autonomic sensations. These may well prove to be valuable tools in evaluating different components of treatment programmes in clinical research aimed at evaluating the newly emerging methods of treating patients with these disorders. However, it seems that different health professionals prefer different levels of analysis, hence physiotherapists writing recently about rehabilitation have tended to focus on general fitness, gait disturbances and positional components, tending to use symptom-based global measures of subjective and objective aspects based on rating scales (Horak *et al.*,

1992; Shepard *et al.*, 1993a). However, where there are multidisciplinary teams consisting of clinical psychologists or audiological scientists and hearing and balance therapists, who additionally address the cognitive activity of these patients, those scales which assess the degree of handicap as discussed by Yardley *et al.* may be of more interest. Clinicians interested in pursuing the relationship of the medical history to prognosis, or treatment response may find the dizziness handicap inventory (Jacobson *et al.*, 1991) of more interest, and so on (see also Cohen, 1992).

It is possible to simplify the assessment for interview purposes by asking about the patient's abilities to perform the activities shown in Table 22.3 and then on finding an activity that is avoided, attempt to ascertain the extent to which this is due to actually experiencing symptoms like dizziness or falling, and whether it always (or just sometimes) happens on performing the activity. This form of assessment is particularly useful for assessing the degree of involvement of paroxysmal attacks, particularly when patients say, 'I only avoid that on bad days'. If an activity has been avoided for some months, but seems to the clinician to be unlikely to cause problems (if compensation seems to have progressed on other movements) then this interview format provides a useful way of introducing the patient to the notion of deliberately trying to make the movements unless they involve a substantial degree of risk.

Table 22.3 Problem activities reported by patients with chronic balance difficulties

Climbing ladders	Bending to pick things up
Shopping in local shops	Shopping in supermarkets
Housework	Job
Doing things around the house	Walking in the street (accompanied)
Going out alone	Walking upstairs
Driving	Playing sports
Using lifts	Using escalators
Dancing	Boarding public transport
Walking (in the light)	Walking (in the dark)
Drinking alcohol	Seeing friends
Running	Walking in open spaces
Going to the cinema/theatre	Getting up (from chair or bed)
Lying down	Sleeping
Turning head suddenly	Walking downstairs
Walking around the house	Walking up slopes
Walking down slopes	

This list of activities provides a useful structure for discussion but, by virtue of the range and complexity of human movements and activity, is not exhaustive. For example, one patient was, in his words, 'perfectly fit' until he examined the underside of his office desk while remaining seated one day. When he achieved this uncomfortable position he discovered he got quite marked positional vertigo. This movement was, however, quite difficult to achieve and he had never performed it before. Hence he was not that motivated to keep doing it in order to retrain his sense of balance. However, recent treatments of benign paroxysmal positional vertigo would lead one to propose a possibly rapid result from making similar atypical movements. Where movements are essential to normal everyday activities it is generally easier to motivate the patient to perform them, and hence important to evaluate them in the process of assessing the need for, or progress through rehabilitation. Different groups may require the development of different types of activity check lists. Arguably, children who regularly climb ropes, do barwork in gymnastics, go canoeing on activity holidays or swim competitively, involving underwater somersaults, would require more careful assessment and counselling (Horak *et al.*, 1988; Ledin, 1992), particularly if the muscular effort involved in these activities generated more severe problems than usual through their also having hyperventilation syndrome (or effort syndrome as it used to be called (Lum, 1976)).

Hence just as adult patients may experience difficulties climbing even a few stairs when they have both dizziness and hyperventilation syndrome (Beyts, 1991) it may be that children who have difficulties with their balance or eye movements after sports lessons could benefit from being allowed to scale down their level of physical activity in gymnastics classes, etc. during the period of treatment for their dizziness, as an overaggressive approach to rehabilitation can cause decompensation (Smith–Wheelock, Shepard and Telian, 1991). This area merits further research.

Before leaving this area it is worth noting that, within the field of psychological treatments for anxiety, there are two main schools of thought concerning the appropriate method of treating stress and hyperventilation-related panic attacks: these are cognitive and behavioural techniques. Hence behaviourists treating agoraphobia would traditionally use a behavioural technique known as systematic desensitization or exposure-based treatments (Ritter, 1969a,b; Lipsedge, 1973; Kennerley, 1991; Marks, 1991), and make behavioural observations to measure treatment effects. More recently, particularly in the psychological management of panic, treatment designed to help patients is aimed at helping them change the way they *think* about their symptoms or problem, and has become more frequently chosen, hence these are termed cognitive techniques. This is because clinical experience showed that some people who do go through graded desensitization to feared objects or stimuli still panic, or retain other anxiety-based behaviour, hence simply relying on habituation or desensitization processes (i.e. behavioural techniques) was not enough (Salkovskis, 1988, 1989b). In this regard, Yardley's (1994) recent study of the role of autonomic sensations, and negative attitudes which

explained an increase in the handicap scores when patients were tested twice on the vertigo handicap questionnaire over a 7-month period, are of interest because they report an effect on handicap scores, caused by the kinds of extreme or catastrophic fears that are also implicated as cognitive factors in panic disorder. Hence this is a direct parallel with the suggestions made by Clarke and Salkovskis (Clark, Salkovskis and Chalkley, 1985; Clark, 1989) and suggests anxiety may be a major factor in the increase of handicap over time, as found by Yardley (1994).

The relationship between autonomic symptoms and negative beliefs about vertigo was observed after controlling for reported illness severity, anxiety, depression and somatization. Yardley (1994) concluded that negative perceptions of physical symptoms may indeed contribute to the psychosocial difficulties of people with vertigo and that the finding that autonomic symptoms are a moderately powerful predictor of residual handicap suggests that the link between handicap and symptoms of anxiety arousal observed by Yardley (1994) is mediated by some causal mechanism. The association between autonomic symptoms, anxiety, and fear of serious disease and social discreditation in patients with vertigo may resemble the cycle of physiological changes and catastrophic fears proposed by Clark, Salkovskis and Chalkley (1985) as an explanation of panic attacks.

Yardley argued that although worsening handicap was predicted by symptoms and beliefs correlated with anxiety, rather than vertigo severity, this does not imply a non-organic aetiology for patient complaints in this study, since illness-related variables contributed significantly to handicap from the onset. Moreover, abnormal balance system test results were obtained in the majority of the sample, and the symptom and psychological profile of the remaining subjects was essentially identical to that of subjects with incontrovertible evidence of vestibular dysfunction. Nevertheless, these findings confirm that psychological factors play a significant role in maintaining or escalating the handicap and distress caused by vertigo. It is for this reason that cognitive and behavioural therapy may usefully complement treatment of vertigo by medication and physiotherapy by helping to promote adjustment and adaptive coping.

In summary, therefore, there has been a considerable change in the way in which subjective reporting of complaint about vertigo is viewed. There is the recognition that the desynchrony between objective measures and complaint (e.g. ENG) particularly in the early stages of Menière's disease (Yardley *et al.*, 1992b), may mean that subjective measures may be more of a guideline for certain management decisions than objective (ENG) measures, particularly when consideration is given to the limitations of objective measures of the vestibular ocular reflex which normally only test the horizontal semicircular canal.

Furthermore, as vertigo and other aspects of

Menière's disease (tinnitus, migraine, aural pressure) are frequently episodic it may be that the objective physical signs are present only during an actual attack, prior to any lesions actually being sustained. Early treatment may therefore depend on reliance on subjective complaint in cases where objective test results contribute little. Certainly it would seem that the WHO definition of handicap would imply that counselling directed at changing negative attitudes about vertigo would be of benefit in the uncompensated patient who is deliberately avoiding many movements. Counselling would also be of use to the type of patient who, despite achieving some progress with vestibular compensation, remains overly restricted in his choice of activities or behaviour through the use of an over-generalized rule that the principle of avoidance of movements is the safest choice available. While this may have simplified decision making during the acute episode or during clusters of major attacks, it is clearly an over-restrictive rule for the compensation period and may actually prevent full recovery. It has been suggested that over-generalized rules feature in the clinical presentation in depression and that techniques like cognitive therapy may be a useful clinical approach (Fennel, 1989).

Hence, when reviewing this literature on subjective complaint, one can conclude that there are many methods of assessing subjective complaints from several new, validated questionnaire scales (detailed above) to simple rating scales of symptoms induced by head and balance exercises which enable the clinician to monitor habituation. It was this type of rating which Norré (1984) recommended initially in the treatment of unilateral hypofunction, and is now part of his vestibular habituation therapy technique (Norré, 1984; Norré and Beckers, 1985). However, in the measurement system shown earlier (see Table 22.1), it is worth noting that, although the observer using the chart is reliant on asking the patient to rate subjective sensations, they are also timing them, which may qualify this latter type of measure as 'objective', if it is carried out carefully.

This type of outcome measure would be most useful with patients who, due to musculoskeletal abnormalities such as arthritis, might show artefactual results on the EquiTest.

Physiotherapeutic management of rehabilitation

Since Margaret Dix's pioneering work in this field with Cawthorne and Cooksey exercises (Table 22.4) which attempted to relate physiotherapeutic management to both diagnostic category and to theoretical considerations, and then empirical evidence (Dix, 1974, 1979), more recent work has had a different emphasis. For example, Dix (1979) saw early treatment with physiotherapy as a means of preventing psychiatric treatment, whereas more recent work has shown an interesting overlap between the disciplines of psychology, psychiatry and physiotherapy. For example, while Jacob *et al.* (1993) proposed a physiological substrate for their observed connections between panic disorder and vertigo, they recommended physiotherapy (for balance rehabilitation) as the appropriate management technique, for patients with vertigo and panic attacks, rather than the treatment of the postulated intermediate condition, namely hyperventilation syndrome (see Salkovskis,

Table 22.4 An example of a handout listing the Cawthorne and Cooksey vestibular retraining exercises

Head and balance exercises	
To be carried out for 15 minutes twice a day (increasing gradually to 30 minutes)	
These exercises may make you dizzy at first, but in the long term should help to prevent further attacks	
Level 1 Eye exercises:	Looking up then down, at first slowly then quickly, 20 times
	Looking from one side to the other at first slowly then quickly, 20 times
	Focus your finger at arm's length then move it in and out 30 cm, 20 times
Level 2 Head exercises:	Bend your head forward and then backward with your eyes open, slowly then quickly, 20 times
	Turn your head from one side to the other slowly then quickly, 20 times
	As the dizziness improves these head exercises should be done with closed eyes
Level 3 Sitting:	Shrug your shoulders 20 times
	Turn your shoulder to right then left 20 times
	Bend forward and pick up objects from the ground, and sit up again, 20 times
Level 4 Standing:	Move from sitting to standing and back again, 20 times with eyes open, then repeat with eyes closed
	Throw a rubber ball from hand to hand above eye level
	Throw the ball from hand to hand under one knee
Level 5 Moving about:	Walk across the room with your eyes open 20 times then repeat with your eyes closed
	Walk up and down steps with your eyes open 10 times then repeat with your eyes closed
	Any game involving stooping or turning is useful in improving balance

After Dix, 1984

Jones and Clark, 1986; Jacob, 1988; Ley, 1988). However, this area of management will be discussed in more detail in a later section.

Within the field of physical therapy for balance disorders, a number of new developments have succeeded in revolutionizing the level of interest in, and importantly the type of treatment received by, these patients in Europe and America. These, broadly speaking, involve recent physiotherapeutic innovations (discussed later), the development of Semont's liberatory manoeuvre or Epley's canalith repositioning procedure, and the use of computerized dynamic posturographic techniques of assessment. These assessment techniques and additional therapeutic instruments giving biofeedback like the Balance Master (Neurocom International), enable a clinician to carry out much more careful and elaborate objective analysis of balance function than was previously possible (Nashner and Peters, 1990).

As a result of the increased interest in this field, the range of positive suggestions and recommendations about methods and modes of vestibular retraining have proliferated, hence only a brief overview is possible here.

In general, definitions of vestibular compensation have included notions of sensory reintegration occurring centrally so as to equalize the vestibular tonus bilaterally over a period of time. The estimate of how long this period is varies between several months to one year and several years (Herdman, 1990, 1991; Pfaltz, 1983), where compensation has not 'naturally' occurred. This latter figure can be assumed, as is the case in studies such as that by Shepard *et al.* (1993a,b) where the mean duration of the symptoms prior to treatment with balance retraining was 5 years. Dix (1986) explained that compensation occurs as a function of suppression and regeneration. 'This is effected by means of release from inhibition of excitatory neurons in the deafferentated nuclei via commissural filters from the nucleus of the intact side (Precht, Shinazu and Markham, 1966)'. She continued, 'the processes whereby long-term regeneration occur are complex, being dependent on the cerebellum (McCabe, 1970), the inferior olivary complex (Llinas and Walton, 1977) and visual mechanisms (Courjon *et al.*, 1977; Putkonnen, Courjon and Jeannerod, 1977)'. She explained that, 'vestibular symptoms abate only when a new intrinsic activity is generated from the nuclei themselves (McCabe, 1970)'. From clinical experience McCabe suggested that it was the provocation of dizziness itself which was responsible for this process, and experimental evidence of this was provided by the work of Lacour, Roll and Appaix (1976). In their studies a series of baboons underwent a unilateral neurectomy, and one group were restrained from movement for 4 days postoperatively by a plaster cast, while the second group were allowed to wander and explore freely. The restrained group showed significant impairment

in recovery rates measured as a function of the number of falls and postural asymmetry over 30 days in comparison with the unrestrained group.

With regard to central pathways, on the basis of her clinical experience, Dix (1974) suggested that diffuse damage of the central vestibular pathways, occurring in conjunction with hair cell damage caused by streptomycin ototoxicity can occasionally make it impossible to rehabilitate the patient. However, for skull fractures and head injuries involving central vestibular pathways she recommended starting the exercises 3 weeks postoperatively for fractures at the base of the skull and other skull fractures as soon as the condition of the patient warrants it.

Hence, within certain limits, habituation is thought to occur to movements made repeatedly which reliably elicit dizziness. As Norré (1984) put it, 'the clinical evolution after a sudden unilateral vestibular loss teaches us that progressively more and more movements become free from vertigo, beginning with the simplest and most frequently executed ones, whereas the rarely executed movements continue to elicit vertigo'. His distinction between positional components and major attacks is useful for both the patient's and physiotherapist's information, although different practices exist for setting limits (see below) to the number of exercises patients should attempt. In this useful chapter (Norré, 1984) he listed all 19 manoeuvres which combine some of Cawthorne and Cooksey's head and balance exercises, with other movements which seem based on the Hallpike manoeuvres.

Norré's approach relied on the assessment of each individual with regard to the movements which elicit disequilibrium or sensations of dizziness and nausea, and individually tailored programmes, as does Smith-Wheelock's (1991). Unlike Dix (1974, 1985), Norré did not specifically advocate a generalization of the balance exercise regimen at a later date to incorporate games which involve bending and stooping such as bowls or skittles which may be termed 'conditioning exercises' (e.g. Horak *et al.*, 1993).

In the more recent papers by physiotherapists in the USA, emphasis on general physical condition or fitness has been incorporated into the physiotherapeutic evaluation, in addition to the range of 'ordinary' movements, gait and posture examinations (Shumway-Cook and Horak, 1989, 1990; Herdman, 1991; Whitney and Blatchly, 1991). Herdman (1991) emphasized the need for rotational and caloric tests prior to the prescription of rehabilitative exercises but did not suggest that, for certain conditions like perilymphatic fistulae, vertebrobasilar artery insufficiency or acute suppurative otitis media, these exercises would be contraindicated. However, Herdman (1991) did recommend some useful adjuncts to the standard Cawthorne and Cooksey exercises which are summarized below.

Vestibular stimulation can be obtained by taping a

business card to the wall in front of the patient at a readable distance. The patient moves the head from side to side at varying speeds while focusing on the card, for 2 minutes without stopping. The exercise is then repeated with the head moved vertically. Both movement patterns are then repeated with a large pattern such as a checkerboard. The aim here is to continue until vision is no longer blurred.

These exercises can be performed while the patient is standing or seated. The rationale behind this approach is that 'adaptation of postural stabilising responses can be induced by altering visual experience' (Gonshor and Melvill Jones, 1980), and points to the constructive cerebral activity that occurs during visual perception, and how it relates to balance.

For oscillopsia, and treatment of a wide-based gait, with decreased head and neck rotation, Herdman suggested that patients may initially require assistive devices to prevent falling. However, she recommended a number of interesting interventions to help train vestibular ocular reflex suppression, including active eye/head movements between two targets, whereby first the eyes move between the two targets, then the head follows. By systematically varying the parameters of eye and head movement, in terms of both direction and speed, she introduced a wide range of simply performed retraining manoeuvres which can be performed while the patient is seated. This range of speed and direction would seem essential to overcome the findings of Collins (1969), that habituation is speed and direction specific.

Herdman went on to suggest a range of exercises not only to enable potentiation of the cervical ocular reflex, involving whole body rotations, but also a very cautious, graded removal of proprioceptive cues. This would involve asking a patient to spend two 10-minute periods a day standing with their feet as close together as they can manage with their hands being removed from the wall for gradually increasing periods as the feet are moved gradually closer together. Precautions have to be taken to prevent the patient from falling as they progress through these increasing challenges, which should be carried out over a period of time, with supervision at first.

It is only after these exercises are tolerated that she recommended walking on foam or walking round in circles with the head turning from side to side. Hence she has devised a system of rehabilitation which can be increased in complexity in small stages, thereby reducing the risk of falling, and which seems to be adaptable to even severely affected bilateral cases. She did not present any data or group comparisons, but did offer creative variations on existing techniques for maximizing visual control of postural mechanisms and the techniques available to enable maximization of the use of somatosensory cues. She suggested that these challenges should only gradually be increased in terms of the degree of task difficulty to which the patient is exposed. These techniques are

therefore easily adaptable to goal planning procedures of the type proposed by McKenna (1987).

Shumway–Cook and Horak (1989) offered a very comprehensive approach to the assessment of the dizzy patient, including objective evaluation of physical status, range of motion, strength of sensation, coordination and pain. They recommended assessing balance control in sitting and standing and using norm-referenced tests (of which computerized dynamic posturography is one category). They also separately assessed gaze stabilization and eye-head coordination. Hence they recommended a general musculoskeletal evaluation, and assessment of pain levels, in static and in movement conditions (Table 22.5). These are examined in addition to vertigo elicited by position changes. They further suggested examining the choice of strategy used by the patient to correct perturbations of balance, namely the ankle strategy, whereby the whole body pivots from the ankle; the hip strategy, where the body bends at the hip; or the stepping strategy where the patient has to take a step to stop himself from falling (see Figure 22.1).

Table 22.5 Functions examined in a rehabilitation assessment

I		*Postural control in sitting/standing/walking*
	A	Musculoskeletal components
		Joint range of motion
		Muscular strength
		Pain
		Sensation
		Alignment
	B	Motor coordination components
		Postural movement strategies
		Adaptation of strategies to task and context
	C	Sensory organization components
		Use of senses to detect centre of mass movement in different sensory contexts
		Perception of stability
II		*Eye-head coordination for gaze stabilization*
	A	Oculomotor control – saccade and smooth pursuit
	B	Gaze stabilization during head motion
	C	Visual modulation of vestibular-ocular responses
III		*Motion perception*
	A	Dizziness questionnaire
	B	Vertiginous positions and movement test
IV		*Physical conditioning*

Reproduced with permission from Shumway-Cook and Horak, *Neurologic Clinics*, **8**, 444, 1990, George Thieme Verlag

It is assumed by various workers in this field that the choice of strategy seems to be unconscious and related to some extent to whether there is unilateral or bilateral vestibular involvement (Black *et al.*, 1988) but, as Balzer (1991) pointed out, the extent to which dynamic platform posturography will actually reveal differences in balance performance will depend in part on the stage of compensation the patient has reached. Hence the dependence on either the hip strategy or the ankle strategy will reduce as compensation proceeds, such that the patient will use whichever strategy is needed in a given surface condition (Nashner and Peters, 1990).

These strategies can be examined using low technology techniques of altering proprioceptive feedback and visual feedback, such as shown below (Shumway-Cook and Horak, 1986, 1989). The more expensive or high technology techniques for assessing these strategies, will be discussed briefly in a later section.

There has been a considerable growth in the number of publications concerning the physiotherapeutic management of balance problems and only a brief review is possible here. Herdman (1990, 1991) suggested innovative strategies for the management of visual symptoms by training vestibular ocular reflex suppression at a variety of head velocities and orientations, and she also proposed some new approaches to help the patient gradually increase his use of somatosensory information. Hamid (1991) looked at patients who reported motion sensitivity while out walking, suggesting a novel adaptation of the notion of standing on foam, namely walking on 18 pillows laid out in a line, slowly adding head movements at a variety of inclinations and velocities. He reported on the effectiveness of this approach with a sample of patients and usefully suggested the strategy of setting 'homework' exercises, once a degree of proficiency has been gained, thus making it possible to use telephone follow ups rather than repeated visits to the clinic. He also proposed that with this group, progress can take as long as 2 years (thus making considerations involving the economic use of costly clinical time through telephone follow ups more salient).

Although it may be technically impossible completely to separate out the effects of the visually-based retraining programmes from those presumed to be based on somatosensory retraining (in the intact human), there are now several new methods of assessing the impact of these retraining approaches using objective measures. Devices for the assessment of sway, including biofeedback devices, have proliferated and present a sometimes bewildering array of possible choices in the best way to provide objective evidence of the numerous changes that occur during vestibular compensation. However, it often seems that studies which look at treatment effects are generally clinically based and observational, rather than formal clinical trials, although there are some notable exceptions, summarized below.

In a study by Horak *et al.* (1993), patients who had positional and/or movement related dizziness for more than 6 months and abnormal posturography were randomly assigned to three treatment groups.

These were described as vestibular rehabilitation, general conditioning exercises, and vestibular suppressant medication. The study was designed to answer a number of long-standing theoretical issues, namely the effects of vestibular suppressant medication (here diazepam and meclozine) as opposed to the effects of a specific balance retraining programme. Their approach to assessment of the dizzy patient is summarized earlier (see Table 21.5) and discussed elsewhere (Shumway–Cook and Horak, 1990) but effectively leads to a quite complex individualized physiotherapy programme. Unlike Shepard's study (Shepard *et al.*, 1993a) where some cases with central lesions were included, patients with CNS involvement, significant cardiac or orthopaedic problems, spontaneously fluctuating vestibular symptoms, or non-compliance with the treatment programme, were dropped from the study, although figures for this dropout rate were not given. The resultant groups consisted of 13 who received vestibular rehabilitation, four who received general conditioning ('keep fit') exercises and eight who received vestibular suppressant medication. Dizziness was assessed in terms of the number of positions which induced dizziness, using an intensity × duration measurement for a range of 12 head movements and positions. A questionnaire was used to assess the patient's estimate of whether their dizziness symptoms had 'improved', 'did not change', or had 'worsened'. Patients were randomly assigned to the three groups, and were not charged for treatment. The vestibular rehabilitation treatment consisted of two weekly one hour physical therapy sessions with specialist physical therapists who taught home exercises addressing the following five areas:

1 Habituation of position and/or movement evoked dizziness.
2 Retraining of sensory and/or motor control of balance.
3 Improvement of eye head coordination for gaze stabilization.
4 General conditioning exercises modified to address problems of dizziness, balance and gaze stabilization.
5 Standard therapeutic intervention for secondary limitations such as back and neck pain, limited joint range and headaches.

Subjects in the general exercises treatment group received the same number of treatments by the same physical therapist. However, they received general exercises, non-specific for the individual patient's symptoms, which were designed to improve strength, range or motion and cardiac function, e.g. stationary bicycle riding, and lifting light weights with the legs and arms. The patients in the medication group received meclozine or diazepam daily as directed by their physician, for 6 weeks or until they were asymptomatic.

The posturographic results indicated that in the

group receiving vestibular rehabilitation there was a significant reduction of postural sway in conditions 5 and 6 in which vestibular information is required for orientation ($P < 0.01$). However, changes in postural sway in all of the six conditions were negligible in the medication condition (Figure 22.5). Results were inconclusive for the group given the general conditioning exercises due to the large variability of results demonstrated in a small group. A further objective posturographic test was used, namely standing on one foot, eyes open and eyes closed, and these improved in both the eyes open and the eyes closed test

conditions for the vestibular rehabilitation group, and in the general exercise group, but not to the same extent. The medication group showed little change on posturographic measures as a result of treatment. All of the groups reported significant symptomatic improvement after 6 weeks of intervention, 92% of the vestibular rehabilitation group (12 out of 13), 75% of the general exercise group (three out of four) and 75% of the medication group (six out of eight). All other patients reported no change with the exception of one (out of eight) in the medication group who reported worse symptoms.

The authors concluded that the only group showing an improvement in balance was therefore that group receiving vestibular rehabilitation. 'Balance' here is presumably defined as the standing on one leg test (which was part of the retraining programme for the vestibular rehabilitation group so may be merely reflective of practice effects) and conditions 5 and 6 of the computerized dynamic posturography tests.

It is of course regrettable that the overall numbers in the three groups were too small to enable firm conclusions to be drawn, although the computerized dynamic posturography data are highly suggestive of their general conclusion being quite correct as to the superiority of the specific vestibular rehabilitation group over the other treatments. It is interesting that all groups showed improvements in the symptoms of dizziness.

Shepard *et al.* (1993) studied 152 patients, and the criteria for inclusion were as follows:

1 History of positional or motion provoked symptoms.
2 Evidence of abnormal postural control as demonstrated by dynamic posturography.
3 Indications of an uncompensated peripheral and or central vestibular system lesion identified physiologically by electronystagmography and rotation chair testing and documented functionally by dynamic posturography.

Earlier research had suggested that vestibular rehabilitation therapy was unsuccessful in patients with only spontaneously occurring events of disequilibrium. If other movement-related dizzy episodes occurred, between the spontaneous spells, then the therapy was found to be unsuccessful if the spontaneous events occurred more frequently than once a month. However, apart from the criterion of excluding patients with *any* spontaneously occurring vestibular episodes, the authors stated that 'no attempt was made to exclude patients on the basis of diagnosis, disease severity, or symptom duration'.

Within the 2 year interval of the study, 63 men and 89 women were enrolled and, after active therapy, they were further enrolled in a 'post therapy maintenance programme'. This involved gentle exer-

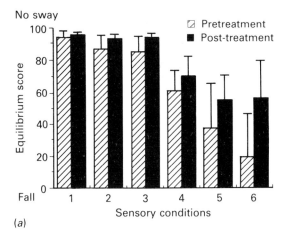

(a)

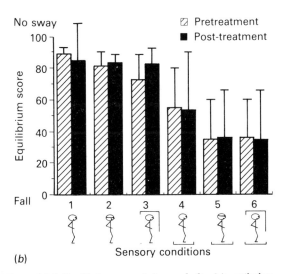

(b)

Figure 22.5 Equilibrium score before and after (*a*) vestibular rehabilitation and (*b*) medication treatment, in six sensory conditions. Equilibrium scores represent a three-trial average of peak-to-peak anterior-posterior body sway measured by surface centre of pressure and normalized for height. (From Horak *et al.*, 1992 with permission of the Publishers, Mosby Year Book, Inc)

cising, taking up golf, walking etc. The age range was 20 to 89 years with a mean age of 52 years. The mean length of time that this group of patients had suffered symptoms was 5 years, and none had experienced symptoms for less than 2 months. The length of active therapy was never less than 2 weeks, with a mean of 10 weeks (s.d. = 6 weeks). Analysis of the site of lesion and balance function studies suggested 58% of patients had unilateral peripheral disease with only 14 patients diagnosed as classic cases of benign paroxysmal positional vertigo. Twenty-three patients had mixed peripheral – central lesions; 8% had pure central vestibulo-ocular pathway involvement, 6% 'undetermined' and 5% had bilateral vestibular paresis.

All patients underwent a full muscular, neuromuscular and vestibular evaluation with specific functional deficits related to motion-provoked symptoms, or to abnormalities of gait and posture control included. These assessments, together with dynamic posturography, were used to develop the customized physiotherapy programmes which were taught to the patients for home use, with the use of infrequent return visits or telephone calls, for follow up.

The programmes devised for each patient had three main aims: habituation therapy for motion-provoked dizziness; correction of functional deficits of balance and gait; and initiation of a general conditioning programme.

The therapy outcome measures were described in detail elsewhere (Smith–Wheelock, Shepard and Telian, 1991). They consisted of two global measures and two specific measures, one related to postural control (dynamic posturography) and one indicative of changes in sensitivity to rapid positioning (motion sensitivity quotient).

The global rating scales consisted of a post-therapy symptom score, and each patient was also allocated a place on a disability scale, the measures of which are detailed below. They were then rated post-therapy, prior to being put on the maintenance programme, which was done when the patient was judged to have reached a plateau with respect to their rate of improvement, with vestibular rehabilitation therapy.

As shown in Figure 22.6, at least 85% of the patients (sum of scores 0, 1 and 2) showed some reduction in symptoms post-therapy compared with pre-therapy. A small percentage showed either no change or that their symptoms had worsened, namely 9% and 6% respectively. Figure 22.7 shows the distribution of disability scores pre- and post-therapy. The mean post-therapy disability score was significantly lower than the pre-therapy levels ($P < 0.001$). While 85% showed some reduction in disability score, the group showing most resistance were those on established long-term sick leave or a disability pension (in category 5).

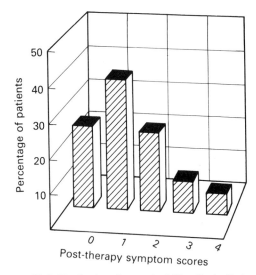

Figure 22.6 Distribution of scores for 152 patients. Post-therapy symptom scores as defined in text indicating percentage of patients (see Table 22.6)

Therapy was longer for those with mixed lesions (Figure 22.8*a*) and those taking suppressive medications (Figure 22.8*b*) and those with indications of prolonged latencies for recovery from induced forward or backward sway (Figure 22.8*c*).

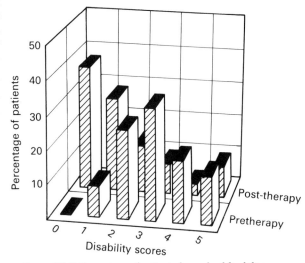

Figure 22.7 Percentage of patients for each of disability rating scores shown for pre-therapy and post-therapy ratings (disability scale explained in text, see Table 22.6)

It would therefore seem that there is now some evidence to suggest that while medication seems to reduce the symptoms of dizziness, it does not lead to

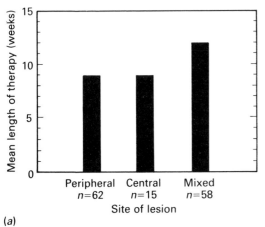

(a)

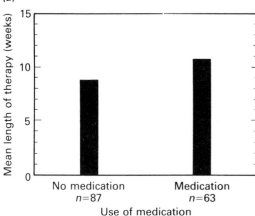

(b)

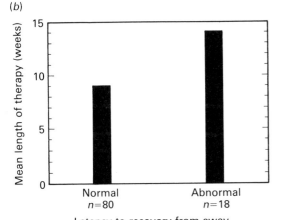

(c)

Figure 22.8 Mean length of active therapy in weeks as function of: (*a*) principal site of lesion as determined by balance function evaluation; (*b*) utilization of vestibular suppressive medication; (*c*) latency to onset of recovery from induced sway, as determined from pre-therapy movement coordination testing from dynamic posturography. Asterisks mark conditions that were statistically long from others at *P* < 0.05 level. (From Shepard *et al.*, 1993a, by kind permission of the authors)

Table 22.6 Global rating scales used to evaluate the effects of vestibular and balance rehabilitation therapy

	Disability scale	*Post-therapy symptom score*
0	No disability Negligible symptoms	No symptoms remaining at the end of therapy
1	No disability Bothersome symptoms	Marked improvement in the symptoms, mild symptoms remain
2	Mild disability Performs usual work duties but symptoms interfere with outside activities	Mild improvement; definite persistent symptoms remaining
3	Moderate disability Symptoms disrupt performance of both usual work duties and outside activities	No changes in symptoms relative to pre-therapy period
4	Recent severe disability On medical leave or had to change job because of symptoms	Symptoms worsened with therapy activities on a persistent basis relative to pre-therapy period
5	Long-term severe disability Unable to work for over one year, or established permanent disability with compensation payments	

Reprinted with permission (Shepard *et al.*, 1993a)

any significant improvement in balancing function over time, unlike the vestibular rehabilitation therapy (Horak *et al.*, 1993). It also seems that medication may marginally increase the time spent in rehabilitation before reaching the 'plateau' (Shepard *et al.*, 1993a) that determined the progression on to the maintenance programme of exercises in their approach. However, the types of medication used by patients in Shepard *et al's*. study were not specified, hence direct comparisons with Horak's results are not possible. Furthermore, the choice of which patient does or does not receive medication may be dependent on an initial assessment of symptom severity but this was not explicitly examined in Shepard's study. It is interesting that those patients who were already on established invalidity benefit or pensions improved less than the other groups, although it would have been helpful to see how symptom severity related to this aspect of socioeconomic status, perhaps through regression or covariate analysis (using analysis of variance).

The other interesting group was those with a history of head injury (with or without loss of consciousness) as they did less well (in terms of both of the outcome measures) than the other groups ($P < 0.004$). The data were also analysed according to the pattern or result on the sensory organization test, and showed that there were significantly poorer results for those patients having a visual vestibular dysfunction or severe dysfunction patterns, in addition to those whose performance on four out of six of the sensory organization tests was poor, and who were thus classified as 'severe'. Thus it seems that the patients with the visual vestibular pattern, who are hypersensitive to destabilizing movements of the platform, when the visual information was normal, are a distinct subgroup with more intractable problems that have a less rapid response to this form of physiotherapy. Again it would be interesting to know more about this group in terms of whether they had ancillary symptoms such as bobbing oscillopsia or visual vertigo, or a history of migraine, in addition to vestibular dysfunction, as this may help in the understanding of these results (Kuritzky, Ziegler and Hassanein, 1981). Hamid's observations regarding the requirement of putting aside 2 years to treat a group of motion-sensitive patients lends further weight to the notion that they might also constitute a distinct subgroup (Hamid, 1992).

Shepard *et al.* (1993b) commented that the relative safety and significant success rate of the therapy programme for the treatment of uncompensated vestibular patients had led to a greater use of this approach (as opposed to nerve sections) as a method of management. They also commented that the management of perilymphatic fistulae (in those patients without hearing complications) had changed, in the direction of using surgical repair only in cases where patients became worse during physiotherapy.

A further aspect of physiotherapeutic management deserves mention, namely the observations reported by Smith–Wheelock, Shepard and Telian (1991) on an 'over enthusiastic or over aggressive approach to physiotherapy'. They described the referral patterns, the types of patients seen, and applications of vestibular rehabilitation therapy, which includes those patients with a 'psychological overlay', although whether these include those patients suffering from panic disorder and vestibular dysfunction is unclear. However, it is an excellent source reference for both basic techniques of physical examination using sensory tests and simple posturographic tests (for which norms are available). They additionally pointed out the relevance of checking on musculoskeletal factors when attempting to isolate the causal factors in determining any asymmetry in the weight distribution. Hence although this clinical team used computerized posturography it also used less technologically-based systems of balance assessment which are described in this useful text. Methods of assessing gait and motion

sensitivity are also outlined, although they did not use the full 19 rapid changes in body position used by Norré (1984).

In terms of the time span required for rehabilitation, the general guidelines given are between 2 weeks and 6 months, and again a distinction was made between balancing training such as standing on one leg and leaning, or practising weight shifts, and habituation training. General conditioning exercises are seen as being necessary in order to counteract the perceived assumption about activity thought to be prevalent in balance patients, namely that 'less is better', and these authors also mention escalating spirals of interactions between lack of activity, loss of fitness, and failure to retrain the sense of balance, although interestingly they leave out all mention of anxiety, worry or stress.

However, these authors emphasized that the conditioning exercises need to be presented with a conservative attitude because, 'An overly aggressive programme can be counterproductive, and quickly make the patient worse. Fatigue can also lead directly to decompensation'. They illustrated these assertions with a case history of a woman who had been accustomed to taking 30-minute daily walks prior to her balance problem so resumed this level of activity at the start of treatment. After 3 months she became frustrated and 'felt much worse'. Very similar observations have led the present author in the past to recommend the use not only of breathing exercises to correct hyperventilation syndrome, but also a graded approach to the reintroduction to greater muscular effort, and greater periods of time spent outdoors (Beyts, 1991). Smith–Wheelock recommended a very cautious and graded reintroduction of muscular effort, with this patient being asked to do 5 minutes walking each day with a 2 minute increase each week. Hence, although physiotherapy is geared towards encouraging greater levels of activity, there are some exceptions to this rule, and a progressive or graded approach may be advisable, particularly with the more chronic patients as chronic stress can affect lactate metabolism (Pitts and McClure, 1967) so that muscular effort is difficult to sustain.

These authors also emphasized the importance of patient counselling. The patients were taught that pacing their activities to avoid fatigue is critical to allow for compensation to take place. This idea of pacing oneself and setting a manageable pace is not dissimilar to the notions of either goal planning (McKenna, 1987) or indeed to the use of systematic desensitization which is merely a guiding framework to allow a sensible pace of progress, albeit based on a pace of stress management. However the postulated delay to habituation caused by high anxiety (Beyts, 1987) is not explicitly part of Smith–Wheelock's more practical approach to management.

Management of benign paroxysmal positional vertigo with the liberatory manoeuvre and the canalith repositioning procedure

Another group of non-invasive treatment interventions which merits discussion is those whose rapid effects are explained in terms of the movement of otolithic debris to a physiologically inert area in the semicircular canals, namely the utricle (Epley, 1992). The work of Brandt and Daroff (1980) which used rapid positioning of the patient from an upright seated position to each side, was thought to be so effective in such a short period because of the mechanical movement of the otolithic debris to the utricle. Hence, Brandt and Daroff (1980), Semont, Freyss and Vitte (1988) and Epley (1992) all described treatments thought to treat the effects of cupulolithiasis in benign paroxysmal positional vertigo.

Benign paroxysmal positional vertigo was first described by Bárány in 1921, and more fully defined by Dix and Hallpike who originated the provocative test now known as the Hallpike manoeuvre, with destructive surgical manoeuvres being the treatment proposed for this condition at that time.

Surgical interventions for the condition were associated with significant postoperative morbidity (Epley, 1992). Hence Epley proposed that these recent non-invasive approaches to management remove these risks. Epley reviewed the evidence for the notion of cupulolithiasis and called his own procedure the canalith repositioning procedure. While it is beyond the scope of this chapter to evaluate fully the evidence for and against cupulolithiasis, the very high success rates reported by Semont, Freyss and Vitte (1988) and Epley (1992) deserve mention.

Epley's procedure relies on applying two forms of vibration during a series of five position changes. First, the affected ear is identified using Hallpike's positioning procedure, and then the angle of the patient's head is raised through a series of positions. This, coupled with the vibration, is thought to move the otolithic debris out of the posterior semicircular canal. In Epley's words (1992): 'The rationale is to use head position and vibration to cause free canaliths (postulated) to migrate by gravitation completely out of the PSC [posterior semicircular canal], by way of the common crus, to the utricle, where they would no longer affect the dynamics of the semicircular canals'. He suggested that the induced nystagmus is usually minimally influenced by visual fixation, so is usually visible to the observer's naked eye. After completion of a treatment session the patient is required to keep his head upright for 48 hours so that loose debris will not gravitate back into the posterior semicircular canal. In this respect the methodology resembles that proposed by Semont, Freyss and Vitte (1988).

Epley (1992) summarized results in 30 cases, where everyone achieved good initial resolution of benign paroxysmal positional vertigo. However, there was a recurrence in nine of these, although repeating the procedure was again highly successful. Epley pointed out that because the canalith repositioning procedure has a low risk and low morbidity, the possibility of recurrence does not significantly degrade its value, so he proposed that this makes it the treatment of choice when compared with a singular neurectomy.

Semont, Freyss and Vitte (1988) similarly reported very high success rates with their liberatory manoeuvre, which they described as an astonishing result. All of these treatment forms rely on the theoretical explanation of moving otolithic debris to a physiologically inert space. Semont *et al.* reported their success rate from 711 patients was 93% with two manoeuvres. The affected ear was identified using the Dix–Hallpike manoeuvre, and then the liberatory manoeuvre is applied. It is described as follows (Semont, Freyss and Vitte, 1988):

'The patient is laid on the ipsilateral side to the sick ear with his head slightly declined. The nystagmus can appear in this condition, but one must wait until it stops. If nothing happens the head is turned to 45° facing up in order to have the cupula in a perpendicular plane to gravity. In this position, after a variable latency, the paroxysmal rotating nystagmus rolling towards the examination table appears. One waits until it has completely stopped and then the patient is left in this position for 2 or 3 minutes. Then holding the patient's head and neck with two hands, he is swung quickly to the opposite side. The speed of the head must be zero at the very moment the head touches the examination table. Then a rotatory nystagmus appears still rolling towards the sick ear which is now the higher one. It must not be an inverted nystagmus. The nystagmus is slightly different: wide amplitude slower frequency, not so paroxysmal as the original one'.

The manoeuvre thus continues through a further two positions, but this section is quoted so as to illustrate some possibly self-evident constraints upon its application, namely that the cervical vertebrae have to be very healthy to cope with this kind of manoeuvre and obese patients or those with spinal degeneration may also be unsuitable candidates. Norré and Beckers (1985) also pointed out these factors in this comparison of the liberatory manoeuvre and vestibular habituation therapy. Herdman (1990) usefully pointed out that a diagnosis which may be confused with that of benign paroxysmal positional vertigo, is cervical vertigo and De Jong and Bles (1986) reported a test to differentiate these, namely that patients with cervical vertigo will fall backwards if they extend their neck with eyes closed. Herdman further suggested that another similar complaint of perilymph fistula may cause similar nystagmus with similar position changes, although other forms of nystagmus also occur (Healy, Strong and Sampogna, 1974; Singleton *et al.*, 1978).

Herdman (1990) was more cautious in her suggestion regarding contraindications for the liberatory manoeuvre than was Norré (1985), saying, 'Elderly patients may be less tolerant of the liberatory manoeuvre than younger patients especially if they move cautiously because of other conditions like arthritis'.

She also pointed out that as in the canalith repositioning procedure, the liberatory manoeuvre requires the patient not to bend the head forwards or backwards for 48 hours afterwards. Cyr (1993) pointed out that, with adequate precounselling and preparation, compliance with this rather constraining requirement of this treatment can be facilitated. Cyr recommended that the patient is advised to avoid being collected from the clinic in a sports car for example, as bending to get in and out of it is contraindicated. He also recommended advising the patient to avoid brushing their hair or cleaning their teeth, all of which requires head movements. Similarly, sleeping in an upright chair with a high back, while wearing a neck collar is also recommended in order to reduce the likelihood of disturbing the repositioned otoliths.

As with other rather new ideas, it is helpful to learn from the practitioners, hence Herdman's paper reviewing diagnostic and management issues is highly recommended. On a more academic level, it is worth emphasizing that despite the impressively high success rates reported by Semont, Freyss and Vitte (1988) and by Epley (1992) for these theoretically similar manoeuvres, they have not been subjected to controlled clinical trials, where a control group is used. This may be vital to confirm these high success rates, for when Norré (1988) compared Semont's manoeuvre to his vestibular habituation therapy, he reported only a 53% success rate compared with Semont's figure of 93%. He also pointed out that the main use for the liberatory manoeuvre had to be with only unilateral cases, the non-obese, and those patients without significant arthritis, while his vestibular habituation therapy remained the main therapeutic treatment for all other diagnostic groups. Hence these psychological and physical effects can be separated out only through the appropriate use of control groups, to exclude type 1 errors and placebo effects.

Just before going to press a controlled trial was reported by Steenerson and Cronin (1996) which suggested little difference in outcomes between canalith repositioning procedures and vestibular habituation exercises, although the untreated group did much less well. They suggest the consideration of combining the two forms of treatment.

Objective measures of balance function

Norré has argued that posturographic measures are more likely to chart progress through vestibular compensation than electronystagmographic measures. This may be because, as proponents of posturographic testing point out, posturography effectively tests how well the balance system is integrating information from all three of the sensory systems involved in the 'sense' of balance (Nashner and Peters, 1990). Furthermore, because subjective reporting of internal physiological processes is likely to be inaccurate (Nisbett and De Camp Wilson, 1977; Frcka *et al.*, 1983) and due to the fact that, for example, hair cell regeneration presumably occurs at levels below that of conscious awareness, it may be that some other aspects of the recovery do as well. This does not mean that the author advocates the choice of subjective versus objective measures (or vice versa) as the 'gold standard' measure of recovery, but that as vestibular compensation is a multilevel process of change, the investigators of such change need to apply thought when selecting an index of change due to the complexities of the processes involved. Furthermore, any desynchrony between awareness of compensation, and the physiological changes that occur during compensation, add to this complexity.

For example, it may be that the brain makes choices as to the use of a hip, or ankle, or stepping strategy in order to remain upright, and these choices occur at preconscious levels and at latencies too rapid to allow for conscious decision-making processes. Similarly, reliance on proprioception versus visual information to correct inaccurate vestibular information presumably occurs at preconscious levels, given the instantaneous nature of the decisions needed when, for example, negotiating a slippery slope. However, changes in the use of such sources of sensory information as a result of balance retraining are best illustrated by case histories, and a brief example is given below. Nevertheless, Hunter and Balzer (1991) discussed the application of computerized dynamic posturography analyses to the understanding of multifactorial balance disorders, as in cases where peripheral neuropathy has occurred or where visual problems have degraded these sources of sensory input, when computerized dynamic posturography analysis is a very useful rehabilitative tool. Hunter and Balzer (1991) and Nashner and Peters (1990) offer very useful reviews of these applications.

Some of the more complex computerized systems for the assessment of balancing are, in fact, biofeedback devices, which reportedly can be very helpful in physiotherapy where central damage has occurred (as in cerebrovascular accidents) or where injury to a limb has affected the patient's weight distribution. However, in vestibular dysfunctions without such complexities there are also a number of low

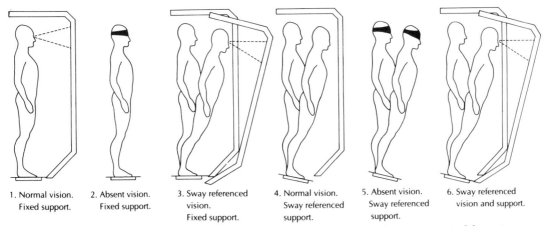

1. Normal vision. Fixed support.   2. Absent vision. Fixed support.   3. Sway referenced vision. Fixed support.   4. Normal vision. Sway referenced support.   5. Absent vision. Sway referenced support.   6. Sway referenced vision and support.

Figure 22.9 The six sensory conditions examined using a dynamic platform posturography or computerized dynamic posturography

technology and low cost alternatives to the computerized systems.

In the computerized dynamic posturography system of assessment generally there are six sensory conditions, summarized in Figure 22.9. These are therefore graded with reference to the degree of difficulty such that in condition 6 the patient is able to rely only on the vestibular information, while visual input is made inaccurate (with movement of the visual surround) and the platform moves, generating a proprioceptive 'challenge'. In condition 5 only the vestibular information is accurate as visual information is removed completely rather than altered. In condition 3 the visual surround is sway referenced while proprioception is unaltered and in condition 4 proprioceptive challenge is present while visual information is accurate. These conditions are therefore analogous to these in the clinical test for sensory interaction in balance developed by Shumway–Cook and Horak (1986), although the patient is not supported by a harness in this latter test (Figure 22.10).

Here, Shumway–Cook and Horak (1986) used rubber foam and a Chinese lantern to provide the altered proprioceptive information and the altered visual information for those sensory challenges. The reader is referred to their texts for further details of their use. Great care must be taken when using this test to avoid falls, in view of the lack of safety harness, as although the patient may successfully employ one of the three strategies (hip, ankle or stepping) to correct their perturbations of balance, they may not be able to stop themselves from falling in the more difficult conditions.

Another low technology method of testing balance and gait has been developed by Fregly and Graybiel (1968) where similar caveats about safety apply. They have timed the performance of various balance tests (e.g. the Romberg test, or standing on one leg with eyes closed) for a variety of different patient

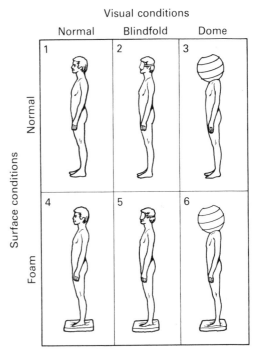

Figure 22.10 The clinical test of sensory interaction in balance (From Shumway-Cook and Horak, 1986, with permission)

groups, so as to provide norms for performance for a wide selection of diagnostic categories. As these require only a line of 12 foot (4 m) taped to the clinic floor, these provide objective measures without the need for a great deal of expenditure – only a stopwatch and 12 foot (4 m) of tape is needed. However, their 'normal' group were Air Force cadets who might arguably be fitter than the general population.

Other posturographic systems exist, and are continually being developed, and hence cannot be reviewed in any depth here. However, in terms of the degree of investigation, the computerized dynamic posturography system has been thoroughly examined (Nashner and Peters, 1990) and provides the basis for the individually structured physiotherapy programme developed by Shepard *et al.* (1993) and Horak *et al.* (1993), which is in wide use.

A case history which illustrates how computerized dynamic posturography can be used in rehabilitation to assess progress involves a young female professional with a stressful job in the legal profession, whose progressive hearing loss caused by endolymphatic hydrops made it more and more difficult for her to cope in the courtroom. Due to the subsequent loss of her job, she decided she wished to make use of the enforced career break to sail round the world. She presented with moderate balance problems in that she had a few positional components on rapid head movement, but her main problem was negotiating stairs. She found she habitually 'froze' at the top of the staircase and had to concentrate to go downstairs, which she did rather slowly. In terms of how she managed when actually sailing, she reported always sailing with her partner and apparently experienced no motion sickness on short trips of up to 2 hours. In an attempt to make the goals of balance rehabilitation realistic, it was suggested that although she could be offered a range of training programmes to develop her sense of balance, it could not be guaranteed that she would be able to sail round the world without experiencing any symptoms. This is partly because anyone with a progressive condition cannot be given unequivocal guarantees which imply that they will never experience major vertigo attacks again. All that can be offered is that the patient will understand how the balance system works such that skills to retrain the sense of balance can be learnt should a further episode of vertigo cause further problems, with positional components or indeed motion sickness.

Following successful resolution in a few weeks of her relatively minor problems with both her positional components and her hyperventilation syndrome, using Innocenti's (1993) approach and the Cawthorne and Cooksey exercises, she was asked to check her endurance for periods at sea with longer boat trips, and to train her use of proprioceptive information without visual information, as she might have to cope in the dark at sea on a long voyage. Hence in the level 5 of the Cawthorne and Cooksey exercises where the patient is required to climb a flight of stairs with eyes open, then progress to eyes closed, she was asked to work on her progress with eyes open, and then to work especially hard on the eyes closed condition, setting goals involving progressive increases in speed, and progressively less dependence on the bannisters. Her initial scores on the EquiTest showed an adapting pattern for use of somatosensory challenges with eye closure, which clearly needed further work (test 5). Similarly she had problems ignoring visual error (test 3).

She was also asked to walk on a mattress positioned near a wall and the solid back of a sofa, after Hamid's technique (Hamid, 1992), so as to provide support in case she staggered. She was asked to practise walking both backwards and forwards on this. Using a combined programme of breathing exercises, habituation training and this somatosensory challenging, she was able to effect quite marked changes over a period of 6 months in terms of both the composite scores from the EquiTest analysis, and on the separate subtests. As the bulk of this type of somatosensory retraining was done in the winter when she was unable to go sailing, it rather suggests that, as Hamid proposed, this form of exposure to a difficult proprioceptive challenge may be quite a useful form of rehabilitation for the vestibular system. Using Computerized Dynamic Posturography it was possible to demonstrate significant improvements on conditions 4 to 6 where somatosensory challenging is used. These improvements were measured by the patients' self reports of improvements in symptoms and balance.

This case illustrates how it is possible to monitor objectively the effects of different types of balance retraining using posturography, which is essential if evaluating these new variations to the Cawthorne and Cooksey exercises. However, as she was both a highly motivated and intelligent patient, she persevered with some exercises involving difficult balance challenges which may be too difficult for the more infirm case. Hence these techniques should only be employed after a thorough assessment of the patient's capabilities, particularly as Herdman's (1991) recommendations for the severe bilateral cases illustrate, some patients have difficulty even with standing with their feet together if they are close to a blank wall with no fixation spot available to stabilize them. Hence there has to be a degree of individual tailoring of the programme specific to the needs of each patient, as recommended by Shepard *et al.* (Shepard, Telian and Smith–Wheelock, 1990; Shepard *et al.*, 1993a,b) and Shumway–Cook and Horak (1989).

It is not really possible at this stage to state categorically that objective measures derived from posturography are more of a 'gold standard' than questionnaire measures, because of the complex changes that occur during compensation, and the wide range of environments an individual may encounter. For example, a pebble beach in the dark may be very difficult for many patients with vestibular disorders because of the somatosensory and visual challenges to remaining upright posed by such an environment. However, as it seems that patients regain greater freedom of choice of the strategy they need to use (hip or ankle) to keep them upright, as they progress through balance training (Nashner and Peters, 1990). They also seem to reduce their overall level of sway, so that the scatter plots of the 'centre of gravity' show less spread, as in the case history given earlier. However, in terms of the definition of handicap given earlier, it may ultimately be irrelevant to some patients whether or not they can negotiate pebble beaches in the dark. Hence both subjective complaint and objective measures of balancing should ideally be used in the setting of treatment goals.

Computerized dynamic posturography cannot localize the lesion in the vestibular system as it is relatively insensitive to compensated unilateral vestibular lesions, so does not provide a substitute for the routine diagnostic tests in the process of differential diagnosis. Similarly, subjective reporting may be of more benefit in assessing how a patient copes in a variety of challenging environmental conditions than posturography. Arguably posturography is less easy to 'fake' than a verbal report, as 'demand characteristics' such as the desire to please the 'nice doctor who helped the patient feel better' are a possible source of error there. Hence there are those who could argue that objective test results overcame the problem of demand awareness, however well designed or well validated the self-report measures are. As yet no one has carried out a sufficiently complex clinical study comparing the two types of measurement to the present author's knowledge, or indeed examined the role of demand awareness on results of a questionnaire measure of rehabilitation, or on computerized dynamic posturography measures of rehabilitation.

Physiologically inconsistent results are easily detected using computerized dynamic posturography. For example, if a patient falls on conditions 1–3 but manages the more difficult conditions 5 and 6 without any problems one might reasonably suspect a degree of exaggeration. Similarly, if a patient reports no problems in walking or driving to the clinical examination, but falls on conditions 1–3 then, again, one might suspect a degree of exaggeration.

In summary, therefore, through computerized dynamic posturography it is now possible to measure objectively the relative contribution of somatosensory, visual, and vestibular inputs to the sense of balance in relation to normative data. Hence for patients with multisensory deficits such as visual or a peripheral neuropathy, these types of posturographic analysis offer a powerful tool enabling the clinician to detect the problem areas and direct the retraining programme to those aspects. As Smith–Wheelock, Shepard and Telian (1991) proposed, the patient should be able to choose flexibly between the hip, ankle or stepping strategies depending on the type of balance challenges posed by a range of environments, e.g. stairs, pebble beaches, slippery slopes etc. They offer a range of techniques to help establish this flexibility of choice in that useful paper.

Hyperventilation syndrome and panic attacks (management of complications)

There is a considerable diversity of opinion in the literature as to the average time it takes for a patient to compensate from a vestibular lesion, ranging from a few hours in the case of a successfully performed liberatory manoeuvre (Semont, Freyss and Vitte, 1988) to 6 months (Horak *et al.*, 1993) or to a year (Pfaltz, 1983) or more. Shepard *et al.* (1993a), Yardley (1994) and Pratt and McKenzie (1958) reported cases where vestibular compensation has not occurred (in the absence of rehabilitation) for several years. Hence opinion as to the degree of disability or handicap experienced by vertiginous patients fluctuates considerably from author to author. One of the primary reasons why compensation may be delayed is because frequent vertiginous episodes may not allow sufficient time for the sensory reintegration to occur. Hence it is interesting to note Shepard's observations concerning treating only those patients with unpredictable episodes of dizziness (major attacks) occurring less than once a month. Even so it is encouraging that 85% of this less florid patient group showed significant improvement with the tailor-made rehabilitation programmes. It is nevertheless probable that other explanations for a failure to compensate exist beyond the possibility of undetected central lesions (Rudge and Chambers, 1982).

Given the complexity of both the balance system itself and the processes of conditioning and habituation involved, I have proposed that the effects of anxiety in reducing the tendency to habituate or the effects of hyperventilation causing cerebral hypoxia through vasoconstriction (Skinhøj, 1973; Gibson, 1979; Wilson and Kim, 1981; Beyts, 1987, 1991) are significant contributing factors to this delay in compensation. Estimates of the prevalence of hyperventilation syndrome in samples of dizzy patients vary from between 30 and 58% (Drachman and Hart, 1972; Theunissen, Huygen and Folgering, 1986). However, recent work by Jacob *et al.* (Jacob, 1983; Jacob *et al.*, 1988, 1989) and Sklare *et al.* (1990) rather suggests that some patients whose presentation is suggestive of panic disorder (a diagnosis used in the USA, from the DSM III system of Psychiatric Classification) in fact frequently suffer from undetected audiovestibular dysfunction. Although the connections between anxiety, 'street neurosis' and various forms of anxiety have a very long history in terms of studies documenting this (Hinchcliffe, 1967; Guraltnick 1973; Stephens, 1975; Hallam, 1985; Hallam and Stephens, 1985), this literature receives scant mention in many recent publications on rehabilitation.

This may be, as Jacob *et al.* (1993) have suggested, because patients with 'psychosomatic disorders' are alexithymic (i.e. dislike discussing emotion) and prefer to be managed within a strictly medical framework and in a non-psychological way. Hence any mention of the stress caused by the complaint may be vigorously denied. Similarly, somatization is considered a process whereby patients with psychological symptoms convert them unintentionally into physical symptoms, and sometimes then begin to persuade themselves that the only way they can possibly get help is to have a 'real' physical symptom, which can occur in cases of chronic hyperventilation syndrome. Such patients, who may have expended considerable time and expense on unsuccessfully seeking a solution for their intractable or bizarre symptoms, can become quite tense or annoyed if any evidence of psychological factors causing appreciable changes is presented to them. This is probably because they feel that the stigma of being chronically physically ill is bad enough without the addition of a further psychological 'label'. Hence, methods of discussing psychological factors have to be very carefully thought out and presented, and one way is simply to state that any recommendations involving psychological techniques used such as relaxation methods are merely borrowed from psychological procedures as a means to an end, namely the notion of using the mind to help the body. Salkovskis (1989b) discussed presenting such attempts to manage health anxiety very diplomatically and, as Jacob *et al.* (1993) proposed, it seems essential to separate these cases from those who are malingering or who have 'insurance disease' (i.e. patients engaged in medico-legal battles where financial compensation is likely). These should be differentiated from health anxiety or somatization as the former behaviours are intentional rather than unintentional (Jacob *et al.*, 1993). Fortunately there are very diplomatic ways of suggesting that the patient tries to adopt a psychological framework (as an experiment) in an attempt to manage their symptoms (Salkovskis, 1989b). Similarly there are also a number of physical and psychological interventions for the treatment of hyperventilation syndrome (which is the probable precursor to the development of panic attacks) which involve no mention of any emotion whatsoever and rely mainly on the use of breathing exercises. Many clinicians may feel in such cases where there is a strong tendency to deny psychological factors, that it is appropriate to try conventional physiotherapy first before considering management of hyperventilation syndrome, should it be present. Hence a multidisciplinary team approach is the most successful framework for these diverse presentations of symptoms.

Hyperventilation syndrome can be very simply tested by asking the patient to overbreathe deliberately at between 40–60 breaths per minute, whereupon either a recording of induced nystagmus can be made (Kayan, 1987) or simply the number and duration of sensations induced can be recorded. There is disagreement in the literature as to whether 1.5 or 3 minutes should be the limit to the induction time

used to check if hyperventilation syndrome is present but, given the wide variety of sensations (which are usually seen by the patient as symptoms) that can be induced, it is a relatively short test of importance to the process of differential diagnosis. However, excluding respiratory disease or cardiac disease may also be necessary with specialist diagnostic tests.

The range of sensations that can be induced is given in Table 22.7.

Table 22.7 Common symptoms in chronic hyperventilation

Cardiac
    palpitations, pericardial pain, 'angina'
Neurological
    dizziness, faintness, visual disturbance, migrainous headache, numbness, 'pins and needles' in face and limbs
Respiratory
    shortness of breath, asthma, chest pain, excessive sighing
Gastrointestinal
    dysphagia, heartburn, burping, air swallowing
Muscular
    cramps, fibrositis pains, tremors, rarely tetany
Psychological
    anxiety, 'unreal' feelings, depersonalization, occasionally hallucinations
General
    weakness, exhaustion, lack of concentration, sleep disturbance, nightmares, emotional sweating, blackouts, faintness

As Innocenti (1993) pointed out, it is sometimes the case that patients with chronic hyperventilation syndrome have undergone numerous medical investigations of the symptoms (or sensations) arising from the effects of respiratory alkalosis, with no abnormalities found. This kind of situation is frustrating for both the patient and the clinician. She discussed this kind of case, describing the respiratory management of the type of patient who has presumably developed an exaggerated ventilatory response (Gorman *et al.*, 1988; Ley, 1988). In this type of patient, the arterial CO_2 is persistently low, and any increase in ventilation drops the CO_2 level further, resulting in more acute symptoms, hence an attempt to encourage the one breath per 6 seconds recommended as the 'normal' rate merely induces more symptoms.

Although Lum (1976) and Salkovskis and Clark (1986) retrained the breathing rate of hyperventilators to the one breath per 6 second level and thereby induced successful management, Innocenti (1993) has usefully described the management of the patients who cannot tolerate even a couple of minutes, breathing at 10 breaths per minute, whose management is considerably more complex.

Innocenti recommended that the patient lies down to receive instruction in a relaxed diaphragmatic breathing pattern, and that initially a recording is made of their resting breathing rate. She described two types of respiration cycle that can be used in treatment: the two-, and the three-phase cycle. In the two-phase version the patient breathes in and then gradually lets the air trickle out to use up the time, while in the three-phase cycle, the patient breathes in and out, but focuses on the gap between breaths as an opportunity to relax. She suggested that either the patient or therapist should monitor chest and abdomen movement by placing their hands on chest and abdomen, as generally the aim of treatment is to re-establish the rhythmic abdominal breathing that characterizes relaxation in the non-hyperventilator (Lum, 1976). Although Lum recommended the monitoring of abdominal and chest movements during training with electrodes (EMG), obviously it is helpful from the point of view of generalizing the therapy effects from the consulting room to the patient's home to have more portable biofeedback devices, and the patients own hands fulfil this function admirably.

In the patient for whom even short periods of paced breathing induce numerous sensations and therefore demonstrate an exaggerated ventilatory response, Innocenti (1993) suggested that the therapist uses the technique of continuous monotonous counting during the breathing cycles while gradually increasing the depth of the breath. The use of a tape recorder is often invaluable at this stage for those who cannot easily carry the memory of the new pattern, and as disturbances of concentration or

memory can occur in chronic hyperventilation the therapist should be wary of appearing over directive in this area. A further complication that can arise is that of relaxation induced tachycardia but this usually fades with perseverance with the relaxation technique and is seen as a habituation phenomenon (Ley, 1988).

Innocenti further suggested a variety of breathing problems demonstrating expiratory and inspiratory phases which are given in Figure 22.11.

Those patients whose periods of relaxation are disrupted by continuous unpleasant thoughts about their dizziness or other symptoms can be encouraged to try simply to redirect their attention back to their breathing rate, or to focus on relaxing their muscles when this occurs. It can also help to make a relaxation tape where, initially, the rationale for relaxation training is given, with particular attention given to a section on paced breathing. However, in the more acute case, the kind of individual breathing retraining suggested by Innocenti may be necessary, rather than a generic tape. This would involve very gradual modifications to the depth and duration of each breath based on modifying the patient's own breathing pattern, which may be one of those described above.

Salkovskis and Clark (1986) described the management of panic attacks using tapes for paced breathing, but added another therapeutic component, namely that of reinterpreting the symptoms as sensations.

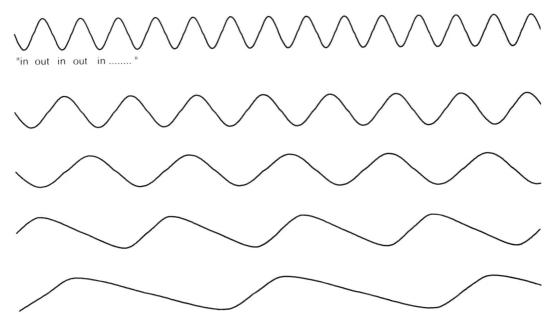

"in out in out in ...."

"in and out two three four and in and out two three four and in and ...."

Figure 22.11 Some suggested breathing patterns demonstrating a regular small tidal volume with various flow rates and periods. (From Innocenti, 1993, by kind permission of the Publishers, Churchill Livingstone)

Their vicious circle model of the factors involved in panic attacks is given in Figure 22.12 (Salkovskis and Clark, 1986).

This illustrates how the threatening stimulus (which can be external or an internal sensation such as dizziness) generates apprehension leading through respiratory alkalosis to increases in body sensations which are then interpreted as catastrophic. Common catastrophic beliefs in dizzy patients are that they will lose control in public, vomit, or fall over (Beyts, 1987; Yardley and Putman, 1992; Yardley *et al.*, 1992a, b). These types of cognitions concerning the potential negative predictive value, or a negative meaning of sensations, are implicated in the increase in measures of handicap caused by balance problems over time demonstrated by Yardley (1994). Hence although cognitive therapy techniques may ultimately be needed to correct any 'resilient' cognitions that do not simply fade as the hyperventilation syndrome responds to this more behavioural form of treatment (e.g. see Salkovskis and Warwick, 1986), for many anxious patients these more behavioural techniques are sufficient to reduce significantly their symptomology (i.e. breathing exercises).

Although the clinical trials of these techniques are not fully complete, the initial clinical impressions of their value with vertigo patients are favourable. So just as Davies, Mckenna and Hallam (1995), Stephens, Hallam and Jakes (1986) and Jakes (see chapter 4) have found that cognitive therapy is useful in challenging irrational or distorted thinking in patients distressed by tinnitus, similar techniques can be applied in this context to symptoms of dizziness and their behavioural and emotional sequelae. Obvi-

ously not all vertiginous patients require these approaches as significant numbers can be helped by tailored physiotherapy programmes, but an awareness of these techniques can make management of even the simpler case more straightforward.

Certainly, knowledge of cognitive restructuring techniques is useful in cases where patients have persistently overrestricted their activities despite achieving some compensation, e.g. take to their beds for weeks after one major vertiginous episode lasting a few hours, in case 'it comes back when I move'. Thus a combination of counselling regarding the mechanisms involved in balance, the need for habituation exercises for positional components, and balance retraining as in taking on mild balance challenges such as those involved in games involving stepping and leaning (and 'conditioning' exercises) may all be sufficient in the majority of cases to alleviate significantly the level of disability and handicap experienced by patients with vestibular dysfunction. In some more handicapped cases, referral for therapy with a clinical psychologist or psychiatrist may be necessary in addition to conventional physiotherapy or counselling, particularly where the secondary depression or anxiety seems too intractable to respond to simpler counselling techniques. However, significant inroads can be made into panic attacks (which is a relatively common secondary complaint) simply by challenging catastrophic fears about sensations actually caused by hyperventilation syndrome and by teaching the appropriate breathing and relaxation exercises. Just as some of the dizzy sensations in the course of habituation retraining become reinterpreted as being related to position changes, and hence become seen

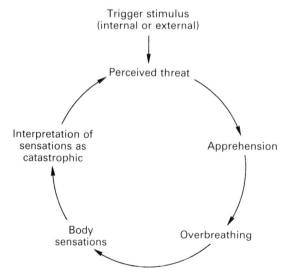

Figure 22.12 A schematic representation of the short-term interaction between cognitive and physiological mechanisms in hyperventilation-related panic attacks. (From Salkovskis and Clark, 1986, In: *Panic and Phobias*, edited by I. Hand and H.U. Wittenden, ch. 10, Berlin: Springer Verlag, reproduced by permission)

as retrainable, other sources of dizzy sensations caused by stress or muscular effort can be reinterpreted as being due to hyperventilation syndrome, or effort syndrome, as it was also termed. So although the counselling approaches may not result in dizzy patients seeing the dizziness 'as their friend' as McCabe (1970) suggested, such therapeutic intervention may result in the patient reinterpreting their sensations in a manner which renders them less catastrophic, and therefore less anxiogenic.

The elderly

There is a wide range of techniques now available to rehabilitate the dizzy patient, within the context of conventional physiotherapeutic or psychological methods of management. In addition there are methods of offering assistance to patients who are unlikely to be able to reduce significantly their risk of falling due either to extensive problems with the CNS, e.g. dementia, cerebrovascular accidents, or extensive musculoskeletal difficulties, e.g. arthritis. These include making alterations to their environment to maximize the salience of visual and proprioceptive cues, e.g. reducing the number of shiny floor surfaces or loose rugs, ensuring areas are always well lit, increasing the number of handrails, and so on. This approach has recently been excellently summarized by Black, Maki and Fernie (1993). Furthermore, training someone to fall safely is an additional potential method of reducing the risks of balance problems causing fractures in the elderly population. Several valuable texts exist on this area, including those by Kataria and Das (1985), and Overstall (1983) which are useful sources of techniques. These can significantly improve the quality of life of the most vulnerable groups, e.g. those with osteoporosis.

However, Smith–Wheelock *et al.* (1990), when reporting on balance training therapy in the elderly, suggested that, as a group, the elderly seemed to suffer less intense subjective dizziness as a result of positional changes, but rely more on movement at the hip joint in situations where movement dominantly at the ankle joint would be more appropriate (Nashner, 1982), for reasons which were not entirely clear. Such situations include standing on a slippery surface, where the coefficient of friction of the ground is insufficient to counteract sheer forces generated by the use of a hip strategy. Hence methods of training found the use of the ankle strategy or stepping one useful here (see Smith–Wheelock *et al.*, 1990; Nashner and Peters, 1990). They further commented that the elderly frequently require more rest breaks between exercises compared with their younger counterparts, and that cognitive factors such as a fear of falling, diminished perception of body position and dementia must all be taken into account in the design of the retraining programme. The elderly may benefit more

from the use of posturography to reveal the multisensory nature of their deficits, and may need somewhat closer supervision of their treatment programmes than the young who, once safety levels have been established, can usually be left safely to follow their individual programmes at home in their homework assignments. Similarly, programmes utilizing the Cawthorne and Cooksey exercises (or indeed the variations by Herdman discussed earlier) have to be carefully supervised in the initial sessions, so as to guard against setting unrealistic goals for homework in terms of levels of safety, poor effort tolerance or a reduced attention span. However, because breathing exercises do not involve significant levels of risk, except in patients with a significant history of cardiac disease (Innocenti, 1993; Gardner, 1994), interventions designed to reduce hyperventilation or anxiety are usually well tolerated in this group. Of necessity the physiotherapist needs also to be aware of the impact of emphysema, or of chronic obstructive airways disease on the type of emphasis required during breathing retraining (Innocenti, 1993; Gardner, 1994).

Conclusions

It has been proposed before that various management techniques are likely to facilitate progress through vestibular rehabilitation (Beyts, 1987, 1991), regardless of the age of the population. These techniques include thorough pre-therapy assessment of the patient's positional dizziness, posturographic performance, and the range of activities that are effectively difficult or impossible to engage in as a result of their complaint. This, coupled with a clear explanation of the rationale behind both habituation therapy and balance retraining of the various forms suggested here, are essential starting points to treatment. In cases where anxiety or panic attacks are occurring it may be necessary to start working mainly on this complication rather than going straight into 'conventional' Cawthorne and Cooksey exercises, although if good goal planning practice is used such that manageable goals are agreed between patient and therapist (McKenna, 1987), it may be preferable to start on some vestibular habituation exercises, running concurrently with the breathing work. During treatment, booklets (with careful regard to clarity of expression and simple explanation) may greatly enhance the patient's comprehension of these various techniques and thereby increase treatment compliance. However, the general principles described in the booklets should always be adapted to apply to the individual requirements, as each case represents its own unique configuration of a number of features.

As Shumway–Cook and Horak (1989, 1990) or Smith–Wheelock *et al.* (1990; Smith–Wheelock, Shepard and Telian, 1991) pointed out, it may also be necessary to manage joint problems such as neck stiffness or a spinal or leg injury concurrently, which all have to be considered prior to suggesting a treatment plan involving balance retraining. Hence, despite the relative complexity of the more recent scientific developments in posturography, or in the fields of psychology and physiotherapy, certain basic clinical management principles endure and survive the test of time, and remain the most important guidelines to remember when constructing a treatment programme. These include using the information gathered from the initial assessment, to construct a treatment programme which has been individually tailored so that there are a number of realistic goals set for homework assignments, which are designed to meet safety levels, and are not likely to exacerbate other problems caused by hyperventilation or joint problems. A programme which is too aggressive should become apparent if the symptom monitoring methods reveal a failure to habituate. Hence the various recording methods, for example of the results of tests for the induction for hyperventilation syndrome (Salkovskis, Jones and Clark, 1986; Beyts, 1987; Innocenti, 1993; Gardner, 1994) and the responses to Cawthorne and Cooksey head and balance exercises (see Table 22.1) and of course the posturographic methods described above, should reveal whether a given programme is too aggressive. Thus, in general terms, follow-up appointments will be needed to monitor a patient's progress over a period of a few months, which may extend into 2 years or so with the more severely affected cases with motion sensitivity (Hamid, 1991), or other complications such as musculoskeletal or psychological problems. Furthermore, changes to levels of handicap and disability can now be assessed using questionnaire measures developed by Yardley *et al.* (Yardley and Putman, 1992; Yardley *et al.*, 1992a, b).

References

ABADI, R. V., CARDEN, D. and SIMPSON, J. (1980) A new treatment for congenital nystagmus. *British Journal of Ophthalmology*, **64**, 2–6

BALZER, G. K. (1991) Clinical contributions of dynamic platform posturography. *Seminars in Hearing*, **12**, 238–247

BÁRÁNY, R. (1921) Diagnose von Krankheitserscheinungen im Bereiche des Otolithenapparatus. *Acta Otolaryngologica*, **2**, 434–437

BECK, A. T. (1976) *Cognitive Therapy and the Emotional Disorders*. New York: New American Library

BECK, A. T., RUSH A. J., SHAW, B. F. and EMERY, G. (1979) *Cognitive Therapy of Depression*. New York: Guildford Press

BEYTS, J. P. (1987) Vestibular rehabilitation. In: *Scott Brown's Otolaryngology*, 5th edn, vol. 2. *Adult Audiology* edited by S. D. G. Stephens and A. G. Kerr. London: Butterworths. pp. 532–537

BEYTS, J. P. (1991) Vestibular rehabilitation. In: *Current Approaches to Vertigo*, edited by J. D. Hood and N. Goeting. Southampton: Duphar Laboratories Ltd. pp. 73–88

BLACK, F. O., SHUPERT, C. L., HORAK, F. B. and NASHNER, L. M. (1988) Abnormal postural control associated with peripheral vestibular disorders. In: *Progress in Brain Research*, edited by O. Pompeiano and J. H. J. Allum. New York: Elsevier Science Publishers. **76**, 263–276

BLACK, S. E., MAKI, B. E. and FERNIE, G. R. (1993) Aging imbalance and falls. In: *The Vestibular-Ocular Reflex and Vertigo*, edited by J. A. Sharpe and H. O. Barber. New York: Raven Press. pp. 317–335

BLANCHARD, E., ANDRASIK, F., NEFF, D., TEDERS, S., PALLMEYER, T., ARENA, J. *et al.* (1982) Sequential comparisons of relaxation training and biofeedback in the treatment of three kinds of headache or the machines may be necessary some of the time. *Behaviour Research and Therapy*, **20**, 469–481

BRANDT, T. and DAROFF, R. B. (1980) Physical therapy for benign positional vertigo. *Archives of Otolaryngology*, **106**, 484–485

CLARK, D. M. (1989) Anxiety states, panic and generalised anxiety. In: *Cognitive Behaviour Therapy for Psychiatric Problems – a Practical Guide*, edited by K. Hawton, P. M. Salkovskis, J. M. Kirk and D. M. Clark. Oxford: Oxford University Press. pp. 52–96

CLARK, D. M., SALKOVSKIS, P. M. and CHALKLEY, A. J. (1985) Respiratory control as a treatment for panic attacks. *Journal of Behaviour Therapy and Experimental Psychology*, **16**, 23–30

CLUFF, R. A. (1984) Chronic hyperventilation and its treatment by physiotherapy. *Journal of the Royal Society of Medicine*, **77**, 855–861

COHEN, H. (1992) Vestibular rehabilitation reduces functional disability. *Otolaryngology – Head and Neck Surgery*, **107**, 638

COLLINS, W. E. (1969) Task control of arousal and the effects of repeated unidirectional angular acceleration on human vestibular responses. *Acta Otolaryngologica Supplementum*, 190

COURJON, J. H., JEANNEROD, M., OSSUZIO, I. and SCHMID, R. (1977) The role of vision in compensation of the vestibulo ocular reflex after hemilabyrinthectomy in the cat. *Experimental Brain Research*, **29**, 235–248

CYR, D. (1993) Presentation on Paediatric Vestibular Rehabilitation given at R.N.T.N.E. Hospital, London

DAVIES, S., MCKENNA, L. and HALLAM, R. S. (1995) Relaxation and cognitive therapy: a controlled trial in chronic tinnitus. *Psychology and Health*, **10**, 129–143

DE JONG, J. M. B. V. and BLES, W. (1986) Cervical dizziness and ataxia. In: *Disorders of Posture and Gait*, edited by W. Bles and T. H. Brandt. Amsterdam: Elsevier. pp. 185–206

DIX, M. R. (1974) Treatment of vertigo. *Physiotherapy*, **60**, 380–384

DIX, M. R. (1979) The rationale and technique of head exercises in the treatment of vertigo. *Acta Oto-Rhino-Laryngologica Belgica*, **33**, 370–384

DIX, M. R. (1984) Rehabilitation of vertigo. In: *Vertigo*, edited by M. R. Dix and J. D. Hood. New York: John Wiley. pp. 457–480

DIX, M. R. (1986) Physical therapy and rehabilitation. In: *Controversial Aspects in Ménière's Disease*, edited by C. R. Pfaltz. Stuttgart: George Thieme Verlag. p. 113

DIX, M. R. and HALLPIKE, C. S. (1952) Pathology, symptomatology and diagnosis of certain disorders of the vestibular system. *Proceedings of the Royal Society of Medicine*, **45**, 341–352

DRACHMAN, D. A. and HART, C. W. (1972) An approach to the dizzy patient. *Neurology*, **22**, 324–334

EPLEY, J. M., (1992) The canalith repositioning procedure: for treatment of benign paroxysmal positional vertigo. *Otolaryngology – Head and Neck Surgery*, **107**, 399–404

FENNEL, M. (1989) Depression. In: *Cognitive Behaviour Therapy for Psychiatric Problems – a Practical Guide*, edited by K. Hawton, P. Salkovskis, J. M. Kirk and D. M. Clark. Oxford: Oxford University Press. Ch. 61. pp. 169–234

FIEBERT, J. M. and BROWN, E. (1979) Vestibular stimulation to improve ambulation after a cerebral vascular accident. *Physical Therapy*, **59**, 423–426

FRCKA, G., BEYTS, J., LEVEY, A. B. and MARTIN, I. (1983) The role of awareness in human conditioning. *Pavlovian Journal of Biological Sciences*, **18**, 69–76

FREGLY, A. R. and GRAYBIEL, A. (1968) An ataxic test battery not requiring the use of rails. *Aerospace Medicine*, **39**, 277–282

GARDNER, W. N. (1994) Diagnosis and organic causes of symptomatic hyperventilation. In: *Behavioural and Psychological Approaches to Breathing Disorders*, edited by B. H. Timmons and R. Ley. New York: Plenum Press. pp. 99–111

GIBSON, T. M. (1979) Hyperventilation in air crew: a review *Aviation, Space and Environmental Medicine*, July, 725–733

GONSHOR, A. and MELVILL JONES, G. (1980) Postural adaptation to prolonged optical reversal of vision in man. *Brain Research*, **192**, 239–248

GORMAN, J. M., FYER, M. R., GOETZ, R., ASKANAZI, J., LIEBOWITZ, M., FYER, A. *et al.* (1988) Ventilatory physiology of patients with panic disorder. *Archives of General Psychiatry*, **45**, 31–39

GURALNICK, M. J. (1973) Behaviour therapy with an acrophobic mentally retarded young adult. *Journal of Behaviour Therapy and Experimental Psychology*, **4**, 263–265

HALLAM, R. S. (1985) *Anxiety, Psychological Perspectives on Panic and Agoraphobia*. New York: Academic Press

HALLAM, R. S. and STEPHENS, S. D. G. (1985) Vestibular disorders and emotional distress. *Journal of Psychosomatic Research*, **29**, 408–413

HALLAM, R. S. and HINCHCLIFFE, R. (1991) Emotional stability – its relationship to confidence in maintaining balance. *Journal of Psychosomatic Research*, **35**, 421–430

HALLAM, R. S., BEYTS, J. P. and JAKES, S. C. (1988) Symptom reporting and objective test results: explorations of desynchrony. *Advances in Audiology*, **5**, 129–136

HAMID, M. A. (1991) Vestibular and postural findings in the motion sickness syndrome. *Otolaryngology – Head and Neck Surgery*, **104**, 135–136

HAMID, M. A. (1992) Vestibular rehabilitation. *Advances in Otolaryngology*, **6**, 27–36

HEALY, G. B., STRONG, M. S. and SAMPOGNA, D. (1974) Ataxia, vertigo and hearing loss. *Archives of Otolaryngology*, **100**, 130–135

HECKER, H. C., HAUG, C. O. and HERNDON, J. W. (1974) Treatment of the vertiginous patient using Cawthorne's vestibular exercises. *Laryngoscope*, **84**, 2065–2072

HERDMAN, S. J. (1990) Treatment of benign paroxysmal positional vertigo. *Physical Therapy*, **70**, 381–388

HERDMAN, S. J. (1991) Management of balance disorders in vestibular deficiency. *Rehabilitation Management*, April/May, 68–73

HINCHCLIFFE, R. (1967) Personality profile in Menière's disease. *Journal of Laryngology and Otology*, **81**, 447–481

HINOKI, M. (1985) Role of the visceral brain in body equilibrium. *Acta Otolaryngologica Supplementum*, **419**, 30–52

HOOD, J. D. (1970) The clinical significance of vestibular habituation. *Advances in Otorhinolaryngology*, **17**, 149–157

HOOD, J. D. (1975) The definition of vestibular habituation. In: *The Vestibular System*, edited by R. F. Naunton. New York: Academic Press. pp. 219–227

HORAK, F. B., SHUMWAY-COOK, A., CROWE, T. K. and BLACK, F. O. (1988) Vestibular function and motor proficiency of children with impaired hearing or with learning disability and motor impairment. *Developmental Medicine and Childhood Neurology*, **30**, 64–79

HORAK, F. B., JONES-RYCEWICZ C., BLACK, O and SHUMWAY-COOK, A. (1993) Effects of vestibular rehabilitation on dizziness and imbalance. *Otolaryngology – Head and Neck Surgery*, **106**, 175–180

HUNTER, L. L. and BALZER, G. K. (1991) Overview and introduction to dynamic platform posturography. *Seminars in Hearing*, **12**, 226–237

IGARASHI, M. (1984) Vestibular compensation. An overview. *Acta Otolaryngologica Supplementum*, **406**, 78–82

INNOCENTI, D. (1993) Hyperventilation. In: *Physiotherapy for Respiratory and Cardiac Problems*, edited by B. A. Webber and J. A. Prior. Edinburgh: Churchill Livingstone. pp. 377–387

JACOB, R. G. (1988) Panic disorder and the vestibular system. In Biologic systems: their relationship to anxiety disorders. *Psychiatric Clinics of North America*, **11**, 361–374

JACOB, R. G., FURMAN, J. M. R., CLARK, D. M., DURRANT, J. D. and BALABAN, C. B. (1993) Psychogenic dizziness. In: *The Vestibular Ocular Reflex and Vertigo*, edited by J. A. Sharpe and H. O. Barber. New York: Raven Press. Ch 25, pp. 305–317

JACOB, R. G., LILIENFELD, S., FURMAN, J. M. R., DURRANT, J. D. and TURNER, S. M. (1989) Space and motion phobia in panic disorder with vestibular dysfunction. *Journal of Anxiety Disorders*, **3**, 117–130

JACOB, R. G., MOLLER, M. B., TURNER, S. M. and WALL, C. (1983) Otoneurological dysfunction in patients with panic disorder or agoraphobia with panic attacks. Paper presented at the 17th Annual Convention, The World Congress on Behaviour Therapy, Washington DC, December 8–11

JACOBSON, G. P., NEWMAN, C. W., HUNTER, L. and BALZER, G. K. (1991) Balance function test correlates of the dizziness handicap inventory. *Journal of the American Academy of Audiology*, **2**, 253–260

KATARIA, M. S. and DAS, S. K. (1985) Gait and falls. In: *Fits, Faints and Falls in Old Age*, edited by M. S. Kataria. Leicester: MTP Press. Ch. 6, pp. 75–83

KATZ, J. R. (1982) The psychological differences between predictable and unpredictable noxious events; subjective, behavioural and autonomic indices. Unpublished doctoral dissertation, University of London

KAYAN, A. (1984) Migraine and vertigo. In: *Vertigo*, edited by M. R. Dix and J. D. Hood, New York: John Wiley. Ch 12. pp. 249–265

KAYAN, A. (1987) Diagnostic tests of balance. In: *Scott-Brown's Otolaryngology*, 5th edn, edited by A. G. Kerr, vol 2 Adult Audiology, edited by D. Stephen. London: Butterworths. pp. 304–367

KAYAN, A. and DERRICK-HOOD, J. (1984) Neuro-otological manifestations of migraine. *Brain*, **107**, 1123–1142

KENNERLEY, H. (1991) *Managing Anxiety*. A Training Manual. Oxford: Oxford Medical Publications

KERR, A. G. (1983) A symptomatic approach to vertigo. *Journal of Laryngology and Otology*, **97**, 813–815

KURITZKY, A., ZIEGLER, D. K. and HASSANEIN, R. (1981) Vertigo, motion sickness and migraine. *Headache*, **21**, 227–231

LACOUR, M., ROLL, J. and APPAIX, R. (1976) Modifications and developments of spinal reflexes in the alert baboon following a unilateral vestibular neurectomy. *Brain Research*, **113**, 255–269

LADER, M. H., GELDER, J. and MARKS, I. M. (1967) Palmar skin conductance measures as predictors of response to desensitization. *Journal of Psychosomatic Research*, **1**, 283–290

LADER, M. H. and WING, L. (1964) Habituation of the psycho-galvanic skin reflex in patients with anxiety states and normal subjects. *Journal of Neurology, Neurosurgery and Psychiatry*, **27**, 210–218

LEDIN, T. (1992) Dynamic posturography in childhood and senescence. In: *Posture and Gait: Control Mechanisms*, Vol. II edited by M. Woollacott and F. B. Horak. Oregon: Eugene University of Oregon Books. pp. 279–282

LEY, R. (1988) Panic attacks during relaxation and relaxation induced anxiety: a hyperventilation interpretation. *Journal of Behaviour Therapy and Experimental Psychology*, **19**, 253–259

LIPSEDGE, M. S. (1973) Systematic desensitisation in phobic disorders. *British Journal of Hospital Medicine*, **9**, 657–664

LLINAS, R. and WALTON, K. (1977) Significance of the olivo-cerebellar system in compensation of labyrinthectomy. In: *Control of Gaze by Brain Stem Neurones*, edited by Baker and Berthoz. Amsterdam: Elsevier. pp. 399–408

LUM, L. C. (1976) The syndrome of habitual chronic hyper-ventilation. In: *Modern Trends in Psychosomatic Medicine*, edited by O. Hill. London: Butterworths. pp. 196–230

MCCABE, B. F. (1970) Labyrinthine exercises in the treatment of diseases characterised by vertigo – their physiological basis and methodology. *Laryngoscope*, **80**, 1429–1433

MCKENNA, L. (1987) Goal planning in audiological rehabilitation. *British Journal of Audiology*, **21**, 5–11

MCKENNA, L., HALLAM, R. S. and HINCHCLIFFE, R. (1991) The prevalence of psychological disturbance in neuro-otology outpatients. *Clinical Otolaryngology*, **16**, 452–456

MARKS, I. (1991) Phobias and related anxiety disorder. *British Medical Journal*, **302**, 1037–1038

NASHNER, L. M. (1982) Equilibrium testing of the disorien-tated patient. In: *Nystagmus and Vertigo: Clinical Approaches to the Patient with Dizziness*, edited by V. Honrubia and Brazier, London: Academic Press. pp. 165–178

NASHNER, L. M. and PETERS, J. F. (1990) Dynamic posturography in the diagnosis and management of dizziness and balance disorders. In: *Neurologic Clinics*, edited by I. K. Arenberg and D. B. Smith. Philadelphia: W. B. Saunders Company. Vol. 8, pp. 331–349

NISBETT, R. E. and DE CAMP WILSON, T. (1977) Telling more than we can know: verbal reports on mental processes. *Psychological Review*, **81**, 231–259

NORRÉ, M. E. (1983) Vestibular compensation and the signifi-cance of rotation tests. *Advances in Otorhinolaryngology*, **30**, 330–333

NORRÉ, M. E. (1984) Treatment of unilateral vestibular hypo-function. In: *Otoneurology*, edited by W. Oosterfeld. New York: John Wiley. pp. 25–39

NORRÉ, M. E. and BECKERS, A. (1985) Comparative study of two types of exercise treatment for paroxysmal positional vertigo. *Advances in Otorhinolaryngology*, **42**, 287–289

O'CONNOR, K. P., HALLAM, R. S., BEYTS, J. P. and HINCHCLIFFE,

R. (1988) Dizziness: behavioural, subjective and organic aspects. *Journal of Psychosomatic Research*, **32**, 291–302

OVERSTALL, P. W. (1983) Rehabilitation of elderly patients with disorders of balance. In: *Hearing and Balance in the Elderly*, edited by R. Hinchcliffe. Edinburgh: Churchill Livingstone. pp. 468–488

PEALTZ, C. R. (1983) Vestibular compensation. *Acta Otolaryn-gologica*, **95**, 402–406

PILGRIM, A. R. (1986) Handling the chronic hyperventilation patient. *Physiotherapy*, **72**, 280–281

PITTS, F. N. and MCCLURE, J. N. (1967) Lactate metabolism in anxiety neurosis. *New England Journal of Medicine*, **277**, 1329–1335

PRATT, R. T. C. and MCKENZIE, W. (1958) Anxiety states following vestibular disorders. *Lancet*, ii, 347–349

PRECHT, W., SHINAZU, H. and MARKHAM, C. H. (1966) A mechanism of central compensation of vestibular function following hemilabyrinthectomy. *Journal of Neurophysiol-ogy*, **29**, 996–1010

PUTKONNEN, P. T. S., COURJON, J. H. and JEANNEROD, M. (1977) Compensation of postural effects of hemilabyrinthectomy in the cat. A sensori-substriatal process. *Experimental Brain Research*, **28**, 249–257

RITTER, B. (1969a) Treatment of acrophobia with contact desensitization. *Behaviour Research and Therapy*, **7**, 41–45

RITTER, B. (1969b) The use of contact desensitization, desensi-tization plus participation, and desensitization alone in the treatment of acrophobia. *Behaviour Research and Therapy*, **7**, 157–164

RUDGE, P. and CHAMBERS, B. R. (1982) Physiological basis for enduring vestibular symptoms. *Journal of Neurology, Neuro-surgery and Psychiatry*, **45**, 126–130

SALKOVSKIS, P. M. (1988) Hyperventilation and anxiety. *Cur-rent Opinion in Psychiatry*, **1**, 76–82

SALKOVSKIS, P. M. (1989a) Somatic problems. In: *Cognitive Behaviour Therapy for Psychiatric Problems – a Practical Guide*, edited by K. Hawton, P. M. Salkovskis, J. M. Kirk and D. M. Clark. Oxford: Oxford University Press. Ch. 7. pp. 235–276

SALKOVSKIS, P. M. (1989b) Cognitive models and interven-tions in anxiety. *Current Opinion in Psychiatry*, **2**, 795–800

SALKOVSKIS, P. M. and CLARK, D. M. (1986) Cognitive and physiological processes in the maintenance and treatment of panic attacks. In: *Panic and Phobias*, edited by I. Hand, and H. U. Wittenden, Berlin: Springer Verlag. Ch. 10. pp. 90–103

SALKOVSKIS, P. M., CLARK, D. M. and JONES, D. R. O. (1986) A psychosomatic mechanism in anxiety attacks: the role of hyperventilation in social anxiety and cardiac neurosis. *Proceedings of the XVth European Conference on Psychoso-matic Research*, edited by J. H. Lacey and D. A. Sturgeon. London: John Libbey. pp. 239–245

SALKOVSKIS, P. M., JONES, D. R. O. and CLARK, D. M. (1986) Respiratory control in the treatment of panic attacks: replication and extension with concurrent measurement of behaviour and PCO_2. *British Journal of Psychiatry*, **148**, 526–532

SALKOVSKIS, P. M. and WARWICK, H. M. C. (1986) Morbid preoccupations, health anxiety and reassurance: a cogni-tive behavioural approach to hypochondriasis. *Behaviour Research and Therapy*, **24**, 597–602

SEMONT, A. G., FREYSS, G. and VITTE, E. (1988) Curing the BPPV with a liberatory manoeuvre. *Advances in Otorhino-laryngology*, **42**, 290–293

SHEPARD, N. T., SMITH-WHEELOCK, M., TELIAN, S. A. and RAJ, A. (1993a) Vestibular and balance rehabilitation therapy. *Annals of Otology, Rhinology and Laryngology*, **102**, 198–204

SHEPARD, N. T., TELIAN, S. A. and SMITH-WHEELOCK, M. (1990) Habituation and balance retraining therapy: a retrospective review. *Diagnostic Neuro-otology in Neurologic Clinics*, **8**, 459–476

SHEPARD, N. T., TELIAN, S. A., SMITH-WHEELOCK, M., KEMINK, J. L. and BOISMIER, T. (1993b) Vestibular rehabilitation therapy: outpatient and post operative programs. In: *The Vestibular Ocular Reflex and Vertigo*, edited by J. A. Sharpe and H. O. Barber. New York: Raven Press. pp. 341–346

SHUMWAY-COOK, A. and HORAK, F. B. (1986) Assessing the influence of sensory interaction in balance. *Physical Therapy*, **66**, 10

SHUMWAY-COOK, A. and HORAK, F. B. (1989) Vestibular rehabilitation, an exercise approach to managing symptoms of vestibular dysfunction. *Seminars in Hearing*, **10**, 196–209

SHUMWAY-COOK, A. and HORAK, F. B. (1990) Rehabilitation strategies for patients with vestibular deficits. *Diagnostic Neuro-otology in Neurologic Clinics*, **8**, 441–457

SINGLETON, G. T., POST, K. N., KARLAN, M. S. and BOCK, D. G. (1978) Perilymph fistulas: diagnostic criteria and therapy. *Annals of Otology*, **87**, 797–803

SKINHØJ, E. (1973) Haemodynamic studies within the brain during migraine. *Archives of Neurology, Chicago*, **29**, 95–98

SKLARE, D. A., STEIN, M. B., PIKUS, A. M. and UHDE, T. W. (1990) Dysequilibrium and audiovestibular function in panic disorder: symptom profiles and test findings. *American Journal of Otology*, **11**, 338–341

SMITH-WHEELOCK, M., SHEPARD, N. T. and TELIAN, S. A. (1991) Physical therapy program for vestibular rehabilitation. *American Journal of Otology*, **12**, 218–225

SMITH-WHEELOCK, M., SHEPARD, N. T., TELIAN, S. A. and BOISMIER, T. (1990) Balance retraining therapy in the elderly. In: *Clinical Geriatric Otolaryngology*, 2nd edn, edited by H. K. Kashima, J. C. Goldstein and F. E. Lecente. New York: B. C. Decker. pp. 71–80

SQUIRES, A. and BAYLISS, D. E. (1985) Rehabilitation of fallers. In: *Fits, Faints and Falls in Old Age*, edited by M. S. Kataria. Lancaster: MTP Press. p. 85

STEENERSON, R. L. and CRONIN, G. W. (1996) Comparison of the canalith repositioning procedure and vestibular habituation training in forty patients with benign paraoxysmal positional vertigo. *Otology – Head and Neck Surgery*, **114**, 61–64

STEPHENS, S. D. G. (1975) Personality tests in Menière's disorder. *Journal of Laryngology and Otology*, **89**, 479–490

STEPHENS, S. D. G., HALLAM, R. S. and JAKES, S. C. (1986) Tinnitus: a management model. *Clinical Otolaryngology*, **11**, 227–238

STEPHENS, S. D. G., HOGAN, S. and MEREDITH, R. (1991) The desynchrony between complaints and signs of vestibular disorders. *Acta Otolaryngologica*, **111**, 188–192

THEUNISSEN, E. J. J. M., HUYGEN, P. L. M. and FOLGERING, H. T. (1986) Vestibular hyperreactivity and hyperventilation. *Clinical Otolaryngology*, **11**, 161–169

THOMPSEN, J., BRETLAU, P., TOS, M. and JOHNSEN, N. J. (1981) Placebo effect in surgery for Menière's disease. *Archives of Otolaryngology*, **107**, 271–277

THOMPSEN, J., BRETLAU, P., TOS, M. and JOHNSEN, N. J. (1983) Menière's disease: a 3-year follow up of patients in a double blind, placebo controlled study of endolymphatic shunt surgery. *Advances in Oto-Rhinolaryngology*, **30**, 350–354

TIWARI, S. and BAKRIS, G. L. (1981) Psychogenic vertigo: a review. *Postgraduate Medicine*, **70**, 69–77

UNTERBERGER, S. (1962) Neue objective registierhare Vestibularis – Drehreaktion, erhalten durch Treten auf der Stelle. *Der Tretreisuch Archiv für Ohren Nasen und Kehlopftheilkunde*, **145**, 473–481

WHITNEY, S. L. and BLATCHLY, C. A. (1991) Dizziness and balance disorders. *Neurology Clinical Management*, **11**, 42–43

WILSON, W. R. and KIM, J. W. (1981) Study of ventilation testing with electronystagmography. *Annals of Otology*, **90**, 56–59

WORLD HEALTH ORGANIZATION (1980) *International Classification of Impairments, Disabilities and Handicaps: a Manual of Classification relating to the Consequences of Disease*. Geneva: WHO

YARDLEY, L. (1991) Orientation perception, motion sickness, beyond the sensory conflict approach. *Journal of Audiology*, **25**, 405–413

YARDLEY, L. (1994) Contribution of symptoms and beliefs to handicap in people with vertigo: a longitudinal study. *British Journal of Clinical Psychology*, **33**, 101–113

YARDLEY, L., TODD, A. M., LACOUDRAYE–HARTER, M. M. and INGRAM, R. (1992a) Psychosocial consequences of vertigo. *Psychology and Health*, **6**, 85–96

YARDLEY, L., GRESTY, M., BRONSTEIN, A. and BEYTS, J. P. (1996) Changes in heart rate and respiration rate following head movements which provoke dizziness. *Journal of Psychosomatic Medicine*.

YARDLEY, L. and PUTMAN, J. (1992) Quantitative analysis of factors contributing to handicap and distress in vertiginous patients: a questionnaire study. *Clinical Otolaryngology*, **17**, 231–236

YARDLEY, L., VERSCHUUR, C., MASSON, E., LUXON, L. and HAACKE, N. (1992b) Somatic and psychological factors contributing to handicap in people with vertigo. *British Journal of Audiology*, **26**, 283–291

Volume index